MEDICAL COMPLICATIONS DURING PREGNANCY

Second Edition

GERARD N. BURROW, M.D.

Sir John and Lady Eaton Professor and
Chairman of the Department of Medicine,
University of Toronto Faculty of Medicine;
Physician-in-Chief, Toronto General Hospital.

THOMAS F. FERRIS, M.D.

Nesbitt Professor and Chairman of the
Department of Medicine, University of
Minnesota Medical School;
Physician-in-Chief, University of
Minnesota Hospitals.

1982

W. B. SAUNDERS COMPANY

Philadelphia   London   Toronto   Mexico City   Rio de Janeiro   Sydney   Tokyo

W. B. Saunders Company: West Washington Square
Philadelphia, PA   19105

1 St. Anne's Road
Eastbourne, East Sussex BN21 3UN, England

1 Goldthorne Avenue
Toronto, Ontario M8Z 5T9, Canada

Apartado 26370—Cedro 512
Mexico 4, D.F., Mexico

Rua Coronel Cabrita, 8
Sao Cristovao Caixa Postal 21176
Rio de Janeiro, Brazil

9 Waltham Street
Artarmon, N.S.W. 2064, Australia

Ichibancho, Central Bldg., 22-1 Ichibancho
Chiyoda-Ku, Tokyo 102, Japan

Library of Congress Cataloging in Publication Data

Main entry under title:

Medical complications during pregnancy.

1. Pregnancy, Complications of.   I. Burrow, Gerard N.   II.
Ferris, Thomas F. [DNLM: 1. Pregnancy complications. WQ
240 M486]

RG571.M4 1982   618.3   81–40692
ISBN 0–7216–2189–9   AACR2

Listed here is the latest translated edition of this book together
with the language of the translation and the publisher.

Spanish (*1st Edition*)—Editorial Medica Panamericana,
Buenos Aires, Argentina

Medical Complications During Pregnancy   ISBN   0–7216–2189–9

Last digit is the print number: 9   8   7   6   5   4   3   2

CONTRIBUTORS

GERALD G. ANDERSON, M.D.
Professor of Obstetrics and Gynecology, Director of Obstetrics and Maternal-Fetal Medicine, The University of Vermont College of Medicine, Burlington, Vermont
Obstetric Management of the High Risk Patient

VINCENT T. ANDRIOLE, M.D.
Professor of Medicine, Co-Chief, Infectious Disease Section, Yale University School of Medicine, New Haven; Attending Physician, Yale-New Haven Hospital, New Haven, Connecticut
Bacterial Infection

IRWIN M. BRAVERMAN, M.D.
Professor of Dermatology, Yale University School of Medicine, New Haven; Attending Dermatologist, Yale-New Haven Medical Center, New Haven; Consultant Dermatologist, West Haven Veterans Administration Hospital, West Haven, Connecticut
The Skin in Pregnancy

GERARD N. BURROW, M.D.
Sir John and Lady Eaton Professor and Chairman of the Department of Medicine, University of Toronto Faculty of Medicine, Toronto; Physician-in-Chief, Toronto General Hospital, Toronto, Canada
Thyroid Diseases; Pituitary, Adrenal, and Parathyroid Disorders

ROBERT L. CAPIZZI, M.D.
Professor of Internal Medicine and Pharmacology, Co-Chief, Division of Hematology/Oncology, University of North Carolina School of Medicine, Chapel Hill; Attending Physician, North Carolina Memorial Hospital, Chapel Hill, North Carolina
Neoplastic Diseases

DONALD R. COUSTAN, M.D.
Associate Professor of Obstetrics and Gynecology, Yale University School of Medicine, New Haven; Attending Perinatologist, Director of Diabetes in Pregnancy Program, Yale-New Haven Medical Center, New Haven, Connecticut
Diabetes Mellitus

DONALD J. DALESSIO, M.D.
Chairman, Department of Medicine, Scripps Clinic, Clinical Professor of Neurology, University of California, San Diego; Physician-in-Chief, Hospital of Scripps Clinic, La Jolla; Attending Physician, University Hospital, San Diego, California
Neurologic Diseases

JOHN W. DOBBINS, M.D.
Associate Professor of Medicine, Yale University School of Medicine, New Haven; Attending Physician, Yale-New Haven Hospital, West Haven Veterans Administration Hospital, New Haven, Connecticut
Gastrointestinal Complications

HAROLD J. FALLON, M.D.
William Branch Porter Professor and Chairman, Department of Internal Medicine, Medical College of Virginia, Richmond; Chairman, Department of Internal Medicine, Medical College of Virginia Hospital, Richmond, Virginia
Liver Diseases

PHILIP FELIG, M.D.
Professor of Medicine, Yale University School of Medicine, New Haven; Attending Physician, Yale-New Haven Hospital, New Haven, Connecticut
Diabetes Mellitus

THOMAS F. FERRIS, M.D.
Nesbitt Professor and Chairman of the Department of Medicine, University of Minnesota Medical School, Minneapolis; Physician-in-Chief, University of Minnesota Hospitals, Minneapolis, Minnesota
Toxemia and Hypertension; Renal Diseases

MARK GIBSON, M.D.
Assistant Professor of Obstetrics and Gynecology, University of Vermont College of Medicine, Burlington; Director, Department of Reproductive Endocrinology, Medical Center Hospital of Vermont, Burlington, Vermont
Obstetric Management of the High Risk Patient

DAFNA D. GLADMAN, M.D., F.R.C.P.(c), F.A.C.P.
Assistant Professor of Medicine, University of Toronto, Department of Medicine, Toronto; Active Staff, Department of Medicine, Women's College Hospital, Toronto; Consultant, Department of Medicine, The Wellesley Hospital, Toronto, Canada
Rheumatic Diseases

JACK HIRSH, M.D.
Professor and Chairman, Department of Medicine, McMaster University Medical School, Hamilton, Ontario, Canada
Venous Thromboembolic Disorders

JOHN C. HOBBINS, M.D.
Professor, Department of Obstetrics/Gynecology and Diagnostic Radiology, Yale University School of Medicine, New Haven; Director of Obstetrics, Yale-New Haven Hospital, New Haven, Connecticut
Obstetric Management of the High Risk Patient

DOROTHY REYCROFT HOLLINGSWORTH, M.D.
Professor of Reproductive Medicine and Medicine, University of California, San Diego, California
The Pregnant Adolescent: A Sociologic Problem with Medical Consequences

DOROTHY M. HORSTMANN, M.D.
Professor of Epidemiology and Pediatrics, Yale University School of Medicine, New Haven; Attending Pediatrician, Yale-New Haven Hospital, New Haven, Connecticut
Viral Infections

JOHN G. KELTON, M.D.
Director, McMaster Medical Centre Blood Bank, McMaster Medical Centre, Hamilton, Ontario, Canada
Venous Thromboembolic Disorders

RICHARD V. LEE, M.D.
Professor of Medicine, State University of New York at Buffalo; Head, Department of Internal Medicine, Children's Hospital of Buffalo, Buffalo; Consultant, Buffalo General Hospital, Veterans Administration Medical Center, South Buffalo Mercy Hospital, Buffalo
Sexually Transmitted Infections; Parasitic Infestations; Drug Abuse

JACK LEVIN, M.D.
Professor of Medicine, The Johns Hopkins University School of Medicine and Hospital, Baltimore; Physician and Physician-in-Charge, Hematology Outpatient Clinic, The Johns Hopkins Hospital, Baltimore; Consultant in Hematology, Loch Raven Veterans Administration Hospital, Baltimore, Maryland
Hematologic Disorders of Pregnancy

JOHN H. McANULTY, M.D.
Associate Professor of Medicine, Oregon Health Sciences University, Portland; Staff, University Hospital, Portland, Oregon
Cardiovascular Disease

JAMES METCALFE, M.D.
Professor of Medicine, Oregon Health Sciences University, Portland; Staff, University Hospital, Portland Veterans Administration Medical Center, Portland, Oregon
Cardiovascular Disease

MALCOLM S. MITCHELL, M.D.
Professor of Medicine and Microbiology, University of Southern California, Los Angeles; Director for Clinical Investigations, Chief of Division of Medical Oncology, University of Southern California Comprehensive Cancer Center, Los Angeles; Attending Physician, Los Angeles County-University of Southern California Medical Center, Hospital of the Good Samaritan, California Hospital Medical Center, Los Angeles, Huntington Memorial Hospital, Pasadena, California
Neoplastic Diseases

ELIZABETH M. SHORT, M.D.
Assistant Professor of Medicine, Associate Dean of Students, Stanford University School of Medicine, Stanford; Attending Physician, Stanford Medical Center, Stanford, California
Genetic Disorders

HOWARD M. SPIRO, M.D.
Professor of Medicine, Yale University School of Medicine, New Haven; Chief of Gastroenterology, Yale-New Haven Hospital, New Haven, Connecticut
Gastrointestinal Complications

KENT UELAND, M.D.
Professor of Gynecology and Obstetrics, Chief, Section of Maternal-Fetal Medicine, Stanford University School of Medicine, Stanford; Attending Staff, Stanford University Medical Center, Stanford, Santa Clara Valley Medical Center, San Jose; Consulting Staff, Kaiser Permanente Medical Center, San Francisco, California
Cardiovascular Disease

MURRAY B. UROWITZ, M.D.
Associate Professor of Medicine, University of Toronto, Department of Medicine, Toronto; Senior Staff Physician, Department of Medicine, The Wellesley Hospital, Rheumatic Disease Unit, Toronto, Canada
Rheumatic Diseases

STEVEN E. WEINBERGER, M.D.
Assistant Professor of Medicine, Harvard Medical School, Boston; Director, Pulmonary Function Laboratory, Beth Israel Hospital, Boston, Massachusetts
Pulmonary Diseases

SCOTT T. WEISS, M.D.
Assistant Professor of Medicine, Harvard Medical School, Boston; Associate Chief, Pulmonary Unit, Beth Israel Hospital, Boston, Massachusetts
Pulmonary Diseases

PREFACE

Diseases occurring during pregnancy pose special problems and opportunities for the physician. The physiologic and biochemical changes that accompany pregnancy may complicate the diagnosis of disease, and therapeutic decisions must always take into account an estimate of fetal risk. At the same time, these changes afford special opportunities for the clinical observer. The self-limited period of gestation provides an opportunity to observe changes before, during, and after pregnancy. Pregnancy is, in effect, a well-designed clinical experiment that should be of interest to all involved in studying normal and pathologic physiology. We became interested in these problems while working at the Medical Complications During Pregnancy Clinic at Yale begun under the late John P. Peters and continued under Franklin H. Epstein. This interest has continued despite our respective moves to Toronto and Minneapolis.

We have been gratified by the acceptance of the first edition of the book, which confirmed our belief that there was a real need to provide the obstetrician with current concepts about the pathophysiology of medical diseases and the medical specialist with the obstetrical experience in treating pregnant patients. A new edition was needed since remarkable medical progress has been made in many areas covered in this text in the six years since the first edition was published. In an effort to bring fresh insights to the second edition, about half of the chapters have been written by different authors; the other chapters have been completely rewritten. In addition, a chapter on medical complications of adolescent pregnancy has been added. The emphasis has remained on the clinical appraisal of available evidence concerning the effect of pregnancy on medical diseases. The object of the book is to provide useful clinical information to the physician who cares for the pregnant woman. It is not intended as a treatment manual but rather as a foundation upon which further clinical findings and therapeutic methods can be based.

We are grateful to Jane Hanes and Linda Bartels for their secretarial assistance. We also wish to express our gratitude to the W. B. Saunders Company and particularly to Mr. Albert E. Meier, Editor-in-Chief, for his encouragement throughout the preparation of both editions.

CONTENTS

OK
But
Better
i?
SCIARRA (?)
Notes

9 PITUITARY, ADRENAL, AND PARATHYROID DISORDERS

Gerard N. Burrow

12   LIVER DISEASES _____ 278

Harold J. Fallon

13   BACTERIAL INFECTION _____ 302

Vincent T. Andriole

18 NEUROLOGIC DISEASES _____ 435

Donald J. Dalessio

Thomas F. Ferris, M.D.

1

TOXEMIA AND HYPERTENSION

Toxemia is a multisystem disease typically occurring in late pregnancy, the usual clinical manifestations being hypertension, proteinuria, edema, and central nervous system irritability. Since convulsions may occur in severe toxemia, the disease has been classified into eclampsia (a synonym for a convulsive disorder used until early in this century) and pre-eclampsia, depending upon whether a seizure has occurred. Although the cause of toxemia remains unclear, great increases in our understanding of the pathophysiology of the disease have occurred in the past 25 years. The changes in cardiovascular physiology and hemostasis that occur in pregnancy and toxemia have provided insights into possible mechanisms of disease in other pathological conditions.

CARDIOVASCULAR CHANGES DURING PREGNANCY

Cardiac output increases in the first trimester of pregnancy and reaches a maximum of 30 to 40 per cent above the nonpregnant level by the 24th week of gestation. The rise in cardiac output is accompanied by an increase in blood volume of approximately 50 per cent, the rise in plasma and red cell volume beginning in the first trimester. The greater increase in plasma volume is responsible for the hemodilution and physiologic anemia of pregnancy. Since arterial blood pressure is the product of cardiac output and peripheral resistance, it is noteworthy that the rise in cardiac output during pregnancy is associated not with an increase, but rather with a reduction, in arterial blood pressure. Vascular resistance strikingly decreases during pregnancy, as is clinically evident from the palmar erythema and spider telangiectases that frequently develop. The development of hypertension in toxemia, as in other hypertensive states, is the result of an increase in vascular resistance. Cardiac output may fall with the development of hypertension in response to autonomic reflexes mediated by carotid baroreceptors. The cause of the increase

in peripheral vascular resistance in toxemia is unknown, but several important factors in the control of vascular resistance in pregnancy have been examined.

RENIN-ANGIOTENSIN-ALDOSTERONE IN PREGNANCY

An extraordinary increase in renin secretion occurs during pregnancy, and an examination of its possible causes provides insight into the physiology of renin in both normal and pathologic states. A brief review of the physiology of renin is necessary for an understanding of the changes that occur with pregnancy.

Renin is an enzyme with a molecular weight of approximately 40,000. It has no vasoconstricting properties but acts upon an alpha-2 globulin, angiotensinogen, to form angiotensin I, a 10–amino acid peptide. Angiotensin I is rapidly converted to the active vasoconstrictor angiotensin II, an octapeptide, by the removal of the two terminal amino acids during circulation through capillary beds, particularly the pulmonary circulation. The enzyme responsible for this conversion is present in endothelial cells and is termed the angiotensin converting enzyme. This enzyme is also responsible for the conversion of bradykinin to inactive metabolites. Inactivation of circulating angiotensin II occurs rapidly through the actions of angiotensinases in tissue and blood. Thus, the level of plasma angiotensin II is dependent upon several factors: release of renin into the circulation, concentration of the substrate angiotensinogen, activity of the converting enzyme, and possibly activity of angiotensinases. Under most circumstances the concentration of renin in plasma is the most important determinant of angiotensin II concentration.

Renin is synthesized in most blood vessels in low concentration, but the source of plasma renin is granules in the afferent arteriole of the renal glomerulus. Tobian first proposed that renin secretion was controlled by stretch receptors in the wall of the afferent arteriole, which act as a baroreceptor responding to changes in renal perfusion pressure.[232] Renin secretion increases with reduction in perfusion pressure and decreases during elevation of perfusion pressure. However, since renal blood flow, like flow to other vascular beds, is relatively constant during changes in perfusion pressure within the autoregulatory range (mean arterial pressure [MAP] approximately 80 to 140 mm Hg), the renal vasculature dilates during a reduction in perfusion pressure. How the renal vasculature remains dilated despite an increase in renin secretion is unclear, but the prevention of vasoconstriction may be due to the concomitant synthesis of vasodilating prostaglandins, either PGI_2 or PGE_2, both of which are synthesized in the kidney. The resistance, or tachyphylaxis, that develops to angiotensin when it is infused into the renal artery is dependent upon renal synthesis of prostaglandin.[162a] This interrelationship between renin and prostaglandin synthesis is important not only in regulation of the renal circulation but, as will be discussed subsequently, in other vascular beds, particularly the uteroplacental circulation.

In addition to a reduction in perfusion pressure, other factors important in the control of renin secretion include the delivery of sodium to the macula densa, a site in the distal tubule that is in continuity with the afferent arteriole; activity of the renal sympathetic nerves; and renal prostaglandin synthesis.[175] When delivery of sodium to the macula densa decreases, renin secretion increases, and conversely, increased sodium delivery to the macula densa decreases renin secretion. Modulation of renin secretion induced by reduction in renal perfusion pressure can be accomplished by altering sodium delivery to the macula densa.

Renal prostaglandin synthesis plays a vital role in renin secretion. Arachidonic acid, the fatty acid substrate for prostaglandin synthesis, increases renin secretion when infused into the renal artery, and renal cortical cells growing in tissue culture are dependent upon prostaglandin synthesis for release of renin into the media.[106, 241] In contrast, prostaglandin-inhibiting drugs like indomethacin or aspirin lower renal renin secretion in vivo and inhibit release of renin from renal cortical cells.[128a, 175]

The sympathetic nervous system is also involved in the control of renin secretion; stimulation of beta-adrenergic receptors in the kidney increases renin secretion, and beta-adrenergic blocking agents like propranolol decrease it.[39]

The unique position of angiotensin II in blood pressure control is that it affects not only vascular resistance but also extracellular volume by stimulating aldosterone secretion. Normally, as extracellular volume expands there is increased renal perfusion pressure, increased delivery of filtered sodium to the distal tubule, and diminished renal sympathetic nerve activity, all of which cause renin secretion to fall. The converse occurs with extracellular volume contraction, and renin secretion increases. The difficulty in understanding renin secretion in pregnancy is that high secretion occurs during expansion of the extracellular volume, increased renal blood flow and glomerular filtration rate (GFR), and presumably increased delivery of sodium to the macula densa. Various suggestions have been made to explain the discrepant increase in renin secretion during pregnancy. One suggestion is that it is due to a salt-losing tendency caused by both an increase in GFR, which necessitates increased tubular reabsorption of sodium and increased progesterone secretion. Progesterone secretion increases early in pregnancy and is an antagonist to aldosterone at the renal tubule.[243] There is, however, no evidence that pregnant women cannot conserve sodium normally. When they are given a 10 mEq sodium intake there is an appropriate rise in plasma renin and aldosterone as urinary sodium falls to the same level as in nonpregnant women.[17] The fact that pregnancy is associated with expansion of the extracellular volume and the frequent presence of edema in pregnancy speak against its being a salt-wasting state. If the persistent increase in renin and aldosterone secretion in pregnancy is necessary to overcome a tendency toward salt wasting, it is of note that neither a 300 mEq Na intake for seven days,[17] nor saline administered intravenously,[243] nor prolonged mineralocorticoid administration[68] suppresses aldosterone secretion to the levels in nonpregnant subjects (Fig. 1–1). The increase in progesterone secretion, although not a cause of salt wasting, may be a factor in the failure of pregnant women to become potassium depleted in spite of high sodium intake and increased aldosterone secretion. The hypokalemia associated with primary aldosteronism[22] has been reported to be ameliorated during pregnancy, and progesterone abolishes a desoxycorticosterone-induced kaliuresis in normal subjects.[68]

Although plasma renin in pregnancy is primarily of renal origin, the high concentration of renin in the uterus, placenta, and amniotic fluid makes them potential sources of plasma renin in pregnancy. The presence of renin in the placenta of pregnant cats was first reported by Stakemann in 1960,[214] and in 1964 Gross et al. reported finding

PLASMA RENIN ACTIVITY &
PLASMA ALDOSTERONE ON 300 mEq Na INTAKE

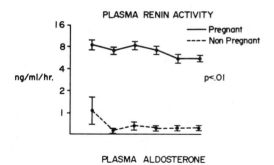

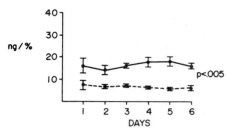

FIGURE 1–1. The effect of 6 days of a 300 mEq sodium intake in pregnant and nonpregnant women. Note the persistent elevation in plasma renin activity and plasma aldosterone in pregnant women. (From Bay and Ferris: Hypertension, 1:410, 1979. Reprinted with permission.)

a renin-like material in rabbit uterus and placenta.[119] Their studies were extended by Ferris et al.[79] and Gorden et al.,[114] who demonstrated that uterine renin persisted for up to 72 hours after nephrectomy and that the concentration in uterus was not altered by variations in sodium intake. Cell cultures of human chorion and uterine muscle synthesize renin.[225] Uterine renin is secreted into the circulation with reduction in uterine perfusion by either ligation of the uterine arteries or hemorrhagic hypotension in nephrectomized pregnant rabbits.[81] Several features of toxemia have been produced in the pregnant dog with induction of uterine hypoperfusion.[1] Whether uterine renin contributes to plasma renin in pregnancy is not clear, but two studies have demonstrated higher renin activity in uterine veins than in uterine arteries in women with toxemia at cesarean section.[144, 211]

The high plasma renin level in pregnant rabbits does not seem to be of uterine origin, since plasma and kidney renin respond appropriately to changes in salt intake whereas uterine renin is not affected by such changes.[114] In pregnant women, plasma renin and aldosterone respond appropriately to changes in sodium intake, but

with a high sodium intake plasma renin and aldosterone do not become suppressed as in nonpregnant women (see Figure 1–1).

Human amniotic fluid has a high renin concentration, mostly in the form of "pro-renin," an inactive renin, which is activated by incubation at an acid pH.[203] Pro-renin appears in amniotic fluid early in pregnancy, and since pro-renin is present in the supernatant of chorionic cell cultures, amniotic pro-renin is probably of chorionic origin. Pro-renin that can be detected in the plasma of pregnant women may be of amniotic origin. Whether pro-renin plays a physiologic role is unclear.

The role of uterine renin in pregnancy is not clear, but according to one hypothesis it is involved in the regulation of uterine blood flow. Angiotensin increases uterine blood flow in the pregnant rabbit,[81] dog,[12] and monkey,[91] and lessens uterine vascular resistance. Angiotensin increases uterine vein PGE_2 concentration,[91] and the increase in uterine PGE_2 synthesis may be the cause of the decrease in uterine vascular resistance and increase in blood flow. Angiotensin is known to release arachidonic acid, the fatty acid substrate necessary for prostaglandin synthesis, from lipid stores, an event that promotes prostaglandin synthesis.

Uterine renin may affect uterine blood flow by control of angiotensin II and PGE synthesis in the uterus. When nephrectomized pregnant rabbits are given prostaglandin synthesis inhibitors, like indomethacin, uterine blood flow decreases,[237] and when they are given the angiotensin I converting enzyme inhibitor captopril, uterine venous PGE concentration falls.[90] This fall in uterine vein PGE concentration appears to be physiologically significant: when captopril was given orally to pregnant rabbits from the 15th day of gestation, fetal survival was 14 per cent compared with 99 per cent fetal survival in controls. Since no change in blood pressure occurred during continued administration of captopril, the reduction in uterine PGE synthesis induced by angiotensin I blockade may be the cause of the high fetal mortality. A high infant mortality in women taking aspirin throughout pregnancy has been reported in one series,[233] although this result was not confirmed by another group.[206] However, in both studies infant size was reduced when women took aspirin during pregnancy. Since several clinical findings suggest that uterine blood flow is reduced in toxemia, factors such as uterine prostaglandin synthesis that may control uterine blood flow are obviously important to our understanding of this disease.

Another determinant of renin secretion is vascular sensitivity to angiotensin. Since upright posture increases renin secretion in both pregnant and nonpregnant women, angiotensin is a factor in maintaining normal blood pressure in the standing subject. However, the level of angiotensin required to elicit a blood pressure response varies with the sensitivity of the vasculature to angiotensin. Vascular sensitivity depends on factors affecting angiotensin receptors in the arterioles. In experimental animals, one can make inferences about angiotensin receptor affinity by determining the amount of angiotensin antibody necessary to block the blood pressure response to an administered dose of angiotensin.[33] If more antibody is needed one can infer that there is greater binding affinity of arteriolar receptors to angiotensin. In contrast, if less antibody is needed, binding affinity of the arteriolar receptors is presumed to have decreased, angiotensin being preferentially bound to the antibody. When hypertension is induced by renal artery constriction, administration of desoxycorticosterone acetate (DOCA), and a high sodium intake, and also in spontaneously hypertensive rats, there is increased arteriolar receptor affinity for angiotensin; more angiotensin antibody is needed to block the hypertensive response to a standard dose of angiotensin. In such circumstances less angiotensin is needed to elicit a rise in blood pressure. When animals are placed on a low sodium diet, arteriolar affinity for angiotensin decreases and more angiotensin must be given to cause a blood pressure response. The factors that control angiotensin sensitivity and receptor affinity are unclear. Changes in arterial wall sodium and calcium concentration or synthesis of angiotensin antagonists like prostaglandins in the blood vessel are thought to be of importance.

Striking changes in angiotensin sensitivity occur during pregnancy. Insensitivity to angiotensin occurs early in the first trimester and persists in normotensive pregnant women throughout pregnancy.[103] Accompanying the decrease in sensitivity, renin secretion increases. Although the threefold to fourfold increase in renin substrate concentration accounts in part for the increase in plasma renin activity (PRA), plasma renin concentration is approximately eight times higher than in nonpregnant women.[246] With the combined rise in renin and substrate concentration, PRA is 15 times higher than in nonpregnant women. Plasma angiotensin is 78 ± 24 picogram/ml in pregnant women compared with a range of 5 to 35 picrogram/ml in nonpregnant women. The elevated angiotensin probably maintains arterial pressure, since in pregnant animals angiotensin blockade with either the angiotensin antagonist Saralasin or the angiotensin I converting enzyme inhibitor captopril causes reduction in arterial pressure.[17] Thus, pregnancy is a state of angiotensin resistance requiring increased secretion of renin to maintain arterial pressure, and this resistance develops early in the first trimester.

PROSTAGLANDIN SYNTHESIS IN PREGNANCY

The potential role of endogenous vasodilators in blood pressure control has been speculated upon for many years. In 1932, von Euler in Sweden and Goldblatt in England discovered a vasodepressor lipid in the seminal vesicle fluid of rams, which they called prostaglandin. There was little interest in this compound until after 1950, when chemical analysis of the various prostaglandins became possible. In the past 20 years, there have been extraordinary developments in our knowledge of the biochemistry of prostaglandins, and although their role in blood pressure control still remains unsettled, several findings suggest a potential role for prostaglandin synthesis in blood pressure control, particularly during pregnancy.

Prostaglandins are 20-carbon fatty acids with a cyclopentane ring (Fig. 1–2). The fatty acid precursor for prostaglandin synthesis is arachidonic acid, which is released from the lipid pool of phospholipids and triglycerides by a phospholipase. Arachidonic acid is then metabolized by a microsomal cyclooxygenase to form an intermediate unstable compound, PGH_2, which is enzymatically converted to one of several biologically active lipids. In blood vessel walls, PGH_2 is converted to PGI_2, or prostacyclin, a vasodilator and antagonist to the vasoconstrictor effect of angiotensin and norepinephrine. PGI_2 has a short half-life, and its rate of synthesis is determined by measurement in plasma or urine of its major metabolite, 6-oxo-PGF_1-alpha. In the kidney, uterus, placenta, and other organs, PGH_2 is converted to PGE_2, PGF_1-alpha, PGD_2, or PGI_2.

The suggestion that prostaglandins are involved in control of blood pressure was derived from early observations of Chanatin and Ferris[41] that partial nephrectomy caused hypertension in rats and Grollman[118] that the renal medulla had an antihypertensive effect in certain forms of experimental hypertension. Muirhead et al.[170] found that transplantation to the peritoneum of renal medullary tissue or renal medullary interstitial cells grown in tissue culture reduced arterial

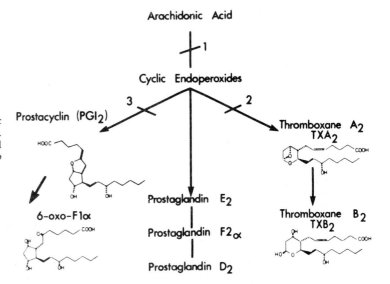

FIGURE 1–2. Conversion of arachidonic acid to prostaglandins and thromboxanes. *1* is the cyclooxygenase step, whereas *2* and *3* are enzymes necessary for conversion to PGI_2 or thromboxane A_2.

blood pressure in rats with various forms of hypertension. This suggested that the antihypertensive effect of the kidney was mediated by liberation of prostaglandins from medullary interstitial cells. A decrease in the lipid granules of medullary interstitial cells has been noted in rats with spontaneous hypertension or hypertension following DOCA administration or after clipping of the renal artery.[232]

In the past, most interest in blood pressure control has centered upon the potential role of renal synthesis of the vasodilator PGE_2. High cyclooxygenase activity is present in the renal medulla, and the granules in renal medullary interstitial cells have a high concentration of arachidonate. Since the renal medulla is strategically located to control the final concentration of sodium and water in collecting tubules, it has been postulated that renal medullary PGE_2 synthesis may also modulate sodium excretion. There is evidence that deep cortical nephrons, whose loops of Henle extend deep into the papilla, are critical in controlling final urinary sodium concentration.[217] However, the role of medullary synthesis of PGE_2 in the control of medullary blood flow or of sodium and water absorption in the loop of Henle is not clear. Infusions of PGE_2 into the renal artery cause natriuresis, a result in part of the renal vasodilation that occurs,[18] but inhibition of sodium transport in isolated collecting tubules by PGE_2 has been demonstrated.[218] In some patients salt retention and edema occur when prostaglandin-inhibiting drugs are given, but this is unusual. Thus, the evidence for a role of renal medullary prostaglandin synthesis in sodium balance remains intriguing but unproved.

If renal secretion of PGE_2 into the circulation is important in blood pressure control, it is striking that approximately 70 per cent of PGE_2 is metabolized to inactive compounds in one passage through the pulmonary capillary bed.[112] This fact seems to make a hormonal role for PGE_2 unlikely. The observation that endothelial cells of blood vessels are capable of synthesizing PGI_2, or prostacyclin, makes that substance a more attractive candidate for control of vascular resistance, both because of its ubiquitous source of synthesis and because it escapes metabolic degradation in the pulmonary vasculature. One could speculate that control of peripheral resistance is dependent upon a balance between circulating vasoconstrictors, such as angiotensin and norepinephrine, and arteriolar synthesis of PGI_2. PGI_2 synthesis increases in endothelial cell cultures in response to angiotensin,[108] so a positive feedback control system may be envisioned.

During pregnancy there is evidence of increased prostaglandin synthesis in several organs. In pregnant rabbits, extraordinary concentrations of PGE_2 have been found in the uterine vein, approximately 150 ng/ml, compared with 0.2 ng/ml in the renal vein of nonpregnant animals.[237] Uterine vein PGE_2 concentration falls following treatment with cyclooxygenase-inhibiting drugs, like indomethacin and meclofenamate, and a reduction in uterine blood flow occurs. In pregnant women, high concentrations of plasma and urinary PGE have been found in the third trimester[17, 237] (Figs. 1–3 and 1–4). Whether the increase in peripheral vein PGE_2 in pregnant women is of uterine or renal origin is not known. Urinary PGE_2 is believed to repre-

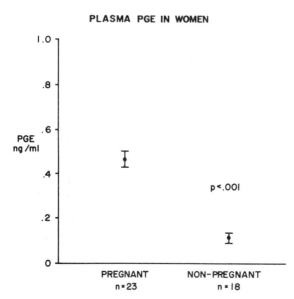

PLASMA PGE IN WOMEN

FIGURE 1–3. Peripheral venous prostaglandin E in 3rd trimester pregnant and in nonpregnant women. (From Venuto et al.: J. Clin. Invest., 55:193, 1975. Reprinted with permission.)

sent renal synthesis of PGE_2, since infusions of PGE_2 into the renal artery do not increase urinary PGE_2 excretion.[96] In addition to an increase in uterine and renal prostaglandin synthesis, recent studies have demonstrated that plasma and urinary 6-oxo-PGF_1-alpha, the major metabolite of PGI_2 synthesis, is elevated in late pregnan-

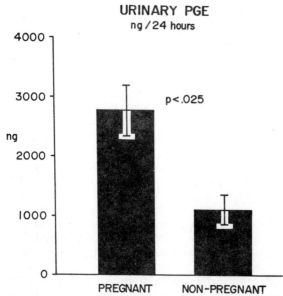

URINARY PGE
ng / 24 hours

FIGURE 1–4. Urinary prostaglandin E excretion in pregnant and in nonpregnant women. (From Bay and Ferris: Hypertension, 1:410, 1979. Reprinted with permission.)

cy.[153] The human myometrium has been demonstrated to synthesize PGI_2,[176] and we have found its metabolite, 6-oxo-PGF_1-alpha, to be approximately ten times higher in uterine vein blood than in the peripheral blood of pregnant rabbits.[77] Gerber et al. have reported high levels of 6-oxo $PGF_1\alpha$ in the uterine vein of pregnant dogs.[1, 106a] In vitro studies have also demonstrated a high capacity for PGI_2 synthesis in human placental and umbilical vascular tissue.[121a, 128a] Thus, there is emerging evidence of increased synthesis of several vasodilating prostaglandins in uterus, kidney, and blood vessels during pregnancy, all of which may be important in the physiological changes in the circulation that occur then.

Pregnancy has many similarities to Bartter's syndrome, a disorder characterized by insensitivity to angiotensin, low to normal blood pressure, high plasma renin level, and elevated urinary PGE_2 excretion.[107] When aspirin or indomethacin is administered to patients with Bartter's syndrome, angiotensin sensitivity increases and renin secretion falls. As in pregnancy, the insensitivity to angiotensin and increase in renin secretion in Bartter's syndrome may be due to increased vascular synthesis of PGI_2 rather than to renal synthesis of PGE_2, since high urinary 6-oxo-PGF_1-alpha excretion is also a characteristic of the syndrome.[120] Thus, the increase in urinary PGE_2 excretion may be a reflection of a generalized increase in prostaglandin synthesis.

Since renal synthesis of PGI_2, probably in the afferent arteriole, increases renin secretion, the elevated renin secretion in Bartter's syndrome and pregnancy may be due to a direct effect of renal PGI_2 synthesis as well as to peripheral antagonism to the pressor effect of angiotensin and norepinephrine induced by PGI_2 synthesis in arterioles. Bartter's original hypothesis was that these patients had a congenital defect in the number or affinity of arteriolar angiotensin receptors with a consequent need for increased secretion of renin to maintain arterial pressure. Fifteen years elapsed before it was appreciated that the angiotensin insensitivity was due to an increase in prostaglandin synthesis.

One feature of Bartter's syndrome that is absent in pregnancy is urinary potassium wasting and potassium depletion. Since potassium depletion in humans, dogs, and rabbits increases renal PGE_2 synthesis, the primary lesion in Bartter's syndrome may be a potassium-losing nephropathy.[100] This would explain why the kaliuresis in Bartter's syndrome persists even after treatment with cyclooxygenase inhibitors. The increased

Variations in angiotensin sensitivity throughout pregnancy

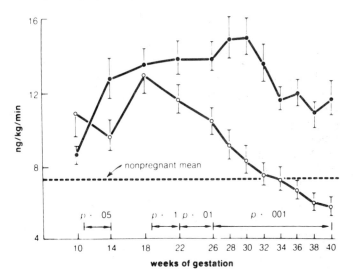

FIGURE 1–5. Comparison of mean angiotensin dose required to cause a 20 mm rise in diastolic blood pressure in 120 primigravidas who remained normotensive (black circles) and 72 primigravidas in whom toxemia occurred (open circles). Nonpregnant mean dose is shown as a broken line. (From Gant et al.: J. Clin. Invest., 52:2682, 1973. Reprinted with permission.)

secretion of progesterone that occurs early in pregnancy may prevent the kaliuresis one ordinarily expects with increased aldosterone secretion and a normal sodium intake.[24]

Angiotensin insensitivity is present in human pregnancy as well as in Bartter's syndrome.[103] The decreased responsiveness to angiotensin that occurs as early as the 10th week of gestation decreases in women destined to develop toxemia as early as the 18th week, in spite of the fact that clinical signs and symptoms of toxemia do not appear until after the 32nd week (Fig. 1–5). In contrast, women who do not develop toxemia maintain insensitivity to angiotensin throughout pregnancy, although a slight increase in sensitivity occurs in all women after the 32nd week. If the resistance to angiotensin in pregnancy is due to increased synthesis of vasodilating prostaglandins, an attractive hypothesis is that the increasing sensitivity in women with toxemia is the result of decreased prostaglandin synthesis. To answer this question, serial determinations of urinary PGE_2 and 6-oxo-PGF_1-alpha throughout pregnancy are needed in a study of women with a high incidence of toxemia.

The increase in sensitivity to angiotensin prior to the onset of toxemia is probably the cause of the positive roll-over test reported by Gant et al.[102] They reported that in pregnant women who ultimately developed toxemia, blood pressure rose excessively when they turned from the lateral recumbent to a supine position. Since lying supine in pregnancy compresses the inferior vena cava, causing reduction in cardiac output, the fall in renal blood flow that occurs

increases renin secretion,[244] and the roll-over test may then function as a measure of endogenous angiotensin sensitivity. Although the clinical reliability of this maneuver as a predictor of toxemia has not been validated in all studies, it probably does measure latent hypertension in women destined to develop toxemia.

Administration of either indomethacin or aspirin to normotensive pregnant women in the last trimester increases sensitivity to angiotensin,[72] which suggests that prostaglandin synthesis is involved in the resistance to angiotensin in pregnancy. However, an increase in sensitivity to angiotensin occurs following the administration of prostaglandin-inhibiting drugs under all circumstances.[171]

Sodium Balance. Although edema occurs in up to 75 per cent of normotensive pregnancies because of compression of the inferior vena cava by the enlarging uterus, dilatation of venous capacitance vessels, and diminished colloid osmotic pressure, the rapid development of edema and a rise in blood pressure usually mark the onset of toxemia. Because of the frequency of edema in pregnancy, the suggestion has been made that edema be disregarded as a clinical sign of toxemia. That would be to deny the most important clinical harbinger of the disease. Edema is benign, provided vascular resistance remains low. However, the onset of edema and a rise in blood pressure are indicative of salt retention during diminished vascular capacity. In these circumstances salt retention is pathologic and is a major factor in causing the hypertension. The failure to recognize the significance of edema in the face of a rising blood pressure prevents recognition of toxemia in its earliest form. Not only does salt retention increase extracellular volume, it also increases sensitivity to angiotensin and may increase peripheral resistance by causing arteriolar swelling.

The cause of the sodium retention with preeclampsia is most likely the reduction in glomerular filtration rate that occurs. Since the renal tubular cells must reabsorb more sodium during pregnancy because of the 50 per cent increase in glomerular filtration rate, a small reduction in glomerular filtration may cause an increase in fractional reabsorption of sodium. The sodium retention is not due to elevated aldosterone secretion, which may fall with the onset of toxemia.[134] Indeed, toxemia with edema has been described in patients with Addison's disease.[143, 149, 173] The renal vasoconstriction that occurs with toxemia may also contribute to the salt retention by preventing the normal natriuretic response to hypertension.

Much has been made of the reduction in plasma volume that occurs in patients with toxemia. The reduction is variable but averages approximately 9 per cent in the published studies of plasma volume in toxemia.[13] This is the same degree of plasma volume contraction reported in patients with essential hypertension.[227] Greater volume depletion is often seen in patients with renal artery stenosis, pheochromocytoma, or malignant hypertension.[53] It reflects constriction of venous capacitance vessels, causing increased capillary hydrostatic pressure. The resulting diminished plasma volume and the low central venous pressure caused by venous constriction have unfortunately been interpreted by some to mean that toxemia is a volume-contracted state that should be treated with volume expansion, utilizing saline or dextran. Such efforts only lead to an increase in blood pressure and the possibility of life-threatening pulmonary edema or cerebral vascular hemorrhage. The use of volume expansion in toxemia has led Nicholas Assali, an eminent obstetrician who has spent a lifetime studying the pathophysiology of toxemia, to state, "These misconceptions would be merely amusing if they did not lead to courses of action that could be devastating to the patient."[13]

The fascination of toxemia to investigators interested in hypertension is that it brings into sharp focus the importance of several factors — salt retention, plasma renin and angiotensin, sensitivity to angiotensin, and prostaglandin synthesis — which play a role not only in toxemia but in all forms of human hypertension.

PATHOLOGY OF TOXEMIA

Liver. Prior to the advent of liver biopsy, studies of hepatic pathology in toxemia were limited to patients with fatal toxemia. In these patients large subcapsular hematomas were found, some of which had ruptured into the peritoneal cavity. The subcapsular hematomas arose either from deep within the liver or from the capsule.[23, 31] Sheehan postulated that the hemorrhagic changes in the liver were due to intense spasm of hepatic arterioles rather than to fibrin deposits.[208] However, in more recent studies utilizing percutaneous liver biopsies of patients with toxemia, patchy areas of necrosis with fibrin deposits have been demonstrated.[9] Of 12 pre-eclamptic women, 2 had focal areas of fibrinoid necrosis with either patchy or extensive necrosis of the liver cells. Immunofluorescence studies of all 12 biopsies showed diffuse sinusoidal staining with antiserum to fibrinogen. In the same areas, mild to moderate fluorescent staining with antiserum to IgG, IgM, and complement were also seen. In biopsies from normal pregnant women, fibrin deposits were not demonstrated. Abnormalities in liver function were found in 7 of the 12 patients with pre-eclampsia in whom elevation in lactic dehydrogenase and glutamic-oxaloacetic transaminase were the most striking observations.

Toxemia may occasionally present with jaundice, particularly when there is clinical and laboratory evidence of a consumptive coagulopathy with hemolysis.[152] Approximately 10 per cent of eclamptic patients are clinically jaundiced, and in some pre-eclamptic women hepatic abnormalities are more prominent than either the hypertension or the proteinuria. It is of note that in many patients with acute fatty liver of pregnancy, there is concomitant evidence of toxemia with proteinuria and diminished renal function. In a review of 49 cases of acute fatty liver of pregnancy, 22 per cent had definite evidence of toxemia preceding the onset of hepatic disease.[126] This figure may be an underestimation of the true incidence of toxemia in acute fatty liver of pregnancy; in several patients the available information was inadequate to exclude the possibility of toxemia. Acute fatty liver has been described following thrombotic thrombocytopenic purpura,[197] in which the pathology is similar. In one patient with toxemia and acute fatty liver, a protein-losing enteropathy developed in a manner consistent with small vessel disease involving the bowel. This case emphasized the generalized nature of the disease.[126]

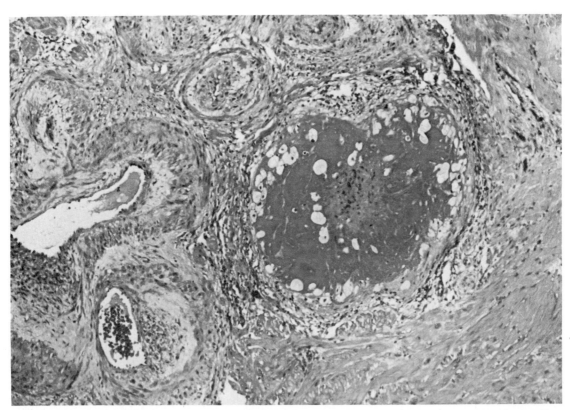

FIGURE 1–6. Placental bed biopsy from a woman with severe toxemia requiring a cesarean section. Note the hyperplastic arteriosclerosis and acute atherosclerosis with reduction in lumen size. Magnification 150×. (Courtesy of Dr. W. B. Robertson.)

Placenta. At 16 weeks of gestation in normal human pregnancy, the spiral arteries in the placental bed progressively lose their musculoelastic tissue and widen, thereby allowing for the increase in blood supply required by the pregnant uterus.[195] In pre-eclampsia these changes may not occur, and a constricting segment of the spiral artery is left. In this narrowed segment, necrosis and filtration of the blood vessels produce the typical picture of acute atherosclerosis (Fig. 1–6). The cause of these changes remains unclear, although Robertson believes they are caused by the hypertension.[195] One is struck by the similarity of these changes to those found in the kidney in postpartum renal failure and scleroderma.

Kidney. Significant changes in the glomeruli in toxemia were first described in 1918 by Lohlein,[155] and in 1920 Fahr called attention to the swelling of the capillary wall.[74] The first electron microscopic study of the glomerulus in toxemia was reported in 1959 by Farquhar, who demonstrated pronounced swelling of the glomerular endothelial cells and deposits of fibrin-like material within and under the endothelial cells.[76]

Spargo et al. confirmed this report and called the lesion *glomerular capillary endotheliosis* (Fig. 1–7).[212] In 1963 Vassalli et al. demonstrated with immunofluorescence staining that the deposits in the glomeruli were fibrinogen or one of its derivatives.[235] Light microscopic studies of renal biopsies demonstrate that the capillary lumen is bloodless and is swollen by endothelial and mesangial cells. The lesion is generalized, usually involving all glomeruli. Endothelial cells not only are swollen but contain large numbers of vacuoles (Fig. 1–8). The basement membrane is not thickened, and there is little proliferation of either endothelial or epithelial cells. Complete resolution of these glomerular changes has been reported to occur as early as four weeks post partum. There is no evidence of immunologic mediated damage to the glomerulus, and the swollen endothelial cells point to endothelial cell injury and resultant local activation of intravascular coagulation. When immunoglobulins have been noted by immunofluorescence in the glomeruli of patients with toxemia, they probably represent nonspecific trapping in injured glomeruli. Although it has been postulated that the

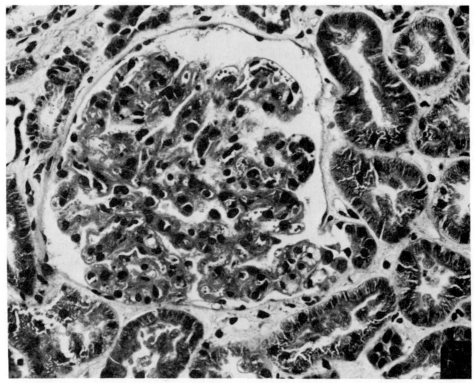

FIGURE 1–7. Glomerulus from a patient with toxemia. Magnification 500×. (Courtesy of Dr. B. Spargo.)

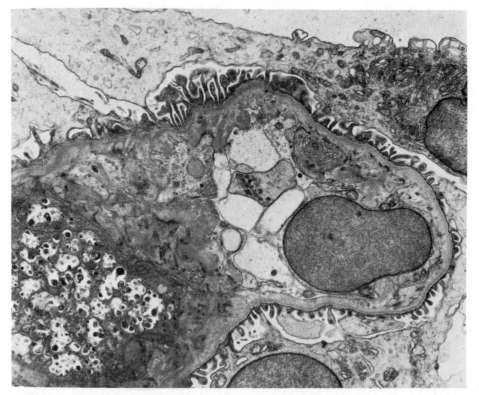

FIGURE 1–8. Electron micrograph of a glomerulus in toxemia. Note the swollen intracapillary cells with lipid-containing lysosomes in the mesangial cell. The endothelial cell is full of clear vacuoles, and there is a trapped platelet. Magnification 10,000×. (Courtesy of Dr. B. Spargo.)

fibrin deposits are due to intravascular coagulation and are similar to lesions produced in experimental animals following thromboplastin infusions,[163] a more complete understanding of local factors involving both platelets and endothelial cells in clot formation suggests that local activation of clotting in response to endothelial cell injury is more likely.

The presence of the glomerular lesion is best correlated with the degree of proteinuria. Proteinuria in toxemia can range from minimal levels, 500 mg/24 hours, to levels that cause the nephrotic syndrome.[84, 85] Some patients with toxemia have severe proteinuria with minimal hypertension, whereas in others the hypertension is more prominent. Hypertension is not the cause of the glomerular pathology; similar glomerular changes are seen in bovine toxemia, in which proteinuria and typical changes in glomerular endotheliosis occur without hypertension.[80] Robson has argued that the changes in toxemia are not unique,[196] but it is interesting that in situations with similar lesions, i.e., the hemolytic-uremic syndrome and following an abruptio placentae, fibrin deposits in the glomeruli, are also involved.

Since toxemia is a description of a clinical disease, it is not surprising that not all biopsies from women with toxemia have the characteristic lesion.[86] In some women, particularly multiparous women with toxemia, hypertension is the prominent feature of the disease, the renal disease being minimal or absent. To restrict the diagnosis of toxemia to a pathologic description of the glomerulus is to deny the clinical and extrarenal manifestations of the disease.

Central Nervous System. The most common cause of death in toxemia is cerebral hemorrhage, which occurs in about 60 per cent of patients who die following eclampsia. The hemorrhages are petechial as well as characterized by large hematomas. Frequently, a large hemorrhage occurs in the white matter and may extend into the subarachnoid space or ventricles. Although cerebral edema following eclampsia was noted frequently by pathologists in the early part of this century, Sheehan and Lynch have disputed these observations on the basis of the average brain weight in patients dying of eclampsia.[208] However, most neuropathologists today rely upon the postmortem appearance of the brain, rather than upon its weight, to document cerebral edema.[64] Cerebral edema occurs frequently in malignant hypertension, but hypertension in toxemia seldom reaches the level where autoregulation of cerebral blood flow is exceeded. That has been found in experimental studies of monkeys to be at a mean arterial pressure of approximately 140 mm Hg, when Pco_2 is normal. Such blood pressures rarely occur with eclampsia. One must look for mechanisms other than pressure alone that cause the central nervous system manifestations of the disease. It is possible that damage to endothelial cells of cerebral capillaries, similar to that occurring in glomeruli and in the liver, causes platelet aggregation and local activation of clotting. Fibrin deposits have been described in the brain of some patients dying of toxemia, but since some dying eclamptic patients have clinical evidence of consumptive coagulopathy, it is difficult to know how much of the cerebral pathology is primary and how much is secondary to the coagulopathy.

An unusual cause of postpartum headache and convulsion is central venous thrombosis. Thrombosis most commonly develops in a vein over the parietal cortex. The convulsions may be indistinguishable from eclampsia. Their cause is unclear but may be related to the hypercoagulable state that occurs post partum and that may also account for postpartum phlebothrombosis and postpartum renal failure. There are over 396 recorded cases of postpartum cerebral findings consistent with a central venous thrombosis. The mortality rate is approximately 40 per cent.[64] Occasionally central venous thrombosis occurs during the pregnancy. Although convulsions mimic eclampsia in these women, the absence of hypertension and proteinuria argues against toxemia.

Coagulation in Pregnancy

Striking changes in coagulation occur in pregnancy with an increase in clotting factors and diminished fibrinolysin activity. Plasma fibrinogen, as well as Factors VII, VIII, X and XIII, increases with pregnancy,[28] and this increase is accompanied by a progressive decrease in the level of plasminogen activator. Pregnancy is associated with a change in the balance of clotting factors toward a state of enhanced coagulability with diminished fibrinolytic activity. Since fibrin deposits occur in the kidney and liver with toxemia, and a fulminant consumptive coagulopathy is present in some patients, intravascular coagulation plays a role in the pathophysiology of toxemia. Although overt evidence of a consumptive coagulopathy is found in only a minority of women with toxemia, there is a great deal of evidence to suggest mild intravascular coagulation. Studies of Factor VIII consumption, estimated by the difference between the levels of

Factor VIII related antigen and Factor VIII clotting activity, show a high correlation with the severity of toxemia and with the increase in plasma urate.[193] In some patients the changes in Factor VIII consumption precede hyperuricemia, a biochemical characteristic of toxemia, and are occasionally seen in the absence of hypertension. Thrombocytopenia occurs with severe toxemia; in one prospective study, a fall in platelet count occurred as early as the 22nd week in women who developed toxemia.[28] A correlation has been reported between hyperuricemia and thrombocytopenia in toxemia, the thrombocytopenia persisting until delivery.[193] In contrast, the platelet count did not change significantly in women with normal levels of plasma urate throughout pregnancy. In addition, studies of platelet function in toxemic women reveal significantly lower maximum aggregation rates in response to collagen, vasopressin, and arachidonic acid, which may indicate that these platelets have undergone aggregation and disaggregation in the circulation.[248] These observations are consistent with the possibility that platelet adherence occurs at the site of endothelial cell damage. It is interesting that thrombocytopenia has been described in babies born of toxemic mothers.[29] Both urinary and serum fibrin degradation products are elevated in pre-eclampsia and remain elevated in the urine for up to seven days post partum.[28]

The demonstration of high plasma 6-oxo-PGF_1-alpha in late pregnancy suggests that the vascular endothelium in pregnancy increases synthesis of PGI_2.[153] Since a balance normally exists between the aggregatory influence of thromboxane production in platelets and the antiaggregatory PGI_2 production in endothelium, one can conceive of platelet aggregation occurring in toxemia if an imbalance between these factors should occur. Although PGI_2 synthesis is elevated in pregnancy, it appears that the balance is shifted toward a state of intravascular coagulation, possibly because of greater platelet thromboxane synthesis. Platelets have been found to be more aggregable in late pregnancy and to contain a higher thromboxane concentration.[253] If the increase in angiotensin sensitivity that occurs in women with toxemia is a manifestation of decreased PGI_2 synthesis, it is intriguing to speculate that this same effect may create a predisposition to aggregation and resultant endothelial cell damage. Recent reports that the fetal and maternal vasculature from toxemic patients synthesize less PGI_2 than normotensive pregnant women are of interest in this regard.[37a, 41, 64, 193a] One can anticipate that investigative efforts in

this area during the next several years will yield a more complete understanding of the factors controlling peripheral resistance and possibly endothelial cell integrity and platelet aggregation during pregnancy. Such studies may give insight not only into the pathophysiology of toxemia but into many other clinical conditions, i.e., hemolytic-uremic syndrome, thrombotic thrombocytopenic purpura, and the Shwartzman reaction following the introduction of endotoxin, wherein a similar pathway with fibrin deposits in kidney, lung, and central nervous system has been demonstrated. It is intriguing that the Shwartzman reaction occurs after one challenge of endotoxin in pregnant animals.

RENAL FUNCTION IN TOXEMIA

There is a reduction in glomerular filtration rate with toxemia, but since an increase in GFR of 50 to 75 per cent occurs in normal pregnancy, GFR with toxemia may remain in the range that is normal for nonpregnant women. The rise in GFR in pregnancy results in a mean blood urea nitrogen of 8.7 ± 1.5 mg per 100 ml, compared with 13 ± 3 mg per 100 ml in nonpregnant women, and in a serum creatinine level of 0.45 ± 0.6 mg per 100 ml compared with 0.67 ± 0.17 mg per 100 ml in nonpregnant women.[185] Bucht found that the inulin clearance increased from 122 ± 24 ml per minute to 170 ± 23 ml per minute from the 8th to the 32nd week of pregnancy, the GFR in toxemic women being about 62 per cent of that in pregnant control subjects.[36] Since for each 50 per cent reduction in GFR, serum creatinine and BUN double, a rise in serum creatinine from 0.5 to 1.0 mg per 100 ml or in BUN from 8 to 16 mg per 100 ml indicates severe reduction in GFR with toxemia. Davison et al. found an increment in GFR five to seven weeks after the last menstrual period in pregnant women.[59] Filtration fraction (the fraction of renal plasma flow that is filtered by the glomerulus) falls during pregnancy, possibly owing to glomerular efferent arteriolar dilatation, but during the last month of pregnancy there is a fall in renal blood flow accompanied by a rise in filtration factor.

Renal blood flow in toxemia falls to 62 to 84 per cent of values in normotensive pregnant controls. In the few studies in which it was measured, filtration fraction was reported to decrease in toxemia, in contrast to the elevation in pregnant patients with essential hypertension. However, studies of renal blood flow and filtration fraction are hampered during toxemia by attempts at determinations of para-amino-hippurate (PAH) clearance during low urine flow rate.[59]

Since 1934 the level of plasma urate has been advocated as an index of the severity of pre-eclampsia.[215] Uric acid clearance increases with pregnancy; the mean urate level in pregnant women is 3.57 ± .7 mg per 100 ml. With the development of toxemia, urate concentration rises, usually prior to any measurable change in the serum creatinine or BUN. There is no increase in urate production with toxemia;[204] the hyperuricemia is due to decreased renal clearance. It was originally suggested that an elevation in serum lactate, which is known to inhibit urate clearance, because of a hypoxic uterus and placenta might be the cause.[122] However, several studies have demonstrated no correlation between arterial lactate and urate clearance in toxemia.[73, 191] Following a seizure, which is known to increase blood lactate, elevated lactate may contribute to the hyperuricemia. A serum urate level greater than 4.5 mg per 100 ml is a strong biochemical indicator of the presence of toxemia, and when it exceeds 5.5 mg per 100 ml the disease is usually severe. The degree of hyperuricemia has correlated well with the severity of toxemia,[73] with the histological lesion found on renal biopsy,[185] and with the fetal prognosis.[191] If the filtration fraction rises in toxemia, such a change in renal hemodynamics might reduce urate clearance. An increase in filtration fraction induced by infusions of angiotensin and norepinephrine has been demonstrated to diminish urate clearance,[78] and an increase in filtration fraction occurs in essential hypertension, wherein hyperuricemia is frequently noted. Since urate clearance is dependent upon tubular secretion, urate clearance may be more dependent upon renal plasma flow than upon GFR. The change in urate clearance is similar to that in patients receiving prolonged diuretic therapy, in whom increased proximal tubular sodium reabsorption occurs and the reduction in urate clearance can be corrected by increasing sodium intake.[216] However, saline loading in pregnant women does not increase urate clearance.[155] The cause of the hyperuricemia in toxemia remains unclear, but it is a valuable biochemical determination to monitor in assessing the severity of the disease.

Plasma osmolality is approximately 10 mOsm/kg of H_2O lower in late pregnancy, the decrease in plasma sodium concentration being approximately 5 mEq/l. In pregnant rats, this change in serum sodium concentration is due in part to a resetting of the release of antidiuretic hormone (ADH) in response to changes in serum tonicity.[67] Since 24 hour urine volumes in human pregnancy increase by about 20 per cent, the increased thirst in pregnant women may also play a role in the hyponatremia. In rats with a hereditary deficiency of ADH, hyponatremia also occurs during pregnancy accompanied by an increase in water intake. Thus, it appears that a change in ADH release and increased water intake both play a role in the hyponatremia of pregnancy. The cause of the increased thirst in pregnancy is not known, but high plasma angiotensin is known to increase thirst in other clinical circumstances.[87]

P_{CO_2} in pregnancy falls to approximately 30 mm Hg, compared with normal values of 40 mm Hg.[24] This hyperventilation causes an increase in the renal excretion of bicarbonate, so plasma bicarbonate in normal pregnancy is approximately 16 to 20 mEq/liter. This compensated respiratory alkalosis has little significance except when a metabolic acidosis, i.e., ketoacidosis, or lactic acidosis supervenes and total buffering capacity is reduced. The cause of the hyperventilation is thought to be a direct effect of increased plasma progesterone on the respiratory center.[159]

CLINICAL FEATURES AND EPIDEMIOLOGY OF TOXEMIA

The incidence of toxemia of pregnancy varies widely. In the United States, the incidence is approximately 7 per cent, but in Scotland Mac-Gillivray et al. found a 24 per cent incidence of hypertension in primigravidas and 8 per cent in multiparous patients.[160] The disease has a bimodal frequency, being most common in young primigravid and older multiparous women. The incidence of the disease obviously depends upon the criteria used for the diagnosis. Data from a collaborative study of over 24,000 pregnancies have demonstrated that blood pressures in excess of 125/75 prior to the 36th week of gestation are associated with significant increases in fetal risk, as are pressures of over 125/85 at term.[93] Among 15,000 pregnant women in another report, the perinatal mortality rate rose progressively with each 5 mm Hg rise in mean arterial pressure (MAP) (diastolic pressure + 1/3 pulse pressure).[178] Those with a MAP of 90 or more (MAP = 93 mm Hg) during the second trimester had a higher risk of stillbirth, fetal growth retardation, and progression into toxemia. Even without proteinuria, a trend towards increased perinatal mortality was found when MAP was greater than 82 mm Hg at midpregnancy or greater than 92 mm Hg at the beginning of the third trimester. MacGillivray accepts a 14 mm Hg rise in diastolic blood pressure during pregnancy as evidence of toxemia. The American Obstetrical Committee has recommended a blood pressure of 130/80 as being the upper limit of normal at any time during pregnancy, a rise of 30 mm Hg systolic or 15 mm Hg diastolic blood pressure during pregnancy being considered abnormal regardless of the absolute values attained. One of the major benefits of prenatal care is the prevention of severe toxemia; prevention is dependent upon awareness by obstetricians of the normal values for blood pressure in pregnancy and recognition that a blood pressure that would not cause concern in a nonpregnant subject indicates pathophysiology during pregnancy. This is evident from the observation of 226 primigravid women on the first visit to an obstetric clinic, in whom blood pressure was found to be 103 ± 11 systolic, 56 ± 10 diastolic when they were sitting and 113 ± 10 systolic, 57 ± 10 diastolic when they were supine.[160] A slight rise in both systolic and diastolic pressure occurs at about the 28th week, interestingly at the time an increase in angiotensin sensitivity has been demonstrated, the blood pressure at term being 109 ± 12/69 ± 9 sitting and 116 ± 10/71 ± 12 supine. There is a tendency for blood pressure to rise post partum; at six weeks post partum blood pressure in these women was 110 ± 12/70 ± 11 sitting and 112 ±

12/67 ± 11 supine. The normal postpartum rise in blood pressure may occasionally result in postpartum hypertension, which has been reported in 5 to 17 per cent of black women following delivery.[62, 219] Most of these women have normal blood pressure one year later, and over half of them have been normotensive during pregnancy.

Although it has been believed that toxemia is more common in blacks, the incidence of toxemia in patients at Kings County Hospital, New York, a hospital serving a primarily black population, is not higher than in whites.[44] Toxemia does have a family prevalence. In the Johns Hopkins series, the incidence of hypertension during pregnancy was 28 per cent in daughters of pre-eclamptic mothers, compared with 13 per cent in daughters of normotensive mothers.[135] This suggests that hypertensive diathesis may be a factor in the development of toxemia. In Chesley's followup study of 270 patients with eclampsia, 26 per cent of the daughters of mothers with eclampsia had toxemia in their first pregnancy compared with 8 per cent of the daughters-in-law. An interesting finding in this study was that systolic pressure was higher in patients who smoked but diastolic pressure was lower. Women who smoked ten or more cigarettes a day had smaller babies compared with nonsmokers, and the incidence of toxemia was higher in women who did not smoke. No explanation of

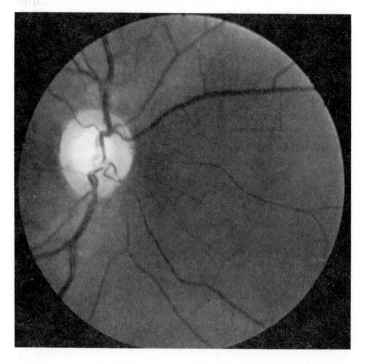

FIGURE 1–9. Retinal photograph from a patient with toxemia. Note the segmental arteriolar narrowing. (Courtesy of Dr. F. Finnerty.)

this finding is apparent, but the smaller babies of smokers may be a factor. However, the adverse effect of heavy smoking during pregnancy on fetal survival[5] outweighs its seemingly protective effect on the development of toxemia.

The presence of underlying essential hypertension or renal disease increases the incidence of toxemia. The association with obesity is less clear, but obesity may be a factor as it is in essential hypertension.

Although much has been written about socioeconomic status and toxemia, in Aberdeen, Scotland, a uniform incidence of toxemia was found throughout all social classes. In the early part of this century, it was believed that toxemia was primarily a disease of the affluent. Death from toxemia, in the United States, is inversely correlated with the average income in various communities, which may be more indicative of inadequate medical care provided to the poor, particularly in rural areas, than of any nutritional or dietary factors.

The clinical onset of toxemia is insidious and may not be accompanied by overt symptoms. The usual sequence is rapid weight gain with edema and a rise in blood pressure followed by proteinuria, although occasionally proteinuria precedes hypertension. Toxemia usually begins after the 32nd week of pregnancy but may begin earlier, particularly in women with pre-existing renal disease or hypertension. When it occurs during the first trimester, it is virtually pathognomonic of a hydatidiform mole. The disease may occur post partum, with hypertension and convulsions usually occurring within 24 to 48 hours after delivery, although it has been reported to occur as late as seven days post partum. Headache, visual disturbances, epigastric pain, and apprehension are frequent symptoms. The physical examination reveals generalized puffy edema, particularly of the face and hands. Diastolic hypertension is prominent, the systolic pressure usually being below 160 mm Hg. A systolic blood pressure greater than 200 mm Hg points to toxemia with underlying essential hypertension. Funduscopic examination will reveal segmental arteriolar narrowing, which can be striking, with a wet glistening appearance indicative of retinal edema (Fig. 1–9). Hemorrhages and exudates are rare, but they may occur in toxemia and are associated with sudden blindness.[101] Detachment of the retina is caused by intraocular edema, and spontaneous reattachment of the retina usually follows diuresis and control of the hypertension. Careful examination of the heart and lungs is always indicated to determine whether congestive heart failure is present; if so, it is usually due to left ventricular failure caused by the hypertension.[221] Left ventricular stroke work is greater in toxemic patients because of the hypertension. However, pulmonary edema may occur in toxemia with normal pulmonary capillary wedge pressure. The mechanism of the pulmonary edema in these instances is probably similar to that occurring in other renal diseases, in which changes in pulmonary capillary permeability cause "uremic pneumonitis." Although fibrin deposits in the pulmonary vasculature have not been described, they may also be a factor in the pulmonary edema, since they have been described in other diseases in which intravascular clotting occurs. Pulmonary edema with normal to low venous pressure should not be interpreted as volume depletion.

Clinical Spectrum of Toxemia

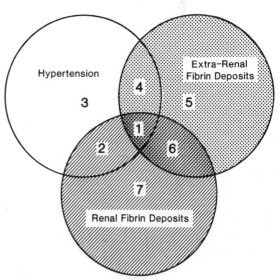

FIGURE 1–10. The variable clinical presentations of toxemia.
1. Fulminant toxemia with convulsions, thrombocytopenia, consumptive coagulopathy, azotemia, and hypertension.
2. Toxemia with hypertension, proteinuria, and reduced glomerular filtration rate but no extrarenal manifestations.
3. Hypertension in pregnancy that disappears post partum.
4. Toxemia with hypertension but with prominent systemic manifestations, i.e., thrombocytopenia, hepatic dysfunction, pancreatitis, central nervous system signs.
5. Systemic manifestations as in number 4 but with minimal hypertension.
6. Systemic manifestations and renal involvement but with minimal hypertension.
7. Nephrotic syndrome with the typical renal lesion of toxemia but with minimal hypertension.

Venous constriction accounts for the normal to low venous pressure and may contribute to the edema of the face and upper extremities as well as to the hemoconcentration. Central nervous system excitability, a useful guide to the severity of neurological involvement, is assessed by careful determination of the spinal reflexes.

Since toxemia is a multisystem disease, it may mimic other conditions in its presentation. This is a relatively common problem. Frequently the internist is called to see the patient because the usual manifestations of toxemia are obscured. Thrombocytopenia may be prominent and may suggest idiopathic thrombocytopenic purpura; if neurologic features are present the diagnosis of thrombotic thrombocytopenic purpura may be entertained.[181, 202] Jaundice and abnormalities of liver function tests may point to hepatitis.[157] Abdominal pain is frequent in toxemia, as it is also in malignant hypertension or with a pheochromocytoma, and is probably pancreatic in origin. Elevation of the serum amylase may be seen in toxemia, in which case the diagnosis of acute pancreatitis may be made. Figure 1–10 shows a diagram accounting for several of the possible presentations of toxemia. It is important that the obstetrician and the internist appreciate the systemic manifestations of toxemia in order for appropriate therapy to be instituted.

POSTULATED MECHANISMS OF TOXEMIA

Figure 1–11 depicts a hypothetical sequence of events that may occur with toxemia. Since there is evidence that PGI_2 synthesis is increased in blood vessels and PGE_2 synthesis increased in uterus and kidney during pregnancy, a reduction in prostaglandin synthesis may occur with toxemia. Since the factors that increase prostaglandin synthesis in pregnancy are not known, it is not possible to speculate on the cause of the decreased synthesis with the development of toxemia. A hormonal effect of pregnancy is an attractive possibility, but we have been unable to demonstrate an effect of estrogen or progesterone on urinary or plasma prostaglandin E_2 in rabbits. However, with reduced prostaglandin synthesis in the uterus, a reduction of uteroplacental blood flow may account for the fetal distress and the increase in fetal mortality. Since the experiments utilizing captopril suggest that uteroplacental prostaglandin E_2 synthesis is dependent upon angiotensin II, a reduction in uterine PGE_2 synthesis may induce an increase in uterine renin synthesis and a possible increase in uterine renin secretion.[90] There is a wide variability in plasma renin activity in toxemia,[226, 245] and some workers have reported plasma angio-

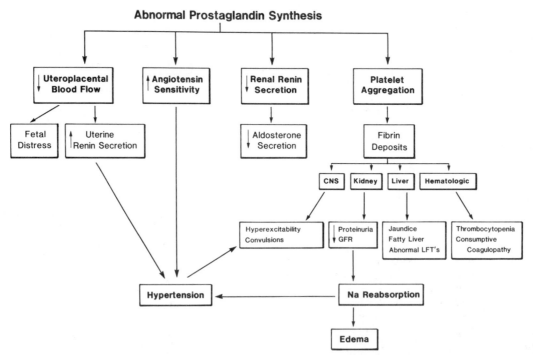

FIGURE 1–11. A hypothesis for the pathophysiology of toxemia.

tensin II to be higher in hypertensive pregnant women.[224] Whether the residual plasma renin with toxemia is of uteroplacental or of renal origin is not known, although higher plasma renin has been reported in the uterine vein in toxemic women.[144, 211] In one patient with an abdominal pregnancy and toxemia, plasma renin activity rose with the development of toxemia.[14]

Regardless of PRA, a decrease in PGI_2 synthesis in blood vessels increases angiotensin sensitivity, and the absolute level of renin or angiotensin is less important than the sensitivity of the arterioles to angiotensin II. Renal renin secretion may decrease owing to diminished prostaglandin synthesis in afferent arterioles, since renin secretion *in vivo* and *in vitro* is dependent upon PGI_2 synthesis. There is also evidence that synthesis of prostaglandins in the adrenal gland is necessary for normal aldosterone secretion,[38, 110] so the fall in aldosterone secretion with toxemia may be due to the fall in renin or may be a direct effect of a fall in prostaglandin synthesis in the adrenal gland. In addition to being involved in the development of hypertension, a derangement in the proportion of PGI_2 synthesis in blood vessels and thromboxane synthesis in platelets could lead to platelet aggregation. This could cause fibrin deposits in the central nervous system, kidney, and liver as well as a consumptive coagulopathy in severe toxemia.

This hypothesis will obviously require much experimental work. It does, however, allow an explanation for the diverse clinical presentations of toxemia. Although hypertension and proteinuria have been the hallmark of the disease, they are not necessarily prominent in every patient. Toxemia may mimic thrombotic thrombocytopenic purpura, idiopathic thrombopenic purpura, and acute fatty liver of pregnancy, and several postpartum diseases such as postpartum renal failure, postpartum cardiomyopathy, and Sheehan's syndrome may be due to thrombosis of small vessels occurring during or immediately after a pregnancy.

PREVENTION AND TREATMENT

The first object of the treatment of toxemia should be its prevention. Proper prenatal care with attention to adequate but not excessive weight gain and careful monitoring of blood pressure reduces the incidence of the disease. Nutritional factors have often been mentioned as being important in causing toxemia, but there is no evidence of a nutritional basis for the disease. Poor blacks in the southern United States have a high incidence of toxemia,[51] but there is no correlation between toxemia and nutrition in India[42] or in Australia.[123] The widely cited decrease in eclampsia in Germany during World War I made popular the doctrine of prevention of toxemia through dietary restrictions. Subsequent studies, however, demonstrated that the decrease in wartime eclampsia was associated with a parallel reduction in total deliveries; after the war the incidence of first births and toxemia increased.[127] The World Health Organization Expert Committee has stated, "There seems to be no scientific basis for believing that deficiency or excess of any essential nutrient predisposes to pre-eclampsia and eclampsia."[251] In many countries, however, the poor suffer a higher incidence of toxemia. In Jerusalem, toxemia in illiterate women is twice that in matched control subjects.[58] The poor are more apt to have children at early and late ages, and this may be a factor explaining the increased incidence.

The most important feature in the prevention and treatment of toxemia is the recognition that a rise in blood pressure greater than 30 mm Hg systolic or 15 mm Hg diastolic during pregnancy is significant and that the development of proteinuria is always an indication for hospitalization. Using 140/90 as the upper limit of normal has no justification in the management of pregnancy. A level of 125/75 before the 32nd week of gestation and 125/85 thereafter is associated with decreased fetal survival and on this basis should be considered abnormal. Although approximately 25 per cent of pregnant women have a blood pressure higher than 125/85 in the last month of pregnancy, it is in these women that toxemia is more apt to occur.

The initial therapy for toxemia is bed rest, preferably with the patient lying on her side. Blood pressure, pulse, respirations, and urine volume are carefully monitored. In the conscious patient there is no need for an indwelling catheter, but in comatose patients or those having convulsions, an indwelling catheter is warranted for the evaluation of urine output. In the patient with mild toxemia, i.e., with blood pressure no higher than 140/90, therapy consists of bed rest; sedation with phenobarbital, 60 mg every six hours, or diazepam (Valium), 10 mg given intramuscularly; salt restriction to 1–2 grams daily; and if edema is present, 50 mg hydrochlorothiazide or 40 mg furosemide orally. These measures usually suffice in controlling the hypertension. Baseline BUN, creatinine, and uric acid are determined, and a 24 hour urine collection for assessing volume and total protein excretion is obtained. Daily weights are a guide to the extent of the diuresis. The level of serum uric acid before the institution of diuretic therapy is a guide to the severity of the toxemia. A uric acid level greater than 4.5 mg per 100 ml is virtually diagnostic of toxemia, and a uric acid level above 5.5 mg per 100 ml is indicative of severe toxemia. Extremely high levels of uric acid can be seen in toxemic patients following a convulsion; the intense muscular effort causes elevation of plasma lactate, which further decreases uric acid clearance. When hypertension develops during pregnancy without the characteristic renal lesion of toxemia, there is usually no change in the serum urate concentration. Thus, a serum uric acid below 4 mg per 100 ml in a pregnant hypertensive woman is most consistent with either essential hypertension or toxemia without renal involvement.

If therapy lowers the blood pressure below 120/80, proteinuria is less than 150 mg per 24 hours, renal function is normal, and there is no evidence of CNS hyperexcitability, the patient can be followed up weekly as an outpatient if further growth of the fetus is desirable. If the patient is at term and there is no concern about fetal viability, delivery is indicated as soon as the patient's clinical status is stable.

When the patient has more severe hypertension, i.e., blood pressure greater than 140/90, more potent antihypertensive therapy should be initiated. Although magnesium sulfate has long been used by American obstetricians (indeed, over a ton of it has been used in one center[187]) it cannot be considered either an antihypertensive or anticonvulsant. Its anticonvulsant effect is dependent on an effect at the neuromuscular junction, where Mg decreases the amount of acetylcholine release by a given motor nerve impulse. There is no evidence that it affects EEG signs of seizure activity. Magnesium concentrations of approximately 3 to 6 mEq per liter are considered to be within the therapeutic range; respiratory failure occurs at higher concentrations. Thus, the disappearance of spinal reflexes with the administration of magnesium sulfate is due to the peripheral action of magnesium and indicates a plasma magnesium concentration of approximately 10 mEq per liter. Convulsions have been reported to occur with "therapeutic" Mg concentrations,[180] and studies have demonstrated no correlation between cerebrospinal fluid concentration of Mg and the serum concentration.[186] Like all smooth muscle relaxants, magnesium sulfate depresses myometrial activity. Now that more potent and safer antihypertensive drugs are available, there seems to be little advantage in magnesium sulfate other than the experience and confidence American obstetricians have in its use.

Hydralazine (Apresoline), a vasodilator, is effective when used in doses of 25 to 50 mg every six hours orally. To prevent the reflex tachycardia that occurs with hydralazine, propranolol, 40 mg every six hours, has been effectively combined with hydralazine in the treatment of essential hypertension. Since propranolol crosses the placenta, it causes fetal bradycardia, which masks one of the clinical markers of fetal distress. Therefore, it has not been used to a great extent in the treatment of acute toxemia, but it and other beta-adrenergic blockers have been used throughout pregnancy in women with essential hypertension and have given excellent results.[70, 99, 198] Methyldopa (Aldomet), an adrenergic blocking drug, also blocks the reflex tachycardia caused by hydralazine and may be given orally in doses of 250 to 500 mg every 6 to 12 hours.

If the diastolic blood pressure is greater than 110 mm Hg, parenteral antihypertensive therapy is indicated. Methyldopa (Aldomet), 500 mg, and furosemide, 40 to 80 mg, may be given intravenously and repeated every 6 hours. Since parenteral methyldopa requires 6 to 8 hours for maximum effect, parenteral hydralazine can be used for immediate control of blood pressure. Hydralazine, 25 mg intramuscularly or 25 to 50 mg dissolved in 50 ml of 5 per cent glucose in water intravenously, usually controls blood pressure rapidly. When given intramuscularly, hydralazine requires frequent administration (at least every 3 to 4 hours), and when it is given intravenously constant monitoring of the blood pressure is necessary. Its effect is rapid, and like all vasodilators it will increase cardiac output and pulse by reflex sympathetic activity. In one report, extreme lowering of maternal diastolic blood pressure to 70 to 90 mm Hg with intravenous hydralazine was noted to cause deceleration of the fetal heart rate when the infant was severely growth retarded.[238] The authors believed their findings indicated that the placenta can maintain blood flow and function following extreme reduction in arterial pressure in toxemia unless severe growth retardation is present, in which case delivery should be carried out. There was, however, no evidence that hydralazine adversely affected fetal survival even when deceleration of the heart rate occurred.

When the diastolic blood pressure is 120 mm Hg or greater, diazoxide, 300 mg intravenously, can be given with 40 to 80 mg of furosemide.

Finnerty treated 60 patients with severe toxemia with diazoxide and furosemide. The treatment resulted in an average diuresis of 16 pounds prior to delivery.[82] Mean arterial pressure fell from 141 to 92 mm Hg. The albuminuria cleared completely in 14 patients and decreased in 47 with treatment of hypertension. There were no maternal deaths and only 4 fetal deaths, an incidence of prematurity of 37 per cent. Fetal mortality was lower in Finnerty's series (6 per cent) than the 11 per cent reported in a series in which hypertension was not treated.[256] Morris et al. used intravenous diazoxide to treat nine patients with severe preeclampsia and three with eclampsia and had an excellent response.[167] Diastolic blood pressure never fell below 50 mm Hg, and significant change in fetal heart rate was observed in only one patient. The only side effect of diazoxide was the cessation of labor in about 50 per cent of the patients, probably as a result of the generalized smooth muscle relaxant effect of the drug. The administration of oxytocic agents immediately restarted labor.

The reluctance of obstetricians to reduce blood pressure is based on the impression that hypertension increases uterine perfusion. There are few studies of the uteroplacental circulation in toxemia, but Assali et al., using the nitrous oxide technique in women with toxemia, demonstrated increased uterine vascular resistance with decreased uterine flow.[11] Utilizing electro-magnetic flow probes applied to one uterine artery in pregnant dogs and ewes, they also reported later that flow to the uterus was increased with increasing perfusion pressure.[12] However, recent studies in pregnant rabbits, in which radioactive microspheres were used to measure uterine blood flow, have demonstrated that uterine blood flow is constant over a range of blood pressure from 75 to 120 mm Hg (Fig. 1–12).[237] Since uterine vasoconstriction may account for the reduction in flow with toxemia, relief of the vasoconstriction may increase perfusion of the uterus, particularly if cardiac output increases. It is known that both hydralazine (Apresoline) and diazoxide increase cardiac output, and methyldopa (Aldomet) reduces blood pressure with little or no change in cardiac output. Diazoxide in the pregnant rabbit increases uterine blood flow,[237] and in pregnant ewes no change in uterine blood flow occurred following diazoxide administration when maternal hypotension did not fall below a MAP of 50 mm Hg. Monitoring of the fetus in these studies revealed no change in fetal pulse even when diazoxide was injected directly into the fetal circulation.[174] In reading the experimental studies of the effect of hypotension on the fetus, one is struck by the tolerance of the fetal circulation to hypotension, a point that has been commented on by Assali.[10] When diazoxide was found to lower uterine blood flow, MAP fell to lower than

PERFUSION PRESSURE & UTEROPLACENTAL BLOOD FLOW

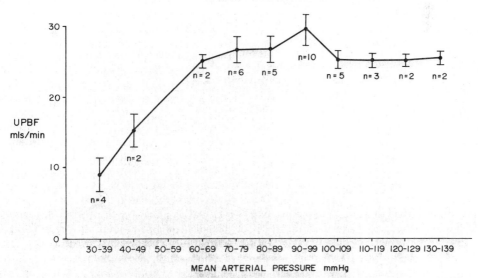

FIGURE 1–12. The effect of varying perfusion on the uterine blood flow of the pregnant rabbit. Arterial pressure was raised by carotid ligation and lowered with antihypertensive drugs. Note the constancy of uterine blood flow over a range of mean arterial pressures ranging from 60–69 mm Hg to 130–139 mm Hg (n = number of observations at each arterial pressure). (From Venuto et al.: J. Clin. Invest., 57:938, 1976. Reprinted with permission.)

TABLE 1–1 CLINICAL CLASSIFICATION OF TOXEMIA

	Mild	Moderate	Severe
Blood Pressure	120/80–140/95	150/100–160/110	>160/110
Clinical	1+ edema Normal reflexes No visual signs	1–2+ edema 1–2+ hyper-reflexia Early visual signs	3–4+ edema 3–4+ hyper-reflexia Convulsion (eclampsia) Congestive heart failure Visual signs
Lab Values BUN Serum creatinine Urate Urinary protein Thrombocytopenia Decreased clotting factors	10 mg/100 ml 1 mg/100 ml <4.5 mg/100 ml 1+ (0.5 gm/24 hr) Absent Absent	10–20 mg/100 ml 1–1.6 mg/100 ml 4.5–6 mg/100 ml 2–3+ (0.5–2 gm/24 hr) Mild Absent	>20 mg/100 ml >1.6 mg/100 ml >6 mg/100 ml 3–4+ (2 gm/24 hr) Present Present occasionally

Treatment
Bed rest, 1–2 gm
   salt diet
Anti-hypertensive drugs
	Chlorothiazide 500 mg
	   QD
		Chlorothiazide 500 mg bid
		   or
		Lasix 40 mg QD
		Hydralazine 50 mg PO
		   Q6H with Aldomet
		   250–500 mg PO Q6H
			Diazoxide 300 mg IV with
			   Lasix 40 mg IV or
			Hydralazine 10–40 mg IV
			   Q3H with Aldomet 500
			   mg IV Q6G

Anti-convulsants	No	Phenytoin 100 mg PO TID	Phenytoin 0.5–1 gm IV in
			   100 ml saline @ 50
			   mg/min
			Diazepam 5 mg IV if
			   convulsion occurred —
			   20 mg IM Q6H thereafter

Delivery	If fetus at term,
	   delivery indicated
	Delay possible if BP
	   and renal function stable
		Delivery usually indicated	Delivery indicated as soon
			   as cardiovascular and
			   CNS signs stable

45 mm Hg.[40] This same study showed that with a slow infusion of diazoxide, 0.02 mg/kg/min for up to four hours, MAP fell only 5 per cent and uterine blood flow increased. In baboons diazoxide has been infused for four hours at 0.06 mg/kg/min with no adverse effects upon the fetal circulation. In some studies, when potent antihypertensive agents are administered to normotensive animals the pressure falls below the autoregulatory range and far below what one strives to attain in the hypertensive subject; it is therefore not surprising that uterine blood flow may fall. Since the major cause of maternal mortality in toxemia is cerebral vascular hemorrhage, one must at all costs prevent this catastrophe, and the evidence is conclusive that antihypertensive agents prevent cerebral vascular accidents in cases of human hypertension.

An outline of a clinical classification and treatment regimen for toxemia is given in Table 1–1. With the present availability of effective antihypertensive drugs there is no reason for not bringing the blood pressure to normal in every patient. The proper utilization of these drugs depends upon cooperation between the obstetrician and an internist with experience in the treatment of hypertension.

After the blood pressure is reduced and the patient's clinical state is stabilized, delivery of the fetus is indicated if toxemia is severe. If fetal survival is unlikely, the pregnancy may be continued, provided blood pressure is controlled and renal function does not deteriorate, but continued hospitalization is required. The patient should be maintained on a 1 to 2 gram sodium diet and diuretics should be given until edema disappears, at which time they should be discontinued. If elevation of the BUN persists in spite of blood pressure control, delivery is indicated, since fetal growth or maturation is not likely to happen in the presence of azotemia.

In patients with severe toxemia and hyperreflexia, anticonvulsant therapy is indicated. Convulsions always indicate severe disease with increased risk of maternal and fetal mortality and are an indication for delivery. For immediate control of seizures diazepam (Valium) 5 mg is administered IV and may be continued at a dose of 20 mg IM every six hours. Diazepam causes immediate cessation of convulsions when given intravenously.[88, 151, 164] The solution should be injected slowly, at least one minute being taken for each 5 mg injected. When any anticonvulsant is used, resuscitative equipment should be readily available. Doses of 5 to 10 mg of diazepam intravenously cause mild transitory tachycardia in the mother but produce no adverse effects on blood pH or PCO_2 in the mother or the newborn.[252] With high dosages of diazepam, particularly when given intravenously to the mother, transient hypotonia has been reported in infants but respiratory depression did not occur.[205] Diazepam has been used extensively in India for treatment of toxemia and has gained wide acceptance, since its hypnotic and sedative effects seem useful in situations where nursing care is limited.

If convulsions appear imminent, phenytoin, 1 gram in 100 ml saline, is given IV at the rate of 50 mg per min. Plasma levels of the drug can be monitored and should not exceed 18 μg per ml. Although intravenous diphenylhydantoin can cause hypotension and respiratory depression, this adverse effect is minimized if the rate of administration of the drug does not exceed 50 mg per minute. Patients developing cardiac arrhythmias with intravenous administration have usually had underlying cardiac disease. Diphenylhydantoin does cross the placenta, and in epileptic mothers receiving both diphenylhydantoin and phenobarbital throughout pregnancy a neonatal coagulation defect has been reported.[169] The defect responds, however, to vitamin K, which should be given to infants of mothers receiving prolonged treatment with anticonvulsants throughout pregnancy. No infants of mothers receiving short-term treatment for toxemia with anticonvulsants have been reported to develop this coagulation defect.

Phenobarbital or diazepam can be used for sedation of the toxemic patient. Diazepam given intramuscularly in a dose of 10 mg is quite effective in allaying anxiety, or phenobarbital can be given orally, 120 to 180 mg every six to eight hours. Following a convulsion, phenobarbital, 200 to 300 mg, may be given intramuscularly and repeated at eight hour intervals. Although phenobarbital crosses the placenta, its margin of safety is high in infants. When it is employed during delivery, varying degrees of central nervous system depression may occur in the newborn, but there is poor correlation between the depth of the depression and the barbiturate level of cord blood.[4]

Since edema is usually prominent in toxemia, diuretics are logical drugs to use. The argument against their use has been based on two findings: the hemoconcentration that may be present in toxemia and the decreased dehydroepiandrosterone clearance caused by diuretics.[105] As was pointed out previously, hemoconcentration is common with all forms of hypertension and is of minimal clinical significance. The 9 per cent reduction in plasma volume is similar to that in nonpregnant subjects with essential hypertension. The dehydroepiandrosterone (DHEA) clearance test was developed by Gant et al. as a measure of uterine blood flow. The clearance of DHEA depends upon placental conversion of DHEA to estrone and estradiol, and this process is reduced approximately 50 per cent in toxemia. As has been pointed out by Clewell and Meschia,[52] the DHEA clearance is not a mathematically acceptable method of measuring uterine blood flow. Human uterine and placental blood flow at term is approximately 500 ml/minute, but the DHEA clearance is only 19 ml/min and falls in toxemia to a value of 11 ml/min. The DHEA clearance may be an indicator of placental function, but it is obviously not a measure of uterine blood flow. No correlation between DHEA clearance and fetal survival has been shown in any of the published studies. Why it is reduced following diuretics and other antihypertensive drugs, including hydralazine, remains unclear at this time.

The largest study of the effect of treatment on fetal prognosis in toxemia was carried out by Friedman and Neff at 14 university hospitals with data on more than 55,000 pregnant women.[93] In women with hypertension but without proteinuria, they noted no difference in fetal survival in women treated with diuretics. However, when hypertension and proteinuria were present, fetal mortality was 1.85 per cent in untreated women compared with 4.43 per cent in women treated with diuretics. However, there was also a significant increase in fetal mortality when any drug was used, whether antihypertensives, narcotics, or anticonvulsants. Since the most frequent complication of toxemia is fetal mortality, this data would be most consistent

Diuretics in Pregnancy

AUTHOR	# PATIENTS	Fetal Mortality %	
		DIURETICS	NO DIURETICS
Flowers, et al (1962)	519	1.79	2.72
Kraus, et al (1966)	1030	2.8	2.8
Cuadros, et al (1964)	1771	1.4	1.7
Finnerty, et al (1966)	3083	.67	4.4
Landesman, et al (1965)	2706	.15	.45
TOTAL	9109	1.36	2.41

FIGURE 1–13. The results of the prophylactic use of thiazides throughout pregnancy in five series of patients.

with the interpretation that with more severe disease fetal mortality is higher and more drugs are used. It does not prove that the drugs caused the higher fetal mortality. In several studies in which diuretics were given throughout pregnancy in an effort to decrease the incidence of toxemia, fetal mortality was no higher in the women given prophylactic diuretics (Fig. 1–13).[56, 83, 87a, 145, 146] In a series of 604 women, Rauramo et al. instituted treatment with diuretics at the first sign of toxemia, i.e., hypertension or proteinuria, and compared the results with a series of patients from the same clinic not treated with diuretics.[189] Severe toxemia developed in 2.3 per cent of the treated women compared with 7.3 per cent in the untreated group, and perinatal mortality was 2.3 per cent in the group treated with diuretics compared with 4.6 per cent in untreated women. Thus, it appears that diuretics are not contraindicated in pregnancy when there is a clinical indication for their use. Since most women with toxemia are edematous, the use of diuretics for their natriuretic and antihypertensive effect is quite appropriate.

The definitive treatment of toxemia is delivery of the fetus, but the question of fetal viability precludes immediate delivery in some instances. Measurements of fetal development may be helpful, utilizing urinary estriol and pregnanediol determinations as well as lecithin:sphingomyelin ratios in amniotic fluid.[234] When toxemia is associated with low urinary estriol excretion, intrauterine growth has probably ceased and delivery of the fetus is indicated. This is probably more feasible today, since neonatal intensive care units allow for optimum care of the premature infant. Delivery by induction of labor or by cesarean section can be accomplished. The uterus of a toxemic patient is very responsive to oxytocic agents, and labor is usually short.

THE REMOTE CONSEQUENCES OF TOXEMIA

It has been argued that the development of both hypertension and renal disease in later life is related to episodes of toxemia during pregnancy. In all series of toxemia patients, subsequent hypertension is more common, but whether toxemia caused the hypertension is open to question.[210] Toxemia, like hypertension induced by contraceptive drugs, may differentiate those women who will ultimately develop essential hypertension from those who will not. The effect of toxemia on the development of hypertension is difficult to evaluate, since many women with underlying renal disease and hypertension are included in every series of toxemic patients. Similarly, the influences of obesity and color, known to be factors in the development of essential hypertension, have been ignored in many studies on the long-term followup of women with toxemia of pregnancy. Bechgaard et al. found the incidence of hypertension in 372 women 15 years after they had suffered from toxemia to be 25 per cent plus an unknown proportion of the 8 per cent who had died in the 15 year period.[18] Epstein found that 37 per cent of his patients were hypertensive 15 years after they had had toxemia, compared with 7 per cent of the control group.[71] Harbert et al. gave an incidence of hypertension after eclampsia of 15 per cent,[124] and Fritzsch et al. in a followup study of 19 eclamptic patients found that 4 were hypertensive, 1 had chronic glomerulonephritis, and 7 had chronic interstitial nephritis.[94]

The two most careful studies of this problem have been done by Chesley et al. and by Epstein.[44, 71] Epstein's study is particularly noteworthy, since he restricted his study to white women with hypertension, proteinuria, and edema. His patients were both primiparous and multiparous. They were examined 15 years after the episodes of toxemia, and the incidence of hypertension (blood pressure greater than 150/90) was three times that in control women of the same age and weight who had had uncomplicated pregnancies. No evidence of residual renal disease or urinary tract infection was found in the toxemic group. Since he found that the incidence of hypertension in siblings was similar in both groups, he concluded that toxemia predisposed women to the development of hypertension.

In contrast, Chesley restricted his study to 270 women surviving eclampsia who were seen over a 20 year period at the Margaret Hague Maternity Hospital. By eliminating pre-eclamptic patients from the study, he believed that essential hypertension during pregnancy was more likely to be excluded as a factor affecting the results. Approximately 40 per cent of hypertensive women have decreased blood pressure during pregnancy, often in the normal range, and the development of hypertension late in pregnancy can be misleading. In Chesley's followup study of white women having eclampsia in the first pregnancy, the remote mortality over 20 years was the same as in unselected women. The frequency distribution curve of diastolic blood pressure was identical in women having had primiparous eclampsia and in women participating in several epidemiologic studies of blood pressure. However, in both black and white multiparous women having eclampsia, the remote mortality was 2.6 to 3.8 times greater than expected. Thus, eclampsia was associated with a higher incidence of subsequent hypertension only in multiparous women.

On followup examination, interestingly, diabetes was five times as common as expected in primiparous women developing eclampsia and ten times the expected rate in multiparous eclamptic women. This increased incidence of diabetes may be related to the fact that prediabetic women have large babies. This possible connection could not be documented because of the absence of recorded infant birth weights for many of Chesley's patients, but it may be an important factor in the development of toxemia.

Some have argued that Chesley's figures are pertinent only to eclamptic women and that pre-eclamptic patients are frequently hypertensive for longer periods and have a greater incidence of subsequent hypertension. This argument presumes that the duration, rather than the severity, of toxemia causes subsequent hypertension and that eclampsia occurs suddenly. The evidence indicates, however, that eclampsia is most often the result of a prolonged and neglected pre-eclamptic state. Although eclamptic patients are rapidly delivered, most have had little or no prenatal care, and how long they have been hypertensive is usually unknown. In Chesley's series, when blood pressure was recorded prior to the episode of eclampsia, in nearly half of the patients pre-eclampsia had been present for at least three weeks and in about 12 per cent it had been present for more than six weeks before convulsions occurred.

In Chesley's 207 primiparous white eclamptic patients, 148 had later pregnancies and 69 suffered recurrent toxemia. Thus, 25 per cent of these patients had at least two toxemic pregnancies, and yet the prevalence of hypertension was not increased over a control population. The recurrence of toxemia with subsequent pregnancies is over 50 per cent in multiparous women but only 25 per cent in women who developed toxemia with the first pregnancy. Singh et al. reported a higher incidence of late hypertension only in women having pre-eclampsia in more than one pregnancy.[209]

Bryans et al. followed up 168 white women and 167 black women for 1 to 44 years after they had suffered from eclampsia and compared their mean blood pressures by age groups with the blood pressures recorded in several epidemiologic studies.[35] The diastolic pressure of primiparous black eclamptic women was no higher than that of control subjects, and the prevalence of hypertension in the white women with eclampsia was not increased when compared with that in most series. Multiparous eclamptic women, however, had a higher prevalence of later hypertension, and blood pressure was higher in relatives of multiparous eclamptic women.

In a review of the 176 patients with the clinical diagnosis of toxemia at the University of Chicago, 54 per cent had the typical renal lesion of toxemia, 21 per cent nephrosclerosis, and 18 per cent a primary renal disease.[86] The prevalence of fixed hypertension in later life in black women with the changes of toxemia was 9.4 per cent, which is similar to age-sex-race adjusted statistics from the national health survey. In women with underlying renal disease or nephrosclerosis, the incidence of subsequent hypertension was 74 per cent. These findings point to the predisposition of some women, usually multiparous and in their thirties, to develop toxemia superimposed on underlying renal disease and probably accounts for the late onset of hypertension in this group.

The development of subsequent hypertension presumes the renal lesion can persist. Biopsy studies indicate that complete resolution of the glomerular changes occurs.[6, 201, 212] One patient reported by Schewitz had two episodes of toxemia with renal biopsies during and after each pregnancy.[201] Although some thickening of the glomerular basement membrane appeared and became more marked during the seven years of followup study, her blood pressure remained normal. Whether these changes were the result of toxemia or of a concomitant renal disease was unclear.

ESSENTIAL HYPERTENSION DURING PREGNANCY

It is becoming clear that the onset of essential hypertension occurs early in life. Children of hypertensive parents have higher blood pressures at all ages than children with normotensive parents,[255] and young individuals who demonstrate labile hypertension frequently develop fixed essential hypertension. Although there is some lability in blood pressure with stress, the development of diastolic pressures greater than 90 mm Hg in nonpregnant patients should be regarded as a premonitory sign of essential hypertension. Essential hypertension accounts for approximately one third of all cases of hypertension during pregnancy. The appearance of hypertension may be the result of the pregnancy or may be simply an indication that many women have their blood pressure taken for the first time during pregnancy. The history frequently reveals hypertension, diabetes, and obesity in other members of the family. Women developing hypertension during the second half of pregnancy without other evidence of toxemia (edema, proteinuria, hyperuricemia) can be regarded as having essential hypertension unmasked by pregnancy, and a high proportion of them remain permanently hypertensive after pregnancy.[3] No intensive work-up of hypertension during preg-

nancy is necessary, but auscultation of the abdomen will determine whether a murmur suggestive of renal artery stenosis is present, and palpation of the femoral arteries will exclude coarctation. Since a pheochromocytoma is associated with high maternal mortality in pregnancy, symptoms suggestive of such a tumor should be elicited. The retina should be examined for evidence of long-standing hypertension, i.e., increased light reflex, arteriolar narrowing, and arteriovenous nicking. An electrocardiogram to determine the presence of left ventricular hypertrophy may also be used as a guide to the chronicity of the hypertension. Retinal hemorrhages and exudates indicate accelerated hypertension, which warrants immediate hospitalization. A baseline serum urate determination should be made; in hypertensive women without toxemia it is usually 4 mg per 100 ml or less.

Because of the proven efficacy of antihypertensive therapy in preventing complications of hypertension, more women receiving antihypertensive drugs are being followed up through pregnancy. Patients with essential hypertension should have their blood pressure maintained below 140/90 with whatever antihypertensive regimen is best suited to them. Table 1–2 depicts the antihypertensive drugs that have been used in pregnant women with essential hypertension. Most patients on long-term therapy for essential hypertension will be receiving a combination either of methyldopa and a diuretic or of propranolol, hydralazine, and a diuretic. The drugs should be continued throughout the pregnancy. In some women reduction of the dose, and in a few elimination of medications, may be necessary during the pregnancy because of a reduction in blood pressure. However, this should be done only with careful monitoring, and the blood pressure should be maintained at a normal level throughout the pregnancy. Diuretics should be continued through the pregnancy, since volume depletion is not present with chronic diuretic administration and their antihypertensive effect is independent of sustained volume depletion. Women on long-term diuretic therapy retain the normal 900 mg of sodium during pregnancy without difficulty.

Although the prognosis for a successful pregnancy in a woman with essential hypertension is excellent, the risks of pregnancy are increased. Hypertension may increase the risk of obstetrical complications, like premature separation of the placenta and abruptio placentae; it predisposes to the development of toxemia,[178] and myocardial infarction is more apt to occur in the hyperten-

TABLE 1–2 ANTIHYPERTENSIVE
MEDICATIONS IN PREGNANCY

Chronic Essential Hypertension	Toxemia
Diuretics	
Thiazide 1–2 tab QD	Thiazide 1–2 tab QD
	Furosemide (Lasix) 40 mg PO or IV
Central Adrenergic Blockers	
Methyldopa (Aldomet) 0.5–3 gm QD	Methyldopa 0.5–2 gm PO QD or
Clonidine (Catapres) 0.2–2 mg QD	0.5 gm IV Q6H
Alpha-Adrenergic Blocker	
Prazosin (Minipress) 2–20 mg QD	Not used
Beta-Adrenergic Blockers	
Propranolol (Inderal) 20–80 mg BID	Not used
Metoprolol (Lopressor) 100–200 mg BID	
Nadolol (Corgard) 80–300 mg QD	
Arteriolar Dilators	
Hydralazine (Apresoline) 25–50 mg QID	Hydralazine 25–50 mg Q6H PO or
	10–40 mg IV Q3H
	Diazoxide 300 mg IV

sive woman during pregnancy if blood pressure is not controlled.[109] The likelihood of toxemia is increased two to seven fold if there is underlying essential hypertension, but essential hypertension is generally associated with an uneventful pregnancy if blood pressure is controlled.[152, 178, 190] Pregnant women with essential hypertension should be treated exactly as if they were not pregnant, the blood pressure being maintained as close to normal as possible with the use of antihypertensive agents.

Chesley and Annitto found that in hypertensive women systolic blood pressure fell 20 mm Hg in 40 per cent and over 40 mm Hg in 11 per cent during the second trimester.[45] A rise in pressure in the second trimester was believed by them to be an indication of placental insufficiency, since only 9 per cent of the infants in this group survived. They believed that the normal physiologic fall in blood pressure in the second trimester had prognostic significance, although more recent studies have demonstrated that even with sustained hypertension in the second tri-

mester the rate of fetal loss is only 16 per cent.[16]

Early studies indicated that approximately two thirds of patients who begin pregnancy with essential hypertension have a rise in blood pressure after the 26th week and that about one half of these women develop proteinuria. Thus, the incidence of toxemia in hypertensive women was thought to be about 30 per cent, five times that in normotensive women, with a rise in blood pressure during pregnancy occurring in 66 per cent. However, in a study of 145 pregnant women with essential hypertension, only 13 per cent developed toxemia.[16] In Dunlop's series of 1220 hypertensive patients in Scotland, toxemia occurred in 11.5 per cent.[65] Thus, the increased incidence of toxemia in essential hypertension is not so high as to preclude pregnancy, particularly if careful control of blood pressure is maintained.[152]

Accidental hemorrhage is thought to be more common in women with essential hypertension because of small blood vessel changes in the uterus and placenta. The incidence was 2 per cent in the series of Barnes but only 0.45 per cent in Dunlop's patients compared with 0.6 per cent in 33,000 normotensive women. Perinatal loss is greater in women with essential hypertension; the figure in most large series is from 8 to 15 per cent. Several factors could cause this increase in perinatal mortality. Women with essential hypertension are usually multiparous in their thirties, and perinatal loss is greater in older multigravida women without hypertension. Frequently the perinatal loss is not associated with toxemia but is the result of intrauterine death in the last two months of pregnancy. When toxemia occurred before the 32nd week of gestation in patients with essential hypertension, older studies revealed fetal loss rising to approximately 75 per cent. According to more recent studies, fetal mortality for women receiving antihypertensive therapy throughout pregnancy is no higher than for normotensive women.[99] However, toxemia, defined as a rise in plasma urate level, occurred with equal frequency in one study that compared treated and untreated hypertensive women.[190]

Patients with essential hypertension should be seen by the physician every two to three weeks during pregnancy and weekly after the 32nd week. The development of proteinuria or a rise in blood pressure is an indication for immediate hospitalization. Although there is no evidence that antihypertensive medication increases urinary estriol excretion,[167] there is evidence that it increases perinatal survival. Kincaid-Smith et al. observed a perinatal mortality of 6.2 per cent in severely hypertensive women treated with methyldopa (Aldomet) throughout pregnancy,[142] and Leather observed, in a randomized series of 100 pregnant hypertensive women with diastolic blood pressure greater than 80 mm Hg prior to the 20th week, that antihypertensive therapy with Aldomet and a diuretic was associated with a significantly better fetal outcome.[152] There were no fetal losses in the treated group compared with five fetal losses in the untreated group. Comparable observations were made by Redman in a larger controlled trial of treatment in which diuretics were not used.[190] Birth weights in the treated group were similar to those in the control group, and there was no evidence of altered fetal growth in the treated group. The condition of the neonates at birth was similar in both groups. In hypertensive women developing toxemia before the 32nd week, delivery is indicated if urinary estriols are low, since the chance for further fetal growth seems slim. In patients with essential hypertension, ergot preparations are contraindicated; oxytocin, which has little pressor activity, should be used to induce labor.

Maternal mortality in women with essential hypertension during pregnancy is under one per cent, and when death does occur it usually is due to a sudden rise in blood pressure and the consequent cerebral hemorrhage, acute left ventricular failure, or malignant encephalography. These complications can now be prevented with antihypertensive agents, and maternal mortality due to hypertension should be virtually eliminated. A woman with hypertension who develops toxemia does not invariably become toxemic with subsequent pregnancies, but if the toxemia occurs early in pregnancy, subsequent pregnancies are more apt to be associated with toxemia.

Malignant hypertension associated with the development of retinal hemorrhages, exudates, or papilledema during the course of pregnancy was an indication for delivery in the past. There was no hope for fetal survival before antihypertensive therapy for malignant hypertension became available; this may not now be the case.

Primary Aldosteronism (Conn's Syndrome). Women with primary aldosteronism have been observed during pregnancy. Biglieri and Slayton reported a woman whose hypokalemia, but not hypertension, disappeared during pregnancy, presumably because of the antagonistic effect of elevated progesterone.[22] Gordon et al. observed suppression of the usual high plasma renin activity of pregnancy in a woman with primary aldosteronism whose adrenal adenoma was removed in early pregnancy because

of extremely high aldosterone secretion.[115] The author has seen one woman with hypertension and polyuria documented since the age of nine, whose severe hypertension in late pregnancy necessitated a cesarean section. Postpartum hypokalemia was detected, and her evaluation revealed primary aldosteronism with adrenal hyperplasia. Thus, the hypokalemia of primary aldosteronism may be relieved during pregnancy, but hypertension persists.

Renal Artery Stenosis. Women with proven renal artery stenosis have undergone pregnancy, and most develop toxemia.[147] Of the nine patients in Landesman's series, five developed toxemia with exacerbation of hypertension during the pregnancy, whereas four developed proteinuria, edema, and hypertension.[147] Although there is evidence in animals that hypertension induced by renal artery constriction improves during pregnancy,[55, 179] hypertension has been induced in pregnant animals with constriction of the renal artery in later pregnancy.[63] The appropriate course would be to maintain normal blood pressure with antihypertensive drugs and to evaluate and possibly operate upon the patient post partum. Hypertension caused by renal artery stenosis can be treated medically as readily as other forms of hypertension. Although the angiotensin I–converting enzyme inhibitors are useful in the treatment of renal hypertension, I consider them to be contraindicated in pregnancy because of their adverse effects on uterine PGE_2 synthesis and their association with fetal mortality in pregnant rabbits.[90]

Coarctation of the Aorta. Coarctation of the aorta is a rare hypertensive complication of pregnancy and is associated with toxemia.[131, 240] Of 10 patients requiring surgical repair for this condition during pregnancy, 9 underwent uncomplicated deliveries with living infants. One patient died in her seventh month of pregnancy of an aneurysm of the aorta at the anastomotic site. The major danger to the pregnant woman with an aortic coarctation is aortic rupture by the cystic medial necrosis often present in the aortic wall. These pathological changes may well be put under stress by the increase in cardiac output of pregnancy, increase in blood pressure during toxemia, or the strain of labor.

Pheochromocytoma. Pheochromocytoma is a potentially lethal condition during pregnancy and is a cause of secondary hypertension that must be diagnosed and treated during pregnancy. It is an extremely rare cause of hypertension; only 93 pheochromocytomas during pregnancy have been reported in the English literature.[89, 128, 200] Severe headache, profuse sweating, palpitations, nausea and vomiting, blurred vision, vertigo, tremulousness, seizures, and general weakness are frequently present. Physical findings suggestive of hyperthyroidism — tachycardia, lid lag, and fine tremor — should alert the obstetrician to the possibility of a pheochromocytoma. In pregnant women with pheochromocytomas, the maternal mortality rate is approximately 50 per cent. The cause of death is usually pulmonary edema or cerebral hemorrhage, with cardiovascular collapse. The tumor should be removed surgically during pregnancy once the diagnosis has been established. Concern about the danger of using x-ray to localize the tumor is inappropriate with this potentially lethal condition.

ANTIHYPERTENSIVE DRUGS

The Food and Drug Administration has developed a system for evaluating the risk to the fetus of all drugs. This system will help resolve the present problem: most drugs have received inadequate testing in pregnant animals, and consequently all drugs are stated to be contraindicated in pregnancy in the package insert or in the Physicians' Desk Reference. The categories to be used in the future are these:

Category A: Controlled studies in women fail to demonstrate a risk to the fetus in the first trimester (and there is no evidence of a risk in later trimesters), and the possibility of fetal harm appears remote.

Category B: Either animal reproduction studies have not demonstrated a fetal risk but there are no controlled studies in pregnant women, or animal reproduction studies have shown an adverse effect (other than a decrease in fertility) that was not confirmed in controlled studies in women in the first trimester (and there is no evidence of a risk in later trimesters).

Category C: Either studies in animals have revealed adverse effects on the fetus (teratogenic or embryocidal effects or others) and there are no controlled studies in women, or studies in women and animals are not available. Drugs should be given only if the potential benefit justifies the potential risk to the fetus.

Category D: There is positive evidence of human fetal risk, but the benefits from use in pregnant women may be acceptable despite the risk (e.g., if the drug is needed in a life-threatening situation or for a serious disease for which safer drugs cannot be used or are ineffective). There will be an appropriate statement in the "warnings" section of the labeling.

Category X: Studies in animals or human beings have demonstrated fetal abnormalities, or there is evidence of fetal risk based on human experience, or both, and the risk of using the drug in pregnant women clearly outweighs any possible benefit. The drug is contraindicated in women who are or may become pregnant. There will be an appropriate statement in the "contraindications" section of the labeling.

Although evaluations have not yet been provided for antihypertensive drugs, it seems from the information available that most will be in the B or C category. As with the use of any drug, a risk/benefit analysis must be made, which in the case of antihypertensive drugs is clearly in favor of their use in the pregnant woman.

Diuretics

Table 1–2 depicts the various pharmacologic categories of drugs that are used in the treatment of hypertension during pregnancy. Some have been used in the acute hypertension of toxemia, whereas others have been used primarily in pregnancy with chronic essential hypertension. All have been widely used in nonpregnant subjects. There are a large number of thiazide preparations, all with essentially the same potency per tablet. They are the first step in the treatment of all hypertensive patients. They not only have intrinsic antihypertensive properties but prevent the refractoriness that develops with the use of other antihypertensive drugs, which usually cause salt retention. Approximately 10 per cent of patients receiving one tablet of thiazide daily develop a serum potassium level below 3.5 mEq/liter, but since the potassium wasting with diuretic therapy is dependent upon aldosterone secretion, hypokalemia below 3.5 mEq/liter will usually suppress aldosterone secretion, and the potassium wasting ceases. Chlorthalidone (Hygroton) is a long-acting thiazide preparation, which causes hypokalemia more often than shorter-acting preparations like chlorothiazide (Diuril) or hydrochlorothiazide (Hydrodiuril). Cardiac arrhythmias in the fetus with maternal hypokalemia have been described,[213] but potassium depletion in pregnancy can be prevented by either the administration of 40 to 60 mEq KCl daily or the addition of a potassium sparing diuretic, e.g., triamterene, to the thiazide. Diazide, the most commonly used diuretic in the treatment of hypertension, represents such a combination of a thiazide and triamterene. In most patients potassium supplementation is not necessary, but if hypokalemia develops it can be readily corrected with oral potassium supplementation. Much has been written in the obstetric literature of the possible adverse complications of diuretics, i.e., pancreatitis, electrolyte disturbances, neonatal thrombocytopenia, and fetal electrocardiogram abnormalities caused by potassium depletion. Considering the fact that diuretics are taken by approximately 15 million Americans for the treatment of essential hypertension, they must be regarded as one of the safest drugs in the pharmacologic armamentarium. Diuretics have been used throughout pregnancy in patients with essential hypertension, and there is no evidence that they increase fetal mortality.

With acute toxemia, the more potent diuretic furosemide should be used when an intravenous diuretic is needed. Furosemide, 40 mg intravenously every four hours, can be given for treatment of severe toxemia, particularly when a vasodilating agent is also used. Vasodilators cause salt retention, and their antihypertensive effects are potentiated by concomitant use of a diuretic. Furosemide has been demonstrated to reduce left ventricular filling pressure prior to the natriuresis by increasing venous capacitance and diminishing venous return.[62] This effect makes the drug particularly helpful to toxemic patients with congestive heart failure. Although cardiac output and extracellular volume fall when diuretic therapy is begun, both return to normal during prolonged diuretic administration but a sustained reduction in peripheral resistance occurs. The mechanism of the reduction in peripheral resistance that occurs with diuretic therapy is not understood. It has been suggested that dilatation of arterioles occurs as a result of altered concentration of sodium and calcium in the vessel walls. The fact that diazoxide, chemically similar to the thiazides, is a potent peripheral vasodilator but not a diuretic suggests a similar action for thiazides independent of natriuresis.

A disadvantage in the use of a diuretic in pregnancy is that elevation of uric acid may occur and obscure the best chemical marker of the development of toxemia. However, urate seldom rises above 6.5 mg per 100 ml with diuretics alone, and higher levels usually indicate toxemia. Serial determination of plasma urate levels in hypertensive women taking a diuretic throughout pregnancy will usually show a rise if toxemia supervenes.

Adrenergic Blocking Drugs

Although the sympathetic depleting agents reserpine and guanethidine were formerly used for the treatment of essential hypertension, they have been replaced by drugs with fewer side effects. Two major drugs that act as adrenergic blockers in the central nervous system are methyldopa (Aldomet) and clonidine (Catapres). Methldopa acts primarily by the build-up within the central nervous system of a false neurotransmitter, alpha-methylnorepinephrine. Its antihypertensive effect is caused by a decrease in peripheral resistance with little change in cardiac output or pulse. Clonidine stimulates central alpha-adrenergic receptors, thereby decreasing sympathetic outflow from the central nervous system and reducing peripheral resistance. Methyldopa may be utilized to lower blood pressure acutely: 500 mg is given intravenously and the dose is repeated at 6 hour intervals. Hypertension usually responds within 6 to 8 hours, and after 24 to 48 hours of parenteral therapy, oral methyldopa in equivalent doses may be substituted. Methyldopa depletes the brain of biogenic amines, which accounts for the somnolence and depression that occurs in some patients. The incidence of a positive Coombs' test in patients receiving methyldopa averages between 10 and 20 per cent, but only rarely does a hemolytic anemia occur. This reaction is not of concern when methyldopa is used for the acute treatment of toxemia. Occasionally fever associated with eosinophilia occurs during the beginning of therapy, and abnormalities of liver function such as elevated alkaline phosphatase and serum transaminase, SGOT, and SGPT have been reported. It has an advantage over other adrenergic blockers in that it rarely causes postural hypotension. The dose varies from 250 mg to 1 gram TID. Fluid retention occurs as with most antihypertensive agents.

The most common side effects of clonidine are sedation and a dry mouth as well as severe hypertension, which may follow abrupt withdrawal of the drug. It reduces cardiac output and pulse, with a decrease in peripheral resistance, and is also used with a diuretic to prevent fluid retention. Both drugs have been used in pregnancy,[152, 190] and followup studies on the children born of mothers taking Aldomet revealed normal mental and physical development. Interestingly, the children born of mothers taking Aldomet throughout pregnancy scored consistently higher than untreated controls on five main indices of intellectual and motor development.[177]

Alpha- and Beta-Adrenergic Blockers. Prazosin (Minipress) acts as a post-synaptic alpha-adrenergic blocking agent. Its hemodynamic effects cause a fall in peripheral resistance with no change in cardiac output. The drug is as potent as Aldomet and can be combined with a beta-adrenergic blocking drug like propranolol to provide a further reduction in blood pressure by lowering cardiac output. The drug can cause severe postural hypotension after the first dose, but this effect is usually a transient phenomenon. No studies of this drug during pregnancy have been reported, but in a woman with hypertension well controlled by prazosin there appears to be no theoretical reason to stop the drug.

Propranolol is a beta-adrenergic blocking drug that lowers blood pressure, primarily by blocking cardiac beta receptors, with a consequent fall in cardiac output and pulse rate. Other actions that might play a role in its antihypertensive effect include inhibition of renin release from the kidney and blockade of beta-adrenergic receptors in the central nervous system, with production of bradycardia and peripheral vasodilatation. Although peripheral beta-adrenergic blockade could theoretically cause peripheral vasoconstriction with Raynaud's phenomenon by unopposed alpha receptor activity, this effect is not usually seen because of the sparsity of peripheral beta-adrenergic receptors. The drug is always combined with a diuretic and usually with a vasodilator. All beta blockers are contraindicated in cases of asthma or obstructive lung disease, but significant side effects have proved to be less a problem than when the central adrenergic blockers are used. Fatigue, depression, cold extremities, and insomnia rarely occur. The use of beta-adrenergic blocking agents during pregnancy is controversial. Adverse effects on the fetus — intrauterine growth retardation, neonatal bradycardia, hypoglycemia — have been reported.[154] However, in a controlled trial comparing the beta blocker oxprenolol with Aldomet there was better fetal growth and improved survival in the group treated with oxprenolol.[99] Since beta blockers cross the placenta and reduce fetal heart rate and cardiac output in the pregnant ewe, there has been fear that beta-adrenergic blockade would mask signs of fetal distress. Also, since beta-adrenergic drugs like isoproterenol suppress myometrial activity and beta-adrenergic blockade enhances uterine activity in experimental animals, premature labor could theoretically be a complication of a beta-adrenergic blocker. However, studies utilizing beta-adrenergic blocking drugs in pregnant women with essential hypertension have not demonstrated an increased rate of premature delivery.[197a] The adverse effects of these drugs have been, for the most part, reported in isolated cases. In the largest series of pregnant women treated for essential hypertension with beta-adrenergic blocking drugs, hydralazine, and

diuretics throughout pregnancy, the perinatal mortality was 1.9 per cent. In contrast, propranolol was reported to be a contributing factor to fetal death in nine patients treated for hypertension and renal disease during pregnancy.[154] At present, a reasonable approach would be to maintain the use of beta-adrenergic blockers throughout pregnancy in women with essential hypertension whose blood pressure is well controlled with these agents, but to await further experience in their use for the treatment of acute toxemia.

Arteriolar Dilators

Several drugs lower blood pressure by a direct vasodilating effect upon arterioles; the most commonly used are hydralazine and diazoxide. Although oral hydralazine is not a potent antihypertensive agent when used alone, the combination of hydralazine and propranolol (Inderal), which prevents the reflex tachycardia that occurs with a vasodilator, together with a diuretic is a common regimen in the treatment of essential hypertension. It controls moderately severe hypertension without side effects. The arteriolar dilator diazoxide (Hyperstat) is a most potent antihypertensive agent when given intravenously. It acts by directly altering the reactivity of arteriole smooth muscle and producing a decrease in peripheral vascular resistance. Like all vasodilators it causes sodium retention and must be used in conjunction with a diuretic. There is an increase in heart rate and cardiac output following the administration of diazoxide owing to a compensatory response of the carotid baroreceptors to the fall in pressure. There is no reduction in renal blood flow or glomerular filtration. The drugs act within 10 to 15 seconds, the maximum effect being achieved within 3 to 40 minutes. The usual dose is 300 mg, given either rapidly (10 to 15 seconds) or in boluses of 50 mg/minute. If a satisfactory fall in pressure does not occur within 5 to 10 minutes, a second dose of 300 mg is given. The effect of the drug usually lasts 3 to 8 hours after injection. It has been used in severe toxemia and is the agent of choice when acute hypertensive emergencies develop during the course of toxemia.[82, 167] Diazoxide induces hyperglycemia when given for a long time and is not useful for the treatment of chronic hypertension. It frequently causes cessation of labor, but this effect can be overcome by an oxytocic agent.

Hydralazine is the most commonly used vasodilator in pregnancy. Its mode of action is not clear, but it may act by inhibiting the movement of calcium into the smooth muscle cells. It causes peripheral vasodilation, with a greater effect on resistance than on capacitance vessels. Accompanying the vasodilation is an increase in heart rate and cardiac output. These compensatory reflexes cause tolerance to hydralazine to develop, but when combined with either a beta-adrenergic blocker like propranolol or a central adrenergic blocker like methyldopa or clonidine, hydralazine becomes quite effective as an antihypertensive agent. No adverse effects have been described in pregnant women given hydralazine, and in studies of pregnant animals hydralazine has been noted to cause an increase in uterine blood flow.

Minoxidil (Loniten), a potent arteriolar dilator, is not used except in severe hypertension that is refractory to other medications. There is no report of its use during pregnancy.

Nitroprusside, another potent vasodilator, is quite effective in controlling hypertensive emergencies, but its use in severe toxemia has not gained favor, since studies in pregnant ewes demonstrated thiocyanate and cyanide accumulation in the fetus.[153a]

The angiotensin blocking agents captopril and Saralasin have not been used in pregnancy, but experiments in pregnant rabbits demonstrate a striking increase in fetal mortality associated with captopril. This drug was found to decrease uterine PGE synthesis, indicating that uterine PGE_2 synthesis in the rabbit is dependent on angiotensin II generation, and this may be the mechanism of its detrimental effect on fetal viability.[90]

References

1. Abitbol, M. M.: Hemodynamic studies in experimental toxemia of the dog. Obstet. Gynecol., 50:293, 1977.
2. Adams, E. M., and Finlayson, A.: Familial aspects of pre-eclampsia and hypertension in pregnancy. Lancet, 2:1375, 1961.
3. Adams, E. M., and MacGillivray, I.: Long term effects of pre-eclampsia on blood pressures. Lancet, 2:1373, 1961.
4. Adamson, K., and Joelsson, I.: The effects of pharmacologic agents upon the fetus and newborn. Am. J. Obstet. Gynecol., 96:437, 1966.
5. Adelstein, P., and Fedrick, J.: Cigarette smoking and pregnancy-induced hypertension. In Bonnar, J., MacGillivray, I., and Symonds, E. M. (eds.): Pregnancy Hypertension. Lancaster, England, MTP Press Ltd., 1980, p. 549.
6. Altchek. A.: Electron microscopy of renal biopsies in toxemia of pregnancy. J.A.M.A., 175:791, 1961.
7. Anderson, K. J., Duncan, S. L., and Lint, R. L.: Advanced abdominal pregnancy with severe pre-eclampsia. Br. J. Obstet. Gynaecol., 83:90, 1976.
8. Anderson, R. C., Herbert, P. N., and Mulrow, P. J.: A comparison of properties of renin obtained from the kidney and uterus of the rabbit. Am. J. Physiol., 215:774, 1968.
9. Arias, F., and Mancilla-Jimenez, R.: Hepatic fibrinogen deposits in pre-eclampsia. N. Engl. J. Med., 295:578, 1976.
10. Assali, N. S., and Brinkman, C. R., III: Disorders of maternal circulatory and respiratory adjustments. In Pathophysiology of Gestational Disorders, Vol. 1. New York, Academic Press, 1972.
11. Assali, N. S., Douglas, R. A., Jr., Baird, W. W., Nicholson, D. B., and Suyemoto, R.: Utero-placental blood flow in toxemic pregnancy. Am. J. Obstet. Gynecol., 66:248, 1953.
12. Assali, N. S., Holm, L. W., and Segal, N.: Regional blood flow and vascular resistance of the fetus in uterine action of vasoactive drugs. Am. J. Obstet. Gynecol., 83:809, 1962.
13. Assali, N. S., and Vaughn, D. L.: Blood volume in pre-eclampsia: Fantasy and reality. Am. J. Obstet. Gynecol., 129:355, 1977.
14. Baehler, R. W., Copeland, W. E., Stein, J. H., and Ferris, T. F.: Plasma renin and aldosterone in an abdominal pregnancy with toxemia. Am. J. Obstet. Gynecol., 122:545, 1975.
15. Baird, D., and Dunn, J. S.: Renal lesions in eclampsia and nephritis of pregnancy. J. Pathol. Bacteriol., 37:291, 1933.
16. Barnes, C. G.: Nontoxemic hypertension. In Medical Disorders in Obstetric Practice, 4th Ed. Oxford, England, Blackwell Scientific Publications, 1974.
17. Bay, W. H., and Ferris, T. F.: Factors controlling plasma renin and aldosterone during pregnancy. Hypertension, 1:410, 1979.

18. Bay, W. H., Mishkind, M. H., Lane, G. E., and Ferris, T. F.: Studies of the mechanism of natriuresis with PGE_2. J. Lab. Clin. Med., 93:78, 1979.
19. Bechgaard, P., Andreassen, C., and Heitel, E.: Ultimate prognosis of hypertension following toxemia. In Morris, N. F., and Browne, J. C. M. (eds.): Nontoxemic Hypertension in Pregnancy. Boston, Little, Brown and Co., 1958.
20. Beller, F. K., Intorp, H. W., Losse, H., Loers, H., Moenpinghoff, W., Schmidt, E. N., and Grundman, E.: Malignant nephrosclerosis during pregnancy and in the post partum period. Am. J. Obstet. Gynecol., 125:633, 1976.
21. Bergstrom, S., Krabisch, L., Samuelsson, B., and Sjovall, J.: Preparation of PGF from PGE. Acta Chem. Scand., 16:969, 1962.
22. Biglieri, E. G., and Slaton, P. E., Jr.: Pregnancy and primary aldosteronism. J. Clin. Endocrinol., 27:1628, 1967.
23. Bis, K. A., and Waxman, B.: Rupture of the liver associated with pregnancy: A review of the literature and report of 2 cases. Obstet. Gynecol. Surv., 31:763, 1976.
24. Blechner, J. N., Cotter, J. R., Stenger, V. G., Hinkley, C. M., and Prystowsky, H.: Oxygen, carbon dioxide and hydrogen ion concentration in arterial blood during pregnancy. Am. J. Obstet. Gynecol., 100:1, 1968.
25. Bodzenta, A., Thompson, J. M., and Poller, L.: Prostacyclin activity in amniotic fluid in pre-eclampsia. Lancet, 2:650, 1980.
26. Bolger, P. M., Eisner, G. M., Ramwell, P. M., and Slotkoff, L. M.: Effect of prostaglandin synthesis on renal function and renin in the dog. Nature, 259:244, 1976.
27. Bonnar, J., MacGillivray, I., and Symonds, M. (eds.): Pregnancy Hypertension. Lancaster, England. MTP Press Ltd., 1980.
28. Bonnar, J., Redman, C. W. G., and Denson, K. W.: The role of coagulation and fibrinolysis in pre-eclampsia. In Lindheimer, M. D., Katz, A. I., and Zuspan, F. P. (eds.): Hypertension in Pregnancy. New York, John Wiley & Sons, 1976, pp. 85–94.
29. Brazy, J. E., Little, V., and Grimm, J.: Neonatal effects of severe maternal hypertension before 36 weeks gestation. Ped. Res., 15:653, 1981.
30. Brown, J. J., Davies, D. L., Doak, P. B., Lever, A. F., Robertson, J. I. S., and Trust, P.: Plasma renin concentration in hypertensive disease of pregnancy. Lancet, 2:1219, 1965.
31. Browne, C. H., Hanson, G. C., DeJude, L. R., and Roberts, P. A.: Rupture of subcapsular haematoma of the liver in a case of eclampsia. Br. J. Surg., 62:237, 1975.
32. Browne, J. C. M., and Veall, N.: The maternal placental blood flow in normotensive women. J. Obstet. Gynaecol. Br. Commonw., 60:141, 1953.
33. Brunner, H. R., Chang, P., Wallach, R., Sealey, J. E., and

Laragh, J. H.: Angiotensin II vascular receptors: Their avidity in relationship to sodium balance, the autonomic nervous system and hypertension. J. Clin. Invest., *51*:58, 1972.

34. Brunner, H. R., Kirschman, J. D., Sealey, J. E., and Laragh, J. H.: Hypertension of renal origin: Evidence for two different mechanisms. Science, *174*:1344, 1971.

35. Bryans, C. I., Jr., Southerland, W. L., and Zuspan, R. B.: Eclampsia: A long term followup study. Obstet. Gynecol., *21*:701, 1963.

36. Bucht, H., and Werko, L.: Glomerular filtration rate and renal blood flow in hypertensive toxemia of pregnancy. J. Obstet. Gynaecol. Br. Emp., *60*:157, 1953.

37. Burstein, R., Alkjaersig, N., and Fletcher, A.: Thromboembolism during pregnancy and the post-partum state. J. Lab. Clin. Med., *78*:838, 1971.

37a. Bussolino, F., Benedetto, C., Massobrio, M., and Camussi, G.: Maternal vascular prostacyclin activity in pre-eclampsia. Lancet, *2*:310, 1980.

38. Campbell, W. B., Gomez-Sanchez, C. E., Adams, B. V., Schmitz, J. M., and Itskovitz, H. B.: Attenuation of angiotensin II and III induced aldosterone release by prostaglandin synthesis inhibition. J. Clin. Invest., *64*:1552, 1979.

39. Campbell, W. B., Graham, R. M., and Jackson, E. K.: Role of renal prostaglandins in sympathetically mediated renin release in the rat. J. Clin. Invest., *64*:448, 1979.

40. Caritis, S., Morishima, H. O., and Stark, R. I.: The effects of diazoxide on uterine blood flow in pregnant sheep. Obstet. Gynecol., *48*:464, 1976.

41. Carreras, L. O., Defryn, G., Van Houtte, E., Vermylen, J., and Van Asche, A.: Prostacyclin and pre-eclampsia. Lancet, *1*:442, 1981.

42. Chanatin, A., and Ferris, E.: Experimental renal insufficiency produced by partial nephrectomy. Arch. Intern. Med., *49*:767, 1932.

43. Chaudhuri, S. K.: Relationship of protein-caloric malnutrition with toxemia of pregnancy. Am. J. Obstet. Gynecol., *107*:33, 1970.

44. Chesley, L. C.: The remote prognosis of eclamptic women. Am. Heart J., *93*:407, 1977.

45. Chesley, L. C.: Hypertension in pregnancy: Definitions, familial factor, and remote prognosis. Kidney Int., *18*:234, 1980.

46. Chesley, L. C., and Annitto, J. E.: Pregnancy in a patient with hypertensive disease. Am. J. Obstet. Gynecol., *53*:372, 1947.

47. Chesley, L. C., Annitto, J. E., and Cosgrove, R. A.: The familial factor in toxemia of pregnancy. Obstet. Gynecol., *32*:303, 1968.

48. Chesley, L. C., Annitto, J. E., and Cosgrove, R. A.: Long term followup study of eclamptic women. Am. J. Obstet. Gynecol., *101*:886, 1968.

49. Christianson, R. E.: Studies on blood pressure during pregnancy. 1. Influence of parity and age. Am. J. Obstet. Gynecol., *125*:509, 1976.

50. Clark, J. F., and Niles, J. H.: Abdominal pregnancy associated with toxemia of pregnancy. J. Natl. Med. Assoc., *52*:22, 1967.

51. Clark, K. E., Farley, D. B., Van Order, D. E., and Brody, M. J.: Role of endogenous prostaglandins in regulation of uterine blood flow and adrenergic neurotransmission. Am. J. Obstet. Gynecol., *127*:455, 1977.

52. Clemendor, A., Sall, S., and Herbilas, E.: Achalasia and nutritional deficiency during pregnancy. Obstet. Gynecol., *33*:106, 1969.

53. Clewell, W., and Meschia, G.: Relationship of metabolic clearance rate of DHEA to placental blood flow. Am. J. Obstet. Gynecol., *125*:507, 1976.

54. Cohn, J. N.: Relationship of plasma volume changes to resistance and capacitance vessel effects of sympathomimetic amine and angiotensin in man. Clin. Sci., *30*:267, 1966.

55. Collins, E., and Turner, G.: Maternal effects of regular aspirin ingestion in pregnancy. Lancet, *2*:335, 1975.

56. Corbit, J. D., Jr.: The effect of pregnancy upon experimental hypertension in the rabbit. Am. J. Med. Sci., *201*:876, 1941.

57. Cuadros, A., and Tatum, H. J.: The prophylactic and therapeutic use of bendroflumethiazide in pregnancy. Am. J. Obstet. Gynecol., *89*:891, 1964.

58. Davies, A. M.: Geographical epidemiology of the toxemias of pregnancy. Isr. J. Med. Sci., *7*:753, 1971.

59. Davies, A. M., Czaczkes, J. W., Sadovsky, E., Prywes, R., Weiskopf, P., and Sterk, V. V.: Toxemia of pregnancy in Jerusalem. Isr. J. Med. Sci., *6*:253, 1970.

60. Davison, J. M., and Dunlop, W.: Renal hemodynamics and tubular function in normal human pregnancy. Kidney Int., *18*:152, 1980.

61. Dawn, C. S., and Sinha, B.: Diazepam therapy in eclampsia. Int. J. Gynaecol., *17*:281, 1979.

62. Dikshit, K., Vyden, J. K., Forrester, J. S., Chatterjee, K., Prakash, R., and Swan, H. H. C.: Renal and extrarenal hemodynamic effects of furosemide in congestive heart failure with acute myocardial infarction. N. Engl. J. Med., *288*:1087, 1973.

63. Donaldson, J. O.: Neurology of Pregnancy. Philadelphia, W. B. Saunders Co., 1978.

64. Downing, I., Shepherd, G. L., and Lewis, P. J.: Reduced prostacyclin production in pre-eclampsia. Lancet, *2*:1374, 1980.

65. Dunlop, J. C. H.: Chronic hypertension and perinatal mortality. Proc. R. Soc. Med., *59*:838, 1966.

66. Dunlop, W., Hill, L. M., Landon, M. J., Oxley, A., and Jones, P.: Clinical relevance of coagulation and renal changes in pre-eclampsia. Lancet, *2*:346, 1978.

67. Durr, J. A., Stamoutsos, B. A., and Lindheimer, M. D.: Plasma osmolality in pregnant rats in the absence of vasopressin (AVP). J. Clin. Invest. (in press, 1981).

68. Ehrlich, E. N., and Lindheimer, M. D.: Effect of administered mineralocorticoids or ACTH in pregnant women. J. Clin. Invest., *51*:1301, 1972.

69. Ekstrom-Jodal, B., Haggendel, E., Linder, L. E., and Wilsson, N. J.: Regulation of cerebral blood flow. Eur. Neurol., *6*:6, 1972.

70. Eliahou, H. E., Silverberg, D. S., Reisin, E., Romen, I., Mashiach, S., and Serr, D. M.: Propranolol for the treatment of hypertension in pregnancy. Br. J. Obstet. Gynaecol., *85*:431, 1978.

71. Epstein, F. H.: Late vascular effect of toxemia of pregnancy. N. Engl. J. Med., *271*:391, 1964.

72. Everett, R. B., Worley, R. J., MacDonald, P. C., and Gant, N. J.: Effect of prostaglandin synthetase inhibition on pressor response to angiotensin II in human pregnancy. J. Clin. Endocrinol. Metab., *46*:1007, 1978.

73. Fadel, H. E., Northrop, G., and Misenheimer, H. R.: Hyperuricemia in pre-eclampsia. A reappraisal. Am. J. Obstet. Gynecol., *125*:640, 1976.

74. Fahr, T.: Über Marenveranderungen bei Eklampsie. Zentral. Gynaekol., *44*:991, 1920.

75. Faith, G. C., and Trump. B. F.: The glomerular capillary wall in human kidney disease: Acute glomerulonephritis, systemic lupus and pre-eclampsia. Lab. Invest., *15*:1682, 1966.

76. Farquhar, M.: Proceedings of the 10th Annual Conference: The Nephrotic Syndrome. New York, National Kidney Disease Foundation, 1959, p. 2.

77. Ferris, T. F.: Unpublished observations. 1981.

78. Ferris, T. F., and Gorden, P.: The effect of angiotensin and norepinephrine upon urate clearance in man. Am. J. Med., *44*:359, 1968.

79. Ferris, T. F., Gorden, P., and Mulrow, P. J.: Rabbit uterus as a source of renin. Am. J. Physiol., *212*:698, 1967.

80. Ferris, T. F., Herdson, P. B., Dunnill, M. S., and Lee, M. R.: Toxemia of pregnancy in sheep: A clinical physiological and pathological study. J. Clin. Invest., *48*:1643, 1969.

81. Ferris. T. F., Stein, J. H., and Kauffman, J.: Uterine blood flow and uterine renin secretion. J. Clin. Invest., *51*:2828, 1972.

82. Finnerty, F. A., Jr.: Hypertensive emergencies. In Laragh, J. H. (ed.): Hypertension Manual. New York, Yorke Medical Books, 1974.

83. Finnerty, F. A., Jr., and Bepko, F. J.: Lowering the perinatal mortality and prematurity rate. J.A.M.A., *195*:429, 1966.

84. First, M. R., Ooi, B. S., Jao, W., and Pollak, V. E.: Pre-eclampsia with the nephrotic syndrome. Kidney Int., *13*:166, 1978.

85. Fisher, K. A., Ahuja, S., Luger, A., Spargo, B. H., and Lindheimer, M. D.: Nephrotic proteinuria with pre-eclampsia. Am. J. Obstet. Gynecol., *129*:643, 1977.

86. Fisher, K. A., Luger, A., Spargo, B. H., and Lindheimer, M. D.: Hypertension in pregnancy: Clinical pathological correlation and remote prognosis. Medicine, *60*:267, 1981.

87. Fitzsimmons, J. T.: The physiological basis of thirst. Kidney Int., *10*:3, 1976.

87a. Flowers, C. E., Grizzle, J. E., Easterling, W. E., and Bonner, O. B.: Chlorothiazide as a prophylaxis against toxemia of pregnancy. Am. J. Obstet. Gynecol., *84*:919, 1962.

88. Flowers, C. E., Rudolph, A. J., and Desmond, M. M.: Diazepam as an adjunct in obstetric analgesia. Obstet. Gynecol., *34*:68, 1969.
89. Fox, L. P., Grandi, J., and Johnson, M. J.: Pheochromocytoma associated with pregnancy. Am. J. Obstet. Gynecol., *104*:288, 1966.
90. Francisco, L. L., and Ferris, T. F.: The effect of Captopril on uterine PGE synthesis and fetal mortality. Circ. Res. (in press).
91. Franklin, G. O., Dowd, A. J., Caldwell, B. V., and Speroff, L.: The effect of angiotensin II intravenous infusion on plasma renin activity and prostaglandins A, E, and F levels in the uterine vein of the pregnant monkey. Prostaglandins, *6*:271, 1974.
92. Freis, E. D.: The treatment of hypertension. Am. J. Med., *52*:664, 1972.
93. Friedman, E. A., and Neff, R. K.: Pregnancy hypertension. Littleton, Mass., PSG Publishing Co., Inc., 1977.
94. Fritzsch, W., Birnbaum, M., Flach, W., and Issel, E. P.: Spatschaden nach Eklampsie. Zentralb Gynaekol., *92*:1009, 1970.
95. Frohlich, J. C., Hollifield, J. W., Michelakis, A. M., Vesper, B. S., Wilson, J. P., Shand, D. G., Seyberth, H. J., Frolich, W. H., and Oates, J. A.: Reduction of plasma renin activity by inhibition of the fatty acid cyclooxygenase in human subjects. Circ. Res., *44*:781, 1979.
96. Frohlich, J. C., and Wilson, T. W.: Urinary prostaglandins: Identification and origin. J. Clin. Invest., *55*:763, 1975.
97. Gallery, E. D. M., Saunders, D. M., Boyce, E. S., and Gyory, A. Z.: Relation between plasma volume and uric acid in the development of hypertension in pregnancy. In Bonnar, J., MacGillivray, I., and Symonds, E. M. (eds.): Pregnancy Hypertension. Lancaster, England, MTP Press Ltd., 1980.
98. Gallery, E. D. M., Saunders, D. M., Gunyor, S. N., and Gyory, A. Z.: Improvement in fetal growth with treatment of maternal hypertension in pregnancy. Clin. Sci. Mol. Med., *55*:359, 1978.
99. Gallery, E. D. M., Saunders, D. M., Hunyor, S. N., and Gyory, A. Z.: Randomized comparison of methyldopa and oxprenolol for treatment of hypertension in pregnancy. Br. Med. J., *1*:1591, 1979.
100. Galvez, O. G., Bay, W. H., Roberts, B. W., and Ferris, T. F.: The hemodynamic effects of potassium deficiency in the dog. Circ. Res., *40*:1, 1977.
101. Gandhi, J., Ghosh, S., and Pillari, V. T.: Blindness and retinal changes with pre-eclamptic toxemia. N.Y. State J. Med., *78*:1930, 1978.
102. Gant, N. F., Chand, S., Worley, R. J., Whalley, P. T., Crosby, V. D., and MacDonald, P. C.: A clinical test useful for predicting the development of acute hypertension in pregnancy. Am. J. Obstet. Gynecol., *120*:1, 1974.
103. Gant, N. F., Daley, G. L., Chand, S., Walley, P. J., and MacDonald, P. C.: A study of angiotensin II pressor response throughout primigravid pregnancy. J. Clin. Invest., *52*:2682, 1973.
104. Gant, N. F., Hutchinson, H. T., Siiteri, P. K., and MacDonald, P. C.: Study of the metabolic clearance rate of dehydroisoandrosterone sulfate in pregnancy. Am. J. Obstet. Gynecol., *111*:555, 1971.
105. Gant, N. F., Madden, J. D., Siiteri, P. K., and MacDonald, P. C.: The metabolic clearance rate of dehydroisoandrosterone sulfate. III. The effect of thiazide diuretics in normal and future preeclamptic pregnancies. Am. J. Obstet. Gynecol., *123*:159, 1975.
106. Gerber, J. G., Keller, R. T., and Nies, A. S.: Prostaglandins and renin release. The effect of PGI_2, PGE_2 and 13,14 dihydro PGE_2 on the baroreceptor mechanism of renin release in the dog. Circ. Res., *44*:796, 1979.
106a. Gerber, J. G., Payne, N. A., Murphy, R. C., and Nies, A. S.: Prostacyclin produced by the pregnant uterus in the dog may act as a circulating vasodepressor substance. J. Clin. Invest., *67*:632, 1981.
107. Gill, J. R.: Bartter's syndrome. Ann. Rev. Med., *31*:405, 1980.
108. Gimbrone, M. A., and Alexander, R. W.: Angiotensin II stimulation of prostaglandin production in cultured human vascular endothelium. Science, *189*:219, 1975.
109. Ginz, B.: Myocardial infarction in pregnancy. J. Obstet. Gynaecol. Br. Commonw., *77*:610, 1970.
110. Glasson, R., Gaillar, R., Riondel, A., and Vallotton, M. B.: Role of renal prostaglandins and relationship to renin, aldosterone, and antidiuretic hormone during salt depletion in man. J. Clin. Endocrinol Metab., *49*:176, 1979.
111. Goldblatt, M. W.: A depressor substance in seminal fluid. J. Soc. Chem. Ind. (London), *52*:1056, 1933.
112. Golub, M., Zia, G., Matsuno, M., and Horton, R.: Metabolism of prostaglandins A_1 and E_1 in man. J. Clin. Invest., *56*:1404, 1975.
113. Goodlin, R. C.: Severe pre-eclampsia: Another great imitator. Am. J. Obstet. Gynecol., *125*:747, 1976.
114. Gorden, P., Ferris, T. F., and Mulrow, P. J.: Rabbit uterus as a possible site of renin synthesis. Am. J. Physiol., *212*:703, 1967.
115. Gordon, R. D., Fishman, L. M., and Liddle, G. W.: Plasma renin activity and aldosterone secretion in a pregnant woman with primary aldosteronism. J. Clin. Endocrinol., *27*:385, 1967.
116. Gordon, R. D., Parsons, S., and Symonds, E. M.: A prospective study of plasma renin activity in normal and toxemic pregnancy. Lancet, *1*:347, 1969.
117. Gordon, R. D., Symonds, E. M., Wilmshurst, E. G., and Pawsey, C. G. K.: Plasma renin activity, plasma angiotensin, and plasma and urinary electrolytes in normal and toxaemic pregnancy, including a prospective study. Clin. Sci., *45*:115, 1973.
118. Grollman, A., Muirhead, E. E., and Vanatta, J.: Role of the kidney in the pathogenesis of hypertension as determined by a study of the effects of bilateral nephrectomy and other experimental procedures on blood pressure in the dog. Am. J. Physiol., *157*:21, 1949.
119. Gross, F., Schaechtelin, G., Ziegler, M., and Berger, M.: A renin-like substance in the placenta and uterus of the rabbit. Lancet, *1*:914, 1964.
120. Gullner, H. G., Bartter, F. C., Cerlette, C., Smith, J. B., and Gill, J. R.: Prostacyclin overproduction in Bartter's syndrome. Lancet, *2*:767, 1979.
121. Gyongyossy, A., and Kelentey, B.: An experimental study of the effect of ischemia of the pregnant uterus on blood pressure. J. Obstet. Gynaecol. Br. Commonw., *65*:617, 1958.
121a. Hamberg, M., Tuoemo, T., Svenson, J., and Jonsson, C. E.: Formation and action of prostacyclin in isolated human umbilical artery. Acta. Physiol. Scand., *106*:289, 1979.
122. Handler, J. S.: The role of lactic acid in the reduced excretion of uric acid in toxemia of pregnancy. J. Clin. Invest., *39*:1526, 1960.
123. Hankin, M. E., and Symonds, E. M.: Body weight, diet and pre-eclamptic toxemia of pregnancy. Aust. N. Z. J. Obstet. Gynaecol., *4*:156, 1962.
124. Harbert, G. M., Clairborne, H. A., McGaughey, H. S., Wilson, L. A., and Thornton, W. N.: Convulsive toxemia. Am. J. Obstet. Gynecol., *100*:336, 1967.
125. Harbert, G. M., Jr., Cornell, G. W., and Thornton, W. N., Jr.: Effect of toxemic therapy on uterine dynamics. Am. J. Obstet. Gynecol., *105*:94, 1969.
126. Hatfield, A. K., Stein, J. H., Greenberger, N. J., Abernathy, R. W., and Ferris, T. F.: Idiopathic acute fatty liver of pregnancy: Death from extrahepatic manifestations. Am. J. Dig. Dis., *17*:167, 1972.
127. Hauch, E., and Lehmann, K.: Investigation into the occurrence of eclampsia in Denmark during the years 1918–1927. Acta Obstet. Gynecol. Scand., *14*:425, 1934.
128. Hendee, A. E., Martin, R. D., and Waters, W. C., III: Hypertension in pregnancy: Toxemia or pheochromocytoma. Am. J. Obstet. Gynecol., *105*:64, 1969.
128a. Henrich, W. L.: Role of prostaglandins in renin secretion. Kidney Int., *19*:822, 1981.
129. Hibbard, B. M., and Rosen, M.: The management of severe pre-eclampsia and eclampsia. Br. J. Anaesth., *49*:3, 1977.
130. Hill, L. M.: Metabolism of uric acid in normal and toxemic pregnancy. Mayo Clin. Proc., *53*:743, 1978.
131. Hillestad, L.: Aortic coarctation and pregnancy. Acta Obstet. Gynecol. Scand., *51*:95, 1972.
132. Horton, E. W.: Prostaglandins at adrenergic nerve endings. Br. Med. Bull., *29*:148, 1973.
133. Howie, P. W., Begg, C. B., Purdie, D. W., and Prentice, C. R.: Use of coagulation tests to predict the clinical progress of pre-eclampsia. Lancet, *2*:323, 1976.
134. Hubl, W., Buchner, M., Bellee, H., Muhlbach, F., and Dorner, G.: Study of plasma aldosterone in normal pregnancy, in pre-eclamptic women and in cord plasma of newborns. Endokrinologie, *73*:162, 1979.

135. Humphries, J.: Occurrence of hypertensive toxemia of pregnancy in mother-daughter pairs. Bull. Johns Hopkins Hosp., *107*:271, 1960.

136. Hyde, E., Joyce, D., Gurevich, V., Flute, P. T., and Barvera, S.: Intravascular coagulation during pregnancy and the puerperium. J. Obstet. Gynaecol. Br. Commonw., *80*:1059, 1973.

137. Hytten, F. E., and Thomson, A. M.: Weight gain in pregnancy. *In* Lindheimer, M., Katz, A., and Zuspan, F. (eds.): Hypertension in Pregnancy. New York, John Wiley & Sons, 1976, p. 179.

138. Karbhari, D., Harrigan, J. T., and Lamagra, R.: The supine hypertensive test as a predictor of incipient pre-eclampsia. Am. J. Obstet. Gynecol., *127*:620, 1977.

139. Kasturilal, R. A., and Shetti, R. N.: Role of diazepam in the management of eclampsia. Curr. Ther. Res., *18*:627, 1975.

140. Khunda, S.: Pregnancy and Addison's disease. Obstet. Gynecol., *39*:431, 1972.

141. Killam, A. P., Dillard, S. H., Patton, R. C., and Peterson, P. R.: Pregnancy induced hypertension complicated by acute liver disease and disseminated intravascular coagulation. Am. J. Obstet. Gynecol., *123*:823, 1975.

142. Kincaid-Smith, P., Bullen, M., and Mills, J.: Prolonged use of methyldopa in severe hypertension in pregnancy. Br. Med. J., *1*:274, 1966.

143. Knowlton, A. I., Mudge, G. H., and Jailer, J. W.: Pregnancy in Addison's disease: A report of four patients. J. Clin. Endocrinol. Metab., *9*:514, 1949.

144. Kokot, F., and Cekanski, A.: Plasma renin activity in peripheral and uterine vein blood in pregnant and non-pregnant women. J. Obstet. Gynaecol. Br. Commonw., *79*:72, 1972.

145. Krauss, G. W., Marchese, J. R., and Yen, S. S. C.: Prophylactic use of hydrochlorothiazide in pregnancy. J.A.M.A., *198*:1150, 1966.

146. Landesman, R., Aguero, O., Wilson, K., LaRussa, R., Campbell, W., and Peralaza, O.: The prophylactic use of chlorthalidine in pregnancy. J. Obstet. Gynaecol. Br. Commonw., *72*:1004, 1965.

147. Landesman, R., Halpern, M., and Knapp, R. C.: Renal artery lesions associated with the toxemias of pregnancy. Obstet. Gynecol., *18*:645, 1961.

148. Landesman, R., Holze, E., and Scherr, L.: Fetal mortality in essential hypertension. Obstet. Gynecol., *6*:354, 1955.

149. Langford, H. G.: Probable toxemia of pregnancy in a patient with Addison's disease. Am. J. Obstet. Gynecol., *91*:296, 1965.

150. Lardner, C. N., Brinkman, C. R., III, and Weston, P. V.: Dynamics of uterine circulation in pregnant and non-pregnant sheep. Am. J. Physiol., *218*:257, 1970.

151. Lean, T. H., Ratnam, S. S., and Sivasamboo, R.: Use of benzodiazepines in the management of eclampsia. J. Obstet. Gynaecol. Br. Commonw., *75*:856, 1968.

152. Leather, H. M., Humphreys, D. M., Baker, P., and Chadd, M. A.: A controlled trial of hypotensive agents in hypertension in pregnancy. Lancet, *2*:488, 1968.

153. Lewis, P. J., Boylan, P., Friedman, L. A., Hensby, C. N., and Dowing, I.: Prostacyclin in pregnancy. Br. Med. J., *280*:1581, 1980.

153a. Lewis, P. E., Cefalo, R. C., Naulty, J. S., and Rodkey, F. L.: Placental transfer and fetal toxicity of sodium nitroprusside. Gynecol. Invest., *8*:46, 1977.

154. Lieberman, B. A., Stirrat, G. M., Cohen, S. L., Beard, R. W., Pinter, G. D., and Belsey, E.: The possible adverse effect of propranolol on the fetus in pregnancies complicated by severe hypertension. Br. J. Obstet. Gynecol., *85*:678, 1978.

154a. Lindheimer, M. D.: Further characterization of the influence of supine posture on renal function in late pregnancy. Gynecol. Invest., *1*:69, 1970.

155. Lohlein, M.: Zur Pathogenese der Nierenkrankherten Nephritis und Nephrose mit besonderer Besichtigung der nephropathia Gravidarum. Dtsch. Med. Wochenschr., *44*:1187, 1918.

156. Long, P. A., Abell, D. A., and Beischer, N. A.: Fetal growth and placental function assessed by urinary estriol excretion before the onset of pre-eclampsia. Am. J. Obstet. Gynecol., *135*:344, 1979.

157. Long, R. G., Scheuer, P. J., and Sherlock, S.: Pre-eclampsia presenting with deep jaundice. J. Clin. Pathol., *30*:212, 1977.

158. Lunell, N. O., Persson, B., Aragon, G., Fredholm, B. B., and Astrom, H.: Circulatory and metabolic effects of acute beta 1–blockade in severe pre-eclampsia. Acta Obstet. Gynecol. Scand., *58*:443, 1979.

159. Lyons, H. A., and Rutonio, R.: The sensitivity of the respiratory center in pregnancy and after the administration of progesterone. Trans. Assoc. Am. Phys., *72*:173, 1959.

160. MacGillivray, I., Rose, G. A., and Rowe, B.: Blood pressure survey in pregnancy. Clin. Sci., *37*:395, 1969.

161. Marshall, G. W., and Newman, R. L.: Roll-over test. Am. J. Obstet. Gynecol., *127*:623, 1977.

161a. McFarlane, C. N.: An evaluation of the serum uric acid level in pregnancy. J. Obstet. Gynaecol. Brit. Commonw., *79*:63, 1963.

162. McFarlane, A., and Scott, J. S.: Pre-eclampsia/eclampsia in twin pregnancies. J. Med. Genet., *13*:208, 1976.

162a. McGiff, J. C., Crowshaw, K., and Itskovitz, H. D.: Prostaglandins and renal function. Fed. Proc., *33*:39, 1974.

163. McKay, D. G.: Disseminated intravascular coagulation and experimental disease models in pregnancy. *In* Lindheimer, M. D., Katz, A. I., and Zuspan, F. P. (eds.): Hypertension in Pregnancy. New York, John Wiley & Sons, 1976, p. 401.

164. Michael, C. A.: The control of hypertension in labor. Aust. N. Z. Obstet. Gynaecol., *12*:48, 1972.

165. Michie, E. A.: Urinary estriol excretion in pregnancies complicated by suspected retarded intrauterine growth or essential hypertension. J. Obstet. Gynaecol. Br. Commonw., *74*:896, 1967.

166. Miyamori, I., FitzGerald, G. A., Brown, M. J., and Lewis, P. J.: Prostacyclin stimulates the renin angiotensin aldosterone system in man. J. Clin. Endocrinol. Metab., *49*:943, 1979.

167. Morris, J. A., Arce, J. J., Hamilton, C. J., Davidson, E. C., Maidman, J. E., Clark, J. H., and Bloom, R. S.: The management of severe preeclampsia and eclampsia with intravenous diazoxide. Obstet. Gynecol., *49*:675, 1977.

168. Morris, R. H., Vassalli, P., Beller, F. K., and McCluskey, R. T.: Immunofluorescent studies of renal biopsies in the diagnosis of toxemia of pregnancy. Obstet. Gynecol., *24*:32, 1964.

169. Mountain, K. R., Hirsh, J., and Gallus, A. S.: Neonatal coagulation defect due to anticonvulsant treatment in pregnancy. Lancet, *1*:265, 1970.

170. Muirhead, E. E., Brown, G. B., Germain, G. S., and Leach, B. E.: The renal medulla as an anti-hypertensive organ. J. Lab. Clin. Med., *76*:641, 1970.

171. Negus, P., Tannen, R. L., and Dunn, M. J.: Indomethacin potentiates the vasoconstrictor actions of angiotensin II in normal man. Prostaglandins, *12*:175, 1976.

172. Nolten, W. E., and Ehrlich, E. N.: Sodium and mineralocorticoids in normal pregnancy. Kidney Int., *18*:162, 1980.

173. Normington, E. A. M., and Davies, D.: Hypertension and edema complicating pregnancy in Addison's disease. Br. Med. J., *2*:148, 1972.

174. Nuwayhid, B., Brinkman, C. R., Katchen, B., Symchowicz, S., Martinek, H., and Assali, N. S.: Maternal and fetal hemodynamic effects of diazoxide. Obstet. Gynecol., *46*:197, 1975.

175. Oates, J. A., Whorton, A. R., and Gerten, J. F.: The participation of prostaglandins in the control of renin release. Fed. Proc., *38*:72, 1979.

176. Omini, C., Folco, G. C., Pasargiklian, R., Fano, M., and Berti, F.: Prostacyclin in pregnant human uterus. Prostaglandins, *17*:113, 1979.

177. Ounsted, M. K., Moor, V. A., Good, F. J., and Redman, C. W. G.: Hypertension during pregnancy with and without specific therapy: The children at the age of 4 years. Br. J. Obstet. Gynaecol., *87*:19, 1980.

178. Page, E. W., and Christianson, R.: The impact of mean arterial pressure in the middle trimester upon the outcome of pregnancy. Am. J. Obstet. Gynecol., *125*:740, 1976.

179. Page, E. W., and Ogden, E.: The physiology of hypertension in eclampsia. Am. J. Obstet. Gynecol., *38*:1939, 1939.

180. Paul, R. H., Koh, K. S., and Bernstein, S. G.: Changes in fetal heart rate — uterine contraction patterns associated with eclampsia. Am. J. Obstet. Gynecol., *130*:165, 1978.

181. Perkins, R. P.: Thrombocytopenia in obstetric syndromes. A review. Obstet. Gynecol. Surv., *34*:101, 1979.

182. Pipkin, F. B., and Symonds, E. M.: The renin-angiotensin system in the maternal and fetal circulation in pregnancy hypertension. Clin. Obstet. Gynaecol., *4*:651, 1977.

183. Pirani, C. L., Pollak, V. E., Lannigan, R., and Folli, G.: The renal glomerular lesions of pre-eclampsia. Am. J. Obstet. Gynecol., 87:1047, 1963.
184. Piver, M. S., Corson, S. L., and Bolognese, R. J.: Hypertension six weeks postpartum in normal patients. Obstet. Gynecol., 30:238, 1967.
185. Pollak, V. E., and Nettles, J. B.: The kidney in toxemia of pregnancy: A clinical and pathologic study based on renal biopsies. Medicine, 39:469, 1960.
186. Pritchard, J. A.: The use of magnesium in the management of eclamptogenic toxemias. Surg. Gynecol. Obstet., 100:131, 1955.
187. Pritchard, J. A.: Management of preeclampsia and eclampsia. Kidney Int., 18:259, 1980.
188. Pritchard, J. A., Cunningham, F. G., and Mason, R. A.: Coagulation changes in eclampsia: Their frequency and pathogenesis. Am. J. Obstet. Gynecol., 124:855, 1976.
189. Rauramo, L., Kivikoski, A., and Salmi, T.: The effect of systematic treatment of toxemia of pregnancy upon fetal prognosis. Ann. Chir. Gynaecol. Fenn., 64:165, 1975.
190. Redman, C. W. G.: Treatment of hypertension in pregnancy. Kidney Int., 18:267, 1980.
191. Redman, C. W. G., and Bonnar, J.: Plasma urate changes in pre-eclampsia. Br. Med. J., 1:484, 1978.
192. Redman, C. W. G., Bonnar, J., and Beilin, L.: Early platelet consumption in pre-eclampsia. Br. Med. J., 1:467, 1978.
193. Redman, C. W. G., Denson, K. W., Beilin, L. J., Bolton, F. G., and Stirrat, G. M.: Factor-VIII consumption in pre-eclampsia. Lancet, 2:1249, 1977.
193a. Remuzzi, G., Marchesi, D., and Mecca, G.: Reduction of fetal vascular prostacyclin activity in pre-eclampsia. Lancet, 2:310, 1980.
194. Roberts, J. M., and May, W. J.: Consumptive coagulopathy in severe pre-eclampsia. Obstet. Gynecol., 48:163, 1976.
195. Robertson, W. B., Brosen, S. I., and Dixon, H. G.: The pathological response of the vessels of the placental bed to hypertensive pregnancy. J. Pathol. Bacteriol., 93:581, 1967.
196. Robson, J. S.: Proteinuria and the renal lesions in pre-eclampsia and abruptio placentae. In Lindheimer, M. D., Katz, A. I., and Zuspan, F. P. (eds.): Hypertension in Pregnancy. New York, John Wiley & Sons, 1976, p. 61.
197. Rosenman, E., Kanter, A., Bacari, R. A., Pirani, C. L., and Pollak, V. E.: Fetal late post-partum intravascular coagulation with acute renal failure. Am. J. Med. Sci., 257:259, 1969.
197a. Rubin, P. C.: Beta blockers in pregnancy. N. Engl. J. Med. 305:1323, 1981.
198. Sandstrom, B. O.: Anti-hypertensive treatment with the adrenergic beta-receptor blocker metoprolol during pregnancy. Gynecol. Invest., 9:195, 1978.
199. Sasaki, C., Nowaczynski, W., Kuchel, O., Chavez, C., Ledoux, F., Gauthier, S., and Genest, J.: Plasma progesterone in normal subjects and patients with benign essential hypertension in normal, low and high sodium intake. J. Clin. Endocrinol. Metab., 34:650, 1972.
200. Schenker, J. G., and Chowers, I.: Pheochromocytoma and pregnancy. Obstet. Gynecol. Surv., 26:739, 1971.
201. Schewitz, L. J., Pirani, C. L., and Pollak, V. E.: Observations of a case of pre-eclampsia with respect to hypertensive vascular disease as a sequel. Obstet. Gynecol., 27:626, 1966.
202. Schwartz, M. L., and Brenner, W. E.: The obfuscation of eclampsia by thrombotic thrombocytopenic purpura. Am. J. Obstet. Gynecol., 131:18, 1978.
203. Sealey, J. E., Atlas, S. A., and Laragh, J. H.: Prorenin and other large molecular weight forms of renin. Endocr. Rev., 1:365, 1980.
204. Seitchik, J.: Observations on the renal tubular reabsorption of uric acid. Am. J. Obstet. Gynecol., 65:981, 1953.
205. Shannon, R. W., Fraser, G. P., Aitken, R. G., and Harper, J. R.: Diazepam in pre-eclamptic toxemia with special reference to its effect on the newborn infant. Br. J. Clin. Pract., 26:271, 1972.
206. Shapiro, S., Monson, R. R., Kaufman, D. W., Suskind, V., Heinonen, O. P., and Slone, D.: Perinatal mortality and birth weight in relation to aspirin taken during pregnancy. Lancet, 1:1375, 1976.
207. Sheehan, H. L.: Renal morphology in pre-eclampsia. Kidney Int., 18:241, 1980.
208. Sheehan, H. L., and Lynch, J. B.: Pathology of Toxaemia of Pregnancy. New York, Longman, Inc., 1973.
209. Singh, M. M., MacGillivray, I., and Mahaffy, R. G.: A study of

210. Sloan, W. C., Florey, C. V., Acteson, R. M., and Kessner, D. M.: Epidemiologic methods in the study of blood pressure in relatives of toxemic primiparas. Am. J. Epidemiol., 91:553, 1970.
211. Smith, R. W., Selinger, H. E., and Stevenson, S. F.: The uteroplacental complex. Am. J. Obstet. Gynecol., 105:1129, 1969.
212. Spargo, B., McCartney, C. P., and Winemiller, R.: Glomerular capillary endotheliosis in toxemia of pregnancy. Arch. Pathol., 68:593, 1959.
213. Speroff, L. G.: Toxemia of pregnancy. Am. J. Cardiol., 32:582, 1973.
214. Stakemann, G.: A renin-like pressor substance found in the placenta of the cat. Acta Pathol. Microbiol. Scand., 50:350, 1960.
215. Stander, H. J., and Cadden, J. F.: Blood chemistry in pre-eclampsia and eclampsia. Am. J. Obstet. Gynecol., 28:856, 1934.
216. Steele, T. H.: Evidence for altered renal urate reabsorption during changes in volume of the extracellular fluid. J. Lab. Clin. Med., 74:288, 1969.
217. Stein, J. H., Osgood, R. W., and Kunau, R. T.: Direct measurement of papillary collecting duct sodium transport in the rat. Evidence for heterogeneity of nephron function during Ringer loading. J. Clin. Invest., 58:767, 1976.
218. Stokes, J. B., and Kokko, J. P.: Inhibition of sodium transport by PGE2 across the isolated perfused rabbit collecting tubule. J. Clin. Invest., 59:1099, 1977.
219. Stout, M. L.: Hypertension six weeks post partum in normal patients. Am. J. Obstet. Gynecol., 27:730, 1934.
220. Strauss, R. G., and Alexander, R. W.: Post-partum hemolytic uremic syndrome. Obstet. Gynecol., 47:169, 1976.
221. Strauss, R. G., Keefer, J. R., Burke, T., and Civetta, J. M.: Hemodynamic monitoring of cardiogenic pulmonary edema complicating toxemia of pregnancy. Obstet. Gynecol., 55:170, 1980.
222. Sturdee, D. W.: Diazepam: Routes of administration and rate of absorption. A study of women with pre-eclampsia. Br. J. Anaesth., 49:1091, 1976.
223. Sullivan, J. M., Palmer, E. T., Schoeneberger, A. A., Jennings, J. C., Morrison, J. C., and Ratts, T. E.: SQ 20,881: Effect on eclamptic–pre-eclamptic women with postpartum hypertension. Am. J. Obstet. Gynecol., 131:707, 1978.
224. Symonds, E. M., Pipkin, F. B., and Craven, D. J.: Changes in the renin-angiotensin system in primigravidae with hypertensive disease of pregnancy. Br. J. Obstet. Gynaecol., 82:643, 1975.
225. Symonds, E. M., Stanley, M. A., and Skinner, S. L.: Production of renin by in vitro cultures of human chorion and uterine muscle. Nature, 217:1152, 1968.
226. Tapia, H. R., Johnson, C. E., and Strong, C. E.: Renin-angiotensin system in normal and in hypertensive disease of pregnancy. Lancet, 2:847, 1972.
227. Tarazi, R. C., Dustan, H. P., and Frohlich, E. D.: Relation of plasma to interstitial fluid volume in essential hypertension. Circulation, 40:357, 1969.
228. Tcherdakoff, Ph., Berrard, E., Kreft, C., and Colliard, M.: Propranolol in hypertension during pregnancy: Ten cases. In Bonnar, J., MacGillivray, I., and Symonds, E. M. (eds.), Pregnancy Hypertension. Lancaster, England, MTP Press Ltd., 1980, p. 467.
229. Templeton, A. A., and Kelman, G. R.: Arterial blood gases in pre-eclampsia. Br. J. Obstet. Gynaecol., 84:290, 1977.
230. Thomson, A. M., Billewecz, W. Z., and Hytten, R. E.: The epidemiology of edema during pregnancy. J. Obstet. Gynaecol. Br. Commonw., 74:1, 1967.
231. Thornton, C. A., and Bonnar, J.: Factor VIII-related antigen and Factor VIII coagulant activity in normal and pre-eclamptic pregnancy. Br. J. Obstet. Gynaecol., 84:919, 1977.
232. Tobian, L.: A viewpoint concerning the enigma of hypertension. Am. J. Med., 52:595, 1972.
233. Turner, G., and Collins, E.: Fetal effects of regular salicylate ingestion in pregnancy. Lancet, 2:338, 1975.
234. Tyson, J. E.: Obstetrical management of the pregnant diabetic. Med. Clin. North Am., 55:961, 1971.
235. Vassali, P., Simon, G., and Rouiller, C.: Production of ultrastructural glomerular lesions resembling those of toxemia of

the long term effects of pre-eclampsia on blood pressure and renal function. J. Obstet. Gynaecol. Br. Commonw., 81:903, 1974.

pregnancy by thromboplastin infusion in rabbits. Nature, *199*:1105, 1963.

236. Venuto, R., Cox, J. W., Stein, J. H., and Ferris, T. F.: Regulation of uterine blood flow in the pregnant rabbit. J. Clin. Invest., *57*:938, 1976.

237. Venuto, R., O'Dorisio, T., Stein, J. H., and Ferris, T. F.: The effect of prostaglandin inhibition on uterine blood flow. J. Clin. Invest., *55*:193, 1975.

238. Vink, G. J., Moodley, J., and Philpott, R. H.: Effects of hydralazine on the fetus in the treatment of maternal hypertension. Obstet. Gynecol., *55*:519, 1980.

239. von Euler, U. S.: Zur Kenntnis der pharmakologischen Wirkungen von Nativsekreten und Extrakten männlicher accessorischer Geschlechtsdrüsen. Arch. Exp. Pathol. Pharmakol., *175*:78, 1934.

240. Wachtel, H. L., and Czarnecki, S. W.: Coarctation of the aorta and pregnancy. Am. Heart J., *72*:251, 1966.

241. Weber, P. C., Larson, C., Anggard, E., Hamberg, M., Covey, E. J., Nicolaou, K. C., and Samuelsson, B.: Stimulation of renin release from rabbit renal cortex by arachidonic acid and prostaglandin endoperoxides. Circ. Res., *39*:868, 1976.

242. Webster, J., Rees, A. J., Lewis, P. J., and Hensby, C. N.: Prostacyclin deficiency in hemolytic-uremic syndrome. Br. Med. J., *281*:271, 1980.

243. Weinberger, M. H., Kramer, N. J., Grim, C. E., and Petersen, L. P.: The effect of posture and saline loading on plasma renin activity and aldosterone concentration in pregnant, non-pregnant, and estrogen-treated women. J. Clin. Endocrinol. Metab., *44*:69, 1977.

244. Weinberger, M. H., Peterson, L. P., Herr, M. J., and Wade, M. B.: The effect of supine and lateral recumbency on plasma renin activity during pregnancy. J. Clin. Endocrinol. Metab., *36*:991, 1973.

245. Weir, R. J., Brown, J. J., Fraser, R., Lever, A. F., et al.: Plasma renin, renin substrate, angiotensin II, and aldosterone in hypertensive disease of pregnancy. Lancet, *1*:291, 1973.

246. Weir, R. J., Doig, A., Fraser, R., Morton, J. J., Parboosingh, J.,

Robertson, J. I. S., and Wilson, A.: Studies of the renin-angiotensin-aldosterone system, cortisol, DOC, and ADH in normal and hypertensive pregnancy. *In* Lindheimer, M., Katz, A., and Zuspan, F. (eds.): Hypertension in Pregnancy. New York, John Wiley & Sons, 1976, p. 251.

247. Whigham, K. A., Howie, P. W., Drummond, A. H., and Prentice, C. R.: Abnormal platelet function in pre-eclampsia. Br. J. Obstet. Gynaecol., *85*:28, 1978.

248. Whigham, K. A., Howie, P. W., Drummond, A. H., and Prentice, C. R.: Abnormal platelet function in pre-eclampsia. *In* Bonnar, J., MacGillivray, I., and Symonds, E. M. (eds.): Pregnancy Hypertension. Lancaster, England, MTP Press Ltd., 1980, p. 397.

249. Whorton, A. R., Misono, K., Hollifield, J., Frolich, J. C., Inagumi, T., and Oates, J. A.: Prostaglandins and renin release: I. Stimulation of renin release from rabbit renal cortical slices by PGI_2. Prostaglandins, *14*:1095, 1977.

250. Wilson, M., Morganti, A., Zervoudakis, I., Letcher, R., Romney, B., Von Oeyon, P., Papera, S., Sealey, J., and Laragh, J. H.: Blood pressure, the renin-aldosterone system and sex steroids throughout normal pregnancy. Am. J. Med., *68*:97, 1980.

251. World Health Organization, Expert Committee on Pregnancy and Lactation: W.H.O. Techn. Rep. Ser., Vol., 302, 1965.

252. Yeh, S. Y., Paul, R. H., Cordero, L., and Hon, E. H.: A study of diazepam during labor. Obstet. Gynecol., *43*:363, 1974.

253. Ylikorkala, O., and Viinikka, L.: Thromboxane A_2 in pregnancy and puerperium. Br. Med. J., *281*:1601, 1980.

254. Young, J.: The aetiology of eclampsia and albuminuria and their relation to accidental hemorrhage. J. Obstet. Gynaecol. Br. Emp., *26*:1, 1914.

255. Zinner, S. H., Levy, P. S., and Kass, E. H.: Familial aggregation of blood pressure in childhood. N. Engl. J. Med., *284*:401, 1971.

256. Zuspan, F. P., and Ward, M. C.: Improved fetal salvage in eclampsia. Obstet. Gynecol., *26*:893, 1965.

2

Philip Felig, M.D.
Donald Coustan, M.D.

DIABETES MELLITUS

Prior to the advent of insulin, the coexistence of diabetes and pregnancy was a rare event and one likely to have fatal consequences for both mother and fetus. In one of the earliest collected series of pregnant diabetic women, Williams, in 1909, reported a maternal mortality rate of 30 per cent and an overall fetal loss rate of 65 per cent.[164] Since 1921 the availability of insulin has markedly improved the outlook for both mother and fetus. Nevertheless, fetal mortality continues at rates of 3 to 5 per cent, considerably above the 1 to 2 per cent rate noted in the general population. In addition, major congenital anomalies occur in 6 to 12 per cent of offspring of diabetic mothers,[48, 98] three to four fold the rate in the general population.[63] Furthermore, the incidence of congenital anomalies has failed to decline despite an overall decline in neonatal mortality.[48] In recent years increasing emphasis has been placed on maintaining maternal fuel metabolism as close to normal as possible so as to reduce neonatal mortality and morbidity to levels comparable with those in the general population. It is now recognized that such efforts may have to extend to the time of conception and the earliest stages of embryogenesis in order to be completely successful.

The improvements in outlook for the fetus that have already been observed are a consequence of intensive methods of insulin administration as well as advances in fetal monitoring and obstetric management. An increased understanding of maternal and fetal fuel metabolism has provided the physiologic principles on which the management of the pregnant diabetic is based.

FUEL AND HORMONE METABOLISM IN NORMAL PREGNANCY

In the normal nondiabetic woman, pregnancy is associated with profound changes in fuel metabolism. The circulating levels of glucose and amino acids are reduced and levels of free fatty acids, ketones, and triglycerides are increased, while the secretion of insulin in response to glucose is augmented. The overall metabolic state has been characterized as one of "accelerated starvation."[48] Pregnancy also has a diabetogenic effect on the mother, as is indicated by (a) the development of diabetes in genetically predisposed women during pregnancy and the reversion to completely normal carbohydrate metabolism post partum (see discussion of gestational diabetes, p. 45), (b) an increase in the upper limits of normal in the 2 hour blood glucose level during glucose tolerance testing,[111] (c) higher postprandial glucose levels after ingestion of a standard meal,[26, 48] and (d) diminished responsiveness to injected insulin. This seeming paradox of coexistence of diabetes with a tendency toward fasting hypoglycemia can best be explained in the context of fetal-maternal-placental fuel-hormone interactions that exist in the fasting, as well as in the fed, state.

Fetal-Maternal Fuel-Hormone Relationships

The fuel requirements of the developing fetus are met primarily, although not exclusively, by glucose.[2, 7] Glucose not only provides the energy necessary for protein synthesis but also is the precursor for the synthesis of fat and the formation of glycogen. The level of glycogen stores in liver and muscle in the fetus, per gram of tissue, is substantially greater than that in the adult. The overall level of glucose uptake required to meet these synthetic and oxidative needs has been estimated at 20 mg per minute at term,[114] representing a glucose utilization rate of 6 mg per kg of body weight per minute. Measurements of the rate of glucose utilization in the human fetus and the lamb fetus have generally yielded similar results.[31, 54] Glucose turnover in the human neonate has been reported to average 4.2 mg per kg per minute.[76] This rate of glucose utilization is in excess of that observed in the normal adult, in whom glucose turnover occurs at a rate of 2 to 2.5 mg per kg per minute.[41]

With respect to the transfer of glucose to the fetus, the level of glucose in fetal blood is generally 10 to 20 mg per 100 ml below that in the maternal circulation, indicating that diffusion per se favors the net movement of glucose from mother to fetus. However, the rate of glucose delivery is more rapid than can be accounted for on this basis, and consequently the process of glucose transfer is described as one of "facilitated diffusion." This process has been shown to be carrier mediated but is not energy dependent.[128] The importance of maternal glucose levels in regulating glucose delivery to the fetus may relate not only to the provision of adequate substrate but also to the avoidance of excess substrate delivery. Teratogenic effects of high concentrations of glucose (500 to 1500 mg per 100 ml) have been observed in rat and mouse embryos maintained in tissue culture.[19, 136] Thus, while glucose delivery is necessary for the growth and development of the fetus, excessive glucose transfer (the expected consequence of maternal hyperglycemia) may alter embryogenesis.

In contrast to the rapid movement of glucose to the fetus, maternal insulin and glucagon fail to traverse the placenta. Fetal glucose utilization is thus not directly dependent on maternal insulin availability. On the other hand, fetal insulin is believed to play a central role in the growth of the conceptus.[153] Insulin is present in the fetus at 9 to 11 weeks of gestation,[92] and its secretion is stimulated, albeit sluggishly, in response to increased glucose availability and even more effectively in response to aminogenic stimulation.[59, 105] The importance of fetal insulin to growth is underscored by the concurrence of macrosomia and hyperinsulinemia in the infants of diabetic mothers.[107, 116] Furthermore, continuous infusion of insulin so as to achieve euglycemic hyperinsulinemia in the rhesus monkey fetus results in macrosomia and organomegaly, including hyperplasia of the liver, heart, spleen, and placenta.[153]

In addition to the transfer of glucose, amino acids are actively transported by the placenta from the maternal to the fetal circulation.[64] Besides the utilization of amino acids for protein synthesis, studies in the fetal lamb suggest that amino acids may also be catabolized and serve as an energy-yielding fuel.[60] Regardless of the ultimate metabolic fate of these amino acids, their transfer results in maternal hypoaminoacidemia.[44] Since amino acids, notably alanine, are key precursors for glucose formation (gluconeogenesis) by the maternal liver in the fasting state,[41] the presence of the fetus causes a drainage of glucose precursors as well as glucose from the mother.[44, 97]

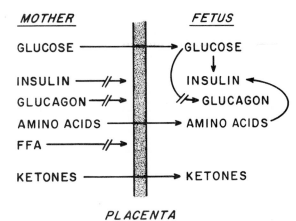

FIGURE 2–1. Maternal-fetal fuel and hormone exchange. Glucose, amino acids, and ketones are transferred from mother to fetus, while insulin and glucagon are not. Free fatty acids are transferred only to a very limited extent. An increase in glucose concentration in the maternal circulation results in fetal hyperglycemia, which stimulates the secretion of insulin and inhibits the secretion of glucagon by fetal islet cells. Amino acids are also potent stimuli of fetal insulin secretion. (From Felig: Med. Clin. North Am. 61:43, 1977.)

With respect to lipid metabolism, transfer of free fatty acids from the maternal to the fetal circulation is limited to the provision of essential fatty acids required for tissue synthesis[68] rather than to the provision of combustible fuels. In contrast, the ketone acids beta-hydroxybutyrate and acetoacetate are readily transferred to the fetus by a diffusion process.[75, 135] Furthermore, the enzymes necessary for ketone oxidation are present in fetal brain tissue[115] as well as in liver.[138]

The overall fetal-maternal fuel-hormone interaction may thus be summarized as follows (Fig. 2–1): Glucose and amino acids are continuously drained by the fetus from the maternal circulation. Fetal insulin availability is not dependent on the transfer of insulin from the mother but is determined by the ambient glucose concentration in the fetus. Hyperketonemia in the mother results in fetal hyperketonemia and ketone utilization by the fetus.

The Fasting State

Nonpregnant Condition. Maintenance of glucose homeostasis in the fasting, postabsorptive state depends on a balance between the production and the utilization of glucose (Fig.

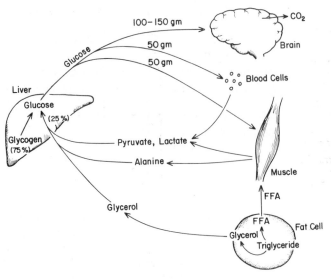

FIGURE 2–2. Glucose turnover in the basal (overnight fasting) resting state in normal, nonpregnant women. Glucose is released by the liver as a consequence of glycogenolysis (75 per cent) and gluconeogenesis (25 per cent). The brain is the major site of glucose utilization, consuming glucose at rates of 100 to 150 gm per day. In pregnancy, glucose utilization is increased as a consequence of uptake by the conceptus. In addition, alanine availability for maternal gluconeogenesis is reduced because of its active transport to the fetus. (From Felig, P.: The endocrine pancreas: Diabetes mellitus. In Felig, P., et al. (eds.): Endocrinology and Metabolism. New York, McGraw-Hill, Inc., 1981. Reprinted with permission.)

2–2). Glucose uptake occurs primarily in the brain and, to a much lesser extent, in the formed elements of the blood and muscle tissue. In each of these sites, glucose consumption during fasting is not insulin dependent. To meet the needs of these tissues, glucose is continuously released by the liver at rates of 2 to 2.5 mg per kg per min (150 to 250 gm/day).[41] The majority of the glucose released, 75 per cent, is derived from the breakdown of glycogen. The remaining 25 per cent represents new glucose production (gluconeogenesis) from lactate, amino acids (principally alanine), and, to a lesser extent, glycerol.[41]

The major hormonal signal regulating the production of glucose by the liver is the fall in circulating insulin levels from concentrations of 50 to 100 microunits per ml in the fed state to 10 to 20 microunits per ml in the fasting condition. The presence of basal concentrations of circulating glucagon (50 to 100 pg/ml) is also necessary for the maintenance of hepatic glucose production.[158] In addition to the need for the proper hormonal milieu, it is evident that glucose precursors, particularly alanine, must be delivered to the liver in adequate concentrations. This is particularly true in circumstances in which hepatic glycogen stores have been depleted and gluconeogenesis is responsible for an increased proportion of total hepatic glucose output.

Pregnancy: Accelerated Starvation. As early as the 15th week of gestation, maternal glucose levels after an overnight, 12 to 14 hour fast are 15 to 20 mg per 100 ml lower than in the nongravid state (Fig. 2–3). The exaggerated decrease in plasma glucose requires a fast of less than 12 to 14 hours to become manifest. Plasma glucose levels are significantly lower during sleep

(11 P.M. to 8 A.M.) in the second and third trimesters compared with the nongravid state.[26] Maternal hypoglycemia is further exaggerated as fasting extends beyond 12 hours and the plasma glucose drops to 40 to 45 mg per 100 ml (Fig. 2–3). The fall in maternal glucose levels results in a decline in the fasting insulin concentration, which in turn leads to an exaggeration of starvation ketosis. Thus, blood levels of beta-hydroxybutyric acid and acetoacetic acid are two to four times higher in pregnancy after no more

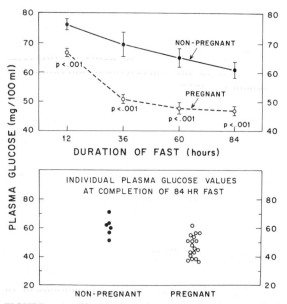

FIGURE 2–3. Plasma glucose levels in pregnant and nonpregnant women during a 3 to 4 day fast. Fasting hypoglycemia characterized the response to starvation in pregnancy. (Based on data of Felig and Lynch, 1970.)

than an overnight fast.[45, 75] The net effect is an exaggeration of the overall response to starvation as indicated by hypoglycemia, hypoinsulinemia, and hyperketonemia.[41] In addition, a more rapid decline in the concentration of alanine, the principal gluconeogenic precursor, is observed in fasting pregnant compared with nonpregnant women.[44, 154a]

The failure to maintain fasting plasma glucose levels during pregnancy at levels comparable to the nongravid state could theoretically be ascribed to (a) a reduction in maternal glucose production; (b) an increase in glucose utilization by the mother, the conceptus, or both; or (c) an increase in the volume of glucose distribution (i.e, the glucose space). The available evidence points strongly away from an impairment in maternal glucose production. Gluconeogenesis by livers removed from pregnant rats is increased.[62a] In fasting pregnant women, alanine administration results in a prompt rise in plasma glucose levels.[44] Furthermore, urine nitrogen excretion, an index of gluconeogenesis, is increased during starvation in human pregnancy.[45] Studies in normal women at term have, in fact, shown a 16 per cent increase in glucose production compared with nongravid women.[75] Interestingly, the decrease in fasting plasma glucose levels in pregnancy is observed in spite of equally augmented rates of glucose utilization and glucose production, suggesting that an increase in the glucose distribution space contributes to the development of hypoglycemia.[75] Furthermore, fasting hypoglycemia is observed in preterm rats even in the absence of an overall rise in glucose turnover.[106] Thus, while increased drainage of glucose and amino acids by the fetus contributes to the "accelerated starvation" of pregnancy,[42] other factors may be operative as well. It is noteworthy that plasma glucose levels during a fast are lower even in nonpregnant women compared with men.[95] The fasting hypoglycemia of pregnancy may therefore reflect an exaggeration of the hormonal or substrate differences or both that exist in females compared with males.

Clinical Implications of Accelerated Starvation. The more rapid development of fasting hyperketonemia in pregnancy may lead to confusion in differentiating starvation ketosis from diabetic ketosis (vide infra). The tendency of the pregnant woman to develop fasting hypoglycemia may also account for the development of severe diabetic ketoacidosis in the absence of marked increases in plasma glucose (<500 mg/100 ml).

The accelerated pattern of starvation may have even more important implications for the fetus. It is noteworthy that in association with maternal ketonemia, ketone bodies accumulate in amniotic fluid[81] and are available to the fetus. The major factor determining ketone utilization by fetal brain and liver is the rate of substrate delivery.[138, 165] It is thus likely that in circumstances of limited glucose availability, ketones synthesized by the maternal liver are transferred to the fetus and serve as an alternative to glucose in meeting fetal fuel requirements. It should be noted, however, that the availability and utilization of ketones by the fetus may not be without risk but may have an adverse effect on neurophysiologic development. Maternal ketonuria, whether due to starvation or to diabetes, has been reported by some, but not all, observers to be associated with a significant reduction in intelligence quotient in offspring tested at age 4.[18, 103, 150] Whether ketones per se or accompanying metabolic aberrations (altered amino acid levels?) are responsible for the effects on brain development has not been established. Nevertheless, these observations indicate that dietary regimens employed in pregnancy should minimize the possibility of maternal ketosis (vide infra).

The Fed State

Nonpregnant Condition. Ingestion of nutrients in the diet is followed by their rapid assimilation and utilization for energy purposes (oxidation to carbon dioxide), storage as fuel (glycogen or triglyceride), or replacement of structural tissues (protein anabolism). The major nutrients in the average diet (carbohydrate, 40 to 45 per cent; fat, 40 per cent; and protein, 15 to 20 per cent) are metabolized or stored in three tissues: liver, adipose tissue, and muscle. The primary hormonal signal regulating the metabolic response to feeding and the tissue utilization of nutrients is insulin. Following the administration of carbohydrate (as in a glucose tolerance test) or the ingestion of mixed meals, plasma insulin levels increase two to ten fold. As a consequence of this hyperinsulinemia, glucose in the diet is taken up in a variety of tissues but most importantly in the liver, where it may be stored as glycogen or converted to fatty acids and triglyceride.[46] In this manner blood glucose excursions during the day are maintained within a very narrow range of 30 to 40 mg per 100 ml despite the intermittent administration of mixed meals.[26, 157] Hyperinsulinemia also facilitates the uptake of amino acids (particularly the

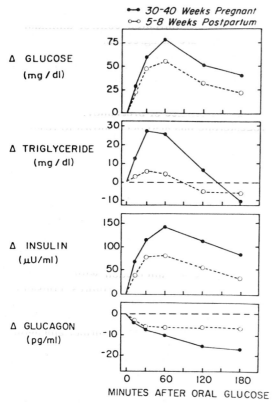

●—● 30-40 Weeks Pregnant
○--○ 5-8 Weeks Postpartum

Δ GLUCOSE (mg/dl)

Δ TRIGLYCERIDE (mg/dl)

Δ INSULIN (μU/ml)

Δ GLUCAGON (pg/ml)

MINUTES AFTER ORAL GLUCOSE

FIGURE 2-4. The effect of oral glucose administration on maternal plasma glucose, triglyceride, insulin, and glucagon concentrations. The data are expressed as changes from the basal concentrations. In pregnancy there are increased levels of glucose, triglyceride, and insulin and enhanced suppression of glucagon. (From Feinkel: Diabetes, 29:1023, 1980. Reprinted with permission.)

branched chain amino acids — valine, leucine, and isoleucine) by muscle tissue, where they are utilized for protein synthesis. It should be noted that plasma glucagon levels are suppressed by the administration of glucose and stimulated by the ingestion of protein.[155] The suppression of glucagon by carbohydrate is not, however, essential for the normal metabolism of this nutrient.[141] On the other hand, protein-stimulated glucagon secretion prevents the hypoglycemia that would otherwise accompany the hyperinsulinemia produced by a pure protein meal.

Pregnancy: Maternal Insulin Resistance. The maternal metabolic response to feeding in pregnancy is characterized by hyperinsulinemia, hyperglycemia, hypertriglyceridemia, and diminished sensitivity to insulin (Fig. 2–4). An increase in plasma insulin levels in pregnancy was demonstrated soon after the availability of a radioimmunoassay for insulin.[149] This hyperinsulinemic effect is most marked in the third trimester and is demonstrable in response to the

administration of glucose or amino acids. The increase in insulin secretion is observed even when blood glucose or amino acid levels are no higher than in control nonpregnant subjects. Thus, a change in the responsiveness of the islets rather than the alteration in the circulating metabolic signal appears to be the responsible factor. Supporting this conclusion is the demonstration that pregnancy is characterized by hypertrophy and hyperplasia of the endocrine pancreas involving primarily the beta (insulin-producing) cells.[156]

It is noteworthy that this increase in insulin secretion cannot be ascribed to augmented secretion of the gastrointestinal hormones that normally influence beta cell function. In fact, a reduction in plasma levels of gastric inhibitory polypeptide is observed in pregnancy.[65]

Despite the hyperinsulinemia observed in pregnancy, the blood glucose response to an oral or intravenous carbohydrate load is higher than in the nonpregnant state[111] (Fig. 2–4). This greater glucose increment necessitates the use of specific, adjusted norms for the glucose tolerance test in pregnancy lest diabetes be overdiagnosed. Studies in healthy human beings have shown that the magnitude of elevation in blood glucose after carbohydrate feeding is a reflection of failure of glucose uptake by the liver and its escape into the systemic circulation.[46] The augmented blood glucose response in the face of hyperinsulinemia thus indicates that the liver is resistant to insulin in pregnancy. Diminished responsiveness to intravenously administered exogenous insulin suggests that peripheral tissues (adipose tissue, muscle) share in this resistance to insulin in pregnancy. Some quantitation of this resistance to insulin may be obtained from studies in which plasma insulin is determined in resonse to a fixed degree of hyperglycemia maintained by a variable glucose infusion ("glucose clamp" technique). In such studies, the rate of glucose infusion divided by the plasma insulin level provides an index of tissue sensitivity. Recent reports of this technique indicate that tissue sensitivity is reduced by as much as 80 per cent in normal pregnancy.[46a] Despite this diminution in tissue responsiveness to insulin in normal pregnancy, during the course of a 24 hour day in which mixed meals are ingested the postprandial increases in blood glucose are variable. The increments may be less than those in nonpregnant subjects or mildly or markedly increased.[26, 48, 157] Maintenance of normal glucose homeostasis in this circumstance is in all instances achieved by a compensatory increase in plasma insulin.

The diminished tissue responsiveness to insulin in the fed state in gravid subjects, coupled with the effects of pregnancy in unmasking diabetes (see gestational diabetes) and in increasing insulin requirements in already manifest diabetes, constitutes the basis for characterizing the effects of pregnancy as "diabetogenic." The factors that may be responsible for these diabetogenic effects of pregnancy are a variety of hormones secreted by the placenta: human placental lactogen (HPL, HCS), progesterone, and estrogen.

A mild but definite impairment in glucose tolerance has been observed following the acute infusion of HPL in nonpregnant subjects over periods of 5 to 12 hours.[9, 78] This is manifest as a small decrease in the rate of glucose utilization despite an increment in circulating insulin levels. HPL, like growth hormone, alters carbohydrate metabolism by diminishing the effectiveness of maternal insulin. It also shares the lipolytic capabilities of growth hormone, causing a marked increase in the mobilization of free fatty acids from peripheral fat depots.

Although the total placental mass is the single most important factor determining HPL secretion, nutrient availability also influences the maternal levels of this hormone. Thus, maternal starvation[81] and insulin hypoglycemia have been demonstrated to cause a rise in HPL levels.[52] In contrast, a small but significant diminution in HPL levels is observed after the intravenous administration of glucose.[52] Despite the known anti-insulin effects of this hormone, it is noteworthy that a consistent relationship has not been observed between maternal HPL levels and insulin requirements during pregnancy in diabetics.[143, 148] Furthermore, maternal HPL levels are not altered by physiologic fluctuations in blood glucose.[143]

Administration of naturally occurring or synthetic estrogen to normal subjects results in a deterioration of oral and intravenous glucose tolerance.[71] An increase in plasma insulin accompanies these abnormalities, suggesting that estrogen acts as an insulin antagonist rather than as an inhibitor of insulin secretion. Complete unanimity of opinion regarding the effects of estrogens on carbohydrate metabolism is, however, lacking.[146] Synthetic estrogens may well produce greater contra-insulin effects than natural estrogens.[146a] It is noteworthy in this regard that while estradiol administration results in hyperinsulinemia, it is accompanied by improvement rather than deterioration in glucose tolerance.[25] Similarly, insulin-stimulated glucose uptake in isolated muscle tissue from rats pretreated with estradiol is augmented rather than reduced compared with with untreated control animals.[139] These findings are in agreement with the ameliorative effect of natural estrogen on diabetes in partially pancreatectomized animals.[67] Thus, it is clear that estrogen may contribute to hyperinsulinemia but is probably not a major factor in the insulin resistance of pregnancy.

Progesterone has also been shown to result in an increase in glucose-stimulated insulin secretion.[77] However, an accompanying diminution in glucose tolerance has not been reported. Nevertheless, the coexistence of hyperinsulinemia and normal glucose tolerance indicates the development of insulin resistance.

While the various hormones of pregnancy have relatively modest effects on glucose tolerance when administered individually, the possibility of synergistic interaction with respect to their contra-insulin effects requires consideration. Synergistic interactions among hormonal antagonists of insulin action have recently been observed in the case of epinephrine, glucagon, and cortisol.[38, 140] The possibility that HPL, estrogen, and progesterone have more than additive effects in antagonizing the action of insulin remains to be explored.

It is of interest that in addition to the exaggerated postprandial rise in plasma insulin, pregnancy is characterized by an exaggerated postprandial suppression of glucagon[32, 85] (Fig. 2–4). Thus, changes in glucagon secretion are not responsible for the insulin resistance of pregnancy.

With respect to the cellular mechanisms of the insulin resistance in pregnancy, studies employing erythrocytes have shown an increase, rather than a decrease, in insulin binding in human pregnancy.[101] An increase in insulin binding to adipocytes and hepatocytes has been observed in pregnant rats.[47] These findings suggest a postreceptor mechanism for the insulin resistance of pregnancy.

Clinical Implications of Maternal Insulin Resistance. The decreased responsiveness of maternal tissues to insulin during normal pregnancy may result in an exaggerated rise in plasma glucose concentrations following mixed meal ingestion, compared with the nongravid state. This may occur even in the absence of gestational or permanent (overt) diabetes.[26, 48] If, as a result of an acquired or inherited defect in beta cell function, maternal insulin secretion fails to keep pace with the exaggerated demands engendered by pregnancy, a further increase in postprandial glucose levels will occur, resulting in the new appearance of diabetes (see gestational diabetes). In the woman who is already diabetic, an increase in insulin requirements will occur, particularly in the second half of pregnancy. However, the presence of increasing insulin resistance in pregnancy cannot be equated with increased brittleness of the diabetic state. Brittleness of diabetes refers to variability, unpredictability, and wide swings in plasma glucose levels, which render clinical control of the plasma glucose concentration very difficult. In pregnant diabetics brittleness may decline, compared with nonpregnant diabetics, despite the increase in insulin resistance.[89] Consequently, the insulin resistance of the pregnant diabetic should not be viewed by the clinician as an impediment to careful metabolic control.

For the fetus, the tendency toward maternal postprandial hyperglycemia increases the likelihood of fetal hyperglycemia and, secondarily, fetal hyperinsulinemia. As noted earlier, marked increases in the glucose concentrations to which the fetus is exposed may of themselves have teratogenic effects.[19, 136] Continuous or intermittent exposure of the fetal pancreatic islets to hyperglycemia also leads to enhancement of the islets' insulin secretory response to glucose.[5, 48] Given the importance of insulin as a growth factor for the fetus, the secondary increases in fetal insulin secretion lead, in turn, to macrosomia.[116] The consequences to the fetus of the diabetogenic effects of pregnancy are thus the risks of fetal exposure to increased levels of glucose (derived from the mother) and increased concentrations of insulin (derived from the fetal islets). These and other effects of maternal diabetes on the fetus are discussed more fully later in this chapter.

THE DIABETIC STATE

Definition and Classification

Diabetes mellitus refers to a chronic disorder of metabolism that is due to an absolute or relative lack of insulin, is characterized by hyperglycemia in the postprandial or fasting state or both, and is accompanied in its most florid form by ketosis and protein wasting. When present for prolonged periods, the disease is complicated by the development of small blood vessel disease, microangiopathy, involving particularly the retina and renal glomerulus; neuropathy; and accelerated atherosclerosis. Clinically, diabetes mellitus may vary from an asymptomatic disorder detected on the basis of an abnormal blood glucose determination to a fulminant, potentially

catastrophic condition in which there is shock, or coma, or both (e.g., diabetic ketoacidosis).

Diabetes has long been classified on the basis of specific clinical features (age of onset, insulin dependence) into two major types: juvenile-onset and maturity-onset diabetes. The large overlap of age of onset among insulin-dependent and insulin-independent diabetics indicates that these descriptive terms, though time-honored, are often inaccurate. In addition, the traditional view that the various clinical forms of spontaneous diabetes represent merely gradations of a single disease process appears not to be true. More recent studies, particularly those examining the role of genetic and acquired factors in the etiology of diabetes, indicate that primary diabetes is not a single disorder but a syndrome that is heterogeneous with respect to its etiology as well as its pathogenesis.[40] These findings suggest that potential etiologic factors such as the presence of islet cell antibodies, specific HLA (histocompatibility) haplotypes, and the concordance rate among identical twins should be considered in the classification process. Accordingly, a new classification was recommended by the National Institutes of Health in July 1979. By this formulation, four major diagnostic classifications are recognized: spontaneous diabetes, which is insulin dependent or insulin independent; secondary diabetes; impaired glucose tolerance; and gestational diabetes (Table 2–1).

In over 90 per cent of cases diabetes is a spontaneous disease that cannot be ascribed to some other more primary disorder. Two major types of spontaneous diabetes are recognized: Type I, or insulin-dependent, diabetes (formerly called juvenile-onset diabetes) and Type II, or insulin-independent, diabetes (formerly called maturity-onset diabetes). Type I diabetes is characterized by an absolute requirement for insulin treatment; a marked tendency to ketosis; an onset generally, but not exclusively, before the age of 40; the absence in most patients of obesity; and the presence in 80 per cent or more of patients of circulating islet cell antibodies at the time of diagnosis. Type II diabetes generally appears after the age of 40; does not lead to ketosis; and often, but not always, does not require treatment with insulin. In 80 per cent of cases the patients are obese, and circulating islet cell antibodies are not present. Recently, attention has been called to a form of insulin-independent diabetes that has been designated maturity-onset diabetes of young people (MODY).[40] In this form of diabetes, which is a variant of Type II diabetes, there is neither ketosis nor insulin dependence, but asymptoma-

TABLE 2–1 CLASSIFICATION OF
DIABETES MELLITUS*

Spontaneous Diabetes Mellitus
Type I, or insulin-dependent diabetes (formerly called
juvenile-onset diabetes)
Type II, or insulin-independent diabetes (formerly
called maturity-onset diabetes)
Secondary Diabetes
Pancreatic disease (pancreoprivic diabetes)
(e.g., pancreatectomy, pancreatic insufficiency,
hemochromatosis)
Hormonal
Excess secretion of contra-insulin hormones
(e.g., acromegaly, Cushing's syndrome, pheochromocytoma)
Drug induced
(e.g., potassium-losing diuretics, contra-insulin hormones, psychoactive agents, diphenylhydantoin)
Associated with complex genetic syndromes
(e.g., ataxia telangiectasia, Laurence-Moon-Biedl
syndrome, myotonic dystrophy, Friedrich's ataxia)
Impaired Glucose Tolerance
Normal fasting plasma glucose and 2 hour value on
glucose tolerance test >140 but <200 mg per 100
ml. Formerly called chemical diabetes, asymptomatic diabetes, latent diabetes, subclinical
diabetes.
Gestational Diabetes
Glucose intolerance that has its onset during pregnancy

*Based on recommendations of the National Institutes of
Health, July 1979.

tic hyperglycemia is observed in children, adolescents, and young adults and is associated with
autosomal dominant transmission. Regardless of
the type of spontaneous diabetes, there is a
progressive increase in vascular and neuropathic
complications as the disease increases in duration.

Secondary diabetes, accounting for less than 5
to 10 per cent of all cases, occurs in patients with
primary pancreatic disease, in those with hypersecretion of hormones antagonistic to insulin,
following the administration of drugs that interfere with carbohydrate metabolism, or in association with complex genetic syndromes in which
hyperglycemia is a characteristic feature (Table
2–1). The clinical spectrum of these secondary
forms of diabetes is quite variable, and an association with long-term complications is often difficult to establish.

Nonpregnant patients in whom an abnormality
in carbohydrate homeostasis is demonstrable
only by determining the glucose tolerance (i.e.,
the fasting plasma glucose level is normal and the

2 hour postprandial plasma glucose level is <200
mg/100 ml) and in whom the elevation in plasma
glucose at the 2 hour point in the glucose tolerance test is <200 mg/100 ml but >140 are classified as having *impaired glucose tolerance*
rather than overt diabetes. The basis for this
separate classification, rather than its inclusion
in Type II diabetes, is the observation that the
development of overt diabetes in such patients
occurs only at a rate of 1 to 5 per cent per year
and that such impairment in glucose tolerance
may not be associated with an increased risk of
long term microangiopathic and neuropathic
complications. The term "impaired glucose tolerance" has replaced a variety of previously
employed but less meaningful designations such
as "chemical diabetes," "latent diabetes,"
"asymptomatic diabetes," and "subclinical diabetes."

When impaired glucose tolerance first appears
in pregnancy it is referred to as *gestational
diabetes*. Unfortunately this term is somewhat
imprecise in that it connotes a postpartum reversion of glucose tolerance to normal, a fact that
can be ascertained only in retrospect. Secondly,
it includes patients with normal as well as elevated fasting plasma glucose levels. A distinction
based on fasting plasma glucose levels may be
important with respect to rates of fetal loss.[96, 109]
Despite these reservations, identification of the
patient with gestational diabetes is important
because the overall risk of fetal death is two to
three fold greater than in the general population,[109] and fetal macrosomia is observed even
when fasting plasma glucose concentrations are
normal.[48] Furthermore, the diagnosis of gestational diabetes has important prognostic implications for the mother. Although all but 2 per cent
of women with gestational diabetes revert to
normal glucose tolerance in the postpartum
period, permanent, overt diabetes will develop in
60 per cent within 16 years.[109] Recent data suggest that the presence of islet cell antibodies in
the plasma of gestational diabetics may predict
those cases in which permanent diabetes will
develop later.[56] As determined by the diagnostic
criteria developed by O'Sullivan, gestational diabetes is observed in 1 to 3 per cent of pregnancies
in the United States.

When diabetes and pregnancy coexist, a special system of classification, originally developed
by Priscilla White, has often been employed
(Table 2–2). This system has been useful in
predicting the outcome of pregnancy in a diabetic
and in individualizing medical and obstetric care.
The various classes take into account the duration as well as the severity of diabetes, as indicat-

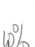

TABLE 2-2 CLASSIFICATION OF DIABETES IN PREGNANCY*

Class	Description
A	Gestational diabetes with normal fasting plasma glucose and postprandial plasma glucose <120 mg/100 ml
B_1	Gestational diabetes with fasting hyperglycemia and/or postprandial plasma glucose >120 mg/100 ml
B_2	Overt diabetes, onset after age 20, and duration less than 10 years
C	Overt diabetes, onset before age 20, or duration 10 to 20 years
D	Overt diabetes, duration more than 20 years or onset before age 10, benign retinopathy
E†	Calcified pelvic vessels
F	Nephropathy (proteinuria, azotemia)
R	Malignant (proliferative) retinopathy (retinitis proliferans)

*Modified from White, P.: Pregnancy and diabetes. In Marbel, A., White, P., Bradley, R. F., and Krall, L. P. (eds.): Joslin's Diabetes Mellitus. 11th ed. Philadelphia, Lea & Febiger, 1971.

†This classification is generally not employed in current practice.

ed by the presence of microangiopathic complications in the form of retinopathy or nephropathy. The Class A diabetics as proposed by White are the patients with "chemical diabetes only"; they have "abnormal blood glucose levels when tested by a glucose load, but fasting values are normal or near normal."[161] A more precise definition, which we prefer, is that Class A diabetics are patients with gestational diabetes, normal fasting plasma glucose levels, and postprandial glucose levels <120 mg/100 ml (Table 2-2). Class B diabetics then include gestational diabetics with elevated fasting plasma glucose levels or postprandial glucose levels >120 mg/100 ml (Class B_1) and overt diabetics with onset after the age of 20 or duration less than 10 years (Class B_2). In Classes D, F, and R there is evidence of benign retinopathy, nephropathy, or proliferative retinopathy, respectively. In general, the incidence of fetal loss (stillbirths and neonatal deaths) increases in proportion to the severity of the diabetes as indicated by White's classification, although some recent data show equivalent rates in Class A and Class D patients. In contrast, excessive birth weight (fetal macrosomia) is more common in Classes A through C than in Classes D through R.

Diagnosis

In the symptomatic patient a diagnosis of diabetes can generally be established on the basis of a fasting plasma glucose value of 140 mg/100 ml or greater or by a 2 hour postprandial value of 200 mg/100 ml or greater. In the asymptomatic patient the diagnosis of gestational diabetes is based upon a glucose tolerance test. Although glucose tolerance testing has recently lost favor as a screening procedure in the nonpregnant population, the prognostic and therapeutic implications of the diagnosis of gestational diabetes dictate its continued use in pregnancy.

Recognizing that glucose tolerance test results in normal pregnant women differ from those observed in normal nonpregnant women, O'Sullivan and Mahan proposed specific criteria for making the diagnosis of impaired glucose tolerance in pregnancy (gestational diabetes).[111] These criteria are based upon a 3 hour, 100 gram oral glucose tolerance test (OGTT) administered to over 750 pregnant women (mainly in the second and third trimesters), with two standard deviations above the mean at each hour being selected as cutoff points defining abnormality. These criteria are presented in Table 2-3. They were validated by long term (2 to 8 years) followup in which 22 per cent of patients with a positive OGTT ultimately manifested permanent diabetes. Subsequent 16 year followup of these patients has revealed diabetes in 60 per cent (O'Sullivan, 1980).[109] Numerous other glucose tolerance test criteria have been proposed, but those just described are the most widely used and extensively validated in the United States. In Europe, 50 and 75 gram glucose loads are commonly employed. Although there has been some sentiment for using the intravenous glucose tolerance test, the oral test is more sensitive, more physiologic, and better standardized. The intra-

TABLE 2-3 CRITERIA FOR ABNORMAL 3 HOUR 100 GRAM ORAL GLUCOSE TOLERANCE TEST IN PREGNANCY

Sample Method	Whole Blood Somogyi-Nelson*	Plasma or Serum Glucose Oxidase†
Fasting	90 mg/100 ml	95 mg/100 ml
1 hour	165 mg/100 ml	180 mg/100 ml
2 hour	145 mg/100 ml	160 mg/100 ml
3 hour	125 mg/100 ml	135 mg/100 ml

*O'Sullivan and Mahan, 1964.
†Coustan and Lewis, 1978.
If any two values are met or exceeded, the test result is abnormal.

venous test, however, may be quite useful for the patient who is unable to tolerate an oral glucose load.

The patient should prepare for the glucose tolerance test by ingesting a diet containing at least 200 grams of carbohydrate per day for the three days prior to the test. If carbohydrate intake is insufficient, falsely elevated values may occur.[163] The test is performed following an overnight fast, the patient being recumbent or seated. After a fasting blood sample has been obtained, 100 grams of glucose dissolved in 200 to 400 ml of water are ingested over no more than 5 minutes. Flavored solutions are commercially available. Blood samples are drawn at 1, 2, and 3 hours. Most laboratories measure glucose in plasma or serum rather than whole blood. In addition, the Somogyi-Nelson method of glucose analysis described in the original report[111] measured approximately 5 mg/100 ml of reducing substances other than glucose, while current methods are more specific. Consequently, the criteria for abnormality have been revised downward by 5 mg/100 ml to correct for changes in methods and upward by 14 per cent to correct for plasma or serum rather than whole blood determinations. These revised criteria appear in Table 2–3.

Traditionally, the indications for performing GTT in pregnancy have included (1) family history of diabetes in a first degree relative, (2) previous delivery of a large infant, (3) a poor obstetric history, or (4) glycosuria during pregnancy. Recent data indicate that it may be valuable to perform a screening test (not a full GTT) even in the absence of such clinical indications. O'Sullivan et al. obtained as a screening test a blood glucose level 1 hour after the ingestion of 50 grams of glucose and also performed a full 3 hour, 100 gram oral glucose tolerance test on 752 unselected pregnant women.[112] Of these 752 women, 19 (2.5 per cent) had positive 3 hour glucose tolerance test results. Clinical history would have identified 12 of these 19 (63 per cent) as being at high risk for gestational diabetes, while 15 of the 19 (79 per cent) had venous whole blood glucose values of 130 mg per 100 ml or above on the 1 hour, 50 gram screening test. Of further interest is the finding that risk factors as revealed by clinical history would have dictated a full GTT for 332 patients (44 per cent), while the screening test would have necessitated the performance of the full GTT on only 109 patients (14.5 per cent). According to another report, if O'Sullivan's screening test criterion of 130 mg/100 ml of whole blood was modified to 147 mg/100 ml of plasma, approximately 40 per cent

of gestational diabetics would be missed.[4] Similarly, it was found that 25 per cent of gestational diabetics would be missed unless the cutoff point on the 1 hour, 50 gram screening test remained at 135 mg/100 ml despite the change to plasma glucose determinations.[14]

It appears reasonable to use the 50 gram, 1 hour test as a primary screening procedure for gestational diabetes. This test is performed at 26 to 28 weeks of pregnancy, late enough for the insulin resistance of pregnancy to have become manifest and early enough for timely administration of the 3 hour GTT if indicated. Since an abnormal screening test result dictates only the performance of a GTT, it is possible to administer the 50 gram glucose challenge even to a nonfasting patient with the assurance that a false positive result will not cause undue harm. At some medical centers all pregnant women are screened with this test. Because the diagnosis of gestational diabetes is less common in women under 25 years of age,[93] and because the implications of that diagnosis are less alarming in younger women,[112] at other centers, including our own, the screening test is performed on all women 25 years old or more and on younger women with the specific indications by history noted earlier.

Since the renal threshold for glucose normally diminishes in pregnancy, glycosuria is not infrequently observed in the presence of normal blood glucose levels. In fact, glucose tolerance testing in asymptomatic patients with antenatal glycosuria reveals a normal response in 75 per cent of cases.[11] Thus, while glycosuria should be further evaluated, the diagnosis of diabetes in pregnancy should never be based solely on the results of the urine tests.

RECOMMENDATION: Perform a 50 gram, 1 hour screening test at 26 to 28 weeks of gestation on all women aged 25 or older and on younger women at high risk for gestational diabetes because of clinical history. If the serum or plasma glucose level is 135 mg per 100 ml or above, perform a 100 gram, 3 hour GTT.

The Course of Diabetes in Pregnancy

Pregnancy is a dynamic state, and the clinical course of diabetes is greatly dependent upon the stage of gestation. It is useful to divide pregnancy into halves rather than trimesters in assessing its influence on diabetes (Fig. 2–5).

During the early stages of pregnancy the dominant factor contributing to altered carbohydrate homeostasis is the transfer of maternal glucose

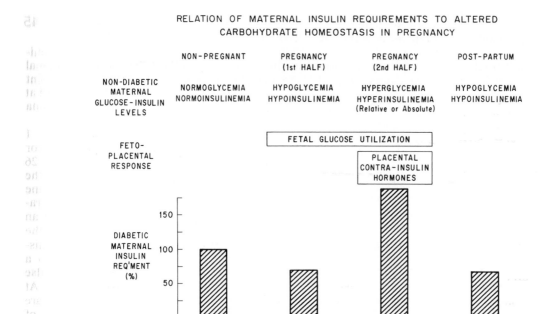

RELATION OF MATERNAL INSULIN REQUIREMENTS TO ALTERED
CARBOHYDRATE HOMEOSTASIS IN PREGNANCY

FIGURE 2–5. Influence of pregnancy on glucose and insulin levels in nondiabetic subjects and on insulin requirements in diabetic subjects. The prepregnancy insulin dose is shown as 100 per cent. The insulin requirement may decline in the first half of pregnancy and in the puerperium and is increased in the second half of pregnancy. (Modified from Tyson and Felig: Med. Clin. North Am., *55*:947, 1971.)

and amino acids to the fetus. This siphoning of substrates by the fetus results in a tendency toward maternal hypoglycemia, which may be symptomatic and frequently necessitates a reduction in insulin dosage. Diminished food intake as a consequence of the nausea and vomiting of early pregnancy may also contribute to a decrement in insulin requirements. The decreased need for insulin thus does not reflect a change in tissue sensitivity but is a consequence of lessened availability of circulating carbohydrate and gluconeogenic substrates. Although it might be postulated that this hypoglycemia is detrimental to the developing fetus, the experiences of White,[161] of the Collaborative Study,[18] and of Drury[36] all fail to demonstrate increased rates of fetal mortality or anomalies with maternal hypoglycemic coma. It has been demonstrated that at least in the subhuman primate, maternal insulin-induced hypoglycemia results in a less marked decrease in fetal plasma glucose and that the fetus may even release glucose to the maternal circulation.[16]

In the second half of pregnancy, the diabetogenic actions of placental hormones outweigh the effects of continuous siphoning of glucose by the fetus. As a consequence, the demand for insulin is increased, necessitating, on the aver-

age, a 186 per cent increase in insulin dosage.[28] Quantitation of the progressive rise in insulin requirements has been particularly feasible with the advent of portable pumps that permit the continuous subcutaneous delivery of insulin and result in normal or near-normal plasma glucose concentrations[134] (Fig. 2–6). Coincident with diminished effectiveness of insulin, there may be an increased tendency to ketoacidosis, particularly in the patient who is not carefully managed. An interesting observation is that brittleness of diabetes was diminished in the second half of pregnancy despite the increase in insulin requirements.[89] Thus, even the very brittle diabetic may achieve good metabolic control at a critical period in pregnancy.

After delivery, as concentrations of HCS, estrogen, and progesterone are falling and growth hormone continues to be suppressed[100] insulin requirements are rapidly reduced to prepregnancy needs or below. Recent studies suggest that virtually no insulin may be required on the day of delivery and for 1 to 2 days thereafter. A contributory factor in this seeming remission of diabetes may be the insulin-like effect of oxytocin,[3] which is generally administered to induce labor. Requirements generally return to prepregnancy levels by 4 to 6 weeks post partum.

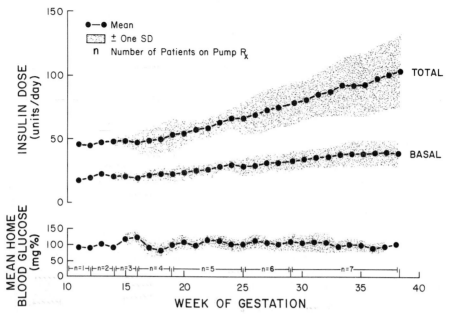

FIGURE 2–6. Increase in 24 hour insulin dose during the course of pregnancy in patients maintained at normoglycemic levels by continuous subcutaneous infusion of insulin with a portable pump. (From Rudolf et al.: Diabetes, *30*:891, 1981. Reprinted with permission.)

COMPLICATIONS OF PREGNANCY IN THE DIABETIC

The course of pregnancy in the diabetic is characterized by an increased incidence of a variety of complications affecting both mother and fetus. Fetal mortality has recently been reduced to ranges of 1 to 3 per cent in perinatal centers where modern team approaches are used, although some observers still report perinatal mortality rates of 12 per cent.[24] Even with ideal management, fetal and neonatal death rates are at least twice those reported in pregnancies uncomplicated by diabetes. On the other hand, maternal mortality is currently negligible, except in mothers with ischemic heart disease.[142] The single largest perinatal problem encountered in the 1970s has been the two to three fold increased incidence of congenital anomalies in infants of diabetic mothers. Rates of spontaneous abortion and infertility appear to be similar to those seen in the general population.[36, 53, 161]

Hydramnios. Hydramnios has been historically associated with maternal diabetes mellitus, but the true incidence of this problem is difficult to document because of a lack of widely applicable criteria for diagnosing it. Although many series do not report the incidence of hydramnios, a sampling of those that do reveals that it is found in 6 to 9 to 13 to 25 per cent of pregnant

diabetics.[36, 94, 124, 144] "Clinically apparent" hydramnios was reported in 31 per cent of pregnant diabetics; 13 per cent of those with hydramnios were delivered prematurely, indicating that the prognosis worsens when this problem is present.[82]

Hypertensive Disorders of Pregnancy. It is generally agreed that hypertensive disorders complicate diabetes with pregnancy more often than they do normal pregnancies; this may be due to underlying diabetic vasculopathy. Preeclampsia is one of Pedersen's "Prognostically Bad Signs in Pregnancy," and is associated with a worsening perinatal outcome. Inconsistent definitions make it difficult to compare the experiences at different centers, but "pre-eclampsia" is reported in 5.8[132] to 25 per cent[36] of pregnant diabetics, with most series reporting an incidence of 12 to 13 per cent.[73, 94, 144] In one report, 5 per cent of diabetics developed preeclampsia, 4 per cent had transient hypertension, and 5 per cent were chronic hypertensives.[82] In another, 13 per cent were pre-eclamptic and an additional 12 per cent were chronically hypertensive.[50]

Maternal Edema. Symptomatic generalized maternal edema has been reported in 10[82] to 22 per cent[28] of cases of overt diabetes with pregnancy. It can be a distressing problem, requiring bed rest and, in some cases, hospitalization. One possible contributing cause is the hypoalbuminemia associated with diabetic nephropathy, but this problem is by no means restricted to Class F diabetics.

Maternal Pyelonephritis. Diabetes is known to be associated with an increase in the incidence of pyelonephritis, which is another one of Pedersen's "Prognostically Bad Signs in Pregnancy." Reported incidences of maternal pyelonephritis in diabetes with pregnancy range from 1.5[73, 82] to 12 per cent.[6, 144]

Intrauterine Fetal Death. Remarkable improvement has occurred in recent years in perinatal mortality among pregnant diabetics. From 1958 through 1969, in New York State exclusive of New York City, 12.3 per cent of pregnancies in diabetics ended with intrauterine fetal death.[104] At the time of the first edition of this book, in 1975, the fetal death rate was quoted at 4 to 12 per cent, three to eight times the stillbirth rate in the general population. In the past few years, most large series have reported stillbirth rates ranging from 1 to 4 per cent.[28, 37, 49, 50, 82, 88, 133, 144] The major exception is a series in which 8.8 per cent of a series of 148 overt diabetics treated in a private hospital from 1968 to 1977 were delivered of stillborns.[24]

The reasons for this dramatic decline in fetal mortality are not yet clear, primarily because the causes of sudden intrauterine death in diabetic pregnancy are poorly understood. To be sure, some were due to poor diabetic control and ketoacidosis,[35] and it may be that increasing emphasis on "tight" metabolic control has contributed greatly to the improvement in outcome. In addition, placental insufficiency in the diabetic mother with vasculopathy may now be detected with the modern perinatal armamentarium of ultrasound, antepartum monitoring, and estriol determination, leading to timely delivery before intrauterine death can occur. Although arbitrary preterm delivery of the diabetic historically lowered the stillbirth rate, an increasing incidence of respiratory distress made this policy a two-edged sword. The subsequent development of amniotic fluid analysis for fetal pulmonic maturity (the L:S ratio and phosphatidyl glycerol) has enabled more rational selection of cases for early delivery.

The incidence of intrauterine fetal death in diabetes with pregnancy is still approximately twice that in the general population, even with the best of prenatal care. Further reduction in the frequency of this tragic outcome awaits further elucidation of the underlying pathophysiology of diabetic fetopathy.

Neonatal Mortality. The above-mentioned reduction in fetal mortality rates has been accompanied by similar decreases in neonatal death. In New York State exclusive of New York City, between 1958 and 1969, 7.3 per cent of liveborn infants of diabetic mothers died during the neonatal period.[104] When the first edition of this book was published in 1975, neonatal mortality rates of 4 to 10 per cent were cited. Most recent large series from perinatal centers report neonatal mortality rates of 1 to 5 per cent.[28, 37, 49, 50, 82, 88, 133, 144] Again, a 6.1 per cent neonatal mortality rate has been reported among patients treated in a private practice between 1968 and 1977.[24]

When the first edition of this book was published, respiratory distress syndrome (RDS) was the major cause of neonatal deaths. In cases of diabetes, this was ascribed to preterm delivery, which was almost universally practiced at the time. The L:S ratio was mentioned as a promising indicator of fetal pulmonic maturity, thus allowing a more logical selection of the appropriate time for delivery. This test and others (phosphatidyl glycerol) are covered elsewhere in this book, but it is worth mentioning that with their widespread use, the incidence of RDS has been reduced from 25 to 30 per cent (cited in the first edition) to current rates of 3 to 10.7 per cent[27, 49, 50, 82, 144] in infants of diabetic mothers. Neonatal deaths from RDS are becoming increasingly rare as well in this group, presumably owing to major improvements in the management of this condition.

Currently, *congenital anomalies are the major single cause of perinatal mortality in diabetic pregnancy.* In recent series, birth defects accounted for 20[37, 82] to 33[49, 50] to 50 per cent[28, 133, 144] or more of all perinatal losses. Birth defects that occur with increased frequency in the offspring of diabetic mothers most commonly involve the heart and the nervous and skeletal systems. Of particular interest is the recent demonstration that such anomalies must occur prior to the 7th week of gestation, given the known dates in pregnancy at which organ development occurs.[99] Furthermore, elevations in glycosylated hemoglobin levels (an index of the integrated plasma glucose level over the period 4 to 6 weeks) at the end of the first trimester have been correlated with an increased incidence of major congenital malformations.[98] These observations suggest that any further reduction in neonatal mortality may require the restoration of a normal metabolic milieu in the diabetic mother from the time of conception.

Neonatal Morbidity

Respiratory Distress Syndrome. Respiratory distress syndrome (RDS), as mentioned earlier, has been a major contributor to neonatal death in infants of diabetic mothers. Although in utero tests for pulmonic maturity have markedly diminished this problem, a significant number of infants of diabetic mothers (IDM's) continue to develop RDS because of maternal or fetal decompensation as a consequence of being delivered early. It has been shown that infants of diabetic mothers are five to six times more likely to develop RDS than are infants of nondiabetic mothers, even when gestational age and route of delivery are taken into account.[129] The reliability of the L:S ratio in diabetes with pregnancy has, however, been questioned. In one report there was an 18 per cent incidence of RDS in IDM's with an L:S ratio of 2.0 or greater, with false positives limited to gestations of less than 38 weeks.[102] In another, there was only a 1 per cent false positive rate in diabetics, similar to that in the normal population.[49, 50] Although the cause of this discrepancy is not clear, it seems reasonable to delay delivery of the diabetic until near term if all indications are that mother and fetus are healthy. Measurements of substances such as phosphatidyl glycerol may also be helpful.[86]

The cause of the increased incidence of RDS in the IDM continues to be unknown. Clearly, prematurity can not be invoked as the explanation.[129] A hypothesis currently under investigation is the possibility that fetal hyperinsulinism secondary to maternal-fetal hyperglycemia may shunt glucose in the fetal lung away from glycerol formation and thus away from surfactant production.[152] If this is true, another reason exists to maintain maternal euglycemia in diabetic pregnancy.

Macrosomia. Fetal macrosomia, or excessive fetal size for gestational age, has long been recognized as a frequent complication of diabetic pregnancy.[53] Infants so affected have a characteristic round, cherubic face and an increase in length proportionate to their weight. The increase in body weight is a consequence of an increase in body fat and visceromegaly, involving particularly the liver and the spleen.[39, 108, 153] In contrast, non–insulin-sensitive tissues such as the brain and the skull are not enlarged. Using serial ultrasound techniques, Ogata et al. recently provided evidence of the existence of evolving macrosomia by demonstrating an increase in the fetal abdominal circumference but no change in biparietal diameters beyond weeks 28 to 32 of gestation in 10 of 23 offspring of diabetic mothers.[107] At the time of birth, these infants did indeed have increased birthweights and excessive subcutaneous fat as determined by skin fold thickness.

Macrosomia is particularly common in Class A through C diabetics and less so in Class D through FR diabetics.[101] A significant increase in birthweight has been documented in the offspring of gestational diabetics with normal fasting plasma glucose levels.[48] The "Pedersen hypothesis" explains fetal macrosomia by noting that maternal hyperglycemia leads to fetal hyperglycemia, which in turn causes the fetal pancreas to produce increased amounts of insulin.[116, 117] It is this fetal hyperinsulinemia that is thought to increase growth in utero.

Evidence in support of the Pedersen hypothesis has come from a number of sources. Infants of diabetic mothers have increased endogenous insulin levels, as measured by C-peptide, compared with normal newborns,[145] and these increased C-peptide levels correlate directly with the presence of macrosomia. Fetal macrosomia has been demonstrated in offspring of rats made mildly diabetic with streptozotocin.[123] This macrosomia could be prevented with insulin treatment during pregnancy. As noted earlier, in a particularly elegant experiment, insulin was administered to rhesus monkey fetuses via a surgically implanted minipump for the last 21 days of pregnancy (approximately one seventh of gestation time).[153] These fetuses, which were hyperinsulinemic but euglycemic (because fetal glucose levels are dependent upon maternal glycemia), were classically macrosomic when compared with untreated and sham-operated controls, undergoing a 34 per cent increase in body weight. These data are very suggestive that fetal insulin is the growth-promoting factor in diabetic offspring. In contrast, marked intrauterine growth retardation is associated with pancreatic agenesis despite normal fetal growth hormone levels.

The lower incidence of fetal macrosomia in diabetics with presumed vasculopathy (Classes D–FR) is usually explained by the vascular disease in uterine vessels, which leads to a decreased availability of nutrients despite maternal hyperglycemia. The result is a small-for-dates infant.

Hypoglycemia. Neonatal hypoglycemia is a common finding in infants of diabetic mothers, occurring in 20 to 60 per cent of such newborns.[23, 27, 49, 50, 82] Because normal neonates usually manifest a dramatic drop in plasma glucose levels shortly after birth, hypoglycemia is usually defined as a glucose level below 30 mg per 100 ml in a term newborn or 20 mg per 100 ml in a premature newborn.

The normal newborn is faced with the task of maintaining a supply of glucose for its brain (which makes up 13% of its body mass compared to 2% in the adult) in the face of a discontinuation of maternal glucose input, immature gluconeogenic enzymes,[125] and a liver not yet fully responsive to the gluconeogenic effects of glucagon.[127] The normal response to the separation from maternal fuel supply consists of a fall in the plasma insulin level,[57] a rise in the glucagon level,[10] mobilization of fat stores,[120] and a rise in the blood ketone level.[120] A decrease in insulin level and rise in glucagon level are of particular importance in stimulating hepatic glucose production in the fetus and the neonate.[57]

In the infant of the diabetic mother, these adaptive mechanisms fail. Neonatal endogenous insulin levels are high[145] and remain so after delivery, while glucagon concentration fails to increase,[10] resulting in an exaggerated fall in plasma glucose concentration. The coexistence of hyperinsulinemia and hypoglucagonemia leads to a reduction in glucose production by the neonate.[76] The high insulin levels also prevent the mobilization of fat stores and ketones. Even in the infant of the Class A diabetic, hypoglycemia correlates with the degree of abnormality in maternal carbohydrate metabolism.[61, 76] It is apparent that the risk of neonatal hypoglycemia can be reduced by careful control of diabetes[27] and by avoiding excessively rapid intravenous glucose administration to the mother during labor.[91]

Hypoglycemia in the infant of the diabetic mother is usually asymptomatic but may occasionally be manifested by tremors, apathy, pallor, apnea, or cyanosis.[122] In low birthweight babies, hypoglycemia has been associated with subsequent neurologic and developmental impairment.[84] In infants of diabetic mothers, Haworth et al. were unable to demonstrate any negative long-term consequences of neonatal hypoglycemia, but the series consisted of only 25 hypoglycemic and 12 nonhypoglycemic IDM's.[62] Clearly hypoglycemia is unlikely to be beneficial to the newborn and consequently should be avoided.

Hyperbilirubinemia. Neonatal jaundice is reported in 15 to 20 per cent of infants of diabetic mothers.[15, 82, 144] The causes are said to include prematurity and high hematocrit levels.

Hypocalcemia. Neonatal hypocalcemia in IDM's has been ascribed to maternal hypercalcemia resulting in fetal parathyroid suppression.[154] In recent series, this complication has been reported in 8 to 22 per cent of the offspring of diabetic mothers.[82, 144]

MANAGEMENT OF THE PREGNANT DIABETIC PATIENT

The cornerstone of management of the pregnant diabetic is adequate metabolic control. This requires frequent measurement of blood glucose, close communication between the patient and her physician, and fairly strict adherence to a schedule of meals and exercise. Most high risk pregnancy centers have found the most effective approach to be that of a team consisting of obstetrician, internist, pediatrician, nurse, nutritionist, and social worker.

Insulin

Except possibly for the Class A diabetic, insulin is required throughout the course of pregnancy. Many protocols exist for insulin administration; most centers find that a single injection of intermediate-acting insulin (NPH or Lente) is not adequate for strict metabolic control. Mixtures of intermediate (NPH) and short-acting (regular) insulin appear to be more satisfactory. A mixture of Lente and regular may also be effective, but this combination may not yield the distinct postprandial insulin peaks desired.[33, 51] Some protocols include multiple premeal doses of short-acting insulin. One particular regimen, based on serum insulin levels monitored throughout the day in nondiabetic pregnant women, calls for a morning insulin dose that is twice the predinner dose. The insulin is administered as a mixture of NPH and regular insulin in a ratio of 2:1 in the morning and 1:1 before the evening meal.[90] Adjustments in individual components are based upon blood glucose levels obtained at appropriate times of the day.

During the first half of pregnancy, insulin requirements may fall slightly, and hypoglycemia tends to be a problem, presumably owing to continuous fetal glucose consumption (see Figure 2–5). In the second half of pregnancy the progressive increase in fetal-placental contra-insulin hormones necessitates an increase in insulin, often to between two and four times the prepregnancy requirements.[27]

The goals for metabolic control continue to be somewhat controversial. Normal nondiabetic pregnant women have fasting plasma glucose values averaging 74 to 88 mg/100 ml and postprandial mean values of 90 to 120 mg/100 ml.[26, 55, 90, 119] Rarely does the plasma glucose level exceed 125 to 130 mg/100 ml. Karlsson and Kjellmer, reporting in 1972 on hospitalized diabetics in the third trimester, found that perinatal mortality rates ranged from 24 per cent if the average blood glucose level was above 150 mg/100 ml to 3.6 per cent if it was below 100 mg/100 ml.[79] Since the publication of that series, many centers have reported perinatal mortality rates below 5 per cent when goals for metabolic control were "tightened."[28, 49, 50, 82, 94, 133]

Although the original series of Karlsson and Kjellmer involved prolonged hospitalization, most of the recent reports were based upon outpatient management, and patients were hospitalized only when specific indications existed. Because no randomized prospective study comparing various levels of metabolic control has yet been reported, it is merely an assumption that the reduced perinatal mortality rates reported are the result of tight control rather than of other recent improvements in perinatal care. However, if tests such as antepartum fetal monitoring and estriol measurement were solely responsible for declining perinatal losses, we would expect that at least 10 to 20 per cent of the surviving babies were delivered because of evidence of deteriorating fetoplacental function. In one recent series, in which 77 per cent of overt diabetics had mean plasma glucose values below 120 mg per 100 ml in the third trimester, only 2.8 per cent of babies were delivered because of abnormal biophysical or biochemical surveillance results.[28] In fact, 51 per cent of the babies were born at or beyond 38 weeks.

Another recent series has raised some doubts about the practicality of extremely tight control during pregnancy. Leveno et al., reporting on a group of 120 diabetics managed with a goal of preprandial plasma glucose levels below 115 mg/100 ml, noted that only 14 per cent met this goal, while the levels in 60 per cent were between 115 and 172 and in 20 per cent, above 172.[188] Perinatal mortality rates were 0/18 in the group receiving the best control, 2/79 (3.5 per cent) in the intermediate group, and 3/24 (12.5 per cent) in the group receiving the worst control. Because these differences did not reach statistical significance, the authors concluded that very tight control is not necessary for a successful perinatal outcome. It should be pointed out that the two fetal deaths in the "intermediate" control group were due to factors not related to maternal diabetes. It should also be pointed out that the important aspect of this series may have been the *attempt* at tight control, with a *goal* of normoglycemia. If, for example, the goal had been set

higher than 115 mg/100 ml, an even larger number of patients probably would have been included in the "poorly controlled" (above 172 mg/100 ml) group, with a possible resultant increase in perinatal mortality. The poor success rate at meeting the goal of 115 mg/100 ml may have been due to patients less motivated than those in other reported series.

Although there is no proof that insulin-induced maternal hypoglycemia has a detrimental effect on the fetus, this complication has often been cited as a reason not to attempt to achieve euglycemia in the pregnant diabetic. In one study, glucose tolerance tests were administered to a group of normal women in the third trimester of pregnancy.[1] Any subject having at least one value below the 5th percentile was considered to be hypoglycemic. Such "hypoglycemic" patients manifested a higher perinatal mortality rate than those patients in whom all values were between the 5th and 95th percentiles. This finding has been considered by some to show a detrimental effect of maternal hypoglycemia on the fetus. It must be pointed out, however, that these patients were not diabetics undergoing exogenous-insulin–induced hypoglycemia but rather "normal" women whose hypoglycemia may have been due to any number of factors influencing postprandial glucose homeostasis. Furthermore, in those women with at least one value on the glucose tolerance test above the 95th percentile there was an even higher perinatal mortality rate than in the "hypoglycemics."[1] The inescapable conclusion from this report is that "normoglycemia" is best and that "hypoglycemia" may be no worse than even mild degrees of "hyperglycemia." In another study, no adverse effect was found of maternal insulin reactions upon subsequent mental and motor function tests of the offspring of diabetic mothers up to the age of 4 years.[17] Roversi et al. administer increasing insulin doses until the patient manifests symptoms of hypoglycemia, then decrease the dose slightly.[133] They maintain their patients throughout pregnancy just on the brink of symptomatic hypoglycemia. The perinatal mortality rate in their patients (3.6 per cent for Classes B through F, corrected to 2.7 per cent when anomalies incompatible with life are excluded) ranks with the lowest in recent series. One factor that makes tight metabolic control practical in the second half of pregnancy is the loss of brittleness that occurs in otherwise brittle diabetics at this time.[89]

The monitoring of metabolic control has undergone considerable modification in the past few years. Urine testing has been supplanted by blood glucose testing in many perinatal centers, and the availability of equipment and supplies for home monitoring of capillary blood glucose levels has made this a practical way of following up pregnant diabetics. Rapid and sustained normalization of plasma glucose levels has been demonstrated with this technique,[74] although other workers have not been as enthusiastic.[151] Home monitoring is more convenient and physiologic and less expensive than frequent trips to the laboratory for the drawing of blood samples. Nevertheless, the use of this technique requires a highly motivated patient. The continuous subcutaneous infusion of insulin with a portable pump[131] is currently being evaluated at many centers for its usefulness in diabetes with pregnancy and offers great promise for the future.

The measurement of plasma glucose concentration defines the adequacy of metabolic control at the instant of measurement, while excursions of glucose at other, nonmeasured times can only be guessed at. The percentage of hemoglobin that has been glycosylated (at the N-terminal amino group of the B chain), i.e., glycosylated hemoglobin or hemoglobin A_{1c} has been shown to correlate with long term plasma glucose control in the diabetic.[13] The glycosylated hemoglobin level provides an integrated index of plasma glucose levels over the 4 to 6 weeks prior to its measurement.[83] Determination of the glycosylated hemoglobin concentration is thus a useful addition in the surveillance of the pregnant diabetic, providing a means of verifying that metabolic control between blood tests is not markedly different from that observed at the times of testing.

Of potential practical importance are two recently reported series of pregnant diabetics, which have shown that mothers with elevated Hb A_{1c} levels at the time of presentation for care are at much greater risk of having babies with major congenital anomalies than are mothers with more nearly normal levels.[87, 98] Thus, even though these gravidas might not have had blood glucose measurements during the critical first 8 weeks of pregnancy, their hyperglycemia left a "fingerprint" that could be evaluated by means of Hb A_{1c} measured at the first visit. This finding has lent credence to the hypothesis that maternal hyperglycemia during the earliest phase of pregnancy is related to the increased malformation rate among IDM's,[99] but further corroboration will be necessary. In the interim, it seems useful to measure glycosylated hemoglobin at the first prenatal visit, and at periodic intervals thereafter, in pregnant diabetics. It is worth noting that recent evidence has suggested that Hb A_{1c} measurement may be confounded by transient hyperglycemia at the time blood is drawn, owing to an unstable temporary bonding of glucose to hemoglobin. This problem can be alleviated by washing the red cells prior to performing the analysis.

RECOMMENDATION: Attempt to attain "tight" metabolic control (plasma glucose <120 mg per 100 ml) prior to and throughout pregnancy by frequent blood glucose monitoring and insulin dosage adjustments. At present, home blood glucose monitoring at least four times daily (fasting and two hours after each meal) may be the most satisfactory approach, particularly in the motivated patient. As further experience is gained, treatment with a portable insulin infusion pump may provide an even more effective approach.[131]

Treatment of the Class A diabetic (gestational diabetes with fasting plasma glucose <105 mg per 100 ml) remains controversial. This form of diabetes is present in 1 to 3 per cent of all pregnancies, being most common in women over the age of 25. Although some recent data[49, 50] have suggested that with appropriate high risk management, perinatal mortality rates are similar to those in nondiabetic pregnant women, problems remain. In practice, many Class A diabetics have few if any plasma glucose determinations once the diagnosis has been established on the basis of a glucose tolerance test, so that the 10 to 20% of gestational diabetics who have fasting or postprandial hyperglycemia are never identified and thus never treated appropriately. In addition, morbidity is clearly higher among infants of Class A diabetic mothers, macrosomia and its attendant complications being the most prominent problem. In a randomized prospective trial, a significant reduction was demonstrated in the incidence of babies over 9 pounds (from 13 to 4.3 per cent) when an arbitrary dose of 10 units of NPH insulin was given each morning to gestational diabetics.[110] No effect on perinatal mortality was evident, and statistics concerning birth trauma and mode of delivery were not presented. A marked reduction was similarly shown in the number of babies weighing more than 8½ pounds (from 50 to 7 per cent) in a random prospective series in which an insulin dose of 20 units NPH and 10 units regular was given each morning.[30] No difference in morbidity or mortality rates was evident. In a recent retrospective series, a significant reduction in macrosomia, operative delivery, and birth trauma was evident when 87 Class A diabetics treated with insulin and diet were compared with 188 treated with diet alone and with 115 untreated patients.[70] Furthermore, a retrospective analysis of O'Sullivan's data revealed an increase in perinatal mortality and an improvement with insulin therapy when maternal age exceeded 25.[113] Thus, on the basis of available data there now is evidence that insulin treatment of Class A diabetics will reduce the incidence of fetal macrosomia and the attendant difficulties in delivery and will possibly reduce perinatal mortality. Further information is necessary in order to establish the critical time for beginning insulin treatment. For the present, it appears that treatment is most effective if started prior to 34 weeks. Problems of insulin-induced hypoglycemia are rare after 28 weeks of gestation. It is, of course, necessary to monitor plasma glucose levels closely in such insulin-treated patients. A set of three values (fasting, two hours after breakfast, and late afternoon) obtained weekly will generally suffice. If fasting plasma glucose levels are above 105 mg/100 ml, or postprandial levels are above 120 mg/100 ml, appropriate increases in insulin dosage are warranted.

RECOMMENDATION: The Class A diabetic should be followed up with a weekly set of three plasma glucose determinations. If the fasting value exceeds 105 mg/100 ml, the postprandial value is above 120 mg/100 ml, or both, insulin therapy should be begun or the insulin dosage increased. Class A diabetics whose fasting and postprandial plasma glucose levels remain below 105 and 120 mg/100 ml, respectively, may also benefit from insulin therapy inasmuch as fetal macrosomia and traumatic delivery will be reduced in frequency by such treatment. A convenient starting dose in a patient beyond 28 weeks is 20 units of NPH and 10 units of regular insulin before breakfast. The newer highly purified insulin preparations are preferable in the gestational diabetic, since they are less antigenic. If insulin therapy is instituted prior to 28 weeks of gestation, hypoglycemia is more likely to occur and a smaller dose of insulin may be necessary.

The avoidance of ketoacidosis in the pregnant diabetic deserves special emphasis, as this complication has been associated with perinatal mortality rates in excess of 50 per cent. However, it is necessary, particularly in pregnancy, to differentiate *starvation ketosis* from *diabetic ketoacidosis*. As mentioned previously, the accelerated metabolic response to starvation in pregnancy results in blood ketone levels that are two to three times greater than those found in the nonpregnant state.[41, 45, 75] Thus, in a pregnant diabetic with ketonuria, low or normal blood glucose levels suggest starvation ketosis, necessitating increased dietary or parenteral carbohydrate. The importance of recognizing and treating starvation ketosis is suggested by the findings of intellectual impairment in children whose mothers manifested acetonuria during pregnancy.[18, 150] However, more recent studies have cast some doubt on the significance of acetonuria,[21, 103] so that the question remains open.

The treatment of diabetic ketoacidosis has in recent years undergone considerable revision; the standard method now is the constant infusion or intermittent administration of insulin at a rate of approximately 2 to 6 units per hour. Copious amounts of hypotonic fluids are given, as are potassium supplements. Bicarbonate treatment is restricted to patients with an arterial pH below 7.25 or a serum bicarbonate concentration below 5 or to those in coma. Plasma glucose levels, blood ketones, and arterial pH are monitored at frequent intervals (2 to 4 hours) to determine the need for changes in the insulin infusion rate or the administration of glucose.

Diet

The cornerstone of management of diabetes in the nonpregnant state in insulin-dependent as well as non–insulin-dependent patients is dietary control.[43, 159] In pregnancy, dietary management is equally important. However, when the goals of diabetic control and adequate fetal nutrition conflict, the needs of the fetus must take precedence.

In diabetes the primary principles of diet management are the following:

1. Regulation of calorie intake in order to achieve ideal body weight. In the obese diabetic (at least 80 per cent of Type II diabetics are obese), this means a reduction in calories. The importance of weight reduction in such patients is predicated upon the finding that following weight loss the demand for insulin is reduced as tissues regain their sensitivity to insulin action. Consequently, glucose tolerance will be improved, as indicated by a reduction or elimination of the need for insulin treatment. In contrast, in the thin, poorly controlled, wasted, Type I diabetic, caloric intake should be increased so as to achieve weight gain and the restoration of normal body fat and protein reserves.

2. Carbohydrate intake should not be dispro-

portionately reduced, but concentrated sweets should be avoided to lessen the likelihood of marked swings in blood glucose concentration. In the average American diet, carbohydrate accounts for 40 to 45 per cent of total calories. Carbohydrate should contribute at least an equal proportion to the diet of the diabetic but should be in the form of complex carbohydrates or starches, such as bread, noodle products, beans, and potatoes. Concentrated sweets, such as candies, pastry, table sugar, and ice cream, are restricted because their rapid absorption results in greater increments of blood glucose than when complex carbohydrates, which are digested and absorbed more slowly, are ingested. It is important to avoid a disproportionate decrease in carbohydrate ingestion, because its replacement by fat may, on a long-term basis, hasten atherogenesis. In addition, some evidence indicates that an isocaloric increase in the carbohydrate content of the diet may improve glucose tolerance.[12] Recent studies suggest that the addition of fiber (nonabsorbable polysaccharides) to the diet may improve blood glucose control in the diabetic.[72]

3. In the insulin-treated diabetic, *regularity of food intake with respect to timing and content of meals and between-meal snacks is of vital importance in reducing the likelihood of insulin reactions*. Whereas food ingestion determines the pattern of insulin secretion in the normal person, injection of insulin dictates the pattern of food ingestion in the diabetic. Thus, it is particularly important that the insulin-dependent diabetic not skip meals and that the total calories taken in be quite similar from day to day. Deviation from such a pattern is likely to result in a severe insulin reaction.

With respect to diet principles in normal pregnancy, it has been shown that normal women allowed to ingest an ad lib diet gained an average of 27.5 lb (12.5 kg) during the course of pregnancy.[69] Since this rate of gain was associated with the lowest overall incidence of pre-eclampsia, prematurity, and perinatal mortality, it is one of the recommended physiologic or desirable norms.[69] The Committee on Maternal Nutrition of the National Research Council recommends a slightly lower average weight gain of 24 lb (10.9 kg) and strongly condemns severe calorie restriction or weight reduction programs during normal pregnancy.[22] The importance of avoiding calorie restriction is apparent from the data presented earlier regarding the acceleration of starvation ketosis in pregnancy[41, 45] and the evidence of transfer of ketones to the fetus.[75, 121, 135] In view of the recent popularity of weight-reducing programs that are based on severe carbohydrate

restriction, the importance of condemning the use of such programs during pregnancy cannot be overstated.[41] Thus, dietary management in normal pregnancy should emphasize avoidance of calorie restriction as well as prevention of excessive (over 26 lb) weight gain. In particular, the physician should stress the need for maintaining a minimal intake of 150 gm of carbohydrate per day, even during brief periods when the patient is attempting to slow her rate of weight gain because of excessive increments.

In the obese pregnant diabetic, obviously the dietary approach that would apply to diabetes per se (hypocaloric intake and weight reduction) cannot be employed during gestation. Nevertheless, a restriction in weight gain to no more than 12 lb had been recommended by the Joslin group in the past.[161] It is our feeling that such weight control can be achieved only at the risk of intermittent severe calorie restriction and its attendant problems of starvation ketosis. Accordingly, we view the accumulation of 8 to 9 lb of maternal fat as a physiologic expression of pregnancy[69] and believe that the optimal weight gain in the pregnant diabetic is in the range of 20 to 24 lb. This is achieved by a diet containing 30 to 35 kcal per kg of actual body weight. Thirty-five to 40 per cent of the calories (equivalent to a minimum of 150 gm) are provided in the form of carbohydrate. The protein content is generally 125 gm per day, and the remainder of the calories are provided as fat (60 to 80 gm).[29] In patients with marked renal glycosuria, an additional 50 gm or more of carbohydrate may have to be provided to make up for urinary losses. As in the nongravid diabetic, the carbohydrate in the diet should be primarily in the form of complex starches rather than concentrated sweets. The importance of regular food intake and between-meal snacks is particularly acute in the pregnant patient treated with multiple doses of insulin.

Other Medications

Although in some clinics oral hypoglycemic agents have been found useful in pregnancy,[20, 153a] we believe that patients not responding to dietary control should be treated with insulin. Oral hypoglycemic agents may cross the placenta and result in stimulation of fetal insulin secretion. The administration of sex steroids (estrogen and progesterone) had been recommended in the past by White.[161] However, there is no evidence of a gestational hormonal deficiency in diabetes.[34] Furthermore, recent studies have shown that the administration of sex steroids may be harmful to the fetus. Consequently, estrogens and progestins should not be administered to pregnant diabetics unless a specific indication exists.

Timing and Management of Delivery

Traditionally, the timing of delivery in diabetic pregnancy has been a compromise between the increasing incidence of stillbirths beyond 36 weeks and the risk of RDS with prematurity. An arbitrary delivery at 36 to 37 weeks of gestation was the initial solution to this dilemma. The advent of fetoplacental function testing allowed for greater individualization, since fetuses about to die in utero could be identified and delivered promptly. The measurement of daily 24-hour urinary total estriol excretion[58] or daily plasma free estriol[162] is generally used to assess fetoplacental endocrine function, a fall of 40 per cent or more from the three previous days' values signifying the possibility of fetal compromise. In at least one series, estriol clearance was shown to be independent of creatinine clearance, and estriol measurement was presumed to be valid even in the presence of diabetic nephropathy.[131] Antepartum biophysical monitoring, in the form of oxytocin challenge testing[126] or nonstress monitoring,[130] is generally considered to be a valid means of evaluating fetoplacental respiratory reserve. Most schemata for management of diabetic pregnancies employ some combination of these two types of tests to assure that the fetus is healthy, thereby obviating the need in most cases for early intervention.

Conversely, as noted earlier, measurement of the lecithin:sphinogomyelin ratio (L:S ratio) in amniotic fluid has offered reassurance that the baby about to be delivered is pulmonically mature and unlikely to develop RDS. The occurrence of a false positive L:S ratio, i.e., in a neonate who develops RDS despite a mature L:S ratio, has been described, most commonly in the diabetic delivered prior to 38 weeks.[102] This has prompted many clinicians to delay elective delivery of the diabetic until at least 38 weeks. The recent description of a "lung profile" (a variety of tests on amniotic fluid to assess pulmonic maturity)[86] offers the possibility of eliminating even those few false positives still reported.

With "tight" metabolic control during pregnancy, the likelihood of intrauterine death or deterioration of fetal status necessitating early intervention is minimal.[28] It is thus generally feasible, in diabetics whose mean plasma glucose during the third trimester is within the range observed in normal nondiabetics, to delay delivery until at least 38 weeks, and longer if the cervix is not ripe for induction. Arbitrary pre-

term delivery is not mandatory in such diabetics, and a greater chance for vaginal delivery exists if intervention is delayed. Nevertheless, primary cesarean section rates of 30 per cent or more are the rule in all recent large series.[28, 49, 50, 82] The mode of delivery should be based on the same obstetric considerations used in managing nondiabetic gravidas. Maternal diabetes is not an a priori indication for cesarean section, although cesarean section may be the most practical way to deliver a particular diabetic at a particular time. For example, the existence of obvious fetal macrosomia may necessitate cesarean section without a trial of labor, in order to avoid the complication of shoulder dystocia.

Hospitalization prior to delivery is no longer routine in all medical centers, although this practice continues at many places. If a diabetic is under excellent metabolic control and is able to comply with requirements for frequent hospital visits for fetoplacental function testing, she may be cared for as an outpatient until spontaneous labor, induction, or planned cesarean section occurs.[28] This is even more practical with the use of home glucose monitoring.[74] Of course, complications such as hypertension, poor compliance, abnormal fetoplacental function tests, or poor metabolic control may dictate admission to the hospital for closer supervision and monitoring.

On the morning of planned induction of labor, food and subcutaneous insulin are withheld and an intravenous infusion line is established. Plasma glucose levels are maintained between 60 and 100 mg per 100 ml by means of a continuous infusion of glucose and insulin.[160] One method involves the administration of 5 per cent dextrose at the rate of 125 ml per hour.[27] An infusion pump is used to maintain this rate. Regular insulin is added to the infusate. A starting concentration commonly used is 10 units of insulin per liter of infusate, giving an approximate insulin dose of 1.25 units per hour. This is approximate because some insulin adheres to the walls of the container and tubing, a fact that is clinically unimportant since the variable of concern is the plasma glucose level, not the insulin dose. A steady state is generally achieved within 4 to 6 hours. Insulin concentration is increased if the plasma glucose level rises above 100 mg per 100 ml and decreased if the glucose level falls below 60 mg/100 ml. The dosage of insulin necessary to achieve euglycemia in labor varies from 0 to 3 units per hour, in our experience, and usually is not higher than 1.5 units per hour. The maintenance of maternal euglycemia during labor is critical in the prevention of neonatal hypoglycemia.[91]

If a diabetic arrives in spontaneous labor,

having recently taken subcutaneous insulin, the procedure just outlined is followed except that insulin is often not necessary and hypoglycemia may result from the combination of the usual insulin dose, the fasting status of the laboring mother, and the possible increase in glucose utilization associated with labor, necessitating increased glucose dosage. The cornerstone of managing any diabetic in labor is the frequent determination of plasma glucose levels. A reflectance meter for glucose measurement with enzyme-impregnated paper strips is a relatively inexpensive and extremely valuable tool for any delivery suite.

The patient undergoing planned cesarean section is managed somewhat differently from the diabetic in labor. If she has been in good metabolic control, her fasting plasma glucose will be below 105 mg/100 ml. On the morning of surgery, food and insulin are withheld and an intravenous infusion of normal saline is started. The cesarean section is performed as early as possible, i.e., around breakfast time. No glucose is given until the baby has been delivered.

Following delivery (either vaginal or cesarean) metabolic control is monitored by frequent blood glucose measurement. In the post–cesarean section patient, who is not allowed to eat for a few days, very little insulin may be required. An intravenous infusion of glucose and insulin may be the most convenient way to manage such patients. Insulin dosage is gradually increased following discharge until a stable state is achieved, usually a few weeks postpartum.

Diabetes is not a contraindication to nursing, but we have observed some difficulty in establishing control in lactating mothers. This is especially true when a "demand" nursing schedule is used and nursing occurs at variable times from day to day. It is probably best for diabetic mothers to attempt a more fixed schedule of nursing.

RECOMMENDATION: 1. Beginning at 28 to 35 weeks, depending upon severity of the diabetes, the presence of obstetric complications, and the presence or absence of evidence of intrauterine growth retardation by ultrasound, begin daily estriol measurement and weekly antepartum biophysical monitoring. The combination of a significant drop in estriol value and a positive oxytocin challenge test dictates immediate delivery.

2. If the patient is in good metabolic control, there are no obstetric or medical complications, and fetoplacental function testing indicates good fetal health, do not perform amniocentesis for pulmonic maturity until 38 weeks.

3. If cesarean section is planned on obstetric grounds, obtain an L:S ratio at 38 weeks and deliver the infant if it is mature. If induction of labor is planned and the cervix is "ripe," induce labor at 38 weeks if the L:S ratio indicates pulmonic maturity.

4. Maintain euglycemia during labor with constant glucose and insulin infusion and frequent blood glucose measurement. For elective cesarean section, operate at breakfast time, withhold food and insulin on the morning of surgery, and give intravenous saline until the baby is born.

Care of the Infant

The neonatal complications observed in diabetic pregnancy have already been described. Morbidity and mortality can be substantially reduced with expert pediatric care. The pediatrician should be present during delivery in order to begin resuscitation immediately if necessary. The baby should be observed in a well-equipped newborn special care unit for signs of respiratory distress. Frequent monitoring of neonatal blood glucose is mandatory, with prompt administration of oral or intravenous glucose if hypoglycemia occurs (below 30 mg/100 ml in a term, or below 20 mg/100 ml in a premature, infant). Occasionally it is necessary, because of inability to establish an intravenous line, to administer glucagon (0.3 mg per kg to a maximum of 1 mg) to mobilize fetal glycogen stores until oral feeding or an intravenous line can be established. It is not appropriate to administer intravenous glucose in a bolus dose to a newborn infant of a diabetic mother, since this is likely to stimulate an exuberant insulin response, leading to reactive hypoglycemia.

Plethora, hyperbilirubinemia, and hypocalcemia are also common problems in such infants and must be watched for. A conscientious search for congenital malformations is necessary, as early diagnosis and treatment may be of critical importance.

INFLUENCE OF PREGNANCY ON LONG-TERM DIABETIC COMPLICATIONS

Although there is little question that pregnancy may exaggerate the metabolic defect in diabetes, less evidence is available concerning the effect of pregnancy on the microangiopathic and neuropathic complications of diabetes. The question is of particular importance in the diabetic with evidence of nephropathy or proliferative retinopathy. Should pregnancy go to completion in these patients or should it be terminated lest severe, rapid progression of vascular changes

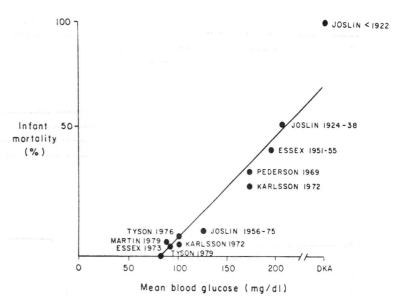

FIGURE 2–7. Relationship of perinatal mortality rate to mean plasma glucose levels over past 60 years. (From Jovanovic and Peterson: Diabetes Care, 3:64, 1980. Reprinted with permission.)

occur? White and her colleagues at the Joslin Clinic noted progression of retinopathy during pregnancy in 30 per cent of a group of 144 diabetic women with pre-existing retinopathy or nephropathy.[161] Control data for a matched non-pregnant group were not presented, however. With respect to renal disease, an elevation in blood urea nitrogen occurred in 26 per cent of White's patients, but there was a prompt decline following delivery, and none developed renal failure with oliguria or anuria.

More recent studies have failed to demonstrate that pregnancy increases the risk to the mother of progression of retinal changes and visual loss.[66] Furthermore, to the extent that metabolic disturbances contribute to the complications of diabetes, the emphasis on intensive metabolic control in pregnancy may lessen the likelihood of progression of microangiopathy. Consequently, we do not believe that any general recommendation can be made regarding the desirability of interrupting pregnancy because of the presence of proliferative retinopathy. The decision in each case must be individualized, taking into account the extent of retinopathy or visual loss or both already present, previous therapy with photocoagulation, the degree or metabolic control, and most importantly the desires of the patient. The physician's responsibility is particularly important in providing the patient with as accurate an assessment of the risks as possible.

OUTCOME OF PREGNANCY

When the first edition of this book was written, perinatal mortality rates of 7.5 to 20 per cent in cases of diabetes with pregnancy were quoted from the recent literature. This rather discouraging outlook has been drastically improved in the past few years, so that at the time of this writing, virtually every major medical center is reporting a perinatal mortality rate below 5 per cent.[28, 37, 49, 50, 82, 88, 133, 144] This trend in perinatal mortality rates is graphically depicted in Fig. 2–7. As a consequence of this reduction in overall perinatal mortality, the proportion of losses due to congenital anomalies has increased dramatically. As outlined earlier in the chapter, major birth defects represent the most pressing problem currently faced in the care of the pregnant diabetic. A large amount of effort is now going into this area of study, and it is hoped that by the time a third edition of this book is necessary, congenital anomalies will be considerably less frequent in infants of pregnant diabetics.

References

1. Abell, D. A., Beischer, N. A., Papas, A. J., and Willis, M. M.: The association between abnormal glucose tolerance (hyperglycemia and hypoglycemia) and estriol execretion in pregnancy. Am. J. Obstet. Gynecol., 124:388, 1976.
2. Adam, P. A. J.: Control of glucose metabolism in the human fetus and newborn infant. Adv. Metab. Disord., 5:183, 1971.
3. Altszuler, N., and Hampshire, J.: Oxytocin infusion increases plasma insulin and glucagon levels and glucose production and uptake in the normal dog. Diabetes, 30:112, 1981.
4. Amankwah, K. S., Prentice, R. L., and Fleury, F. J.: The incidence of gestational diabetes. Obstet. Gynecol., 49:497, 1977.

5. Asplund, K.: Effect of intermittent glucose infusions in pregnant rats on the functional development of the foetal pancreatic β-cells. J. Endocrinol., *59*:285, 1973.

6. Ayromlooi, J., Mann, L. I., Weiss, R. R., Tejani, N. A., and Paydar, M.: Modern management of the diabetic pregnancy. Obstet. Gynecol., *49*:137, 1977.

7. Battaglia, F. C., and Meschia, G.: Principal substrates of fetal metabolism. Physiol. Rev., *58*:499, 1978.

8. Beard, A., Cornblath, M., Gentz, J., Kellum, M., Perssou, B., Zetterstrom, R., and Haworth, J. C.: Neonatal hypoglycemia: A discussion. J. Pediatr., *79*:314, 1971.

9. Beck, P., and Daughaday, W.: Human placental lactogen: Studies of its acute metabolic effects and disposition in man. J. Clin. Invest., *46*:103, 1967.

10. Bloom, S. R., and Johnston, D. I.: Failure of glucagon release in infants of diabetic mothers. Br. Med. J., *4*:453, 1972.

11. Brundenell, M., and Beard, R.: Diabetes in pregnancy. Clin. Endocrinol. Metab., *1*:673, 1972.

12. Brunzell, J. D., Lerner, R. L., Hazzard, W. R., Porte, D., Jr., and Bierman, E. L.: Improved glucose tolerance with high carbohydrate feeding in mild diabetes. N. Engl. J. Med., *284*:521, 1971.

13. Bunn, H. F., Haney, D. N., Kawin, S., Gabbay, K. H., and Gallop, P. M.: The biosynthesis of human hemoglobin in vivo. J. Clin. Invest., *57*:1652, 1976.

14. Carpenter, M., and Coustan, D. R.: Screening test criteria for gestational diabetes (submitted for publication).

15. Cassar, J., Gordon, H., Dixon, H. G., Cummins, M., and Joplin, G. F.: Simplified management of pregnancy complicated by diabetes. Br. J. Obstet Gynaecol., *85*:585, 1978.

16. Chez, R. A., Mintz, D. H., Horger, E. O., and Hutchinson, D. L.: Factors affecting the response to insulin in the normal subhuman pregnant primate. J. Clin. Invest., *49*:1517, 1970.

17. Churchill, J. A., and Berendes, H. W.: Intelligence of children whose mothers had acetonuria during pregnancy. *In* Perinatal factors affecting human development, Scientific publication No. 185. Washington, D. C., Pan American Health Organization, 1969.

18. Churchill, J. A., Berendes, H. W., and Nemore, J.: Neuropsychological deficits in children of diabetic mothers. Am. J. Obstet. Gynecol., *105*:257, 1969.

19. Cockroft, D. L., and Coppola, P. T.: Teratogenic effects of excess glucose on head-fold rat embryos in culture. Teratology, *16*:141, 1977.

20. Coetzee, E. J., and Jackson, W. P. U.: Metformin in management of pregnant insulin-independent diabetics. Diabetologia *16*:241, 1979.

21. Coetzee, E. J., Jackson, W. P. U., and Berman, P. A.: Ketonuria in prenancy with special reference to calorie restricted food intake in obese diabetics. Diabetes, *29*:177, 1980.

22. Committee on Maternal Nutrition: Maternal nutrition and the course of pregnancy. Washington, D.C., National Academy of Sciences, 1970.

23. Cornblath, M., and Schwartz, R.: Disorders of Carbohydrate Metabolism in Infancy. Philadelphia, W. B. Saunders, 1976, p. 157.

24. Corwin, R. S.: Pregnancy complicated by diabetes mellitus in private practice: A review of ten years. Am. J. Obstet. Gynecol., *134*:156, 1979.

25. Costrini, N. V., and Kalkhoff, R. K.: Relative effects of pregnancy, estradiol, and progesterone on plasma insulin and pancreatic islet insulin secretion. J. Clin. Invest., *50*:992, 1971.

26. Cousins, L., Rigg, L., Hollingsworth, D., Brink, G., Aurand, J., and Yen, S. S. C.: The 24-hour excursion and diurnal rhythm of glucose, insulin and c-peptide in normal pregnancy. Am. J. Obstet. Gynecol., *136*:483, 1980.

27. Coustan, D. R.: Recent advances in the management of diabetic pregnant women. Clin. Perinatol., *7*:299, 1980.

28. Coustan, D. R., Berkowitz, R. L., and Hobbins, J. C.: Tight metabolic control of overt diabetes in pregnancy. Am. J. Med., *68*:845, 1980.

29. Coustan, D. R., and Lewis, S. B.: Clinical approaches to diabetes in pregnancy. Contemp. OB/GYN, *7*:27, 1976.

30. Coustan, D. R., and Lewis, S. B.: Insulin therapy for gestational diabetes. Obstet. Gynecol., *51*:306, 1978.

31. Crenshaw, C., Jr.: Fetal glucose metabolism. Clin. Obstet. Gynecol., *13*:579, 1970.

32. Daniel, R. R., Metzger, B. E., Freinkel, N., et al.: Carbohydrate metabolism in pregnancy. XI. Response of plasma glucagon to overnight fast and oral glucose during normal pregnancy and in gestational diabetes. Diabetes, *23*:771, 1974.

33. Deckert, T.: Intermediate-acting insulin preparations: NPH and lente. Diabetes Care, *3*:623, 1980.

34. DeHertogh, R., Thomas, K., Hoet, J. J., and Vanderheyden, I.: Plasma concentrations of unconjugated estrone, estradiol-17β and estriol, and HCS throughout pregnancy in diabetics and gestational diabetics. Diabetologia, *12*:455, 1976.

35. Delaney, J. J., and Ptacek, J.: Three decades of experience with diabetic pregnancies. Am. J. Obstet. Gynecol., *106*:550, 1970.

36. Drury, M. I.: Diabetes mellitus and pregnancy — the nine month experiment. Postgrad. Med. J., *55*(Suppl. 2): 36, 1979.

37. Drury, M. I., Greene, A. T., Stronge, J. M.: Pregnancy complicated by clinical diabetes mellitus. Obstet. Gynecol., *49*:519, 1977.

38. Eigler, N., Sacca, L., and Sherwin, R. S.: Synergistic interactions of physiologic increments of glucagon, epinephrine, and cortisol in the dog. A model of stress-induced hyperglycemia. J. Clin. Invest., *63*:114, 1979.

39. Enzi, G., Inelmen, E. M., Caretta, F., Villani, F., Zanardo, V., and DeBiasi, F.: Development of adipose tissue in newborns of gestational-diabetic and insulin-dependent diabetic mothers. Diabetes, *29*:100, 1980.

40. Fajans, S. S., Cloutier, M. C., and Crowther, R. L.: Clinical and etiologic heterogeneity in idiopathic diabetes mellitus. Diabetes, *27*:1112, 1978.

41. Felig, P.: Maternal and fetal fuel homeostasis in human pregnancy. Am. J. Clin. Nutr., *26*:998, 1973.

42. Felig, P.: Body fuel metabolism and diabetes mellitus in pregnancy. Med. Clin. North Am., *61*:43, 1977.

43. Felig, P.: The endocrine pancreas: Diabetes mellitus. *In* Felig, P., Baxter, J., Broadus, A., and Frohman, L., (eds.): Endocrinology and Metabolism. New York, McGraw-Hill, 1981, p. 761.

44. Felig, P., Kim, Y. J., Lynch, V., and Hendler, R.: Amino acid metabolism during starvation in human pregnancy. J. Clin. Invest., *51*:1195, 1972.

45. Felig, P., and Lynch, V.: Starvation in human pregnancy: Hypoglycemia, hypoinsulinemia, and hyperketonemia. Science, *170*:990, 1970.

46. Felig, P., Wahren, J., and Hendler, R.: Influence of oral glucose ingestion on splanchnic glucose and gluconeogeneic substrate metabolism. Diabetes, *24*:468, 1975.

46a. Fisher, P. M., Sutherland, H. W., and Bewsher, P. D.: Insulin response to glucose infusion in normal human pregnancy. Diabetologia, *19*:15, 1980.

47. Flint, A. J.: Changes in the number of insulin receptors of isolated rat hepatocytes during pregnancy and lactation. Biochim. Biophys. Acta, *628*:322, 1980.

48. Freinkel, N.: Of pregnancy and progeny. Diabetes, *29*:1023, 1980.

49. Gabbe, S. G., Mestman, J. H., Freeman, R. K., Anderson, G. V., and Lowensohn, R. I.: Management and outcome of class A diabetes mellitus. Am. J. Obstet. Gynecol., *127*:465, 1977.

50. Gabbe, S. G., Mestman, J. H., Freeman, R. K., Goebelsmann, U. T., Lowensohn, R. I., Nochimson, D., Cetrulo, C., and Quilligan, E. J.: Management and outcome of pregnancy in diabetes mellitus, classes B to R. Am. J. Obstet. Gynecol., *129*:723, 1977.

51. Galloway, J. A., Spradlin, C. T., Nelson, R. L., Wentworth, S. M., Davidson, J. A., and Swarner, J. L.: Factors influencing the absorption, serum insulin concentration, and blood glucose responses after injections of regular insulin and various insulin mixtures. Diabetes Care, *4*:366, 1981.

52. Gaspard, V. J., Sandront, H. M., Luyckx, A. S., et al.: The control of human placental lactogen (HPL) secretion and its interrelation with glucose and lipid metabolism in pregnancy. *In* Camerini-Davalos, R. A., and Cole, H. S., (eds.): Early Diabetes in Early Life. New York, Academic Press, 1975.

53. Gellis, S. S., and Hsia, D. Y.: The infant of the diabetic mother. J. Dis. Child., *97*:1, 1959.

54. Gennser, G., and Nilsson, E.: Plasma glucose concentration in human midterm foetus. Biol. Neonate, *17*:135, 1971.

55. Gilmer, M. D. G., Oakley, N. W., and Brooke, F.: Metabolic profiles in pregnancy. Isr. J. Med. Sci., *11*:601, 1975.

56. Ginsberg-Fellner, F., Mark, E. M., Nechemias, C., Hausknecht, R. U., Rubinstein, P., Dobersen, M. J., and Notkins, A. L.: Islet cell antibodies in gestational diabetics. Lancet, *2*:362, 1980.

57. Girård, J. R., Cuendet, G. S., Marliss, E. B., Kervran, A., Rieutort, M., and Assan, R.: Fuels, hormones, and liver metabolism at term and during the early postnatal period in the rat. J. Clin. Invest., 52:3190, 1973.

58. Goebelsmann, U., Freeman, R. K., Mestman, J. H., Nakamura, R. M., and Woodling, B. A.: Estriol in pregnancy. Am. J. Obstet. Gynecol., 115:795, 1973.

59. Grasso, S., Saporito, N., Messina, A., et al.: Serum insulin response to glucose and amino acids in the premature infant. Lancet, 2:755, 1968.

60. Gresham, E. L., James, E. J., Raye, J. R., Battaglia, F. C., Makowski, E. L., and Meschia, G.: Production and excretion of urea by the fetal lamb. Pediatrics, 50:372, 1972.

61. Haworth, J. C., and Dilling, L. A.: Relationships between maternal glucose intolerance and neonatal blood glucose. J. Pediatr., 89:810, 1976.

62. Haworth, J. C., McRae, K. N., and Dilling. L. A.: Prognosis of infants of diabetic mothers in relation to neonatal hypoglycaemia. Dev. Med. Child Neurol., 18:471, 1976.

62a. Herrera, E., Knopp, R. H. and Freinkel, N.: Carbohydrate metabolism in pregnancy. VI. Plasma fuels, insulin, liver composition, gluconeogenesis and nitrogen metabolism during late gestation in the fed and fasted rat. J. Clin. Invest., 18:2260, 1969.

63. Holmes, L. B.: Congenital malformations. In Cloherty, J. P., and Stark, A. R., (eds.): Manual of Neonatal Care. Boston, Little, Brown, 1980, p. 91.

64. Holzman, H. R., Lemons, J. A., Meschia, G., and Battaglia, F. C.: Uterine uptake of amino acids and placental glutamine-glutamate balance in the pregnant ewe. J. Dev. Physiol., 1:137, 1979.

65. Hornnes, P. J., Kuhl, C.,and Lauritsen, K. B.: Gastrointestinal insulinotropic hormones in normal and gestational-diabetic pregnancy. Diabetes, 30:504, 1981.

66. Horvat, M., MacLean, H., Goldberg, L., and Crock, G. W.: Diabetic retinopathy in pregnancy: A 12-year prospective survey, Br. J. Ophthalmol., 64:398, 1980.

67. Houssay, B. A., Foglia, V. G., and Rodriquez, R. R.: Acta Endocrinol., 17:146, 1954.

68. Hull, D., and Elphick, M. C.: Evidence for fatty acid transfer across the human placenta. In Pregnancy Metabolism, Diabetes and the Fetus. Ciba Foundation Symposium No 63. Amsterdam, Excerpta Medica, 1979, p. 71.

69. Hytten, F. E., and Thomson, M. A.: Maternal physiological adjustments. In Committee on Maternal Nutrition: Maternal Nutrition and the Course of Pregnancy. Washington, D.C., National Academy of Science, 1970.

70. Imarah, J., and Coustan, D. R.: Insulin prophylaxis in the gestational diabetic reduces operative delivery and birth trauma (submitted for publication).

71. Javier, Z., Gershberg, H., and Hulse, M.: Ovulatory suppressants, estrogens, and carbohydrate metabolism. Metabolism, 17:443, 1968.

72. Jenkins, D. J. A., Taylor, R. H., Nineham, R., Goff, D. V., Bloom, S. R., Sarson, D., and Alberti, K. G. M. M.: Combined use of guar and acarbose in reduction of postprandial glycemia. Lancet, 2:924, 1979.

73. Jervell, J., Moe, N., Skjaeraasen, J., Blystad, W., Egge, K.: Diabetes mellitus and pregnancy — management and results at Rikshopitalet, Oslo, 1970–1977. Diabetologia, 16:151, 1979.

74. Jovanovic, L., Peterson, C. M., Saxena, B. B., Dawood, M. Y., and Saudek, C. D.: Feasibility of maintaining normal glucose profiles in insulin-dependent pregnant diabetic women. Am. J. Med., 68:105, 1980.

75. Kalhan, S. C., D'Angelo, L. J., Savin, S. M., and Adam, P. A. J.: Glucose production in pregnant women at term gestation. J. Clin. Invest., 63:388, 1979.

76. Kalhan, S. C., Savin, S. M., and Adam, P. A. J.: Attenuated glucose production rate in newborn infants of insulin-dependent diabetic mothers. N. Engl. J. Med., 296:375, 1977.

77. Kalkhoff, R. K., Jacobson, M., and Lemper, D.: Progesterone, pregnancy and the augmented plasma insulin response. J. Clin. Endocrinol., 31:24, 1970.

78. Kalkhoff, R. K., Richardson, B. L., and Beck, P.: Relative effects of pregnancy, human placental lactogen and prednisone on carbohydrate tolerance in normal and subclinical diabetic subjects. Diabetes, 18:153, 1969.

79. Karlsson, K., and Kjellmer, I.: The outcome of diabetic pregnancies in relation to the mother's blood sugar level. Am. J. Obstet. Gynecol., 112:213, 1972.

80. Kim, Y. J., and Felig, P.: Plasma chorionic somatomammotropin levels during starvation in mid-pregnancy. J. Clin. Endocrinol., 32:864, 1971.

81. Kim, Y. J., and Felig, P.: Maternal and amniotic fluid substrate levels during caloric deprivation in human pregnancy. Metabolism, 21:507, 1972.

82. Kitzmiller, J. L., Cloherty, J. P., Younger, M. D., Tabatabaii, A., Rothchild, S. B., Sosenko, I., Epstein, M. F., Singh, S., and Neff, R. K.: Diabetic pregnancy and perinatal morbidity. Am. J. Obstet. Gynecol., 131:560, 1978.

83. Kjaergaard, J. J., and Ditzel, J.: Hemoglobin as an index of long-term blood glucose regulation in diabetic pregnancy. Diabetes, 28:694, 1979.

84. Koivisto, M., Blanco-Sequeiros, M., and Krause, U.: Neonatal symptomatic and asymptomatic hypoglycaemia: A follow-up study of 151 children. Dev. Med. Child. Neurol., 14:603, 1972.

85. Kuhl, C., and Holst. J. J.: Plasma glucagon and the insulin-glucagon ratio in gestational diabetes. Diabetes, 25:16, 1976.

86. Kulovich, M. V., and Gluck, L.: The lung profile. II. Complicated pregnancy. Am. J. Obstet. Gynecol., 135:64, 1979.

87. Leslie, R. D. G., John, P. N., Pyke, D. A., and White, J. M.: Haemoglobin A in diabetic pregnancy. Lancet, 2:958, 1978.

88. Leveno, K. J., Hauth, J. C., Gilstrap, L. C., and Whalley, P. J.: Appraisal of "rigid" blood glucose control during pregnancy in the overtly diabetic women. Am. J. Obstet. Gynecol., 135:853, 1979.

89. Lev-Ran, A., and Goldman, J..A.: Brittle diabetes in pregnancy. Diabetes, 26:926, 1977.

90. Lewis, S. B., Murray, W. K., Wallin, J. D., Coustan, D. R., Daane, T. A., Tredway, D. R., and Navins, J. P.: Improved glucose control in nonhospitalized pregnant diabetic patients. Obstet. Gynecol., 48:260, 1976.

91. Light, I. J., Keenan, W. J., Sutherland, J. M.: Maternal intravenous glucose administration as a cause of hypoglycemia in the infant of the diabetic mother. Am. J. Obstet. Gynecol., 113:345, 1972.

92. Like, A., and Orci, L.: Embryogenesis of the human pancreatic islets: A light and electron microscopic study. Diabetes, 21:511, 1972.

93. Macafee, C. A. J., and Beischer, N. A.: The relative value of the standard indications for performing a glucose tolerance test in pregnancy. Med. J. Aust., 1:911, 1974.

94. Martin, T. R., Allen, A. C., and Stinson, D.: Overt diabetes in pregnancy. Am. J. Obstet. Gynecol., 133:275, 1979.

95. Merimee, T. J., and Tyson, J. E.: Stabilization of plasma glucose during fasting: Normal variations in two separate studies. N. Engl. J. Med., 291:1275, 1974.

96. Mestman, J. H.: Outcome of diabetes screening in pregnancy and perinatal morbidity in infants of mothers with mild impairment in glucose tolerance. Diabetes Care, 3:447, 1980.

97. Metzger, B. E., Hare, J. W., and Freinkel, N.: Carbohydrate metabolism in pregnancy. IX: Plasma levels of gluconeogenic fuels during fasting in the rat. J. Clin. Endocrinol., 32:864, 1971.

98. Miller, E., Hare, J. W., Cloherty, J. P., Dunn, P. J., Gleason, R. E., Soeldner, S., and Kitzmiller, J. L.: Elevated maternal hemoglobin A in early pregnancy and major congenital anomalies in unfants of diabetic mothers. N. Engl. J. Med., 304:1331, 1981.

99. Mills, J. L., Baker, L., and Goldman, A. S.: Malformations in infants of diabetic mothers occur before the seventh gestational week. Diabetes, 28:292, 1979.

100. Mintz, H. D., Stock, R., Finster, J., and Taylor, A.: The effects of normal and diabetic pregnancies on growth hormone responses to hypoglycemia. Metabolism, 17:54, 1968.

101. Moore, P., Kolterman, O., Weyant, J., and Olefsky, J. M.: Insulin binding in human pregnancy: Comparisons to the postpartum, luteal and follicular states. J. Clin. Endocrinol. Metab., 52:437, 1981.

102. Mueller-Heubach, E., Caritis, S. N., Edelstone, D. I., Turner, J. H.: Lecithin/sphingomyelin ratio in amniotic fluid and its value for the prediction of neonatal respiratory distress syndrome in pregnant diabetic women. Am. J. Obstet. Gynecol., 130:28, 1978.

103. Naeye, R. L., Chez, R. A.: Effects of maternal acetonuria and low pregnancy weight gain on children's psychomotor development. Am. J. Obstet. Gynecol., *139*:189, 1981.

104. North, A. F., Mazumdar, S., and Logrillo, V. M.: Birth weight, gestational age, and perinatal deaths in 5471 infants of diabetic mohhers. J. Pediatr., *90*:444, 1977.

105. Obenshain, S. S., Adam, P. A. J., King, K. C., et al: Human fetal insulin response to sustained maternal hyperglycemia. N. Engl. J. Med., *283*:566, 1970.

106. Ogata, E. S., Metzger, B. E., and Freinkel, N.: Carbohydrate metabolism in pregnancy. XVI. Longitudinal estimates of the effects of pregnancy on D-6^{3}H glucose and D-(6-^{14}C) glucose turnovers during fasting in the rat. Metabolism, *30*:487, 1981.

107. Ogata, E. S., Sabbagha, R., Metzger, B. E., Phelps, R. L., Depp, R., and Freinkel, N.: Serial ultrasonography to assess evolving fetal macrosomia, J.A.M.A., *243*:2405, 1980.

108. Osler, M.: Body fat of newborn infants of diabetic mothers. Acta Endocrinol., *34*:277, 1960.

109. O'Sullivan, J. B.: Establishing criteria for gestational diabetes. Diabetes Care, *3*:437, 1980.

110. O'Sullivan, J. B., Gellis, S. S., Dandrow, R. V., and Tenney, B. O.: The potential diabetic and her treatment in pregnancy. Obstet. Gynecol., *27*:683, 1966.

111. O'Sullivan, J. B., and Mahan, C. M.: Criteria for the oral glucose tolerance test in pregnancy. Diabetes, *13*:278, 1964.

112. O'Sullivan, J. B., Mahan, C. M., and Dandrow, R. V.: Screening criteria for high-risk gestational diabetic patients. Am. J. Med., *116*:895, 1973.

113. O'Sullivan, J. B., Mahan, C. M., and Dandrow, R. V.: Medical treatment of the gestational diabetic. Obstet. Gynecol., *43*:817, 1974.

114. Page, E. W.: Human fetal nutrition and growth. Am. J. Obstet. Gynecol., *104*:378, 1969.

115. Page, M. A., and Williamson, D. H.: Enzymes of ketone-body utilization in human brain. Lancet, *2*:66, 1971.

116. Pedersen, J.: The Pregnant Diabetic and Her Newborn. Baltimore, Williams & Wilkins, 1977.

117. Pedersen, J., Bojsen-Moller, B. M., and Poulsen, H.: Blood sugar in newborn infants of diabetic mothers. Acta Endocrinol., *15*:33, 1954.

118. Pedersen, J., Molsted-Pedersen, L., and Andersen, B.: Assessors of fetal perinatal mortality in diabetic pregnancy. Diabetes, *23*:302, 1974.

119. Persson, B.: Treatment of diabetic pregnancy. Isr. J. Med. Sci., *11*:609, 1975.

120. Persson, B., and Gentz, J.: The pattern of blood lipids, glycerol and ketone bodies during the neonatal period, infancy and childhood. Acta Paediatr. Scand., *55*:353, 1966.

121. Persson, B., and Tunnell, R.: Influence of environmental temperature and acidosis on lipid mobilization in the human infant during the first two hours after birth. Acta Paediatr. Scand., *60*:385, 1971.

122. Pildes, R. S.: Infants of diabetic mothers. N. Engl. J. Med., *289*:902, 1973.

123. Pitkin, R. M., Plank, C. J., Filer, J., et al.: Fetal and placental composition in experimental maternal diabetes. Proc. Soc. Exp. Biol. Med., *138*:163, 1971.

124. Queenan, J. T., and Gadov, E. C.: Polyhydramnios: Chronic versus acute. Am. J. Obstet. Gynecol., *108*:349, 1970.

125. Raiha, N. C., and Lindros, K. O.: Development of some enzymes involved in gluconeogenesis in human liver. Ann. Med. Exp. Biol. Fenn., *47*:146, 1969.

126. Ray, M., Freeman, R., Pine, S., and Hesselgesser, R.: Clinical experience with the oxytocin challenge test. Am. J. Obstet. Gynecol., *114*:1, 1972.

127. Reisner, S. H., Aranda, J. V., Colle, E., Papgedrigov, A., Schiff, D., Scriver, C. R., and Stern, L.: The effect of I.V. glucagon on plasma amino acids in the newborn. Pediatr. Res., *7*:184, 1973.

128. Rice, P., Rourke, J., and Nesbitt, R. E. L., Jr.: In vitro perfusion studies of the human placenta. Am. J. Obstet. Gynecol., *133*:649, 1979.

129. Robert, M. F., Neff, R. K., Hubbell, J. P., Taeusch, H. W., and Avery, M. E.: Association between maternal diabetes and the respiratory distress syndrome in the newborn. N. Engl. J. Med., *294*:357, 1976.

130. Rochard, F., Schifrin, B. S., Goupil, F., Legrand, H., Blottiere, J., and Sureau, C.: Nonstressed fetal heart rate monitoring in the antepartum period. Am. J. Obstet. Gynecol., *126*:699, 1976.

131. Rothchild. S. B., Tulchinsky, D., Fencl, M. D., Metcalf, W., and Frigoletto, F. D.: Estriol determinations in diabetic pregnancies complicated by nephropathy. Am. J. Obstet. Gynecol., *134*:772, 1979.

132. Roversi, G. D., Canussio, V., Gargiulo, M., and Candiani, G. B.: The intensive care of perinatal risk in pregnant diabetics (136 cases): A new therapeutic scheme for the best control of maternal disease. J. Perinat. Med., *1*:114, 1973.

133. Roversi, G. D., Gargiulo, M., Nicolini, U., Pedretti, E., Marini, A., Barbarani, V., and Peneff, P.: A new approach to the treatment of diabetic pregnant women. Am. J. Obstet. Gynecol., *135*:567, 1979.

134. Rudolf, M. C. J., Coustan, D. R., Sherwin, R. S., Bates, S. E., Felig, P., Genel, M., and Tamborlane, W. V.: Efficacy of the insulin pump in the home treatment of pregnant diabetics. Diabetes, *30*:891, 1981.

135. Sabata, V., Wolf, H., and Lausmann, S.: The role of fatty acids, glycerol, ketone bodies and glucose in the energy metabolism of the mother and fetus during delivery. Biol. Neonate, *13*:7, 1968.

136. Sadler, T. S.: Effects of maternal diabetes on early embryogenesis: I. The teratogenic potential of diabetic serum. Teratology, *21*:339, 1980.

137. Senior, B.: Neonatal hypoglycemia. N. Engl. J. Med., *289*:790, 1973.

138. Shambaugh, G. E., III, Mrozak, S. C., and Freinkel, N.: Fetal fuels. I. Utilization of ketones by isolated tissues at various stages of maturation and maternal nutrition during late gestation. Metabolism, *26*:623, 1977.

139. Shamoon, H., and Felig, P.: Effects of estrogen on glucose uptake by rat diaphragm. Yale J. Biol. Med., *47*:227, 1974.

140. Shamoon, H., Hendler, R., and Sherwin, R. S.: Synergistic interactions among anti-insulin hormones in the pathogenesis of stress hyperglycemia in humans. J. Clin. Endocrinol. Metab., *52*:1235, 1981.

141. Sherwin, R. S., Fisher, M., Hendler, R., et al: Hyperglucagonemia and blood glucose regulation in normal, obese and diabetic subjects. N. Engl. J. Med., *294*:455, 1976.

142. Silfen, S. L., Wapner, R. J., and Gabbe, S. G.: Maternal outcome in class H diabetes mellitus. Obstet. Gynecol., *55*:749, 1980.

143. Soler, N. G., Nicholson, H. O., and Malins, J. M.: Serial determinations of human placental lactogen in the last half of normal and complicated pregnancies. Am. J. Obstet. Gynecol., *120*:214, 1974.

144. Soler, N. G., Soler, S. M., and Malins, J. M.: Neonatal morbidity among infants of diabetic mothers. Diabetes Care, *1*:340, 1978.

145. Sosenko, I. R., Kitzmiller, J. L., Loo, S. W., Blix, P., Rubenstein, A. H., and Gabbay, K. H.: The infant of the diabetic mother. N. Engl. J. Med., *301*:859, 1979.

146. Spellacy, W. N.: A review of carbohydrate metabolism and the oral contraceptives. Am. J. Obstet. Gynecol., *104*:448, 1969.

146a. Spellacy, W. N., Buhi, W. C., and Birk, S. A.: The effect of estrogens on carbohydrate metabolism: Glucose, insulin and growth hormone studies on one hundred and seventy-one women ingesting Premarin, mestranol, and ethinyl estradiol for six months. Am. J. Obstet. Gynecol., *114*:378, 1972.

147. Spellacy, W. N., Buhi, W. C., Birk, S. A., et al: Distribution of human placental lactogen in the last half of normal and complicated pregnancies. Am. J. Obstet. Gynecol., *120*:214, 1974.

148. Spellacy, W. N., and Cohn, J. E.: Human placental lactogen levels and daily insulin requirements in patients with diabetes mellitus complicating pregnancy. Obstet. Gynecol., *42*:330, 1973.

149. Spellacy, W. N., and Goetz, F. C.: Plasma insulin in normal late pregnancy. N. Engl. J. Med., *268*:988, 1963.

150. Stehbens, J. A., Baker, G. L., Kitchell, M.: Outcome at age 1, 3 and 5 years of children born to diabetic women. Am. J. Obstet. Gynecol., *127*:408, 1977.

151. Stubbs, S. M., Pyke, D. A., Brudenell, J. M., and Watkins, P. J.: Management of the pregnant diabetic: Home or hospital, with or without glucose meters? Lancet *2*:1122, 1980.

152. Stubbs, W. A., and Stubbs, S. M.: Hyperinsulinism, diabetes

mellitus, and respiratory distress of the newborn: "A common link." Lancet, 2:308, 1978.

153. Susa, J. B., McCormick, K. L., Widness, J. A., Singer, D. B., Oh, W., Adamsons, K., and Schwartz, R.: Chronic hyperinsulinemia in the fetal rhesus monkey. Diabetes, 28:1058, 1979.

153a. Sutherland, H. W., Stowers, J. M., Cormack, J. D., and Bewsher, P. D.: Evaluation of chlorpropamide in chemical diabetes diagnosed during pregnancy. Br. Med. J., 3:9, 1973.

154. Tsang, R. C., Kleinman, L. I., Sutherland, J. M., Light, I. J.: Hypocalcemia in infants of diabetic mothers. J. Pediatr., 80:384, 1972.

154a. Tyson, J. E., Austin, K. L., Farinholt, J. W., and Fiedler, A. J.: Endocrine metabolic response to acute starvation in human gestation. Am. J. Obstet. Gynecol., 125:1073, 1976.

155. Unger, R. H., and Orci, L.: Glucagon and the A cell; physiology and pathophysiology. N. Engl. J. Med., 304:1518, 1981.

156. Van Aasche, F. A., and Aerts, L.: Morphologic and ultrastructure modifications in the endocrine pancreas in pregnant rats. In Camerini-Davalos, R. A., and Cole, H. S., (eds.): Early Diabetes in Early Life. New York, Academic Press, 1975.

157. Victor, A.: Normal blood sugar variation during pregnancy. Acta Obstet. Gynecol. Scand., 53:37, 1974.

158. Wahren, J., Efendic, S., Luft, R., Hagenfeldt, L., Bjorkman, O., and Felig, P.: Influence of somatostatin on splanchnic glucose metabolism in postabsorptive and 60-hour fasted humans. J. Clin. Invest., 59:299, 1977.

159. West, K. M.: Diet therapy of diabetes; An analysis of failure. Ann. Intern. Med., 79:425, 1973.

160. West, T. E. T., and Lowy, C.: Control of blood glucose during labour in diabetic women with combined glucose and low-dose insulin infusion. Br. Med. J., 1:1252, 1977.

161. White, P.: Pregnancy and diabetes. In Marbel, A., White, P., Bradley, R. F., and Krall, L. P., (eds.): Joslin's Diabetes Mellitus, 11th Ed. Philadelphia, Lea & Febiger, 1971.

162. Whittle, M. J., Anderson, D., Lowensohn, R. I., Mestman, J. H., Paul, R. H., and Goebelsmann, U.: Estriol in pregnancy. VI. Experience with unconjugated plasma estriol assays and antepartum fetal heart rate testing in diabetic pregnancies. Am. J. Obstet. Gynecol., 135:764, 1979.

163. Wilkerson, H. L., Hyman, H., Kaufman, M., McCuistion, A. C., and Francis, J. O'S.: Diagnostic evaluation of oral glucose tolerance tests in nondiabetic subjects after various levels of carbohydrate intake. N. Engl. J. Med., 262:1047, 1960.

164. Williams, J. W.: The clinical significance of glycosuria in pregnant women. Am. J. Med. Sci., 137:1, 1909.

165. Williamson, D. H.: Regulation of the utilization of glucose and ketone bodies by brain in the perinatal period. In Camerini-Davalos, R. A., and Cole, H. S., (eds.): Early Diabetes in Early Life. New York, Academic Press, 1975.

3

Jack Levin, M.D.

HEMATOLOGIC DISORDERS OF PREGNANCY

THE ANEMIAS OF PREGNANCY

Physiologic Alterations Associated with Pregnancy

The major hematologic alterations produced by pregnancy result from the need for increased circulation to the vascular placenta and to the growing breast mass.[21] Plasma volume increases approximately 50 per cent, starting at 3 months of gestation.[25] The maximal plasma volume occurs during the 9th month and increases 1000 ml in a single fetus pregnancy.[27] It may decrease slightly at term and then returns to normal by 3 weeks post partum. The stimulus for the increase of plasma volume may be placental lactogen, causing increased aldosterone secretion.[21] The total red cell volume and hemoglobin mass increase by 25 per cent, starting at 6 months and peaking at term;[25] they return to normal by 6 weeks post partum. The stimulus for the 300 to 350 ml increase in red cell mass may result from the interrelationship between maternal hormones and the increased levels of erythropoietin found in pregnancy.[2, 21] The increase in red cell mass is not sufficient to compensate for the marked increase in plasma volume; thus hemoglobin and hematocrit values are significantly lower than in the nongravid state. Hemoglobin levels of 10 to 10.4 gm per 100 ml may be observed in normal pregnant women.[9, 12] Hemoglobin and hematocrit values begin to decrease at 3 to 5 months of gestation, reach their lowest values at 5 to 8 months, rise slightly at term, and return to nor-

The preparation of this chapter was supported in part by Training Grant T32 HL 07377 from the National Heart, Lung, and Blood Institute, National Institutes of Health, Bethesda, Maryland.

The author wishes to thank Drs. Samuel Charache, Paul Ness, William Zinkham, Haig Kazazian, and John Phillips for reviewing various sections of this chapter.

This chapter has excluded white cell disorders and hematologic malignancies, which are discussed elsewhere in this book.

mal 6 weeks post partum.[8, 12, 25, 32] Serum iron levels decrease but remain within normal limits during a pregnancy not complicated by iron deficiency.[5, 12, 14] The total iron binding capacity is increased in 15 per cent of pregnant women without evidence of iron deficiency.[5]

The total leukocyte count is slightly elevated in pregnant women.[26] Myelocytes and metamyelocytes can be seen in the peripheral blood in association with normal and increased numbers of leukocytes.[22] Döhle bodies, blue inclusions in the cytoplasm of neutrophils, may be observed during all 3 trimesters and for 6 to 8 weeks post partum.[1]

Platelet counts during pregnancy have been reported to be increased,[24] decreased,[26, 34] or similar to nongravid values.[4] During labor the platelet count falls, and in the early postpartum period it rises sharply.[4, 24, 34] However, none of the alterations in levels of circulating platelets result in significant thrombocytopenia or thrombocytosis.

As many as 56 per cent of pregnant women are anemic, depending on the geographic and socioeconomic group studied.[10] The signs and symptoms are those common to anemia: pallor, fatigue, anorexia, weakness, lassitude, dyspnea, and edema. The major causes are iron deficiency, folate deficiency, or a combination of the two; the predominant type depends on the population studied. Pernicious anemia is rare.[33] Hemoglobin concentrations greater than 6 gm per 100 ml are not associated with increased fetal morbidity, but lower concentrations are associated with an increase in stillborn and premature infants.[3] Folate deficiency has been suspected of bringing about a predisposition to abnormal placentation and thus to an increased frequency of abruptio placentae,[35] but this suspicion has not been confirmed by other studies.[29]

Serum B_{12} concentrations decrease below the values normal in nonpregnant women as pregnancy progresses, reaching their nadir in the 3rd trimester. Some concentrations are in the range seen in pernicious anemia but invariably return to normal during the postpartum period.[23] Few definite cases of pernicious anemia have been reported in pregnancy.[21]

Iron Deficiency

Because of menstruation, premenopausal women maintain a tenuous iron balance, and many are iron deficient without being anemic. Iron stores in adult females contain 2 gm, of which 60 to 70 per cent is in circulating red cells. Ten to 30 per cent is storage iron, located primarily in the liver, spleen, and bone marrow.[19, 25] The increased red cell mass of the gravid patient requires approximately 450 mg of iron. The fetus, placenta, and cord require an additional 360 mg of iron,[39] and approximately 190 mg is lost during an uncomplicated, single fetus vaginal delivery.[27] During the postpartum period, 0.5 to 1 mg per day of iron is necessary for lactation.[19] Thus, if iron stores are initially reduced, the pregnant patient easily becomes iron deficient, since the fetus can accumulate iron even from an iron deficient mother.[29, 37] Therefore, iron requirements are increased and may not be met by normal dietary habits, despite the increased iron absorption that occurs in pregnancy and provides 1.3 to 2.6 mg per day.[14, 37, 39] After each pregnancy, up to 2 years of a normal diet is required to replenish iron stores that were lost during the pregnancy.[39] As a result of these factors, primary iron deficiency is responsible for up to 77 per cent of nonphysiologic anemias during pregnancy[10] (Table 3–1).

The first changes that occur during the development of iron deficiency are depletion of liver, spleen, and marrow iron stores, followed by a decrease in serum iron and an increase in serum total iron binding capacity. Finally, anemia occurs.[17] The red cells are classically described as hypochromic and microcytic, but these characteristic morphologic changes may not occur until the hematocrit value has fallen far below normal levels. Microcytosis precedes hypochromia. Owing to the lack of iron, the reticulocyte count is low for the degree of anemia. The platelet count is frequently increased, and occasional hypersegmented neutrophils are seen.[17]

A serum iron level below 60 μg per 100 ml and less than 16 per cent saturation of transferrin is suggestive of iron deficiency, provided that other causes of decreased serum iron are ruled out.[12]

TABLE 3–1 MATERNAL AND FETAL IRON BALANCE*

Maternal Iron Stores (including hemoglobin)	2000 mg
Losses and Requirements	
Increased Red Blood Cell Mass of Gravid Patient	450 mg
Fetus and Cord	275 mg
Obligatory Iron Loss/day (gastrointestinal tract, skin, etc.)	0.7 mg/day (196 mg/280 days)
Delivery Losses (including placenta and lochia)†	250 mg
Lactation	0.5–1 mg/day
Intake‡	1.3–2.6 mg/day

*Derived from De Leeuw et al., 1966; Holly, 1965; Pritchard, 1965; Wallerstein, 1973; and Zuspan et al., 1971.

†Delivery of twins or a cesarian section results in an *additional* loss of approximately 140 mg of iron.

‡De Leeuw et al. (1966) estimated that a pregnant woman requires more than 4 mg of iron per day, an amount that exceeds that absorbed from a normal diet, even if a person is iron deficient.

Serum ferritin levels have been shown to reflect iron stores quantitatively.[20] The normal concentration in women is approximately 35 ng per ml. There is a correlation between saturation of transferrin and the serum ferritin level in women; a serum ferritin concentration of less than 10 ng per ml is associated with a transferrin saturation of less than 16 per cent.[20] During pregnancy, serum ferritin, along with serum iron and transferrin saturation, falls to an iron deficient level in the third trimester and remains reduced unless supplemental iron is administered.[14] Iron therapy results in a less marked decline in ferritin levels during the initial 28 weeks of pregnancy. However, it remains surprisingly unclear whether the reduced levels of ferritin and low transferrin saturation, observed in pregnant women who did not receive iron during gestation, are associated with lower hemoglobin concentrations and reduced mean corpuscular volume (MCV) at term.[14, 31] Similarly, there is disagreement whether reduction of iron stores in mothers results in reduced iron stores in their newborn children.[14, 31] If the diagnosis of iron deficiency is suspected but the laboratory data are equivocal, bone marrow aspiration is diagnostic if stainable iron is absent. A hypochromic, microcytic anemia also can be found in thalassemia trait, but it can be differentiated from iron deficiency by a normal serum iron level, stainable iron in the marrow, and elevated hemoglobin A$_2$. All pregnant women with hematocrit values less than 33 ml per 100 ml or hemoglobin levels less than 11 gm per 100 ml should be hematologically evaluated.

Prophylaxis and Treatment. Iron deficiency, while rarely a cause of mortality or significant morbidity, detracts from the gravid woman's general state of well-being. For this reason, oral iron supplements are recommended during gestation, especially for those who are prone to deficiency states such as those caused by poor dietary intake, frequent pregnancies, or prior iron depletion. One 300 mg tablet of ferrous sulfate provides 60 mg of elemental iron, of which approximately 10 per cent is absorbed normally. Therefore, this is an appropriate dose for prophylaxis.[25] However, if iron deficiency exists, 300 mg of ferrous sulfate three times daily is necessary. Iron should be administered 30 to 45 minutes before meals to assure maximum absorption. The hydremia or "physiologic" anemia of pregnancy is not due to iron deficiency, since if iron stores are adequate, supplemental iron does not increase the hematocrit value.[14, 32]

Folic Acid Deficiency

Folic acid deficiency is *the* cause of megaloblastic anemia during pregnancy and the puerperium, since pernicious anemia in pregnancy is very rare.[33] Although folic acid deficiency can exist as a single deficiency state, it is found more commonly in association with iron deficiency.[6] The frequency, which varies from 0.5 to 26 per cent, depends upon nutrition in particular regions and among various groups.[33] Maternal folate deficiency is probably not a cause of increased fetal mortality and morbidity, since the needs of the fetus are usually met despite severe maternal deficiency.[28]

Folate stores, located primarily in the liver, are normally sufficient for 6 weeks.[17] Eighteen weeks of a folic acid–deficient diet are necessary for the development of megaloblastic anemia. The first change that occurs during the development of folic acid deficiency is a fall of serum folate levels below normal after 3 weeks of a deficient diet. Hypersegmentation of marrow neutrophils is noted at 5 weeks. Red cell folate levels fall at 17 weeks. At 18 weeks the marrow becomes megaloblastic, anemia develops, and urinary excretion of formiminoglutamic acid (FIGLU) is abnormally elevated after an oral histidine load.[17] In the gravid state, this sequence is probably hastened owing to the increased

folate demands of pregnancy.[7] However, none of 440 pregnant women not receiving supplementary folic acid developed detectable folic acid deficiency.[13, 14]

In the nonpregnant state, 50 μg per day of folic acid is required, but in the gravid female the daily folate requirement for maintenance of a positive folate balance increases to 150 to 300 μg per day.[8, 33, 38] This increase is due to decreased gastrointestinal absorption of folic acid in pregnancy[7, 15, 16] and to increased maternal requirements and fetal parasitism.[6, 33]

Folate deficiency in pregnancy is chiefly due to increased fetal and maternal demands and inadequate oral intake, but non-nutritional causes may also play a part. Chronic hemolytic anemia and states of ineffective erythropoiesis, including hemoglobinopathies, in which red cell turnover is increased, can deplete folate stores by increasing the production of red blood cells. Twin pregnancies double the fetal folate requirement and are associated with an increased frequency of megaloblastosis. Acute infectious processes can precipitate a megaloblastic state. Malabsorptive states, including sprue, may compromise the pregnant patient's folate balance and thus precipitate folic acid deficiency. Anticonvulsant drugs, such as diphenylhydantoin, may block folic acid absorption.[6, 33] Finally, dihydrofolate reductase inhibitors, such as methotrexate, may block conversion of folic acid to tetrahydrofolic acid (THFA) and may thus promote megaloblastosis.[17]

Fifty per cent of the megaloblastic anemias of pregnancy develop during gestation and the remainder in the puerperal period. Almost all that occur before term become evident after 31 weeks of gestation. Before 30 weeks of gestation, megaloblastic anemias usually develop only in women with unusually high folate requirements, i.e., those with twin pregnancies, infections, or malabsorptive states; Dilantin users; and those with increased red cell turnover secondary to peripheral or intramedullary destruction. In the puerperium, megaloblastic anemias develop because of the need for an additional 60 μg per day of folic acid for breast milk production.[33]

The diagnosis of folate deficiency is best established by detection of the characteristic megaloblastic changes in the peripheral blood or marrow. Since the peripheral changes may be subtle or may be masked by iron deficiency, and bone marrow aspiration is uncomfortable for the pregnant patient, alternative diagnostic methods have been sought. Serum THFA is decreased below normal levels in up to 60 per cent of pregnant, nonanemic patients, and thus this measurement is of value only if normal.[6] Red blood cell or whole blood folate levels may be more representative, but similarly, some normal pregnancies are associated with low values.[6, 13, 30] These phenomena may be secondary to the increased clearance of folate from the blood in pregnancy.

Excretion of FIGLU has been used to diagnose folate deficiency. THFA is necessary to degrade this normal product of histamine metabolism to glutamic acid. Thus, when folate is deficient, urinary excretion of this metabolite increases. Folate stores can be tested by the oral administration of 15 mg of histidine and the collection of an 8 hour urine specimen for a FIGLU measurement.[33] Unfortunately, FIGLU excretion is increased in one third of normal pregnant women owing to delayed gastrointestinal absorption of histidine and increased glomerular filtration with decreased tubular resorption, which result in increased excretion of FIGLU by the gravid woman. Therefore, the results of this test may be misleading.[6, 33] Lobe counts of neutrophils have been used as a diagnostic aid in folic acid deficiency. Seventy-five per cent of folate deficient patients have more than 5 per cent of neutrophils with five lobes or greater, but so do 25 per cent of normal pregnant women.[18, 36] The white blood cell and platelet count may be decreased below normal values. The decrease in platelets may be sufficient to cause bleeding.[21] Since all of these observations may be difficult to interpret, a bone marrow aspiration should be performed in anemic patients when the cause is unclear, despite the inconvenience.

Prophylaxis and Treatment. The increased requirement for folate during pregnancy and the inadequate intake by members of certain socioeconomic groups have led to the suggestion that supplements of 100 to 300 μg per day of folic acid be provided during gestation and the puerperal period.[9, 11] Although this may result in the administration of excessive amounts of folic acid to a large proportion of the pregnant population, it also prevents significant maternal morbidity in populations in which folate deficiency is prevalent. High doses of folic acid may ameliorate the anemia of pernicious anemia but allow subacute combined degeneration to progress. However, at the dosage indicated, folic acid will not correct the hematologic abnormalities of pernicious anemia.[17, 21]

The treatment of established anemia secondary to folic acid deficiency should be directed at the administration of folic acid adequate to produce maximal hematologic response, replenish body stores, and provide the minimum daily requirement. Five hundred μg to 1 mg per day,

given orally or parenterally, is sufficient to fulfill those needs and will produce an initial reticulocyte response within 4 days followed by maximum reticulocytosis at 1 week.

Combined Iron and Folate Deficiency

Many folate deficient patients lack iron stores, and for this reason a mixed anemia is relatively common. A complete hematologic response does not occur unless both folic acid and iron are provided. A mixed anemia may be difficult to detect because of equivocal laboratory data and the lack of diagnostic red blood cell changes. For this reason, when significant anemia of undetermined cause exists and only a partial response to a single hematinic occurs, bone marrow aspiration is mandatory to assess both iron stores and the presence of megaloblastic changes.

HEMOLYTIC DISEASE OF THE NEWBORN

Hemolytic disease of the newborn results from maternal sensitization to fetal red blood cell antigens and transfer of the resultant antibodies to the fetus. Most cases involve destruction of fetal red cells that are Rh incompatible owing to the $Rh_o(D)$ antigen. ABO maternally incompatible cells, usually group A and occasionally group B, also may result in hemolytic disease. The antibody is either an induced anti-$Rh_o(D)$ or the IgG component of a pre-existent major blood group isoagglutinin, anti-A or anti-B. Isoantibodies to neonatal white cells or platelets may occur in maternal sera, but their clinical manifestations are less frequent than are those of the antibodies that cause hemolytic disease of the newborn.

More than 95 per cent of cases of Rh hemolytic disease of the newborn are caused by the D antigen. The administration of high titer anti-D immunoglobulin (produced from hyperimmune $Rh_o(D)$ negative volunteers) to $Rh_o(D)$ negative mothers results in prevention of immunologic processing of $Rh_o(D)$ cells.[44, 48, 49, 51] ABO incompatibility due to naturally occurring isoagglutinins cannot be prevented, but it rarely results in hydrops fetalis and does not require exchange transfusions as often as does Rh incompatibility.

Anti-D immunoglobulin apparently prevents sensitization in approximately 98 per cent of patients when given up to 72 hours post partum, despite possible sensitization earlier in pregnancy.[42, 43] The use of antenatal prophylaxis re-

500 ug — 1 mg/DAY

mains unsettled.[43, 47] If supplies of anti-D immunoglobulin were more abundant, treatment could be instituted earlier in pregnancy, thus preventing the occasional case of sensitization that occurs in spite of postpartum administration.

Because of the risk of sensitization in induced, threatened, or incomplete abortions and following amniocentesis in $Rh_o(D)$ negative patients, most investigators have advocated the use of anti-D immunoglobulin under these circumstances.[40, 43, 44, 45, 50] The administration of anti-D immunoglobulin during pregnancy does not cause fetal or maternal morbidity; there is only discomfort at the site of injection.[42, 43, 46] The use of anti-D immunoglobulin will decrease the proportion of cases of hemolytic disease of the newborn due to $Rh_o(D)$ incompatibility, and what now are considered minor blood group incompatibilities will account for a higher proportion of these cases.

THE HEMOGLOBINOPATHIES

The application of certain general principles in the care of pregnant patients with hemoglobinopathies is important in minimizing morbidity and mortality. An accurate diagnosis, including hemoglobin electrophoresis (which should be performed in all patients at risk), is essential. Family studies are valuable. The previous clinical history provides important insights into the potential risks for a patient and guidelines for therapy. Finally, scrupulous attention to details and anticipation of possible adverse signs or symptoms may prevent the development of serious complications in both the mother and the child. Increasing anemia must be evaluated thoroughly, and causes other than the underlying hemoglobinopathy must be considered. Deficiency of folic acid or iron may contribute to a worsening hematologic status, particularly because the requirement for the former is increased in patients with chronic hemolytic disorders. Since some patients with sickling disorders are severely affected by pregnancy, this group requires the most deliberate and continuous observation during gestation and the postpartum period.

Sickle Cell Anemia (SS)

Sickle cell anemia has some of the most deleterious effects on the pregnant woman and fetus of all of the major forms of hemoglobinopathies (Table 3–2). However, as in the case of the other abnormal hemoglobins, reports have to be inter-

TABLE 3–2 PREGNANCY IN SICKLE CELL ANEMIA PATIENTS NOT RECEIVING PROPHYLACTIC TRANSFUSION THERAPY (245 Pregnancies)*

Complication	Sickle Cell Anemia Per Cent	Normal Controls† Per Cent
Maternal deaths	1.6	0
Pulmonary problems	16.9	0.003
Preeclampsia	17.4	5.2
Surviving infants	67.8	97.0
Spontaneous abortions	24.0	10.8
Neonatal deaths	6.7	1.1
Stillborn	9.3	1.4
Weight <2500 g	31.4	14.8

*Modified from Charache et al., 1980, and based on six reported series.
†Based on 2377 pregnancies at the Johns Hopkins Hospital in 1977.

preted in relationship to the patient populations and the areas of the world in which the studies were performed. For example, the 18 per cent mortality rate reported in pregnant Nigerian patients with homozygous sickle cell anemia[69] is clearly not present in similarly affected patients in the United States, where the mortality rate now approaches zero.[53, 57, 62, 65, 68, 72, 82, 88, 90] Nevertheless, maternal morbidity may be severe and the frequency of complications high. Anemia becomes more severe, reflecting in part the hemodilution associated with pregnancy.[53, 68, 69, 72, 90] Sickle cell crises may occur more frequently, and those involving the bones may result in bone marrow emboli.[53, 62, 69, 70, 72, 88, 90] Pulmonary complications, often diagnosed as pneumonitis, may reflect the occurrence of pulmonary infarctions due either to aggregates of sickled cells within the pulmonary vessels or to bone marrow emboli. Infections are more common than in normal women.[57, 64, 65, 69, 72, 90] Since infections can precipitate both sickle crises and aplastic crises, their increased frequency is an important factor in the evaluation of these serious episodes. Congestive heart failure and toxemia also occur more commonly.[57, 68, 72, 88] In some women, fertility is decreased.[62, 68, 69, 74]

There is no disagreement about the deleterious effects on the fetus that result from maternal sickle cell anemia (Table 3–2). The rate of abortion is markedly increased.[57, 62, 67, 68, 69, 72, 74, 82, 88] In some series it is as high as 25 per cent.[57, 68, 88] In addition, perinatal mortality (often associated with prematurity) is increased, resulting in a high level of fetal loss.[53, 57, 62, 64, 65, 67, 68, 69, 72, 80, 82, 88]

In some of the reports cited, overall fetal loss was as high as 50 per cent. Infarction of the placenta may account for some of these complications.

Treatment. Careful observation and prompt therapy for complications as they arise are important. A decrease in hematocrit value below 20 to 25 ml per 100 ml is usually considered an indication for transfusion.[68, 90] Because of the risk of precipitating congestive heart failure, red blood cells should probably be administered in association with diuretic therapy. Exchange transfusion has also been used to correct clinical problems caused by severe anemia and attendant hypoxemia. The administration of adequate amounts of folic acid (see discussion of folic acid deficiency) will prevent the development of megaloblastic anemia.

Exchange transfusion to reduce the proportion of circulating red blood cells that contain hemoglobin S may interrupt a cycle of sickle crises[56] and in some instances has been used effectively to prevent crises during the latter part of the last trimester.[88, 91] Exchange transfusion allows maintenance of an adequate red blood cell mass and concomitant reduction of the proportion of hemoglobin S while decreasing the risk of congestive failure or increased viscosity. Fetal monitoring should be performed during exchange transfusion. Prophylactic transfusions have been reported to reduce maternal morbidity and increase fetal salvage.[61, 83] The frequency of perinatal mortality can apparently be reduced. For the prevention of crises, the concentration of hemoglobin S should be reduced to ≤ 50 per cent of the total hemoglobin in circulating red blood cells and prevented from increasing above 50 per cent for the duration of the pregnancy. Buffy coat–poor, washed red blood cells should be used, if available. However, trials of prophylactic transfusions in association with concomitant controls have not yet been reported, and therefore transfusions should probably be administered for specific indications (e.g., severe anemia or development of a crisis). It is important to emphasize that despite prophylactic transfusions, the intrauterine environment remains deficient and transfusion reactions, hepatitis, and alloimmunization can occur.[83, 85]

Hypoxia should be avoided during the administration of anesthetic agents, and therefore conduction anesthesia should be used when possible. An exchange transfusion should be considered if general anesthesia is required for a cesarian section. However, it is important not to attribute all abnormal signs and symptoms to SS disease; common conditions should be considered.[81] The distinction between pneumonitis and pulmonary infarction is difficult but important. Infections, congestive heart failure, and toxemia should be treated in the usual manner.

In the management of crises, precipitating causes should be treated. Analgesia and adequate hydration are important.[56] Concurrent infections should be treated. Although a wide variety of therapies have been recommended, their efficacy remains unproved. The use of urea solutions to treat crises or of sodium cyanate to prevent crises has not been demonstrated to be effective and safe,[59, 60, 81, 89] and these solutions have not been approved for use during pregnancy. When the risk of embolization from bone crises is high, some physicians have administered heparin.[69, 88, 90] Controlled studies are not available, and the risk of hemorrhage is considerable unless anticoagulation is carefully monitored.

The great variation in reported mortality and morbidity has resulted in disagreement about the appropriateness of sterilization, but this procedure has been advocated by some.[61, 67, 68] Therapeutic abortion also has been recommended or made available.[61, 72] Hypertonic saline should not be used to induce abortion because of the risk of precipitating a sickle crisis. However, improved prenatal and perinatal care and the judicious use of transfusion therapy have improved the outcome during the past decade.

Hemoglobin SC Disease

Although some studies have indicated that SC disease is associated with a higher risk to the pregnant woman than SS disease,[62, 72] it now appears that maternal morbidity and mortality are not greater in this disorder.[53, 57, 67, 68, 80, 82, 88] As in SS disease, fertility is probably decreased, and there is increased incidence of infection (including pyelonephritis), pulmonary disease, crises, and toxemia.[53, 57, 62, 67, 68, 72, 80, 90] The studies just cited have also noted the worsening of anemia in many of these patients. Pulmonary infarction, secondary to crises involving bone and marrow, may be fatal.[88, 90] The frequency of postpartum hemorrhage and infection has been stressed.[68, 80, 88, 90]

The abortion rate is significantly greater than normal and probably is similar to that observed in SS disease.[62, 67, 68, 82, 88] Similarly, there is a high degree of overall fetal loss.[62, 67, 68, 80, 82, 88] However, one study reported a relatively high salvage rate.[90]

Treatment. The treatment of patients with SC disease is essentially the same as for persons with SS hemoglobin. The risk to the mother and the fetus is increased, as in SS disease, and careful observations and continuous evaluation are required.[53, 68, 82, 88, 90] Particular attention is needed during labor and the puerperium, and the increased risk of pulmonary infarction must be considered during evaluation of bone crises or pulmonary symptoms.[63] The potential risk to the mother is sufficient for some physicians to have recommended abortion and sterilization for women with SC disease.[67, 68, 72] However, as has been the case for sickle cell anemia, the outcome of pregnancy in women with SC disease has improved.

Sickle Cell–Beta Thalassemia (S-β Thal)

This condition is appropriately considered to be a syndrome with great variety in hemoglobin pattern and clinical expression. Classically, S-β Thal is associated with a higher proportion of hemoglobin S than of A in the red blood cells. The lower the proportion of hemoglobin S, the less the likelihood of maternal complications or fetal loss, which in most series are relatively infrequent.[54, 57, 62, 70, 88] However, maternal mortality and the abortion rate may be slightly increased.[77, 90, 92] During the 3rd trimester, bone pain, increasing anemia, infection, and embolism may occur.[77, 90]

Therapy. The care of patients with these disorders is similar to that required for patients with SS or SC disease. It is important to distinguish patients with S-β Thal from those with iron deficiency anemia; the peripheral blood smears in both groups of patients contain hypochromic red blood cells.[54, 66, 86]

Sickle Cell Trait (AS)

Approximately 8 per cent of American Negroes have sickle trait. It is fortunate that the concurrence of pregnancy and AS is not associated with deleterious side effects on either the mother or the fetus.[55, 65, 70, 79, 87, 88, 90, 94] However, one report indicated an increased abortion rate.[68] All series indicate an increased incidence of bacteriuria and perhaps (in some of these patients) of pyelonephritis, presumably secondary to previous subclinical damage to the kidneys similar to that which causes an increased incidence of hyposthenuria in this disorder.[55, 68, 70, 88, 94] It has been stated that perhaps the major risk is the mating of a woman and man who both have sickle trait (AS), resulting in the birth of a child with sickle cell anemia (SS).[90] Genetic counseling is essential in this situation.

Treatment. Except for the administration of adequate iron and folic acid, no special therapy is required. However, continued evaluation of hematuria when it occurs and the detection of bacteriuria are important in these patients. The risks of anesthesia are much lower than in sickle cell anemia or hemoglobin SC disease, but oxygenation should be carefully maintained if inhalation anesthesia is used.

Hemoglobin C Disease (CC)

This relatively rare disorder may be associated with a slight increase in fetal loss.[68] The degree of anemia may worsen during pregnancy.[70,76,88] However, there is no increase in maternal mortality,[62, 68] and pregnancy produces no other significant adverse effects on the hemoglobinopathy.[53a, 62, 76]

Treatment. Since the major potential problem in pregnant women with CC disease is increasing anemia, careful attention should be paid to the hematocrit or hemoglobin level, and iron and folate deficiency should be prevented.

Hemoglobin C Trait (AC)

Except for urinary tract infections, patients with hemoglobin C trait apparently have normal pregnancies and there is no adverse effect on the fetus.[68, 88] One report has suggested that the number of premature infants is increased.[80]

Treatment. Careful evaluation of urinary tract signs and symptoms is required. The development of anemia suggests iron or folic acid deficiency.[80]

Other Hemoglobinopathies

β-thalassemia trait (thalassemia minor) is probably not associated with a significant increase in maternal or fetal morbidity.[66, 86, 88] However, one report indicated that the abortion rate increased[71] and another that the severity of anemia worsened in some patients.[84] Inappropriate administration of iron to patients with thalassemia trait can lead to iron overload.

The variability and relative rarity of the other types of thalassemia, and the even rarer reports of these interactions with abnormal hemoglobins other than S, make additional specific comments unwarranted.[54, 70, 80, 93] It appears that patients with hereditary persistence of fetal hemoglobin (HPFH) or hemoglobin S-HPFH are unaffected by pregnancy.[58, 70, 73, 78]

Prenatal Diagnosis of Hemoglobinopathies

It is now possible, by use of either fetal red blood cells or amniotic fluid cells (amniocytes), to diagnose nearly all hemoglobinopathies. The first technique requires the sampling of fetal blood during the second trimester, by fetoscopy or placental aspiration. Sonography should be first performed to localize the placenta. To insure that fetal rather than maternal blood has been obtained, a small portion of the sample can be studied with a particle size analyzer. Since fetal erythrocytes are markedly macrocytic compared with maternal erythrocytes, the proportion of fetal and maternal erythrocytes can be determined. Subsequently, the acid elution method of Kleihauer and Betke can be used to confirm the degree of contamination of the sample by maternal red blood cells.

The proportion of various globin chains, newly synthesized by reticulocytes, is measured by radioisotopic labeling followed by chromatographic separation of the proteins. Abnormal or variant hemoglobin chains are detected by their altered elution patterns, and β thalassemia by decreased β globin chain synthesis (i.e., a reduced β/γ ratio).[52] Contamination of fetal blood samples by maternal blood can be monitored as described earlier, and, if needed, selective lysis of maternal cells can be used to enrich the sample for fetal cells. A recent review of the application of this method indicated a diagnostic error in only 2 per cent of 481 adequate samples.[52] However, the technique is complex, and the rate of fetal loss was 9 per cent in a combined series of 524 cases. In approximately 8 per cent of cases, a satisfactory sample could not be obtained.

The second technique uses DNA isolated from amniotic fluid cells to diagnose disorders associated with gene deletions (e.g., $\delta\beta$ thalassemia, most types of α thalassemia) or point mutations (e.g., sickle cell anemia, S-O Arab disease, most types of β-thalassemia). Fetal amniocytes, obtained by amniocentesis at approximately 16 to 18 weeks of gestation, are cultured, although sometimes culture is not required. DNA extracted from amniocytes is incubated with restriction endonucleases, which cleave the DNA at specific sites, recognized because of specific nucleic acid sequences. The cleaved DNA is then subjected

to molecular hybridization and gene mapping.[52] Fragments of DNA produced following cleavage of DNA by these enzymes can be detected after hybridization (by means of autoradiography) to radioisotopically labeled, specific DNA probes for globin gene sequences.

The presence of an abnormal globin gene can be detected, in rare instances, because the mutation affects a restriction endonuclease cleavage site (e.g., $\beta^{0\ Arab}$) or by linkage analysis using restriction sites outside the gene (e.g., β^S, β^C, β-thalassemia). In the case of sickle cell anemia, a complete diagnosis of AA, AS, or SS or an exclusion of SS is possible in over 90 per cent of pregnancies, using multiple restriction endonuclease analysis. This same approach can provide complete diagnosis of the beta-thalassemia status or exclude the disorder in approximately 75 per cent of pregnancies at risk.[75] This technique is much safer for the fetus, since fetal loss following amniocentesis is probably not greater than the spontaneous abortion rate, and amniotic fluid is more easily obtained than fetal blood. Importantly, this technique requires linkage analysis of the parents and appropriate family members to determine whether gene map patterns indicate that restriction endonculeases can be effectively used diagnostically.[75] Therefore, family studies should be performed before pregnancy or during the early stages, so that results are available in time to permit amniocentesis during the 16th to 18th week of pregnancy. Currently, major centers are recommending DNA testing of parents and affected children, followed by amniocentesis if appropriate. Amniocentesis is readily available, and the amniotic fluid can be sent to a laboratory that performs this evaluation.

For couples whose pregnancy outcomes cannot be determined by the present DNA technique, fetoscopy and its increased risk (in order to obtain fetal blood for studies of hemoglobin synthesis) remains an alternative. For a large portion of such couples, DNA analysis may nevertheless determine the risk of an affected fetus to be 50 per cent, owing to detection of at least one abnormal gene. The increased likelihood of a significant clinical abnormality in the children of the latter subset of patients makes the increased risk of fetoscopy more acceptable. If the patient needs fetoscopy, she can be referred to a specialized center for this procedure. However, as methods improve it should be possible to use amniocentesis to provide prenatal diagnosis of most hemoglobinopathies. It is to be hoped that methods based on linkage analysis of DNA will soon be supplanted by methods that directly assay for the mutation, such as β^S. This achievement should result in techniques applicable to all pregnancies at risk.

DISORDERS OF BLOOD COAGULATION AND PLATELETS

Evaluation of Hemorrhagic Disorders

A thoughtful history and physical examination can provide much information, indicate whether a disorder of blood coagulation, platelets, or blood vessels is likely to be present, and suggest the laboratory tests that are most appropriate. It is important to first establish whether a disorder of hemostasis is lifelong (i.e., inherited) or acquired. If the former, the family history may indicate whether an autosomal or X-linked disorder is present. Only hemophilia A (Factor VIII deficiency) and hemophilia B (Factor IX deficiency) are X-linked. They are the only two inherited disorders of blood coagulation characterized by spontaneous soft tissue bleeding and hemarthroses in males. Acquired disorders suggest the possible development of an underlying disease that causes derangement of coagulation factors, platelets, or blood vessels, including the presence of a circulating anticoagulant.

The physical examination can play an important role in discriminating between coagulation, platelet, and vascular disorders. Abnormal hemostasis due to a deficient blood coagulation mechanism is associated with ecchymoses and hematomas. Platelet disorders sufficient to cause hemorrhage produce petechiae of the skin and mucous membranes. Thrombocytopenia produces small, relatively fine petechiae. Since these lesions result from extravasations of red blood cells through the walls of small blood vessels, they will not blanch under pressure but do fade and disappear after 3 to 5 days. This characteristic distinguishes them from small vascular malformations, such as telangiectases, that may blanch but do not disappear. Nonthrombocytopenic purpura usually consists of larger, more discrete lesions, with strikingly symmetrical distributions on the extremities. These lesions, which result from a platelet or vascular disorder, may itch and be palpable, two features that are *not* characteristic of thrombocytopenic purpura. Petechial lesions are not produced by disorders of blood coagulation. Corticosteroids produce a form of nonthrombocytopenic purpura that is indistinguishable from senile purpura (the latter is presumably due to defective connective tissue support of small blood vessels). Neither of

the latter two forms of nonthrombocytopenic purpura is of clinical importance, although they may concern the patient cosmetically.

The combination of clinical history and physical signs will almost always correctly indicate whether an abnormality of coagulation or of platelets is the cause of a hemorrhagic diathesis. A drug history is particularly important if the disorder is of recent or sudden onset; drugs are capable of affecting coagulation factors, platelets, or blood vessels. If abnormal coagulation seems likely, screening tests such as the prothrombin and partial thromboplastin times are initially appropriate. A disseminated intravascular coagulopathy will be suggested by the combination of abnormal bruising and oozing from venipuncture sites in an appropriate clinical setting (see discussion of disseminated intravascular coagulopathy). If petechiae are present, a blood smear or a platelet count will immediately distinguish between thrombocytopenic and nonthrombocytopenic purpura. There is no purpose in the performance of a bleeding time or tourniquet test if petechiae are present, the platelet count is markedly reduced, or a coagulation disorder is suspected (except for von Willebrand's disease, vide infra).

Inherited Disorders of Plasma Coagulation Factors

Accurate diagnosis of any patient suspected of having a coagulation disorder is important, since unanticipated bleeding can occur either spontaneously or secondary to trauma. For this reason, any woman suspected of having a coagulation disorder or whose family has a history of an inherited disorder of blood coagulation should be carefully studied before pregnancy occurs. It is well recognized that levels of many coagulation factors increase during pregnancy.[108, 143, 160, 167, 185] Therefore, accurate diagnosis is difficult, particularly after the first trimester. Interesting exceptions are Factors XI and XIII, which apparently decrease during pregnancy to levels of 50 to 70 per cent of normal at term.[114, 165] These decreases are not associated with a hemorrhagic tendency.

A normal clotting time never rules out a disorder of blood coagulation; the test is helpful only if the time is prolonged. Similarly, commonly used screening tests, the prothrombin time (which measures Factors II, V, VII, and X) and the partial thromboplastin time (which is sensitive in different degrees to deficiencies of all recognized factors except VII and XIII), indicate

TABLE 3-3 LABORATORY ABNORMALITIES IN SOME HEMORRHAGIC DISORDERS*

Disorder (Factor)	Clotting Time	Partial Thromboplastin Time	Prothrombin Time	Bleeding Time
Afibrinogenemia (I)	Infinite	Infinite	Infinite	Variable
Hypoprothrombinemia (II)	Variable	Variable	Long	Normal†
Parahemophilia (V)	Long	Long	Long	Normal†
Proconvertin deficiency (VII)	Normal	Normal	Long	Normal†
Hemophilia A (VIII)	Variable	Long	Normal	Normal†
von Willebrand's disease (VIII)	Variable	Variable	Normal	Long
Hemophilia B (IX)	Variable	Long	Normal	Normal†
Stuart-Prower Factor deficiency (X)	Variable	Long	Long	Normal†
PTA deficiency (XI)	Variable	Long	Normal	Variable
Hageman deficiency (XII)	Long	Long	Normal	Normal
Fibrin-stabilizing Factor deficiency (XIII)	Normal	Normal	Normal	Normal

*These data have been compiled from a variety of sources and represent an attempt to summarize many conflicting descriptions.

†Some patients with these disorders have been reported to have prolonged bleeding times.

potential diagnoses only if abnormal. Table 3-3 summarizes the laboratory abnormalities in some hemorrhagic disorders. All three tests are non-specific. In an appropriate family setting, or if a history of significant hemorrhage is present, additional specific factor assays should be performed to adequately rule out significant abnormalities of blood coagulation. A prolonged bleeding time in a patient with a history of a hemorrhagic disorder, but in whom blood coagulation and platelet counts are normal, suggests a qualitative abnormality of platelets. Underlying disorders such as uremia, a dysproteinemia, or a rare inherited qualitative disorder of platelets should be considered and appropriate tests of platelet function performed.

Although typical female carriers of hemophilia A or B are not clinically affected, rare carriers with unusually low Factor VIII or IX levels (10 to 30 per cent) may experience abnormal bleeding after trauma or surgery. Therefore, it is important to identify carriers prior to pregnancy, not only to provide potentially helpful genetic counseling but to anticipate the possibility of abnormal bleeding in those rare women with very low levels. This problem is more likely to occur in carriers of X-linked Factor IX deficiency than of Factor VIII deficiency. Fortunately, as in the case in normal women, the level of the deficient factor in carriers tends to rise during pregnancy,[103] and thus abnormal bleeding is unlikely to occur in carriers of hemophilia A or B who have become pregnant.

In addition to measurement of coagulation factors with traditional procoagulant assays, the use of immunologic methods to detect Factor VIII (antihemophilic globulin, or AHG) or Factor VIII–related antigen has increased the rate of carrier detection in hemophilia A.[103, 104] In normal persons, the levels of Factor VIII, measured as procoagulant or antigen, are identical (i.e., the ratio of activity to antigen is 1),[189] whereas female carriers of hemophilia A produce approximately only 50 per cent as much functional Factor VIII as antigenic material.[104] This abnormal ratio (1:2) persists during pregnancy, and therefore detection not only is more accurate but theoretically can be carried out at any time during gestation. Similar techniques for the detection of carriers of hemophilia B are currently limited, since only some families demonstrate discordant Factor IX procoagulant and antigen levels.

Prenatal diagnosis of X-linked hemophilia A is now possible if a sample of fetal plasma can be obtained by fetoscopy during the second trimester.[125] Immunologic measurement of the procoagulant portion (VIIIC:Ag) of the Factor VIII molecule discriminates between normal and affected children, since VIIIC:Ag is markedly reduced in affected males.

VON WILLEBRAND'S DISEASE

This illness accounts for approximately 10 per cent of all inherited disorders of blood coagulation. However, since the more common disorders, hemophilia A and B, are X-linked, recessive diseases, von Willebrand's disease is the most common clinically significant abnormality of blood coagulation in women.

Von Willebrand's disease is characterized by

TABLE 3-4 LABORATORY DIAGNOSIS OF VON WILLEBRAND'S DISEASE

Factor VIII (AHG) procoagulant deficiency (VIII:C)
Decreased Factor VIII related antigen (VIIIR:Ag)
Prolonged bleeding time*
Positive tourniquet test*
Decreased platelet adhesiveness*
Decreased platelet agglutination with Ristocetin (VIIIR:VW)*
Unique delayed response to plasma with production of new Factor VIII in vivo

---

*These abnormalities are presumably due to a deficiency or abnormality of the von Willebrand factor (VIII:VWF or VIIIR:VW)

In some patients not all of these abnormalities are detectable.

epistaxis, menorrhagia, easy bruising following trauma, gastrointestinal bleeding, and postoperative hemorrhage. Tooth extractions may result in significant hemorrhage. Hemarthroses are rare. Important laboratory abnormalities are summarized in Table 3-4. Von Willebrand's disease is the only inherited disorder of blood coagulation commonly associated with a prolonged bleeding time. However, the bleeding time often correlates poorly with other laboratory abnormalities.[139, 150] Although abnormalities in platelet adhesiveness and agglutination in the presence of ristocetin are commonly present in vitro, there is no evidence of an intrinsic defect in the platelets. The diagnosis of von Willebrand's disease rests primarily on the clinical and family history, reduction in levels of Factor VIII measured as procoagulant activity (VIII:C) or in assays that do not depend on coagulation (VIIIR:Ag or

FACTOR VIII COMPLEX

VIIIC: Procoagulant } M.W. 293,000
VIIIC, Ag: Immunol./human antibody } X-chromosome

VIIIR: von Willebrand Factor (bleeding time, ristocetin aggregation) } M.W. 220,000 (Δ polymers) Autosome
VIIIR, Ag: Immunol./heterologous antibody }

VIIIC + VIIIR = Complex
(M.W. > 1 x 10⁶)

FIGURE 3-1. The Factor VIII Complex. Various components and functions of the Factor VIII molecule are measured as indicated in Table 3-4. The indicated molecular weights are approximations. Both VIIIC:Ag and VIIIR:Ag are reduced in typical von Willebrand's disease, whereas VIIIR:Ag is normal or elevated in X-linked hemophilia A.

VIIIR:VW) (Figure 3-1 and Table 3-4), and the response to transfusion that is characteristic of this disorder.

Studies that have measured Factor VIII both as a procoagulant, i.e., VIII:C (in a standard coagulation assay) and as an antigen, i.e., VIII:Ag (using heterologous rabbit anti-human Factor VIII) have indicated that in both test systems, Factor VIII or Factor VIII-like material is reduced in classical von Willebrand's disease[189] (see Table 3-4). In contrast, patients with X-linked hemophilia A, while demonstrating reduced levels of Factor VIII (AHG) measured as a procoagulant, have normal levels of the antigen that reacts with rabbit anti-human AHG (see Figure 3-1).[189]

Pregnancy. Although there is no evidence that the presence of von Willebrand's disease results in either increased maternal mortality or fetal loss, there is an increased risk of postpartum hemorrhage.[137, 158, 187] The relatively low frequency of complications during pregnancy and delivery may reflect the relatively benign nature of this disorder in many patients, moderate rather than severe deficiencies of Factor VIII in many patients, and the tendency of levels of Factor VIII to rise during pregnancy, so that at the time of birth, Factor VIII levels almost reach or achieve normality.[122, 130, 143, 155, 158, 183] However, it appears that more severely affected women do not demonstrate striking elevations of Factor VIII.[158, 186, 187, 188] Nevertheless, postpartum hemorrhage may not occur, even when Factor VIII levels are low.

Since there is great variability in von Willebrand's disease, and postpartum hemorrhage is unpredictable, a careful history and evaluation of the effects of previous trauma and childbirth and measurement of Factor VIII levels during gestation are most important in determining whether prophylactic replacement therapy is required during labor and delivery. If the level of Factor VIII is greater than 30 per cent, therapy is probably not required for a normal delivery.

Treatment. Patients with von Willebrand's disease respond typically to the transfusion of plasma or certain plasma components with the production of new Factor VIII in vivo. Apparently, any fraction of plasma that contains the antigen detected by rabbit antihuman Factor VIII (VIIIR:Ag) is capable of producing this response. However, the production of new Factor VIII does not depend upon the presence of functional, procoagulant Factor VIII in the donor material, since plasma from patients with hemophilia A is capable of producing the same response as that seen with normal plasma.

The administration of 3 units (bags) of fresh frozen plasma or 6 units (bags) of cryoprecipitate probably produces the maximum response of which a given patient is capable.[103] However, since the response is variable, Factor VIII levels should be monitored carefully to determine the peak levels obtained and the duration of response. When measurements of the effects of previous transfusions are not available, and if clinically indicated, a trial transfusion of 3 units of fresh frozen plasma is warranted in order to determine the time of maximum response (usually 4 to 12 hours after transfusion), the maximum level achieved, and the duration of the elevation of Factor VIII levels. In many instances, one transfusion per day may be sufficient to maintain hemostatically adequate levels of Factor VIII. Concentrates of Factor VIII should not be used except in emergency situations in which an immediate and marked increase in levels of Factor VIII is required, because purified concentrates of Factor VIII may lack the "von Willebrand's stimulating factor" that is responsible for the production of new Factor VIII in vivo.

Maximum levels of 30 to 50 per cent are probably adequate to stop bleeding from the uterus or from an episiotomy in the absence of obstetric or local causes of bleeding. Therapy should be continued for approximately 3 to 5 days after cessation of postpartum bleeding and for 5 to 7 days following gynecological surgery. However, prophylactic therapy during labor to *prevent* abnormal bleeding probably does not have to be continued for more than 24 hours after successful completion of labor and delivery, if hemostasis has been normal. Although emphasis has been placed on correction of Factor VIII levels, the temporary and often erratic correction of the prolonged bleeding time by transfusion may also play a role in the clinical response to transfusional therapy. Evaluation of postpartum bleeding must include consideration of the possibility that the cause is unrelated to the underlying hemorrhagic disorder.[120, 133, 188]

Thrombocytopenia

The normal platelet count is 150,000 to 400,000 per cu mm (150–400 × 10^9/l) of blood, but hemorrhage secondary to thrombocytopenia usually does not occur until the platelet count has fallen to levels of less than 50,000 per cu mm. In fact, spontaneous bleeding is unlikely to occur until the platelet count has fallen to less than 20,000 to 30,000 per cu mm, unless there are other contributory causes or the decrease in platelet levels has been acute. Thrombocytopenia is character-

ized by bleeding from the small blood vessels of the skin and mucous membranes. Petechiae, which are minute hemorrhagic lesions, are the hallmark of thrombocytopenic purpura in contrast to the ecchymotic lesions that are characteristic of disordered blood coagulation. Patients with clinically significant thrombocytopenia usually also have prolonged bleeding times, decreased clot retraction, and positive tourniquet tests. Intracranial bleeding is the leading cause of death secondary to severe thrombocytopenia.

Evaluation of thrombocytopenia includes examination of the peripheral blood and bone marrow. Although platelet counts are important to accurately monitor platelet levels, examination of a smear of the peripheral blood is adequate to determine if the platelet count is markedly or moderately reduced, normal, or elevated. Examination of the bone marrow provides a means of determining if the marrow is cellular and whether megakaryocytes are present. The presence of megakaryocytes in association with severe peripheral thrombocytopenia strongly suggests that the thrombocytopenia is secondary to peripheral destruction or sequestration of platelets. However, it is important to interpret hematologic alterations in the context of the clinical problem.

Thrombocytopenia secondary to decreased production of platelets occurs in disorders associated with decreased numbers of or functionally suppressed megakaryocytes. Therefore, replacement of normal marrow by tumor is commonly associated with thrombocytopenia (as well as with anemia and leukopenia). Deficiencies of vitamin B_{12} or folate often are associated with thrombocytopenia; this has been discussed elsewhere in this chapter. Rare congenital disorders of megakaryocytopoiesis cause thrombocytopenia. Bacterial and viral infections can result in thrombocytopenia, probably both by suppression of marrow function and by increased peripheral destruction. However, the commonest cause of clinically significant thrombocytopenia *secondary to bone marrow depression* is probably the administration of cytotoxic drugs. Following the administration of these agents, the platelet count gradually falls; after a single dose, the lowest count occurs at 10 to 14 days.[149a]

Thrombocytopenia in the absence of leukopenia or anemia usually indicates the peripheral destruction of platelets. Drug-induced and immunologically mediated thrombocytopenia, disseminated intravascular coagulopathy, and infection are the chief causes of an increased rate of platelet destruction. Idiosyncratic reactions to drugs are common.[149a] Therefore, the development of thrombocytopenia is an indication for the discontinuation of all medications, unless another obvious cause is present or a medication is critically important for the well-being of the particular patient *and* is not known to cause thrombocytopenia. Even in the latter instance, the marked specificity of the immunological reaction that results in drug-induced thrombocytopenia makes it likely that discontinuation of the drug with the administration of a closely related compound will be tolerated and that the episode of thrombocytopenia will be terminated.[149a] Rechallenge of a sensitive individual with the offending drug results in recurrent thrombocytopenia and should not be undertaken.

If significant hemorrhage persists after discontinuation of a drug suspected of causing thrombocytopenia, corticosteroids may be helpful until the platelet count returns to an adequate level. If life-threatening bleeding continues despite the administration of steroids, platelet transfusions may provide adequate numbers of platelets for hemostasis or exchange transfusion may be used to sufficiently lower the concentration of the drug to decrease the rate of platelet destruction.

Other causes of acute thrombocytopenia without suppression of thrombopoiesis are summarized in Table 3–5. Infection (usually with gram-negative organisms), malignancy, and hemolytic reactions to blood transfusions can result in intravascular coagulation that produces both thrombocytopenia and hypofibrinogenemia.[116a, 157a, 174b] Endotoxin or red cell stroma from incompatible red cells may be the precipitating triggers of the first and last examples,[116a, 174b] but the mechanisms by which some tumors produce intravascular coagulation remain unclear. In some instances, turbulent blood flow in vascular tumors is believed to result in sequestration and destruction of platelets sufficient to produce systemic thrombocytopenia.[184a] The rapid transfusion of large volumes of blood that do not contain viable platelets can produce thrombocytopenia by diluting circulating platelets.[139a] In rare instances, the production of antibodies against *donor* platelets can result in delayed thrombocytopenia (post-transfusion purpura). It has been postulated that this occurs when antigen-antibody complexes, containing donor platelets or fragments thereof, adhere to the platelets of the recipient.[111a, 188a, 205a]

Immunologic Thrombocytopenic Purpura (ITP). This designation refers to a heterogeneous group of patients with thrombocytopenia in whom known causes of thrombocytopenia have not been detected after careful evaluation. Historically, they have been said to have idiopathic thrombocytopenic purpura, a term that should be abandoned. Many patients in this group are women of childbearing age. In some, the development of thrombocytopenia is a prelude to another underlying disorder, such as systemic lupus erythematosus or a lymphoma. Occasionally there is a history of a preceding viral illness. Interestingly, there appears to be an increased frequency of thyroid disease.[117, 156] The chronicity and natural course of the illness cannot be predicted. The spleen is not palpable. The bone marrow is essentially normal, although an increased proportion of megakaryocytes has been reported. There is no evidence that platelet production is decreased in this syndrome; available information indicates that platelet production is significantly increased in ITP and that peripheral thrombocytopenia results from a rate of destruction for which the bone marrow cannot adequately compensate.

It has been demonstrated that the plasma of affected patients contains a factor, shown to be an IgG immunoglobulin, that produces thrombocytopenia when transfused into normal recipients. Presumably, transplacental transfer of this factor accounts for the occurrence of thrombocytopenia in some of the children born to mothers with ITP. The immunoglobulin causes damage to the platelets, which then are sequestered and destroyed in the reticuloendothelial system, i.e., the spleen, and in some patients with high antibody titers, the liver. Recently, techniques that measure small concentrations of immunoglobulins have demonstrated increased levels of platelet-associated IgG, in over 90 per cent of patients with ITP.[156] There is a correla-

TABLE 3–5 PRODUCTION OF ACUTE THROMBOCYTOPENIA WITHOUT SUPPRESSION OF THROMBOPOIESIS

Agent	Mechanism
Quinidine*	Immunologic
Blood transfusion	Immunologic (post-transfusion purpura)
Blood transfusion	Intravascular coagulation (hemolytic transfusion reaction)
Infection	Intravascular coagulation (endotoxin ?)
Malignancy	Intravascular coagulation
Blood transfusion	Dilution of circulating platelets

*Many other drugs also produce thrombocytopenia by this mechanism.

Find underlying cause

tion between the amount of IgG detected on the platelets of patients with ITP and the degree of thrombocytopenia.[112, 156]

Treatment. A thorough attempt should be made to identify any underlying cause or additional factor that may contribute to the degree of thrombocytopenia. In the absence of a treatable underlying disease, therapy should be based on the severity of the hemorrhagic diathesis. The platelet count per se should not be treated. In the absence of petechiae or other forms of hemorrhage, corticosteroids should not be used. Some patients tolerate platelet counts of less than 20,000 per cu mm without difficulty. However, careful and continuous evaluation is necessary, since the appearance of petechiae, particularly involving the mucous membranes, may herald the development of more severe visceral or intracranial bleeding. The initial dose of corticosteroid is 60 to 80 mg of prednisone; when a response occurs, it is usually observed within 1 to 2 weeks.[117] However, even in the absence of a change in platelet levels, corticosteroids may improve hemostasis and fresh petechiae may no longer appear. Whether or not a response has been observed in the platelet count, corticosteroids should be tapered off slowly after 2 to 3 weeks (approximately 10 to 20 mg per week until a dose of 30 mg per day has been reached, then 5 mg per week until 20 mg per day has been reached, and 2.5 mg/week subsequently) until the lowest dose compatible with adequate hemostasis has been attained. A rapid decrease in the dose of steroids may result in recurrence of hemorrhage that can be avoided by more judicious tapering. Another advantage of slowly decreasing the dose of corticosteroids is that recurrence of symptoms can be accurately related to the most recent decrease in dose, and the medication can be appropriately increased one or two steps. Platelet counts should be monitored carefully during this period.

A significant proportion of patients respond satisfactorily to corticosteroids, and although the platelet count may not return to normal levels, the increase may be sufficient to provide normal hemostasis. Relapses can occur, even in patients who initially remained in remission after corticosteroids had been discontinued. The mechanism by which corticosteroids exert their effect is unclear, but improvement probably results in part from inhibition of phagocytosis by the reticuloendothelial system or from antibody binding.[156]

Splenectomy should be considered for patients who do not respond satisfactorily to corticosteroids or in whom the dose of prednisone produces unacceptable side affects. Splenectomy is not indicated as the initial therapy unless intracranial bleeding is present. Approximately 75 per cent of patients with ITP respond to splenectomy with a rise in platelet count that results in cessation of bleeding.[95, 117] However, relapses often occur after an initial response. Corticosteroids remain necessary for some patients, but usually at lower dose than before splenectomy. Performance of a splenectomy presents problems in pregnancy, which are discussed later in this chapter.

Immunosuppressive agents have recently been recommended for the treatment of this disorder in patients who have not responded to either steroids or splenectomy.[156] However, the effectiveness of this mode of therapy has not been satisfactorily established, and no controlled studies are yet available.[111, 124, 166] The use of toxic drugs should be considered only after corticosteroids and splenectomy have failed and if serious bleeding persists.

The use of platelet transfusions is not recommended except in the most life-threatening situations, since platelets are rapidly destroyed by the circulating antiplatelet antibodies present in these patients. Platelet transfusions are not necessary for the management of patients with ITP during splenectomy.[95] Even severely thrombocytopenic persons tolerate this procedure amazingly well without platelet transfusions. Oral contraceptive agents may be helpful in controlling menstrual bleeding in women with thrombocytopenic purpura.

Pregnancy. There is no evidence that pregnancy worsens the clinical manifestations of ITP.[131, 134, 141, 161, 163, 182] Although older reports indicated an increased mortality rate in pregnant women who had not undergone splenectomy prior to pregnancy,[131, 182] a review revealed that the maternal mortality rate decreased from 14 per cent between 1949 and 1953 to 5 per cent between 1954 and 1961.[96] These early studies have to be interpreted in the context of more recent reports that indicate no increase in maternal mortality.[141, 149, 159, 162] More extensive consideration of splenectomy during pregnancy, for this and other hematologic disorders, is presented later in this chapter. Potential improvement in the pregnant woman must be balanced against increased fetal loss following splenectomy.[162] The indications for and response to corticosteroids are similar to those in nonpregnant individuals.

Although there is an increased frequency of postpartum bleeding from perineal trauma in thrombocytopenic patients, there is no increase in uterine bleeding, because contraction of the uterus is apparently the primary basis of hemostasis after delivery.[131, 134, 162, 163]

Many children born to mothers with ITP have thrombocytopenia and purpura at the time of birth;[131, 134] in some series more than 50 per cent of the neonates are thrombocytopenic.[121, 149, 163, 182, 184] Fetal morbidity and mortality are increased, and perinatal mortality ranges from 15 to 25 per cent,[134, 149, 161, 162, 163, 182] although two recent studies reported no neonatal deaths,[141, 159] and in another, fetal death due to hemorrhage occurred in only 8 per cent.[162] Death is usually due to intracranial bleeding. The administration of steroids to the mother apparently does not prevent development of thrombocytopenia in the fetus.[135, 141] The failure of corticosteroids to prevent or lessen thrombocytopenia in the fetus may reflect the common use of prednisone, the active metabolite of which is prednisolone. It has been shown that the concentration of prednisolone in cord blood is only approximately 10 per cent of its concentration in maternal blood after administration of either prednisone or prednisolone to the mother.[100] Perhaps the use of betamethasone or dexamethasone, both of which have been shown to produce maternal/fetal concentration ratios of 3:1,[98, 128] would be more effective for the treatment of immune thrombocytopenia in *both* the mother and the fetus. Administration of one of the latter corticosteroids to a thrombocytopenic mother should be particularly considered during the 1 to 3 week period preceding delivery.

When present, purpura is usually evident at the time of birth but in some cases does not develop until the neonate is at least a few days old.[131, 141, 162] Although some reports suggest that children born of thrombocytopenic mothers have a higher frequency of thrombocytopenia,[141, 162, 163, 182, 184] a clear relationship has not been established between the maternal platelet count or the presence or absence of the maternal spleen and the occurrence of thrombocytopenia in the newborn.[159, 175] It has been observed that women in complete remission, with and without prior splenectomy, bore children who were thrombocytopenic.[134, 162, 182] These observations support the concept that ITP is associated with a humoral factor that is capable of transplacental transfer.

Although an overall correlation between maternal and neonatal platelet counts may exist, there are sufficient data suggesting a poor correlation[159, 175] that does not warrant making arbitrary guidelines for the performance of a cesarian section, based solely on maternal platelet levels or the presence or absence of the maternal spleen.[162, 175] Cesarian section will not prevent the more than 50 per cent of fetal deaths during pregnancy in ITP that occur before the onset of labor. Furthermore, less than 50 per cent of fetal deaths can be attributed to hemorrhage.[162] Serious neonatal hemorrhage is unlikely to occur unless the neonate's platelet count is less than 50,000 per cu mm.[175] It is important to emphasize that most thrombocytopenic newborns will not have significant hemorrhage.[159, 162, 175] In one report, only 8 per cent of 113 live children required treatment.[162] Therefore, many recent reports have stressed the need to individualize management and have recommended against prophylactic cesarian sections.[159, 162, 175]

Currently, although good management includes serial measurements of the maternal platelet count, maternal thrombocytopenia per se is probably not an adequate basis for cesarian section. However, since the platelet count in a sample of scalp blood has been shown, in a small series, to adequately indicate the presence of thrombocytopenia,[175] and as neonatal platelet counts over 50,000 per cu mm are not associated with serious hemorrhage, the use of scalp blood to determine the platelet count at the onset of labor appears to be worthwhile. If the fetal scalp blood platelet count is over 50,000 per cu mm, vaginal delivery should be used. If the count is less than 50,000 per cu mm, a cesarian section probably should be performed and in most instances can be performed safely.[142]

Thrombocytopenia in newborn infants gradually improves and usually disappears within 2 to 4 months.[96] Treatment is required for a minority of patients. It is important to observe the newborn carefully for the delayed onset of thrombocytopenic purpura. Corticosteroid therapy is helpful in controlling significant bleeding. Platelet transfusions should be used in these infants only in life-threatening situations, since they are unlikely to be effective and may lead to the development of additional antiplatelet antibodies. Exchange transfusions may be effective in removing circulating antiplatelet antibodies.

Aspirin. Aspirin should not be administered to patients with deficiencies of Factors VIII or IX (and probably other deficiencies as well) or to patients with thrombocytopenia or qualitative platelet disorders. This agent interferes with platelet function and thereby creates an additional hemostatic defect in these persons. One 300 mg tablet of aspirin (acetylsalicylic acid) is adequate to acetylate all platelets in the circulation, an effect that persists for the lifetime of the platelets. Since 65 per cent of a series of 50,282 pregnant women were reported to ingest aspirin at some time during gestation, the potential for inappropriate use of aspirin is considerable.[132]

Disseminated Intravascular Coagulopathy

A group of seemingly unrelated disorders is occasionally responsible for the derangement of blood coagulation known as disseminated intravascular coagulopathy (DIC). The word "coagulopathy" has been deliberately used here, rather than "coagulation," to emphasize that hemorrhage rather than thrombosis is the major clinical manifestation of DIC. Only in relatively few patients, usually those with a malignancy, is DIC associated with thrombotic or thromboembolic complications. Table 3–6 lists the major causes of DIC in pregnant women; those unique to pregnancy will be discussed in detail. The diagnosis of DIC is confirmed by abnormalities in some, but not necessarily all, of the laboratory tests listed in Table 3–7.[101, 113, 118, 157]

Elevation of various coagulation factors during pregnancy and the alterations in levels during normal labor and delivery make important the careful interpretation of tests of blood coagulation at the termination of pregnancy. Fibrinogen and Factor VIII levels fall, but they do not fall below normal, nonpregnant levels.[108, 126, 146] Fibrinolytic activity temporarily decreases during delivery, and levels of fibrinogen degradation products (FDP) and fibrin degradation products (fdp) increase to the upper limit of the normal range.[108, 146] These observations have been interpreted as indicating that minor "physiologic defibrination" is normally associated with the termination of pregnancy[146, 176] and that labor and delivery are associated with the possible release of thromboplastic materials from the uterus into the systemic circulation. However, the platelet count, thrombin time, prothrombin time, and partial thromboplastin time remain within nor-

TABLE 3–6 ACQUIRED HYPOFIBRINO-GENEMIA DURING PREGNANCY

Premature separation of the placenta
Intrauterine death with retained dead fetus
Amniotic fluid embolism
Septic abortion
Retained placenta
Toxemia
Transfusion reaction
Malignancy
Septicemia
Intra-amniotic injection of hyperosmolar urea or hypertonic saline

TABLE 3–7 LABORATORY EVALUATION OF CONSUMPTION COAGULOPATHY

Clot observation
Peripheral blood smear
Fibrinogen concentration
Platelet count
Fibrinogen-fibrin degradation products (FDP-fdp)
Thrombin time
Prothrombin time
Partial thromboplastin time

mal limits during delivery. Altered blood coagulation tests gradually revert to normal within the first few postpartum weeks.[107, 126, 146]

Premature Separation of the Placenta. Separation of the placenta from the uterus before delivery is often associated with DIC. Severe hypofibrinogenemia occurs in approximately 25 per cent of patients with this obstetric complication, usually within 8 hours of the onset of symptoms.[136, 169] However, not all of these women bleed, and maternal mortality is fortunately low.[99, 136, 169] Although local utilization of fibrinogen in the hematoma that forms between the placenta and uterus has been considered to play a role in the development of hypofibrinogenemia in this disorder, it is most likely that systemic DIC accounts for the clinical and laboratory abnormalities.[168, 173] A correlation between placental separation severe enough to kill the fetus and significant hypofibrinogenemia has been reported.[169] Thrombocytopenia is common but not necessarily marked.[146, 168]

In one study there was a correlation between elevated FDP-fdp levels and postpartum hemorrhage in women who had developed hypofibrinogenemia.[99] Women with both hypofibrinogenemia and elevated levels of FDP-fdp had a higher frequency of bleeding than those with comparably low levels of fibrinogen in the absence of circulating FDP-fdp.

Intrauterine Death, with Retained Dead Fetus. Gradual development of clinically significant DIC occasionally occurs in women who have retained a dead fetus for more than one month.[168, 176] It has been presumed that thromboplastic material from the degenerated placenta, or perhaps absorbed amniotic fluid, accounts for the changes in blood coagulation observed in approximately 30 per cent of these women. The fall in plasma fibrinogen concentration is gradual and should be carefully monitored to determine whether clinically significant hypofibrinogenemia is impending.[146] The onset of bruising or bleeding should be immediately reported. Perhaps because of the subacute nature of the process, many of these patients have normal prothrombin, partial thromboplastin, and thrombin times.[146] Severe thrombocytopenia is unusual.[146, 168] Careful clinical observations support the concept that hypofibrinogenemia is secondary to coagulation and not fibrinogenolysis.[140]

Amniotic Fluid Embolism. The entrance of amniotic fluid into the maternal circulation is associated with respiratory distress and cardiovascular collapse and commonly with acute, severe hemorrhage.[116] Particulate matter (including meconium) in the fluid may contribute significantly to these complications.[116, 168] Amniotic fluid has been shown to contain procoagulant activity, although perhaps not in concentrations sufficient to produce generalized activation of coagulation mechanisms.[164] The combination of the acuteness and the severity of this disorder results in an 80 per cent mortality rate.[116] A dead fetus increases the risk to the mother.

Septic Abortion. Septicemia associated with an abortion is only rarely associated with DIC. When sepsis is caused by gram-negative organisms, it is postulated that endotoxin initiates intravascular coagulation. In patients in whom *Clostridium perfringens* sepsis is associated with severe hemolysis, the latter phenomenon has been proposed as the direct cause of DIC.[168] However, it is well recognized that gram-positive organisms also are associated with DIC. It has been suggested that the susceptibility of pregnant women to the effects of endotoxin is related to a decreased clearance of endotoxin or related antigen-antibody complexes by the reticuloendothelial system.

Effects of Hypertonic Saline. The intra-amniotic injection of hypertonic saline for the production of abortion is associated with a fall in fibrinogen levels and platelet counts, although both remain within normal limits.[148, 178, 180] The FDP-fdp remains elevated until 18 hours after delivery,[178, 180] and in 20 to 24 hours the results of laboratory evaluation are again normal. Prothrombin, partial thromboplastin, and thrombin times generally remain normal in asymptomatic women. There are inconsistent decreases in other specific coagulation factors.[147, 178] It appears that the greatest risk occurs from 2 to 12 hours after injection, although clinically significant bleeding is rare and self-limited.[178]

It has been suggested that intra-amniotic infusion of hypertonic saline results in transfer of amniotic fluid into the maternal circulation, with initiation of a mild coagulopathy.[181] Physiologic-ally significant alterations of serum sodium or potassium do not occur, and therefore systemic hypernatremia does not appear a likely mechanism.[147] Hyperosmolar urea also produces similar alterations in levels of fibrinogen, platelets, and FDP-fdp, but in a smaller proportion of patients than when hypertonic saline is used. Clinically significant hemorrhage is even more rare than with the use of hypertonic saline. The actual mechanisms remain unknown.[102, 148] The use of prostaglandin $F_2\alpha$ is not associated with changes in blood coagulation or fibrinolysis, and therefore this agent is safer to use in patients with an abnormality of blood coagulation.[102, 110]

Eclampsia and Pre-eclampsia. Eclampsia is the occurrence of convulsions in a woman with pregnancy-induced or pregnancy-aggravated hypertension. The possible pathophysiology of this clinical syndrome is discussed in Chapter 1. The deposition of fibrinogen (or fibrin) in the kidneys of some women with fatal eclampsia and its detection in liver biopsy specimens from some women with pre-eclampsia,[97] in association with laboratory abnormalities suggestive of deranged hemostasis, have led to the concept that "low grade" disseminated intravascular coagulopathy plays a role in the production of the clinical abnormalities observed in this syndrome. Vasospasm may result in local injury that in the presence of DIC provides the pathologic settings for deposition of fibrinogen or fibrin in various organs.

However, laboratory data indicative of DIC in pre-eclampsia or eclampsia are often minimal or conflicting. Although increased levels of FDP-fdp[106, 109, 138] and thrombocytopenia[106, 109, 138, 145, 170, 172] have been reported, the abnormalities are usually minor. Interestingly, an increase in FDP-fdp *after* seizures has been reported.[109] Prolonged thrombin times have been observed.[119, 170, 172] In contrast to most disorders in which DIC is generally agreed to be present, fibrinogen concentrations are usually normal.[97, 106, 109, 129, 138, 145, 151] Furthermore, although some studies have reported a correlation between abnormalities of blood coagulation and clinical severity,[129, 151, 174a] others have not.[106, 119] Therefore, the question has often been raised whether there is any cause and effect relationship between DIC, if present, and eclampsia.[106, 109, 119, 151, 170]

Treatment. Since DIC always results from an underlying disorder, the cornerstone of therapy is correction of the primary pathologic condition. The importance of this approach is demonstrated by the occurrence of chronic DIC in patients with malignancies; lack of successful therapy is usually associated with persistence or recurrence of the coagulopathy. In contrast, successful treatment of sepsis is associated with cessation of DIC. When present, hemorrhage, anoxia, and shock must be treated promptly and aggressively, especially in the presence of premature separation of the placenta[99] or amniotic fluid embolism.[116]

Usually the complications of pregnancy associated with DIC are susceptible to therapy (see Table 3–6), and therefore their proper management is essential for the effective treatment of DIC. Emptying of the uterus in cases of premature separation of the placenta, intrauterine death, or septic abortion apparently results in immediate cessation of accelerated coagulation.[99, 136, 140, 146, 168, 176] Within 24 hours after the uterus has been emptied, levels of coagulation factors are usually adequate for hemostasis, even in the absence of agents specifically directed at correction of abnormal coagulation.[113, 146, 168, 169] Normal levels of coagulation factors and FDP-fdp are usually achieved in 1 to 3 days. Although the platelet count may not rise to normal levels for 3 to 5 days, this does not appear to be a critical factor post partum. It is well recognized that normal uterine contractions are adequate to provide hemostasis in that organ, and therefore subsequent attention must be paid to ensure that good contractions and subsequent retraction occur.[99, 116, 136, 176] In most instances, *no other therapy* is required for the treatment of DIC.

Criteria for the use of heparin to interrupt a coagulopathy remain somewhat controversial. As already indicated, correction of the underlying obstetric complication usually ends the DIC, and uterine contractions control hemorrhage. Therefore, in most instances vaginal delivery of the fetus and the placenta can be accomplished without the use of heparin (or fibrinogen). Once the uterus has been emptied, there is even less indication for therapy unless bleeding persists in the *absence* of recognized obstetric or traumatic causes. Heparin should not be given to a patient who is not bleeding, no matter how deranged are the tests of blood coagulation. Therapy must be individualized and the patient, not the tests, treated.[118, 136] Since DIC is a continuously changing pathologic state, laboratory abnormalities must be interpreted cautiously and in relationship to the clinical findings. Similar patterns of laboratory abnormalities may occur in both bleeding and nonbleeding patients.

Since heparin can exaggerate the problem for which it is being administered, i.e., hemorrhage, its use should probably be limited to helping achieve stabilization of a patient until a definitive

obstetric procedure can be performed. In this regard, it is probably most effective in temporarily correcting hypofibrinogenemia associated with a retained dead fetus, until the uterus has been emptied. However, this should only be done under carefully controlled conditions.[168] Because of the dangers involved and the changing state of the hemostatic mechanism, in these circumstances heparin should be administered intravenously, preferably in a constant infusion, so that maximum continuous control of effective dosage can be maintained. The maternal circulatory system must be intact in order for this to be a feasible approach. The value of heparin for the treatment of DIC associated with premature separation of the placenta or amniotic fluid embolism is unproved; heparin in such a case may be dangerous.[116, 168] There is no evidence that heparin improves survival in patients with DIC.[101, 115, 152]

The temporary correction of hypofibrinogenemia with replacement therapy has been successful in some patients but probably should be undertaken in association with heparin to prevent the possibility that administration of fibrinogen in the presence of ongoing DIC will only perpetuate the process.[113, 157] There is essentially no indication for replacement of fibrinogen once the uterus has been emptied, although normal or near-normal fibrinogen levels probably play a role in helping provide adequate hemostasis for those women who require surgical intervention, e.g., hysterectomy or cesarian section. Fibrinogen concentrations of 100 to 150 mg per 100 ml provide adequate levels. Cryoprecipitate is the most effective source of fibrinogen currently available. If necessary, fresh frozen plasma can be used, although its effect on fibrinogen levels is limited.

Because of laboratory evidence of fibrinogenolysis and fibrinolysis, epsilon aminocaproic acid (EACA, an inhibitor of the conversion of plasminogen to plasmin) has occasionally been suggested as an agent for treatment of DIC. However, because of the current belief that primary fibrinolysis is rare and that inhibition of fibrinolysis in a patient with ongoing DIC may precipitate thrombotic episodes, and because treatment of the underlying disorder is primary, as is the case with heparin and fibrinogen, EACA and other inhibitors of plasmin formation are not recommended for the treatment of DIC, especially in association with obstetric complications.[113, 136, 144, 146, 157, 168] However, in rare instances when severe hypofibrinogenemia and hemorrhage persist *after* the uterus has been emptied, with overt lysis of blood clots and failure to respond to therapy with heparin or heparin together with a source of fibrinogen, this agent may be indicated.[99, 169]

The controversy concerning the potential role (if any) of DIC in eclampsia and pre-eclampsia, and a report of the successful treatment without the use of heparin of 154 cases of eclampsia with no maternal deaths,[171] provide strong justifications not to use heparin for the treatment of women with this syndrome.

Circulating Anticoagulants

Circulating anticoagulants are acquired inhibitors of blood coagulation, most examples of which are inhibitors of Factor VIII (AHG). More rarely, inhibitors against Factors V, IX, XI, and XIII have been reported. In addition, the abnormal proteins in some patients with dysglobulinemia, such as those with multiple myeloma, apparently inhibit coagulation by complexing with one or more of the coagulation factors.

Inhibitors against Factor VIII have been reported in a variety of clinical conditions (Table 3–8), and when studied they have usually been shown to be IgG immunoglobulins.[123, 174] Occasionally a circulating anticoagulant to Factor VIII appears in a woman post partum, after the birth of one or more children.[123, 154]

The onset may occur at any time during the year following parturition but usually is first detected within a few months after termination of the first pregnancy.[177] There may be ecchymoses, soft tissue bleeding, hematuria, or bleeding following trauma or surgery. Hemarthroses are uncommon. The bleeding can be severe and fatal; however, it also may abate despite the continued presence of the inhibitor. The mechanism by which women develop inhibitors against Factor VIII during the postpartum period remains unknown. In about one half of the cases, the anticoagulant disappears spontaneously and does not necessarily recur during subsequent pregnancies. Such an inhibitor also has been detected prior to delivery; however, the male child had a normal level of Factor VIII at birth.[153] In another patient who had developed an inhibitor following the birth of her first child, the second pregnancy was associated with a series of hemorrhagic episodes during the last trimester and in the postpartum period. The circulating anticoagulant was present in the blood of her male child, but he had no signs of abnormal bleeding and the inhibitor disappeared after approximately 4 months.[127] The development of an anticoagulant directed against Factor VIII is a rare complication of systemic lupus erythematosus, in contrast to the more common development in SLE of an inhibitor of the activation of prothrombin.[123, 174, 177]

The spontaneous development of a Factor VIII inhibitor in nonhemophiliacs is often characterized by the concurrent presence of reduced but detectable levels of both Factor VIII and the inhibitor. In contrast, in hemophiliacs who have developed inhibitors, no Factor VIII procoagulant activity is demonstrable.

Detection of Circulating Anticoagulants. Any patient in whom the result of a screening test for blood coagulation is abnormal should be examined for the presence of a circulating anticoagulant. Such an evaluation is particularly indicated when the abnormal test result is associated with the development of a hemorrhagic disorder in a previously normal patient. Initial evaluation of the possible presence of a circulating anticoagulant is easily performed by utilizing the test for blood coagulation that yielded an abnormal result in the particular patient. An equal volume of the patient's plasma is mixed with normal plasma, and the test is repeated with appropriate controls. In the absence of a significant titer of circulating anticoagulant, the mixture of patient's and normal plasma will result in a normal test result. However, if a circulating inhibitor is present, the mixture of plasma will still result in a prolonged (abnormal) time. The sensitivity of this procedure may be increased by preincubation of the mixture at 37° C for 1 hour. If a circulating anticoagulant is believed to be present, more specific assays should then be performed to determine the factor or factors against which the circulating inhibitor is directed. It is important to include appropriate controls in these tests to compensate for any deterioration of coagulation factors in normal plasma that may occur during the incubation period.

Therapy. A variety of therapeutic approaches have been used in the treatment of patients with circulating anticoagulants. Evalua-

TABLE 3–8 OCCURRENCE OF INHIBITORS OF FACTOR VIII (AHG)

Hemophilia A

Postpartum period

Various immunologic disorders, including rheumatoid arthritis, ulcerative colitis, systemic lupus erythematosus

Absence of detectable underlying disease

tion of the effectiveness of these modes of therapy has been difficult because of the lack of controlled studies and because of the vagaries in the natural history of circulating anticoagulants. In some instances, exchange transfusion, combined with replacement therapy, has been used for the treatment of acute hemorrhagic episodes. Since administration of Factor VIII, the antigen against which the circulating anticoagulant is directed, often results in increased titers of the inhibitor (antibody), this type of therapy should only be used in life-threatening situations.[123, 153] While attempts to elevate levels of a particular factor in the presence of an inhibitor may be unsuccessful, there may nevertheless be a salutary effect on hemostasis. Replacement therapy should be based on firm knowledge of the specificity of the anticoagulant being treated. Certain preparations of Factor IX concentrates are reportedly effective for the correction of the hemostatic abnormality produced by inhibitors of Factor VIII.[179] In some instances, adrenocorticosteroids have been used to treat patients with a circulating anticoagulant; but except in those with systemic lupus erythematosus, this therapy has generally been unsuccessful.

Immunosuppressive agents have also been used, particularly in the treatment of patients with inhibitors directed against Factor VIII.[174, 177] Although some good results have been reported, this mode of therapy should be considered experimental and particularly dangerous during pregnancy.

Systemic Lupus Erythematosus. Five to 10 per cent of patients with systemic lupus erythematosus (SLE) develop a circulating anticoagulant. These patients also commonly have other serologic abnormalities, including a biologic false-positive test for syphilis. The typical anticoagulant of SLE, either an IgG or IgM immunoglobulin, inhibits the conversion by prothrombin activator of prothrombin to thrombin.[123, 154, 177] It has also been detected in a variety of patients with other types of autoimmune disease.

Typically, the prothrombin time is moderately prolonged, as are the whole blood clotting time and partial thromboplastin time. Some of the patients have a markedly prolonged prothrombin time; it is believed that these patients have not only a circulating anticoagulant but also a deficiency of Factor II (prothrombin) activity.[123]

Most patients with this anticoagulant do not bleed abnormally. Therefore, there is no correlation between the titer of the lupus anticoagulant and clinical hemorrhage. In some instances, these patients have undergone major surgery without abnormal bleeding. In general, patients in whom the lupus anticoagulant was present in association with a hemorrhagic diathesis have also had either concomitant thrombocytopenia or decreased levels of prothrombin activity in their plasma.

The anticoagulant usually persists, but activity may decrease or disappear during the course of therapy (such as the administration of corticosteroids) directed against some of the other manifestations of SLE. Since the lupus anticoagulant is not necessarily associated with pathologic hemorrhage, its presence per se is not an indication for therapy.

ANTICOAGULATION

It is the purpose of this section to discuss not the indications for anticoagulation but rather the means by which it can most appropriately be accomplished. Long-term anticoagulation presents problems during pregnancy because both coumarin compounds and heparin create major risks for both the mother and the fetus.[195, 205] A major review of the outcome of pregnancies in which the mother received either coumarin compounds (418 cases) or heparin (136 cases) indicated that only approximately two thirds of the pregnancies resulted in full-term, normal infants.[195] An embryopathy characterized by nasal hypoplasia, with depression of the bridge of the nose and stippled epiphyses, occurred in 4 per cent of the children of women who had received warfarin during the sixth to ninth week of gestation. Another 1 per cent had central nervous system or ophthalmologic abnormalities associated with maternal ingestion of the drug during the second and third trimesters. This study confirms previous reports that coumarin compounds might cause fetal abnormalities if administered during the first trimester[198, 200, 207] and result in fetal hemorrhage (particularly at birth) because of their ability to cross the placenta.[194, 203, 207] Since heparin does not cross the placenta,[194, 197, 201] its administration is not associated with fetal hemorrhage or malformation.

Lack of adequate control during the administration of anticoagulants also may contribute to fetal mortality and maternal morbidity.[193, 194, 197, 207] Some authors have concluded that hemorrhagic complications can be avoided if therapy is carefully monitored.[193, 195, 197, 207, 208] However, a 10 per cent frequency of maternal hemorrhage when heparin was administered has been reported[195] in contrast to only 1 per cent with coumarin compounds. In addition, heparin has been shown to produce thrombocytopenia in

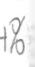

approximately 14 per cent of recipients.[190] The mechanism remains unknown. This poses another potential danger to recipients of heparin, although fortunately hemorrhage is rarely observed with this side effect. Because of the considerable risk to both mother and fetus, anticoagulants should be administered only when there are definite indications for their use, such as venous thrombosis, pulmonary embolism, or prosthetic heart valves.[196] The diagnosis of venous thrombosis or pulmonary embolism should be established by appropriate radiologic and other objective evaluations and should not depend solely upon physical examination and clinical history. Underlying hemorrhagic disorders, in particular thrombocytopenia, should be ruled out before the administration of these drugs.

If anticoagulation is required during the first trimester, heparin is the drug of choice. If that is not feasible, an oral anticoagulant* can be used but with the recognition that there is an increased risk of fetal malformation. After the first trimester, coumarins can be administered (although a lesser risk of malformation persists), but they probably should be discontinued 1 to 3 weeks before labor is anticipated. If anticoagulant therapy is still required, treatment with heparin should be begun at the time the coumarin is discontinued, but heparin probably should not be administered during delivery.[196] Coumarin or heparin may be reinstituted during the puerperium if necessary.

Patients receiving oral anticoagulants should be monitored frequently with prothrombin times. Therapeutic levels are indicated by prothrombin times that are 15 to 25 per cent of normal (approximately twice the control time). Liver disease and decreased absorption of vitamin K increase responsiveness to the coumarins; pregnancy decreases the response. If prolongation of the prothrombin time indicates an activity level of less than 15 per cent, the drug should be discontinued until the prothrombin time returns to the therapeutic range. Markedly prolonged prothrombin times or abnormal bleeding require treatment with vitamin K_1, plasma, or both. Concentrates of plasma that contain the vitamin K–dependent coagulation factors should be used only if life-threatening hemorrhage cannot be controlled with vitamin K_1 and plasma. It is important to consider the effects of other drugs on the metabolism of coumarins and to anticipate the possibility of untoward drug interactions.[199] Among other drugs, barbiturates, glutethimide, and griseofulvin inhibit the anticoagulant effects of oral anticoagulants; chloramphenicol, phenylbutazone, and large doses of salicylates potentiate them. Although coumarin compounds may appear in the milk of nursing mothers, their administration is not associated with hemorrhage or prolongation of the prothrombin time in breast-fed infants.[191, 201] However, an episode of postoperative hemorrhage has been reported in a 5 week old infant who was being breast-fed while his mother was receiving phenindione.[192] His prothrombin and partial thromboplastin times were both prolonged.

Heparin should be administered intravenously, in a continuous manner if possible (approximately 25,000 to 40,000 units per day or 350 to 700 units per kg per day). Clotting times are the only established means of determining that the dose is appropriate. The use of the partial thromboplastin time to monitor the dose of heparin and to indicate that appropriate antithrombotic levels of heparin have been achieved cannot be justified on the basis of currently available data.[202, 204, 206] After regulation of the dose, the clotting time should be determined daily and maintained at two to three times normal, but in no instance less than 20 or greater than 40 minutes. Since the half-life of heparin is only 90 minutes, discontinuation of the intravenous administration of this agent results in a rapid decrease in the blood level and diminution of anticoagulation. However, if therapy with heparin is associated with significant hemorrhage or if its effects must be immediately reversed, protamine sulfate, which effectively neutralizes heparin, can be administered intravenously.

SPLENECTOMY FOR HEMATOLOGIC DISORDERS DURING PREGNANCY

Splenectomy is often performed to cure or ameliorate hematologic conditions that can occur simultaneously with pregnancy, e.g., autoimmune thrombocytopenic purpura, thrombotic thrombocytopenic purpura, hereditary spherocytosis, autoimmune hemolytic anemia, Hodgkin's disease, myelofibrosis and myeloid metaplasia, aplastic anemia, thalassemia major, severe red cell enzyme deficiencies, Felty's syndrome, and Gaucher's disease.[212]

Splenectomy appears to result in a predisposition to premature labor and fetal death when performed during pregnancy but may be necessary for maternal welfare. When it is performed, the commonest cause of fetal loss is surgical

---

*Although only coumarins have been discussed in this section because they are the most commonly used group of oral anticoagulants, the same considerations apply to derivatives of indan-1,3,-dione, the other class of oral anticoagulants.

induction of premature labor.[215] Owing to the technical difficulties of performing a splenectomy during pregnancy, maternal morbidity is increased compared with splenectomy in nonpregnant women.[216, 223, 225]

Immunologic thrombocytopenic purpura (ITP) is the most common disease for which splenectomy is undertaken during pregnancy. However, corticosteroids are the treatment of choice for patients with ITP. Only if an adequate clinical response does not occur should splenectomy be considered. Splenectomy for ITP has been reported to be associated with a fetal loss rate of 25 to 30 per cent[224, 226] compared with 15 to 25 per cent in women with this condition who do not require a splenectomy while pregnant.[217, 219, 223, 225] However, recent reports indicate that splenectomy may be safer than was previously described.[217, 219, 223]

Thrombotic thrombocytopenic purpura (TTP), a syndrome that includes thrombocytopenic purpura, hemolytic anemia with fragmented red blood cells, fever, and neurologic and renal dysfunction, has been observed during pregnancy[209, 209a, 220, 221, 222] and in some cases appears to be related to eclampsia.[221] When performed early in the clinical course, splenectomy combined with pharmacologic doses of corticosteroids[214] or

with corticosteroids and dextran 70[213] has been reported to be either curative or palliative in some patients with this disorder. Other studies have failed to demonstrate the efficiency of splenectomy per se.[210, 218] Nevertheless, since the mortality rate has been 60 to 70 per cent in TTP,[209, 218] splenectomy is justified *if indicated to save the mother,* despite any potential adverse effects on the fetus.

However, recent advances in the treatment of TTP, including exchange transfusion, infusion of fresh frozen plasma, or administration of drugs that interfere with platelet function, have reduced the mortality rate and provided therapeutic alternatives.[210, 211]

Reports of the effects of splenectomy performed during gestation for other hematologic disorders are not readily available, since relatively few splenectomies have been required during pregnancy for the other problems indicated previously. The potential benefit to the mother, as well as the risk of fetal loss, must be carefully weighed before a splenectomy in pregnancy is attempted. Splenectomy should be considered only in life-threatening clinical situations that have not responded to corticosteroids or other medical attempts to control the underlying disease.

References

THE ANEMIAS OF PREGNANCY

1. Abernathy, M. R.: Döhle bodies associated with uncomplicated pregnancy. Blood, 27:380, 1966.
2. Ball, E. W., and Giles, C.: Folic acid and vitamin B_{12} levels in pregnancy and their relation to megaloblastic anemia. J. Clin. Pathol., 17:165, 1964.
3. Beischer, N. A.: The effects of maternal anemia upon the fetus. J. Reprod. Med., 6:21, 1971.
4. Bonnar, J., McNicol, G. P., and Douglas, A. S.: Fibrinolytic enzyme system and pregnancy. Br. Med. J., 3:387, 1969.
5. Carr, M. C.: Serum iron/TIBC in the diagnosis of iron deficiency anemia during pregnancy. Obstet. Gynecol., 38:602, 1971.
6. Chanarin, I.: Diagnosis of folate deficiency in pregnancy. Acta Obstet. Gynecol. Scand., 46:39, 1967.
7. Chanarin, I., MacGibbon, B. M., O'Sullivan, W. J., and Mollin, D. L.: Folic acid deficiency in pregnancy: The pathogenesis of megaloblastic anemia of pregnancy. Lancet, 2:634, 1959.
8. Chanarin, I., Rothman, D., and Berry, V.: Iron deficiency and its relation to folic acid status in pregnancy: Results of a clinical trial. Br. Med. J., 1:480, 1965.
9. Chanarin, I., Rothman, D., Ward, A., and Perry, J.: Folate status and requirement in pregnancy. Br. Med. J., 2:890, 1968.
10. Chopra, J., Noe, E., Matthew, J., Dhein, C., Rose, J., Cooperman, J. M., and Luhby, A. L.: Anemia in pregnancy. Am. J. Public Health, 57:857, 1967.
11. Cooper, B. A., Cantlie, G. S. D., and Brunton, L.: The case for folic acid supplements during pregnancy. Am. J. Clin. Nutr., 23:848, 1970.
12. De Leeuw, N. K. M., Lowenstein, L., and Hsieh, Y. S.: Iron deficiency and hydremia of normal pregnancy. Medicine, 45:291, 1966.
13. Ek, J.: Plasma and red cell folate values in newborn infants and their mothers in relation to gestational age. J. Pediatr., 97:288, 1980.
14. Fenton, V., Cavill, I., and Fisher, J.: Iron stores in pregnancy. Br. J. Haematol., 37:145, 1977.
15. Giles, C.: An account of 335 cases of megaloblastic anemia of pregnancy and the puerperium. J. Clin. Pathol., 19:1, 1966.
16. Giles, C., and Ball, E. W.: Iron and folic acid deficiency in pregnancy. Br. Med. J., 1:656, 1965.
17. Harris, J. W., and Kellermeyer, R. W.: The Red Cell: Production, Metabolism, Destruction: Normal and Abnormal. Cambridge, Mass., Harvard University Press, 1970, pp. 64–148 and 334–444.
18. Hibbard, B. M., and Hibbard, E. D.: Neutrophil hypersegmentation and defective folate metabolism in pregnancy. J. Obstet. Gynaecol. Br. Commonw., 78:776, 1971.
19. Holly, R. G.: Dynamics of iron metabolism in pregnancy. Am. J. Obstet. Gynecol., 93:370, 1965.
20. Jacobs, A., Miller, F., Worwood, M., Beamish, M. R., and Wardrop, C. A.: Ferritin in the serum of normal subjects and patients with iron deficiency and iron overload. Brit. Med. J., 4:206, 1972.
21. Kitay, D. Z.: Folic acid deficiency in pregnancy. Am. J. Obstet. Gynecol., 104:1067, 1969.
22. Kuvin, S. F., and Brecher, G.: Differential neutrophil counts in pregnancy. N. Engl. J. Med., 266:877, 1962.
23. Lowenstein, L., Labonde, M., Deschenes, E. B., and Shapiro, L.: Vitamin B_{12} in pregnancy and the puerperium. Am. J. Clin. Nutr., 8:265, 1960.
24. Mor, A., Yang, W., Schwarz, A., and Jones, W. C.: Platelet counts in pregnancy and labor. Obstet. Gynecol., 16:338, 1960.
25. Pitkin, R. M.: Nutritional influences during pregnancy. Med. Clin. North Am., 61:3, 1977.
26. Pitkin, R. M., and Witte, D. L.: Platelet and leukocyte counts in pregnancy. J.A.M.A., 242:2696, 1979.
27. Pritchard, J. A.: Changes in the blood volume during pregnancy and delivery. Anesthesiology, 26:393, 1965.
28. Pritchard, J. A., Scott, D. E., Whalley, P. J., and Haling, R. F.

Jr.: Infants of mothers with megaloblastic anemia due to folate deficiency. J.A.M.A., *211*:1982, 1970.

29. Pritchard, J. A., Whalley, P. J., and Scott, D. E.: The influence of maternal folate and iron deficiencies on intrauterine life. Am. J. Obstet. Gynecol., *104*:388, 1969.

30. Rae, P. C., and Robb, P. M.: Megaloblastic anemia of pregnancy: A clinical and laboratory study with particular reference to the total and labile serum folate levels. J. Clin. Pathol., *23*:379, 1970.

31. Rios, E., Lipschitz, D. A., Cook, J. D., and Smith, N. J.: Relationship of maternal and infant iron stores as assessed by determination of plasma ferritin. Pediatrics, *55*:694, 1975.

32. Robertson, J. G.: The blood in pregnancy. Br. J. Clin. Pract., *18*:667, 1964.

33. Rothman, D.: Folic acid in pregnancy. Am. J. Obstet. Gynecol., *108*:149, 1970.

34. Shaper, A. G., Kear, J., Macintosh, D. M., Kyobe, J., and Njama, D.: The platelet count, platelet adhesiveness and aggregation and the mechanism of fibrinolytic inhibition in pregnancy and the puerperium. J. Obstet. Gynaecol. Br. Commonw., *75*:433, 1968.

35. Streiff, R. R., and Little, A. B.: Folic acid deficiency in pregnancy. N. Engl. J. Med., *276*:776, 1967.

36. Varadi, S., Abbott, D., and Elwis, A.: Correlation of peripheral white cell and bone marrow changes with folate levels in pregnancy and their clinical significance. J. Clin. Pathol., *19*:33, 1966.

37. Wallerstein, R. O.: Iron metabolism and iron deficiency during pregnancy. Clin. Haematol., *2*:453, 1973.

38. Willoughby, M. L. N., and Jewell, F. J.: Investigation of folic acid requirements in pregnancy. Br. Med. J., *2*:1568, 1966.

39. Zuspan, F. P., Long, W. N., Russell, J. K., Stone, M. L., and Tarlov, A. R.: Anemia in pregnancy. J. Reprod. Med., *6*:13, 1971.

HEMOLYTIC DISEASE OF THE NEWBORN

40. Aicken, D. R.: Rhesus immunization before delivery of the first baby. Aust. N. Z. J. Obstet. Gynaecol., *10*:93, 1970.

41. Bowman, J. M.: Rh erythroblastosis fetalis 1975. Semin. Hematol., *12*:189, 1975.

42. Bowman, J. M., Chown, B., Lewis, M., and Pollock, J. M.: Rh isoimmunization during pregnancy: Antenatal prophylaxis. Can. Med. Assoc. J., *118*:623, 1978.

43. Davey, M. G., and Zipursky, A.: McMaster conference on prevention of Rh immunization. Vox Sang., *36*:50, 1979.

44. Edwards, R. F.: The place for anti-D gamma globulin in abortion. Aust. N. Z. J. Obstet. Gynaecol., *10*:96, 1970.

45. Godel, J. C., Buchanan, D. I., Jarosch, J. M., and McHugh, M.: Significance of Rh-sensitization during pregnancy: Its relation to a preventive programme. Br. Med. J., *4*:479, 1968.

46. Mollison, P. L.: Clinical aspects of Rh immunization. Am. J. Clin. Pathol., *60*:287, 1973.

47. Nusbacher, J., and Bove, J. R.: Rh immunoprophylaxis: Is antepartum therapy desirable? N. Engl. J. Med., *303*:935, 1980.

48. Pollack, W., Gorman, J. G., Freda, V. J., Ascari, W. Q., Allen, A. E., and Baker, W. J.: Results of clinical trials of RhoGAM in women. Transfusion, *8*:151, 1968.

49. Sussman, L. N., Romeo, U. Y., and Berk, H.: The prophylaxis of Rh hemolytic disease with Rh immunoglobulin. Am. J. Clin. Pathol., *50*:287, 1968.

50. Visscher, R. D., and Visscher, H. C.: Do Rh-negative women with an early spontaneous abortion need Rh immune prophylaxis? Am. J. Obstet. Gynecol., *113*:158, 1972.

51. World Health Organization: The suppression of Rh immunization by passively administered human immunoglobulin (IgG) anti-D (anti-Rh$_0$). Bull. W.H.O., *37*:483, 1967.

THE HEMOGLOBINOPATHIES

52. Alter, B. P.: Prenatal diagnosis of hemoglobinopathies and other hematologic diseases. J. Pediatr., *95*:501, 1979.

53. Anderson, M., Went, L. N., MacIver, J. E., and Dixon, H. G.: Sickle-cell disease in pregnancy. Lancet *2*:516, 1960.

53a. Anderson, M., Bluestone, R., and Milner, P. F.: Pregnancy and homozygous haemoglobin C disease. J. Obstet. Gynaecol. Br. Commonw., *74*:694, 1967.

54. Beaven, G. H., Dixon, G., and White, J. C.: Studies on thalassaemia-like anemias in pregnant immigrants in London. Br. J. Haematol., *12*:777, 1966.

55. Blank, A. M., and Freedman, W. L.: Sickle cell trait and pregnancy. Clin. Obstet. Gynecol., *12*:123, 1969.

56. Charache, S.: The treatment of sickle cell anemia. Arch. Intern. Med., *133*:698, 1974.

57. Charache, S., Scott, J., Niebyl, J., and Bonds, D.: Management of sickle cell disease in pregnant patients. Obstet. Gynecol., *55*:407, 1980.

58. Conley, C. L., Weatherall, D. J., Richardson, S. N., Shepard, M. K., and Charache, S.: Hereditary persistence of fetal hemoglobin: A study of 79 affected persons in 15 Negro families in Baltimore. Blood, *21*:261, 1963.

59. Cooperative Urea Trials Group: Clinical trials of therapy for sickle cell vaso-occlusive crises. J.A.M.A., *228*:1120, 1974.

60. Cooperative urea trials group: Treatment of sickle cell crisis with urea in invert sugar. A controlled trial. J.A.M.A., *228*:1125, 1974.

61. Cunningham, F. G., and Pritchard, J. A.: Prophylactic transfusions of normal red blood cells during pregnancies complicated by sickle cell hemoglobinopathies. Am. J. Obstet. Gynecol., *135*:994, 1979.

62. Curtis, E. M.: Pregnancy in sickle cell anemia, sickle cell-hemoglobin C disease, and variants thereof. Am. J. Obstet. Gynecol., *77*:1312, 1959.

63. Davey, R. J., Esposito, D. J., Jacobson, R. J., and Corn, M.: Partial exchange transfusion as treatment for hemoglobin SC disease in pregnancy. Arch. Intern. Med., *138*:937, 1978.

64. Eisenstein, M. I., Posner, A. C., and Friedman, S.: Sickle-cell anemia in pregnancy. A review of the literature with additional case histories. Am. J. Obstet. Gynecol., *72*:622, 1956.

65. Fiakpui, E. Z., and Moran, E. M.: Pregnancy in the sickle hemoglobinopathies. J. Reprod. Med., *11*:28, 1973.

66. Fleming, A. F., and Lynch, W.: Beta-thalassaemia minor during pregnancy, with particular reference to iron status. J. Obstet. Gynaecol. Br. Commonw., *76*:451, 1969.

67. Fort, A. T., Morrison, J. C., Berreras, L., Diggs, L. W., and Fish, S. A.: Counseling the patient with sickle cell disease about reproduction: Pregnancy outcome does not justify the maternal risk. Am. J. Obstet. Gynecol., *111*:391, 1971.

68. Freeman, M. G., and Ruth, G. J.: SS disease, SC disease, and CC disease — obstetric considerations and treatment. Clin. Obstet. Gynecol., *12*:134, 1969.

69. Hendrickse, J. P. de V., Harrison, K. A., Watson-Williams, E. J., Luzzatto, L., and Ajabor, L. N.: Pregnancy in homozygous sickle-cell anaemia. J. Obstet. Gynaecol. Br. Commonw., *79*:396, 1972.

70. Hendrickse, J. P. de V., and Watson-Williams, E. J.: The influence of hemoglobinopathies on reproduction. Am. J. Obstet. Gynecol., *94*:739, 1966.

71. Hocking, I. W., and Ibbotson, R. N.: The effect of the beta thalassaemia trait on pregnancy with particular reference to its complications and outcome. Med. J. Aust., *2*:397, 1966.

72. Horger, E. O., III: Sickle cell and sickle cell-hemoglobin C disease during pregnancy. Obstet. Gynecol., *39*:873, 1972.

73. Jacob, G. F., and Raper, A. B.: Hereditary persistence of foetal haemoglobin production, and its interaction with the sickle-cell trait. Br. J. Haematol., *4*:138, 1958.

74. Jimenez, C. T., Scott, R. B., Henry, W. L., Sampson, C. C., and Ferguson, A. D.: Studies in sickle cell anemia. XXVI. The effects of homozygous sickle cell disease on the onset of menarche, pregnancy, fertility, pubescent changes, and body growth in Negro subjects. Am. J. Dis. Child, *111*:497, 1966.

75. Kazazian, H. H., Jr., Phillips, J. A., III, Boehm, C. D., Vik, T. A., Mahoney, M. J., and Ritchey, A. K.: Prenatal diagnosis of β-thalassemias by amniocentesis: Linkage analysis using multiple polymorphic restriction endonuclease sites. Blood, *56*:926, 1980.

76. Kitay, D. Z., and Perrin, E. V.: Homozygous hemoglobin C disease and pregnancy. Obstet. Gynecol., *32*:657, 1968.

77. Laros, R. K., Jr., and Kalstone, C. E.: Sickle cell β-thalassemia and pregnancy. Obstet. Gynecol., *37*:67, 1971.

78. MacIver, J. E., Went, L. N., and Irvine, R. A.: Hereditary persistence of foetal hemoglobin: A family study suggesting allelism of the F gene to the S and C haemoglobin genes. Br. J. Haematol., *7*:373, 1961.

79. Mason, V. C., and West, G. A.: The hemoglobinopathies and the sickling phenomenon in pregnancy. J. Natl. Med. Assoc., *55*:538, 1963.

80. McCurdy, P. R.: Abnormal hemoglobins and pregnancy. Am. J. Obstet. Gynecol., 90:891, 1964.
81. Milner, P. F.: The sickling disorders. Clin. Haematol., 3:289, 1974.
82. Milner, P. F., Jones, B. R., and Döbler, J.: Outcome of pregnancy in sickle cell anemia and sickle cell–hemoglobin C disease. Am. J. Obstet. Gynecol., 138:239, 1980.
83. Morrison, J. C., Schneider, J. M., Whybrew, W. D., Bucovaz, E. T., and Menzel, D. M.: Prophylactic transfusions in pregnant patients with sickle hemoglobinopathies: Benefit versus risk. Obstet. Gynecol., 56:274, 1980.
84. Necheles, T.: Obstetric complications associated with haemoglobinopathies. Clin. Haematol., 2:497, 1973.
85. Orlina, A. R., Unger, P. J., and Koshy, M.: Post-transfusion alloimmunization in patients with sickle cell disease. Am. J. Hematol., 5:101, 1978.
86. Pakes, J. B., Cooperberg, A. A., and Gelfand, M. M.: Studies on beta thalassemia trait in pregnancy. Am. J. Obstet. Gynecol., 108:1217, 1970.
87. Pearson, H. A., and Vaughan, E. O.: Lack of influence of sickle cell trait on fertility and successful pregnancy. Am. J. Obstet. Gynecol., 105:203, 1969.
88. Perkins, R. P.: Inherited disorders of hemoglobin synthesis and pregnancy. Am. J. Obstet. Gynecol., 111:120, 1971.
89. Peterson, C. M., Tsairis, P., Ohnishi, A., Lu, Y. S., Grady, R., Cerami, A., and Dyck, P. J.: Sodium cyanate induced polyneuropathy in patients with sickle-cell disease. Ann. Intern. Med., 81:152, 1974.
90. Pritchard, J. A., Scott, D. D., Whalley, P. J., Cunningham, F. G., and Mason, R. A.: The effects of maternal sickle cell hemoglobinopathies and sickle cell trait on reproductive performance. Am. J. Obstet. Gynecol., 117:662, 1973.
91. Ricks, P.: Exchange transfusion in sickle cell anemia and pregnancy. Obstet. Gynecol., 25:117, 1965.
92. Sternberg, H.: Sickle cell–thalassemia and pregnancy. Aust. N. Z. J. Obstet. Gynaecol., 5:198, 1965.
93. van Enk, A., White, J. M., and Lehmann, J.: Benign obstetric history in women with sickle-cell anaemia associated with α-thalassaemia. Br. Med. J., 4:524, 1972.
94. Whalley, P. J., Pritchard, J. A., and Richards, J. R., Jr.: Sickle cell trait and pregnancy. J.A.M.A., 186:1132, 1963.

DISORDERS OF BLOOD COAGULATION AND PLATELETS

95. Ahn, Y. S., and Harrington, W. J.: Treatment of idiopathic thrombocytopenic purpura (ITP). Ann. Rev. Med., 28:299, 1977.
96. Anthony, B., and Krivit, W.: Neonatal thrombocytopenic purpura. Pediatrics, 30:776, 1962.
97. Arias, F., and Mancilla-Jimenez, R.: Hepatic fibrinogen deposits in pre-eclampsia. N. Engl. J. Med., 295:578, 1976.
98. Ballard, P. L., Granberg, P., and Ballard, R. A.: Glucocorticoid levels in maternal and cord serum after prenatal betamethasone therapy to prevent respiratory distress syndrome. J. Clin. Invest., 56:1548, 1975.
99. Basu, H. K.: Fibrinolysis and abruptio placentae. J. Obstet. Gynaecol. Br. Commonw., 76:481, 1969.
100. Beitins, I. Z., Bayard, F., Ances, I. G., Kowarski, A., and Migeon, C. J.: The transplacental passage of prednisone and prednisolone in pregnancy near term. J. Pediatr., 81:936, 1972.
101. Bell, W. R.: Disseminated intravascular coagulation. Johns Hopkins Med. J., 146:289, 1980.
102. Bell, W. R., and Wentz, A. C.: Abortion and coagulation by prostaglandin. J.A.M.A., 225:1082, 1973.
103. Bennett, B., and Ratnoff, O. D.: Changes in antihemophilic factor (AHF, Factor VIII) procoagulant activity and AHF-like antigen in normal pregnancy, and following exercise and pneumoencephalography. J. Lab. Clin. Med., 80:256, 1972.
104. Bennett, B., and Ratnoff, O. D.: Detection of the carrier state for classic hemophilia. N. Engl. J. Med., 288:342, 1973.
105. Bennett, B., Ratnoff, O. D., and Levin, J.: Immunologic studies in von Willebrand's disease. J. Clin. Invest., 51:2597, 1972.
106. Birmingham Eclampsia Study Group: Intravascular coagulation and abnormal lung-scans in pre-eclampsia and eclampsia. Lancet, 2:889, 1971.
107. Bonnar, J., McNichol, G. P., and Douglas, A. S.: Fibrinolytic enzyme system and pregnancy. Br. Med. J., 3:387, 1969.
108. Bonnar, J., McNichol, G. P., and Douglas, A. S.: Coagulation and fibrinolytic mechanisms during and after normal childbirth. Br. Med. J., 2:200, 1970.
109. Bonnar, J., McNichol, G. P., and Douglas, A. S.: Coagulation and fibrinolytic systems in pre-eclampsia and eclampsia. Br. Med. J., 2:12, 1971.
110. Brenner, W. E., Fishburne, J. I., McMillan, C. W., Johnson, A. M., and Hendricks, C. H.: Coagulation changes during abortion induced by prostaglandin $F_2\alpha$. Am. J. Obstet. Gynecol., 117:1080, 1973.
111. Caplan, S. N., and Berkman, E. M.: Immunosuppressive therapy of idiopathic thrombocytopenic purpura. Med. Clin. North Am., 60:971, 1976.
111a. Cimo, P. L., and Aster, R. H.: Post-transfusion purpura. Successful treatment by exchange transfusion. N. Engl. J. Med., 287:290, 1972.
112. Cines, D. B., and Schreiber, A. D.: Immune thrombocytopenia. N. Engl. J. Med., 300:106, 1979.
113. Colman, R. W., Robboy, S. J., and Minna, J. D.: Disseminated intravascular coagulation (DIC): An approach. Am. J. Med., 52:679, 1972.
114. Coopland, A., Alkjaersig, N., and Fletcher, A. P.: Reduction in plasma factor XIII (fibrin stabilizing factor) concentration during pregnancy. J. Lab. Clin. Med., 73:144, 1969.
115. Corrigan, J. J., Jr., and Jordan, C. M.: Heparin therapy in septicemia with disseminated intravascular coagulation. Effect on mortality and on correction of hemostatic defects. N. Engl. J. Med., 283:778, 1970.
116. Courtney, L. D.: Amniotic fluid embolism. Obstet. Gynecol. Surv., 29:169, 1974.
116a. Deykin, D.: The clinical challenge of disseminated intravascular coagulation. N. Engl. J. Med., 283:636, 1970.
117. DiFino, S. M., Lachant, N. A., Kirshner, J. J., and Gottlieb, A. J.: Adult idiopathic thrombocytopenic purpura. Am. J. Med., 69:430, 1980.
118. Dixon, R. E.: Disseminated intravascular coagulation: A paradox of thrombosis and hemorrhage. Obstet. Gynecol. Surv., 28:385, 1973.
119. Dube, B., Bhattacharya, S., and Dube, R. K.: Blood coagulation profile in Indian patients with pre-eclampsia and eclampsia. Br. J. Obstet. Gynaecol., 82:35, 1975.
120. Dubois, J., Morel, H., and Le Guen, C.: Accouchement d'une femme atteinte d'une maladie de Willebrand. Bull. Féd. Soc. Gynecol. Obstét., 19:361, 1967.
121. Epstein, R. D., Lozner, E. L., Cobbey, T. S., Jr., and Davidson, C. S.: Congenital thrombocytopenic purpura. Purpura hemorrhagica in pregnancy and in the newborn. Am. J. Med., 9:44, 1950.
122. Evans, P. C.: Obstetric and gynecologic patients with von Willebrand's disease. Obstet. Gynecol., 38:37, 1971.
123. Feinstein, D. I., and Rapaport, S. I.: Acquired inhibitors of blood coagulation. Prog. Hemostasis Thromb., 1:75, 1972.
124. Finch, S. C., Castro, O., Cooper, M., Covey, W., Erichson, R., and McPhedran, P.: Immunosuppressive therapy of chronic idiopathic thrombocytopenic purpura. Am. J. Med., 56:4, 1974.
125. Firshein, S. I., Hoyer, L. W., Lazarchick, J., Forget, B. G., Hobbins, J. C., Clyne, L. P., Pitlick, F. A., Muir, W. A., Merkatz, I. R., and Mahoney, M. J.: Prenatal diagnosis of classic hemophilia. N. Engl. J. Med., 300:937, 1979.
126. Fletcher, A. P., Alkjaersig, N. K., and Burstein, R.: The influence of pregnancy upon blood coagulation and plasma fibrinolytic enzyme function. Am. J. Obstet. Gynecol., 134:743, 1979.
127. Frick, P. G.: Hemophilia-like disease following pregnancy with transplacental transfer of an acquired circulating anticoagulant. Blood, 8:598, 1953.
128. Funkhouser, J. D., Peevy, K. J., Mockridge, P. B., and Hughes, E. R.: Distribution of dexamethasone between mother and fetus after maternal administration. Pediatr. Res., 12:1053, 1978.
129. Galton, M., Merritt, K., and Beller, F. K.: Coagulation studies on the peripheral circulation of patients with toxemia of pregnancy: A study for the evaluation of disseminated intravascular coagulation in toxemia. J. Reprod. Med., 6:78, 1971.
130. Gelman, S. R., O'Leary, J. A., and Feldman, M.: von Willebrand's disease and pregnancy. South. Med. J., 65:897, 1972.
131. Goodhue, P. A., and Evans, T. S.: Idiopathic thrombocytopenic purpura in pregnancy. Obstet. Gynecol. Surv., 18:671, 1963.
132. Heinonen, O. P., Slone, D., and Shapiro, S.: Birth Defects and Drugs in Pregnancy. Littleton, Mass., Publishing Sciences Group, Inc., 1977, p. 457.

133. Henrion, R.: La maladie de Willebrand en obstétrique et en gynécologie. Rev. Fr. Gynécol. Obstét., 60:587, 1965.
134. Heys, R. F.: Child bearing and idiopathic thrombocytopenic purpura. J. Obstet. Gynaecol. Br. Commonw., 73:205, 1966.
135. Heys, R. F.: Steroid therapy for idiopathic thrombocytopenic purpura during pregnancy. Obstet. Gynecol., 28:532, 1966.
136. Hibbard, B. M., and Jeffcoate, T. N. A.: Abruptio placentae. Obstet. Gynecol., 27:155, 1966.
137. Hill, C., and Taylor, J. J.: von Willebrand's disease in obstetrics and gynaecology. J. Obstet. Gynaecol. Br. Commonw., 75:453, 1968.
138. Howie, P. W., Prentice, C. R. M., and McNicol, G. P.: Coagulation, fibrinolysis and platelet function in pre-eclampsia, essential hypertension and placental insufficiency. J. Obstet. Gynaecol. Br. Commonw., 78:992, 1971.
139. Italian Working Group: Spectrum of von Willebrand's disease: A study of 100 cases. Br. J. Haematol., 35:101, 1977.
139a. Jackson, D. P., Krevans, J. R., and Conley, C. L.: Mechanism of the thrombocytopenia that follows multiple whole blood transfusions. Trans. Assoc. Am. Phys., 69:155, 1956.
140. Jimenez, J. M., and Pritchard, J. A.: Pathogenesis and treatment of coagulation defects resulting from fetal death. Obstet. Gynecol., 32:449, 1968.
141. Jones, R. W., Asher, M. I., Rutherford, C. J., and Munro, H. M.: Autoimmune (idiopathic) thrombocytopenic purpura in pregnancy and the newborn. Br. J. Obstet. Gynecol., 84:679, 1977.
142. Jones, W. R., Storey, B., Norton, G., and Neische, F. W., Jr.: Pregnancy complicated by acute idiopathic thrombocytopenic purpura. J. Obstet. Gynaecol. Br. Commonw., 81:330, 1974.
143. Kasper, C. K., Hoag, M. S., Aggeler, P. M., and Stone, S.: Blood clotting factors in pregnancy: Factor VIII concentrations in normal and AHF-deficient women. Obstet. Gynecol., 24:242, 1964.
144. Kazmier, F. J., Bowie, E. J. W., Hagedorn, A. B., and Owen, C. A., Jr.: Treatment of intravascular coagulation and fibrinolysis (ICF) syndromes. Mayo Clin. Proc., 49:665, 1974.
145. Kitzmiller, J. L., Lang, J. E., Yelenosky, P. F., and Lucas, W. E.: Hematologic assays in pre-eclampsia. Am. J. Obstet. Gynecol., 118:362, 1974.
146. Kleiner, G. J., Merskey, C., Johnson, A. J., and Markus, W. B.: Defibrination in normal and abnormal parturition. Br. J. Haematol., 19:159, 1970.
147. Laros, R. K., Jr., Collins, J., Penner, J. A., Hage, M. L., and Smith, S.: Coagulation changes in saline-induced abortion. Am. J. Obstet. Gynecol., 116:277, 1973.
148. Laros, R. K., Jr., and Penner, J. A.: Pathophysiology of disseminated intravascular coagulation in saline-induced abortion. Obstet. Gynecol., 48:353, 1976.
149. Laros, R. K., Jr., and Sweet, R. L.: Management of idiopathic thrombocytopenic purpura during pregnancy. Am. J. Obstet. Gynecol., 122:182, 1975.
149a. Levin, J.: Chemotherapy and thrombopoiesis. In Brodsky, I., Kahn, S. B., and Conroy, J. F. (eds.): Cancer Chemotherapy III. New York, Grune and Stratton, 1978, pp. 313–325.
150. Lian, E. C-Y., and Deykin, D.: Diagnosis of von Willebrand's disease. Am. J. Med., 60:344, 1976.
151. Lopez-Llera, M., de la Luz Espinosa, M., de Leon, M. D., and Rubio Linares, G.: Abnormal coagulation and fibrinolysis in eclampsia. Am. J. Obstet. Gynecol., 124:681, 1976.
152. Mant, M. J., and King, E. G.: Severe, acute disseminated intravascular coagulation. A reappraisal of its pathophysiology, clinical significance and therapy based on 47 patients. Am. J. Med., 67:557, 1979.
153. Marengo-Rowe, A. J., Murff, G., Leveson, J. E., and Cook, J.: Hemophilia-like disease associated with pregnancy. Obstet. Gynecol., 40:56, 1972.
154. Margolius, A., Jackson, D. P., and Ratnoff, O. D.: Circulating anticoagulants: A study of 40 cases and a review of the literature. Medicine, 40:145, 1961.
155. McCammon, R. E.: Pregnancy complicated by pseudohemophilia (von Willebrand's disease). J. Indiana State Med. Assoc., 60:1363, 1967.
156. McMillan, R.: Chronic idiopathic thrombocytopenic purpura. N. Engl. J. Med., 304:1135, 1981.
157. Merskey, C.: Diagnosis and treatment of intravascular coagulation. Br. J. Haematol., 15:523, 1968.
157a. Merskey, C., Johnson, A. J., Kleiner, G. J., and Wohl, H.: The defibrination syndrome: Clinical features and laboratory diagnosis. Br. J. Haematol., 13:528, 1967.
158. Noller, K. L., Bowie, E. J. W., Kempers, R. D., and Owen, C.

A., Jr.: Von Willebrand's disease in pregnancy. Obstet. Gynecol., 41:865, 1973.
159. Noriega-Guerra, L., Aviles-Miranda, A., de la Cadena, O. A., Espinosa, L. M., Chavez, F., and Pizzuto, J.: Pregnancy in patients with autoimmune thrombocytopenic purpura. Am. J. Obstet. Gynecol., 133:439, 1979.
160. Nossel, H. L., Lanzkowsky, P., Levy, S., Mibashan, R. S., and Hansen, J. D. L.: A study of coagulation factor levels in women during labour and in their newborn infants. Thromb. Diath. Haemorrh., 16:185, 1966.
161. O'Reilly, R. A.: Problems of haemorrhage and thrombosis in pregnancy. Clin. Haematol., 2:543, 1973.
162. O'Reilly, R. A., and Taber, B-Z.: Immunologic thrombocytopenic purpura and pregnancy. Obstet. Gynecol., 51:590, 1978.
163. Peterson, O. H., and Larson, D.: Thrombocytopenic purpura in pregnancy. Obstet. Gynecol., 4:454, 1954.
164. Phillips, L. L., and Davidson, E. C., Jr.: Procoagulant properties of amniotic fluid. Am. J. Obstet. Gynecol., 113:911, 1972.
165. Phillips, L. L., Rosano, L., and Skrodelis, V.: Changes in factor XI (plasma thromboplastin antecedent) levels during pregnancy. Am. J. Obstet. Gynecol., 116:1114, 1973.
166. Picozzi, V. J., Roeske, W. R., and Creger, W. P.: Fate of therapy failures in adult idiopathic thrombocytopenic purpura. Am. J. Med., 69:690, 1980.
167. Preston, A. E.: The plasma concentration of factor VIII in the normal population. I. Mothers and babies at birth. Br. J. Haematol., 10:110, 1964.
168. Pritchard, J. A.: Haematological problems associated with delivery, placental abruption, retained dead fetus and amniotic fluid embolism. Clin. Haematol., 2:563, 1973.
169. Pritchard, J. A., and Brekken, A. L.: Clinical and laboratory studies on severe abruptio placentae. Am. J. Obstet. Gynecol., 97:681, 1967.
170. Pritchard, J. A., Cunningham, F. G., and Mason, R. A.: Coagulation changes in eclampsia: Their frequency and pathogenesis. Am. J. Obstet. Gynecol., 124:855, 1976.
171. Pritchard, J. A., and Pritchard, S. A.: Standardized treatment of 154 consecutive cases of eclampsia. Am. J. Obstet. Gynecol., 123:543, 1975.
172. Pritchard, J. A., Ratnoff, O. D., and Weisman, R., Jr.: Hemostatic defects and increased red cell destruction in pre-eclampsia and eclampsia. Obstet. Gynecol., 4:159, 1954.
173. Reid, D. E.: Acquired coagulation defects in pregnancy. Obstet. Gynecol. Surv., 20:431, 1965.
174. Robboy, S. J., Lewis, E. J., Schur, P. H., and Colman, R. W.: Circulating anticoagulants to factor VIII. Immunochemical studies and clinical response to factor VIII concentrates. Am. J. Med., 49:742, 1970.
174a. Roberts, J. M., and May, W. J.: Consumptive coagulopathy in severe preeclampsia. Obstet. Gynecol., 48:163, 1976.
174b. Rock, R. C., Bove, J. R., and Nemerson, Y.: Heparin treatment of intravascular coagulation accompanying hemolytic transfusion reactions. Transfusion, 9:57, 1969.
175. Scott, J. R., Cruikshank, D. P., Kochenour, N. K., Pitkin, R. M., and Warenski, J. C.: Fetal platelet counts in the obstetric management of immunologic thrombocytopenic purpura. Am. J. Obstet. Gynecol., 136:495, 1980.
176. Scott, J. S.: Coagulation failure in obstetrics. Br. Med. Bull., 24:32, 1968.
177. Shapiro, S. S., and Hultin, M.: Acquired inhibitors to the blood coagulation factors. Semin. Thromb. Hemostas., 1:336, 1975.
178. Shaw, S. T., Jr., and Ballard, C. A.: Subclinical coagulopathy following amnioinfusion with hypertonic saline. Am. J. Obstet. Gynecol., 118:1081, 1974.
179. Sonoda, T., Solomon, A., Kraus, S., Cruz, P., Jones, F. S., and Levin, J.: Use of prothrombin complex concentrates in the treatment of a hemophilic patient with an inhibitor of Factor VIII. Blood, 47:983, 1976.
180. Spivak, J. L., Spangler, D. B., and Bell, W. R.: Defibrinogenation after intra-amniotic injection of hypertonic saline. N. Engl. J. Med., 287:321, 1972.
181. Talbert, L. M., Adcock, D. F., Weiss, A. E., Easterling, W. E., Jr., and Odom, M. H.: Studies on the pathogenesis of clotting defects during salt-induced abortions. Am. J. Obstet. Gynecol., 115:656, 1973.
182. Tancer, M. L.: Idiopathic thrombocytopenic purpura and pregnancy. Am. J. Obstet. Gynecol., 79:148, 1960.
183. Telfer, M. C., and Chediak, J.: Factor-VIII-related disorders and their relationship to pregnancy. J. Reprod. Med., 19:211, 1977.
184. Territo, M., Finklestein, J., Oh, W., Hobel, C., and Kattlove,

H.: Management of autoimmune thrombocytopenia in pregnancy and in the neonate. Obstet. Gynecol., *41*:579, 1973.

184a. Thatcher, L. G., Clatanoff, D. V., and Stiehm, E. R.: Splenic hemangioma with thrombocytopenia and afibrinogenemia. J. Pediatr., *73*:345, 1968.

185. Todd, M. E., Thompson, J. H., Jr., Bowie, E. J. W., and Owen, C. A., Jr.: Changes in blood coagulation during pregnancy. Mayo Clin. Proc., *40*:370, 1965.

186. van Creveld, S., Kloosterman, G. J., Mochtar, I. A., and Koppe, J. G.: Interchange between blood of mother and fetus in vascular hemophilia. Biol. Neonate, *4*:379, 1962.

187. Walker, E. H., and Dormandy, K. M.: The management of pregnancy in von Willebrand's disease. J. Obstet. Gynaecol. Br. Commonw., *75*:459, 1968.

188. Winckelmann, G., Groh, R., Schneider, J., and Huber, P.: Pregnancy and childbirth in von Willebrand's disease. Ger. Med. Monthly, *12*:208, 1967.

188a. Zeigler, Z., Murphy, S., and Gardner, F. H.: Post-transfusion purpura. A heterogeneous syndrome. Blood, *45*:529, 1975.

189. Zimmerman, T. S., Ratnoff, O. D., and Powell, A. E.: Immunologic differentiation of classic hemophilia (Factor VIII deficiency) and von Willebrand's disease. J. Clin. Invest., *50*:244, 1971.

ANTICOAGULATION

190. Bell, W. R., and Royall, R. M.: Heparin-associated thrombocytopenia: A comparison of three heparin preparations. N. Engl. J. Med., *303*:902, 1980.

191. Brambel, C. E., and Hunter, R. E.: Effect of dicumarol on the nursing infant. Am. J. Obstet. Gynecol., *59*:1153, 1950.

192. Eckstein, H. B., and Jack, B.: Breast-feeding and anticoagulant therapy. Lancet, *1*:672, 1970.

193. Fillmore, S. J., and McDevitt, E.: Effects of coumarin compounds on the fetus. Ann. Intern. Med., *73*:731, 1970.

194. Finnerty, J. J., and MacKay, B. R.: Antepartum thrombophlebitis and pulmonary embolism. Obstet. Gynecol., *19*:405, 1962.

195. Hall, J. G., Pauli, R. M., and Wilson, K. M.: Maternal and fetal sequelae of anticoagulation during pregnancy. Am. J. Med., *68*:122, 1980.

196. Hirsh, J., Cade, J. F., and Gallus, A. S.: Anticoagulants in pregnancy: A review of indications and complications. Am. Heart J., *83*:301, 1972.

197. Hirsh, J., Cade, J. F., and O'Sullivan, E. F.: Clinical experience with anticoagulant therapy during pregnancy. Br. Med. J., *1*:270, 1970.

198. Kerber, I. J., Warr, O. S., III, and Richardson, C.: Pregnancy in a patient with a prosthetic mitral valve. J.A.M.A., *203*:223, 1968.

199. Koch-Weser, J., and Sellers, E. M.: Drug interactions with coumarin anticoagulants. N. Engl. J. Med., *285*:487, 547, 1971.

200. Kronick, J., Phelps, N. E., McCallion, D. J., and Hirsch, J.: Effects of sodium warfarin administered during pregnancy in mice. Am. J. Obstet. Gynecol., *118*:819, 1974.

201. O'Reilly, R. A., and Aggeler, P. M.: Determinants of the response to oral anticoagulant drugs in man. Pharmacol. Rev., *22*:35, 1970.

202. Poller, L., Thomson, J. M., and Yee, K. F.: Heparin and partial thromboplastin time: An international survey. Br. J. Haematol., *44*:161, 1980.

203. Saidi, P., Hoag, M. S., and Aggeler, P. M.: Transplacental transfer of bishydroxycoumarin in the human. J.A.M.A., *191*:761, 1965.

204. Shapiro, G. A., Huntzinger, S. W., and Wilson, J. E., III: Variation among commercial activated partial thromboplastin time reagents in response to heparin. Am. J. Clin. Pathol., *67*:477, 1977.

205. Shaul, W. L., and Hall, J. G.: Multiple congenital anomalies associated with oral anticoagulants. Am. J. Obstet. Gynecol., *127*:191, 1977.

205a. Shulman, N. R.: A mechanism of cell destruction in individuals sensitized to foreign antigens and its implications in autoimmunity. Ann. Intern. Med., *60*:506, 1964.

206. Ts'ao, C-H., Galluzzo, T. S., Lo, R., and Peterson, K. G.: Whole-blood clotting time, activated partial thromboplastin time, and whole-blood recalcification time as heparin monitoring tests. Am. J. Clin. Pathol., *71*:17, 1979.

207. Villasanta, U.: Thromboembolic disease in pregnancy. Am. J. Obstet. Gynecol., *93*:142, 1965.

208. Wingfield, J. G.: Anticoagulation for antenatal thrombo-embolic disease. J. Obstet. Gynaecol. Br. Commonw., *76*:518, 1969.

SPLENECTOMY FOR HEMATOLOGIC DISORDERS DURING PREGNANCY

209. Amorosi, E. L., and Ultmann, J. E.: Thrombotic thrombocytopenic purpura: Report of 16 cases and review of the literature. Medicine, *45*:139, 1966.

209a. Bernard, R. P., Bauman, A. W., and Schwartz, S. I.: Splenectomy for thrombotic thrombocytopenic purpura. Ann. Surg., *169*:616, 1969.

210. Bukowski, R. M., Hewlett, J. S., Reimer, R. R., Groppe, C. W., Weick, J. K., and Livingston, R. B.: Therapy of thrombotic thrombocytopenic purpura: An overview. Semin. Thromb. Hemostas., *7*:1, 1981.

211. Byrnes, J. J.: Plasma infusion in the treatment of thrombotic thrombocytopenic purpura. Semin. Thromb. Hemostas., *7*:9, 1981.

212. Crosby, W. H.: Splenectomy in hematologic disorders. N. Engl. J. Med., *286*:1252, 1972.

213. Cuttner, J.: Splenectomy, steroids, and dextran 70 in thrombotic thrombocytopenic purpura. J.A.M.A., *227*:397, 1974.

214. Goldenfarb, P. B., and Finch, S. C.: Thrombotic thrombocytopenic purpura: A ten year study. J.A.M.A., *226*:644, 1973.

215. Goodhue, P. A., and Evans, T. S.: Idiopathic thrombocytopenic purpura in pregnancy. Obstet. Gynecol. Surv., *18*:671, 1963.

216. Heys, R. F.: Childbearing and idiopathic thrombocytopenic purpura. J. Obstet. Gynaecol. Br. Commonw., *73*:205, 1966.

217. Jones, R. W., Asher, M. I., Rutherford, C. J., and Munro, H. M.: Autoimmune (idiopathic) thrombocytopenic purpura in pregnancy and the newborn. Br. J. Obstet. Gynaecol., *84*:679, 1977.

218. Kennedy, S. S., Zacharski, L. R., and Beck, J. R.: Thrombotic thrombocytopenic purpura: Analysis of 48 unselected cases. Semin. Thromb. Hemostas., *6*:341, 1980.

219. Laros, R. K., Jr., and Sweet, R. L.: Management of idiopathic thrombocytopenic purpura during pregnancy. Am. J. Obstet. Gynecol., *122*:182, 1975.

220. Mitch, W. E., Spangler, D. B., Spivak, J. L., and Bell, W. R.: Thrombotic thrombocytopenic purpura presenting with gynaecological manifestations. Lancet, *1*:849, 1973.

221. Moon, E. C., and Kitay, D. Z.: Hematologic problems in pregnancy. II. Thrombotic (thrombohemolytic) thrombocytopenic purpura. J. Reprod. Med., *9*:212, 1972.

222. Neame, P. B.: Immunologic and other factors in thrombotic thrombocytopenic purpura (TTP). Semin. Thromb. Hemostas., *6*:416, 1980.

223. O'Reilly, R. A., and Taber, B-Z: Immunologic thrombocytopenic purpura and pregnancy. Obstet. Gynecol., *51*:590, 1978.

224. Paul, J. D., Jr., Pranckun, P. P., and Grosh, J. L.: Splenectomy for thrombocytopenic purpura in pregnancy. Obstet. Gynecol., *28*:236, 1966.

225. Peterson, O. H., Jr., and Larson, P.: Thrombocytopenic purpura in pregnancy. Obstet. Gynecol., *4*:454, 1954.

226. Tancer, M. L.: Idiopathic thrombocytopenic purpura and pregnancy. Am. J. Obstet. Gynecol., *79*:148, 1960.

Gerald G. Anderson, M.D.
Mark Gibson, M.D.
John C. Hobbins, M.D.

4

OBSTETRIC MANAGEMENT OF THE HIGH RISK PATIENT

The explosion of new information in the field of maternal-fetal medicine in the last decade has been fueled by the application of basic science discoveries to clinical practice and has been aided by technologic advances. The percentage of patients classified as "high risk" in any obstetric population generally varies from 10 to 25 per cent depending upon the institution and the economic status of the population. Approximately half of these have medical complications, such as hypertension or diabetes, while the remainder have purely obstetric complications, such as premature labor or incompetent cervix. Although we will be discussing care of the patient with medical complications, the surveillance procedures are generally the same. The focus of most tests is the fetus (i.e., the fetoplacental unit), which is often adversely affected by maternal medical complications.

In 1950, the maternal and perinatal mortality rates were 83.3 per 100,000 and 39.7 per 1000,

respectively. In 1978, these rates had declined to 9.9 per 100,000 and 10.6 per 1000 nationally.[113] The 1979 perinatal mortality rate in Vermont was at a record low of 7.3 per 1000.[146] This progress is due most recently to the procedures to be described here and to improved neonatal care. The procedures include surveillance techniques, therapeutic approaches, and intervention routines, which together constitute the means to maternal safety and neonatal well-being.

ENDOCRINE SURVEILLANCE

Human pregnancy is accompanied by a progressive increase in levels of estrogen in fetal and maternal blood, maternal urine, and amniotic fluid. At term, unconjugated estrogen in the maternal compartment comprises estrone, estradiol, and estriol in roughly equivalent proportions.[143]

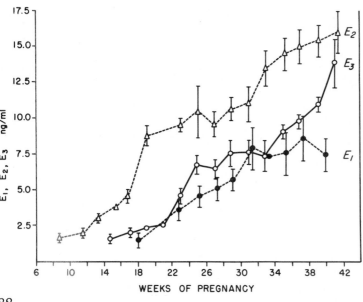

FIGURE 4-1. Mean plasma estrogen levels during human pregnancy. (From Tulchinsky et al.: Am. J. Obstet. Gynecol., 112:1095, 1972. Reprinted with permission.)

Estriol

Estriol is by far the most plentiful circulating estrogen of the conjugated species[52, 53] (Fig. 4–1, Table 4–1). Estrogen in pregnancy arises primarily from the placental aromatization of androgens produced by the fetal adrenal. The combined fetal and placental origin of estrogens, particularly estriol, is embodied by the concept of a fetal-placental endocrine unit, as introduced by Diczfalusy.[29] The dependence of maternal estrogens, particularly estriol, upon fetal viability prompted empirical application of estriol measurements as a test of fetal well-being.[56] The value of this approach has been confirmed in a variety of clinical circumstances. However, these estriol determinations are now only one element in an array of antepartum fetal assessment methods dominated by biophysical techniques discussed elsewhere in this chapter.

Androgen substrate for estrogen formation originates in both the fetal and the maternal adrenal glands. The principal adrenal androgen, dehydroepiandrosterone sulfate (DS), is secreted by the maternal adrenal in amounts approximating 40 mg per day during pregnancy. The rate of metabolic disposition of this substance increases tenfold during pregnancy.[7, 144] One third of DS in the maternal compartment is subjected to placental aromatization and is recoverable as estradiol. Metabolism of another one third of maternal DS to 16-hydroxydehydroepiandrosterone sulfate (16-OH DS) allows a direct maternal contribution to substrate for estriol synthesis.[93] However, the ultimate contribution of maternal androgens to the synthesis of estriol is relatively small. Androgens from the maternal pool are responsible for one half the estrone and estradiol found in the maternal circulation but are responsible for only 10 per cent of estriol production.

The fetal adrenal, possessing a relative impairment in 3β-ol-dehydrogenase, Δ^{4-5} isomerase, secretes an estimated 75 mg of DS per day. This striking production of adrenal androgen by the specialized fetal zone of the fetal adrenal cortex provides 90 per cent of the precursor for the synthesis of estriol. Hydroxylation at the 16 position of fetal DS occurs in the fetal liver to form 16-hydroxydehydroepiandrosterone sulfate (16-OHDS). 16-OHDS then sequentially undergoes desulfation (to 16-hydroxydehydroepiandrosterone), A-ring isomerization and reduction (to 16-hydroxyandrostenedione), aromatization (to 16-hydroxyestrone), and reduction of the oxygen function on the 17 carbon (to form estriol) within the placental compartment.[29]

Estriol thus formed in the placenta is preferentially secreted into the maternal circulation,[141] where it undergoes a variety of conjugation transformations and eventual excretion either into the urine or as a participant in the enterohepatic circulation.[3] The principal metabolic steps in the maternal compartment include conjugation with glucuronic acid at the 16 or 3 position, and 3 sulfoconjugation.[52] There are four principal conjugates in the maternal plasma: estriol-16-glucuronide (E_3-16G), estriol-3-glucuronide (E_3-3G), estriol-3-sulfate (E_3-3S), and estriol-3-sulfate-16-glucuronide (E_3-3S-16G) (Table 4–1). Biliary or urinary disposition of estriol varies from conjugate to conjugate; sulfates are preferentially found in bile entering the enterohepatic circulation, while the glucuronides are readily excreted in the urine, the renal clearance of estriol-16-glucuronide approaching that of PAH (Table 4–1).[156]

Estriol production correlates very well with fetal size,[90, 91] apparently reflecting the fact that fetal-adrenal production of dehydroepiandrosterone sulfate is a function of fetal size. In addition to a progressive rise throughout gestation, a surge in plasma unconjugated estriol is inconsistently seen at 36 weeks.[75] The fall in estriol excretion that accompanies fetal compromise in a variety of circumstances is poorly understood. In contrast to the adult, in whom

TABLE 4–1 ESTRIOL IN HUMAN PREGNANCY AT TERM*

Species	Plasma Concentration NG/ML	Renal Clearance ML/MIN	Average Urine Excretion MG/DAY
Estriol — unconjugated	7	–	–
Estriol-3-sulfate	15	30	1
Estriol-16-glucuronide	25	400	21
Estriol-3-glucuronide	10	133	5
Estriol-3-sulfate, 16-glucuronide	50	28	3

*Derived from Young, B.K., Jirku, H., Kadner, S., and Levitz 1976; and Aldercreutz, H., 1974.

stress may increase production of all adrenal steroids, there is little evidence that DS production in the fetal compartment or estriol production by the entire fetal-placental unit ever increases in the face of metabolic or physiologic challenge to the fetus.[55]

Variations in Estriol Determinations. While the usefulness of measurement of estriol in its various forms and in various compartments has been an accepted clinical dictum, it is well recognized that significant imprecision is manifest as variation in daily, hourly, or more frequent samples and can be laid in part to sampling errors and assay variance. Also, the variability in estriol measurements reflects the complex physiology of estriol production, conjugation, and disposition by various routes in the maternal compartment.[72] Disturbances in maternal physiology affecting renal function, hepatic function, and the enterohepatic circulation will introduce variability in assessment of estriol production by the fetal-placental unit. A given change may induce opposing errors in the assessment of fetal-placental estriol production in different compartments. For example, an acute decrease in renal function might result in falling urinary estriol measurements while plasma estriol would simultaneously rise. Finally, fetal ACTH levels responsible for fetal DS synthesis vary according to the amount of maternal cortisol transferred into the fetal compartment; thus, variation in maternal corticoid production (as in stress) may generate variability in fetal androgen substrate availability independently of that resulting from fetal health.[95] Other unknown factors may also affect fetal androgen synthesis aside from uteroplacental compromise; those known to affect assessment of estriol production are listed in Table 4-2.

Fetal central nervous system abnormalities or maternal glucocorticoid therapy both result in diminished estriol production because of the dependency of the fetal adrenal cortex upon ACTH for synthesis of DS. A similar effect is noted in congenital hypoplasia. Placental sulfatase deficiency is an X-linked disorder associated with dramatic reduction of estriol excretion during pregnancy.[37, 39, 108] The deficiency, well described in both whole patient and in vitro studies, is accompanied by diagnostic elevation of sulfate androgen precursors in the fetal and amniotic fluid compartments. Maternal renal compromise variably affects urinary and plasma estriol determinations.[17] Published reports of clinical experience suggest that simple generalizations cannot be made about the impact of severe renal impairment upon estriol determinations, while mild to moderate renal disease appears to affect estriol dynamics very little. In the face of significant renal impairment or changing renal function, simultaneous assessment of plasma and urinary estriol is necessary to prevent erroneous interpretation of data. Gastrointestinal disease may also affect estriol measurements.[140] Estriol excretion is lower in patients who have undergone colectomies, presumably owing to loss of reabsorptive surface for the enterohepatic circulation of estriol.[107] The impact of antibiotic therapy on estriol excretion is well known. In this instance impaired hydrolytic activity of gut flora results in diminished reabsorption of free estriol from the gastrointestinal tract, and gastrointestinal loss of this steroid is increased at the expense of urinary loss.[3] Finally, substances in the urine such as excessive glucose or the urinary antiseptic Mandelamine result in destruction of estriol during the hydrolysis steps routinely used in most urinary assays.

Despite multiple physiologic and pathophysiologic factors that may affect estriol levels, a large body of clinical data attests to the usefulness of estriol measurements in monitoring the status of

TABLE 4-2 FACTORS AFFECTING ESTIMATION OF FETO-PLACENTAL ESTRIOL PRODUCTION

Locus	Conditions
Low fetal ACTH	Maternal stress
	Maternal glucocorticoid therapy
	Anencephaly
Impaired fetal androgenesis	Congenital adrenal hypoplasia
Liberation of sulfate precursors	Placental sulfatase
Maternal renal function	Severe renal compromise
Maternal gastrointestinal	Colectomy
	Antibiotic therapy
Direct interference with assay	Mandelamine ⎱ applies to methods involving
	Glucose ⎰ hydrolysis of urinary conjugates only.

the fetus at risk.[28, 30] Clinical circumstances in which estriol measurements have been applied with success include pregnancy with diabetes,[30, 44, 51] pregnancy with hypertension,[46, 63] postdate pregnancy,[46] and intrauterine growth retardation.[91] In each of these settings the reliability of estriol measurement has been questioned. False positive decreases in serial estriol determinations are not uncommon,[28, 30, 46] and falsely reassuring values prior to fetal loss have also been seen.[128] In certain clinical circumstances, like erythroblastosis fetalis, estriol measurements are of no use whatsoever in assessing fetal well-being.[63]

Assessing Estriol Production. Several different methods of assessing estriol production are available.[53, 60] Determination of unconjugated estriol in the plasma by radioimmunoassay represents the most direct and immediate access to placental secretion of the free compound. It must be borne in mind that this measurement still depends upon the balance between secretion and disposition into a variety of compartments. Additionally, there is considerable short-term variability in unconjugated estriol levels in the plasma; an apparent diurnal variation may reflect diurnal renal function changes.[22, 72] The 95 per cent confidence limits for a single plasma estriol determination with respect to concurrent mean levels is as high as 42 per cent.[15] Assays of immunoreactive estriol in unextracted, diluted plasma measure the unconjugated species as well as the three sulfate and the three glucuronide conjugates. (These constitute about one half the total plasma estriol.)[53]

Immunoreactive estriol represents a less labile pool, whose levels represent an integral of recent estriol production. The theoretical advantage of immunoreactive as opposed to unconjugated estriol determination from the plasma has not been demonstrated to be important in clinical use.[53, 77]

Twenty-four hour urinary estriol determination is the oldest clinically applied method for assessment of fetal-placental estriol production. Classically, this method involves hydrolysis of urinary conjugates (dominated by the 16-glucuronide) and subsequent fluorometric analysis. Recent methods have eliminated the hydrolytic and extraction steps and employed direct radioimmunoassay of urinary conjugates, particularly the 16-glucuronide.[60] These methods of direct immunoassay greatly simplify the assessment of urinary estriol and theoretically provide for increased precision with fewer steps that introduce error. The 24 hour urinary estriol measurement theoretically eliminates the problem of short-term variation by integrating fetoplacental production. Disadvantages include the potential for error in the face of significantly changing or significantly impaired renal function (frequently an element of concern in a high risk obstetric patient), 24 hour lag time in assessment, and potential errors in sample collection. The adequacy of sample collection can be checked by a simultaneous assessment of creatinine excretion over the same period of time.[51] The 24 to 36 hour lag between the beginning of the collection and the receipt of a laboratory determination has prompted introduction of spot urinary estriol/creatinine ratios.[6, 92] Such measurements provide for more rapid estimation of estriol production, show excellent correlation with 24 hour values over the same period, and may vary less than plasma measurements.[77]

The appropriate frequency of estriol determination for assessment of fetal status is determined by (1) the amount of time between the fall in estriol production and fetal critical status or demise and (2) the anticipated pace of the underlying process that threatens pregnancy well-being. In the management of diabetes mellitus, daily measurements are required if estriol determinations are to be relied upon to guarantee timely intervention.[51] When the underlying deterioration is perceived to be gradual, as in postmaturity, sampling is required less frequently.[43]

In few centers today would estriol measurements alone be relied upon for assessment of fetal status; increasingly, they are used as a screen to direct the application of biophysical methods of assessment of fetal status.[28] In isolated instances, however, biochemical monitoring may prove more sensitive than standard biophysical methods.[121] Interpretation of estriol measurements must take into consideration the various sources of error just discussed. Because of the wide variability of this measurement, which cannot be attributed to alterations in fetal well-being, a decline in individual values of plasma or urinary estriol amounting to a 40 per cent fall from previously established means is required before fetal compromise is suspected.[30, 51, 77] Lesser declines from previously established means may indicate the need to increase surveillance.

Estetrol

Estetrol, or 15-hydroxyestriol, is an estrogen that is even more associated with the fetus than estriol and is found in all major compartments.

Measurements in maternal urine or blood have been applied to high risk pregnancy in much the same manner as estriol. Except possibly in cases of erythroblastosis,[63] these measurements have shown no significant advantage over those of estriol.[82, 106, 142] Measurement of the conversion of DS into estradiol in the maternal compartment, employing either tracer or bulk loading techniques, has been employed as a test of placental function.[81, 144] Although this test appears to correlate relatively well with fetal well-being, it theoretically bypasses the role of fetal androgen precursor in the genesis of falling estriol levels. Further, the test is cumbersome and complex and offers little advantage over simpler methods of biochemical monitoring. Such techniques will remain of value as research tools.[7, 45]

Steroids Other Than Estrogen

Interest in fetal glucocorticoid production is based on evidence that fetal cortisol increases at term to precipitate a series of events leading to labor[86] as well as the apparent importance of corticoids in lung maturation.[48] Studies of fetal cortisol production are made difficult by the ready placental exchange of cortisol between maternal and fetal circulations. According to observations, corticosterone sulfate of fetal origin is measurable in the maternal circulation, and there may indeed be a surge in fetal corticoid synthesis prior to labor.[36]

Amniotic Fluid Alpha-Fetoprotein (AFP)

Alpha-fetoprotein is produced by the fetal yolk sac and liver. Levels of this feto-specific protein in fetal serum and amniotic fluid fall rapidly throughout the second trimester. In open neural tube defects, AFP leaks through the exposed meninges into the amniotic fluid in very high concentrations. Spina bifida, for instance, is associated with amniotic fluid AFP levels that are more than 5 standard deviations above the mean for gestation. Other fetal abnormalities, such as intestinal obstruction, omphalocele,[103] and congenital nephrosis, are associated with high levels of amniotic fluid AFP.[11, 12, 127] By using amniotic fluid AFP alone, one can detect neural tube defects in approximately 90 per cent of those tested. In the remaining 10 per cent the defect is closed, and the AFP is unable to leak across an intact integument.

Maternal serum AFP increases slowly until the 30th week, after which the levels decline.[1] Maternal serum AFP (MSAFP) reflects the AFP level in amniotic fluid, so in cases of open neural tube defect the serum AFP is markedly elevated (more than 2.5 multiples above the median). Mass screening of the serum AFP of pregnant women during the second trimester should result in a substantial increase in the diagnosis of neural tube defects.[24] A problem encountered when using serum AFP is the high percentage of false positive results — about 95 per cent. Each patient found to have a high serum AFP must be scanned and tapped in order to identify those pregnancies truly complicated by neural tube anomaly. This type of screening will result in an appreciable increase in scans and amniocenteses. For example, for every 1000 patients screened with MSAFP, approximately 50 to 75 patients will have two elevations of more than 2.5 multiples above the mean. Only 20 of these patients will require amniocentesis, since the remaining patients will be found on ultrasound evaluation to have erroneous dating, intrauterine demise, or multiple gestation, all resulting in falsely high MSAFP levels. Only 1 to 2 patients of the 20 requiring amniocentesis will have an amniotic fluid elevation of more than 5 SD's above the mean for gestation. In many cases a thorough ultrasound examination by an operator experienced in the diagnosis of neural tube defects should enable the lesion to be characterized with regard to the location and extent of the spinal defect. Also, surgically correctable defects such as upper GI obstruction and omphalocele can be identified.

The cost, benefits, and risks (not the least of which is unnecessary patient anxiety) have been the topic of heated debate. However, in view of the fact that over 80 per cent of neural tube defects can be identified in the second trimester, it is likely that mass screening of MSAFP will become a reality.

Some investigators[127, 148] have found that many patients in whom elevations of maternal serum AFP are not associated with amniotic fluid elevations of AFP are at greater risk for fetal death, prematurity, and abruptio placentae. Even though the correlation is not invariable, one should consider monitoring fetal growth and condition in those patients whose fetuses do not have neural tube defects but in whom serum AFP levels were elevated. Since AFP values are increased in patients with twins, mass AFP screening in the second trimester should result in early identification by ultrasound of twin gestations.

Human Placental Lactogen (HPL)

Human placental lactogen, a polypeptide exhibiting extensive amino acid homology with prolactin and growth hormone, was identified in the early 1960s.[76, 122] Despite a short circulating half-life, maternal serum levels of HPL are unusually high and increase throughout pregnancy, reflecting an enormous placental production rate (1 to 3 grams per day at term).

HPL has weak somatotropic and lactogenic properties, and the growth hormone–like activity may contribute importantly to the ketogenic (lipolytic), insulin resistant, glucose-sparing tendencies of maternal energy metabolism.[119] In this regard HPL enhances maternal fat utilization and oxidation during fasting to spare carbohydrate fuel for placental transfer to the fetus. The brisk fall in insulin requirement following loss of pituitary function in pregnant diabetics (Houssay phenomenon) shows that other factors in the maternal milieu are also important to the maintenance of the maternal ketogenic, glucose-sparing state.[70]

Regulation of HPL production is poorly understood; there are no known trophic factors. Severe hypoglycemia and prolonged fasting are followed by increases in circulating levels, which may result from changes in production or in metabolic clearance of HPL.[111, 132]

HPL levels have been used to predict the outcome of threatened abortion with limited success. However, HPL determinations are easily superseded in accuracy and immediacy by ultrasound techniques, and it is unlikely that this application of HPL measurement will achieve widespread use.

HPL measurements have been employed for the evaluation of the fetus at risk in the third trimester and in some settings have found specific useful applications. Levels in the latter part of pregnancy fluctuate significantly, accounting for some of the imprecision found in single determination predictions of fetal outcome.[147] In general, there is a rough correlation between HPL levels and placental size,[46, 78, 94, 123] and in diabetes HPL levels may actually be higher than in normal pregnancy.[145]

HPL measurements are useful mainly as a screening tool. They have no utility as an on-line biochemical assessment, as is the case with estriol.[82] It is therefore not surprising that HPL fails to enhance the management of postdate pregnancy.[8] By contrast, early third trimester HPL determinations are useful in identifying fetuses at risk from advanced stages of diabetes and from hypertension.[46, 78, 100, 134] In both of these examples HPL contributes to management principally by identifying fetuses at risk from intrauterine growth retardation (IUGR). HPL screening can identify fetuses with idiopathic IUGR as well. Because IUGR frequently escapes clinical detection, the routine use of HPL may identify an otherwise unsuspected population of fetuses at risk. Such a program of routine screening can improve perinatal outcome.[130]

The accuracy of HPL screening for IUGR will vary with the population studied, the assay employed, and the definitions of normal. Low HPL levels will identify 20 to 40 per cent of fetuses with IUGR while falsely incriminating only 15 per cent of normally growing fetuses in the same population.[100, 129]

The current primacy of biophysical monitoring techniques in high risk pregnancy seems to have eclipsed any place earned by HPL measurement in the last few years. However, the test remains of interest as a one-time third trimester screening procedure for clinically occult abnormalities (usually manifest as IUGR). Its ultimate role in routine and high risk obstetrics is unclear.

ULTRASOUND

There has been a remarkable improvement in ultrasound imagery over the past few years, and the field of obstetrics has been significantly affected by these engineering triumphs to a point where most obstetricians would be uncomfortable managing high risk patients without access to ultrasonically derived information.

It has been estimated that 30 to 50 per cent of pregnant patients will be scanned. The most commonly reported examinations include (1) determination of fetal age by measurement of the biparietal diameter (BPD), (2) localization of the placenta, and (3) diagnosis of multiple gestation. In addition, ultrasound is particularly useful in monitoring fetal growth and in diagnosing congenital anomalies.

Dating. Most of the literature pertaining to the obstetric use of ultrasound has been devoted to the fetal head. In the first trimester the fetal head can be distinguished as being separate from the body, but measurement of the BPD is rarely possible until after the 12th week of gestation. The precision of estimating fetal age diminishes as pregnancy progresses. For instance, a carefully obtained BPD measurement at 18 weeks of gestation should be within ± 6 days of the true gestational age. The reason for the diminished accuracy of later examinations is the fact that in a near-term fetus there is much greater biological variation of head size than in the second trimester. Also, there is a plateau in incremental growth of the BPD in late gestation. As a result, the standard error of the method would affect the accuracy more when head growth has slowed. Validation of the patient's dates is particularly important in high risk patients, since the timetable of events scheduled for these patients is based on gestational age.

It has been estimated that 15 per cent of patients cannot recall the time of their last menstrual period (LMP). In another 15 per cent, the date given is misleading because the patient has ovulated late. Consequently, an appropriately timed BPD should be of great benefit in firmly establishing the dates of the high risk patient.

If the BPD is obtained before the 26th week of gestation, and the measurement indicates a mean gestational age that is less than 1 to 1½ weeks from the patient's dates, the dates should be considered valid. If there is more than a 1 to 1½ week difference between BPD and dates, then another ultrasound examination should be obtained at least 1 month later. In most cases, this measurement either will be colinear with the original ultrasound determination or will more closely approximate the patient's dates. In the former case, the patient's dates should be abandoned in favor of the ultrasound dating, and in the latter case the first ultrasound date should be discarded and the patient's dates accepted.

It is a common misconception that a BPD measurement is easy to perform. The measurement must be precisely performed in the proper plane or an incorrect measurement, varying by 3 to 4 mm from the proper reading, can result. Examinations performed in a cavalier manner can sometimes result in disastrous consequences.

Monitoring Fetal Growth. In the development of obstetric ultrasound it was thought that insufficient fetal growth would result in a plateau in incremental BPD growth. Indeed, the literature appearing in the early 1970s suggested that this was true. Current reports, however, have indicated that in most cases of IUGR, slowing of BPD growth is barely perceptible. Apparently, intrauterine deprivation affects the fetal body first, and the head is relatively spared. BPD growth is curtailed when the fetus is symmetrically small as a result of fetal anomalies, as seen in viral infections, chromosomal abnormalities, or renal dysplasia; symmetrical IUGR can also occur when a fetus has been subjected to deprivation for a prolonged period. In most cases, however, the fetus will have a BPD measurement that is appropriate for dates but a body measurement that is far less than expected. For this reason, investigators have found measurements of abdominal circumference (AC) to be particularly useful when compared with head circumference (HC) measurements (HC/AC ratio).[16, 66] In IUGR the head-to-body ratio is often in the 95th percentile. It is also possible to estimate fetal weight utilizing a formula dependent upon BPD and AC.[150] Since IUGR is based on weight, the deficit can be quantified by comparing estimated fetal weight with expected mean weight for gestation.

We have found estimation of total intrauterine volume (TIUV) to be a very useful screening test in the diagnosis of IUGR.[54] This is a rather simple test to perform and indirectly reflects the relative sizes of the fetus and placenta. Since oligohydramnios is the rule in IUGR and the placenta is most often smaller than expected for gestation, a TIUV measurement that is within one SD of the mean for gestation should preclude IUGR if the patient's dates are valid. Conversely, a TIUV value of more than one SD below the mean may reflect IUGR, and further evaluation is indicated.

Placental Localization. In patients with vaginal bleeding, ultrasound can be used to rule out placenta previa. When the placenta clearly is free of the cervical os, placenta previa can be excluded with assurance. On the other hand, in some cases the placenta can appear to cover the cervical os and later in pregnancy the placenta will seem to have an attachment away from the cervix. We have noted, for example, that in about 20 per cent of second trimester scans the placenta appears to be in contact with the cervix, and yet placenta previa is only found in 5 per cent of those patients afterwards. There is an explanation for this mysterious shifting of the placenta. An artificial placenta previa can be created by overdistention of the patient's bladder, thus compressing the lower uterine segment. In addition, it is often difficult to identify the exact location of the endocervical os. In some cases, the placenta actually may be touching the cervix in early pregnancy, but as pregnancy progresses, the lower segment lengthens, carrying the placenta with it. This "relative placental migration" can be demonstrated with serial scans. Since the relationship between the placenta and the lower uterine segment can change markedly in a few weeks, any patient in whom placenta previa is diagnosed weeks before term should have another scan before a decision is made empirically to perform a cesarean section.

Multiple Gestation. Twins should be easily identified with ultrasound. In fact, today a twin delivery should rarely be a surprise to the obstetrician. Early identification of a multiple gestation will often alter the management of the pregnancy.

It is now possible to diagnose the potentially lethal phenomenon of twin-to-twin transfusion. In this pathologic situation, the twins share the same blood supply and one twin donates a small but essential portion of its blood volume to the recipient. The donor becomes growth retarded, and the recipient eventually suffers from cardiac overload. Both fetuses can die before term if the vascular communication is significant. The ultrasound diagnosis of twin-to-twin transfusion can be made when a marked discrepancy is noted between the two fetal bodies and, in some cases, their heads. Once the condition is diagnosed, the twins' lives can be saved by judicious timing of delivery.

Congenital Anomalies. Centers with experience in prenatal diagnosis of fetal defects are now receiving referrals for ultrasound evaluation of many patients who have been delivered of a child with a fetal deformity or whose pregnancies are complicated by conditions known to be associated with fetal anomalies.[67]

Up until the 16th week of gestation intracranial structures such as cerebral hemispheres appear to be floating in fluid. After the 17th week of gestation, the outer margins of the lateral ventricles should not extend more than halfway between the falx and the outer skull outline. In hydrocephaly, abnormal dilation of the lateral ventricles precedes distention of the calvarium, and our experience to date suggests that in most cases this phenomenon occurs in the second trimester. Therefore, in patients at risk for hydrocephaly, ultrasound examination before the 24th week of gestation should be extremely informative. In third trimester patients the diagnosis of hydrocephaly is not difficult to make once the head circumference has attained abnormal proportions. If the fetal head circumference at any time in gestation is more than 50 cm, or if there is significant shift of midline structures, or if the cortical thickness is less than 1 cm, the prognosis is poor. Because of significant improvement in results from shunting techniques used on the neonate, the tendency today is to deliver these fetuses by cesarean section to minimize trauma to the fetal head.

Ultrasound examinations of the spine are time-consuming and require significant operator experience. However, the determination of alpha-fetoprotein levels in serum, amniotic fluid, or both, combined with careful ultrasound examination, should enable diagnosis of spina bifida to be made in more than 90 per cent of second trimester cases. Ultrasound diagnosis depends upon demonstration of a wedge-shaped defect in the fetal spine on transverse scan. It is now feasible to characterize the defect with regard to its location and extent, thereby giving patients useful information concerning the potential neurologic status of the fetus.

The heart is a clearly discerned landmark, which has become a rich source of perinatal information. Today, with high resolution real-time and M-mode ultrasound, it is possible to visualize chambers, specific valves, and great vessels. For example, the ability to diagnose tricuspid atresia, hypoplastic right ventricle, and an A-V tunnel defect (associated with Down's syndrome) has recently been reported.[79]

Obstruction to the gastrointestinal tract proximal to the distal ileum is most often associated with polyhydramnios. The diagnosis of esophageal atresia may be difficult with ultrasound, because in many cases amniotic fluid may be diverted around the obstruction through the trachea, and the fetal stomach is still visualized. However, obstruction distal to the stomach and proximal to the distal ileum is associated with marked distention of the fetal stomach. Duodenal atresia classically presents as a double echo-spared area within the upper fetal abdomen. Ileovolvulus can present with a similar picture. Other conditions associated with multiple dilated loops of bowel include imperforate anus, congenital megacolon, and meconium ileus.

The finding of oligohydramnios should alert the physician to investigate a renal cause for this abnormality. Diminution of amniotic fluid associated with nonfunctioning kidneys or obstruction to the lower urinary tract results in fetal crowding and a markedly contracted uterine cavity. Both kidneys at the level of the umbilical vein should not occupy more than one third of the intraabdominal area. Kidney diameters increase linearly as pregnancy progresses, but the ratio of mean kidney circumference to abdominal circumference is remarkably constant throughout gestation. A variety of anomalous conditions can affect the fetal kidneys, and many result in bilateral or unilateral kidney enlargement. Infantile polycystic kidney disease is one such condition; multicystic kidney disease and renal dysplasia are others. Obstruction to the urinary tract will produce ultrasound findings that vary according to the level of obstruction. Urethral strictures will result in a massively enlarged bladder and hydronephrotic kidneys, for instance.

Most forms of skeletal dysplasia affect the

fetal limbs by the 20th week of gestation. Since fetal limb measurements can now be made with ultrasound measurements of long bones in the second trimester, this technique should enable the diagnosis of these conditions to be made.

AMNIOTIC FLUID

Because the fetus sheds cells into the amniotic fluid, excretes metabolic by-products into it, and also exhales small amounts of this fluid, investigators have used amniotic fluid as a potent source of information about fetal condition, development, and maturity.

Amniocentesis. In 1956, Bevis described the analysis of bilirubin pigments in amniotic fluid in Rh-sensitized pregnancies.[9] In the mid 1960s, reports began to emerge concerning the use of components of amniotic fluid in the third trimester to predict fetal maturity. In 1973, the potential to culture fetal cells from second trimester amniotic fluid specimens was realized.[89] This established the feasibility of karyotypic analysis in fetuses at risk for chromosome disorders. Recently, more specific tests have been designed to detect phospholipids involved in fetal pulmonic maturation. In view of the justifiably heightened interest in the study of amniotic fluid constituents, we estimate that at present about 20 per cent of "high risk" patients will have an amniocentesis in the third trimester, and a majority of second trimester patients over 35 years of age (and therefore at greater risk of having a fetus with Down's syndrome) will be referred for an amniocentesis.

In 1968, a study by Creasman suggested that a third trimester amniocentesis is a relatively safe procedure.[26] Since then there have been other studies to support the earlier impressions concerning the safety of the technique in the second and third trimesters.[102, 116] With the advent of ultrasound, however, the element of chance has been removed from amniocentesis. Armed with ultrasound information, the physician can determine the exact position of the intrauterine contents and choose a pocket of amniotic fluid away from fetal vital parts and, in most cases, the placenta. In our experience we have found that with ultrasound the procedure is easier, fewer needle insertions are required, and the incidence of bloody taps is decreased. It also simply makes sense for the operator to know the location of the fetus, umbilical cord, and placenta before approaching the uterus with a sharp needle. The incidence of premature labor or fetal injury in third trimester amniocentesis has recently been

estimated to be about 1 per cent (although in our experience it is significantly lower). Procedure-related fetal death and abortion are reported to be between 0.5[116] and 1 to 2 per cent[154] in second trimester taps.

Analysis of Fetal Condition. Since the introduction of Rh-immune globulin, the incidence of erythroblastosis fetalis has diminished appreciably. Nevertheless, tertiary centers are still receiving referrals of Rh-sensitized patients who either received insufficient dosage of the anti-immune globulin in a previous pregnancy, were first pregnant before this substance became available, or became sensitized as a result of a silent feto-maternal transfusion during a previous pregnancy or abortion. Also, other antibodies, such as Kell, C^w, C, and E, are capable of causing erythroblastosis fetalis, for which there is no means of prophylaxis.

In this potentially lethal condition the mother, after sensitization, develops antibodies against fetal erythrocytes. The antibody, which is a 7S globulin, crosses the placenta, ultimately resulting in the removal of red cells from the fetal circulation because of decreased red cell survival. The anemic fetus attempts to compensate by activating erythropoiesis in the spleen, liver, and placenta. As a result of red cell destruction, indirect bilirubin accumulates in the amniotic fluid, through an unknown mechanism. This can be indirectly quantified by spectrophotometric analysis of amniotic fluid. Indirect bilirubin is absorbed at a wave length of 450 mμ. The amount of indirect bilirubin can be indirectly measured by assessing the degree of absorption at 450 mμ compared with an expected reading at this wavelength (ΔOD).

Liley designed a graph to simplify management of Rh disease.[88] If the ΔOD falls into Zone I, the fetus either is in excellent condition or is Rh negative and not affected with the disease. A ΔOD low in Zone II suggests that the fetus is affected but tolerating the condition well. A high Zone II reading is cause for concern, and, depending upon the slope of the ΔOD rise and how close the value is to Zone III, the patient should be retapped in one week, or delivered within a few days, or an intrauterine transfusion should be performed. A ΔOD$_{450}$ value in Zone III indicates a severely compromised fetus that will die unless delivered or transfused within a week.

Generally, amniocentesis is utilized in previously unsensitized patients whose antibody titers (Coombs) rise above 1:8 or in those whose previous infants were shown to have erythroblastosis fetalis. Amniocenteses, once initiated, are usually performed every 2 weeks until delivery unless the results indicate the desirability of more frequent intervals.

Fetal Maturity. The respiratory distress syndrome (RDS) consists of progressive atelectasis of the lungs of a newborn infant caused by an increase in surface tension. Normally, the pulmonary alveoli are lined with a surface-active phospholipid-protein complex, called pulmonary surfactant, which decreases surface tension, thereby facilitating lung expansion and preventing atelectasis. In full-term infants, surfactant is present at birth in sufficient amounts to permit adequate lung expansion and normal breathing. In premature infants, however, surfactant is present in lesser amounts, and when it is insufficient, postnatal lung expansion and ventilation are frequently impaired, presenting as the clinical stigmata of the respiratory distress syndrome.

Phosphatidylcholine (lecithin) has been identified as a major lipid of the surfactant complex.[50] Beginning at 20 to 22 weeks of pregnancy, a less stable and less active lecithin, palmitoylmyristoyl lecithin, is formed. Hence, a premature infant does not always develop respiratory distress syndrome; however, in addition to the lesser activity of this lecithin, its synthesis is more susceptible to stress and acidosis, making the premature infant more vulnerable to respiratory distress syndrome. At about the 35th week of gestation, there is a sudden surge of dipalmitoyl lecithin, the major surfactant lecithin, which is stable and very active. Since the fetal lungs contribute to the formation of amniotic fluid, and the sphingomyelin concentration of amniotic fluid changes relatively little throughout pregnancy, measurement of the lecithin/sphingomyelin (L/S) ratio indicates the change that occurs at approximately 34 to 36 weeks of pregnancy, when the great increase in dipalmitoyl lecithin takes place.

Gluck began analyzing amniotic fluid for the presence of lecithin.[49] Since the concentration of any substance is dependent upon the amount of diluent, lecithin values theoretically would be affected by the amniotic fluid volume. In an effort to diminish the effect of polyhydramnios or oligohydramnios, Gluck began his investigation by comparing the lecithin concentration with that of sphingomyelin, another phospholipid. The latter compound was used as an internal standard, and the two values were expressed as a ratio of L to S.

A specimen of amniotic fluid is centrifuged at 5000 rpm as soon as possible, precipitated with methanol, and extracted with chloroform. The chloroform extract is dried, and cold acetone is added to concentrate that portion of the total lecithin which is surface-active. After centrifugation and draining of the acetone, the precipitate is taken up with chloroform and spotted on a silica gel H thin-layer chromatography plate with a 5 per cent ammonium sulfate binder. Quantification of the lecithin and sphingomyelin spots is best achieved by a densitometer, although some laboratories utilize area measurements obtained by calipers or planimeter.

Initially Gluck and coworkers correlated L/S ratio results with the pregnancy outcome with regard to the presence or absence of RDS.[49] They found that the concentration of sphingomyelin tended to drop as pregnancy progressed, while lecithin levels began to rise steeply after the 32nd week of gestation. Before the 28th week of gestation, the L/S ratio was less than 1:1, but the mean ratio rose to 2:1 at about 35 weeks (Fig. 4–2). The investigators also noted in their initial study that if an infant was delivered before the critical ratio was attained, the infant did develop RDS. This report generated much excitement, and other investigators initiated testing with Gluck's original method. Their expanded data confirmed the strong correlation between an L/S ratio above 2:1 and the absence of RDS. L/S ratios below 2:1, however, were by no means consistent predictors of pulmonic immaturity. In fact, more recent collaborative data

FIGURE 4–2. The mean L/S ratios throughout normal pregnancy, illustrating the rise to a mature level (greater than 2.0) at 34 to 36 weeks of pregnancy. (From Gluck and Kulovich, Am. J. Obstet. Gynecol., *115*:539, 1973. Reprinted with permission.)

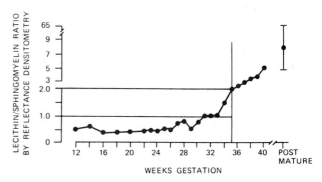

WEEKS GESTATION

indicate that an L/S ratio between 1.5:1 and 1.9:1 (intermediate or transitional ratio) is associated with only a 20 per cent chance of RDS when infants are delivered within a few days after the tap. Ratios of less than 1.5:1 are associated with a 78 per cent chance of RDS, and 50 per cent of these infants die. From these and other data one could conclude that the lower the ratio, the higher the chances of RDS. Despite a very tight correlation between an L/S ratio of 2:1 or greater and pulmonic maturity, there were exceptions to this relationship. In some studies, RDS occurred in up to 3 per cent of infants when delivery was preceded by an L/S ratio greater than 2:1. Many of these falsely predictive results were in diabetic patients and in those whose pregnancies were complicated by intrapartum asphyxia.

One group reported a 0 per cent incidence of RDS in infants of diabetics with L/S ratios of 2:1 or more if the infants were delivered at 38 weeks of gestation or later.[101] The spurious results occurred only when the infant was delivered before 37 weeks of gestation.

The L/S ratio must be precisely performed, and studies that show a poorer predictive correlation than just stated usually involve a modification of the original method. These less-than-ideal results should be attributed not to the test itself but to the modification of the method.

Blood and meconium contamination of the amniotic fluid specimen will alter the L/S ratio. Since meconium has an unpredictable effect on the ratio, it is unwise to make judgments based on L/S ratios performed on meconium-stained fluid. The L/S ratio of maternal blood is about 1.49:1, so if the fetus is pulmonically mature, the addition of this blood will tend to decrease the ratio. Therefore, an L/S ratio greater than 2:1 in a blood-stained specimen should be a valid prediction of pulmonic maturity. A ratio below 1.4:1 in blood-stained amniotic fluid should be suggestive evidence of pulmonic immaturity, since the addition of blood in this case would tend to raise the L/S ratio artificially.[14]

PHOSPHATIDYL GLYCEROL (PG). Two other phospholipids have been identified in amniotic fluid, phosphatidyl glycerol (PG) and phosphatidyl inositol (PI). PG generally appears after 36 weeks, and PI begins to rise at about 30 weeks and will fall toward term. PG does not, by itself, affect surface tension in the alveoli, but it dramatically potentiates the surface tension lowering effect of lecithins (phosphatidyl choline). For this reason Gluck has found that if PG is present in amniotic fluid, the chances of an infant developing RDS are zero.[59] PI, on the other hand, may often be present in pregnancies resulting in neonatal RDS.

The advantages of testing amniotic fluid for the presence or absence of PG, a process that requires two-dimensional thin layer chromatography, are these: (1) blood and meconium have no effect on the analysis, and (2) the incidence of false negatives is virtually nonexistent. The obvious disadvantages of the method include (1) the more complicated technique required to identify and quantify the lipid and (2) the fact that it is an even poorer predictor of pulmonic immaturity than is the L/S ratio. In any case the method should be used in conjunction with the L/S ratio.

OTHER AMNIOTIC FLUID CONSTITUENTS AS INDICATORS OF FETAL MATURITY. Mandelbaum et al. studied the 450 mμ spectrophotometric bilirubin peak in amniotic fluid specimens obtained at various stages of gestation in 83 patients and found that the concentrations decreased significantly throughout pregnancy and that no patient with a zero reading was less than 36 weeks pregnant.[96] Pitkin and Zwirek studied creatinine levels in 120 amniotic fluid specimens at various stages of gestation and found a gradual rise.[110] They noted that no fetus at 37 weeks gestation had a creatinine content in amniotic fluid of less than 2 mg per 100 ml. Brosens and Gordon reported a simple test involving a drop each of 0.1 per cent Nile blue sulfate and amniotic fluid on a slide.[13] After the preparation has been heated for 1 to 2 minutes, microscopic examination of 500 cells for orange or blue color is performed and the color is compared with the following index: less than 32 weeks, less than 1 per cent orange cells; 34 to 38 weeks, 1 to 10 per cent orange cells; 38 to 40 weeks, 10 to 50 per cent orange cells; and more than 40 weeks, more than 50 per cent orange cells.

The above tests have suffered in popularity simply because each of the above amniotic fluid components as a marker of organ (or enzymatic) maturity is an imperfect predictor of RDS. The L/S ratio, on the other hand, specifically assesses the status of the fetal lung. Since the premature baby generally dies of RDS, all tests of other organ systems must be put in proper perspective.

FETAL MONITORING

Electronic fetal monitoring (EFM), which was pioneered by Edward Hon,[68, 69] has become the leading diagnostic procedure in obstetrics. Used both ante partum (stress test) and during labor, EFM yields myriad pieces of information concerning the response of the fetus to its environ-

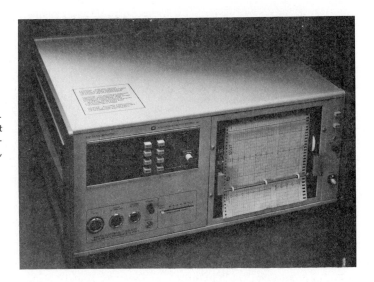

FIGURE 4–3. A typical monitoring device capable of computing and plotting fetal heart rate and uterine pressure. (Courtesy of Corometrics Medical Systems, Inc., Wallingford, Ct.)

ment. The basic instrument (Fig. 4–3) receives input of fetal cardiac activity via Doppler ultrasound, phonocardiography, or electrocardiograph leads placed upon the maternal abdomen. In labor, when the cervix is dilated and the membranes are ruptured, a direct lead can be applied to the fetus with a dermal spiral electrode. The fetal heart rate (FHR) is computed beat by beat and is printed as a continuous line on a strip chart moving at a slow rate of 3 cm per minute. A second channel records uterine contraction input either from the maternal abdominal wall by a plunge gauge tocodynamometer ante partum or via an open-ended catheter inserted through the cervix into the amniotic cavity during labor. Recordings from the abdominal wall are relative, while the intrauterine catheter allows exact pressure measurement (mm Hg). The real time relationships between various FHR patterns and uterine activity are of prime importance in interpretation.

Uteroplacental Insufficiency

The central aim of EFM is to identify fetal hypoxia. The hypoxia may be due to prolonged oxygen deprivation associated with maternal microvascular disease (e.g., hypertension or lupus) or to acute causes such as maternal hypotension secondary to hemorrhage. In this instance the recognizable FHR pattern is a *late deceleration* due to uteroplacental insufficiency (*UPI*). As noted in Figure 4–4, the "lateness" of the nadir of the deceleration is in relation to the peak of the uterine contraction. The fetal heart decelerates in response to a declining tissue PO_2 and pH. During a uterine contraction, uterine blood flow

essentially ceases. This interval is tolerated by a healthy fetus because gas exchange can still take place from the pool of oxygenated maternal blood in the intervillous space of the placenta. If the fetus is already compromised, however, oxygen lack becomes apparent as soon as the intravillous space pool is consumed, thus accounting for the occurrences of the late decelerations and neonatal morbidity.[40] When microvascular disease has resulted in scarring and contracture of the placenta, the surface for gas exchange and the potential intervillous pool space can be severely compromised. Before conditions have deteriorated to the point of late decelerations, the FHR may accelerate to a higher baseline rate (i.e., the basal average rate between contractions). The normal FHR ranges between 120 and 160 beats per minute (BPM). Thus a baseline rate of 170 BPM may be the earliest sign of fetal hypoxia and may represent efforts by the fetus to clear its acidosis. This is especially true if the baseline exhibits little beat-to-beat variability.[139] With hypoxia, the fetus appears to lose the fine tuning of the sympathetic-parasympathetic control system, and the baseline FHR appears noticeably smooth.[115] However, the most common cause of fetal tachycardia is infection, usually amnionitis. The fetus normally uses the umbilical circulation as its main resource for divesting itself of metabolic heat. Thus, when maternal temperature rises, fetal tachycardia is invoked to hasten the work of losing heat.

Two other patterns are noted in Figure 4–4. The *early deceleration* or head compression pattern appears to be due to CNS compression during labor but is not associated with fetal acidosis or a poor outcome. Its importance lies in

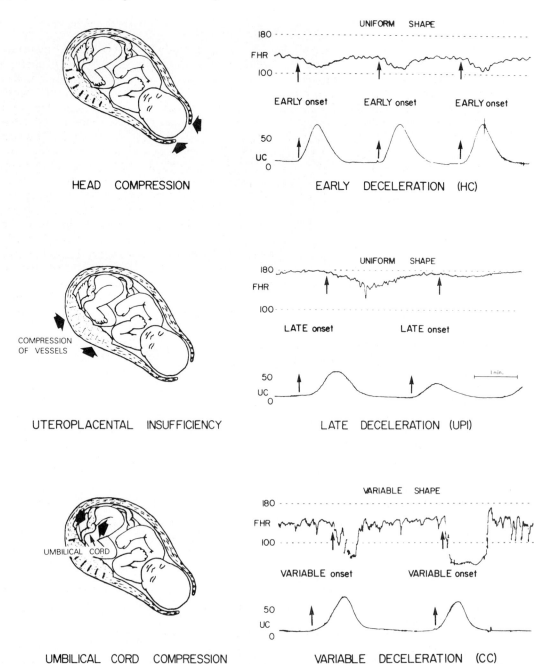

FIGURE 4–4. The *head compression pattern* has an early onset and inversely mimics the uterine contraction. The rate of peak deceleration is usually above 100 beats per minute. The *uteroplacental insufficiency pattern* has a later onset. The severity is judged by the number of beats per minute below base line at peak deceleration, a drop of more than 40 beats per minute being considered a *severe* pattern. Also note the high, smooth base line associated with this pattern. These are two additional indicators of fetal distress. The uteroplacental insufficiency pattern indicates that the fetus is experiencing some degree of hypoxia. The *cord compression pattern* is thought to be associated with mechanical interference of umbilical cord blood flow. This pattern is present to some degree in nearly all labors and is also called a *variable deceleration pattern* because it is variable in time of onset as well as in shape. A mild pattern is considered clinically insignificant, while a severe pattern (greater than 60 seconds and below 70 beats per minute) is associated with fetal hypoxia. (Courtesy of Edward H. Hon, M.D.)

its similarity to the ominous late deceleration pattern, for which it could be mistaken except for the time relationship to the uterine contraction. In this case the deceleration coincides with the uterine contraction, thus the "early" deceleration. The third pattern, the *variable deceleration*, is more important and the most common of all of the patterns. It is also called a "cord compression" pattern, reflecting its etiology. The variable patterns are usually jagged and swift and are shaped like a V, U, or W. The term "variable" applies not just to varying shapes but to the time relationship to uterine contractions. The decelerations can occur early, late, or between contractions. The beat-to-beat variability of the baseline is often increased. Obviously, when umbilical blood flow is impeded by either prolapse through the cervix or entanglement about the fetus, oxygenation is impeded. The depth and duration of the decelerations are indicators of the relative impedance. Cardiovagal impulses stimulated by interference with the umbilical circulation cause the deceleration by producing a functional heartblock.[155] Thus, mild variable decelerations are not primarily associated with fetal hypoxia. More severe variable decelerations, if not relieved by changes in maternal position in attempts to decompress the cord, may require immediate delivery.

Stress Tests. In high risk pregnancies associated with such conditions as severe diabetes or hypertension, in which there is the risk of stillbirth and its precursor intrauterine growth retardation, antepartum EFM in the form of stress testing is employed. Stress tests are sometimes used as early as the 28th week in these pregnancies. The oxytocin challenge test (OCT), now more widely known as the contraction stress test (CST), can be administered on an outpatient basis. The patient is placed in bed in the semi-Fowler's position and slightly wedged to her left side. This position minimizes the potential for uterine compression of the maternal vena cava, leading to supine hypotension, or of the internal iliacs, leading to reduced uterine blood flow. The EFM devices are applied to her abdomen and the strip recorder is activated. The tocodynamometer not only senses uterine contractions but may also detect abrupt fetal movements. When the fetus moves, it reacts with a sudden burst of tachycardia of at least 15 BPM lasting at least 15 seconds. It has been shown that reactive tachycardia occurring three times in a 20 minute period is usually associated with a nonstressed fetus.[34] This initial portion of the test is the *nonstress test* (NST), so called because no stress (contraction) has yet been induced. Fetal movements are random events dependent upon sleep-wake states, maternal glucose and medication levels, and other imponderables. Movements may be stimulated by deep abdominal palpation. Thus, a "reactive" NST has greater specificity than a "nonreactive" one. During the second portion of the test, the CST, dilute oxytocin is delivered by an infusion pump, starting at a rate

of 0.5 ml per minute and doubling every 15 minutes until three contractions occur within a 10 minute period.[71] In addition to the occurrence of late decelerations (positive CST), other important information may be obtained. The baseline FHR may suggest the presence of infection or hypoxia if tachycardic; hypoxia, sleep state, or maternal medication if smooth; or severe hypoxia or heart block if bradycardic. The stress of contractions may stimulate a previously quiet fetus into movement, with or without accompanying accelerations. Frequent or severe variable decelerations are often seen with oligohydramnios, which is associated with intrauterine growth retardation and cord compression, and may indicate that labor would not be tolerated. If late decelerations do not occur, the test is generally repeated weekly. If the test is positive it is taken as a major determinant, with other factors, in intervention decisions. If the NST is nonreactive and the CST is positive, labor is a virtual impossibility for the fetus.

Some workers are suggesting the exclusive use of the NST as the routine screening test;[151] however, the information obtained from both portions of the test is useful and should be obtained in the high risk pregnancy. It is rather difficult to determine the sensitivity and specificity of stress testing because the outcome variables are affected by interventions. Evertson, among others, observed an incidence of fetal death of 0.5 to 1 per cent within one week of a negative CST (false negative).[33] The "false negative" rate of the CST averages 25 per cent;[71] thus, other test results, history and physical findings, duration of pregnancy, and other variables are evaluated before intervention is begun. Often a trial of labor is attempted, especially if the L/S ratio is 2:1 or greater. A recent national collaborative study of nearly 20,000 stress tests is now being processed and should clarify many of the issues that are impossible to evaluate statistically in any one institution.[41]

Intrapartum Monitoring. During labor, intrapartum monitoring evaluates the same end points that were discussed earlier. In this case, however, the stress to the fetus is prolonged, and a better quality of recording can be obtained with internal direct application of the electrode and pressure catheter. Exact measurement of the intensity of uterine contractions allows a precise diagnosis of both uterine hyperactivity that causes fetal hypoxia and inadequate contractions that may require oxytocin stimulation. Which patients are monitored? Certainly all high risk patients. A frequently used screening procedure is to apply external EFM to all patients on admission to the labor ward for a 20 minute period. If abnormal tracing is observed and if there are no risk factors, a stethoscope is used periodically for the remainder of labor. The worth of EFM during labor is intellectually obvious and widely accepted.[5] However, a nationally rising cesarean section rate has raised questions concerning its impact on this intervention.[61] It has been shown that judicial use of *fetal scalp blood sampling* (FSB) helps to discriminate between fetuses that require immediate delivery and those that can be monitored during labor, thus modifying the intervention rate.[157] The scalp (or buttock) blood sample is collected in a heparinized glass tube from a small dermal puncture site and is obtained under direct vision through a dilated cervix — obviously, membranes must be ruptured. A pH determination of less than 7.2 is compatible with a diagnosis of biochemical fetal distress, although trends may be more important.[97] Because uterine blood flow is dependent upon maternal blood pressure, one must be certain that relative maternal hypotension, or another temporary and potentially correctable cause, is not present.

Other electronic means of assessing fetal well-being include recording fetal movements,[118] respiratory excursions,[109] and responses to noxious stimuli.[114] Because of the random periodicity of these events, alterations are less meaningful in individual cases than are changes in the nonrandom FHR.

If *induction of labor* is the selected intervention, oxytocin is administered by infusion pump as described earlier. EFM is used at all times, both to monitor the fetus and to gauge the uterine contractile response. Whether cesarean section or vaginal delivery is planned, in certain situations consultation with or the presence of an internist, a pediatrician, or both may be helpful.

THERAPEUTIC ABORTION

When pregnancy is a threat to the mother's life or the fetus is congenitally abnormal, therapeutic abortion may be recommended. During the first trimester (up to 12 weeks from the last menstrual period), suction curettage is the recommended procedure. Suction curettage may be performed on an outpatient basis under local paracervical block analgesia and has both a low acute and a low chronic morbidity rate.[99] Aspirated tissue can be used for chromosomal, but not morphologic, studies.

Second trimester abortions (13 to 20 + weeks) entail higher morbidity and mortality rates and can be performed surgically or medically. In the earlier portion of the second trimester, a dilation and evacuation (D & E) procedure can be performed. This is a form of dilation and curettage (D & C) in which the products of conception are removed via instrumentation.[57] Another surgical approach is the hysterotomy, actually a mini-cesarean section. Both surgical procedures are rapid and definitive but can subject the patient to traumatic short- and long-term complications (e.g., uterine scar, incompetent cervix). Medical approaches are concerned with the premature stimulation of labor with prostaglandins. Although various prostaglandins can be administered by several routes, at present the most acceptable and safest routine appears to be the use of vaginal PGE_2 suppositories.[23] Twenty-milligram suppositories are inserted every 4 hours until abortion occurs. Alternative methods include intra-amniotic instillations of prostaglandins, saline, urea, and combinations thereof. The selection of the proper technique obviously also depends upon the patient's physical condition and desires.

TREATMENT IN UTERO

Diet

Little attention has been given to nutrition in the curricula of medical schools and in didactic teaching in residency programs. Yet, an enlightened approach to nutrition in the pregnant patient is very worthwhile, since recent studies have demonstrated impressive decreases in rates of toxemia, prematurity, and perinatal mortality when nutrition is improved.

For many years it was ingrained into obstetric teaching that excessive weight gain was associated with a much higher complication rate and that if a woman curtailed her weight gain she would be rewarded with a healthier baby and a pregnancy devoid of complications. No recent study has borne this out.

It is difficult to determine from the literature what is an ideal weight gain for different women in pregnancy. Eastman and Jackson have indicated that the total of all physiologic components of a normal pregnancy is 24 pounds.[31] In Aberdeen, Scotland, the average weight gain of healthy pregnant patients with the lowest complication rate was 27 pounds.[138] The corresponding healthy group in Philadelphia, Pennsylvania, had an average weight gain of 24 pounds.[138] Perhaps the question of even greater importance is, what is the danger of "excessive" weight gain? In Aberdeen, even patients who gained over 30 pounds had a complication rate no higher than normal.

In general, patients with higher prepregnancy weights or those who gain more weight have larger babies.[104] Those with lower prepregnancy weights and those who gain little weight have smaller babies. Patients who weigh more than 5 per cent below a weight calculated "normal" for themselves have higher rates of toxemia and prematurity when they do become pregnant.[112] All this suggests that the energy that has been directed in the past toward scolding the "overindulgent" patient would be better used to determine why a patient is *not* gaining weight.

Calories. Caloric requirements increase with each trimester of pregnancy. Variables such as age, activity level, prepregnant weight, and nutritional state must be considered before the patient's needs are estimated. A teenager 13 to 15 years of age needs 2600 kilocalories a day when she is not pregnant. A woman 16 to 19 years of age needs about 2400 kilocalories.[112] We recommend for a pregnant patient, over 20 years of age, weighing 110 to 120 pounds, engaging in moderate activity, an intake of about 2200 kilocalories a day. For every 10 pounds of starting weight over 120 pounds, up to 160 pounds, one should add 50 kilocalories. A very active individual may need an extra 100 kilocalories.

An adequate caloric intake dispersed evenly throughout the day should protect a patient from periods of hypoglycemia. A pregnant woman is relatively hypoglycemic between meals because of her baby's dependence upon glucose; an inadequate caloric intake will exaggerate this trend. Maternal hypoglycemia may adversely affect the fetus in two ways: (1) Lowered blood sugar levels stimulate a lipolytic response, and maternal ketonemia has been associated with developmental abnormalities.[20] (2) Hypoglycemia stimulates catecholamine release, which can decrease placental perfusion.

Protein and Other Nutrients. Fetal aminoacid levels are significantly higher than maternal levels, and transfer of amino acids across the placenta requires active transport. A rather commonly accepted concept was that protein was intimately involved in fetal growth and that maternal protein malnutrition would result in small for gestation age (SGA) infants. In fact, in the laboratory animal one could produce a symmetrically growth retarded fetus with a protein poor diet.[153] There was certainly a suggestion from experience during the 1944–45 famine in Holland

that lack of protein was intimately involved in IUGR.

In fact, Heller noted that there was increased fetal growth in patients in whom a protein preparation was injected intra-amniotically.[64] This rather bold investigation suggested that fetal growth could be effected by circumventing the placenta in patients having insufficient fetal growth. Certainly, it has been demonstrated that the fetus swallows substantial amounts of amniotic fluid per day and has the capability to assimilate the protein contained within. However, other investigations, including human studies in Guatemala[58] and a recent, carefully controlled study in New York City,[117] in which populations at risk for IUGR were supplemented separately with protein and calories, suggest that the growth-limiting factor in the fetus is probably glucose and not protein. The effect of protein on fetal growth is an unsettled issue, but it makes sense that the quality of the product of conception will be affected by the protein available to the fetus.

In many countries protein malnutrition is common, but in North America the intake of protein by most mothers exceeds 30 grams per day. It is recommended, however, that more than 60 grams per day be consumed in order to satisfy maternal and fetal requirements.

It is generally recommended that because of the gradual depletion of iron stores in the menstruating female and the greatly increased iron requirements during pregnancy, iron supplementation be undertaken in pregnancy. Most diets are probably adequate in the essential vitamins, with the possible exception of folic acid, but most physicians prescribe supplemental vitamins based on the premise that it is difficult to determine whose diets are vitamin deficient, and there is no evidence that vitamins in the usual dosage cause harm.

Two vitamins, however, A and D, have been shown to affect the fetus adversely if taken in dosages of over 6000 USP units and 400 USP units by causing teratogenic effects and hypervitaminosis D, respectively.

Minerals. It is recognized that retention of water and sodium is a physiologic readjustment in pregnancy. There are two strong physiologic tendencies toward sodium depletion in pregnancy: (1) a 50 per cent increase in glomerular filtration rate, accounting for a theoretical filtered sodium load of 10,000 to 15,000 mEq daily; and (2) a steady increase in progesterone, which exerts a natriuretic effect by antagonizing aldosterone. Consequently, the pregnant woman must counter these salt-losing influences with significant adjustments in the components of the renin-angiotensin-aldosterone system. Fluid makes up about 60 per cent of the normal weight gain during pregnancy, and this is reflected in the 30 to 50 per cent increase in maternal blood volume. Inadequate intake of sodium decreases the blood volume at a time when the capacity of the vascular compartment has been maximally expanded by the decrease in resistance in the capillary beds and placental circulation.

The use of a low salt diet is no longer encouraged in obstetrics. We believe this measure was used routinely in the misguided notion that it was prophylactic in toxemia, but instead this type of therapy interfered with a normal and necessary physiologic development of pregnancy.

Recent investigation has been directed to the role played in pregnancy by copper, zinc, and certain trace elements. Zinc, for instance, is an essential component of amniotic fluid and is intimately involved in the inherent bacteriostatic abilities of this fluid.[84]

Maternal Activity

It has been demonstrated in numerous studies that rest in the lateral recumbent position can improve uterine blood flow dramatically. In patients diagnosed at Yale–New Haven as having IUGR, spurts of fetal growth have been noted by serial assessment of fetal BPD, AC, and TIUV when activity has been restricted and liberal amounts of rest in the lateral recumbent position have been prescribed. In some cases fetal weight has risen far above the 10th percentile when this simple regimen has been utilized.

In normal patients who are athletically inclined and in whom there is no indication of impaired fetal growth, there is no evidence that exercise has a deleterious effect in the first and second trimester. Strenuous activity should probably be limited in the third trimester, however, when fetal demands are greater and when the logistics of weight-bearing predispose patients to injury.

Physiologic edema, mainly due to increased venous pressure in the lower limbs, usually appears at the end of the day and is associated with nocturia (nighttime diuresis). A patient with symptomatic fluid retention is best treated with bed rest. Increasing the time a patient spends lying down increases the time when venous return and cardiac output are increased, and as a result, renal blood flow and water and electrolyte excretion are increased. Therefore, bed rest in a lateral position is the treatment of choice in symptomatic edema. It is not uncommon for a diuresis of 3 to 6 pounds to occur with bed rest alone over a 24 hour period.

Medications

Corticoids to Stimulate Fetal Lung Maturity. Since Liggins observed early labor and survival of premature lambs following the administration of cortisol to the fetus,[85] investigation into the acceleration of pulmonary maturity with corticosteroids has been pursued further. It is now clear that injection of corticosteroids directly into a fetus accelerates the appearance of surface activity and increases the viability of the fetus in various animals. Indeed, Liggins published a clinical trial for the prevention of respiratory distress syndrome.[87] Betamethasone was injected into patients in whom premature delivery was threatened or planned, and there was a significant decrease in the neonatal mortality rate in the group of infants treated with steroids more than 24 hours before delivery. In his expanded experience Liggins has found the efficiency of steroids to be greatest in the fetus at 32 to 34 weeks and no statistical difference in fetuses after 34 weeks. Spellacy et al. demonstrated a significantly greater rate of rise of the L/S ratio obtained from amniocenteses performed at 2 week intervals in pregnant women between 28 and 32 weeks of gestation who were given 0.5 mg dexamethasone four times daily for the 2 week period.[131]

These studies have led some practitioners to utilize steroid treatment before its full safety has been established. Cortisol-treated rabbits exhibit a reduced cell number in their lungs,[18] and large doses of steroid in rats can produce permanent neurologic deficits.[120]

Longer followup of those infants treated prenatally is necessary before this important question can be answered. An evaluation of school performance as well as the general health will be important data in the followup.

These data are accumulating, and some answers will be available soon. Even though corticoids have been used clinically for at least 5 years, questions concerning the risk/benefit ratio in various clinical situations are still unanswered. Therefore, it is recommended that the drugs be used only when there is a clear indication and under rigid protocols.

Diuretics. The majority of diuretic agents employed in obstetrics are thiazide derivatives, and there is no doubt that thiazide produces a significant natriuresis in the pregnant patient. In fact, a patient receiving 0.5 gm of chlorothiazide daily may lose almost a third of her total exchangeable sodium in only 3 days.[38] Indeed, the pregnant patient is especially prone to the development of sodium and potassium depletion when treated with diuretic agents. In addition, thiazide drugs are not without side effects in both the infant (hyponatremia, thrombocytopenia) and the mother (hyperuricemia, impaired glucose tolerance, acute hemorrhagic pancreatitis). A case has been described of heart block in the fetus associated with maternal hypokalemia.[4]

In view of these observations, the use of diuretics in the treatment of hypertension in pregnancy has become a highly controversial issue. Proponents of diuretics cite their beneficial effect in lowering blood pressure through an effect on blood volume and their potentiating action with other antihypertensive agents. Opponents point out that in toxemia of pregnancy the blood volume is often contracted and that the blood pressure lowering effect produced by diuretics will decrease uterine blood flow and potentially exacerbate the problem by producing placental ischemia. This concept has validity in view of the fact that investigators have reported success in treating toxemia with plasma expanders.

There are many pregnant patients with chronic hypertension in whom a different mechanism is responsible for their elevated pressures, who would benefit from diuretic therapy. In the acutely hypertensive patient, however, some assessment of the patient's blood volume should be attempted before diuretic therapy is empirically initiated.

PREMATURE LABOR

Premature birth is still responsible for most neonatal deaths and is more common in the high risk patient. Many drugs and treatment regimens have been used for stopping premature labor (tocolysis) through the years, though none have been completely efficacious or without side effects. These include, among others, alcohol,[42] isoxsuprine (Vasodilan),[27] terbutaline,[73] and magnesium sulfate.[135] Of these, the beta agonists appear most successful. Recently ritodrine (Yutopar) has become the first drug approved by the Federal Drug Administration for tocolysis. Ritodrine is a beta-adrenergic agonist with a preference for beta-2 receptors. The drug is effective in halting premature labor in most indicated cases; however, side effects can be bothersome and serious.[10, 98] The known cardiovascular effects of beta-mimetic drugs and their various metabolic effects[133] may contraindicate their use in some medical conditions. The most severe complication involves pulmonary edema when corticosteroids, given for the induction of fetal lung maturity, are given with beta-mimetics.[32, 136] Ritodrine is initially given intravenously, starting at 100 mcg per minute and increasing 50 mcg every 10 minutes to a maximum of 350 mcg per minute or to tolerance. The infusion is continued for 12 hours after labor has stopped, when a graded oral dosage regimen is recommended.

Despite the availability of ritodrine, the search for an effective safe tocolytic agent continues.

References

1. Adinolfi, A., Adinolfi, M., and Lessof, M. H.: Alpha-fetoprotein during development and in disease. J. Med. Genet., 12:138, 1975.
2. Adinolfi, M.: Human alpha-fetoprotein in 1956–1978. In Harris, H., and Hirschhorn, K. (eds.): Advances in Human Genetics. New York, Plenum, 1979.
3. Adlercreutz, H., Martin, F., Pulkkinen, M., Decker, H., Rimer, U., Sjoberg, N. O., and Tikkunen, M. J. Intestinal metabolism of estrogens. J. Clin. Endocrinol. Metabl., 43:497, 1976.
4. Anderson, G. G., and Hanson, T. M.: Chronic fetal bradycardia: Possible association with hypokalemia. Obstet. Gynecol., 44:896, 1974.
5. Antenatal Diagnosis. Report of a consensus development conference. NIH publication #79–1973. Washington, D.C., U.S. Government Printing Office, 1979.
6. Aubry, R. H., Rourke, J. E., Guenca, V. G., and Marshall, L. D.: The random urine estrogen/creatinine ratio: A practical and reliable index of fetal welfare. Obstet. Gynecol., 46:64, 1975.
7. Belisle, S., Osathanondh, R., and Tulchinsky, D.: The effect of constant infusion of unlabeled dehydroepiandrosterone sulfate on maternal plasma androgens and estrogens. J. Clin. Endocrinol. Metab., 45:544, 1977.
8. Berkowitz, R. L., and Hobbins, J. C.: A reevaluation of the value of hCS determination in the management of prolonged pregnancy. Obstet. Gynecol., 49:156, 1977.
9. Bevis, D. C. A.: Blood pigments in hemolytic disease of the newborn. J. Obstet. Gynaecol. Br. Commonw., 63:68, 1956.
10. Bordon, T. P., Peter, J. B. and Merkatz, I. R.: Ritodrine hydrochloride: A betamimetic agent for use in preterm labor. Obstet. Gynecol., 56:1, 1980.
11. Brock, D. J. H.: Protein measurements in the early prenatal diagnosis of spina bifida. Hum. Hered., 26:401, 1976.
12. Brock, D. J. H., and Sutcliffe, R. G.: Alpha fetoprotein in the antenatal diagnosis of anencephaly and spina bifida. Lancet, 2:197, 1972.
13. Brosens, I., and Gordon, H.: The estimation of maturity by cytological examination of liquor amnii. J. Obstet. Gynaecol. Br. Commonw., 73:88, 1966.
14. Buhi, W. C., and Spellacy, W. N.: Effects of blood or meconium on the determination of the amniotic fluid lecithin/sphingomyelin ratio. Am. J. Obstet. Gynecol., 121:321, 1975.
15. Buster, J. E., Meis, P. J., Hobel, C. J., and Marshall, J. R.: Subhourly variability of circulating third trimester maternal steroid concentrations as a source of sampling error. J. Clin. Endocrinol. Metab., 46:907, 1978.
16. Campbell, S.: Ultrasound measurement of the fetal head to abdomen circumference ratio in assessment of growth retardation. Br. J. Obstet. Gynecol., 84:165, 1977.
17. Carrington, E. R., Oesterling, M. J., and Adams, F. M.: Renal clearance of estriol in complicated pregnancies. Am. J. Obstet. Gynecol., 106:1131, 1970.
18. Carson, S. H., Taeusch, H. W., Jr., and Avery, M. E.: Inhibition of cell division associated with accelerated differentiation in lungs of hydrocortisone-treated fetal rabbits. Fed. Proc., 31:154, 1972. (abstract)
19. Chard, T., Kitau, M. J., Ledward, R., Coltart, T., Embury, S.,

and Seller, M. J.: Elevated levels of maternal plasma alpha-fetoprotein after amniocentesis. Br. J. Obstet. Gynaecol., 83:33, 1976.

20. Churchill, J. A., and Berendes, H. N.: Intelligence of children whose mothers had acetonuria during pregnancy. In Perinatal Factors Affecting Human Development. Washington, D.C., Pan American Health Organization, Scientific publication no. 185, 1969.

21. Cohen, H., Graham, H., and Lau, H. L.: Alpha-1 fetoprotein in pregnancy. Am. J. Obstet. Gynecol., 115:881, 1973.

22. Compton, A. A., Kirkish, L. S., Parra, M. J., Stoecklein, S., Barclay, M. L., and McCann, D. S.: Diurnal variations in unconjugated and total plasma estriol levels in late normal pregnancy. Obstet. Gynecol., 53:623, 1979.

23. Corson, S. L., and Bolognese, R. J.: Vaginally administered prostaglandin E_2 as a first and second trimester abortifacient. J. Reprod. Med., 14:43, 1975.

24. Cowchock, F. S.: Use of alpha-fetoprotein in prenatal diagnosis. Clin. Obstet. Gynecol., 19:871, 1976.

25. Cowchock, F. S., and Jackson, L. G.: Diagnostic use of maternal serum alpha-fetoprotein levels. Obstet. Gynecol., 47:63, 1976.

26. Creasman, W. T., Lawrence, R. A., and Thiede, H. A.: Fetal complications of amniocentesis. J.A.M.A., 204:91, 1968.

27. Csapo, A. I., and Herczeg, J.: Arrest of premature labor by isoxsuprine. Am. J. Obstet. Gynecol., 129:482, 1977.

28. Curet, L. B., and Olson, R. W.: Oxytocin challenge tests and urinary estriols in the management of high-risk pregnancies. Obstet. Gynecol., 55:296, 1980.

29. Diczfalusy, E., and Mancuso, S.: Oestrogen metabolism in pregnancy. In Klopper, A., and Diczfalusy, E. (eds.): Foetus and Placenta. Oxford, Blackwell, 1969, pp. 191–248.

30. Distler, W., Gabbe, S. G., Freeman, R. K., Mestman, J. H., and Goebelsmann, U.: Estriol in pregnancy. Am. J. Obstet. Gynecol., 130:424, 1978.

31. Eastman, N., and Jackson, E.: Weight relationships in pregnancy. Obstet. Gynecol. Surv., 23:1003, 1968.

32. Elliot, H. R., Abdullah, U., and Hayes, P. J.: Pulmonary oedema associated with ritodrine infusion and betamethasone administration in premature labor. Br. Med. J., 2:799, 1978.

33. Evertson, L. R., Gauthier, R. J., and Collea, J. V.: Fetal demise following negative contraction stress tests. Obstet. Gynecol., 51:671, 1978.

34. Evertson, L. R., Gauthier, R. J., Schifrin, B. S., and Paul, R. H.: Antepartum fetal heart rate testing. I. Evolution of the nonstress test. Am. J. Obstet. Gynecol., 133:29, 1979.

35. Fal, D., Nuchoff, S., Lilling, M. I., and Taucer, M. L.: False negative oxytocin challenge test. Am. J. Obstet. Gynecol., 133:111, 1979.

36. Fencl, M., Stillman, R. J., Cohen, J. C., and Tulchinsky, D.: Direct evidence of sudden rise in fetal corticoids late in human gestation. Nature, 287:225, 1980.

37. Fliegner, J. R. H., Schindler, I., and Brown, J. B.: Low urinary estriol excretion during pregnancy associated with placental sulfatase deficiency. Obstet. Gynecol. Br. Commonw., 79:810, 1972.

38. Flowers, C. E., Grizzle, J. E., and Easterling, W. E.: Chlorothiazide as a prophylaxis against toxemia of pregnancy, a double blind study. Am. J. Obstet. Gynecol., 84:919, 1962.

39. France, J. T., and Liggins, G. C.: Placental sulfatase deficiency. J. Clin. Endocrinol. Metab., 29:138, 1969.

40. Freeman, R. K.: The use of the oxytocin challenge test for antepartum evaluation of uteroplacental respiratory function. Am. J. Obstet. Gynecol., 121:481, 1975.

41. Freeman, R. K., and Anderson, G. G.: Personal communication.

42. Fuchs, F.: Prevention of prematurity. Am. J. Obstet. Gynecol., 126:809, 1976.

43. Gabbe, S. G., and Hagerman, D. D.: Clinical application of estriol analysis. Clin. Obstet. Gynecol., 21:353, 1978.

44. Gabbe, S. G., Mestman, J. H., Freeman, R. K., Goebelsmann, U. T., Lowensohn, R. I., Nochimson, D., Cetrulo, C., and Quilligan, E. J.: Management and outcome of pregnancy in diabetes mellitus, classes B to R. Am. J. Obstet. Gynecol., 129:723, 1977.

45. Gant, N. F., Hutchinson, H. T., Siiteri, P. K., and MacDonald, P. C.: Study of the metabolic clearance rate of dehydroisoandrosterone in pregnancy. Am. J. Obstet. Gynecol., 111:555, 1971.

46. Garoff, L., and Seppala, M.: Toxemia of pregnancy: assessment of fetal distress by urinary estriol and circulating human placental lactogen and alpha-fetoprotein levels. Am. J. Obstet. Gynecol., 126:1027, 1976.

47. Garoff, L., and Seppala, M.: AFP and HPL levels in maternal serum in multiple pregnancies. J. Obstet. Gynaecol Br. Commonw., 80:695, 1973.

48. Giannopoulos, G., and Tulchinsky, D.: The influence of hormones on fetal lung development. In Tulchinsky, D., and Ryan, K. J. (eds.): Maternal-Fetal Endocrinology. Philadelphia, W. B. Saunders, 1980.

49. Gluck, L., and Kulovich, M. V.: Lecithin/sphingomyelin ratios in amniotic fluid in normal and abnormal pregnancy. Am. J. Obstet. Gynecol., 115:539, 1973.

50. Gluck, L., Kulovich, M. V., Borer, R. C., Brenner, P. H., Anderson, G. G. and Spellacy, W. N.: Diagnosis of respiratory distress syndrome by amniocentesis. Am. J. Obstet. Gynecol., 109:440, 1971.

51. Goebelsmann, U., Freeman, R., Mestman, J., Nakamura, R., and Woodling, B.: Estriol in pregnancy. II. Am. J. Obstet. Gynecol., 115:795, 1973.

52. Goebelsmann, U., and Jaffe, R. B.: Oestriol metabolism in pregnant women. Acta Endocrinol., 66:679, 1971.

53. Goebelsmann, U., Katagiri, H., Stanczyk, F. Z., Cetrulo. C. L., and Freeman, R. K.: Estriol assays in obstetrics. J. Steroid Biochem., 6:703, 1975.

54. Gohari, P., Berkowitz, R. L., and Hobbins, J. C.: Prediction of intrauterine growth retardation by determination of total intrauterine volume. Am. J. Obstet. Gynecol., 127:225, 1977.

55. Goldkrand, J.: Unconjugated estriol and cortisol in maternal and cord serum and amniotic fluid in normal and abnormal pregnancy. Obstet. Gynecol., 52:264, 1978.

56. Greene, J. W., and Touchstone, J. C.: Urinary estriol as an index of placenta function. Am. J. Obstet. Gynecol., 85:1, 1963.

57. Grimes, D. A., and Cates, W.: Gestational age limit of twelve weeks for abortion by curettage. Am. J. Obstet. Gynecol., 132:207, 1978.

58. Habitch, J.: Guatemala study. In Nutritional Supplementation and the Outcome of Pregnancy. Proceeding of a workshop. Washington, National Academy of Sciences, 1973, pp. 93–104.

59. Hallman, M., Kulovich, M., Kirkpatrick, E., Sugarman, R., and Gluck, L.: Phosphatidylinositol and phosphatidylglycerol in amniotic fluid: Indices of lung maturity. Am. J. Obstet. Gynecol., 125:613, 1976.

60. Haning, R., Orczyk, G. P., Caldwell, B. V., and Behrman, H. R.: Plasma estradiol, estrone, estriol and urinary estriol glucuronide. In Jaffe, S., and Behrmann, H. (eds.): Methods of Hormone Radioimmunoassay. New York, Academic Press, 1979, pp. 675–697.

61. Haverkamp, A. D., Orleans, M., Langendoerfer, S., McFee, J. G., Murphy, J., and Thompson, J. E.: A controlled trial of the differential effects of intrapartum fetal monitoring. Am. J. Obstet. Gynecol., 134:399, 1979.

62. Hay, D. M., Forrester, P. I., Hancock, R. L., and Lorscheider, F. L.: Maternal serum alpha-fetoprotein in normal pregnancy. Br. J. Obstet. Gynaecol., 83:534, 1976.

63. Heikkila, J., and Luukkainen, T.: Urinary excretion of estriol and 15-alpha-hydroxyestriol in complicated pregnancies. Am. J. Obstet. Gynecol., 110:509, 1971.

64. Heller, L.: Intrauterine amino acid feeding of the fetus. In Bode, H. H., and Warshaw, J. B. (eds.): Advances in Experimental Medicine and Biology. New York, Plenum, 1974, pp. 206–218.

65. Hertz, J. B., Larsen, J. F., Svenstrup, B., and Johnson, S. G.: Estradiol, estriol and human placental lactogen in serum in threatened abortion. Acta Obstet. Gynecol. Scand., 58:365, 1979.

66. Hobbins, J. C., Berkowitz, R. L., and Grannum, P. A. T.: Diagnosis and antepartum management of intrauterine growth retardation. J. Reprod. Med., 21:319, 1978.

67. Hobbins, J. C., Mahoney, M. J., Berkowitz, R. L., Grannum, P., and Silverman, R.: Use of ultrasound in diagnosing congenital anomalies. Am. J. Obstet. Gynecol., 135:331, 1979.

68. Hon, E. H.: The electronic evaluation of the fetal heart rate. Preliminary report. Am. J. Obstet. Gynecol., 75:1215, 1958.

69. Hon, E. H.: Electronic evaluation of the fetal heart rate. Am. J. Obstet. Gynecol., 83:333, 1962.

70. Houssay, B. A.: Carbohydrate metabolism. N. Engl. J. Med., 214:971, 1936.

71. Huddleston, J. F., and Freeman, R. K.: The use of the oxytocin challenge test for the management of pregnancies at risk for

uteroplacental insufficiency. *In* Bolognese, R. J., and Schwarz, R. J. (eds.): Perinatal Medicine. Baltimore, Williams & Wilkins, 1977, p. 68.

72. Hull, M. G. R., Monro, P. P., and Gillmer, M. D. G.: Plasma unconjugated oestriol in late pregnancy: Circadian variation and the effect of meals and a glucose load. Br. J. Obstet. Gynaecol., *85*:645, 1978.

73. Ingemarsson, I.: Effect of terbutaline on premature labor. Am. J. Obstet. Gynecol., *125*:520, 1976.

74. Ishiguro, T., and Nishimuro, T.: Radioimmunoassay of maternal serum alpha-fetoprotein associated with pregnancy. Am. J. Obstet. Gynecol., *116*:27, 1973.

75. Johnson, T. R. B., Compton, A. A., Kirkish, L. S., Bozynski, M. E. A., Barclay, M. L., and McCann, D. S.: Plasma estriol in the elevation of third-trimester gestational age. Obstet. Gynecol., *55*:621, 1980.

76. Josimovich, J. B., and MacLaren, J. A.: Presence in the human placenta and term serum of a highly lactogenic substance immunologically related to pituitary growth hormone. Endocrinology, *71*:209, 1962.

77. Katagiri, H., Distler, W., Freeman, R. K., and Goebelsmann, U.: Estriol in pregnancy. IV. Am. J. Obstet. Gynecol., *124*:272, 1976.

78. Kelly, A. M., England, P., Lorimer, J. D., Ferguson, J. C., and Govan, A. D. T.: An evaluation of human placental lactogen levels in hypertension of pregnancy. Br. J. Obstet. Gynaecol., *82*:272, 1975.

79. Kleinman, C. S., Hobbins, J. C., Jaffe, C. C., Lynch, D. C., and Talner, N. S.: Echocardiographic studies of the developing human fetus — a technique for the prenatal diagnosis of congenital heart disease and cardiac dysrhythmias. Pediatrics, *65*:6, 1980.

80. Kloza, E. M., and Haddow, J. E.: Maternal serum alpha-fetoprotein screening (Letter). Am. J. Obstet. Gynecol., *136*:145, 1980.

81. Korda, A. R., Challis, J. J., Anderson, A. B., and Turnbull, A. A.: Assessment of placental function in normal and pathologic pregnancies by estimation of plasma estradiol levels after injection of dehydroepiandrosterone sulfate. Br. J. Obstet. Gynaecol., *82*:656, 1975.

82. Kundu, N., Carmody, P. J., Didolkar, S. M., and Petersen, L. P.: Sequential determination of serum human placental lactogen, estriol, and estetrol for assessment of fetal morbidity. Obstet. Gynecol., *52*:513, 1978.

83. Kunz, J., and Keller, P. J.: HCG, HPL, oestradiol, progesterone and AFP in serum in patients with threatened abortion. Br. J. Obstet. Gynaecol., *83*:640, 1976.

84. Larsen, B., Schlievert, P., and Galask, R.: The spectrum of antibacterial activity of human amniotic fluid by scanning electron microscopy. Am. J. Obstet. Gynecol., *119*:895, 1974.

85. Liggins, G. C.: Premature parturition after infusion of corticotropin or cortisol into fetal lambs. J. Endocrinol., *43*:323, 1968.

86. Liggins, G. C., Fairclough, R. J., Grieves, S. A., Kendall, J. Z., and Knox, B. S.: The mechanism of initiation of parturition in the ewe. Recent Prog. Horm. Res. *29*:111, 1973.

87. Liggins, G. C., and Howie, R. N.: A controlled trial of antepartum glucocorticoid treatment for prevention of the respiratory distress syndrome in premature infants. Pediatrics, *50*:515, 1972.

88. Liley, A. W.: Liquor amnii analysis in the management of the pregnancy complicated by rhesus sensitization. Am. J. Obstet. Gynecol., *82*:1359, 1961.

89. Littlefield, J. W.: Recent experience with prenatal genetic diagnosis. *In* Genetics and the Perinatal Patient. Mead Johnson Symposium on Perinatal and Developmental Medicine, No. 1, 1973.

90. Loriaux, D. L., Ruder, H. J., Knab, D. R., and Lipsett, M. B.: Estrone sulfate, estrone, estradiol and estriol plasma levels in human pregnancy. J. Clin. Endocrinol. Metab., *35*:887, 1972.

91. Low, J. A., Galbraith, R. S., and Boston, R. W.: Maternal urinary estrogen patterns in intrauterine growth retardation. Obstet. Gynecol., *42*:325, 1973.

92. Luther, E. R., MacLeod, S. C., and Langan, M. J.: The value of single-specimen estriol/creatinine determinations during pregnancy. Am. J. Obstet. Gynecol., *116*:9, 1973.

93. Madden, J. D., Gant, N. F., and MacDonald, P. C.: Study of the kinetics of conversion of maternal plasma dehydroisandros-

terone sulfate to 16-alpha-dehydroisandrosterone sulfate, estradiol and estriol. Am. J. Obstet. Gynecol., *132*:392, 1978.

94. Magiste, M., Von Schenck, H., Sjöberg, N-O., Thorell, J. I., and Aberg, A.: Screening for detecting twin pregnancy. Am. J. Obstet. Gynecol., *126*:697, 1976.

95. Maltau, J. M., Eielsen, O. V., and Stokke, K. T.: Effect of stress during labor on the concentration of cortisol and estriol in maternal plasma. Am. J. Obstet. Gynecol., *134*:681, 1979.

96. Mandelbaum, B., LaCroix, G. C., and Robinson, A. R.: Determination of fetal maturity by spectrophotometric analysis of amniotic fluid. Obstet. Gynecol., *29*:471, 1967.

97. Mann, L. I.: Intrapartum fetal monitoring: Scalp blood pH is a useful tool. Contemp. OB/GYN, *11*:25, 1978.

98. Merkatz, I. R., Peter, J. B., and Borden, T. P.: Ritodrine hydrochloride: A beta-mimetic agent for use in preterm labor. Obstet. Gynecol., *56*:7, 1980.

99. MMWR: Abortion-related mortality — United States, 1977. Center for Disease Control Morbidity and Mortality Weekly Report, *28*:301, 1979.

100. Morrison, I., Green, P., and Oomen, B.: The role of human placental lactogen assays in antepartum fetal assessment. Am. J. Obstet. Gynecol., *136*:1055, 1980.

101. Mueller-Heubach, E., Caritis, S. N., Edelstone, D. I., and Turner, J. H.: L/S ratio in amniotic fluid and its value for prediction of neonatal respiratory syndrome in pregnant diabetic women. Am. J. Obstet. Gynecol., *130*:28, 1978.

102. N.C.H.D. Study Group Report. J.A.M.A., *236*:1471, 1976.

103. Nevin, N. C., and Armstrong, M. J.: Raised alpha-fetoprotein levels in amniotic fluid and maternal serum in a triplet pregnancy in which one fetus had an omphalocoele. Br. J. Obstet. Gynaecol., *82*:826, 1975.

104. Niswander, K. R., and Gordon, M. (eds.): The Women and Their Pregnancies: The collaborative perinatal study of the National Institute of Neurological Diseases and Stroke. Philadelphia, W. B. Saunders, 1972, p. 240.

105. Norgaard-Pedersen, B., and Gaede, P.: Serial maternal serum alpha-1 fetoprotein in amniotic fluid. Acta Obstet. Gynecol. Scand., *53*:37, 1974.

106. Notation, A. D., and Tagatz, G. E.: Unconjugated estriol and 15 alpha-hydroxyestriol in complicated pregnancies. Am. J. Obstet. Gynecol., *128*:747, 1977.

107. Osathanondh, R., Fencl, M., Schiff, I., Himmel, M., and Tulchinsky, D.: Reduced urinary and serum total estriol levels in pregnancies after colectomy. Obstet. Gynecol., *53*:664, 1979.

108. Osathanondh, R., Ganick, J., Ryan, K. J., and Tulchinsky, D.: Placental sulfatase deficiency: A case study. J. Clin. Endocrinol. Metab. *43*:208, 1976.

109. Patrick, J., Campbell, K., Carmichael, L., Natale, R., and Richardson, B.: Patterns of human fetal breathing during the last 10 weeks of pregnancy. Obstet. Gynecol., *56*:24, 1980.

110. Pitkin, R. M., and Zwirek, S. J.: Amniotic fluid creatinine. Am. J. Obstet. Gynecol., *98*:1135, 1967.

111. Prieto, J. C., Cifuentes, I., and Serrano-Rios, M.: HCS regulation during pregnancy. Obstet. Gynecol., *48*:297, 1976.

112. Primrose, T., and Higgins, A.: Study in human antepartum nutrition. J. Reprod. Med., *7*:257, 1971.

113. Pritchard, J. A., and MacDonald, P. C. (eds.): Williams Obstetrics, 16th Ed. New York, Appleton-Century-Crofts, 1980, pp. 5–6.

114. Read, J. A., and Miller, F. C.: Fetal heart rate acceleration in response to acoustic stimulation as a measure of fetal well-being. Am. J. Obstet. Gynecol., *129*:512, 1977.

115. Renou, P., Newman, W., and Wood, C.: Automatic control of fetal heart rate. Am. J. Obstet. Gynecol., *105*:949, 1969.

116. Rome, R. M., Glover, I. I., and Simmons, S. C.: Benefits and risks of amniocentesis for assessment of fetal lung maturity. Br. J. Obstet. Gynaecol., *82*:662, 1975.

117. Rush, D., Stein, Z., and Suffer, M.: Diet in pregnancy: Randomized controlled trial of nutritional supplements. *In* March of Dimes Birth Defects original article series, Vol XVI:3, New York, Allen R. Liss, Inc., 1980.

118. Sadovsky, E., and Polishak, W. Z.: Fetal movements in utero. Obstet. Gynecol., *50*:49, 1977.

119. Samaan, N., Yen, S. C. C., Gonzalez, D., and Pearson, O. H.: Metabolic effects of placental lactogen (HPL) in man. J. Clin. Endocrinol. Metab., *28*:485, 1968.

120. Schapiro, S.: Some physiologic, biochemical, and behavioral consequences of neonatal hormone administration, cortisol and thyroxin. Gen. Comp. Endocrinol., *10*:214, 1968.

121. Schmidt, P. L., Thorneycroft, I. H., and Goebelsmann, U.: Fetal distress following a reactive nonstress test. Am. J. Obstet. Gynecol., 136:960, 1980.

122. Sciarra, J. J., Kaplan, S. L., and Grumbach, M. M.: Histology — localization of anti-human growth hormone serum within the human placenta: Evidence for a human chorionic "growth hormone prolactin." Nature, 199:1005, 1963.

123. Sciarra, J. J., Sherwood, L. M., Varma, A. A., and Lundberg, W. B.: Human placental lactogen (HPL) and placental weight. Am. J. Obstet. Gynecol., 101:413, 1968.

124. Seller, M. J., Creasy, M. R., and Alberman, E. D.: Alpha-fetoprotein levels in amniotic fluid from spontaneous abortions. Br. Med. J., 2:542, 1974.

125. Seppala, M.: Alpha-fetoprotein in the management of high-risk pregnancies. Clin. Perinatol., 1:293, 1974.

126. Seppala, M., and Ruoslahti, E.: Alpha-fetoprotein in maternal serum: a new marker for detection of fetal distress and intrauterine death. Am. J. Obstet. Gynecol., 115:48, 1973.

127. Seppala, M., and Unnerus, H. A.: Elevated amniotic fluid alpha-fetoprotein in fetal hydrocephaly. Am. J. Obstet. Gynecol., 119:270, 1974.

128. Shaxted, E. J.: Critical evaluation of 24-hour urinary oestriol estimation in clinical practice. Br. Med. J., 280:684, 1980.

129. Spellacy, W. N., Buhi, W. C., and Birk, S. A.: Human placental lactogen and intrauterine growth retardation. Obstet. Gynecol., 47:446, 1976.

130. Spellacy, W. N., Buhi, W. C., and Birk, S. A.: The effectiveness of human placental lactogen measurements as an adjunct in decreasing perinatal deaths. Am. J. Obstet. Gynecol., 121:835, 1975.

131. Spellacy, W. N., Buhi, W. C., Riggall, P. C., and Holsinger, K. L.: Human amniotic fluid lecithin/sphingomyelin ratio changes with estrogen or glucocorticoid treatment. Am. J. Obstet. Gynecol., 115:216, 1973.

132. Spellacy, W. N., Buhi, W. C., Schram, J. D., Birk, S. A., and McCreary, S. A.: Control of human chorionic somatomammotropin levels during pregnancy. Obstet. Gynecol., 37:567, 1971.

133. Spellacy, W. N., Cruz, A. C., Buhi, W. L., and Birk, S. A.: The acute effects of ritodrine infusion on maternal metabolism: Measurement of levels of glucose, insulin, glucagon, triglycerides, cholesterol, placental lactogen, and chorionic gonadotropin. Am. J. Obstet. Gynecol., 131:637, 1978.

134. Spellacy, W. N., Teoh, E. S., Buhi, W. C., Birk, S. A., and McCreary, S. A.: Value of human chorionic somatomammotropin in managing high-risk pregnancies. Am. J. Obstet. Gynecol., 109:588, 1971.

135. Steer, C. M., and Petrie, R. H.: A comparison of magnesium sulfate and alcohol for the prevention of premature labor. Am. J. Obstet. Gynecol., 129:1, 1977.

136. Stubblefield, P. G.: Pulmonary edema occurring after therapy with dexamethasone and terbutaline for premature labor. A case report. Am. J. Obstet. Gynecol., 132:341, 1978.

137. Thomson, A., and Billewicz, W.: Br. Med. J., 5013:243, 1957.

138. Tompkins, W. T., Weihl, D. G., and Mitchell, R. M.: The underweight patient as an increased obstetrical hazard. Am. J. Obstet. Gynecol., 36:48, 1955.

139. Trierweiler, M. W., Freeman, R. K., and James, J.: Baseline fetal heart rate characteristics as an indicator of fetal status during the antepartum period. Am. J. Obstet. Gynecol., 125:619, 1976.

140. Trolle, D., Pedersen, S. N., and Gaede, P.: Estriol concentrations in urine and serum in patients with various intestinal diseases. Acta Obstet. Gynecol. Scand., 56:345, 1977.

141. Tulchinsky, D.: Placental secretion of unconjugated estrone, estradiol and estriol into the maternal and the fetal circulation. J. Clin. Endocrinol. Metab., 36:1079, 1973.

142. Tulchinsky, D., Frigoletto, F. D., Ryan, K. J., and Fishman, J.: Plasma estetrol as an index of fetal well-being. J. Clin. Endocrinol. Metab., 40:560, 1975.

143. Tulchinsky, D., Hobel, C. J., Yeager, E., and Marshall, J.: Plasma estrone, estradiol, estriol, progesterone and 17-hydroxyprogesterone in human pregnancy. Am. J. Obstet. Gynecol., 112:1095, 1972.

144. Tulchinsky, D., Osathanondh, R., and Finn, A.: Dehydroepiandrosterone sulfate loading test and the diagnosis of complicated pregnancies. N. Engl. J. Med., 294:517, 1976.

145. Ursell, W., Brudenell, M., and Chard, T.: Placental lactogen levels in diabetic pregnancy. Br. Med. J., 2:80, 1973.

146. Vermont State Health Department, Burlington, Vermont, 1979.

147. Vigneri, R., Squatrito, S., Pezzino, V., Cinquerui, E., Proto, S., and Montoneri, C.: Spontaneous fluctuations of human placental lactogen during normal pregnancy. J. Clin. Endocrinol. Metab., 40:506, 1975.

148. Wald, N. J., Cuckle, H., Brock, J. H., et al.: Maternal serum alpha-fetoprotein measurement in antenatal screening for anencephaly and spina bifida in early pregnancy. Lancet, 1:1323, 1977.

149. Wald, N., Cuckle, G. M., Stirrat, M. J., Bennett, M. I., and Turnbull, A. C.: Maternal serum alpha-fetoprotein and low birth weight. Lancet, 2:268, 1977.

150. Warsof, S. L., Gohari, P., Berkowitz, R. L., and Hobbins, J. C.: The estimation of fetal weight by computer-assisted analysis. Am. J. Obstet. Gynecol., 128:881, 1977.

151. Weingold, A. B., Yonekura, M. L., and O'Kieffe, J.: Nonstress testing. Am. J. Obstet. Gynecol., 138:195, 1980.

152. Whyly, G. A., Ward, H., and Hardy, N. R.: Alpha-fetoprotein levels in pregnancies complicated by rhesus isoimmunization. J. Obstet. Gynaecol. Br. Commonw., 81:459, 1974.

153. Winnick, M.: Cellular growth in intrauterine malnutrition. Pediatr. Clin. North Am., 17:69, 1970.

154. Working Party on Amniocentesis: An assessment of the hazards of amniocentesis. Br. J. Obstet. Gynaecol., 85(Suppl. 2):1, 1978.

155. Yeh, M. N., Marishima, H. O., Niemann, W. H., and James, S. L.: Myocardial conduction defects in association with compression of the umbilical cord. Am. J. Obstet. Gynecol., 129:951, 1975.

156. Young, B. K., Jirku, H., Kadner, S., and Levitz, M.: Renal clearance of estriol conjugates in normal human pregnancy at term. Am. J. Obstet. Gynecol., 126:38, 1976.

157. Zalar, R. W., and Quilligan, E. J.: The influence of scalp sampling on the cesarean section rate for fetal distress. Am. J. Obstet. Gynecol., 135:239, 1979.

Elizabeth M. Short, M.D.

5

GENETIC DISORDERS

In a sense, the physician caring for the pregnant woman is more concerned with genetics than any other medical specialist, for he is privileged to deal with young couples at the time when they are transmitting their genetic inheritance to the next human generation. He is present at the creation of new lives, each of which (except identical twins) is a unique combination of genes. As this chapter will make clear, the field of genetic diseases is one in which scientific understanding and technologic advances are occurring so rapidly that no one person can remain completely up-to-date on each new breakthrough. The goal of the practicing physician must be to be aware of areas of development that may benefit his patients and to identify those families and pregnancies for which the new genetic knowledge is critical to successful reproduction. Once this is done, a vast array of services and specialists exists to assist in diagnosis, management, or referral of the genetic high risk couple.

These genetic services are best used to help the patient before her pregnancy and during the first trimester. Since therapy of genetic diseases is as yet very limited, prevention is a keystone of management. High risk couples can be identified who may wish to have carrier testing performed and to receive genetic counseling about their risk of having a child with a disease common to their ethnic background or their own family. Such testing can lead to wise reproductive planning for those who are at risk. Alternatives such as artificial insemination and, in future, preconception sex selection may be the right preventive measures for some couples. Perhaps more important, carrier testing can relieve anxiety in the majority of couples, who will find they are not at risk for offspring with diseases such as Tay-Sachs disease or sickle cell anemia. Such testing can be arranged through a center that provides genetic counseling to interpret the test results.

Couples who are closely related (e.g., first cousins) or those in which one member has been exposed to a potential mutagen (e.g., therapeutic radiation) may benefit from genetic counseling at a center where experts can calculate the specific increase in risk to the health of future children that may result from these circumstances.

Genetic disorders that affect the mother-to-be should be evaluated thoroughly before she becomes pregnant, since her health may be threatened by the pregnancy and since the intrauterine growth conditions for her fetus may be compromised by her disease. Information about reproductive success in various genetic disorders is growing, and this is an area in which treatment of the mother, the infant, or both before conception and early in gestation may lead to a successful pregnancy. Even fathers with genetic diseases, before they commit themselves to childrearing, may benefit from a discussion of the prognosis of their disease as well as the risks that their children will inherit it.

The physician may first identify a genetic disorder in the context of studying a couple that has not been able to have children. Some genetic diseases are associated with reproductive difficulties, causing either infertility or repeated spontaneous abortion. Proper diagnostic evaluation can enable such a couple to consider adoption, artificial insemination, or sterilization as realistic alternatives.

Once a genetic high risk couple is identified, either by parental screening or by the birth of a child with the disease, many such couples will undertake pregnancy only with the support of prenatal diagnosis by amniocentesis. The list of diseases that can be diagnosed in the fetus increases steadily. As of 1980, 160 fetal maladies had been successfully identified in utero, and it is safer for the practicing physician to assume that a diagnosis might be possible for any disease and refer the patient to those major genetic centers that maintain contact with the latest research laboratory capabilities. Such a referral or telephone consultation is appropriate even if no prenatal diagnosis was possible with the patient's last pregnancy, since scientific advances in this field are rapid. Ideally, counseling about the risks and benefits of monitoring future pregnancies with diagnostic amniocentesis is best carried out before the pregnancy is under way. There are couples who would rather not have children once they understand these risks and options.

Realistically, the obstetrician often first sees the patient to confirm a diagnosis of pregnancy and must then quickly determine whether amniocentesis is indicated in this pregnancy, because the procedure should be performed at 15 to 16 menstrual weeks. Still, since the vast majority of diagnostic amniocenteses are performed in older women because of the increasing risk of fetal chromosome abnormalities with increasing maternal age, these patients could be identified and counseled before pregnancy. The stress of diagnostic amniocentesis and the choice of midpregnancy abortion of an affected child are not acceptable alternatives for some couples, who might prefer the obstetrician's advice about reliable methods of birth control.

Finally, it remains true that a major way of identifying a family at risk for genetic disease is through the unexpected birth of an affected child. Here again, it is the obstetrician who must be aware of the implications of this birth for the future children. If the infant survives to reach a neonatal intensive care unit, the responsibility for diagnosis can be shifted to a team, which will often include a neonatologist, a pediatric geneticist, and/or a pediatric dysmorphologist. But the primary responsibility for organizing the diagnostic effort falls squarely on the obstetrician when such an infant is spontaneously aborted, is stillborn, or is not vigorously resuscitated because of severe congenital abnormalities. Such an infant may be lost, but the key to successful management of future pregnancies is to obtain an accurate diagnosis. Often key specimens to facilitate such a diagnosis must be obtained immediately. Heparinized blood for future chromosome analysis, a skin biopsy, and tubes of plasma and serum for potential biochemical tests are easy to obtain at delivery and are sometimes of irreplaceable value in diagnosis. Any deceased infant whose anatomic features or uterine environment were abnormal (e.g., oligohydramnios) warrants full necropsy, if possible by a pathologist who will obtain external photographs, skeletal x-rays, and any other permanent documentation possible, in addition to a description of gross and microscopic organ anatomy. Such documentation makes future consultation with regional or national diagnostic resources possible. A diagnosis in this infant is one of the positive steps that parents in mourning can take towards the future.

This chapter will deal in turn with each of these areas of genetic obstetrics:

1. Identification of high risk couples
2. Prenatal diagnosis of genetic or chromosomal disease in the fetus
3. Diagnostic amniocentesis and fetal ultrasonography
4. The obstetric patient with genetic disease
5. Genetic/chromosomal evaluation of the dead fetus or neonate

The many genetic diseases are each so rare in the obstetric population (although each will be common in the family at risk) that only a nationwide network of genetics centers that deal exclusively with such problems can be expected to command the requisite depth and breadth of knowledge and services to support the obstetrician in the management of particular families. That network exists, and it exists to serve the local obstetrician and his patient with the least interruption possible in their relationship but with the shared goal of a successful pregnancy and the birth of a healthy infant.

CATEGORIES OF GENETIC DISEASES

Genetic diseases are those which result from detrimental change in the number or composition of individual genes or entire chromosomes. These changes affect the copy of the human genome contained in the germ cells and are therefore heritable. The human genome is composed of enough DNA for 5 million average-sized genes contained in 23 paired chromosomes. It is likely that much of this DNA is redundant, and it has been estimated that there are perhaps 60 thousand to 100 thousand key structural genes. Two similar, but not necessarily identical, copies (called alleles) of each gene are present in the same position (locus) on each pair of chromosomes. Figure 5–1 illustrates the conventional arrangement of the human chromosomes from a cell nucleus, called a karyotype. The chromosome pairs are arranged by size. Each newly created fetus obtains one member of each chromosome pair (and thus one of each pair of genes) from the germ cell of each parent. Twenty-two of the chromosomal pairs (and their gene pairs) are called autosomes, and evidence indicates that both members of each gene pair function and contribute to the phenotype (appearance) of the individual. The 23rd pair, the sex chromosomes, contains genes that are crucial in determining sex phenotype. The X chromosome also contains key genes that are not involved in sexual phenotype but that are sex-linked (X-linked), while the Y may have only male-determining genes. The human karyotype is written as 46XY for males and 46XX for females, specifying the composi-

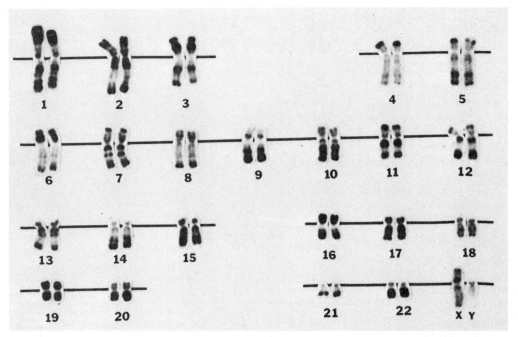

FIGURE 5–1. Human chromosome karyotype. R (reverse) banded cell. Four major banding techniques have been described (Q, G, C, R). R, Q, and G banding permit distinctive identification of each chromosome pair and detection of small abnormalities. They should be used routinely for cytogenetic studies and especially for antenatal studies.

tion of the 23rd, nonhomologous pair of chromosomes.

New change in a single gene, called a point mutation, is estimated to occur once per million genes per generation or approximately five mutations per newly created human genome. Many mutational changes may not affect structural genes or are not deleterious but serve to introduce heritable genetic variation to the human species. Those which lead to heritable diseases are collectively called mendelian diseases, because such mutations henceforth are inherited according to the laws of single gene inheritance first proposed by Gregor Mendel in 1865. Genetic diseases resulting from mutation to one member of a single gene pair are called dominant; those caused by mutation of both members of a pair, recessive; and those due to damage to a gene on the X chromosome, sex-linked. Diseases caused by visible damage to a chromosome, thus involving large numbers of genes, are called cytogenetic diseases, as are diseases resulting from an abnormal number of chromosomes (aneuploidy). An individual with significant abnormalities in chromosome number or structure invariably suffers physical deformities and usually mental retardation as well. Such chromosome damage is heritable if it has occurred in the parental germ cell chromosomes or at conception so that the new individual's germ cell chromosomes are affected.

Cytogenetic/Chromosome Disorders

Any individual who suffers from chromosomal aneuploidy or damage is at high risk of passing this abnormal chromosome constitution to offspring. Since chromosome disorders can be detected prenatally, the goal is to identify those couples at risk for such a child. Three types of chromosomal abnormalities can occur that will result in an abnormal fetal karyotype.

Postmitotic or Postconceptional Chromosome Damage. Major damage to chromosomes of the fertilizing sperm or egg or the early zygote itself will result in a fetus with acquired chromosome damage, which cannot be predicted a priori. Loss of chromosomal material (e.g., cri du chat syndrome, in which a portion of one chromosome 5 is deleted) is most common; such a deletion would be heritable only if the affected child reproduced.[83] Appropriate chromosome diagnostic studies in such an affected stillbirth or infant may well include studies of the parental karyotypes to prove that the chromosome damage is de novo and did not result from the balanced rearrangement of chromosome material in one parent. For instance, in cri du chat syndrome, while 85 to 90 per cent of cases are de novo, 10 to 15 per cent of cases result from a situation in which one parent has a normal overall genetic constitution although material from one chromosome 5 has been deleted and added

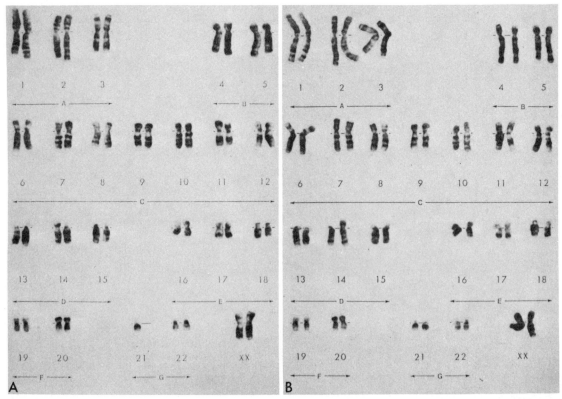

FIGURE 5–2. *A,* Karyotype of a parent who carries a balanced translocation with chromosome 21 fused to the proximal end of chromosome 14. *B,* The child's karyotype includes a normal 14 and 21 from the normal parent *and* the translocated 14/21 as well as the normal 21 from the carrier parent. The child thus has genetic material from three number 21 chromosomes and has translocation Down's syndrome. (G-banded, courtesy of S. Sakaguchi, Stanford Cytogenetics Laboratory.)

to another chromosome (translocated). Such parents are at risk for a recurrence of an abnormal karyotype in future offspring.

Translocation. It is possible for a normal person to carry a balanced rearrangement of chromosomal material that causes no ill effects because all genes are present. The most common example is 14/21 translocation, shown in Figure 5–2*A.* However, during the reduction division (meiosis), which yields a sperm or egg with half the parental chromosome constitution, it is clear that the germ cell of such a balanced translocation carrier parent could receive one of several possible assortments of the number 14 and 21 pairs. If the parental germ cell to be fertilized receives the normal chromosomes 14 and 21, the resulting offspring will be normal; if it receives the 14/21 translocation chromosome, the child will be an unaffected translocation carrier. However, should any other of four possible separations of these two pairs occur, the resulting offspring will be monosomic or trisomic for either 14 or 21 (Fig. 5–3). Of these possible combinations, only translocation Down's syndrome (Fig. 5–2*B*) is compatible with survival. The

child will be phenotypically indistinguishable from a child with standard Down's syndrome, for it too has the genetic equivalent of three number 21 chromosomes. But the recurrence risk for the translocation carrier parent will be high. It varies from 2 to 10 per cent depending upon the type of translocation and the sex of the carrier parent.[72] A parental chromosome translocation is the cause of 3.3 per cent of all cases of Down's syndrome,[31] and the probability is 2 per cent that one of the parents of a child with Down's syndrome born to a mother under age 30 is a translocation carrier. In any family in which one normal person has been identified as a balanced translocation carrier, all first-degree relatives should have chromosome studies to determine who else may carry the translocation and be at risk for the birth of children with an unbalanced karyotype.

Nondisjunction. The most common chromosomal error in offspring results from the failure of a pair of parental chromosomes to separate during the meiotic, or reduction, division of egg or sperm. This event, called nondisjunction, leads to a parental gamete with both members or

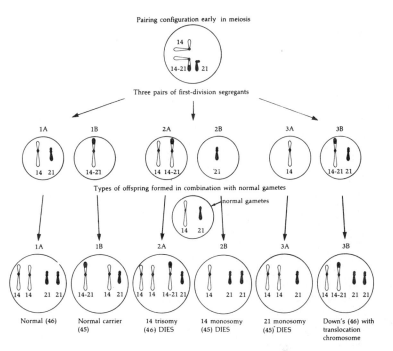

Pairing configuration early in meiosis

Three pairs of first-division segregants

1A 1B 2A 2B 3A 3B

14 21   14-21   14 14-21   2i   14   14-21 21

Types of offspring formed in combination with normal gametes

normal gametes

14 21

1A 1B 2A 2B 3A 3B

14 14   21 21   14-21   14 21   14 14   14-21 21   14   21 21   14 14   21   14 14-21   21 21

Normal (46)   Normal carrier (45)   14 trisomy (46) DIES   14 monosomy (45) DIES   21 monosomy (45) DIES   Down's (46) with translocation chromosome

FIGURE 5–3. Outcome of the first meiotic division in the germ cell of a 14/21 translocation carrier parent. Six possible gametes are shown, as are the final combinations for chromosomes 14 and 21 that would appear in offspring. (From Genetics, Evolution, and Man by W. F. Bodmer and L. L. Cavalli-Sforza. W. H. Freeman and Company. Copyright 1976.)

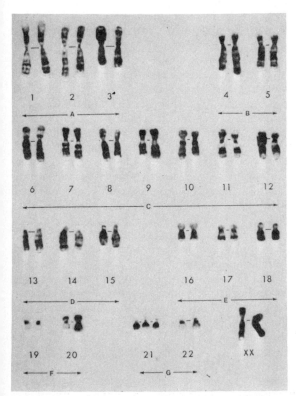

1	2	3	4	5
A			B	

6 7 8 9 10 11 12

C

13 14 15 16 17 18

D E

19 20 21 22 XX

F G

FIGURE 5–4. Karyotype of a child with trisomy 21 (Down's syndrome) resulting from nondisjunction of the 21 chromosome pair during gamete formation in either mother or father. In offspring of parents under age 30, the extra 21 is paternal in origin in 25 per cent of the cases; it is maternal in origin in most infants with trisomy 21 born to women over age 35. (G-banded, courtesy of S. Sakaguchi, Stanford Cytogenetics Laboratory.)

neither member of a chromosome pair and, if fertilized, to an aneuploid fetus. The aneuploid fetus will have either one or three copies of the particular chromosome involved. Down's syndrome, with its constellation of typical facial features, mental retardation, and high frequency of cardiac and intestinal malformations, is the most common aneuploidy in liveborns. It is caused by trisomy for chromosome 21 (Fig. 5–4). Absence of an entire autosome results in spontaneous miscarriage of the affected fetus. Turner's syndrome, in which one of the pair of sex chromosomes is missing (45X0), is the only human monosomy compatible with survival, and even so, it is estimated that 75 per cent of such fetuses are spontaneously aborted. Liveborn infants with three copies of a chromosome pair (trisomy) have been recorded for a number of pairs. Trisomy for 13, 18, 21, and the sex chromosomes is most common, but even in these cases, recent studies of aborted fetuses show that spontaneous abortion is the most common outcome (see Table 5–16, p. 130). The risk of nondisjunction is present in each meiosis of parental gemetes; the absolute rate of its occurrence is difficult to determine because selection against the survival of such conceptuses is so strong. However, statistics show that for the most common trisomy (trisomy 21, Down's syndrome) the risk of nondisjunction increases sharply with increasing maternal age at conception. While the exact molecular basis of nondisjunction is not known, its increasing incidence in offspring of older mothers corresponds with the aging of maternal egg cells, which were formed originally during fetal ovarian development.

Single Gene Genetic Disorders

Dominant Diseases. Humans carry two copies of each gene located on their 22 pairs of autosomal chromosomes. Mutation in one of these paired genes (alleles) can affect the appearance or health of the individual. Such gene mutations are called dominant. A person with a dominant gene mutation is himself affected by it and, since he passes one of those two genes at random to each of his children, each child has a 1:2 (50 per cent) chance of inheriting the mutant gene and also being affected. Thus, identification of a dominant gene mutation in either parent places that couple at a high risk for transmitting that disease to their children. Successful genetic management in this situation calls for the identification of this disease in the parent first.

Recessive Diseases. Even in the presence of a mutant gene, the second gene of each pair is likely to be normal and to function normally. In most gene pairs this functioning gene provides enough product so that the person is not physically altered or diseased. Thus, there is no obvious physical (phenotypic) evidence that this person carries one mutant gene, and the mutant gene is said to be recessive or hidden. To place this phenomenon in perspective, it has been estimated that each of us carries one or two recessive deleterious mutations. Thus, every potential parent is a carrier of deleterious genes; the key to responsible genetic management is to determine whether both members of a couple carry the *same* recessive mutation. Only then do they become a high risk couple with a 1:4 (25 per cent) chance that each child will inherit the mutant gene from each parent and suffer the full effects of a complete absence of the normal product of this gene. Such a child is referred to as an affected homozygote; that is, both alleles of the gene pair are mutated. Each parent is a heterozygote, possessing two alleles for that gene pair that are different. At some future time we may all be "genotyped," as we now have our blood type determined, and carry a card that reminds us which deleterious mutant genes we carry; at present such generalized prospective heterozygote identification is not technically feasible.

X-Linked Diseases. The identification of women who carry X-linked recessive disease genes is also of importance. The 23rd pair of chromosomes, the sex chromosomes, differs in males and females. A male has only one X chromosome, which he inherits from his mother, since he is male by virtue of the Y sex chromosome he inherited from his father. Each female possesses two X chromosomes, one from each parent, but each cell in her body randomly inactivates one of the two X's, and thus male and females have similar amounts of X-gene products. A male's X-gene products all come from the genes he inherited from his mother; a female's are a random mixture of product from the genes of each parent. Because a woman possesses two X chromosomes, she can be a recessive carrier for X-linked diseases, which will affect her sons. Her risk is 1:2 (50 per cent) of giving birth to affected sons regardless of her spouse's genetic makeup. The presence of a male with an X-linked disease, such as hemophilia, anywhere in the maternal line should lead to the testing of all women in the family as possible carriers.

Multifactorial Diseases

Several congenital malformations and diseases show a significant risk of recurrence within the same family, although the risk is not as high as the 25 to 50 per cent incidence expected from diseases caused by inheritance of single gene mutations of large effect. These diseases are presumed to be due either to the inheritance of several genes of cumulative detrimental effect or to the inheritance of genes that result in increased susceptibility to environmental hazards. Empiric recurrence risks for such conditions are known and can be used to counsel families and to identify those pregnancies in which the risk warrants attempts at prenatal diagnosis (see Table 5–5, p. 117). The neural tube defects anencephaly and spina bifida are examples of such a multifactorial malformation syndrome in which the population risk is 1 to 3 per 1000 for a child with a neural tube defect but 4 to 5 per cent for the next child in a family with one affected sibling and 12 to 15 per cent for a third case in a family with two affected siblings.[11, 65]

THE HIGH RISK COUPLE

Ideally, identification of a couple at high risk for a genetic disorder should occur a priori rather than after the birth of an affected child. The idea that genetic and chromosomal disease are so rare that they can be dismissed from consideration is a common misconception. A number of human diseases caused by single gene mutations are

TABLE 5–1 INCIDENCE, PREVALENCE, AND MORBIDITY OF GENETIC DISORDERS

Estimated Incidence at Birth of Diseases with a Major Heritable Component

Disorder	Per cent of all births
Chromosomal abnormalities at birth	0.5–1.0
Most common single gene disorders	1–2
Major congenital anomalies (3 per cent of births) with a genetic component	1.2
Nonspecific mental retardation (3 per cent of births) with a genetic component	1.8
TOTAL:	4.5–6

Estimated Prevalence of Morbidity and Mortality Due to Genetic Diseases

Perinatal Morbidity and Mortality	Per cent of all cases
Chromosome disorders	
Spontaneous abortions	50
Stillbirths/neonatal deaths	5
Surviving livebirths	0.5
Genetic disorders	
Genetic variation potentially handicapping — liveborn	10

Late Morbidity

Pediatric hospital admissions attributable to Single gene / Chromosomal / Multifactorial } diseases	12
Pediatric hospital admissions attributable to multifactorial congenital malformations	18
Adult hospital admissions with a significant genetic component	12
Severe mental retardation with a significant genetic component	60
15 per cent single gene	
45 per cent genetic component	

Data derived from Scriver, 1978; based on CDC, 1974; Childs, 1972; Day, 1973; Marden, 1964; and Opitz, 1977.

each rare, but in the aggregate, single gene or multi-gene (chromosomal) abnormalities account for a significant proportion of human disease. As illustrated in Table 5–1, there is an aggregate likelihood of 4 to 6 per cent for the birth of a child with a specific genetic or chromosomal disease. In any one family the risk may vary from 1 to 50 per cent. The key to prospective identification of such couples is a family history.

Family History

The five features of a thorough family history designed to search for evidence of heritable

TABLE 5–2 THE FAMILY HISTORY

Consanguinity

Ethnic/racial background

Present age

Medical illnesses/physical abnormalities
  Each parent
  Previous children of either parent

Unexpected deaths, rare diseases, known genetic diseases in any family member

diseases or deformities are outlined in Table 5–2. General questions in each of these important areas and the goals of these questions follow:

Consanguinity

Questions: Are you and your spouse related? Are there similar surnames on both sides of the family? Have both sides of the family come from the same town or geographic area in past generations?

Goal: Couples with close blood relationships share large groups of identical genes, thus increasing the risk that they will share similar mutant genes. Table 5–3 illustrates the genetic relationships and the risk. Consanguinity increases the general risk of miscarriage and the risk of rare recessive genetic diseases in offspring.

TABLE 5–3 PARENTAL RELATIONSHIPS AND RISK OF DISEASE IN OFFSPRING

Parental Relationships	a priori Risk of Deleterious Recessive Disease* Per Cent	Overall Risk of Infant Morbidity/ Mortality Per Cent
Incest parent-child brother-sister	12.5–25	33
Consanguinity aunt-nephew uncle-niece	6.25–12.5	15
First cousins	3.1–6.25†	6–8
Second cousins	0.8–1.6	4–6
Unrelated	.001	2–4

*Calculated on the assumption that every person is heterozygous for 1–2 genetic traits that would be deleterious in homozygous combination.

†The empiric risk figure for documented recessive disease in offspring of first-cousin marriages in families with no prior history of recessive gene traits is ≤ 1 per cent (Fraser, 1976).

TABLE 5–4   EXAMPLES OF INHERITED DISORDERS THAT OCCUR WITH
INCREASED FREQUENCY IN SPECIFIC ETHNIC GROUPS

Ethnic Group	Inherited Disorders
African blacks	Hemoglobinopathies, especially Hb S, Hb C, persistent Hb F, α and β thalassemias Glucose 6-phosphate dehydrogenase deficiency Adult lactase deficiency
Armenians	Familial Mediterranean fever
Ashkenazi Jews	Abetalipoproteinemia Bloom's syndrome Dystonia musculorum deformans (recessive form) Familial dysautonomia (Riley-Day syndrome) Gaucher's disease (adult form) Neimann-Pick disease Tay-Sachs disease
Chinese	α thalassemia Glucose 6-phosphate dehydrogenase deficiency Adult lactase deficiency
Eskimos	Pseudocholinesterase deficiency Adrenogenital syndrome Amyloidosis
Finns	Congenital nephrosis
French Canadians	Tyrosinemia Morquio syndrome
Japanese	Acatalasemia
Mediterranean peoples (Italians, Greeks, Sephardic Jews)	β thalassemia Glucose 6-phosphate dehydrogenase deficiency Familial Mediterranean fever Glycogen storage disease, type III
Northern Europeans	Cystic fibrosis Hemochromatosis
Scandinavians	α_1-Antitrypsin deficiency LCAT (lecithin:cholesterol acyltransferase) deficiency
South African whites	Porphyria variegata

(Excerpted from McKusick, V. A.: Mendelian Inheritance in Man, 5th Ed. Baltimore and London, Johns Hopkins University Press, 1978.)

Ethnicity

Questions: What is your ethnic background? Your spouse's? Do you and your spouse share a common racial or ethnic background? Are your ancestors from the same country?

Goal: Certain genetic diseases occur with increased frequency in specific ethnic groups. Table 5–4 lists such diseases. Americans who trace their ancestry to these specific groups share the increased risk of these diseases. When both members of the couple share the same ethnic background, screening may be possible to determine whether they both carry a mutant gene for a recessive disease common in their racial or ethnic background (see Carrier Detection, p. 118).

Parental Age

Question: How old are you and your husband?

Goal: With increasing maternal age, risks for offspring with chromosomal abnormalities rise from 1/750 at age 20 to 1/10 at age 45 (see Figure 5–9, p. 120). At maternal age 35 the risk reaches 1 per cent and exceeds the risk of the amniocentesis procedure used to detect such abnormalities. Older fathers are at increased risk for offspring with a de novo single gene mutation resulting in a dominant disease. Although a specific figure is not available, this risk is much less than 1 per cent. Advanced paternal age at conception is not associated with *significantly* increased risk of a chromosome abnormality in the fetus.[40]

Medical Illnesses and Physical Abnormalities

EACH PARENT

Questions: In the context of traditional medical history–taking, diseases afflicting either parent should be readily uncovered. A reference identifying those human disorders for which a risk of inheritance of 25 to 50 per cent is documented or suspected is the book Mendelian Inheritance in Man.[53] Over 3800 diseases and traits are catalogued in the 5th edition. Several atlases are available that catalogue those diseases and traits producing physical malformations. The Birth Defects Compendium[5] and Recognizable Patterns of Human Malformation[83] each detail available information on the inheritance of each malformation they describe.

A parent with any suspected heritable condition or physical trait often benefits from referral for diagnostic evaluation. Counseling about inheritance must be based on a definite diagnosis. A number of apparently similar traits are heterogeneous, and inheritance varies with the subtype. It is often necessary, in the case of biochemical and metabolic disorders, to establish a firm understanding of the molecular basis of the disorder in the family before attempting prenatal diagnosis.

Goal: An established diagnosis of a genetic disease in either parent pinpoints a high risk couple who should receive appropriate counseling concerning the risk of transmitting that disease to their children and the possibilities for prenatal diagnosis.

PREVIOUS CHILDREN

Questions: The medical history of all siblings and half-siblings of the future child is crucial. Many congenital malformations and some serious chronic diseases of childhood have a significant risk of recurrence in future siblings.

Goal: Identification of a rare genetic disease in a previous sibling is the most certain means of identifying a genetic high risk couple. While homocystinuria may be extremely rare in the population at large, this diagnosis in their child poinpoints a couple as carriers. Each subsequent child has a 25 per cent risk of inheriting the disease. Common congenital malformations also have a higher risk of recurrence in the family where one has already been born than in the general population, as shown in Table 5–5. Inability to conceive or repeated spontaneous miscarriage also may be a clue to a genetic disorder that has thus far limited reproduction but that could lead, in a future pregnancy, to the survival of an abnormal child until birth.

TABLE 5–5 RECURRENT RISKS FOR COMMON CONGENITAL MALFORMATIONS

Malformation	Percentage of Risk for Each Subsequent Child
Cleft lip with or without cleft palate*	
One affected child	4
Two affected children	9
One affected parent	4
One affected parent and one affected child	17
Cleft palate only	
One affected child	2
Two affected children	10
One affected parent	6
One affected parent and one affected child	15
Neural tube defects (anencephaly, myelomeningocele, encephalocele)	
One affected child	4–5
Two affected children	12–15
Congenital heart disease	
Ventricular septal defect	5
Atrial septal defect	3
Patent ductus arteriosus	4
Pulmonic stenosis	3
Aortic stenosis	2
Tetralogy of Fallot	3
Transposition of great vessels	2
Coarctation of aorta	2
Clubfoot	3
Congenital hip dislocation	4–5
Pyloric stenosis	
One affected child	3
Mother affected	16
Father affected	5

*All the risk figures are somewhat increased if affected individuals are female or if cleft is severe.

(From Nadler, H. L., and Burton, B. K.: Genetics. *In* Quilligan, E. J., and Kretchmer, N. (eds.): Fetal and Maternal Medicine. New York, John Wiley & Sons, 1980.)

CLOSE RELATIVES

Questions: A history of significant medical illnesses and physical deformities in all close relatives is critical information. First-degree relatives of the couple are their parents and siblings. These relatives have 25 per cent of their genes in common with the future baby. A careful listing of diseases and unexplained or early deaths can be a clue to genetic diseases. A woman who is an unsuspected carrier of hemophilia may give the only clue to this diagnosis in noting that her mother had two brothers who died in infancy with bleeding trouble. Careful documentation of

TABLE 5-6 EXAMPLES OF DOMINANT GENETIC DISORDERS OF LATE CLINICAL ONSET WITH SERIOUS MORBIDITY/MORTALITY

Disorder	Risk for Children of an Affected Parent *Per Cent*
Familial hypercholesterolemia	50
Adult polycystic kidney disease	50
Familial breast cancer	50
Familial colon polyposis/cancer	50
Hereditary hemorrhagic telangiectasia	50
Huntington's chorea	50
Acute intermittent porphyria	50
Marfan's syndrome	50
Neurofibromatosis	50
Myotonic dystrophy	50

the health of all known male relatives of the potential mother may be the only clue to X-linked genetic diseases that can reappear in her sons.

Genetic Diagnosis in the Family

Any family history that reveals even one member with a suspected genetic disease is sufficient grounds for referral of that member for diagnostic evaluation. Only a firm diagnosis can form the basis for proper assumptions about the risk to other members of the family of inheriting this disease. Proper diagnosis cannot be overemphasized, and it can occur at any age. It may be only as your patient considers having her second child that her father, after a premature heart attack, is identified as having familial hypercholesterolemia, or that her mother develops renal failure at age 45 and genetic adult polycystic kidney disease is diagnosed. Serious genetic diseases of late onset can pose a significant future health risk for the patient herself (Table 5–6). Her future plans for reproduction may be altered if such a disease is detected in a parent, aunt, or uncle on either side of the family. It is advisable that family members delay reproduction while the possibility of a genetic disease is being evaluated in the family. Often it will be possible within a short time to decide whether the branch of the family that includes your patient is at any risk of having or transmitting the disease, and the necessary diagnostic studies sometimes cannot be done on pregnant women.

Detection of Carriers of Genetic Diseases

Genetic carrier testing identifies those phenotypically normal individuals who carry a muta-

tion in one of their two alleles at one genetic locus. Such persons are heterozygotes and, in theory, have half the normal amount of gene product or gene activity measurable in a genotypically normal person. Today, carrier testing can be performed for only a small fraction of known genetic diseases because of several theoretical and technical limitations. The basic molecular genetic defect must be elucidated, the normal gene product or its activity must be accessible to measurement, the quantitative ranges must discriminate normal subjects from heterozygotes, and an individual laboratory must have sufficient experience with a rare disease before carrier testing for the disease is feasible. Three genetic diseases illustrate these problems with carrier detection. Heterozygotes for sickle cell anemia (1:12 American blacks) can be identified by a simple biochemical determination, the metasulfide test for sickle hemoglobin. A more complex test, which exploits the difference in thermal stability between two hexosaminidase isoenzymes present in serum, can be used to identify carriers of Tay-Sachs disease (1:27 American Ashkenazi Jews), who produce less of isoenzyme A. Heterozygotes for cystic fibrosis (1:20 American Anglo-Saxons) cannot be detected because the molecular defect in this common disease has not been elucidated.

Detection of Autosomal Recessive Disease Carriers. Detection of healthy parents who each carry one mutant copy of the same gene presently occurs in two ways. The commonest and most tragic is through the birth of a child with a recessive genetic disease. That child identifies its parents as obligate heterozygote carriers with a 25 per cent chance in every future pregnancy of giving birth to another affected child. Formal carrier testing to prove that each parent carries that mutant gene is rarely done. However, if such carrier testing is possible, it would be appropriate for the new spouse of either of these parents should they divorce and remarry. Because each parent is a carrier, it would be appropriate to prove that the new spouse (or semen donor in artificial insemination) is not a carrier, thus reducing the risk for affected offspring from 25 per cent to zero.

The second method of heterozygote detection is prospective; individuals with a high likelihood of being carriers of a specific genetic disease are identified because of their ethnic background or because of the presence of an affected patient in another branch of the family. Table 5–4 (page 116) lists examples of diseases for which carrier frequency is high in a definable subgroup of the population. To date, Tay-Sachs disease is the only disease for which a high-carrier-risk ethnic subgroup has participated voluntarily in a large-

TABLE 5–7 FREQUENCY OF THREE GENETIC DISEASES AND OF CARRIER STATE IN ETHNIC SUBGROUPS COMPARED WITH FREQUENCY IN ENTIRE POPULATION

Disease	Ethnic Subgroup	General Population
Tay-Sachs Disease		
Disease frequency	1/3600	1/360,000
Carrier frequency	1/30	1/300
Couples at risk	1/900	1/90,000
Sickle Cell Anemia		
Disease frequency	1/625	1/6.25 million
Carrier frequency	1/12.5	1/1250
Couples at risk	1/156	1/1.56 million
Galactosemia		
Disease frequency	—	1/180,000
Carrier frequency	—	1/212
Couples at risk	—	1/45,000

scale carrier testing program. Uniquely, such couples may be able to arrive for their first prenatal visit secure in the knowledge that they are *not* at risk of having an infant with Tay-Sachs disease. As simpler carrier tests are devised this practice will become more common.

At present, attempts to test for heterozygous carriers are limited to situations in which the risk is high a priori. Three rare but serious genetic diseases illustrate this concept. In Tay-Sachs disease, absence of a lysosomal catabolic enzyme, hexosaminidase A, results in progressive accumulation of the sphingolipid GM_2-ganglioside in brain and viscera, causing progressive mental retardation, blindness, and paralysis; death occurs in early childhood. In sickle cell anemia, a mutation in the structure of hemoglobin A leads to irreversible sickling of red blood cells in areas of low oxygen tension, causing infarction of the tissues and anemia. In galactosemia, absence of functioning hexose-1-PO_4-uridyltransferase enzyme leads to progressive toxicity from unmetabolized galactose and to subsequent cataracts, liver disease, mental retardation, and failure to thrive. Accurate carrier testing is available for all three of these recessive diseases,[25, 42] but, as Table 5–7 makes clear, the risk that both members of a couple will be heterozygotes for one of these diseases is the product of the two individual carrier risks. This risk is so low for couples in the general population that routine carrier testing is not recommended. However, if one member of the couple is in a high risk ethnic subgroup or from a family with a known case of the disease, that person should have carrier testing. Carrier testing in recessive disease can be done for the higher risk spouse

first; only if this spouse is a carrier need the partner be tested. As the figures in Table 5–7 make clear, even when carriers are common, couples at risk are rare. For each mendelian recessive genetic disease, every tenth person in the population would need to be a carrier before even 1 per cent of couples were at risk for affected children. The incidence of the genetic disease itself would be 1:400, or 2.5 per 1000. Most genetic diseases are much less common than that.

Thus carrier detection serves two purposes. For most couples, the tests provide reassurance that although they are from a high risk ethnic subgroup, they themselves are not at risk. Even when one member of such a couple is a known carrier, it is most likely that the other is *not* (e.g., for sickle cell trait, the chance is 92 per cent or 11:12). For those rare couples at risk, prospective identification may enable them to make use of prenatal diagnosis to identify the 1:4 infants who are affected, so that treatment may be provided, as with galactosemia, or elective abortion performed, as with Tay-Sachs disease.

Detection of X-linked Disease Carrier Females. Table 5–8 lists some X-linked diseases for which a carrier test is possible. However, there are limits to our ability to detect women with a mutant gene on one of their two X chromosomes. Since a woman inactivates one of her two X chromosomes at random, it is possible for her to have inactivated enough of the X's

TABLE 5–8 EXAMPLES OF GENETIC DISEASES FOR WHICH CARRIER TESTING IS POSSIBLE

Autosomal Recessive Diseases
Prospective mother tested first; only if she is a carrier need father be tested. Only if both are carriers is there a risk (25 per cent) for affected children.

  Tay-Sachs disease
  Gaucher's disease
  Phenylketonuria
  Galactosemia
  Sickle cell anemia
  Thalassemia
  Hurler's disease

X-linked Disease
Prospective mother tested; if she is a carrier the risk is 50 per cent for sons to be affected and 50 per cent for daughters to be carriers.

  Hemophilia A and B
  Fabry's disease
  G6PD deficiency
  Lesch-Nyhan syndrome
  Hypophosphatemic rickets
  Ornithine transcarbamylase deficiency
  Duchenne muscular dystrophy
  Hunter's syndrome

carrying the mutant gene to appear normal in a carrier test. For example, modern carrier testing for hemophilia A measures a ratio of all the antihemophilia globulin (AHG) produced (antigen) to all of that which is functional (activity). This activity/antigen ratio discriminates carriers from normals and detects 94 per cent of carrier women.[45] This test cannot detect the 6 per cent of carriers whose normal gene is active in so many of their cells that they produce mostly functional AHG. Such carrier women have the same 50 per cent chance as their more easily identifiable sisters of passing the X chromosome with the mutant gene to their sons.

Females heterozygous for X-linked disorders should be prospectively identified if possible; for them each pregnancy has a high risk for affected offspring. Half of their daughters will be carriers and half of their sons will suffer the disease. A number of X-linked diseases can be diagnosed by prenatal studies. Even in cases where such diagnosis is not yet possible, fetal sex can be determined, and some families would prefer termination of all male pregnancies to the 50 per cent risk of a son with hemophilia or muscular dystrophy.

PRENATAL DIAGNOSIS OF GENETIC DISEASES

Throughout this book, techniques for prenatal evaluation of the health of a developing fetus are discussed in many contexts. Fetal medicine represents one of the most exciting areas of advancing medical knowledge in this decade. In this chapter, I will restrict discussion to aspects of prenatal diagnosis that are concerned with detection of cytogenic, biochemical, genetic, and some multifactorial diseases in the fetus. At present, prenatal diagnostic testing for such diseases is restricted by the specific technologic limitations of various tests. Tests that are elaborate, costly, time-consuming, and personnel-intensive and that present a significant risk to the successful continuation of the pregnancy should be used only when the risk of fetal genetic disease is high enough to justify the procedure. Midtrimester amniocentesis is an example of such a technique. However, we are on the verge of technical innovations that will revolutionize our approach to fetal medicine. For example, when high resolution ultrasonography becomes widely available at low risk and low cost, it will be possible to screen all pregnancies for certain severe fetal malformations even when the a priori risk for such abnormalities is low.

Presently available techniques for evaluation of genetic diseases in the fetus include

TABLE 5–9 TECHNIQUES FOR PRENATAL DIAGNOSIS OF GENETIC DISEASE IN THE MIDTRIMESTER FETUS

Techniques	Risk of Fetal Loss (Per Cent Increase Over Controls)
Maternal blood studies	0
Diagnostic fetal ultrasonography	0
Midtrimester amniocentesis	0.2–0.5
Fetoscopy	4–5
Fetal blood sampling	
Fetoscopy	4–5
Placental aspiration	3–10

1. Maternal blood studies
2. Diagnostic fetal sonography
3. Midtrimester amniocentesis
4. Fetoscopy
5. Fetal blood sampling

The indications, risks, and limitations of each of these techniques will be discussed. In Table 5–9 each diagnostic technique and the risk from the test itself to the successful outcome of the pregnancy is outlined.

Maternal Blood Studies

Fetal diagnostic studies based on maternal blood samples are of low risk to the pregnancy and permit widespread pregnancy screening. Diffusible fetal metabolites and proteins cross into the maternal circulation through the placenta and can be measured directly. Recent research studies have documented that a small number of fetal cells (probably leukocytes) can be detected in the maternal circulation at 20 weeks gestation as well.[78] These studies raise the hope that in the future much of the prenatal diagnosis of chromosomal and biochemical disorders can be accomplished by utilizing samples obtained from maternal serum.

At present, only a few maternal serum tests are in widespread use and can be applied to all pregnancies. A well-established example is the routine test for maternal Rh (anti-D) antibodies in Rh negative mothers to detect pregnancies at risk for erythroblastosis fetalis.

Maternal Serum Rh Determination. Rh incompatibility represents a model example of a fetal genetic disease whose diagnosis has passed into the realm of routine obstetric care and in which maternal prophylaxis in high risk couples can prevent a fetal health risk.

Maternal serum Rh determination involves the following steps: (1) High risk couples are easily identified by blood typing, beginning with the mother. Only if the mother is Rh negative (15 per cent chance) is there a risk of erythroblastosis, and then only if the paternal blood type is Rh positive (85 per cent chance). (2) Monitoring high risk pregnancies with monthly maternal antibody titer measurements provides assurance that sensitization has not occurred. (3) Prophylactic treatment of the mother with proper use of Rh immune globulin in the postpartum period prevents sensitization of the mother if the newborn is Rho (D) or Du positive. (4) Treatment of the affected fetus is possible. Even if Rh sensitization should occur, amniocentesis and intrauterine transfusion can be utilized to treat the fetus affected with a hemolytic anemia because of its genotype.

This disease has been so well managed that we have almost forgotten its historic importance as one of the first genotypic disorders affecting the human fetus that could be detected and treated before birth and in which identification of high risk couples led to prophylatic treatment to prevent risk of recurrence in future siblings.

Maternal Serum Alpha-Fetoprotein Determination. For one group of congenital malformations we stand on the verge of having a simplified maternal screening program applicable in all pregnancies and having the potential for eliminating this group of birth defects. Neural tube defects (NTD) are a group of major fetal central nervous system malformations that are among the most common major congenital malformations in the United States. They result from a fundamental defect in the closure of the developing fetal nervous system, which normally occurs during the first weeks of embryonic life. The defects range in severity from anencephaly, in which the brain does not develop, to spina bifida. While anencephaly is incompatible with extrauterine fetal life, it represents a high burden disease of pregnancy because the fetus is often carried to term and there is slow progression of labor. Spina bifida varies in severity, depending upon the location of the closure defect along the spinal axis, but usually there is some paraplegia and a lack of bladder and bowel control as well as a risk of mental retardation and hydrocephalus. The overall risk of neural tube defects in the United States is approximately 2 per 1000 live births. In the Northwest United Kingdom, the overall rate is 6 to 8 per 1000.

Women who have had a previous child with any neural tube defect have a significant risk of recurrence, ranging from 1.7 to 6 per cent in different ethnic groups. Amniocentesis for determination of amniotic fluid alpha-fetoprotein and ultrasound examination of the fetal nervous system are utilized in such subsequent pregnancies (see Chapter 4). However, 90 per cent of all children born with neural tube defects each year will be delivered into families with no previous case.[49]

Alpha-fetoprotein of fetal origin is increased in amniotic fluid and in maternal serum in the presence of an open neural tube defect. The experience in England makes it clear that screening for neural tube defects can be accomplished with maternal serum samples.[87] Since fetal alpha-fetoprotein (AFP) measurable in the maternal circulation increases from the 7th week in normal singleton gestations, the radioimmunoassay test result must be carefully correlated with duration of gestation (Figure 5–5). Several model screening programs have been established in the United States,[60] and more are planned in the near future depending upon the development of reliable lab-

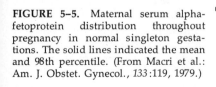

FIGURE 5–5. Maternal serum alpha-fetoprotein distribution throughout pregnancy in normal singleton gestations. The solid lines indicated the mean and 98th percentile. (From Macri et al.: Am. J. Obstet. Gynecol., *133*:119, 1979.)

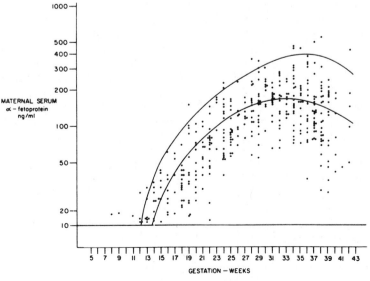

oratory standards for the maternal serum assay procedure in this country. Physicians are cautioned that previously developed AFP assays (for use in cancer programs) that do not have reliable pregnancy standards and controls should not be used.

Experience in the United Kingdom and with the initial United States screening programs has defined the uses and pitfalls of this screening test. The optimal sampling time is 16 to 18 weeks gestation, and blood samples should be taken apart from uterine manipulation, amniocentesis, or other procedures. If the AFP is abnormally high (by the standards of the testing laboratory) the test should be repeated immediately. In a New York screening program, 7.4 per cent of women had abnormal serum AFP levels. On repeat testing within 1 to 2 weeks, the AFP of 4.4 per cent remained elevated and led to further study of the fetus.[49] By contrast, in Milunsky's assay system using 2.5 standard deviations above the median as the cutoff point, 2.5 per cent of first samples were classified as abnormal.[62]

False positive results should be an accepted part of any screening test. The goal of a screening procedure is to include all possible cases, which can then be restudied by more specific methods to make an accurate diagnosis. All women with test results above the 95th percentile should undergo a repeat test. The false negative risk in maternal serum AFP tests, that is, the risk of missing a case of NTD, is real but low. Ferguson-Smith reported 16 false negative results in 11,585 cases; 3 infants with open and 13 with closed spina bifida born to mothers whose serum AFP levels were normal.[18]

The 2 to 4 per cent of women with two serum AFP results above normal should undergo a diagnostic ultrasound procedure for determination of fetal gestational age and twinning. Gestational age discrepancies between sonogram and calendar dates can lead to a determination that the maternal AFP value was in the normal range for the actual gestational age. Twinning is associated with increased serum AFP, as are a number of other conditions, outlined in Table 5–10. Once these causes have been eliminated, the remaining women with elevated serum AFP have a 3 to 8 per cent chance of having an infant with NTD. They should be offered diagnostic amniocentesis and ultrasonography, since the risk of a NTD exceeds the risk of harm from the procedures. Amniocentesis for determination of amniotic fluid AFP concentration and detailed ultrasonography of the fetal neural axis together can accurately diagnose 95 to 99 per cent of such cases. Elevated amniotic fluid AFP is present in 90 per cent of all fetuses with NTD, but the

TABLE 5–10 DISORDERS THAT MAY BE ASSOCIATED WITH AN ELEVATED MATERNAL SERUM ALPHA-FETOPROTEIN

Multiple gestation
Threatened abortion
Intrauterine fetal distress or death
Rh disease
Ectopic pregnancy
Maternal or neonatal hepatitis
Maternal hepatoma, GI cancer, tumor metastatic to liver
Maternal herpes infection
Fetal congenital cirrhosis
Fetal tyrosinosis
Fetal major malformations, e.g. omphalocele nephrosis esophageal atresia
Pre-eclampsia/toxemia
Fetal growth retardation

concentration of protein does not correlate with the severity of the lesion. Closed NTD (with overlying skin) may not cause elevated amniotic fluid AFP, and AFP may return to normal levels after 24 weeks gestation even in fetuses with open NTD. The false positive rate for amniotic fluid samples is 0.1 per cent, the most common cause being fetal blood contamination of the sample. Research laboratories performing this assay routinely assay all samples with elevated AFP values for fetal hemoglobin. Thus, a bloody amniotic tap is not suitable for NTD diagnosis by AFP determination. If amniotic fluid AFP is elevated above +3 SD and there is no fetal blood contamination, then the likelihood is high that *some* serious fetal disorder such as those mentioned in Table 5–10 is present. Figure 5–6 illustrates the dramatic elevations in amniotic fluid AFP that are present in cases of fetal NTD.

Ultrasonic Prenatal Diagnosis

As technologic capability advances, it is likely that ultrasound scanning will soon be employed to screen all pregnancies for certain fetal anomalies. The virtues of this technique include its lack of risk to mother and fetus, the ability to obtain motion films or static views that can be used for consultation, and the potential ability of this visual technique to identify fetal malformations that will never be detectable by amniocentesis (see Chapter 4).

Sonography is increasingly employed by the obstetrician to evaluate the course of pregnancies with discrepancy between uterine-fetal size and calendar dates. The preliminary sonographic "diagnoses" for such date-size discrepancies may be (1) multiple gestations, (2) oligohydramnios, (3) polyhydramnios, (4) discrepant fetal head size, and (5) intrauterine growth retardation.

These obstetric diagnoses may be confirmed by simple sonograms, but a diagnostic opportunity is missed if such findings are not accompanied by careful efforts to evaluate fetal structure, since each of these situations is associated with significant likelihood of congenital malformations in the fetus. Diagnostic ultrasonography at 15 to 20 weeks gestation is also indicated for these genetic indications: (1) a previous child with a neural tube disorder, (2) a previous child with a major congenital anomaly, (3) elevated maternal serum or amniotic fluid alpha-fetoprotein, and (4) parents at genetic risk (recessive or dominant) for a child with a disease accompanied by prenatal physical abnormalities (Table 5–11). Ideally, such studies are performed before 24 weeks gestation so that the option of elective abortion remains open to the parents should a

TABLE 5–11 INDICATIONS FOR FETAL SONOGRAPHY BEFORE 24 WEEKS GESTATION TO DETECT MAJOR FETAL MALFORMATIONS

Obstetric Indications
Discrepancy between uterine size and dates
Oligohydramnios (renal anomalies)
Polyhydramnios (18–20 per cent associated with fetal anomalies)
Intrauterine growth retardation
Multiple gestations
Small fetal head to palpation

Genetic Indications
Previous child with neural tube defect
Previous child with congenital anomalies
Maternal serum and/or amniotic fluid elevation of alpha-fetoprotein
Parent with dominant genetic disease associated with prenatal physical deformity
Parents both carriers of a recessive genetic disease associated with prenatal physical deformity

major abnormality be detected. Ultrasonographic standards for normal fetal anatomy between 14 and 24 weeks gestation are still being developed at major university diagnostic centers; crown-rump length and biparietal head diameter are well standardized.[77] Standards for abdominal girth, limb length and proportionate ratios of long bones, and even fetal echocardiographic standards for cardiac chamber size, ejection fraction, and valve appearance are presently being developed.[10, 36]

Individual case reports documenting a sonographic diagnosis of a fetal structural abnormality confirmed at delivery or elective abortion are accumulating daily. The collected experience of prenatal diagnosis at major centers is now appearing and documents that major types of fetal anomalies can be visualized in the second trimester. Such detectable defects presently fall in the major anatomic categories outlined in Table 5–12. This list makes clear that the future potential of ultrasound for defining fetal anatomy is a major advance in prenatal diagnosis.

Such studies should be done before 24 fetal weeks to provide maximum utility; however, in conditions diagnosed after 24 fetal weeks in which there is no possibility of successful extrauterine survival, prompt termination of the pregnancy may still be indicated to spare the patient the stress of carrying a fatally deformed fetus for weeks. In still other cases, advance knowledge of specific fetal abnormalities may alter management of labor or lead to arrangements for delivery of a high risk fetus at an institution where skilled neonatologists and pediatric surgeons may provide immediate therapy (see Chapter 4).

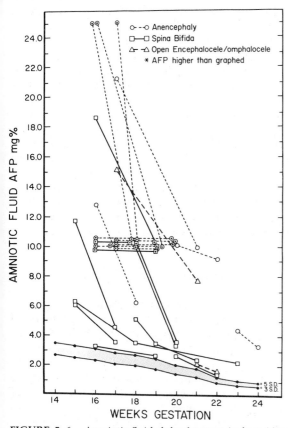

FIGURE 5–6. Amniotic fluid alpha-fetoprotein from 14 to 24 weeks in singleton gestations. The shaded area represents the range for values +3 to +5 SD above the normal mean, and individual data points represent values obtained in fetuses with neural tube defects. (From Milunsky, A.: unpublished data, 1980.)

TABLE 5–12 EXAMPLES OF ULTRASOUND DIAGNOSIS OF CONGENITAL ANOMALIES IN SECOND TRIMESTER FETUSES*

Cranium
 Anencephaly
 Hydrocephalus
 Encephalocele (Meckel's)
 Microcephaly
 Cystic hydroma
 Lymphangiectasia
 Holoprosencephaly
 Iniencephaly

Face
 Robert's syndrome
 Treacher Collins syndrome (T)
 Achondroplasia (T)
 Thanatophoric dysplasia (T)

Spine
 Meningomyelocele
 Sacrococcygeal teratoma
 Spina bifida

Thorax
 Diaphragmatic hernia
 Thoracic cyst
 Thanatophoric dysplasia (T)
 Thoracic asphyxiating dystrophy (T)
 Chondroectodermal dysplasia (T)
 Osteogenesis imperfecta
 Hypophosphatasia (T)

Abdomen
 Duodenal atresia
 Omphalocele
 Ascites
  "prune belly" syndrome
  chylous ascites
  multiple anomaly syndromes
 Ileal volvulus
 Esophageal atresia (T)

GU Tract
 Ureteral obstruction/hydronephrosis
 Infantile polycystic kidney disease
 Renal agenesis
 Unilateral multicystic kidney disease
 Dysplastic kidneys
 Urethral obstruction
 Reliable sex determination before 24 weeks is *not* presently possible with sonography

Extremities
 Rhizomelic dwarfism (e.g., achondroplasia) (T)
 Mesomelic dwarfism (e.g., Ellis-Van Creveld syndrome)
 Acromelic dwarfism (e.g., Grebe syndrome) (T)
 Bowing of long bones
  camptomelic dysplasia (T)
  osteogenesis imperfecta congenita (T)
  thanatophoric dwarfism
 Fanconi's syndrome (T)
 Radial aplasia–thrombocytopenia (T)

Heart
 Tricuspid atresia
 Hypoplastic RV
 Hypoplastic LV (T)
 Total anomalous venous return (T)
 Tetralogy of Fallot (T)
 Ventricular septal defects (T)

*This table features *examples* of midtrimester diagnoses that have already been made in affected fetuses or are theoretically possible (T). Prenatal diagnosis by ultrasonography is *not* limited to the examples on this list.
(Data from Campbell, 1979; Hobbins, 1979; Hobbins and Venus, 1979.)

Radiologic Prenatal Diagnosis

Ultrasonographic image resolution has improved so rapidly that it should always be the first technique employed for visualization of fetal malformations. However, it is worthwhile to remember that other techniques are available should fetal sonograms raise more questions than they answer. Radiologic fetal diagnosis can be very useful in diagnosing bony malformations, from anencephaly (absent calvarium) to various forms of dwarfism. If such severe diseases are suspected, the exposure of a second trimester fetus to diagnostic quantities of radiation becomes justifiable.[30] Radiographic views must be well planned. A fetus of 18 weeks gestation is usually in a transverse position in the true pelvis, and a prone maternal film may best reveal fetal bony structures, while a 24 week fetus may have assumed the vertex position and a 45 degree prone compression oblique film would be best. An experienced radiologist should be present who understands the visualization desired. Ultrasound scanning may be employed to locate the fetus and confirm the utility of the exposure, thereby reducing the necessity for repeated films.

Amniography, the introduction of water-soluble contrast material into the amniotic fluid, may aid in outlining fetal soft parts, and 24 to 48 hours after amniogram a standard x-ray will often reveal a fetal "GI series" owing to concentration of swallowed contrast material in the fetal intestinal tract. These techniques have been used to document fetal intestinal obstruction in association with polyhydramnios. In the third trimester, fetography can provide sharp x-ray outlines of soft tissue by absorption of an oily contrast material to the vernix caseosa over 24 hours. The contrast material has a high iodine content, which may affect the fetus (see Chapter 8). These x-ray techniques are more hazardous to the pregnancy because of the risks associated with amniocentesis for instillation of contrast material, but they may be indicated to confirm a diagnosis that will result in elective abortion. These techniques, and even direct fetoscopy (see page 135), should be used to confirm an equivocal ultrasound diagnosis in order to avoid any risk of aborting an unaffected infant. Several cases have been reported in which, because of an elevated amniotic fluid alpha-fetoprotein value and a normal-appearing ultrasound image, amniography was employed to confirm the diagnosis of meningomyelocele prior to abortion.[93] Since in several reported instances an apparently normal fetus has been aborted because of

elevated amniotic fluid alphafetoprotein,[44] diagnostic sonography, radiography, and even fetoscopy to confirm the presence of a neural tube defect before abortion seems indicated.[30]

Midtrimester Amniocentesis

Diagnostic amniocentesis for prenatal detection of genetic disease is performed at 14 to 16 menstrual weeks to obtain amniotic fluid and fetal skin fibroblasts for analysis. It is desirable to perform the test as early as possible so that diagnosis of disease in a fetus can be obtained before 24 menstrual weeks if elective abortion is to be performed. Amniocentesis before 14 weeks is often unsuccessful owing to the small volume of amniotic fluid present (Fig. 5–7). On the other hand, 3 to 6 weeks must be allowed for fetal cell culture before a diagnosis can be determined.[23, 68, 70]

Risks. Four major North American studies are now available examining the outcome in over 7000 cases where diagnostic amniocentesis was performed at 14 to 18 menstrual weeks. The experience of these studies (nationwide collaborative trials in the United States and Canada and single center experiences in Boston and San Francisco) is summarized in Table 5–13. Results from all of these studies are remarkably consistent and show that this procedure carries a low risk of danger to the fetus or mother when properly performed either in the obstetrician's

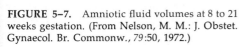

FIGURE 5–7. Amniotic fluid volumes at 8 to 21 weeks gestation. (From Nelson, M. M.: J. Obstet. Gynaecol. Br. Commonw., 79:50, 1972.)

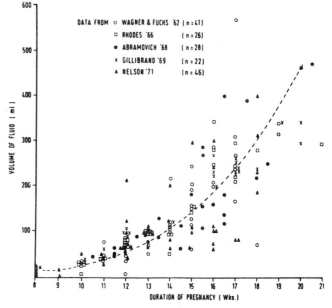

TABLE 5-13 DATA ON MIDTRIMESTER DIAGNOSTIC AMNIOCENTESIS FROM LARGE-SCALE STUDIES IN NORTH AMERICA

Data	United States Collaborative Study 1976	MRC Study Canada 1976	Milunsky et al. Boston 1979	Golbus et al. San Francisco 1979	Controls United States Collaborative Study 1976
Cases studied	1040	1020	1995	3000	992
Twins	13 (1:80)	13 (1:78)	23 (1:87)	36 (1:83)	12 (1:83)
Normal outcome	942 (90.6%)	870 (85.3%)	1831 (91.8%)	—	927 (93.5%)
Prenatal diagnosis affected fetus	34 (3.3%)	39 (3.8%)	38 (1.9%)	106 (3.8%)	—
male at risk for X-linked disease	11 (1.1%)	23 (2.3%)	13 (0.7%)	23 (0.8%)	—
Errors in diagnosis	6 (0.6%)	7 (0.7%)	2 (0.1%)	14 (0.5%)	—
Elective abortion	39 (3.8%)	55 (5.4%)	41 (2.1%)	113(3.8%)	1 (0.1%)
Fetal loss week of test	(0.1%)	3 (0.2%)	10 (0.5%)	* (1.2%)	—
14–24 fetal weeks	24 (2.3%)	18 (1.7%)	51 (2.6%)	42 (1.5%)	21 (2.1%)
14–44 fetal weeks	36 (3.5%)	33 (3.3%)	72 (3.6%)	—	32 (3.2%)
Neonatal deaths	8 (0.8%)	10 (1.0%)	7 (0.4%)	—	5 (0.5%)

*1.2 per cent spontaneous fetal loss the week of the test for women who were scheduled for amniocentesis but had *not* yet had the test.
(Data from NICHD, 1976; Simpson et al. MRC 1976; Milunsky, 1979 [Ref. no. 57]; Golbus, 1979.)

TABLE 5–14 MATERNAL COMPLICATIONS AFTER MIDTRIMESTER AMNIOCENTESIS

Complications	US Study*	Canadian Study†
Vaginal fluid leakage	12	16
Vaginal bleeding	11	3
Abortion	1	3
Amnionitis	1	—
Uterine contractions	2	5
Abdominal tenderness	—	11
Other	—	6
Total complications	27	44
Total amniocenteses	1195	1223
% complications	2.3	3.6

*within 1 week
†within 72 hours

office or in a major university center. However, the procedure is not risk free, and since a risk must be estimated and balanced against the risk of a specific genetic disorder, Milunsky estimates this risk at 0.2 per cent (1/500)[57] and Golbus at 0.5 per cent (1/200).[28]

As Table 5–13 makes clear, recognized intrauterine demise in close proximity to amniocentesis is rare (0.1 to 0.5 per cent), and little evidence has accumulated to show that such events are due to needle trauma to the placenta or the fetus. Unexplained fetal death during the procedure has been observed (0.7/1000 cases).[29] Rare cases of amnionitis, skin puncture (1/929 infants in the United States study), chronic amniotic fluid leakage, ileocutaneous abdominal fistula, and gangrenous arm in an anencephalic fetus have been reported.[57] Maternal complications have included vaginal bleeding or fluid leakage, abortion, and amnionitis (Table 5–14).

Significant fetomaternal hemorrhage after midtrimester amniocentesis can occur if the placenta is punctured. Thus, there is a risk that an Rh negative mother carrying an Rh positive fetus could be sensitized and could develop antibodies following the procedure. For this reason, the American College of Obstetricians and Gynecologists[1a, 53a] recommends routine RhoGAM prophylaxis following amniocentesis. However, a prospective study of safety, efficacy, and need has not been done. The safety of prophylaxis at 28 to 34 fetal weeks has been established and routine administration to *all* Rh negative mothers in midgestation is recommended.[1a, 53a] Although the risk to the fetus of

treatment at 14 weeks has not been well studied, earlier reports of increased fetal death rates in women treated with 300 μg following amniocentesis[54] have not been confirmed by recent reports, especially those from centers administering a 100 μg dose.[43] Debate continues concerning the need for such therapy. Postamniocentesis prophylaxis does reduce the isoimmunization rate to 0.2 per cent, well below the spontaneous sensitization rates during pregnancy of 1.6 per cent for primigravidas and 2.2 per cent for multigravidas.[53a] Reports of a risk of isoimmunization ranging from 2.7 to 4.3 per cent following amniocentesis suggest that treatment is warranted.[27, 43, 48a, 54] However, Golbus notes that with the advent of concurrent ultrasound use and greater technical experience with the procedure, the isoimmunization rate is declining.[27] He questions whether routine prophylaxis is necessary if the sensitization rate following amniocentesis (2.1 per cent) does not exceed the spontaneous sensitization rate.

The informed consent for prenatal amniotic cell culture reproduced in Figure 5–8 makes clear the major limitations of which the patient and her obstetrician should be aware. At 16 weeks gestation there are about 12,000 cells per ml in amniotic fluid, but only 1:2000, or 6 per ml, are viable. It is necessary to culture the cells obtained to select for viable cells, to obtain chromosome spreads, and to insure adequate numbers of cells for biochemical diagnostic procedures. A recent worldwide survey reports a culture failure rate of 3.2 per cent even after repeated amniocenteses.[57] If poor culture viability is evident in the first 14 days, then a second sample should be obtained. A second sample was necessary in 2 to 3 per cent of cases in Milunsky's series, but it provided the necessary back-up cells to enable a diagnosis to be obtained in 1000 consecutive cases.

Chromosome analysis may prove inaccurate under the following circumstances: (1) maternal skin cells contaminating the culture, (2) an undetected chromosome mosaicism in the fetus, and (3) abnormal chromosome karyotype of which the clinical significance is yet unknown. An overall error rate of 0.4 per cent has been reported; half of these errors are attributable to maternal cell contamination resulting in incorrect sex assignment. Most important, a normal karyotype and normal alpha-fetoprotein level do not guarantee a normal newborn. Many major birth defects and causes of mental retardation (3 to 4 per cent of all births) cannot be diagnosed by chromosome karyotype or AFP determination.

STANFORD UNIVERSITY HOSPITAL
Stanford Medical Center
Stanford, California 94305

CONSENT FOR PRENATAL
DIAGNOSTIC TESTING

addressograph

I.   I, the undersigned, request and authorize Doctor _____ and associates to perform a genetic test(s) on my unborn child:

    A.   Test(s) to determine if there is anything abnormal about the chromosomes: _____
                              (Initials)

    B.   Test(s) to determine the level of alpha-fetoprotein in amniotic fluid, with the understanding that this test is effective in detecting certain defects in the tube enclosing the brain and spinal column: _____
                         (Initials)

    C.   Test(s) to determine the presence of the following genetic disorder (s): _____
    _____
                        (Initials)

II.   I consent to the use of ultrasound examination prior to amniocentesis as an aid to determine location of the placenta and placement of the needle, to detect twins, and to detect condition(s) which might be relevant to amniocentesis and/or genetic tests.

III. I understand that the genetic test(s) to be performed on my unborn child require tests on the fluid, and cells contained in it, which surrounds the unborn child in the uterus (womb). I understand that a specimen of fluid is removed by amniocentesis which involves the penetration of the mother's abdominal and uterine walls by a hollow needle.

IV.   I acknowledge that the above described procedure(s) has/have been thoroughly explained to me, including, without limitation, the following important points:

    A.   That there may be slight pressure or discomfort when the needle is introduced.

    B.   That, although transabdominal amniocentesis is a proven technique, there is a small risk of less than one-half of one percent that the procedure may cause a complication in the mother or fetus. Minor complications may include: cramping, bloody spotting or leakage of amniotic fluid from below, and soreness at the site of the needle puncture. More rarely, serious complications may occur which may include initiation of premature labor resulting in spontaneous abortion, hemorrhage, infection or injury to the fetus.

    C.   That, in the case of twins, the results provided may pertain only to one of the pair.

    D.   That, although over 90% of the time sufficient amniotic fluid is obtained at the first attempt, occasionally a repeat amniocentesis will be necessary. Repeat amniocentesis is successful over 94% of the time. However, very rarely, all attempts may be unsuccessful.

    E.   That, although 99% of the time a diagnosis can be made, occasionally a diagnosis may not be possible because a tissue culture from amniotic cells may be unsuccessful or because the chromosome preparations may be of poor quality or unusable. Any special test(s) which may be attempted may also be unsuccessful.

    F.   That, although 99% of the time the diagnosis is accurate and, in this case, the likelihood of misinterpretation is considered to be extremely small, a complete and correct diagnosis of the condition of the fetus based on the test(s) performed cannot be guaranteed.

    G.   That any and all abnormal findings will be explained to me. Should a serious abnormality be diagnosed in my unborn child, the decision to continue or end this pregnancy is entirely mine.

    H.   That normal results for the tests which are to be performed on my unborn child do not eliminate the possibility that the child may have illnesses, birth defects or mental retardation because of other causes.

    I.   That my participation in this diagnostic procedure is wholly voluntary and is not a prerequisite to eligibility for, or receipt of, any other service or assistance from, or participation in, any other program. If I wish to withdraw from the procedure at any time, my medical care will not be affected.

V.   I have had my questions freely answered, and recognize and accept the possible hazards and limitations of the techniques and interpretations involved in the genetic test(s) of my unborn child.

15-394 (2/81)

MOTHER: _____   WITNESS: _____

FATHER: _____   DATE: _____
(optional)

FIGURE 5-8.   Consent form for prenatal diagnostic studies on amniotic fluid and cell specimens.

TABLE 5–15   GENETIC INDICATIONS FOR
MIDTRIMESTER AMNIOCENTESIS

Chromosomal Indications
Maternal age > 35 years at conception
Previous child with chromosomal abnormalities
Either parent a translocation chromosome carrier
Mother a carrier for X-linked disease
    fetal sex determination
    diagnosis in male fetus (if possible)

Sex Determination
Mother a carrier for X-linked disease
    fetal sex determination
    diagnosis in male fetus (if possible)

Mendelian Genetic Indications
Either parent affected with a dominantly inherited
    disease that can be detected in utero, e.g.,
    porphyria
Both parents known carriers for detectable
    recessive disease, e.g., sickle cell anemia
Mother a carrier for X-linked disease
    fetal sex determination
    diagnosis in male fetus (if possible)

Multifactorial Disease Indications
Maternal serum alpha-fetoprotein elevated
Previous child with neural tube defect
Maternal medical disease that increases risk of de-
    tectable fetal abnormality, e.g., hypothyroidism

Indications for Amniocentesis.   The indications for genetic prenatal diagnosis by amniocentesis are given in Table 5–15. The vast majority
of these procedures are performed for cytogenetic studies in the fetuses of women over the age
of 35 at conception. A smaller number are intended to detect neural tube defects when a
previous child has been afflicted (recurrence risk
2 to 6 per cent) or when maternal serum alpha-
fetoprotein is elevated (1 to 2 per cent of
screened women) or to examine fetal chromosomes when a previous child has been born with
chromosomal aneuploidy to a young mother (recurrence risk 1 to 1.5 per cent). Detection of
mendelian genetic disorders or fetal sexing for
X-linked disorders currently represents a complicated but small proportion of amniocenteses.

This procedure is *not* indicated in healthy
young women with no family history indicating a
high risk of genetic disease merely to assuage
general anxiety that the baby is abnormal or
because of a vague worry about exposure to
environmental teratogens. For women under the
age of 35 without a specific indication, the risk of
fetal loss is much greater than that of a detectable
disorder in a liveborn child.

Cytogenetic Diagnosis at Amniocentesis

Competently performed cytogenetic study of
chromosome structure from cultured amniotic
fluid fetal cells enables detection of a wide range
of potential chromosomal disorders. Abnormal
numbers of chromosomes (aneuploidy) are easily
identified, and translocations, deletions, and
other structural abnormalities are also detectable. Mosaicism, in which fetal tissues are
derived from two cells of differing chromosome
constitutions, can be identified if both cell lines
are represented in the cells available for culture.
However, ability to predict the physical appearance or medical problems of a fetus with abnormal chromosomes is based on experience with
liveborn fetuses of similar karyotype. For the
most common trisomies such clinical data are
readily available, but for subtle or previously
unreported abnormalities of chromosome structure the phenotypic outcome is not always easy
to predict. Families with rare chromosomal abnormalities require special counseling concerning the limits of prediction in prenatal cytogenetic diagnosis.

Since most prenatal cytogenetic studies are
performed because of advanced maternal age,
fetuses with abnormal numbers of chromosomes
will be detected most frequently. Such aneuploidy arises because of nondisjunction of chromosome pairs during meiosis, an event that
occurs with increasing frequency in the aging
ovum. The exact age-specific risk for a chromo-
somally abnormal offspring is important information for a woman and her obstetrician in their
decision to perform amniocentesis. At present
such information is not fully available for several
reasons. Data on chromosome abnormalities at
amniocentesis and at birth were initially grouped
by five-year maternal age intervals before it was
appreciated that the risk rises rapidly and that
such average risk figures can be misleading.
More recently, pooled data from cytogenetic
studies of first trimester abortuses and midtrimester amniocentesis have provided evidence
of an underappreciated biologic phenomenon.[37, 38] Throughout gestation, strong selective
forces work against the survival of aneuploid
fetuses. A representative study of the chromosome constitution of 234 consecutive spontaneous abortuses (Table 5–16) shows that 47 per
cent are abnormal irrespective of maternal
age.[32, 33] Amniocentesis data on the karyotypes
of midtrimester fetuses of mothers 35 years or
older have also shown a higher prevalence of
cytogenetic abnormalities than was anticipated

TABLE 5–16 INCIDENCE OF CHROMOSOMAL ABNORMALITIES IN SPONTANEOUS FIRST TRIMESTER ABORTUSES

Chromosomes of Abortus	Per Cent	
Normal karyotypes 46XX XY	53	
Abnormal karyotypes	47	
	Per Cent of all abortuses	Per Cent of abnormal karyotypes
45 XO	11.5	25
47 + 1	21.4	45.9
48 + 2	1.3	2.7
69 (3n)	6.4	13.8
92 (4n)	2.6	5.5
Deletions, mosaics, other	3.5	7.3

(Data from Hassold et al., 1978.)

from the frequency of such abnormalities at birth. These findings suggest that spontaneous loss of such fetuses continues at a high rate throughout gestation. Exact maternal-age–specific rates for *liveborn* infants with chromosomal abnormalities are not readily available in the United States; such data are confounded by underreporting, ascertainment bias, and a possible increase in the true incidence within the last decade.[46] Amniocentesis data may also suffer from a bias toward performing the procedure in women with a higher risk (e.g., those with multiple previous miscarriages). Studies are under way to obtain unbiased prevalence figures for livebirths, and amniocentesis data must continue to be pooled, since the number of older women studied is still very small. Eventually unbiased maternal-age–specific risk figures will be available for the risk of conception, survival to midtrimester, and livebirth of fetuses with different cytogenetic abnormalities. The general trend is obvious already. As Figure 5–9 shows, the chance of detecting an aneuploid fetus at amniocentesis is higher than any risk of the procedure (<1 per cent) by maternal age 35. Data by 2 year maternal age intervals show that the chance of detecting fetal aneuploidy of all types (Fig. 5–9A) and of detecting the most common form of aneuploidy, Down's syndrome (Fig. 5–9B), rises steadily.[28] Numbers of women in the two older age groups are small, and in fact so few women over age 45 have been studied that an exact risk

figure is not available (NA). Figure 5–9B also shows, in the cross-hatched portion of each bar graph, the risk for livebirth of a child with Down's syndrome. These risk figures are from Swedish data on Down's syndrome births by single year maternal age groups.[39] Such data are not available for the prevalence of all liveborn infants with any variety of chromosomal aneuploidy.

This discordance between the rates of chromosome abnormalities diagnosed prenatally and those diagnosed at birth has raised questions concerning counseling of women in these age groups. Should amniocentesis be recommended only for those women whose risk of an abnormal liveborn infant is greater than risks from the procedure? Preliminary estimates indicate that from 25 to 50 per cent of fetuses with Down's syndrome detected by 20 weeks gestation will be subsequently lost. Presumably, late fetal loss is even greater in aneuploidy associated with more severe physical defects (e.g., trisomy 13), but clearly the risk of a severely affected liveborn infant is real. When exact and unbiased data are

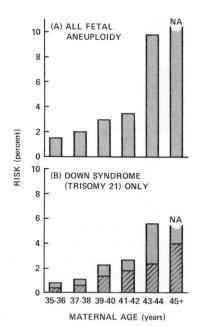

FIGURE 5–9. *A*, Per cent risk for an aneuploid fetus at midtrimester amniocentesis based upon maternal age (data from Golbus, 1979). *B*, Per cent risk for detection of a fetus with Down's syndrome (trisomy 21) at amniocentesis (entire shaded bars) and for livebirth of an infant with trisomy 21 (hatched areas) based upon maternal age (data from Hook and Lindsjo, 1978; Milunsky, 1979; Golbus, 1979). NA indicates accurate risk estimate not available. Risk is presumed to be at least equal to that of the previous age group.

available on the prevalence of affected liveborns, it is still likely that the risk will exceed risk from the procedure performed on women over age 34. These older women can be advised that there is a difference between midtrimester prevalence and newborn prevalence risk data.[69] Women who would choose amniocentesis and elective abortion of a cytogenetically abnormal infant will act on midtrimester risk data; women who do not wish amniocentesis or who would not abort an abnormal fetus may find some comfort in the lower risk for a surviving infant.

Infants with sex chromosome aneuploidy deserve special mention in this discussion. They are included in the overall risk figures for detection of aneuploidy at amniocentesis. These disorders are frequent in the population; Klinefelter's syndrome (47XXY karyotype) affects 1:600 males, Turner's syndrome (45X with or without mosaicism) is present in 1:3000 newborn females, and the 47XYY karyotype is present in 1:1000 newborn males, irrespective of maternal age. These three conditions are also more common in offspring of older mothers, although exact, year-specific risk figures are not available. In 2404 amniocenteses in women over age 34, 14 per cent of the fetuses with cytogenetic abnormalities had sex chromosome aneuploidy.[28] As with the rarer autosomal trisomies, specific discussion of the phenotype expected if such a child is liveborn is best done in individual counseling of a couple whose fetus has one of these abnormalities. Some couples will choose not to abort a fetus with abnormal sex chromosome constitution.

Prenatal cytogenetic diagnosis is also indicated in women of any age who have borne a previous child with aneuploidy. The chance of detecting an aneuploid fetus at amniocentesis is 1 to 1.4 per cent in several studies of younger mothers. For mothers past the age of 35, the age-related risk is greater than 1 per cent and determines the total risk. Recurrent nondisjunction may not involve the same chromosome pair in subsequent infants; one study of trisomy 21 revealed that only 50 per cent of detected abnormalities in siblings involved chromosome 21.[58]

Any parent with an abnormal karyotype has a risk of having children with cytogenetic abnormalities that may involve any chromosome pair. A parent carrying a balanced translocation has an increased risk of early spontaneous abortion and of midtrimester detection of a fetus with an abnormal karyotype. The risk for a liveborn child of unbalanced karyotype is 10 to 11 per cent in families that already have one such child. The risk of abnormal progeny is lower in families ascertained through a balanced carrier. The risk may be 4 per cent if the mother is the carrier and 2 per cent if the father is; the reason for this sex difference is not known. Amniocentesis is indicated in all families with a translocation carrier parent. Other abnormal parental karyotypes that increase the risk of fetal cytogenetic abnormality include Down's syndrome and fertility with sex chromosome aneuploidy (XXX, XYY, or mosaic Klinefelter's or Turner's syndrome).

Cytogenetic prenatal diagnosis may be indicated in women with thyroid disease, because several retrospective studies suggest an increased risk of nondisjunction in progeny of such women.[58] The reason is unknown.

Whether prenatal diagnosis has any benefit in couples with habitual abortion (consecutive loss of three or more conceptions) is a difficult decision. If the pregnancy of such a couple is successfully carried to 16 or 18 weeks, they may not wish to undertake any procedure with even a low risk to the continuation of the pregnancy unless they have a high risk for livebirth of an abnormal child. Parental karyotyping is indicated in the diagnostic evaluation of such couples; if no parental chromosome abnormality is detected, then prenatal cytogenetic studies are not indicated, although the rare possibility of parental gonadal abnormality has not been strictly excluded. The likelihood of finding a *parental* abnormality has ranged from 0 to 5 per cent in various studies.[26, 90] This variation is attributable to unrecognized differences in the cause of fetal loss. Cytogenetic studies on the abortuses would clearly define a subgroup of parents with a higher risk for recurrent cytogenetic abnormalities, but it is easier to do parental karyotypes after the fact and at least detect parents with mosaicism, translocations, and other predisposing causes. The study has not yet been done that would tell us whether a young mother with first trimester fetal loss due to nondisjunction (aneuploid abortus) has as high a recurrence risk as the young woman who has given birth to such a child (1 per cent).

Several genetic disorders are associated with chromosomal breakage or abnormalities that may be detected prenatally. These include Fanconi's syndrome, Bloom's syndrome, ataxiatelangiectasia, and a newly described syndrome of X-linked mental retardation associated with a fragile site on the X-chromosome. Despite the use of special cytogenetic culture techniques when such diagnoses are suspected, it is not possible to detect all cases prenatally.

TABLE 5–17 MENDELIAN INHERITANCE IN MAN*

Trait	1958	1966	1968	1971	1975	1978
Autosomal Dominant	285	837	793	943	1218	1489
Autosomal Recessive	89	531	629	783	947	1117
Sex-Linked	38	119	123	150	171	205
Totals	412	1427	1545	1876	2336	2811

*Includes totals of proposed and proven assignments of traits and diseases to the three patterns of inheritance. (Adapted from McKusick, 1978.)

Mendelian Genetic Diagnosis at Amniocentesis

Single gene disorders are each quite rare, but collectively they are present in about 1 per cent of livebirths. Table 5–17, adapted from McKusick's comprehensive catalogues of those human diseases and traits with a proposed or proved monogenic pattern of inheritance, shows that 2811 mendelian traits had been identified by 1978.[53] Successful prenatal diagnosis of monogenic disease is presently limited to (1) diseases resulting in fetal dysmorphology that can be visualized by ultrasonographic, radiographic, or fetoscopic techniques; (2) diseases whose unique biochemical features permit a diagnosis from analysis of amniotic fluid, uncultured or cultured amniotic cells, or fetal blood samples; and (3) X-linked diseases of such severity in affected males that even when no diagnosis is possible, families desire fetal sex determination and plan to abort all male fetuses. Prenatal diagnoses of genetic disorders by fetal visualization techniques or fetal sex determination are discussed in other sections of this chapter. This section focuses on those genetic disorders whose detection is based on biochemical techniques. While over 100 such monogenic disorders can be diagnosed in utero, these successes are still limited to less than 10 per cent of genetic disorders, and active research in molecular genetics will continue to expand this list.

A specific discussion of the techniques for prenatal diagnosis in each such disease is beyond the scope of this chapter; even the list of those disorders whose diagnosis is possible has now exceeded the format of simple tables and requires yearly updating. Midtrimester pregnancies cannot be screened for such diseases; any attempt at prenatal diagnosis of an inborn error of metabolism requires intense efforts by specialized research laboratories and is targeted to those pregnancies with a 25 to 50 per cent risk of an affected fetus. Thus, only those pregnancies in which one parent has the disease (autosomal dominant), both parents (autosomal recessive) or the mother (X-linked) are carriers of one mutant gene, or a previous sibling has been born with the disease are candidates for attempted prenatal diagnosis.

A fundamental limitation in prenatal diagnosis of metabolic disorders is that diagnosis must be made in those fetal materials that are accessible for study during early pregnancy. Amniotic fluid, fetal fibroblasts, and small fetal blood samples can be obtained. If the genetic defect produces a detectable abnormality in these fetal products, diagnosis can be attempted. However, there are some diseases in which, although the molecular defect is understood, a prenatal diagnosis cannot be made because the defect is expressed only in liver, brain, or other inaccessible tissues. Because the entire genomic DNA is present in each fetal fibroblast, it is possible that the newer techniques of molecular genetics will eventually enable us to study any genetic locus in any cell from an individual even if we are studying a tissue in which that genetic locus is not active in vivo.

For the present, Table 5–18 illustrates categories of genetic metabolic diseases for which prenatal diagnosis is feasible or has already been accomplished. Present techniques of molecular genetic diagnosis exploit any significant and reproducible difference between tissues from an affected fetus and those from normal controls. Such differences range from unexplained but reproducible "bystander" phenomena to direct measurement of the gene itself and include, in order of ascending specificity, these determinations:

1. Measurement of any difference between homozygote and normal control cells. The difference may be distantly related, if at all, to the basic genetic defect, but it is reliably detectable. Example: attempts to diagnose cystic fibrosis in utero by a broad-based search for abnormalities in cellular enzymes, cell viability, or response to various drugs in amniotic cells from affected fetuses.[48]

2. Measurement of excess amounts of a metabolite present because of the genetic defect.

TABLE 5–18 CATEGORIES OF BIOCHEMICAL DISORDERS FOR WHICH PRENATAL DIAGNOSIS IS FEASIBLE; EXAMPLES OF SPECIFIC DISORDERS

Amino Acid Metabolic Disorders
Argininosuccinic aciduria
Maple syrup urine disease
Methylmalonic acidemia
Proprionyl-CoA carboxylase deficiency
Cystinosis
Homocystinuria
Carbohydrate Metabolic Disorders
Galactosemia
Glycogen storage diseases — Types II, III, IV
Glucose-6-phosphate dehydrogenase deficiency
Mucolipidoses — Types I–IV
Lipid Metabolic Disorders

Lipidosis Group
Gaucher's disease
Fabry's disease (XL)
Tay-Sachs disease
Sandhoff's disease
GM_1-gangliosidosis
Krabbe's disease
Metachromatic leukodystrophy
Niemann-Pick disease
Farber's disease

Other Lipid Disorders
Familial hypercholesterolemia (AD)
Cholesterol ester storage disease
Refsum's syndrome
Wolman's disease
Mucopolysaccharide Metabolic Disorders
Hurler's syndrome
Hunter's syndrome (XL)
Sanfilippo's syndrome
Scheie's syndrome
Morquio's syndrome
B-glucuronidase deficiency
Miscellaneous Disorders
Orotic aciduria
Lesch-Nyhan syndrome (XL)
Testicular feminization (XL)
Xeroderma pigmentosa
Hypophosphatasia (AR or AD)
Combined immunodeficiency disease (AR and XL)
Congenital adrenal hyperplasia
Porphyrias (AR and AD)
Sickle cell anemia
Thalassemia

Mode of inheritance: Autosomal recessive (AR) except when noted AD (autosomal dominant) or XL (X-linked).

Example: cystinosis, in which, although the exact genetic defect has not been elucidated, homozygotes can be detected in utero because of the accumulation of excesses of the amino acid cystine in their amniotic fluid cells.

3. Measurement of absence of activity of the mutant gene. Example: Tay-Sachs disease, in which the activity of the enzyme hexosaminidase A is measured in cultured amniotic fluid cells and found to be virtually absent in affected fetal cells.

4. Direct measurement demonstrating absence of a gene product. Example: hemophilia A, in which immunoradiometric measurement of Factor VIII coagulant antigen demonstrates absence or severe deficiency of the gene product in fetal plasma samples from affected males.

5. Direct measurement of an abnormal gene product synthesized by the mutant gene. Example: sickle cell anemia, in which the abnormal sickle hemoglobin can be detected in fetal blood samples.

6. Direct measurement of the absence (deletion) of a gene itself. Example, alpha-thalassemia, in which new molecular hybridization techniques can probe the amniotic fluid cell DNA directly and document the absence of the alpha-globin genes in affected fetuses.

7. Use of fortuitous linkage of the mutated gene locus to another locus that is polymorphic and can be measured. Example: sickle cell anemia, in which the polymorphism of a restriction endonuclease site near the beta-globin gene site can be used for linkage analysis in some families to detect fetuses that must have inherited the sickle genes. In families in which both carrier parents have the linked restriction site mutation and the sickle mutation, homozygous infants can be identified by detecting the former mutation easily and quickly in amniotic fluid cells. Direct assay of fetal blood for the presence of sickle hemoglobin is no longer necessary, and the higher risk fetoscopy and fetal blood sampling procedures are avoided. Further examples include myotonic dystrophy, in which the affected gene locus is linked to the ABH secretor locus, and nail-patella syndrome, with linkage of the affected gene locus to the ABO locus.

Autosomal Biochemical Disorders. These disorders are, with few exceptions, severe and life-threatening whether in childhood (e.g., Tay-Sachs disease) or in later life (e.g., myotonic dystrophy). A description of the diagnostic features of individual diseases is beyond the scope of this chapter, as are the specifics of prenatal diagnosis where this is possible. However, these diseases share certain features, which provide the impetus for attempts at prenatal diagnosis. Some, such as Tay-Sachs disease, are untreatable, involve severe morbidity, and are ultimately fatal. Many couples who have experienced this course of events with a previous child would have no further children rather than run the 1:4

risk of recurrence, and most couples would elect midtrimester abortion of a similarly affected child if prenatal diagnosis were available. Some, such as maple syrup urine disease, are treatable,[14] but the treatment regimen is so difficult and the outcome so uncertain that many parents who have had an affected child would elect abortion of another such fetus. For a few of the autosomal recessive metabolic disorders, it has been shown or is suspected that treatment of an affected infant would be improved if therapy were begun during pregnancy, and these cases provide the greatest impetus for prenatal diagnosis. Galactosemia and vitamin B_{12}–responsive methylmalonic acidemia are examples of metabolic genetic diseases in which prenatal therapy has been beneficial.[1, 20] For most of the metabolic genetic disorders it is assumed that the relevant maternal enzyme, though present at heterozygote concentration (50 per cent), can maintain a normal metabolic environment for both mother and fetus and that the homozygous affected infant will experience the metabolic effects of his inheritance only after birth.

Sex Determination: X-linked Diagnosis. There are about 200 X-linked genetic disorders, many of which are associated with mental retardation, serious physical morbidity, or death. Because prenatal sex determination is readily available, these disorders represent an underutilized area of prenatal diagnosis. In families at risk for such serious and ultimately fatal diseases as Duchenne muscular dystrophy, it is possible to identify and abort all male fetuses, since only males are at risk for the disease. For families who would have no children unless some form of diagnosis were available, sex determination offers a guarantee that they can have normal girls.

Four methods for determining fetal sex have been employed. These are (1) demonstration of the inactive X-chromosome chromatin (Barr body), (2) Y-chromosome fluorescence, (3) determination of fetal karyotype, and (4) determination of amniotic fluid testosterone. Determining the full fetal karyotype with specific identification of all chromosomes including the sex chromosomes, using cultured amniotic fluid cells, is the most reliable method. However, it is the most time-consuming as well, and studies have been done to see if either the inactive second X of a female (Barr body) or the Y of a male can be identified in uncultured amniotic fluid cells. These methods are not reliable enough and are not recommended for prenatal genetic diagnosis. Amniotic fluid testosterone measurement is more accurate, and there is little overlap in values for the two sexes between 11 and 20 weeks gestation. Values obtained earlier or later in the pregnancy do not discriminate as clearly between the sexes. Since female serum testosterone in either the mother or a female fetus is higher than amniotic fluid testosterone in a male gestation, contamination of the amniotic fluid sample with either fetal or maternal blood could result in a false positive prediction of a male fetus.

When prenatal diagnosis is undertaken for serious genetic indications and identification of a male fetus may lead to midtrimester abortion or further invasive studies such as fetoscopy, both amniotic cell culture for fetal karyotype and amniotic fluid testosterone determination should be performed. The latter provides a second means of confirming a sex diagnosis, serves as backup in case of a cell culture failure, and provides a clue to the possibility of maternal fibroblast contamination of the amniotic cell culture. Since maternal cell admixture is the most common source of error in fetal sex determination by cultured cell karyotype and may occur in 2 to 3 of every 1000 amniocenteses, Milunsky recommends routine determination of the maternal karyotype in cases involving X-linked diagnosis.[61] Comparison of chromosome heteromorphisms can establish that a female karyotype is indeed both female and of fetal origin.

At present only a minority of X-linked disorders can be specifically diagnosed in utero. Some of the more common of these disorders for which prenatal diagnosis is either feasible or has already been accomplished are listed in Table 5–19. If prenatal diagnosis can be made from cultured amniotic fluid cells, fetal cells are grown

TABLE 5–19 SELECTED X-LINKED DISORDERS FOR WHICH PRENATAL DIAGNOSIS IS FEASIBLE

Amniotic Fluid Cell Culture
Adrenoleukodystrophy
Androgen resistance/receptor deficiency
Combined immunodeficiency disease
Fabry's disease
G-6-PD deficiency
Hunter's syndrome
Lesch-Nyhan syndrome
Menkes' disease
Steroid sulfatase deficiency/X-linked ichthyosis
X-linked mental retardation/fragile X chromosome

Fetal Blood Samples
Chronic granulomatous disease
Duchenne muscular dystrophy
Hemophilia A
Hemophilia B
Wiskott-Aldrich syndrome

in tandem for sex determination and biochemical diagnosis should this prove necessary. If specific determination that a fetus is affected requires assay of fetal blood samples, diagnostic efforts begin with amniocentesis at 16 menstrual weeks for amniotic fluid testosterone and amniotic cell karyotype studies. Once a male fetus has been diagnosed, plans are made for fetal blood sampling at 18 to 20 weeks gestation.

Thus, a couple at risk for an X-linked fetal disease faces a series of decisions, which should be made after counseling with the prenatal genetics group that will perform the procedures. The a priori risk for an affected fetus is 1:4 (25 per cent). Fetal sex determination will identify the 50 per cent of all such pregnancies that are not at risk because the fetus is female. For those pregnancies with a male fetus, the risk is now 50:50. The fetus either has the disease or is completely normal. If no prenatal diagnosis is available for the disease, a couple must then decide whether to keep or abort a male pregnancy at this juncture — a difficult decision, involving the twin realizations that the aborted male is as likely to have been normal as affected and that the decision means the couple will have no male offspring. If prenatal diagnosis is to be performed on samples already obtained at amniocentesis, the couple will be able to await the final decision concerning abortion of an affected male with the 50:50 likelihood that the tests will identify a normal male. If fetal blood sampling is necessary to reach a diagnosis, the couple must decide to undergo this risk to the fetus and the continuation of the pregnancy as well as the further difficulties and costs associated with travel to one of the few prenatal diagnosis centers where the procedure can be performed. These risks (discussed in detail in the section on fetoscopy) may range from 3 to 5 per cent for fetal loss and 9 per cent for premature birth.[51a]

Fetoscopy and Fetal Tissue Sampling

The techniques discussed here provide a major and exciting extension of the possibilities of prenatal diagnosis and treatment of numerous conditions affecting the fetus. Even in experienced hands, these procedures carry a significant risk of fetal demise, miscarriage, or later pregnancy complications such as amniotic fluid leakage or premature delivery, and so they have first come into use for genetic diagnosis where the a priori risk of fetal disease ranges from 25 to 50 per cent. Their widespread application in fetal medicine is likely in the near future; this discussion is restricted to their use in genetic diseases.

The techniques presently in use include transabdominal endoscopy with rigid or flexible fiberoptic endoscopes, which permit direct visualization of specific aspects of fetal anatomy with good success. A general examination of surface anatomy is not feasible. The cannula sheath (2 to 3 mm in diameter) permits introduction of a biopsy forceps or blood sampling needle from which fetal samples for diagnosis can be obtained. Skin biopsies (1 mm) can be obtained from fetal scalp or flank with minimal trauma. Blood samples are obtained from fetal vessels on the chorionic plate of the placenta or the cord under direct visualization. Aspiration through such thin-gauge needles is difficult, and fetal blood samples are often mixed with amniotic fluid, maternal blood or both. Postpuncture bleeding usually stops spontaneously, and blood loss is estimated at 1 to 3 ml, representing no more than 3 per cent of the fetal and placental blood volume at 18 to 20 weeks gestation. Fetal blood can also be obtained by placental aspiration without fetoscopy. This technique requires that each sample be tested immediately for the presence of fetal blood. Repeated aspirations beneath the chorionic plate are performed blindly until fetal blood is obtained. Such samples may be mixed with maternal blood or interstitial fluid but are less likely to contain amniotic fluid. Fetoscopy for anatomic diagnosis is performed between 15 and 18 weeks, when the fetus is small and the amniotic fluid clear. Fetal blood sampling is done between 18 and 20 weeks gestation, when the fetal blood volume is large enough. The procedures are always done in conjunction with ultrasound scanning to document fetal age, fetal lie, placental location, and fetal viability before and after the procedure. These procedures can be performed under local anesthesia, and the mother is observed overnight following the procedure.[51]

The risks from these invasive procedures are difficult to estimate, since few procedures have been done and variables such as technical talent and experience will affect risk statistics. To date fetoscopic examination carries a risk of fetal death or miscarriage of at least 3 per cent in those pregnancies that were not electively aborted because of the fetal diagnosis.[51a] Fetal exsanguination, placental abruption, early labor, and amnionitis have been reported. Chronic amniotic fluid leakage (8 per cent) and premature delivery (9 per cent) are further complications. The risk of Rh sensitization is undoubtedly greater than in routine amniocentesis, and RhoGAM is recommended unless the fetal blood type was obtained and proved Rh negative. Placental aspiration carries similar risks of acute fetal death and Rh sensitization, with an overall fetal loss of 10 per cent, and has been abandoned in those university centers where direct fetoscopy is available.

Anatomic Diagnosis. Endoscopic visualization of fetuses at risk for genetic diseases causing morphologic abnormalities that cannot be seen by ultrasound scan has been successful. To date, the procedure is most successful if a single, severe surface defect can be seen in a limited portion of the anatomy. This defect may be a marker for the entire birth defect syndrome, although not itself the most devastating of the defects. For instance, Ellis–van Creveld syndrome, a recessive disorder with dwarfism, congenital heart disease, and polydactyly, has been diagnosed by visualization of the postaxial sixth digit at 17 weeks gestation.[50] A number of genetic syndromes causing fetal dysmorphology, which at present cannot be detected before birth by any other means, could potentially be diagnosed by combined use of ultrasound scans and fetoscopy. Such disorders include anophthalmia and the Apert's, Crouzon's, Cockayne's, de Lange's, Coffin's, Fanconi's, Meckel's, Lawrence-Moon-Biedel, leprechaun, Noonan's, Lowe's, Robert's, Seckel's, Smith-Lemli-Opitz, and Treacher Collins syndromes.

Biopsy Diagnosis. Direct fetal skin biopsy provides tissue for enzymatic or karyotype diagnosis and can be used if amniotic fluid cells cannot provide a diagnosis. In future, biochemical, immunologic, or morphologic analysis of skin may enable us to diagnose diseases of collagen, keratin, or epidermis. It is even conceivable that biopsies of fetal muscle or liver by microtechniques will someday be feasible and will permit diagnosis of genetic diseases expressed only in these organs. For instance, ornithine transcarbamylase deficiency, in which absence of a urea cycle enzyme leads to lethal neonatal hyperammonemia in affected males, can be diagnosed only from enzyme assay in liver tissue.

Fetal Blood Sampling. In theory many of the genetic diseases that can be diagnosed from peripheral blood samples after birth could be diagnosed before 20 fetal weeks. A number of practical limitations now exist, which can be overcome in time. Normal standards for each test at 20 fetal weeks will be necessary, but they will be slow in coming because the risks preclude performing fetal sampling in normal pregnancies. Normal fetal developmental schedules for various enzymes and metabolic processes are not known, nor is it known whether some metabolic effects of a genetic disease can be measured in fetal plasma despite placental clearance. The technology necessary to aspirate a pure fetal blood sample will be very helpful, since some assays will never be possible in the presence of contaminating interstitial fluid, amniotic fluid, or maternal blood cells or plasma.

Diseases that could be diagnosed from fetal red cells include the hemoglobinopathies — sickle cell anemia and alpha- and beta-thalassemia. Abnormal hemoglobins such as the sickle beta-globin, as well as absent or reduced rates of globin chain synthesis in the thalassemias, can be detected. However, recent advances in molecular genetics now permit diagnosis of alpha-thalassemia, beta-thalassemia, and 60 to 80 per cent of cases of sickle cell anemia in fetuses from amniotic fluid cell assays, so that fetal blood need not be obtained in these cases. Diseases involving red cell enzyme deficiencies (argininemia, pyruvate kinase deficiency) can also be diagnosed from fetal red cells.

Hemophilia A can be diagnosed from fetal plasma samples by use of an immunoradiometric assay, which reveals normal concentrations of Factor VIII–related-antigen and absence or severe deficiency of Factor VIII coagulant-antigen in affected males. Measurement of Factor VIII coagulant activity, the standard diagnostic test in newborns, has proved unreliable in fetal samples mixed with amniotic fluid.[19] Hemophilia B potentially can be diagnosed by similar means. Attempts to diagnose Duchenne muscular dystrophy by assay of fetal plasma CPK have been partially successful; not all affected fetuses have shown CPK elevation by 20 weeks gestation.

Studies of fetal leukocytes, platelets, and B and T lymphocytes should permit diagnosis of several heritable defects in these cell lines. Chronic granulomatous disease of childhood has already been diagnosed by the demonstration of abnormal white cell function in fetal cells, and Chédiak-Higashi syndrome (abnormal polys), Wiskott-Aldrich syndrome (abnormal platelets), agranulocytosis, agammaglobulinemia (absent B cells), and combined immunodeficiency disease (absent B and T cells) should be detectable.

In short, fetoscopy and fetal tissue sampling extend the range of genetic prenatal diagnosis and enable us to detect anatomic abnormalities and abnormalities in fetal tissues accessible to the sampling tools (such as components of blood or skin) that are not detectable in any other way. The risk of these invasive procedures is balanced against the high risk for an affected infant (25 to 50 per cent) and the severity of the disease when decisions are made about the use of these tests to reach a prenatal diagnosis. Possibly, these same techniques will soon provide the fetal access necessary to treat such a disease once diagnosed.

PREGNANCY IN GENETIC DISEASES

The effect of individual maternal genetic diseases on the course and successful outcome of pregnancy is an area of increasing interest and developing knowledge. The most obvious area of future interest is the management of pregnancy in those women who have been successfully treated for genetic metabolic disorders and who are now reaching childbearing age. In addition, our increasing clinical sophistication in recognizing a spectrum of severity within genetic disorders has led to an appreciation of the need to define risks and prognosis for pregnancy within each disorder in relation to the severity of expression of the maternal genetic disease rather than in terms of general caveats. Recommendations concerning reproduction should be based on as accurate a prognosis for both mother and fetus as can be determined prospectively and should not confuse the separable components of the prognosis. Most of this chapter deals with the clinical situation when the mother is presumed to be clinically normal and capable of a normal pregnancy and delivery. Recommendations concerning reproduction are based on the risk of a fetal genotype that will lead to clinical abnormalities in the fetus either from conception or after birth. The opposite extreme along the spectrum of maternal-fetal interaction is the situation in which the mother's genetic disease is so clinically severe that it precludes her carrying even a normal fetus successfully. Those few maternal genetic diseases that preclude successful reproduction will be reviewed in this section. However, the usual clinical situation in maternal genetic diseases is more subtle and complex than either of the extremes, and several individual variables as well as their interaction must be considered in predicting pregnancy outcome. These variables include

1. Genotypes — the fetal and maternal genotypes and their respective contributions to the fetomaternal environment
2. Genetic therapy — the ability to directly treat the genetic disease in the mother, the fetus, or both
3. Medical therapy — the clinical severity of the maternal disease and the ability to treat maternal medical complications
4. Unique pregnancy complications — unique complications of pregnancy, labor, or lactation due to the genetic disease or unique effects of these biologic processes on the maternal disease

Clinical data bearing on these variables are available for some maternal genetic diseases, but these data are often anecdotal or suffer from ascertainment bias because workers in centers that see the most severe cases publish the clinical reviews. For only a few diseases do we have sufficient unbiased data on pregnancy outcome to make secure prognoses, and even in these situations, improvements in treatment of the disease or its complications are altering those prognoses yearly. No systematic, collated body of information yet exists that reviews what is known about *pregnancy* in each genetic disease, although such compilations exist for the diseases themselves.[5, 53] Before proceeding to discussion of those genetic diseases in which substantial evidence of pregnancy outcome has been compiled, the types of variables involved merit brief review.

Genotypes. The maternal and fetal genotypes will have individual and combined effects on the pregnancy. For example, in chromosomal diseases we have assumed in previous discussion that the risk in a pregnancy is the risk of *conceiving* a child with an abnormal karyotype and that only the fetal phenotype will affect the pregnancy outcome. In considering pregnancy in a woman with Down's syndrome we have focused on the high risk (50 per cent) that the fetus will be aneuploid. But even if the fetus had a normal karyotype, fetal outcome might be compromised. Our increasing appreciation of the biochemical effects of the triple dose of each gene on chromosome 21 and how these gene dosages contribute to the maternal disease[92] should lead us to realize that these effects might reach the fetus and cause developmental abnormalities that could not be offset by a normal fetal karyotype.[84]

Historically, we have assumed for all genetic diseases that a genetically normal fetus can compensate for a maternal disease and that a genetically normal mother not only can maintain her health while carrying a fetus of abnormal genotype but can compensate for the fetus so that the fetus suffers the full effect of its genotype only after birth. The degree to which mother and fetus can compensate or aggravate each other's genetic deficiencies is crucial to pregnancy outcome, and it is worthy of review apart from specific diseases so that we are aware of the range of genotype-genotype combinations and interactions possible. This review can clarify certain unspoken assumptions and the subtle differences in combined genetic environment that might affect outcome. To illustrate, let us examine the situation in a metabolic genetic disease due to autosomal recessive inheritance of an enzyme deficiency. Nine maternal-fetal genotypic combinations could theoretically occur (Fig. 5–10). A normal maternal-fetal combination (N) needs no

FETAL GENOTYPE

AUTOSOMAL
RECESSIVE
DISEASE

	HOMOZYGOUS AFFECTED (Ho)	HETEROZYGOUS CARRIER (He)	NORMAL (N)
HOMOZYGOUS AFFECTED (Ho)	Ho - Ho 0/4 alleles at this locus normal <div align="right">3</div>	Ho - He ¼ alleles normal 1 fetal <div align="right">4</div>	X <div align="right">1</div>
HETEROZYGOUS CARRIER (He)	He - Ho ¼ alleles normal 1 maternal <div align="right">5</div>	He - He 2/4 alleles normal 1 maternal 1 fetal <div align="right">6</div>	He - N 3/4 alleles normal 1 maternal 2 fetal <div align="right">7</div>
NORMAL (N)	X <div align="right">2</div>	N - He 3/4 alleles normal 2 maternal 1 fetal <div align="right">8</div>	N

MATERNAL GENOTYPE

FIGURE 5–10. The nine fetomaternal genotypic combinations that are theoretically possible in a recessive genetic disease.

further discussion. Two genotypic combinations could not occur unless the allele inherited by the fetus from the mother had undergone spontaneous mutation back to normal (X, box 1) or to the mutation inherited from the father (X, box 2), and these possibilities are so remote that we dismiss them a priori. But from this dismissal comes one important realization. A mother affected with this disease will *never* carry a genetically normal fetus; the fetus will be an obligate carrier of the mutation and may have a limited ability to compensate for the maternal disease.

Consider next the genotypes Ho-Ho (box 3). This genotypic combination cannot occur because of the mother's disease; it occurs only if the father is a carrier of the same genetic mutation. Yet, covert assumptions about this genotypic combination underlie two extremes of prognostic advice. Physicians confronted with a woman with a recessive genetic disease may incorrectly tell her she cannot have children because they will have the disease and the combination would be lethal. At the other extreme, advice is based on the assumption that the chance of the father's being a carrier of the same mutation is so remote that this combination will never arise. In fact, the maternal genotype is homozygous recessive, and the fetal genotype at that locus is already at least heterozygous for the mutation. Thus the carrier rate for this mutation in the relevant population becomes the key variable determining the risk that an affected mother could be carrying an affected child. For several recessive genetic diseases now compatible with maternal survival and conception, the spousal carrier rate is not trivial. For instance, in sickle cell anemia, an affected black woman has a 10 per cent risk that her black spouse is a carrier and thus a 5 per cent risk that both mother and fetus will have sickle cell anemia. Carrier testing of the spouses of women with recessive genetic diseases is an important aspect of determining pregnancy prognosis.

The remaining combinations of maternal-fetal genotypes are those we encounter most frequently. If the mother herself suffers from the recessive disease, then at best her fetus is a carrier and between them they have only one normal allele at the locus in question (Ho-He, Fig. 5–10, box 4). The normal allele is fetal and may well have a developmental schedule for its expression that leaves the fetus vulnerable. This genetic situation could well account for the inability of women with untreated phenylketonuria or homocystinuria to bear normal children. If the mother is a heterozygous carrier, she may carry a fetus who is affected (box 5), heterozygous (box 6), or normal (box 7), depending upon the allele inherited from the father. We assume that the health of mother and infant will be normal until birth in all three of these genotypic combinations, but systematic studies to examine outcome in these three situations have not been done. The one normal maternal allele is assumed to be capable of both keeping the mother well and compensating for either the homozygous or the heterozygous fetal genotype without distinction. The final possible combination (box 8) is also assumed to be normal.

For X-linked recessive diseases the same considerations apply, with the further complications that (1) the sex of the fetus alters risk, since an affected male has only one mutated allele at the locus in question, (2) the contribution of the normal and abnormal maternal alleles cannot be predicted a priori, since random inactivation of the two maternal X chromosomes will make the mother a mosaic of these alleles and their products, and (3) a heterozygous mother carrying a heterozygous daughter creates a maternal-fetal combination in which the ratio of normal to mutated alleles expressed in each mosaic contributes to the final amount of normal gene product available to sustain fetal development.

Autosomal dominant diseases create yet other maternal-fetal conditions. For instance, studies are now under way to determine whether infants with dominant diseases such as neurofibromatosis, myotonic dystrophy, or Marfan's syndrome are more severely affected if they have an affected mother and not only inherited her mutated allele but also developed in an abnormal maternal milieu. It is possible that severe congenital myotonia results when a mother with autosomal dominant myotonic dystrophy carries a fetus with an inherited mutated allele.[91]

Genetic Disease Therapy. Ability to treat the genetic disease directly has clear implications for pregnancy outcome, and such therapy is becoming more possible. For instance, in genetic diseases that can be treated by dietary restriction, it is possible that treatment of maternal disease before conception and throughout pregnancy will permit normal intrauterine development. In galactosemia, galactose restriction during pregnancy has prevented mental retardation and cataracts in homozygous affected infants carried by heterozygous mothers. Such therapy may also work for heterozygous or homozygous infants carried by affected mothers.[20] In phenylketonuria, successful therapy through dietary phenylalanine restriction has led to normal development of affected women who are now in their childbearing years. A recent analysis of pregnancies in such women has shown a high rate of spontaneous abortion as well as microcephaly and mental retardation in offspring of women who did not resume their dietary therapy during pregnancy. Even resumption of therapy during pregnancy did not prevent these fetal problems, and it is not yet known whether maternal dietary restriction before conception as well as throughout pregnancy will be successful.[47]

Medical Therapy. The clinical severity of the maternal disease and the ability to treat its medical complications may be the determinants of successful pregnancy outcome in some settings. Ability to control anemia and avoid sickle crises will affect pregnancy outcome in sickle cell anemia; prevention of hemorrhagic complications due to deficiencies in platelet number or function would be important in adult Gaucher's disease or Glanzman's thrombasthenia.[41] These situations involve medical judgments about the mother's health, the ability to treat complications of her disease, and the effect of pregnancy on the mother's medical condition.

Unique Pregnancy Complications. The biologic process of pregnancy, labor, delivery, and lactation may pose unique hazards in certain maternal genetic diseases. For instance, anecdotal reports suggest that some women affected with Types III or IV Ehlers-Danlos syndrome may be at increased risk for spontaneous rupture of major arteries during pregnancy and delivery.[3] Women with porphyria may suffer acute attacks.[9] Alternatively, the genetic disease itself may complicate the pregnancy or delivery. For example, in X-linked ichthyosis a carrier mother and affected infant have placental steroid sulfatase deficiency resulting in low concentrations of urine and serum estriol during pregnancy and failure to enter labor.[80] Table 5–20 lists some of the reported unique complications of pregnancy in genetic diseases.

Specific Genetic Disorders and Pregnancy

Metabolic Disorders. Genetic disorders that lead to an abnormal maternal metabolic environment could be expected to expose the fetus to potentially toxic deficiency or excess of key metabolic products at a developmental stage when the fetal enzyme systems are not able to compensate for this exposure.

PHENYLKETONURIA. Successful treatment of this recessive disorder has taught us that phenylalanine excess is toxic to the developing brain.

TABLE 5–20 UNIQUE COMPLICATIONS OF PREGNANCY AND LABOR IN GENETIC DISEASES*

Premature Birth
    fetal Ehlers-Danlos syndrome
    fetal or maternal Marfan's syndrome
    maternal myotonic dystrophy

Arrested Labor
    fetal X-linked adrenal hypoplasia
    fetal X-linked steroid sulfatase deficiency
    maternal myotonic dystrophy

Indications for Possible Cesarean Section
Cephalopelvic disproportion
        maternal achondroplasia
        maternal dwarfism — various types
Tissue fragility
        fetal osteogenesis imperfecta congenita
        maternal Ehlers-Danlos syndrome
Bleeding diathesis
        hemophilia A or B
        Glanzmann's thrombasthenia
        Von Willebrand's disease
        Gaucher's disease with thrombocytopenia

Lactation
Maternal metabolic disorder
        hypercholesterolemia — excess cholesterol in milk
        hypophosphatemia — deficient phosphate in milk
Infant metabolic disorder
        phenylketonuria — requires phenylalanine restriction
        hypercholesterolemia — requires cholesterol restriction
        urea cycle disorders — require protein restriction

Effect of Pregnancy on Maternal Disease
Maternal disease may improve
        hereditary angioneurotic edema
        hemochromatosis
        familial Mediterranean fever
Maternal disease may worsen
        retinitis pigmentosa
        porphyrias
        sickle cell anemia
        Refsum's syndrome
        cutaneous collagenoma

*Examples of disorders are listed; this table is not comprehensive.

Affected infants are normal at birth because of maternal compensation. If treated in childhood with dietary phenylalanine restriction, they reach a stage of mental developmental maturity at which hyperphenylalaninemia can be tolerated without mental deterioration and the diet can be abandoned. However, when such women become pregnant, the toxic effects of hyperphenylalaninemia during intrauterine development include an increased risk of spontaneous abortion as well as of microcephaly, mental retardation, and congenital heart disease in their offspring. A recent study of 524 pregnancies in 155 such women has demonstrated the correlation of these fetal defects with the degree of maternal phenylalanine excess. Dietary restriction reinstituted at varying times during gestation did not prevent fetal abnormalities; in three pregnancies, treatment was resumed before conception, and two fetuses were normal and one microcephalic. Further study with carefully monitored early treatment is necessary.[47]

HOMOCYSTINURIA. Women with cystathionine-β-synthetase deficiency have abnormalities including lens dislocation, scoliosis, osteoporosis, mental retardation, and vascular thromboemboli, but are fertile. Pregnancies in 15 such women have resulted in 11 spontaneous abortions or fetal deaths, 1 hydrocephalic infant, and 3 apparently normal infants. Of these three, one was born to a woman on vitamin B_6 therapy who had had five spontaneous abortions before treatment. It is possible that women with the B_6-responsive enzyme mutation have greater reproductive success with therapy; it is clear that the spectrum of reproductive fitness in this disease is not yet defined.[8, 64, 75]

GALACTOSEMIA. The hepatic failure and cataracts characterizing patients with galactose transferase enzyme deficiency can be prevented by dietary galactose restriction. Since the syndrome is present at birth in affected infants, dietary restriction during pregnancy is recommended in heterozygous mothers[16] and should be recommended during pregnancy in affected women themselves. Reproductive experience in successfully treated galactosemic women is not yet available.

UREA CYCLE DISORDERS. Five distinct biochemical diseases result from deficiency of different enzymes in the hepatic urea cycle. Various metabolites preceeding the blocked step may accumulate, but the serious neurologic toxicity that can occur seems related to the degree of hyperammonemia that ensues when dietary nitrogen cannot be fixed to form urea. Restriction of dietary protein intake has been successful in preventing severe brain damage in these patients, and careful dietary treatment to protect the fetuses of such women may be needed, because the effect of chronic modest hyperammonemia on fetal development is not yet known.

WILSON'S DISEASE. This recessive disease of progressive copper storage leads to toxic damage to the liver and basal ganglia. It can now be treated by chelation and removal of copper stores with D-penicillamine and is thus compatible with survival to adulthood and reproduction. Copper chelation therapy must be lifelong, and attempts to avoid penicillamine treatment during pregnancy have permitted rapid maternal copper reaccumulation and can result in an acute toxic hemolytic anemia. Despite the potential dangers of penicillamine treatment during pregnancy, there has been no clear-cut evidence of reproductive difficulties or fetal impairment from pregnancy in treated maternal Wilson's disease.[81, 89]

PORPHYRIAS. Women with the dominantly inherited hepatic porphyrias (variegate, acute intermittent, and coproporphyria) are at risk for exacerbation of their disease during pregnancy. In one series of 50 patients, 54 per cent had an acute attack during pregnancy or the puerperium; total fetal loss was 13 per cent, and there was one maternal death. Infants born to mothers who experienced an acute attack were smaller than those of porphyric women without such gestational relapses.[9]

Many genetic metabolic disorders are so rare that adequate experience with fertility, reproductive fitness, special risks or complications of pregnancy, and fetal outcome are not available to aid in estimating a prognosis for an individual woman affected by one of these diseases. Further, experience with successful treatment of such diseases is limited, and few treated patients have reached their reproductive years. In counseling of such rare patients, the metabolic nuances of each patient's own disease as well as the available collective experience must be considered and reviewed with the prospective mother.

Connective Tissue, Skeletal, and Muscular Disorders. These disorders may limit childbearing, depending upon the clinical severity of the mother's condition.

MARFAN'S SYNDROME. Women affected with this dominant disorder have ectopia lentis and skeletal and cardiovascular abnormalities. There is a broad spectrum of clinical severity, and anecdotal reports of aortic dissection in association with pregnancy portray a rare complication. Since the maternal risks in pregnancy as well as the diminished life expectancy in this disease are related to cardiovascular complications, prospective studies of early detection and propranolol treatment may alter these risks.[74] A recent review of pregnancy in Marfan's syndrome revealed one maternal death in 106 pregnancies of 26 affected women. This death was due to endocarditis in a woman with known mitral regurgitation before pregnancy. Other maternal medical complications were no different from those of unaffected mothers carrying infants with Marfan's syndrome, but the rates of spontaneous abortion (21 per cent) and premature birth (12 per cent) were higher. Thus, the chance for unsuccessful pregnancy outcome may be higher than the risk of severe complications of the maternal disease during childbearing.[73]

EHLERS-DANLOS SYNDROMES. This group of collagen diseases is heterogeneous; the classic form causes skin and joint hyperelasticity and fragile, easily bruised skin with poor wound healing. In some of the seven distinguishable subtypes, spontaneous arterial or intestinal rupture has occurred, but reports of rupture during pregnancy are rare and no accurate risk is calculable.[3] Complications that clearly occur include premature birth when the infant has Ehlers-Danlos syndrome,[2] complications of labor and delivery related to skin fragility and hyperextensibility, and postpartum uterine prolapse.[4]

OSTEOGENESIS IMPERFECTA. The congenital form of this collagen disorder causes severe bone fragility with fractures in utero and during delivery. It is an indication for cesarean section.[76] Women with the dominant form of osteogenesis imperfecta, while subject to risk of bone fractures with little trauma, do not have undue difficulty during pregnancy.

SKELETAL DISORDERS. Various genetic forms of dwarfism lead to maternal pelvic deformities, which may necessitate cesarean section delivery. Achondroplasia is chief among these, but in any of the rarer skeletal dysplasias estimates can be made of anticipated cephalopelvic disproportion, assuming that the infant will be of normal size.

MYOTONIC DYSTROPHY. Women affected with this dominant muscle disease have progressive myotonia, muscle weakness, cardiac involvement, and ovarian dysfunction and fibrosis. Thus, fertility is impaired, but in those women who do become pregnant the obstetric complications include spontaneous abortion, hydramnios, premature labor, uterine atony, and postpartum hemorrhage as well as neonatal death due to severe congenital myotonia. The latter may be an example of the detrimental effect of the maternal genetic disease on infants who have inherited the myotonia gene.[91]

Hematologic Disorders. Many genetic disorders cause severe anemia, thrombocytopenia, platelet dysfunction, clotting disorders, or white cell dysfunction. Management of maternal or fetal complications during pregnancy, delivery, and the puerperium is generally related to the ability to manage particular medical complications and is reviewed in Chapter 3.

GENETIC HEMOGLOBINOPATHIES AND HEMOLYTIC ANEMIAS. Successful management of pregnancy in a patient with sickle cell anemia or sickle–hemoglobin C anemia is very challenging (see Chapter 3). Heterozygotes for sickle trait may have isosthenuria and an increased incidence of urinary tract infections during pregnancy but are not at increased risk for other complications.[6] Hemolytic anemia occurring during pregnancy may be the first clue to a previously undiagnosed genetic disorder.[63]

CLOTTING DISORDERS. In treatment of hemophilia A and B, consideration must be given to the ability of the carrier mother to maintain hemostasis during labor and delivery, because her random balance of active and inactive X chromosomes may limit her ability to synthesize adequate amounts of these X-linked clotting factors. Women with Von Willebrand's disease also require special attention to the risk imposed by their prolonged bleeding times, and in all the genetic clotting disorders the safe delivery of an affected infant may require cesarean section. Genetic abnormalities of platelets, such as Glanzmann's thrombasthenia, may require platelet transfusions to prevent maternal bleeding or cesarean delivery of an affected infant. Several genetic disorders of catabolic pathways lead to storage of unmetabolized compounds in the reticuloendothelial system, the bone marrow, or both and cause hypersplenism and thrombocytopenia. Adult Gaucher's disease[41] and Von Gierke's disease[17] are examples of such disorders, in which therapy is directed at medical management of bleeding problems.

In short, modern techniques for medical management of various hematologic disorders are applicable to the management of pregnancy in a woman with a genetic hematologic disorder and are the key determinants of a successful pregnancy outcome.

GENETIC DIAGNOSIS IN ABORTIONS AND STILLBIRTHS

Genetic disease may be the cause of spontaneous abortion or stillbirth, and despite loss of the present pregnancy, an accurate diagnosis may have important implications for counseling, parental testing, and prenatal diagnosis in subsequent pregnancies. Since miscarriage in the first trimester is a common event, occurring in 15 to 20 per cent of all pregnancies, one or two early spontaneous abortions in a couple with no other evidence of abnormality do not warrant extensive investigation. However, recurrent unexplained fetal loss or the loss of physically abnormal fetuses does call for further diagnostic studies.

Recurrent early miscarriage may be a clue to a balanced chromosome translocation in either parent. Chromosome studies on both parents using the new banding techniques may reveal a parental translocation in 1 to 10 per cent of such couples (see translocation, p. 112). Such a diagnosis would permit more accurate counseling of the couple concerning the risk of miscarriage in subsequent pregnancies and the need for diagnostic amniocentesis and fetal chromosome studies in any pregnancies that reach 16 weeks.

When a pregnancy is lost later in gestation or the infant is stillborn, a range of diagnostic studies might assist in determining whether the present fetal loss was caused by a genetic disease with a risk of recurrence in future pregnancies. Full autopsy should be encouraged in all such cases, especially if any external physical abnormalities are present. Helpful adjuncts to the necropsy dissection are external photographs and full body skeletal radiographs, which can later be reviewed by specialists in pediatric dysmorphology. As all obstetricians know, a diagnosis of Down's syndrome can be difficult to make in a newborn, let alone in a macerated fetus. Static morphologic features should be fully documented, but even more critical are the key samples for diagnosis that must be obtained from viable tissues. A heparinized cord or fetal blood sample can be used to examine fetal chromosome karyotype. A small sample of fetal skin (1 to 2 mm.) placed in tissue culture medium can be used to grow fetal cells for both chromosomal and biochemical genetic diagnosis. Fetal serum and plasma samples may be frozen and may ultimately prove useful in the attempt to document a diagnosis of an inborn error of metabolism. If a specific biochemical diagnosis is strongly suspected a priori, preparations can be made in advance to obtain key fetal tissues rapidly and quick-freeze (liquid nitrogen) or transport them for specific enzyme studies. Such tissue samples are not routinely obtained but would be the only ones useful in diagnosing metabolic genetic disorders that are not detectable in amniotic fluid cell or skin fibroblast cultures.

If a midtrimester abortion is induced because of a prenatal diagnosis of genetic disease in the fetus, then it is important to obtain all the morphologic and tissue assay evidence necessary to confirm the original diagnosis. This diagnostic confirmation serves two purposes. It is very consoling for the couple that made the agonizing decision to interrupt a pregnancy at 20 weeks gestation because of the evidence from one brief needle sample of amniotic fluid, and it is important in advancing our scientific understanding in the relatively new area of prenatal diagnosis. The geneticists who make the diagnosis will be able to instruct the obstetrician in techniques for obtaining diagnostic fetal tissue samples.

References

1a. American College of Obstetricians and Gynecologists Technical Bulletin 61, 1981. The selective use of Rho(D) immune globulin (RhIg).

1. Ampola, M. G., Mahoney, M. J., Nakamura, E., et al.: Prenatal therapy of a patient with vitamin B_{12} responsive methylmalonic acidemia. N. Engl. J. Med., *293*:313, 1975.

2. Barabas, A. P.: Ehlers-Danlos syndrome associated with prematurity and premature rupture of foetal membranes. Br. Med. J., *2*:682, 1966.

3. Barabas, A. P.: Vascular complications of the Ehlers-Danlos syndrome with special reference to the "arterial type" or Sack's syndrome. J. Cardiovasc. Surg., *13*:160, 1972.

4. Beighton, P.: Obstetrical aspects of the Ehlers-Danlos syndrome. J. Obstet. Gynaecol. Br. Commonw., *76*:97, 1969.

5. Bergsma, D. (ed.): Birth Defects Compendium, (2nd Ed.) New York, A. R. Liss, Inc., 1979.

6. Blattner, P., Dar, H., and Nitowsky, H. M.: Pregnancy outcome in women with sickle cell trait. J.A.M.A., *238*:1392, 1977.

7. Boughman, J. A., Caldwell, R. J., and Nance, W. E.: Genetic counseling in retinitis pigmentosa. Am. J. Hum. Genet., *32*:100A, 1980.

8. Brenton, D. P., Cusworth, D. C., Biddle, S. A., Garrod, P. J., and Lasley, L.: Pregnancy and homocystinuria. Ann. Clin. Biochem., *14*:161, 1977.

9. Brodie, M. J., Moore, M. R., Thompson, G. G., Goldberg, A., and Low, R. A.: Pregnancy and the acute porphyrias. Br. J. Obstet. Gynaecol., *84*:726, 1977.

10. Campbell, S.: Diagnosis of fetal abnormalities by ultrasound. *In* Milunsky, A. (ed.): Genetic Disorders and the Fetus. New York, Plenum Press, 1979, pp. 431–467.

11. Carter, C. O.: Genetics of common single malformations. Br. Med. Bull., *32*:21, 1979.

12. Center for Disease Control: Congenital Malformations Surveillance. Annual Summary, 1974.

13. Childs, B., Miller, S. M., and Bearn, A. G.: Gene mutation as a cause of human disease. *In* Sutton, H. E., and Harris, M. I. (eds.): Mutagenic Effects of Environmental Contaminants. New York, Academic Press, 1972, p. 3.

14. Dancis, J., and Levitz, M.: Abnormalities of branched-chain amino acid metabolism. *In* Stanbury, J. B., Wyngaarden, J. B., and Fredrickson, D. S. (eds.): The Metabolic Basis of Inherited Disease. New York, McGraw-Hill, 1978, p. 397.

15. Day, N., and Holmes, L. B.: The incidence of genetic disease in a university hospital population. Am. J. Hum. Genet., *25*:237, 1973.

16. Donnel, G. N., Koch, R., and Bergren, W. R.: Observations on results of management of galactosemic patients. *In* Hsia, D. Y. (ed.): Galactosemia. Springfield, Illinois, Charles C Thomas, 1969.

17. Farber, M., Knuppel, R. A., Binkiewicz, A., and Kennison, R. D.: Pregnancy and von Gierke's Disease. Obstet. Gynecol., *47*:226, 1976.

18. Ferguson-Smith, N. A., Rawlinson, H. A., May, H. M., et al.: Avoidance of anencephalic and spina bifida births by maternal serum alph-fetoprotein screening. Lancet, *1*:1330, 1978.

19. Firsheim, S., Hoyer, L. W., Lazarchick, J., et al.: Prenatal diagnosis of classic hemophilia. N. Engl. J. Med., *300*:937, 1979.

20. Fishler, K., Donnell, G. N., Bergren, W. R., et al.: Intellectual and personality development in children with galactosemia. Pediatrics, *50*:412, 1972.

21. Fraser, F. C., and Biddle, C. J.: Estimating the risks for offspring of first cousin matings. An approach. Am. J. Hum. Genet., *28*:522, 1976.

22. Frigoletto, F. D., and Umansky, I.: Diagnosis, treatment and prevention of isoimmune hemolytic disease of the fetus. *In* Milunsky, A. (ed.): Genetic Disorders and the Fetus. New York, Plenum Press, 1979, pp. 557–568.

23. Fuchs, F.: Genetic amniocentesis. Sc. Am., *242*:47, 1980.

24. Gerald, P.: X-linked mental retardation and an X-chromosome marker. N. Engl. J. Med., *303*:696, 1980.

25. Gilbert, F., and Mellman, W. T.: Genetic heterogeneity: Problems of allelic diversity in heterozygote detection and in the determination of gene frequency. *In* Kelly, S., Hook, E. B., Janerich, D. T., and Porter, I. H. (eds.): Birth Defects: Risks and Consequences. New York, Academic Press, 1976, pp. 281–287.

26. Glass, R. H., and Golbus, M. S.: Habitual abortion. Fertil. Steril., *29*:257, 1978.

27. Golbus, M. S., Cann, H. M., and Mann, J.: Rh isoimmunization following genetic amniocentesis. Prenat. Diag., in press, 1982.

28. Golbus, M. S., Caughman, W. D., Epstein, C. J., Halbasch, G., Stephens, J. D., and Hall, B. D.: Prenatal diagnosis in 3000 amniocenteses. N. Engl. J. Med., *300*:157, 1979.

29. Deleted in press.

30. Griscom, N. T.: Radiographic fetal diagnosis. *In* Milunsky, A. (ed.): Genetic Disorders and the Fetus. New York, Plenum Press, 1979, pp. 469–499.

31. Hall, B.: Mongolism in newborn infants. Clin. Pediatr., *5*:4, 1966.

32. Hassold, T. J.: A cytogenetic study of repeated spontaneous abortions. Am. J. Hum. Genet., *32*:723, 1980.

33. Hassold, T. J., Matsuyama, A., Newlands, I. M., Matsuura, J. S., Jacobs, P. A., Manuel, B., and Tsuei, J.: Cytogenetic study of spontaneous abortions in Hawaii. Ann. Hum. Genet., *41*:443, 1978.

34. Henry, G., Wexler, P., and Robinson, A.: Rh immune globulin after genetic amniocentesis. Obstet. Gynecol., *48*:557, 1976.

35. Hobbins, J. C., Grannum, P. A., Berkowitz, R. L., Silverman, R., and Mahoney, M. J.: Ultrasound in the diagnosis of congenital anomalies. Am. J. Obstet. Gynecol., *134*:331, 1979.

36. Hobbins, J. C., and Venus, I.: Congenital anomalies. *In* Hobbins, J. C. (ed.): Diagnostic Ultrasound in Obstetrics. New York, Churchill Livingstone, 1979, pp. 95–122.

37. Hook, E. B.: Differences between rates of trisomy 21 (Down Syndrome) and other chromosome abnormalities diagnosed in livebirths and in cells cultured after second trimester amniocentesis. Proceedings of the 1977 Birth Defects Conference, Memphis. *In* Bergsma, D., and Summitt, R. L. (eds.): Birth Def. Orig. Art. Ser. New York, A. R. Liss, Inc., 1978.

38. Hook, E. B.: Spontaneous deaths of fetuses with chromosome abnormalities diagnosed prenatally. N. Engl. J. Med., *299*:1036, 1978.

39. Hook, E. B., and Lindsjo, A.: Down Syndrome in live births by single year maternal age interval in a Swedish Study: Comparison with results from a New York State study. Am. J. Hum. Genet., *30*:19, 1978.

40. Hook, E. B., Regal, R. R., Cross, P. K., Lamson, S. H., Liss, S. M., Baird, P. A., and Uh, S. H.: Paternal age and Down's syndrome. Am. J. Hum. Genet., *32*:111A, 1980.

41. Houlton, M. C., and Jackson, M. B.: Gaucher's disease and pregnancy. Obstet. Gynecol., *51*:619, 1978.

42. Kaback, M. M., Rimoin, D. D., and O'Brien, J. S. (eds.): Tay-Sachs Disease: Screening and Prevention. New York, A. R. Liss, Inc., 1977.

43. Kaback, M. M., and Bantock, H.: International Workshop on Amniocentesis and Prenatal Diagnosis. Montreal, 1978. Personal communication, 1982.

44. Kjessler, B., Hemmingsson, A., and Nilsson, B. A.: Early diagnosis of trophoblastic disease and fetal maldevelopment by alphafetoprotein, human chorionic gonadotrophin, and amniography. Acta. Obstet. Gynecol. Scand. Suppl., *69*:83, 1977.

45. Klein, H. G., Aledort, L. M., Bouma, B. N., Hoyer, L. W., Zimmerman, T. S., and DeMets, D. L.: A cooperative study for the detection of the carrier state of classic hemophilia. N. Engl. J. Med., *296*:959, 1977.

46. Lamson, S. H., and Hook, E. B.: A simple function for maternal age specific rates of Down Syndrome in the 20–40 year age range and its biologic implications. Am. J. Hum. Genet., *32*:743, 1980.

47. Lenke, R. R., and Levy, H. L.: Maternal phenylketonuria and hyperphenylalaninemia. An international survey of the outcome of untreated and treated pregnancies. N. Engl. J. Med., *303*:1202, 1980.

48. Littlefield, J. W.: Research on cystic fibrosis. N. Engl. J. Med., *304*:44, 1981.

48a. Loeffler, F. E. (ed.): An assessment of the hazards of amniocentesis. Br. J. Obstet. Gynecol. *85*(suppl 2):1, 1978.

49. Macri, J. N., Haddow, J. E., and Weiss, R. R.: Screening for neural tube defects in the United States. Am. J. Obstet. Gynecol., *133*:119, 1979.

50. Mahoney, M. J., and Hobbins, J. C.: Prenatal diagnosis of chondroectodermal dysplasia (Ellis–van Creveld syndrome) using fetoscopy and ultrasound. N. Engl. J. Med., *297*:258, 1977.

51. Mahoney, M. J., and Hobbins, J. C.: Fetoscopy and fetal blood sampling. *In* Milunsky, A. (ed.): Genetic Disorders and the Fetus. New York, Plenum Press, 1979, pp. 501–526.

51a. Mahoney, M. J., Venus, I. H., and Hobbins, J. C.: Six years' experience with clinical fetoscopy. Am. J. Hum. Genet., *33*: 84A, 1981.

52. Marden, P. M., Smith, D. W., and McDonald, M. J.: Congenital anomalies in the newborn infant, including minor variations. J. Pediatr., *64*:357, 1964.

53. McKusick, V. A.: Mendelian Inheritance in Man, 5th Ed. Baltimore and London, Johns Hopkins University Press, 1978.

53a. McMaster Conference on Prevention of Rh Iso immunization. Vox. Sang., *36*:50, 1979.

54. Miles, J. H., and Kaback, M. M.: Rh immune globulin after genetic amniocentesis. Clin. Res., *27*:103A, 1978.

55. Miller, O. J., and Breg, W. R.: Current concepts in genetics: Autosomal chromosome disorders and variations. N. Engl. J. Med., *294*:596, 1976.

56. Milunsky, A. (ed.): Genetic Disorders and the Fetus. New York, Plenum Press, 1979.

57. Milunsky, A.: Amniocentesis. *In* Genetic Disorders and the Fetus. New York, Plenum Press, 1979, pp. 19–46.

58. Milunsky, A.: Prenatal diagnosis of chromosomal disorders. *In* Genetic Disorders and the Fetus. New York, Plenum Press, 1979, pp. 93–156.

59. Milunsky, A.: Prenatal diagnosis of hereditary biochemical disorders of metabolism. *In* Genetic Disorders and the Fetus. New York, Plenum Press, 1979, pp. 209–367.

60. Milunsky, A.: Prenatal diagnosis of neural tube defects. *In* Genetic Disorders and the Fetus. New York, Plenum Press, 1979, pp. 379–430.

61. Milunsky, A.: Sex chromosome and X-linked disorders. *In* Genetic Disorders and the Fetus. New York, Plenum Press, 1979, pp. 157–208.

62. Milunsky, A., Alpert, E., Neff, R. K., and Frigoletto, F. D.: Prenatal diagnosis of neural tube defects. IV. Maternal serum alpha-fetoprotein screening. Obstet. Gynecol., *55*:60, 1980.

63. Mintz, U., Moohr, J. W., and Ultmann, J. E.: Hemolytic anemias during pregnancy and the reproductive years. J. Reprod. Med., *19*:243, 1977.

64. Mudd, S. H., and Levy, H. L.: Disorders of transsulfuration. *In* Stanbury, J. B., Wyngaarden, J. B., and Fredrickson, D. S., (eds.): Metabolic Basis of Inherited Disease, 4th Ed. New York, McGraw-Hill, 1978.

65. Nadler, H. L., and Burton, B. K.: Genetics. *In* Quilligan, E. J., and Kretchmer, N. (eds.): Fetal and Maternal Medicine. New York, John Wiley & Sons, 1980, Chapter 3, pp. 59–107.

66. Nelson, M. M.: Amniotic fluid volumes in early pregnancy. J. Obstet. Gynaecol. Br. Commonw., *79*:50, 1972.

67. NICHD National Amniocentesis Study Group: Midtrimester amniocentesis for prenatal diagnosis: Safety and accuracy. J.A.M.A., *236*:1471, 1976.

68. NIH Consensus Development Conference on Antenatal Diagnosis. Clin. Pediatr., *18*:454, 1979.

69. Oakley, G. P.: Natural selection, selection bias and the prevalence of Down's Syndrome. N. Engl. J. Med., *299*:1068, 1978.

70. Omenn, G. S.: Prenatal diagnosis of genetic disorders. Science, *200*:952, 1978.

71. Opitz, J. M.: Diagnostic genetic studies in severe mental retardation. *In* Lubs, H. A., and de la Cruz, F. (eds.): Genetic Counseling. New York, Raven Press, 1977, p. 417.

72. Palmer, C. G., Wallace, M., Breg, W. R., Hook, E. B., Magenis, E., Pasztor, L., and Summitt, R.: Risk in reciprocal translocation families: Data from the interregional cytogenetics registry system. Am. J. Hum. Genet., *32*:82A, 1980.

73. Pyeritz, R. E.: Results and maternal risks of pregnancy in the Marfan Syndrome. Am. J. Hum. Genet., *32*:124A, 1980.

74. Pyeritz, R. E., and McKusick, V. A.: The Marfan Syndrome: Diagnosis and management. N. Engl. J. Med., *300*:772, 1979.

75. Rassin, D. K., Fleisher, L. D., Muir, A., Desnick, R. J., and Gaull, G. E.: Fetal tissue amino acid concentrations in argininosuccinicaciduria and in "maternal homocystinuria." Clin. Chim. Acta, *94*:101, 1979.

76. Roberts, J. M., and Solomons, C. C.: Management of pregnancy in osteogenesis imperfecta: New perspectives. Obstet. Gynecol., *45*:168, 1975.

77. Sabbagha, R. E.: The use of ultrasound in defining gestational age. *In* Hobbins, J. C. (ed.): Diagnostic Ultrasound in Obstetrics. New York, Churchill Livingstone, 1979, pp. 23–39.

78. Schroder, J., and Herzenberg, L. A.: Fetal cells in the maternal circulation. *In* Milunsky, A. (ed.): Genetic Disorders and the Fetus. New York, Plenum Press, 1979, pp. 541–555.

79. Scriver, C. R., Clow, C. L., and Fraser, F. C.: Genetics in medicine: An evolving relationship. Science, *200*:946, 1978.

80. Shapiro, L. J., Cousins, L., Fluharty, A. L., Stevens, R. L., and Kihara, H.: Steroid sulfatase deficiency. Pediatr. Res., *11*:894, 1977.

81. Sheinberg, I. H., and Sternlieb, I.: Pregnancy in penicillamine-treated patients with Wilson's disease. N. Engl. J. Med., *293*:1300, 1975.

82. Simpson, N. E., Dallaire, L., Miller, J. R., Siminovich, L., Hamerton, J. L., Miller, J., and McKeen, C.: Prenatal diagnosis of genetic disease in Canada: Report of a collaborative study. Can. Med. Assoc. J., *115*:739, 1976.

82a. Singer, N., Shapiro, L. R., and Mannor, S. M.: Immediate and unexplained fetal demise during mid-trimester amniocentesis. Am. J. Hum. Genet., *33*:91A, 1981.

83. Smith, D. W.: Recognizable Patterns of Human Malformation: Genetic, Embryologic and Clinical Aspects, 2nd Ed. Philadelphia, W. B. Saunders Co. 1976.

84. Smith, G. F., and Berg, J. M.: Down's Anomaly, 2nd Ed. New York, Churchill Livingstone, 1976, p. 224, Table 93.

85. Trimble, B. K., and Doughty, J. H.: The amount of hereditary disease in human populations. Ann. Hum. Genet., *38*:199, 1974.

86. Tsang, R. C., Glueck, C. J., McLain, C., Russell, P., Joyce, T., Bove, K., Mellies, M., and Steiner, P. M.: Pregnancy, parturition and lactation in familial homozygous hypercholesterolemia. Metabolism, *27*:823, 1978.

87. U.K. Collaborative study on alpha-fetoprotein in relation to neural tube defects. Maternal serum alpha-fetoprotein measurement in antenatal screening for anencephaly and spina bifida in early pregnancy. Lancet, *1*:1323, 1977.

88. Verma, R., and Lubs, H.: A simple R banding technic. Am. J. Hum. Genet., *27*:110, 1975.

89. Walshe, J. M.: Pregnancy in Wilson's disease. Q. J. Med., *46*:73, 1977.

90. Ward, B. E., Henry, G. P., and Robinson, A.: Cytogenic studies in 100 couples with recurrent spontaneous abortions. Am. J. Hum. Genet., *32*:549, 1980.

91. Webb, D., Muir, I., Faulkner, J., and Johnson, G.: Myotonica dystrophica: Obstetric complications. Am. J. Obstet. Gynecol., *132*:265, 1978.

92. Weil, J., and Epstein, C. J.: The effect of trisomy 21 on the patterns of polypeptide synthesis in human fibroblasts. Am. J. Hum. Genet., *31*:478, 1979.

93. Weiss, R. R., Macri, J. N., and Balsam, D.: Amniography in the prenatal diagnosis of neural tube defects. Obstet. Gynecol., *51*:299, 1978.

John H. McAnulty, M.D.
James Metcalfe, M.D.
Kent Ueland, M.D.

6

CARDIOVASCULAR DISEASE

GENERAL CONSIDERATIONS

In considering the implications of pregnancy for a woman with heart disease, several general categories of concern can be defined. First, the hemodynamic changes of normal pregnancy may result in her disability or death. Pregnancy is particularly dangerous in the presence of some specific cardiac lesions, including Eisenmenger's syndrome,[72, 98] primary pulmonary hypertension,[172] Marfan's syndrome,[140] and hemodynamically significant mitral stenosis.[172, 173] Second, pregnancy may permanently aggravate pre-existing maternal heart disease. There is some evidence that rheumatic fever is more likely to recur during pregnancy, occasionally resulting in severe symptoms or even death.[15, 37, 94, 109, 183] Additionally, endocarditis associated with labor and delivery may cause further injury to a deformed valve. Third, pregnancy may cause maternal heart disease. Though uncommon, a peripartal cardiomyopathy may develop in individuals with previously normal hearts.[24, 46, 47]

In addition to these considerations, fetal health may be jeopardized by maternal heart disease. Although maternal well-being must predominate in our consideration of management, the well-being of the fetus is sometimes critical in decision-making. Fetal health depends on an adequate and continuous supply of well-oxygenated maternal blood to the uterus. When this supply is limited, as it appears to be when there is severe maternal heart disease, the risk of abnormal fetal development or death is significant, exceeding 50 per cent in women with some congenital lesions.[70, 72, 117, 172] Further, if either parent has congenital heart disease, the fetus has an increased likelihood of being born with a cardiac deformity. Additionally, if the mother is the affected parent, her heart lesion may limit uterine blood flow, thereby adding an environmental handicap to the genetic risk.

Finally, despite remarkable advances in the detection, definition, and management of heart disease, its presence in women of childbearing age is associated with a life expectancy significantly less than normal. The likelihood of premature death of the mother is important in considering the implications of maternal heart disease and pregnancy.

HEMODYNAMIC CHANGES ASSOCIATED WITH PREGNANCY

Maternal physiology is dramatically changed during pregnancy, and some of the alterations affect the cardiovascular system. In women with cardiac abnormalities, the hemodynamics of normal pregnancy can be life-threatening. Even in women without heart disease, these changes may result in symptoms and signs that are difficult to distinguish from those associated with heart disease.

Changes in Fluid Balance

Retention of sodium and water during pregnancy has important hemodynamic consequences. Total body water increases steadily, achieving an increase of 6 to 8 liters in a normal pregnancy, most of the water being located in the extracellular space.[95] Excess sodium accumulation reaches 500 to 900 mEq by the time of delivery.

Maternal blood volume rises by an average of 40 per cent above nonpregnant levels, with extremely wide individual variations.[68] The rise begins in the first trimester and plateaus after the 30th week.[136] Some workers have observed a slight fall (on the average) with the approach of term,[68] but this has not been uniformly recorded.[136]

Total red cell volume increases steadily throughout pregnancy. The increment ranged from 20 to 40 per cent of nonpregnant values in one series, the mean attaining 1635 ml compared with a nonpregnant value of 1290 ml.[135] The expansion of blood volume is mainly due to an

145

increase in plasma volume. As a result, hemodilution occurs and is manifested by a decreased hematocrit, which is sometimes referred to as "the physiologic anemia of pregnancy." The lowest hematocrit values range from 33 to 38 per cent in the series of Hytten and Leitch.[67] Blood hemoglobin concentration falls to between 11 and 12 gm per 100 ml in late pregnancy from levels of 13.5 to 14 gm per 100 ml in nonpregnant women. According to Hytten and Thomson, the fall in blood hemoglobin concentration cannot be prevented by iron administration;[69] however, women treated with oral iron in the last trimester of pregnancy show a significant rise in blood hemoglobin concentration compared with a control group treated with a placebo.[34] The evidence indicates that iron supplementation significantly improves the oxygen-carrying capacity of maternal blood during pregnancy.[28, 137]

The increment in plasma volume that occurs during normal pregnancy is greater in multigravidas than in primigravidas,[2] and its magnitude does not correlate well with maternal weight.[68] In a large series of primigravidas, the increase in maternal blood volume correlated with the birth weight of the infant.[68] In patients with twin pregnancies, the plasma volume increased progressively until term, achieving an average maximum of 67 per cent above normal. It rose an average of 48 per cent in women with single pregnancies, plateauing for the last eight weeks before term.[150]

Studies of the distribution of the increased blood volume that accompanies pregnancy show significant changes depending upon body position. In late pregnancy, supine recumbency for 1 hour decreased the plasma volume measured by T-1824 and resulted in slower mixing of the dye, presumably by trapping blood in the legs.[33] Perhaps because adequate precautions regarding maternal body position have not been taken, studies of central blood volume have given conflicting results. Decreased pressures in the pulmonary artery, the right atrium, and the right ventricle in pregnancy as well as a decrease in pulmonary blood volume have been reported.[87, 189] However, two other studies have shown an increased central blood volume during pregnancy.[2, 152]

Venous pressure is not elevated in the arms but is considerably above normal in the lower extremities.[108] The increment in venous pressure in the legs is attributed in large part to the mechanical impediment to blood flow in the inferior vena cava by the enlarged uterus,[78] but it is undoubtedly due in part to venous return from the maternal uterine circulation. Finger plethysmography indicates that venous distensibility is considerably increased during pregnancy,[105] a change that has also been observed in studies of the larger venous bed.[192]

The mechanisms responsible for the profound alterations in fluid balance that accompany pregnancy have not been completely defined. Plasma renin activity and blood aldosterone levels both increase. The rise in plasma renin activity has been attributed to estrogenic stimulation of renin substrate production by the liver.[175] Increased plasma renin activity may play a part in encouraging sodium retention by stimulating aldosterone secretion.[96] Additionally, progesterone has been shown to inhibit the sodium-retaining action of aldosterone on the cells of the renal tubules,[89, 90] and the administration of progesterone to normal human volunteers produced a rise in plasma aldosterone levels, an effect that probably depends upon a sodium diuresis secondary to the aldosterone blocking action of progesterone.[170] Estrogens and progesterone both act to increase plasma aldosterone levels and thereby to promote sodium retention[99] and an increase in total body water.[161] The degree of retention, however, is importantly magnified by the distensibility of the venous system and the increased venous capacity that is apparent in the uterine veins at cesarean section delivery.

Cardiac Output

Hemodynamically, the most significant change occurring in the maternal circulation is an increase in cardiac output. In the average woman, the increment attains 40 per cent above the nonpregnant resting value.[181] This remarkable change has several unexpected features. First, the majority of the changes occur early in pregnancy. As shown in Figure 6–1, resting maternal cardiac output reaches its highest levels halfway through gestation, by 20 to 24 weeks. A second important observation is that the resting cardiac output fluctuates markedly with changes in body position during pregnancy. Consideration of Figure 6–1 shows that when the supine position is assumed, cardiac output falls from levels observed when the patient is sitting down or in lateral recumbency. Finally, the resting cardiac output tends to decline in the last 8 weeks of pregnancy. As Figure 6–1 shows, resting cardiac output is even lower at the 38th to 40th week of gestation than it is 6 to 8 weeks post partum when studies are made in the supine position. This decrement is attributed to compression of the inferior vena cava by the enlarged uterus, a

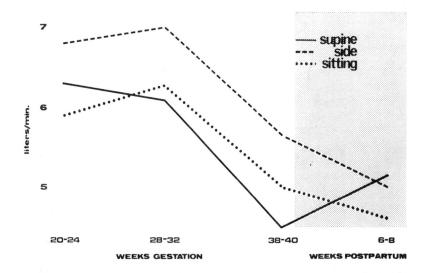

FIGURE 6–1. Maternal cardiac output was measured three times during pregnancy and once post partum in 11 normal women. At each study, measurements were made with the patient sitting, supine, and in left lateral recumbency. Near term, assumption of the supine position causes cardiac output to fall below the postpartum value. (From Ueland et al.: Am. J. Obstet. Gynecol., 104:856, 1969. Reprinted with permission.)

tamponade that results in decreased venous return even in women with demonstrably enlarged venous collaterals. In a few women, presumably those whose collateral vessels are not well developed, maintenance of the supine position results in hypotension and bradycardia, a vasovagal syndrome that has been called the "supine hypotensive syndrome of pregnancy."[78, 79] This syndrome can be promptly relieved by placing the patient in lateral recumbency. According to the measurements illustrated in Figure 6–1, maternal cardiac output tends to decline slightly during the last 10 weeks of pregnancy, even in the sitting and lateral recumbent positions, presumably owing to increased abdominal pressure.

Maternal cardiac output has been studied in patients with twin and triplet pregnancies.[151] The change in cardiac output (above the nonpregnant control) was larger in these women than the average for patients with a single fetus. Although the peak cardiac output was only slightly greater in women with more than one fetus, the fall in cardiac output as pregnancy proceeded was smaller and the cardiac index was 15 per cent above nonpregnant control values at term, whereas the cardiac index of women with single pregnancies had fallen almost to the average in nonpregnant women. Unfortunately, the body position in which the cardiac output measurements were made is not stated in the report.[151]

The increase in resting cardiac output that occurs early in pregnancy is mainly due to an increase in stroke volume, as shown in Figure 6–2. This hemodynamic variable declines later in pregnancy. As pregnancy advances, heart rate increases (Fig. 6–3), and stroke volume falls concurrently to values within the normal nonpregnant range at term. Indeed, the resting stroke volume in the supine position is lower at term than in the postpartum period.[114] Because resting cardiac output increases before a significant rise in maternal oxygen consumption occurs, the arteriovenous oxygen difference declines early in pregnancy. As resting oxygen consumption rises progressively with the advance of pregnancy, achieving a level 20 per cent above the nonpregnant state at term,[114] peripheral oxygen extraction gradually increases. By the end of gestation, arteriovenous oxygen difference exceeds nonpregnant values, even in lateral recumbency.

The physiologic mechanism responsible for these hemodynamic changes has not been entirely explained. They are not related to the metabolic needs of the mother and the fetus in any obvious way. Early in pregnancy, when the fetus is still small, resting maternal cardiac output has already reached its highest point. As pregnancy advances toward term the maternal cardiac output declines while fetal size increases exponentially. The mother's oxygen consumption at rest (which includes that of her fetus) increases progressively.[67] Most of the increase is undoubtedly due to the metabolic needs of the fetus, but some must be due to the increased work and metabolic needs of the mother's heart and respiratory muscles.

Burwell recognized in 1938 the discrepancy between the increments in cardiac output and oxygen consumption associated with pregnancy and drew an analogy between the circulation of the pregnant woman and that of a patient with an arteriovenous fistula.[26] Hemodynamically, the analogy is appropriate because peripheral vascular resistance declines in the pregnant woman. This is manifest by a wide pulse pressure (due to

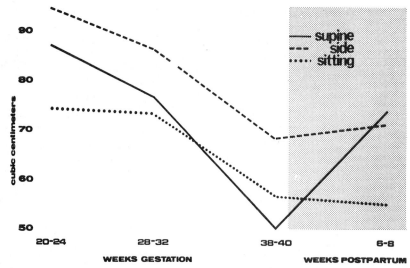

FIGURE 6-2. Stroke volume of the maternal heart increases early in pregnancy and declines, particularly in the supine position, as pregnancy advances. Most of the increase in cardiac output at the 20th week of pregnancy is due to an increasing stroke volume. Near term, stroke volume is *below* the postpartum value with the patient supine and is not higher than postpartum values with the patient seated or in lateral recumbency. (From Ueland et al.: Am. J. Obstet. Gynecol., *104*:856, 1969. Reprinted with permission.)

a fall in the diastolic value), and mean arterial pressure falls despite the rise in cardiac output. In pregnant dogs, declines in heart rate, central venous pressure, and cardiac output occur immediately when the uterine arteries are occluded, while systolic and diastolic arterial blood pressure rise.[56] These changes are identical with those produced by occlusion of an arteriovenous fistula. Burwell's hypothesis implied that the fall in uterine vascular resistance was due to erosion of the maternal endometrial vessels by the invasive fetal trophoblast. More recently, however, it has been recognized that the vascular resistance of the pregnant uterus falls strikingly even in those species, like the ungulates, in which no

erosion of the maternal uterine vessels occurs.[112] This is additional evidence that the changes in vascular resistance occurring as part of normal pregnancy are based upon hormonal actions. The administration of estrogens to nonpregnant sheep has been shown to produce an increased cardiac output and a reduced vascular resistance,[186] and estrogenic steroids have been shown to act upon the uterine vascular bed to produce vasodilation.[58] However, the changes in uterine blood flow do not explain the changes in maternal cardiac output. Uterine blood flow increases to only 100 ml per min at the end of the first trimester and reaches 200 ml per min by the 28th week and 500 ml per min at term.[6, 13] This

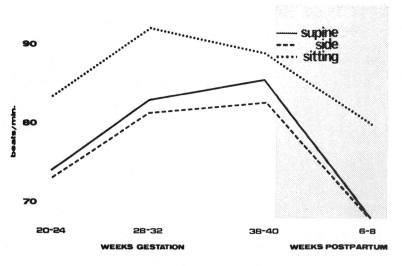

FIGURE 6-3. Maternal heart rate increases slightly early in pregnancy and continues to rise as pregnancy advances and stroke volume (Fig. 6-2) falls. At term, any increment in cardiac output above postpartum values is due to the relative tachycardia. (From Ueland et al.: Am. J. Obstet. Gynecol., *104*:856, 1969. Reprinted with permission.)

progressive rise in uterine blood flow is clearly out of phase with the augmentation of resting maternal cardiac output and accounts for only a portion of the increment in cardiac output observed by the 20th week of pregnancy.

Neither can the augmented cardiac output be attributed to the increase in circulating blood volume, because the filling pressures of the heart are not elevated during pregnancy.[7, 87, 132, 189]

Prolactin, a protein hormone produced by the anterior pituitary during pregnancy, has been invoked to explain the changes in maternal hemodynamics. When it was given in doses of 250 μg per day to female rats, a fall in blood pressure and an increase in blood volume were observed. In larger doses, 2.5 mg per animal per day, the effects were more pronounced and the recipients became hyporesponsive to infused angiotensin.[22]

In addition to their effects upon vascular resistance, the steroid hormones of pregnancy appear to affect the myocardium directly. Oral contraceptives containing both estrogenic and progestational compounds cause an increase in cardiac output, entirely because of an increase in stroke volume.[187] Estrogens may alter the actomyosin-ATPase relationships in the myocardium, thereby increasing myocardial contractility.[40] Ventricular actomyosin-ATPase is significantly reduced in rats after ovariectomy and can be restored by estrogen administration.[80]

Measurements of systolic time intervals have been made in pregnant human volunteers. Early in gestation, the pre-ejection period of left ventricular systole is reduced, and this alteration becomes more marked in the second trimester.[25] The change in ventricular dynamics may reflect a change in myocardial performance brought about by direct action of steroid hormones upon the myocardium.[174] Alternatively, the reduction in pre-ejection period may result from the decrease in diastolic aortic pressure that occurs in early pregnancy. Echocardiographic assessment of left ventricular performance has shown no consistent change in either the extent or the velocity of dimensional shortening during gestation. End-diastolic dimension increases progressively during gestation without a change in end-systolic dimension.[76, 88, 153] These data suggest that ventricular enlargement, rather than an increase in intrinsic myocardial performance, is the predominant mechanism for the increase in stroke volume that occurs early in pregnancy. Our present hypothesis for explaining the augmentation of maternal cardiac output that occurs early in pregnancy is that changes in circulating steroid hormones not only affect venous distensibility

and arteriolar tone but also cause relaxation of the connective tissue "skeleton" of the maternal heart. This change allows end-diastolic volume to increase without an increased filling pressure, evoking the augmented stroke volume of early human pregnancy.[66, 122]

The increment in maternal cardiac output is not uniformly distributed. Changes in the vascular resistance of specific tissues cause a distribution of maternal blood flow, which changes as pregnancy advances. The progressive rise in uterine blood flow has already been described. Early in pregnancy, renal blood flow increases to levels approximately 30 per cent above those found in controls.[32, 97] Subsequently, renal blood flow remains unchanged or declines as gestation advances. Engorgement of the breasts begins early in human pregnancy, and there is visible dilation of the veins in the overlying skin. It is therefore reasonable to assume that mammary blood flow is increased throughout pregnancy, but quantitative studies on human subjects have not been reported.

There is circumstantial evidence that female sex hormones also produce structural changes in blood vessels. The appearance of spider angiomas in early pregnancy is well documented, and the growth of a pre-existing arteriovenous fistula of an extremity has been reported in association with pregnancy.[27] Histologic changes in the wall of the aorta have also been described[100] and disputed in a later study.[31] Arterial aneurysms occur four to five times more commonly in women than in men. Ruptures of aneurysms of the splenic artery occurring before the age of 45 are also more common in females than in males, and the majority of ruptures occur during pregnancy, usually between the 7th and 9th months.[1]

During labor, cardiac output increases significantly during each uterine contraction, the magnitude of the increase depending upon body position.[182] Venous return is augmented by blood squeezed out of the uterine vasculature during each contraction. The resultant increase in cardiac output is most dramatic when the woman is supine, but a lesser increment is detectable in lateral recumbency (Fig. 6–4). The contracting uterus also partially obstructs the abdominal aorta, so that the augmented cardiac output is diverted to the upper portions of the body during uterine contraction. A transient bradycardia accompanies each contraction and is attributed to the rise in arterial blood pressure that occurs secondary to the increases in venous return and cardiac output.

The hemodynamic changes of later labor and

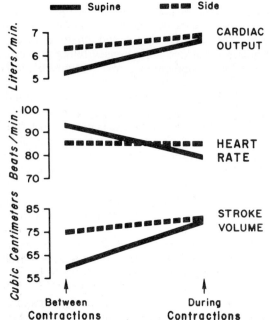

FIGURE 6–4. Changes in maternal cardiac output, heart rate, and stroke volume that occur during uterine contractions compared with values between contractions. Each uterine contraction appears to squeeze maternal blood out of the uterus, resulting in increased return to the heart (central venous pressure rises) and a rise in cardiac output. This causes arterial blood pressure to increase, eliciting a reflex fall in heart rate. The hemodynamic effects of uterine contractions are more marked in supine recumbency, because venous obstruction (between contractions) is more pronounced in that position than in lateral recumbency. (From Metcalfe and Ueland: Prog. Cardiovasc. Dis., *16*:363, 1974. Reprinted with permission.)

delivery are influenced by anesthesia and analgesia. Marked variations among several anesthetic agents and techniques have been demonstrated. Cardiac output increases progressively as labor advances under local anesthesia. This change is of lesser magnitude when caudal anesthesia is used, a difference that may be attributable to better relief of pain with caudal anesthesia.[182]

Cesarean section delivery performed before the onset of labor prevents the transient hemodynamic changes that accompany uterine contractions, but abdominal delivery is associated with the hemodynamic consequences of apprehension, anesthesia, and surgical manipulation. Figure 6–5 summarizes hemodynamic studies in a series of normal patients undergoing cesarean section delivery at term under spinal anesthesia, epidural anesthesia without epinephrine in the local anesthetic solution, epidural anesthesia with epinephrine, or balanced general anesthesia (pentothal, nitrous oxide/oxygen, and succinylcholine). With both spinal anesthesia and epidural anesthesia with epinephrine, significant falls in both cardiac output and blood pressure occurred prior to the onset of surgery. With balanced general anesthesia, marked transient changes in cardiac output, heart rate, and blood pressure accompanied tracheal intubation and extubation and awakening of the patient postoperatively. Those patients who received epidural anesthesia without epinephrine showed remarkable hemodynamic stability throughout the entire surgical procedure and a very small rise in cardi-

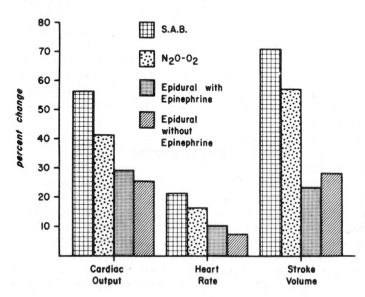

FIGURE 6–5. Maximum hemodynamic changes during cesarean section delivery, comparing supine preanesthesia values to values obtained immediately after the surgical procedure. Studies were performed during spinal anesthesia (SAB), nitrous oxide-oxygen and succinylcholine ($N_2O–O_2$), epidural anesthesia with epinephrine in the anesthetic solution, and epidural anesthesia without epinephrine. (From Metcalfe and Ueland: Prog. Cardiovasc. Dis., *16*:363, 1974. Reprinted with permission.)

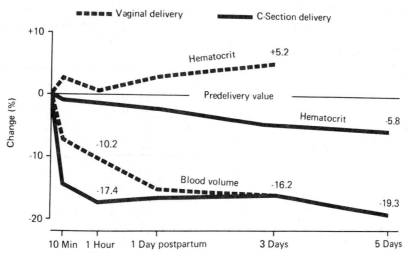

FIGURE 6–6. Serial estimations of blood volume and venous hematocrit in patients undergoing vaginal or cesarean section delivery. Values are expressed as percentage changes from results obtained immediately before delivery. The greater loss of blood associated with cesarean section delivery is apparent by the 17 per cent fall in blood volume measured one hour after delivery, compared with a fall of only 10 per cent one hour after vaginal delivery. By 3 days post partum, blood volume has declined by 16 per cent in both groups of women, but the decrease is due to diuresis in those delivered vaginally, as is shown by the difference in the hematocrits of the two groups. (From Metcalfe and Ueland. *In* Fowler, N. O. (ed.): Cardiac Diagnosis and Treatment, 3rd ed. Hagerstown, Md., Harper & Row, 1980, p. 1159. Reprinted with permission.)

ac output at delivery. All the patients undergoing cesarean section under epidural anesthesia with epinephrine required some form of therapy to correct preoperative hypotension. Treatment consisted of uterine displacement, rapid infusion of intravenous fluids, compression bandaging of the lower extremities, or some combination of these measures, in addition to the intravenous administration of a vasopressor (ephedrine) in over half the patients. These procedures, of course, modified the maternal hemodynamic responses.[178, 179, 180, 182]

Immediately following vaginal delivery, the cardiac output often increases by as much as 60 per cent above predelivery values. This is attributed to the removal of vena caval obstruction and the presence of augmented blood volume with decreased venous capacity secondary to uterine contraction and involution. A relative bradycardia accompanies the elevated cardiac output, but these changes regress within two weeks of delivery as sodium and water balance return to nonpregnant levels. Changes in blood volume and hematocrit following delivery are shown in Figure 6–6. Cesarean section, which on the average is accompanied by a maternal blood loss of 1 liter (compared with 500 cc for vaginal delivery), may be followed by a transient decrease in maternal cardiac output and blood pressure.[178, 180]

Maternal Exercise

So far, we have considered only those changes observed in the mother at rest. The cardiovascular responses to exercise are also altered during gestation. At a standard "moderate" level of sitting exercise, pregnant women have a greater increase in oxygen consumption[184] and a relatively smaller widening of the arteriovenous oxygen difference than when they perform the same exercise in the postpartum state. The maximum cardiac output is reached at lower levels of exercise in pregnancy because the pregnant woman starts from a higher level of cardiac output than when she is not pregnant.[60] In animal models, maternal exercise is associated with a fall in uterine blood flow,[92, 111, 149] but the functional significance of this diversion is not clear.

THE RECOGNITION OF HEART DISEASE DURING PREGNANCY

Pregnancy increases the difficulty of recognizing and defining heart disease. The changes in blood volume and hemodynamics that accompany normal pregnancy are associated with symptoms and signs suggestive of heart disease. Easy fatigability, chest discomfort, dyspnea, orthopnea, palpitations, peripheral edema, and syncope may all occur during normal pregnancy. However, dyspnea severe enough to limit activity, progressive orthopnea, and paroxysmal nocturnal dyspnea each require cardiac evaluation. Hemoptysis cannot be considered normal (although nosebleeds are more frequent during pregnancy and may mimic hemoptysis), and syncope during or immediately following exertion demands careful definition. Chest pain that is associated with activity, anxiety, or anger or that is typical of myocardial ischemia in distribution and relief by rest should also be investigated because myocardial ischemia occurs occasionally in pregnant women.[3, 13, 36, 71, 162]

Cardiovascular findings on physical examination are altered during pregnancy. Peripheral edema is found in as many as 80 per cent of normal pregnant women. A third heart sound occurs normally in individuals under 30 years of age. It is more common during normal pregnancy and does not suggest a cardiac abnormality. Systolic murmurs are common in normal pregnancy, but a systolic murmur of Grade III intensity or more deserves evaluation. Although a diastolic murmur attributed to increased flow across the atrioventricular valve orifices has been described in association with normal pregnancy,[42] it is so unusual that any diastolic murmur deserves expert cardiologic evaluation. Care must be taken to exclude bruits originating in the internal mammary artery (the mammary souffle) and venous hums, both of which have diastolic components and are common in pregnancy. Pulsations of the neck veins are prominent in normal pregnancy, but persistent neck vein distention lasting throughout the cardiac cycle requires evaluation for heart disease, particularly when it is associated with hepatomegaly or peripheral edema. Cyanosis may, of course, be due to causes other than heart disease, but its cause should be defined, and the same is true of digital clubbing. Similarly, pulmonary rales that do not clear with deep inspiration warrant further evaluation.

MANAGEMENT OF HEART DISEASE DURING PREGNANCY

Some general principles can be applied to the management of all pregnant women with heart disease.

Preconception Counseling

Every young woman with heart disease should be aware of the potential problems associated with pregnancy. She should be advised about the risks to herself and to her child, during both the pregnancy and the years to follow. Such counseling requires a definition of the specific cardiac lesion involved and its functional severity as well as knowledge of the recorded experience with pregnancy in other women with a similar lesion. Evaluation for surgery should be completed before pregnancy. In the case of congenital heart disease, counseling requires knowledge of genetic and environmental components in the causation of heart disease. Most of all, effective counseling requires supportive explanation. Optimism about pregnancy is more justifiable in patients with an understanding of their disease than in uninformed individuals.

Management During Pregnancy

All pregnant women with heart disease should be seen at least once during pregnancy by a cardiologist familiar with the hemodynamics of pregnancy and with the desirability of various diagnostic and therapeutic interventions (including surgery). Some of these increase the risk to both mother and child, many give misleading information if the changes of normal pregnancy are not understood, and all are unjustifiably expensive unless they are indicated and correctly interpreted.

Maternal health has the highest priority during pregnancy. The responsible physician should recognize that some drugs, diagnostic studies, and surgery jeopardize fetal health. Sometimes safer alternatives such as restriction of maternal activity will accomplish the desired result. However, diagnostic or therapeutic interventions that are required for optimal maternal safety should be employed.

Pregnancy diminishes the cardiac reserve and jeopardizes the health and life of a few women with heart disease. In such women, restriction of other hemodynamic burdens during pregnancy is an important principle for maximizing the chances of successful childbearing. The principle of medical management is "to make a place in the patient's cardiac budget for the expenditures of pregnancy by eliminating equivalent amounts of other expenditures."[27]

Some of the variables that impose a significant hemodynamic burden on the heart can be modified during pregnancy. These include maternal activity, infections, anxiety, and anemia.

Most women limit their activity to some extent during pregnancy, especially in the early months and again near term. When heart disease evokes symptoms, further restriction of maternal activity is justified. In an occasional patient, hospitalization for weeks or months near term may be necessary for maximum safety.

The risk of urinary tract infections should be minimized by proper hygienic procedures. Any bacterial infection must be treated vigorously, but it must be remembered that some antibiotics should be avoided during pregnancy. If a viral infection occurs, its hemodynamic consequences should be minimized by restriction of maternal activity.

It is important to prevent as many infections as possible by the use of appropriate immunizations. Once pregnancy has begun, vaccination with live organisms in inadvisable.[143]

Anxiety results in significant hemodynamic changes. Attempts to relieve it by counseling and by manipulation of the maternal environment are appropriate. Sustaining optimism is always justified and is more successful than tranquilizing medications.

Anemia evokes an increase in cardiac output, further lessening the reserve of the pregnant woman. Most anemia is avoided by prophylactic administration of iron and folic acid. If anemia occurs despite these measures, prompt diagnosis and definitive treatment are essential, especially in women with heart disease.

DIAGNOSTIC DEFINITION OF HEART DISEASE

In applying these general principles to the management of the individual patient, a clear definition of the hemodynamic abnormalities in that patient is essential. For this purpose, the diagnostic classification of the New York Heart Association (adopted by the American Heart Association) serves admirably. It consists of the following components:

Etiologic Diagnosis. The etiology of the lesion under consideration is important in considering the natural history of the disease, the possible genetic consequences, and the necessity for prophylaxis against recurrent rheumatic fever or bacterial endocarditis.

Anatomic Diagnosis. The pathologic anatomy of the lesion plays a large role in determining its hemodynamic consequences.

Physiologic Classification. This component details the presence of such complications as arrhythmia, pulmonary hypertension, or venous congestion.

Functional Classification or Cardiac Status. Traditionally, this has depended upon the symptomatic state of the patient. Class I patients are asymptomatic at all degrees of activity. Class II patients develop symptoms with greater than ordinary activity. Class III patients are symptomatic during ordinary activity, and patients in Class IV are symptomatic at rest. In recent years, "cardiac status" has been substituted for "functional classification" in an attempt to introduce objective criteria rather than depending entirely upon symptomatology. According to this newer classification, the patient is designated as (1) uncompromised, (2) slightly compromised, (3) moderately compromised, or (4) severely compromised.

Therapeutic Classification or Prognosis. When a patient requires digitalis or diuretic therapy in order to achieve and maintain a given functional classification, her prognosis is generally less good than that of a patient in the same functional class without medications. Recently, "prognosis" has been recommended as a replacement for the older "therapeutic classification." The recommended prognostic categories are (1) good, (2) good with therapy, (3) fair with therapy, and (4) guarded despite therapy.

USEFUL QUESTIONS FOR THE PHYSICIAN

In addition to the discipline imposed by insistence upon accurate diagnostic classification, it is useful for the physician to ask a series of questions in evaluating the condition of each patient at each visit.

Is the patient's hemodynamic status optimal?

This requires a review of symptoms, blood pressure, and pulse rate, and blood hemoglobin concentration. If any of these are unsatisfactory, diagnostic and therapeutic plans are made.

Is antibiotic prophylaxis against endocarditis indicated?

Although the efficacy of antibiotic prophylaxis against infective endocarditis has not been proved, the recommendations of the American Heart Association are, in our view, applicable during pregnancy.[74] We recommend prophylaxis during labor and delivery in women with valve abnormalities and with some congenital lesions. We recognize that the benefit of this approach has not been documented, but the low risk associated with antibiotic prophylaxis in a woman hospitalized for delivery make it appropriate. This caution is particularly applicable in women with prosthetic valves because of the high mortality associated with prosthetic valve endocarditis.

In summary, prophylaxis during genitourinary surgery or instrumentation consists of 2,000,000 units of aqueous crystalline penicillin G given intramuscularly or intravenously and 1.5 mg per kg (not exceeding 80 mg) of gentamycin intramuscularly or intravenously given at the time of delivery.[74] These doses are repeated every 8 hours for two additional doses. Ampicillin in a dose of 1 g intramuscularly or intravenously can be substituted for penicillin G. Streptomycin (1 g intramuscularly) can be substituted for gentamycin, but when streptomycin is used, the drugs are repeated every 12 hours for two additional doses. For patients who are allergic to penicillin, vancomycin (1 g intravenously over a 1-hour period) plus streptomycin (1 g intramuscularly) is given at delivery, and the same doses of both drugs are repeated in 12 hours. Any of these regimens will be modified in the presence of obstetric complications and in patients with compromised renal function.

Is antibiotic prophylaxis against rheumatic fever required?

The regimens recommended by the American Heart Association[75] should be used in patients with a history of rheumatic fever, especially those with rheumatic heart disease. A monthly intramuscular injection of benzathine penicillin G (1,200,000 units) is the most effective method of prophylaxis against rheumatic fever recurrence. When inconvenience or the pain of injection jeopardizes patient acceptance of this program, oral sulfadiazine, 1 g daily, or penicillin G, 200,000 units twice daily, may be taken orally. For the exceptional patient who is sensitive to both penicillin and sulfonamides, erythromycin, 250 mg twice a day orally, is suggested.[75]

Is anticoagulation required?

Because of the high incidence of thromboembolic events in patients with heart disease, the issue of anticoagulation must be repeatedly reviewed. Anticoagulants are required in all individuals with mechanical valve prostheses and are recommended in those with valve disease who have a history of systemic emboli. The issue is more difficult during pregnancy, however, because the warfarin derivatives cross the placenta and increase the dangers of abnormal fetal development and hemorrhage. For this reason, heparin therapy should be substituted for oral anticoagulation whenever possible in pregnant women. Because the dangers of inducing a fetal abnormality are greatest early in pregnancy, warfarin is contraindicated in women who are planning to become pregnant.

Are the presenting symptoms attributable to heart disease?

This question is worth considering whenever symptoms arise in a patient with heart disease. As an example, musculoskeletal complaints are common, especially during pregnancy. In the presence of valve disease, endocarditis should be considered as a possible cause; as many as 25 per cent of patients with endocarditis have musculoskeletal complaints as their presenting symptoms.[35]

Should diagnostic or therapeutic plans be changed because the patient is a woman of childbearing age?

As an example of the importance of this question, if a woman with mitral stenosis is planning to become pregnant, it is prudent to consider an earlier commissurotomy even if her symptomatic limitation is minimal. Similarly, if a woman requires a prosthetic valve, the possibility of a future pregnancy may argue in favor of a heterograft prosthesis, with the lower need for anticoagulation, rather than a mechanical prosthetic valve, which is presently the more common choice for a young person.

SPECIFIC FORMS OF CARDIOVASCULAR DISEASE IN PREGNANCY

Rheumatic Fever

Active rheumatic fever is disappearing in the United States,[16, 85, 190] but it remains a problem throughout much of the world[85] and is still the most common cause of heart disease encountered in pregnancy. There is some evidence that rheumatic fever is more likely to occur during pregnancy,[15, 37, 94, 109, 183] and the resultant myocarditis may be associated with fetal and maternal mortality.[172] Historically, chorea is more apt to recur during pregnancy,[37, 94] may be especially severe in the pregnant woman, and has been associated with maternal death, spontaneous miscarriage, premature labor, and intrauterine death of the fetus. It may occasionally be an indication for termination of pregnancy.[11] The diagnosis of rheumatic fever should be considered when a pregnant woman develops an unexplained fever, joint pains, chest pains, or evidence of congestive heart failure. Antibiotic prophylaxis against rheumatic fever is indicated in all women with rheumatic heart disease, and it should be continued during pregnancy.

Valve Deformities

Mitral Stenosis. This lesion is more common in women than in men and is caused almost exclusively by rheumatic fever. The stenotic valve (and perhaps associated myocardial changes) severely restricts cardiac output, causing fatigue, the most common symptom. The obstruction to left atrial outflow leads to pressure elevations in the left atrium, pulmonary veins, and pulmonary capillaries. This sequence results in pulmonary vascular congestion and the associated symptoms of dyspnea, orthopnea, and paroxysmal nocturnal dyspnea. The left atrium enlarges, and in the presence of sluggish blood flow, there is increased likelihood of thrombus development. As a result, a systemic arterial embolus may cause the first symptoms in a patient with mitral stenosis. Distention of the left atrium predisposes to atrial fibrillation, resulting in a further decrease in cardiac output and an increased likelihood of thrombus formation. Pulmonary arteriolar resistance increases and may cause right-sided heart failure with peripheral edema, hepatomegaly, abdominal distention, and distention of the neck veins.

Accentuation of the first heart sound is often the first recognizable physical finding of mitral stenosis. The other classic findings of mitral stenosis are the "opening snap," an early diastolic sound heard best at the lower left sternal border, and an apical diastolic rumbling murmur with a presystolic accentuation. Most patients with significant mitral stenosis have a palpable right ventricular lift, and many have evidence of associated mitral regurgitation. Some have involvement of other valves. Although the history and physical observations are often adequate for establishing the diagnosis, an electrocardiogram may be helpful in determining the severity of the lesion. The presence of atrial fibrillation or of right ventricular hypertrophy suggests that the disease is advanced in its natural history. A chest x-ray that shows left atrial or right ventricular enlargement has the same implication. In women of childbearing age, the chest x-ray is unlikely to show valve calcification. The echocardiographic findings are specific for mitral stenosis and will differentiate it from the rare left atrial myxoma, which presents with symptoms and physical findings indistinguishable from those of mitral steno-

sis. This procedure is of particular value for patients early in pregnancy, when x-ray exposure should be avoided.

The increased cardiac output, tachycardia, and fluid retention that accompany pregnancy may cause deterioration in functional classification. Symptoms occur in as many as 25 per cent of patients with mitral stenosis during pregnancy.[172, 173] Symptoms of pulmonary congestion usually are apparent by the 20th week and usually do not worsen after the 30th week of pregnancy, but an exacerbation may occur at the time of delivery if there is prolonged tachycardia.

In the presence of significant mitral stenosis, cardiac output is maintained to some degree by elevation of left atrial pressure. Because the pregnant woman is especially liable to sudden shifts in the distribution of her blood volume, she is at increased risk of sudden decline in venous return. This may be the explanation for the reported deaths of women with mitral stenosis without a previous history of pulmonary congestion.[173]

Management of the patient with mitral stenosis in pregnancy should include rheumatic fever prophylaxis,[75] since the condition is almost invariably due to previous rheumatic fever.[146] We recommend antibiotic prophylaxis during labor and delivery to avoid bacterial endocarditis. When severe mitral stenosis is identified prior to pregnancy, mitral commissurotomy should be undertaken before conception. The active, asymptomatic woman with mitral stenosis requires no definitive treatment. If symptoms of pulmonary congestion develop, restriction of activity to minimize heart rate and cardiac output is appropriate. If the symptoms persist, cautious diuretic therapy is required. The onset of atrial fibrillation has important hemodynamic consequences. If evidence of pulmonary congestion or a dangerous fall in cardiac output is present, electrical DC cardioversion should be performed promptly. If the hemodynamic state is stable, digitalis should be used to slow the ventricular rate prior to cardioversion, and digitalis administration is continued to insure a reasonably slow ventricular rate should atrial fibrillation recur. If recurrence does occur, maintenance quinidine therapy is justified. When symptoms of pulmonary congestion are unrelenting despite medical therapy, mitral commissurotomy during pregnancy should be considered as a possibility.[11, 27, 55, 115, 146, 172] Open-heart surgery with valve replacement can be performed during pregnancy, but fetal loss may be as high as 33 per cent.

If a thromboembolic complication develops,

anticoagulation is required, but warfarin derivatives are avoided because of danger to the fetus.[63, 168] Although heparin is not devoid of complications, it is currently the preferred anticoagulant during pregnancy and it can be administered at home after instruction in the hospital.

Mitral Regurgitation. This lesion may be due to rheumatic fever, to a previous endocarditis, or to redundancy of the valve with prolapse during systole. Mitral valve prolapse is found in as many as 10 per cent of young adults and may be the most common cause of mitral regurgitation. Regurgitation occurs rarely as a result of spontaneous rupture of the chordae tendineae, secondary to endocarditis or cardiac trauma. Papillary muscle dysfunction or rupture may also result in mitral regurgitation, but it is usually due to coronary artery disease and thus is very uncommon in pregnant women. Spatial disorientation of the papillary muscles occurs with left ventricular enlargement and may result in mitral regurgitation in patients with cardiomyopathy. Finally in patients with idiopathic hypertrophic subaortic stenosis, the mitral valve may be pulled open during systole with resultant mitral regurgitation.

The symptoms and signs of mitral regurgitation are well explained by its pathophysiology. Fatigue secondary to a decrease in effective left ventricular output (some portion of left ventricular output regurgitates into the left atrium) is the most common early symptom. Elevations in left atrial, pulmonary venous, and pulmonary capillary pressures are frequently less severe in patients with chronic mitral regurgitation and appear later than in patients with mitral stenosis. When elevated left atrial pressure occurs, symptoms of pulmonary congestion develop together with a propensity for atrial fibrillation and for the formation of thrombi in the left atrium. Pulmonary arteriolar resistance may also increae, resulting in right-sided heart failure with its associated peripheral edema, hepatomegaly, and abdominal distention.

An apical holosystolic murmur radiating to the left axilla is the hallmark of mitral regurgitation on physical examination. If the murmur is preceded by one or more clicks in midsystole or late systole, mitral valve prolapse is the likely diagnosis. If there is associated evidence of mitral stenosis, the regurgitant lesion is almost certainly due to rheumatic fever. In the absence of both of these causes, the possibility of idiopathic hypertrophic subaortic stenosis should be specifically considered. The electrocardiogram may show left atrial enlargement, atrial fibrillation, and evidence of hypertrophy of one or both ventricles. The chest x-ray usually shows cardiomegaly when mitral regurgitation is significant, and there may be evidence of pulmonary vascular congestion. An echocardiogram may help in determining the cause by showing evidence of bacterial endocarditis, rheumatic mitral stenosis, prolapse of the mitral valve, or idiopathic hypertrophic subaortic stenosis.

Patients with mitral regurgitation often remain asymptomatic for many years. The lesion is generally well tolerated during pregnancy. When there is evidence of rheumatic fever as the cause, antibiotic prophylaxis against streptococcal infection is indicated. Prophylaxis against bacterial endocarditis at the time of labor and delivery is recommended. Symptoms of congestive heart failure or arrhythmia developing in association with pregnancy are rare, and in our experience, surgery for mitral regurgitation has not been necessary during pregnancy.

Aortic Stenosis. More common in males than in females, aortic stenosis is encountered infrequently during pregnancy. When severe, this obstruction to left ventricular outflow decreases cardiac output enough to cause fatigue and even cerebral ischemia sufficient to cause syncope. Exertion is particularly likely to evoke these symptoms. Left ventricular work increases, the left ventricle hypertrophies, and the oxygen requirement of the heart rises. These changes, together with a decreased coronary blood flow caused by a reduced cardiac output, can result in angina pectoris, even when the coronary arteries are normal. In order to fill the thick-walled left ventricle adequately, left atrial pressure increases, often to a level that causes pulmonary vascular congestion and dyspnea.

The classic physical sign of aortic stenosis is a harsh systolic ejection murmur heard at the base of the heart, radiating to the carotid arteries. Because a similar murmur is common in persons without a significant hemodynamic abnormality, other evidence of left ventricular outflow obstruction should be assessed. A slowly rising and prolonged carotid arterial pulse, a fourth heart sound, and a second heart sound that is single or paradoxically split can be taken as evidence of significant obstruction. In these patients, an electrocardiogram will demonstrate left ventricular hypertrophy, and a chest x-ray will show dilation of the ascending aorta. Aortic valve calcification is uncommon in young women with aortic stenosis.

Patients with aortic stenosis rarely experience pulmonary congestion during pregnancy. The critical problem with aortic stenosis, occurring long in advance of congestive heart failure, is the inability of the heart to maintain an adequate output with an increased filling pressure. Any significant reduction in venous return may result in a dramatic drop in cardiac output, causing cerebral or cardiac ischemia. Maternal mortality rates as high as 17 per cent have been reported in patients with aortic stenosis.[5] The mortality is highest, approaching 40 per cent when the pregnancy is interrupted, presumably because hypovolemia is apt to occur in association with the procedure.[5] A fetal mortality rate of 32 per cent has been noted in women with aortic stenosis.[5]

If hemodynamically severe aortic stenosis is diagnosed prior to pregnancy, surgical correction before conception is advisable. In most young women, a commissurotomy will produce the desired result. If a prosthesis must be used, the need for long-term anticoagulation in a woman contemplating pregnancy weighs heavily in favor of the use of a heterograft rather than a mechanical prosthesis. When pregnancy occurs in a woman with severe aortic stenosis, measures to avoid hypovolemia and to restrict physical activity are important. If symptoms develop and are not controlled by restriction of activity, aortic valve surgery during pregnancy must be considered because of the reportedly high maternal mortality rate associated with interruption of pregnancy.

Prophylaxis against bacterial endocarditis at the time of labor and delivery is recommended in women with aortic stenosis.

Aortic Regurgitation. This lesion is more common than aortic stenosis in women of childbearing age. It may be the result of a congenital abnormality of the valve, or the valve may be damaged by rheumatic fever, endocarditis, or a systemic vasculitis such as rheumatoid arthritis or systemic lupus erythematosus. When aortic regurgitation results from rheumatic fever, mitral valve damage is almost always associated with it. Aortic regurgitation may also result from dilation of the aortic root. This, or aortic dissection, is the mechanism of the regurgitation in patients with Marfan's syndrome.

As a result of the valve's incompetence, a portion of the left ventricular output returns to the left ventricle during diastole. To compensate, the left ventricle dilates and its stroke volume increases, although usually not enough to maintain normal levels of cardiac output. In order to fill the enlarged left ventricle adequately, left atrial pressure rises, resulting in pulmonary congestion.

The initial symptom of aortic regurgitation is usually fatigue, which is attributed to diminished cardiac output. Syncope, chest pain, and dyspnea on exertion are late and ominous symptoms.

The physical signs of aortic regurgitation are detected on palpation of the carotid pulse, which shows a rapid upstroke and a rapid decline. Often a double systolic component is felt, the bisferious pulse. The classic murmur of aortic regurgitation is a high-pitched, blowing diastolic decrescendo murmur heard best along the left sternal border at the end of a forced expiration, with the patient sitting upright. The electrocardiogram may show left ventricular hypertrophy and left atrial enlargement, and the chest x-ray usually shows left ventricular cardiomegaly. Echocardiographic demonstration of fluttering of the mitral valve leaflets during diastole supports the diagnosis of aortic regurgitation. Rarely, vegetations are detected on the aortic valve by echocardiography, establishing the diagnosis of endocarditis.

Like mitral regurgitation, aortic regurgitation is usually well tolerated during pregnancy. If pulmonary congestion develops, restriction of activity is essential, and treatment with digitalis and diuretics is indicated. At the time of labor and delivery, antibiotic prophylaxis against bacterial endocarditis is advised. When aortic regurgitation results from active endocarditis, early surgery should be considered if the infection is not rapidly controlled or if progressive hemodynamic deterioration occurs, despite the hazard to pregnancy. Mortality with medical therapy alone is high in these patients.[103, 134, 142, 191]

Pulmonary Valve Disease. Hemodynamically significant abnormalities of the pulmonary valve are uncommon. Stenosis is a congenital anomaly, which occasionally goes unrecognized or untreated through childhood. When severe, it may result in chest pain, dyspnea, fatigue, or syncope. Physical examination shows evidence of right ventricular hypertrophy with a parasternal lift and a systolic murmur along the left sternal border associated with an ejection click. The electrocardiogram shows evidence of right ventricular hypertrophy, and the chest x-ray often shows poststenotic dilation of the pulmonary artery. When pulmonary stenosis produces symptoms prior to pregnancy, commissurotomy is indicated if the hemodynamic severity is confirmed by right-heart catheterization. If severe symptoms develop during pregnancy, pulmonic valve commissurotomy should be considered. Antibiotic prophylaxis against endocarditis is appropriate during labor and delivery.

Pulmonary regurgitation is very uncommon except when it occurs secondary to pulmonary hypertension.

Tricuspid Valve Disease. Although lesions of the tricuspid valve are uncommon, the incidence of tricuspid regurgitation may be increasing because of the use of intravenous drugs with resultant right-sided endocarditis. Tricuspid regurgitation is recognized by evidence of right-sided heart failure with large V waves in the neck veins, a pulsatile enlarged liver, and pedal edema. In general, the lesion is tolerated asymptomatically during pregnancy, and no special therapy is indicated except prophylaxis against bacterial endocarditis.

Congenital Heart Disease and Pregnancy

Increasing numbers of women who were born with congenital heart disease are reaching the childbearing age. Many of them are capable of conception. Some have had complete surgical correction of their deformity; others have undergone partial correction and have a residual hemodynamic defect that predisposes them to bacterial endocarditis.

Each abnormality has unique implications for pregnancy (Table 6–1), but some generalizations apply in all cases. First, some deformities carry an increased risk of maternal morbidity and mortality during pregnancy. Second, the presence of a congenital cardiac abnormality in either parent or a sibling significantly increases the risk of cardiac and other congenital abnormalities in the fetus. Third, there is increased risk of fetal death, depending upon the hemodynamic effects of the maternal lesion.

Congenital heart disease is recognized in 0.8 per cent of all live births in the United States.[119, 130, 145] When one of the parents has congenital heart disease, the first offspring has a 2 to 4 per cent chance of having a cardiac abnormality.[130] When the abnormality is transmitted as an autosomal dominant trait, as is the case with idiopathic hypertrophic subaortic stenosis, the child has a 50 per cent chance of developing the same abnormality.

As with other congenital defects, congenital heart disease is due to both genetic and environmental factors. In 8 per cent of children born with congenital heart disease, the primary cause appears to be genetic (5 per cent attributable to chromosomal damage and 3 per cent to "point" mutations). In another 1 to 2 per cent, the congenital deformity results from a detectable environmental factor, the most apparent of which is rubella occurring in the first trimester of pregnancy. The large residual number of cases is attributable to an interaction between genetic and environmental factors (including inadequate

TABLE 6–1   CARDIOVASCULAR DISEASE AND RATES OF MATERNAL/FETAL MORTALITY AND FETAL HEART DISEASE

Maternal Lesion	Maternal Mortality Per Cent	Fetal Mortality Per Cent	Fetal Heart Disease Per Cent
CONGENITAL DEFECTS			
Ventricular septal defect*	0– 1	25	4
Patent ductus arteriosus*	0– 1	10	4
Atrial septal defect*	0– 2	15	3
Pulmonary stenosis	0– 5	20	4
Tetralogy of Fallot	5–10	30–40	4
Aortic valve disease	10–20	30	4
Coarctation of the aorta	0– 5	20	2
Eisenmenger's syndrome	50	50	?
"DEVELOPMENTAL" ABNORMALITIES			
Marfan's syndrome	?	?	50
Idiopathic hypertrophic subaortic stenosis	0	?	50
Prolapsing mitral valve	0	?	10–20

*Uncomplicated by pulmonary hypertension
(These figures were compiled from many different sources [Jones and Howitt, 1965; Szekely and Snaith, 1974; Meyer, et al., 1964; Nora and Nora, 1978; Burwell and Metcalfe, 1958; Arias and Pineda, 1978; Deal and Wooley, 1973; Devereux et al., 1976; Oakley et al., 1979; Murdoch et al., 1972; Kahler, 1975; Cannell and Vernon, 1963; Copeland et al., 1963; Schaefer et al., 1968; Neilson et al., 1970], and the compilation should be accepted with reservation. The data were collected over different time periods in the last 30 years by different workers under different conditions and sometimes without regard to variables known to be important, such as the severity of the maternal abnormality, the presence and degree of cyanosis, and the presence of associated abnormalities.)

uterine blood flow or defective fetal oxygen supply secondary to maternal cyanosis).

In order to minimize the likelihood of congenital heart disease in the fetus, potential teratogens should be avoided, especially by the woman with congenital heart disease. Abstention from alcohol and from tobacco[51] must be advised. All drugs should be avoided unless clearly indicated, an interdiction which applies not only to drugs sold in a pharmacy but to "street" drugs as well.[4, 147] Exposure to rubella is dangerous, and live rubella vaccine is contraindicated because the virus may persist for months after injection.

In general, corrective surgery should be performed prior to pregnancy, not only for the well-being of the mother but to provide the best possible intrauterine environment for fetal development. Any residual or inoperable lesions require careful definition before pregnancy is undertaken.

Prophylaxis against endocarditis is indicated in patients with lesions that render them susceptible to this complication.

LEFT-TO-RIGHT SHUNTS

Left-to-right shunting occurs through an atrial septal defect, a ventricular septal defect, or a parent ductus arteriosus. Some women with these lesions reach adulthood without previous recognition of their disease, and some lesions are discovered for the first time during pregnancy. Most patients born with these lesions will have undergone surgical correction prior to pregnancy, but a residual defect may persist. The degree of shunting is influenced by the relative resistances in the systemic and pulmonary vascular circuits. Both of these decline during normal pregnancy to a similar degree,[114] so that no significant alteration in the degree of shunting results from pregnancy. When complicating pulmonary vascular disease has developed, however, the normal fall in pulmonary vascular resistance may not occur with pregnancy, a circumstance that tends to diminish the degree of left-to-right shunting. Although these lesions increase the chance of pulmonary hypertension, right ventricular failure, arrhythmias, and emboli, it is not clear that these complications are made more likely by pregnancy.

Atrial Septal Defect. The most common form of atrial septal defect, the ostium secundum defect, occurs more often in females than males and is more easily missed on physical examination than other cardiac abnormalities. For these reasons, it may occur in women of childbearing age. Additionally, patients with this defect are often asymptomatic or may have vague complaints of malaise and fatigue. The first symptoms may not occur until atrial arrhythmia or pulmonary hypertension develops.

On physical examination, the classic sign is a persistently split second heart sound associated with a systolic ejection murmur, which is heard best at the base of the heart. The electrocardiogram generally shows rightward displacement of the QRS axis with delayed right ventricular forces, and the chest x-ray may show evidence of increased pulmonary blood flow.

Pregnancy is well tolerated by patients with an uncomplicated atrial septal defect, and no specific treatment is recommended. Bacterial endocarditis is rare, and prophylactic antibiotics are not required. Although there may be an increased risk of thromboembolic phenomena, the routine use of anticoagulation is not warranted. Fetal loss approaches 15 per cent.[73] In couples of which either parent has an atrial septal defect, 2.6 per cent of the children have the same lesion, an incidence 30 times the frequency in unaffected subjects.[130]

Ostium primum defects are no more likely to result in difficulty during pregnancy than secundum lesions, but they are more often associated with other congenital abnormalities that may increase the risk of pregnancy.

Ventricular Septal Defect. Defects of the ventricular septum are more common than atrial septal defects, but over half of them close spontaneously in infancy and childhood, and those that do not close are usually easily detected and are frequently corrected by surgery prior to the childbearing age. Most patients with this lesion are asymptomatic, but fatigue or symptoms of pulmonary congestion occasionally occur.

On physical examination, a loud holosystolic murmur is heard along the left sternal border, and there is often an associated thrill. Occasionally, an apical diastolic rumble is heard secondary to the increased blood flow traversing the mitral valve. The second heart sound is usually normally split.

Patients with a ventricular septal defect generally tolerate pregnancy well. The lesion predisposes to bacterial endocarditis, so antibiotic prophylaxis is appropriate. Maternal mortality has only been described in those with complicating pulmonary hypertension, but occasionally pregnancy precipitates heart failure or arrhythmias, each of which is managed as in nonpregnant patients. Fetal loss may approach 25 per cent[73] (Table 6–1), and the child of a parent with a ventricular septal defect has approximately a 4 per cent chance of being born with the same cardiac abnormality.[130]

Patent Ductus Arteriosus. Patency of the ductus arteriosus is usually recognized and treated in childhood. When diagnosed, the lesion usually causes no symptoms, although occasionally fatigue or dyspnea on exertion occurs. classic machinery murmur, a continuous, harsh, to-and-fro murmur, is heard best at the base of the heart, particularly along the upper left sternal border and under the left clavicle, and is sometimes accompanied by a palpable thrill. The arterial pulse pressure is wide. Chest x-ray may show increased pulmonary vascular markings, and the electrocardiogram may show left ventricular hypertrophy. This lesion, like atrial and ventricular septal defects, is well tolerated by pregnant women, the only maternal deaths occurring in patients with complicating pulmonary hypertension. The fetal loss approximates 7 per cent, and a child of a parent with a patent ductus arteriosus has a chance of approximately 4 per cent of having the same abnormality. The patent ductus tends to become infected, so antibiotic prophylaxis at the time of labor and delivery is indicated.

RIGHT-TO-LEFT SHUNTS

Right-to-left shunting occurs through an atrial or ventricular septal defect or a patent ductus arteriosus when pulmonary vascular resistance rises to exceed peripheral vascular resistance or when an organic obstruction to right ventricular outflow exists. These patients develop cyanosis and clubbing and show evidence of right ventricular hypertrophy on physical examination, chest x-ray, and electrocardiogram. The risk of fetal mortality increases progressively with the severity of maternal cyanosis as judged by the degree of elevation of the maternal hematocrit. Even when born alive, the offspring of cyanotic mothers are unusually small.[126]

The most common cause of right-to-left shunting is tetralogy of Fallot, a combination of ventricular septal defect, pulmonary valve stenosis, right ventricular hypertrophy, and rightward displacement of the aortic root. Affected persons are cyanotic from childhood, show clubbing, and suffer from occasional "spells" of dyspnea, tachypnea, and loss of consciousness. Pulmonary vascular resistance is usually normal. In these patients, surgical correction of the heart lesion should be undertaken before pregnancy occurs. If correction is not feasible, or if the patient is already pregnant when the disease is recognized, pregnancy can be carried to term, although there is an increased risk of maternal and fetal morbidity and mortality.[70, 117] Maintenance of venous return, especially near term and post partum, is of critical importance in order to maintain pulmonary blood flow.

When right-to-left shunting results from the Eisenmenger syndrome (the development of high pulmonary vascular resistance in a patient with previous left-to-right shunting), pregnancy is a dangerous undertaking. Maternal mortality rates range from 30 to 70 per cent,[72, 128, 134, 172] death occurring either during gestation or in the postpartum period.[41, 72] Fetal mortality exceeds 40 per cent even when the mother survives. If pregnancy occurs in a woman with Eisenmenger's syndrome, we recommend interruption of pregnancy. If this recommendation is not accepted, management should include measures to avoid central hypovolemia, especially during and after delivery. Any sudden fall in venous return jeopardizes the ability of the right ventricle to force blood through the fixed pulmonary vascular resistance.

In addition to its occurrence as a component of Eisenmenger's syndrome, pulmonary hypertension may be "primary" (with no recognizable cause) or secondary to drug abuse or to recurrent pulmonary emboli. Symptoms include chest pain, syncope, and dyspnea, but some patients are asymptomatic. The condition should be suspected in any patient with evidence of right ventricular hypertrophy manifest by a left parasternal lift, a loud pulmonic component of the second heart sound, and right ventricular hypertrophy shown by the electrocardiogram or chest x-ray.

Whatever its cause, pulmonary hypertension is a contraindication to pregnancy. Maternal mortality rates approach 50 per cent even in women with primary pulmonary hypertension and no intrinsic cardiac defect.[49, 104, 129] If pregnancy occurs in a woman with pulmonary hypertension, interruption is recommended. Venous return must be carefully maintained at all times.

COARCTATION OF THE AORTA

This lesion is uncommon in association with pregnancy. It is usually located at the level of the left subclavian artery and is recognized by hypertension in the right arm without hypertension in the left arm or the legs. The presenting symptoms may be chest pain, or leg fatigue from inadequate blood flow when the coarctation is severe. As many as 25 per cent of patients with this lesion have an associated bicuspid aortic valve, which may result in aortic stenosis and regurgitation. Collateral blood flow may be recognized by palpable pulsations or audible bruits over the ribs posteriorly, and notching of the inferior surface of the ribs may be noted on chest x-ray.

These patients are at risk of aortic dissection, bacterial endocarditis, cerebral hemorrhage due to rupture of associated intracranial aneurysms, and the complications of prolonged hypertension. The risk of these events occurring during pregnancy is even higher than at other times, with an overall maternal mortality rate ranging from 3 to 8 per cent,[45, 172] and cardiac complications are common in those who survive pregnancy.[8, 121]

Correction of the coarctation, when possible, should be accomplished before pregnancy is undertaken. When pregnancy occurs in a patient with coarctation, treatment of the hypertension is indicated. Major swings in blood pressure should be avoided, and prophylactic antibiotics are indicated at labor and delivery to obviate the risk of bacterial infection of the lesion. Fetal loss in these patients approximates 11 per cent,[73] and offspring have a 2 per cent chance of developing the same congenital abnormality if one parent is affected.[130]

COMPLEX CONGENITAL HEART LESIONS

Any combination of congenital cardiac defects may occur. Usually they include an atrial or ventricular septal defect or a patent ductus arteriosus. In general, the more complex the lesion, the higher are the maternal and fetal morbidity and mortality rates. Surgical correction of complex cardiac lesions should be considered prior to pregnancy in order to decrease maternal and fetal risk. The more complex and severe the maternal lesion, the greater is the chance that the child will have congenital heart disease.[130]

Developmental Abnormalities

These lesions have been arbitrarily designated as "developmental" rather than "congenital."

Mitral Valve Prolapse. Found in 5 to 10 per cent of young adults, mitral valve prolapse is encountered frequently in pregnant women. Although this abnormality has a familial occurrence,[10, 21, 43, 48, 101, 138, 144, 164] there is no clear genetic pattern of inheritance. Most individuals with the syndrome are asymptomatic, but some have arrhythmias, chest pain atypical of myocardial ischemia, syncope, or peripheral emboli. The diagnosis is made on auscultation when one or more midsystolic-to-late systolic clicks, often followed by a systolic murmur, are heard at the lower left sternal border or cardiac apex. These signs are variable between individuals and in the same individual from day to day. The chest x-ray and electrocardiogram are usually normal. Echocardiography usually shows characteristic abnormal mitral valve motion in systole. Pregnancy may change the physical signs, either enhancing or diminishing them, depending on changes in vascular resistance and blood volume.[61] There is no evidence that the rare complications are more likely to occur during pregnancy,[48, 61, 156] and no treatment is required except the use of prophylactic antibiotics during labor and delivery.

Idiopathic Hypertrophic Subaortic Stenosis. This condition is inherited as an autosomal dominant trait with variable penetrance and is associated with an increased risk of sudden death and with dyspnea, chest pain, and arrhythmias. The latter provide the presenting symptoms, and on physical examination a brisk rise in the carotid pulse is noted, occasionally with a bisferious quality. The left ventricular impulse may be double or triple on precordial palpation, and a systolic ejection murmur is heard, usually along the left sternal border, radiating poorly to the carotids and to the left axilla. The murmur varies greatly in intensity, increasing dramatically with conditions that cause a decrease in left ventricular volume, such as the Valsalva maneuver or assumption of the standing position. There is often associated mitral regurgitation producing an apical holosystolic murmur. The echocardiogram is diagnostic, showing marked thickening of the ventricular septum and abnormal systolic movement of the mitral valve. Left ventricular hypertrophy with large septal Q waves is frequently noted on the electrocardiogram. The chest x-ray is usually normal.

Pregnancy may cause important alterations in the hemodynamics associated with idiopathic hypertrophic subaortic stenosis. A sudden decrease in venous return due to obstruction of the inferior vena cava or to blood loss at delivery, combined with the fall in peripheral vascular resistance that accompanies pregnancy, compounds the severity of outflow tract obstruction. This may be aggravated further by increases in the circulating levels of catecholamines during labor and delivery. On the other hand, the increased blood volume of pregnancy tends to lessen the degree of outflow obstruction. Although several authors have recorded an increase in symptomatology in patients during pregnancy, maternal death has not been recorded.[19, 83, 131, 171, 177]

Medical management of this condition during pregnancy should be directed toward maintaining blood volume and venous return to the heart and diminishing the force of myocardial contraction by avoidance of excitement, anxiety, and strenuous activity. Propranolol should be used in those with symptoms. If blood loss at delivery is associated with evidence of increased obstruction, volume replacement and vasopressor agents should be used immediately. Propranolol has been used at the time of labor and delivery,[83] but no convincing evidence of its benefit has been presented.

Marfan's Syndrome. Although the fundamental biochemical defect is still not defined, Marfan's syndrome results from a weakness of connective tissue that leads to dislocation of the ocular lenses, joint deformities, and dangerous weakness of the aortic root and aortic wall.[107, 140] Affected persons are classically tall with disproportionately long extremities. Arachnodactyly and lax joints are salient features. Scoliosis may develop anywhere in the thoracolumbar spine, and other evidence of weakness of connective tissue is spontaneous joint dislocations and a high incidence of inguinal hernias.

The cardiovascular manifestations are the most dangerous. Over half of the affected individuals have evidence of a mitral or aortic valve abnormality by auscultation, and 25 per cent have detectable aortic regurgitation. The incidence of mitral valve prolapse may be as high as 90 per cent depending upon the criteria used for diagnosis.[20] The chest x-ray may show dilatation of the ascending aorta.

In a woman with this syndrome, pregnancy raises several problems. First, half of her offspring will be affected with the syndrome. Second, the expected life span of affected individuals is reduced to about half normal, implying that her years of motherhood will be limited.[123] Third, although statistics are not available, there is evidence of an increased risk of aortic dissection and rupture during pregnancy.[116] For these reasons, we advise women with Marfan's syndrome to avoid pregnancy. If the diagnosis is definite, interruption of pregnancy is recommended. If the parents elect to continue the pregnancy, efforts should be made to reduce pulsatile forces on the aortic wall. Maternal activity should be restricted and propranolol given to decrease the force of myocardial contraction. Education for childbirth and adequate analgesics should be employed, and prophylactic antibodies should be administered during labor and delivery to avoid endocarditis.

Congestive Cardiomyopathies

Cardiomyopathy may occur in the peripartum period.[24, 46, 47] The cause of this syndrome is unclear, but it resembles other congestive cardiomyopathies. In the United States, it is seen almost exclusively in black women, especially those who are multiparous, older than average, and pregnant (or recently pregnant) with twins.[24] Those whose pregnancy has been complicated by hypertension are also at increased risk.[46, 47] Mural thrombi in the left ventricle may give rise to peripheral emboli.

In most patients, heart size returns to normal soon after delivery. If cardiomegaly persists beyond six months, the prognosis is poor and further pregnancies are contraindicated. Indeed, we advise against pregnancy in all women with a past history of any congestive cardiomyopathy.

Infant mortality is close to 10 per cent in pregnant patients with congestive heart failure. Treatment includes limitation of activity, restriction of sodium, and the use of diuretics and digoxin. Anticoagulants are required when thromboembolic complications occur.

Cardiac Arrhythmias

Several authors have suggested that tachyarrhythmias, particularly atrial tachyarrhythmias, occur more frequently in pregnant women,[14, 109, 172] but data to support this belief have not been published. It is clear, however, that arrhythmias occur commonly during pregnancy. As in nonpregnant individuals, management involves reassurance, the elimination of stimulants, and the avoidance of fatigue and anxiety. Every effort should be made to avoid drug treatment. When drugs are required, standard medications should be used. If cardioversion is necessary, it can be employed without apparent danger to the mother or to the child.[159] Drug treatment of asymptomatic premature beats is not justified.

Bradyarrhythmias occur during pregnancy[38, 109] but do not require treatment unless they compromise maternal hemodynamics. Even complete heart block, usually of congenital origin in these young women, is compatible with successful pregnancy.[12, 77]

PREGNANCY AFTER CARDIAC SURGERY

Surgical repair and commissurotomy of heart valves are valuable procedures, but they seldom restore heart function to normal. The condition of patients who have had the benefit of these procedures should be evaluated in the same way as that of other patients with valve disease. Before pregnancy is undertaken, those who remain symptomatic despite surgery should be carefully studied and further surgery considered. Some patients will not obtain sufficient improvement from surgery to permit a safe pregnancy.

Patients who undertake pregnancy following valve surgery should be managed like other patients with valve disease. Antibiotics are advised at labor and delivery, and when the valve lesion is rheumatic in origin, long-term antibiotics should be taken to prevent rheumatic recurrences.

Women with prosthetic heart valves have increased risks during pregnancy, although some are delivered without complications.[30] Patients with mechanical prostheses require anticoagulation. Because warfarin derivatives cross the placenta and endanger the fetus,[63, 168] heparin therapy should be substituted for oral anticoagulation when pregnancy is planned or undertaken. The avoidance of oral anticoagulants is particularly important during fetal organogenesis, but the risks of fetal hemorrhage and uterine hemorrhage remain high throughout pregnancy.

The mortality rate from prosthetic valve endocarditis exceeds 40 per cent,[81, 103, 166] so antibiotic prophylaxis is mandatory during dental and surgical procedures and during labor and delivery. Drugs that protect against genitourinary organisms should be used.[74] If prosthetic endocarditis develops during pregnancy, vigorous antibiotic treatment must be instituted at once; replacement of the prosthesis is indicated if the infection is not brought under control immediately.[142, 166, 191]

Patients with heterograft prostheses are also at risk of developing bacterial endocarditis and require antibiotic prophylaxis; however, those with heterografts have a lower susceptibility to thrombosis and thromboembolic events than do those with mechanical prostheses. Nevertheless, patients with aortic heterografts suffer a 1 to 3 per cent incidence of systemic emboli per year when they do not receive anticoagulants. The corresponding figures for mitral heterografts are 3 to 5 per cent per year,[82, 124] and the incidence increases further in the presence of atrial arrhythmias or left atrial enlargement. If an embolic event occurs in a patient with a heterograft, anticoagulant therapy (heparin during pregnancy) must be given at once. Against this background, there is a logical argument for employing heterograft prostheses in young women who are contemplating pregnancy. The patient should recognize that valve replacement will probably be required in subsequent years and that the dangers of thromboembolism are not completely avoided by this course.

The risks of pregnancy after surgery for congenital heart lesions depend upon the residual anatomic and hemodynamic defects. When pulmonary hypertension persists, pregnancy is dangerous for both mother and fetus. If a patch, an artificial conduit, or a valve prosthesis has been inserted, or if closure of the defect has been incomplete, antibiotics are indicated for prophylaxis against bacterial infection.

DIAGNOSTIC PROCEDURES FOR HEART DISEASE

Some diagnostic procedures carry risks to the pregnant woman and her child. Unless the normal changes of pregnancy are recognized, a diagnosis of heart disease may be mistakenly made with consequent anxiety, apprehension, and unnecessary expense. Electrocardiography is safe, but it is only useful when indicated. Nonspecific changes have been reported, including a shift in the electric axis, but these observations have not been universally accepted.[160]

All x-ray procedures should be avoided, especially in early pregnancy. In most patients, chest x-rays do not yield useful information.[17, 102, 155] A cardiac ultrasound evaluation carries no apparent risk, but it is expensive and should be performed only when required to answer a specific question.

Cardiac catheterization should be avoided because of the dangers of fluoroscopic exposure and the potentially adverse effects of introducing foreign material into the cardiovascular system. It is important to emphasize that any woman who is about to undergo x-ray examination or cardiac catheterization should be questioned about the possibility of being pregnant. When there is a clear indication for the performance of x-ray examination, it should be carried out with maximum shielding.

CARDIOVASCULAR DRUGS AND PREGNANCY

As previously stated, no medication should be used during pregnancy unless there is clear justification.

Diuretics. The use of thiazide diuretics for prophylaxis against toxemia[54] is not generally accepted.[57, 84] When congestive heart failure is uncontrolled by restriction of activity and sodium intake, diuretics should be given, with careful monitoring of electrolyte and water balance.

Inotropic Agents. Pregnancy does not change the indications for digitalis therapy.[18] However, because both digoxin and digitoxin cross the placental barrier and because of the expansion of body water during pregnancy, a given dose of these drugs results in lower circulating levels during pregnancy than in the nonpregnant state. Accordingly, if the desired clinical effect is not apparent, blood levels should be determined.[148] Digitalis may exert an effect on the myometrium similar to its inotropic effect on the myocardium, acting to shorten gestation and labor.[188]

Standard intravenous inotropic and vasopressor agents (dopamine, norepinephrine, dobutamine) all decrease uterine blood flow and may stimulate uterine contractions.[18] Their use during pregnancy is justified only when the mother's survival is at stake.

Adrenergic Receptor Blockade. These agents are used with increasing frequency for the treatment of hypertension and tachyarrhythmias. Beta-blocking agents have been used for the treatment of gestational hyperthyroidism without apparent ill effects[18, 23, 91] despite evidence from animal work that propranolol lowers umbilical blood flow.[33a] The drugs should be used with caution during pregnancy because they have the potential for initiating premature labor through the beta-blocking action on the uterus.[9] The sustained increase in uterine tone induced by propranolol could potentially lead to a small and infarcted placenta and a low birth weight infant as suggested by some investigators.[154] The drug has been used successfully in the treatment of dysfunctional labor.[120] A large dose administered intravenously to the mother shortly before delivery may result in delayed respiration by the newborn.[18, 176] When a beta-blocking agent is required, fetal heart rate should be monitored and the infant should be closely watched with regard to heart rate, blood glucose concentration, and respiratory status.[44, 62, 83, 139]

Blocking of the alpha-receptor sites with phentolamine or phenoxybenzamine may be required during pregnancy for control of pheochromocytoma.[18, 59, 158]

Antiarrhythmic Agents. Quinidine has been used frequently during pregnancy without clear adverse effects,[65] but occasional problems are encountered with procainamide or disopyramide.[93, 106, 163] We believe that it is best to treat arrhythmias without drugs whenever possible, but these agents may be used when necessary.

Anticoagulants. Patients taking therapeutic doses of warfarin derivatives have a 1 to 5 per cent chance per year of a significant bleeding episode, and the risk of a minor hemorrhage is as high as 10 per cent per year. These substances cross the placenta, and fetal exposure during the first two months is associated with a 15 to 25 per cent incidence of malformations.[136, 141, 165, 168] Even after the first trimester, warfarin increases the chance of fetal bleeding or maternal intrauterine hemorrhage.[165, 168] and the risk of hemorrhage persists at the time of labor and delivery. Although pregnancy is sometimes successful despite these handicaps,[30, 53] we advise avoidance of warfarin derivatives whenever possible. In some patients, especially those with prosthetic heart valves or with a history of recurrent embolic episodes, heparin anticoagulation must be substituted for oral anticoagulants. Heparin does not cross the placental barrier, but some evidence of increased maternal and fetal death has been reported.[63, 110, 168]

OBSTETRIC DRUGS WITH CARDIAC EFFECTS

Drugs That Stimulate the Uterus. The injection of hypertonic solutions into the uterus to produce abortion may result in hypervolemia and, if saline is used, in hypernatremia. Prostaglandins E_2 and $F_2\alpha$ when employed in the small doses necessary to induce therapeutic abortion of labor at term do not produce significant hemodynamic effects.

Drugs That Quiet the Uterus. Ethyl alcohol has important effects on the myocardium, especially in patients with heart disease.[118] When administered intravenously in hypertonic concentrations to avert premature labor, substantial alterations in fluid balance and ventricular function result.

Ritodrine, isoxsuprine hydrochloride, terbutaline, and other beta-sympathomimetic amines are used with increasing frequency to stop premature labor. All these agents cause maternal tachycardia and are hazardous to patients with mitral stenosis. Terbutaline should not be used in the presence of hypertension or heart disease. The use of ritodrine and terbutaline at term has been associated with maternal pulmonary edema,[50, 169] usually when corticosteroids are being administered concurrently to promote fetal lung maturation. The mechanism of this pulmonary edema is unclear, but it responds promptly to cessation of the beta-sympathomimetic amine.

Drugs Used at Delivery. Adequate analgesia during labor and delivery reduces anxiety and pain and minimizes the danger of pulmonary edema precipitated by tachycardia. The anesthetic technique employed for delivery should depend upon the training and competence of the anesthesiologist. Scopolamine should not be used because it evokes restlessness and tachycardia, and atropine should be used cautiously.

A term delivery in a well-managed patient offers the best hope of a successful outcome for the mother with heart disease. Term cesarean section has historically been associated with a high maternal mortality in women with mitral stenosis, but the method utilizing pentothal, nitrous oxide, and succinylcholine by intravenous drip[52] raises the possibility that cesarean section delivery should be reevaluated. With modern techniques and in skilled hands, it may be preferable to labor for the rare patient who is close to pulmonary edema despite the best management.

Synthetic oxytocin (pitocin) is preferable to the natural product for patients with heart disease because it is free of pressor agents. It is given slowly to minimize blood loss after delivery because a bolus injection of 5 to 10 units causes marked, though transient, hypotension.[64] Both ergonovine and methylergonovine maleate should be avoided in patients who are in danger of pulmonary congestion.[64]

The administration of intravenous fluids during labor and the postpartum period should be closely monitored, especially in women with heart disease. After delivery, we recommend early ambulation and carefully fitted elastic stockings to lessen the danger of thromboembolism.

References

1. Abramovich, D. R., Francis, W., and Helsby, C. R.: Two cases of ruptured aneurysm of splanchnic arteries in pregnancy with comment on the lesser sac syndrome. J. Obstet. Gynaecol. Br. Commonw., 76:1037, 1969.
2. Adams, J. Q.: Cardiovascular physiology in normal pregnancy: Studies with the dye dilution technique. Am. J. Obstet. Gynecol., 67:741, 1954.
3. Ahronheim, J. H.: Isolated coronary periarteritis: Report of a case of unexpected death in a young pregnant woman. Am. J. Cardiol., 40:287, 1977.
4. Amarose, A. P.: Chromosome aberrations in the mother and the newborn from drug addiction pregnancies. J. Reprod. Med., 20:323, 1978.
5. Arias, F., and Pineda, J.: Aortic stenosis and pregnancy. J. Reprod. Med., 20:229, 1978.
6. Assali, N. S., Rauramo, L., and Peltonen, T.: Measurements of uterine blood flow and metabolism. VIII. Uterine and fetal blood flow and oxygen consumption in early human pregnancy. Am. J. Obstet. Gynecol., 79:86, 1960.
7. Bader, R. A., Bader, M. E., Rose, D. J., and Braunwald, E.: Hemodynamics at rest and during exercise in normal pregnancy as studied by cardiac catheterization. J. Clin. Invest., 34:1524, 1955.
8. Barash, P. G., Hobbins, J. C., Hook, R., Stansel, H. C., Jr., Whittmore, R., and Hehre, F. W.: Management of coarctation of the aorta during pregnancy. J. Thorac. Cardiovasc. Surg., 69:781, 1975.
9. Barden, T. P., and Stander, R. W.: Myometrial and cardiovascular effects of an adrenergic blocking drug in human pregnancy. Am. J. Obstet. Gynecol., 101:91, 1968.
10. Barlow, J. B., and Pocock, W. A.: The problem of nonejection systolic clicks and associated mitral systolic murmurs: Emphasis on the billowing mitral leaflet syndrome. Am. Heart J., 90:636, 1976.
11. Barnes, C. G.: Medical Disorders in Obstetric Practice, 3rd Ed. Oxford, Blackwell Scientific Publications, 1970.
12. Barton, R. M., and LaDue, C. N.: Complete heart block in a case of pregnancy. Am. J. Med., 4:447, 1948.
13. Beary, J. F., Summer, W. R., and Bulkley, B. H.: Postpartum acute myocardial infarction: A rare occurrence of uncertain etiology. Am. J. Cardiol., 43:158, 1979.
14. Bellet, S.: Essentials of Cardiac Arrhythmias: Diagnosis and Management. Philadelphia, W. B. Saunders Co., 1972.
15. Beresford, O. D., and Graham, A. M.: Chorea gravidarum. J. Obstet. Gynaecol. Br. Emp., 57:616, 1950.
16. Bland, E. F.: Declining severity of rheumatic fever: A comparative study of the past four decades. N. Engl. J. Med., 262:599, 1960.
17. Bonebrake, C. R., Noller, K. L., Loehnen, C. P., Muhm, J. R., and Fish, C. R.: Routine chest roentgenography in pregnancy. J.A.M.A., 240:2747, 1978.
18. Brinkman, C. R., III, and Woods, J. R., Jr.: Effects of cardiovascular drugs during pregnancy. Cardiovasc. Med., 1:231, 1976.

19. Brown, A. K., Doukas, N., Riding, W. D., and Jones, E. W.: Cardiomyopathy and pregnancy. Br. Heart J., 29:387, 1967.
20. Brown, O. R., DeMots, H., Kloster, F. E., Roberts, A., Menashe, V. D., and Beals, R. K.: Aortic root dilatation and mitral valve prolapse in Marfan's syndrome. An echocardiographic study. Circulation, 52:651, 1975.
21. Brown, O. R., Kloster, F. E., and DeMots, H.: Incidence of mitral valve prolapse in the asymptomatic normal. Circulation, 52(suppl II):77, 1975.
22. Bryant, E. E., Douglas, B. H., and Ashburn, A. D.: Circulatory changes following prolactin administration. Am. J. Obstet. Gynecol., 115:53, 1973.
23. Bullock, J. L., Harris, R. E., and Young, R.: Treatment of thyrotoxicosis during pregnancy with propranolol. Am. J. Obstet. Gynecol., 121:245, 1975.
24. Burch, G. E.: Heart disease and pregnancy. Am. Heart J., 93:104, 1977.
25. Burg, J. R., Dodek, A., Kloster, F. E., and Metcalfe, J.: Systolic time intervals in pregnancy. Clin. Res., 20:365, 1972.
26. Burwell, C. S.: The placenta as a modified arteriovenous fistula considered in relation to the circulatory adjustments to pregnancy. Am. J. Med. Sci., 195:1, 1938.
27. Burwell, C. S., and Metcalfe, J.: Heart Disease and Pregnancy: Physiology and Management. Boston, Little, Brown & Co., 1958.
28. Butler, E. F.: The effect of iron and folic acid on red cell and plasma volume in pregnancy. J. Obstet. Gynaecol. Br. Commonw., 75:497, 1968.
29. Cannell, D. E., and Vernon, C. P.: Congenital heart disease and pregnancy. Am. J. Obstet. Gynecol., 85:744, 1963.
30. Casanegra, P., Avilés, G., Maturana, G., and Dubernet, J.: Cardiovascular management of pregnant women with a heart valve prosthesis. Am. J. Cardiol., 36:802, 1975.
31. Cavanzo, F. J., and Taylor, H. B.: Effect of pregnancy on the human aorta and its relationship to dissecting aneurysms. Am. J. Obstet. Gynecol., 105:567, 1969.
32. Chesley, L. C.: Renal functional changes in normal pregnancy. Clin. Obstet. Gynecol., 3:349, 1960.
33. Chesley, L. C., and Duffus, G. M.: Posture and apparent plasma volume in late pregnancy. J. Obstet. Gynaecol. Br. Commonw., 78:406, 1971.
33a. Chez, R. A., Ehrenkranz, R. A., Oakes, G. K., Walker, A. M., Hamilton, L. A., Jr., Brennan, S. C., and McLaughlin, M. K.: Effects of adrenergic agents on ovine umbilical and uterine blood flows. In Longo, L. D., and Reneau, D. D. (eds.): Fetal and Newborn Cardiovascular Physiology, Vol. 2, Fetal and Newborn Circulation. New York, Garland STPM Press, 1978.
34. Chisholm, M.: A controlled clinical trial of prophylactic folic acid and iron in pregnancy. J. Obstet. Gynaecol. Br. Commonw., 73:191, 1966.
35. Churchill, M. A., Geraci, J. E., and Hunder, G. G.: Musculoskeletal manifestations of bacterial endocarditis. Ann. Intern. Med., 87:754, 1977.

36. Ciraulo, D. A., and Markovitz, A.: Myocardial infarction in pregnancy associated with a coronary artery thrombus. Arch. Intern. Med., *139*:1046, 1979.

37. Clinch, J.: Chorea gravidarum. Hosp. Med., *2*:317, 1967.

38. Copeland, G. D., and Stern, T. N.: Wenckebach periods in pregnancy and puerperium. Am. Heart J., *56*:291, 1958.

39. Copeland, W. E., Wooley, C. F., Ryan, J. M., Runco, V., and Levin, H. S.: Pregnancy and congenital heart disease. Am. J. Obstet. Gynecol., *86*:107, 1963.

40. Csapo, A.: Actomyosin formation by estrogen action. Am. J. Physiol., *162*:406, 1950.

41. Cutforth, R., Catchlove, B., Knight, L. W., and Dudgeon, G.: The Eisenmenger syndrome and pregnancy. Aust. N.Z. J. Obstet. Gynaecol., *8*:202, 1968.

42. Cutforth, R., and MacDonald, C. B.: Heart sounds and murmurs in pregnancy. Am. Heart J., *71*:741, 1966.

43. Darsee, J. R., Mikolich, J. R., Nicoloff, N. B., and Lesser, L. E.: Prevalence of mitral valve prolapse in presumably healthy young men. Circulation, *59*:619, 1979.

44. Datta, S., Kitzmiller, J. L., Ostheimer, G. W., and Schoenbaum, S. C.: Propranolol and parturition. Obstet. Gynecol., *51*:577, 1978.

45. Deal, K., and Wooley, C. F.: Coarctation of the aorta and pregnancy. Ann. Intern. Med., *78*:706, 1973.

46. Demakis, J. G., and Rahimtoola, S. H.: Peripartum cardiomyopathy. Circulation, *44*:964, 1971.

47. Demakis, J. G., Rahimtoola, S. H., Sutton, G. C., Meadows, W. R., Szanto, P. B., Tobin, J. R., and Gunnar, R. M.: Natural course of peripartum cardiomyopathy. Circulation, *44*:1053, 1971.

48. Devereux, R. B., Perloff, J. K., Reichek, N., and Josephson, M, E.: Mitral valve prolapse. Circulation, *54*:3, 1976.

49. Dresdale, D. T., Schultz, M., and Michtom, R. J.: Primary pulmonary hypertension. I. Clinical and hemodynamic study. Am. J. Med., *11*:686, 1951.

50. Elliott, H. R., Abdulla, U., and Hayes, P. J.: Pulmonary oedema associated with ritodrine infusion and betamethasone administration in premature labour. Br. Med. J., *2*:799, 1978.

51. Elliott, J.: Maternal smoking and the fetus: One fear buried but others arise. J.A.M.A., *241*:867, 1979.

52. Ferraris, G., and Gambotto, C.: Cesarean section as the method of choice for patients with cardiac decompensation. Minerva Ginecol., *14*:198, 1962.

53. Fillmore, S. J., and McDevitt, E.: Effects of coumarin compounds on the fetus. Ann. Intern. Med., *73*:731, 1970.

54. Finnerty, F. A., and Bepko, F. J., Jr.: Lowering the perinatal mortality and the prematurity rate; the value of prophylactic thiazides in juveniles. J.A.M.A., *195*:429, 1966.

55. Gilchrist, A. R.: Cardiological problems in younger women, including those of pregnancy and the puerperium. Br. Med. J., *1*:209, 1963.

56. Glaviano, V. V.: Evidence for an arteriovenous fistula in the gravid uterus. Surg. Gynecol. Obstet., *117*:301, 1963.

57. Gray, M. J.: Use and abuse of thiazides in pregnancy. Clin. Obstet. Gynecol., *11*:568, 1968.

58. Greiss, F. C., Jr., and Anderson, S. G.: Effect of ovarian hormones on the uterine vascular bed. Am. J. Obstet. Gynecol., *107*:829, 1970.

59. Griffith, M. I., Felts, J. H., James, F. M., Meyers, R. T., Shealy, G. M., and Woodruff, L. F.: Successful control of pheochromocytoma in pregnancy. J.A.M.A., *229*:437, 1974.

60. Guzman, C. A., and Caplan, R.: Cardiorespiratory response to exercise during pregnancy. Am. J. Obstet. Gynecol., *108*:600, 1970.

61. Haas, J. M.: The effect of pregnancy on the midsystolic click and murmurs of the prolapsing posterior leaflet of the mitral valve. Am. Heart J., *92*:407, 1976.

62. Habib, A., and McCarthy, J. S.: Effects on the neonate of propranolol administered during pregnancy. J. Pediatr., *91*:808, 1977.

63. Hall, J. G., Pauli, R. M., and Wilson, K. M.: Maternal and fetal sequelae of anticoagulation during pregnancy. Am. J. Med., *68*:122, 1980.

64. Hendricks, C. H., and Brenner, W. E.: Cardiovascular effects of oxytocic drugs used postpartum. Am. J. Obstet. Gynecol., *108*:751, 1970.

65. Hill, L. M., and Malkasian, G. D., Jr.: The use of quinidine sulfate throughout pregnancy. Obstet. Gynecol., *54*:366, 1979.

66. Hohimer, A. R., Morton, M. J., and Metcalfe, J.: Maternal hemodynamics during guinea pig pregnancy. Physiologist, *23*:148, 1980 (abstract).

67. Hytten, F. F., and Leitch, I.: The Physiology of Human Pregnancy. Philadelphia, F. A. Davis Co., 1964.

68. Hytten, F. F., and Paintin, D. B.: Increase in plasma volume during normal pregnancy. J. Obstet. Gynaecol. Br. Commonw., *70*:402, 1963.

69. Hytten, F. E., and Thomson, A. M.: Maternal physiological adjustments. *In* Assali, N. S. (ed.): Biology of Gestation. New York, Academic Press, 1968.

70. Jacoby, W. J., Jr.: Pregnancy with tetralogy and pentalogy of Fallot. Am. J. Cardiol., *14*:866, 1964.

71. Jewett, J. F.: Two dissecting coronary-artery aneurysms post partum. N. Engl. J. Med., *298*:1255, 1978.

72. Jones, A. M., and Howitt, G.: Eisenmenger syndrome in pregnancy. Br. Med. J., *1*:1627, 1965.

73. Kahler, R. L.: Cardiac disease. *In* Burrow, G. N., and Ferris, T. F. (eds.): Medical Complications During Pregnancy, 1st Ed. Philadelphia, W. B. Saunders Co., 1975.

74. Kaplan, E. L., Anthony, B. F., Bisno, A., Durack, D., Houser, H., Millard, H. D., Sanford, J., Shulman, S. T., Stillerman, M., Taranta, A., and Wenger, N.: Prevention of bacterial endocarditis. Circulation, *56*:139A, 1977.

75. Kaplan, E. L., Bisno, A., Facklam, R., Gordis, L., Houser, H. B., Jackson, W. H., Millard, H. D., Shulman, S. T., Taranta, A. V., and Wannamaker, L. W.: Prevention of rheumatic fever. Circulation, *55*:1, 1977.

76. Katz, R., Karliner, J. S., and Resnik, R.: Effects of a natural volume overload state (pregnancy) on left ventricular performance in normal human subjects. Circulation, *58*:434, 1978.

77. Kenmore, A. C. F., and Cameron, A. J. V.: Congenital complete heart block in pregnancy. Br. Heart J., *29*:910, 1967.

78. Kerr, M. G.: The mechanical effects of the gravid uterus in late pregnancy. J. Obstet. Gynaecol. Br. Commonw., *72*:513, 1965.

79. Kerr, M. G., Scott, D. B., and Samuel, E.: Studies of the inferior vena cava in late pregnancy. Br. Med. J., *1*:532, 1964.

80. King, T. M., Whitehorn, W. V., Reeves, B., and Kubota, R.: Effects of estrogen on composition and function of cardiac muscle. Am. J. Physiol., *196*:1282, 1959.

81. Kloster, F. E.: Infective prosthetic valve endocarditis. *In* Rahimtoola, S. H. (ed.): Infective Endocarditis. New York, Grune and Stratton, Inc., 1978.

82. Kloster, F. E.: Complications of artificial heart valves. J.A.M.A., *241*:2201, 1979.

83. Kolibash, A. J., Ruiz, D. E., and Lewis, R. P.: Idiopathic hypertrophic subaortic stenosis in pregnancy. Ann. Intern. Med., *82*:791, 1975.

84. Kraus, G. W., Marchese, J. R., Yen, S. S. C.: Prophylactic use of thiazides in pregnancy. J.A.M.A., *198*:1150, 1966.

85. Krause, R. M.: The influence of infection on the geography of heart disease. Circulation, *60*:972, 1979.

86. Krugman, S.: Rubella immunization: Progress, problems and potential solutions. Am. J. Public Health, *69*:217, 1979.

87. Lagerlöf, H., and Werkö, L.: Studies on the circulation in man. II. Normal values for cardiac output and pressure in the right auricle, right ventricle, and pulmonary artery. Acta Physiol. Scand., *16*:75, 1949.

88. Laird-Meeter, K., Van de Ley, G., Bom, T. H., Wladimiroff, J. W., and Roelandt, J.: Cardiocirculatory adjustments during pregnancy. An echocardiographic study. Clin. Cardiol., *2*:328, 1979.

89. Landau, R. L., Bergenstal, D. M., Lugibihl, K., and Kascht, M. E.: The metabolic effects of progesterone in man. J. Clin. Endocrinol. Metab., *15*:1194, 1955.

90. Landau, R. L., and Lugibihl, K.: Inhibition of the sodium-retaining influence of aldosterone by progesterone. J. Clin. Endocrinol. Metab., *18*:1237, 1958.

91. Langer, A., Hung, C. T., McAnulty, J. A., Harrigan, J. T., and Washington, E.: Adrenergic blockade: A new approach to hyperthyroidism during pregnancy. Obstet. Gynecol., *44*:181, 1974.

92. Leduc, B.: The effect of hyperventilation on maternal placental blood flow in pregnant rabbits. J. Physiol., *225*:339, 1972.

93. Leonard, R. F., Braun, T. E., and Levy, A. M.: Initiation of uterine contractions by disopyramide during pregnancy. N. Engl. J. Med., *299*:84, 1978.

94. Lewis, B. V., and Parsons, M.: Chorea gravidarum. Lancet, *1*:284, 1966.

95. Lindheimer, M. D., and Katz, A. I.: Sodium and diuretics in pregnancy. N. Engl. J. Med., *288*:891, 1973.

96. Lipsett, M. B., Combs, J. W., and Seigel, D. G.: Problems in contraception. Ann. Intern. Med., *74*:251, 1971.

97. Little, B.: Water and electrolyte balance during pregnancy. Anesthesiology, *26*:400, 1965.

98. Loffer, F. D.: Eisenmenger's complex and pregnancy. Obstet. Gynecol., *29*:235, 1967.

99. MacGillivray, I., and Buchanan, T. J.: Total exchangeable sodium and potassium in non-pregnant women and in normal and pre-eclamptic pregnancy. Lancet, *2*:1090, 1958.

100. Manalo-Estrella, P., and Barker, A. E.: Histopathologic findings in human aortic media associated with pregnancy: A study of 16 cases. Arch. Pathol., *83*:336, 1967.

101. Markiewicz, W., Stoner, J., London, E., Hunt, S. A., and Popp, R. L.: Mitral valve prolapse in one hundred presumably healthy young females. Circulation, *53*:464, 1976.

102. Mattox, J. H.: The value of a routine prenatal chest x-ray. Obstet. Gynecol., *41*:243, 1973.

103. McAnulty, J. H., and Rahimtoola, S. H.: Surgery for infective endocarditis. J.A.M.A., *242*:77, 1979.

104. McCaffrey, R. N., and Dunn, L. J.: Primary pulmonary hypertension in pregnancy. Obstet. Gynecol. Surv., *19*:567, 1964.

105. McCausland, A. M., Human, C., Winsor, T., Trotter, A. D., Jr.: Venous distensibility during pregnancy. Am. J. Obstet. Gynecol., *81*:472, 1961.

106. McCrum, I. D., and Guidry, J. R.: Procainamide-induced psychosis. J.A.M.A., *240*:1265, 1978.

107. McKusick, V. A.: Hereditable Disorders of Connective Tissue. 4th Ed. St. Louis, C. V. Mosby Co., 1972.

108. McLennan, C. E.: Antecubital and femoral venous pressure in normal and toxemic pregnancy. Am. J. Obstet. Gynecol., *45*:568, 1943.

109. Mendelson, C. L.: Cardiac Disease in Pregnancy. Philadelphia, F. A. Davis Co., 1960.

110. Merrill, L. K., and VerBurg, D. J.: The choice of long-term anticoagulants for the pregnant patient. Obstet. Gynecol., *47*:711, 1976.

111. Metcalfe, J., Hohimer, A. R., Bissonnette, J., and Lawson, M.: Exercise reduces uterine blood flow in the pregnant pygmy goat. Physiologist, *23*:49, 1980 (abstract).

112. Metcalfe, J., and Parer, J. T.: Cardiovascular changes during pregnancy in ewes. Am. J. Physiol., *210*:821, 1966.

113. Metcalfe, J., Romney, S. L., Ramsey, L. H., Reid, D. E., and Burwell, C. S.: Estimation of uterine blood flow in normal human pregnancy at term. J. Clin. Invest., *34*:1632, 1955.

114. Metcalfe, J., and Ueland, K.: Maternal cardiovascular adjustments to pregnancy. Prog. Cardiovasc. Dis., *16*:363, 1974.

115. Metcalfe, J., and Ueland, K.: The heart and pregnancy. *In* Hurst, J. W. (ed.): The Heart. 4th Ed. New York, McGraw-Hill, 1978.

116. Metcalfe, J., and Ueland, K.: Heart disease and pregnancy. *In* Fowler, N. O. (ed.): Cardiac Diagnosis and Treatment, 3rd Ed. Hagerstown, Md., Harper and Row, 1980.

117. Meyer, E. C., Tulsky, A. S., Sigmann, P., and Silber, E. N.: Pregnancy in the presence of tetralogy of Fallot. Observations on two patients. Am. J. Cardiol., *14*:874, 1964.

118. Mitchell, J. H., and Cohen, L. S.: Alcohol and the heart. Mod. Concepts Cardiovasc. Dis., *39*:109, 1970.

119. Mitchell, S. C., Korones, S. B., and Berendes, H. W.: Congenital heart disease in 56,109 births: Incidence and natural history. Circulation, *43*:323, 1971.

120. Mitrani, A., Oettinger, M., Abinader, E. G., Sharf, M., and Klein, A.: Use of propranolol in dysfunctional labor. Br. J. Obstet. Gynaecol., *82*:651, 1975.

121. Mortensen, J. D., and Ellsworth, H. S.: Coarctation of the aorta and pregnancy. Obstetric and cardiovascular complications before and after surgical correction. J.A.M.A., *191*:596, 1965.

122. Morton, M. J., Hohimer, A. R., and Metcalfe, J.: Maternal left ventricular adaptations to pregnancy. Clin. Res. *28*:11A, 1980 (abstract).

123. Murdoch, J. L., Walker, B. A., Halpern, B. L., Kuzma, J. W., and McKusick, V. A.: Life expectancy and causes of death in the Marfan syndrome. N. Engl. J. Med., *286*:804, 1972.

124. Murphy, E. S., and Kloster, F. E.: Late results of valve replacement surgery. I. Clinical and hemodynamic results. Mod. Concepts Cardiovasc. Dis. *48*:53, 1979.

125. Murphy, E. S., and Kloster, F. E.: Late results of valve replacement surgery. II. Complications of prosthetic heart valves. Mod. Concepts Cardiovasc. Dis., *48*:59, 1979.

126. Neill, C. A., and Swanson, S.: Outcome of pregnancy in congenital heart disease. Circulation, *24*:1003, 1961 (abstract).

127. Neilson, G., Galea, E. G., and Blunt, A.: Congenital heart disease and pregnancy. Med. J. Aust., *1*:1086, 1970.

128. Neilson, G., Galea, E. G., and Blunt, A.: Eisenmenger's syndrome and pregnancy. Med. J. Aust., *1*:431, 1971.

129. Nielsen, N. C., and Fabricius, J.: Primary pulmonary hypertension with special reference to prognosis. Acta Med. Scand., *170*:731, 1961.

130. Nora, J. J., and Nora, A. H.: The evolution of specific genetic and environmental counseling in congenital heart diseases. Circulation, *57*:205, 1978.

131. Oakley, G. D. G., McGarry, K., Limb, D. G., and Oakley, C. M.: Management of pregnancy in patients with hypertrophic cardiomyopathy. Br. Med. J., *1*:1749, 1979.

132. Palmer, A. J., and Walker, A. H. C.: The maternal circulation in normal pregnancy. J. Obstet. Gynecol. Br. Emp., *56*:537, 1949.

133. Pauli, R. M., Madden, J. D., Kranzler, K. J., Culpepper, W., and Port, R.: Warfarin therapy initiated during pregnancy and phenotypic chondrodysplasia and punctata. J. Pediatr., *88*:506, 1976.

134. Pelletier, L. L., Jr., and Petersdorf, R. G.: Infective endocarditis: A review of 125 cases from the University of Washington Hospitals, 1963–1972. Medicine, *56*:287, 1977.

135. Pritchard, J. A.: Hematologic aspects of pregnancy. Clin. Obstet. Gynecol., *3*:378, 1960.

136. Pritchard, J. A.: Changes in the blood volume during pregnancy and delivery. Anesthesiology, *26*:393, 1965.

137. Pritchard, J. A.: Anemias complicating pregnancy and the puerperium. *In* Committee on Maternal Nutrition, Food and Nutrition Board, National Research Council (eds.): Maternal Nutrition and the Course of Pregnancy, Washington, D.C., National Academy of Sciences, 1970.

138. Procacci, P. M., Savran, S. V., Schreiter, S. L., and Bryson, A. L.: Prevalence of clinical mitral-valve prolapse in 1,169 young women. N. Engl. J. Med., *294*:1086, 1976.

139. Pruyn, C. S., Phelan, J. P., and Buchanan, G. C.: Long-term propranolol therapy in pregnancy: Maternal and fetal outcome. Am. J. Obstet. Gynecol., *135*:485, 1979.

140. Pyeritz, R. E., and McKusick, V. A.: The Marfan syndrome: Diagnosis and management. N. Engl. J. Med., *300*:772, 1979.

141. Raivio, K. O., Ikonen, E., Saarikoski, S.: Fetal risks due to warfarin therapy during pregnancy. Acta Paediatr. Scand., *66*:735, 1977.

142. Richardson, J. V., Karp, R. B., Kirklin, J. W. and Dismukes, W. E.: Treatment of infective endocarditis: A 10-year comparative analysis. Circulation, *58*:589, 1978.

143. Rimland, D., McGowan, J. E., and Shulman, J. A.: Immunization for the internist. Ann. Intern. Med., *85*:622, 1976.

144. Rizzon, P., Biasco, G., Brindicci, G., and Mauro, F.: Familial syndrome of midsystolic click and late systolic murmur. Br. Heart J., *35*:245, 1973.

145. Roberts, N.: A predictive study of congenital heart disease and need for care. West. J. Med., *129*:19, 1978.

146. Roberts, W. C., and Perloff, J. K.: Mitral valvular disease. A clinicopathologic survey of the conditions causing the mitral valve to function abnormally. Ann. Intern. Med., *77*:939, 1972.

147. Robinson, D. S.: Evaluation of drugs used in pregnancy and pediatric age groups. Ann. Intern. Med., *82*:841, 1975.

148. Rogers, M. C., Willerson, J. T., Goldblatt, A., Smith, T. W.: Serum digoxin concentrations in human fetus, neonate and infant. N. Engl. J. Med., *287*:1010, 1972.

149. Roman-Ponce, H., Thatcher, W. W., Caton, D., Barron, D. H., and Wilcox, C. J.: Effects of thermal stress and epinephrine on uterine blood flow in ewes. J. Anim. Sci., *46*:167, 1978.

150. Rovinsky, J. J., and Jaffin, H.: Cardiovascular hemodynamics in

pregnancy. I. Blood and plasma volumes in multiple pregnancy. Am. J. Obstet. Gynecol., *93*:1, 1965.

151. Rovinsky, J. J., and Jaffin, H.: Cardiovascular hemodynamics in pregnancy. II. Cardiac output and left ventricular work in multiple pregnancy. Am. J. Obstet. Gynecol., *95*:781, 1966.

152. Rovinsky, J. J., and Jaffin, H.: Cardiovascular hemodynamics in pregnancy. III. Cardiac rate, stroke volume, total peripheral resistance, and central blood volume in multiple pregnancy: Synthesis of results. Am. J. Obstet. Gynecol., *95*:787, 1966.

153. Rubler, S., Damani, P. M., and Pinto, E. R.: Cardiac size and performance during pregnancy estimated with echocardiography. Am. J. Cardiol., *40*:534, 1977.

154. Sabom, M. B., Curry, C., Jr., and Wise, D. E.: Propranolol therapy during pregnancy in a patient with idiopathic hypertrophic subaortic stenosis: Is it safe? South. Med. J., *71*:328, 1978.

155. Sagel, S. S., Evens, R. G., Forrest, J. V., and Bramson, R. T.: Efficacy of routine screening and lateral chest radiographs in a hospital-based population. N. Engl. J. Med., *291*:1001, 1974.

156. Sasse, L.: Systolic clicks and murmurs. Am. Heart. J., *94*:265, 1977.

157. Schaefer, G., Arditi, L. I., Solomon, H. A., and Ringland, J. E.: Congenital heart disease and pregnancy. Clin. Obstet. Gynecol., *11*:1048, 1968.

158. Schenker, J. G., and Chowers, I.: Pheochromocytoma and pregnancy: Review of 89 cases. Obstet. Gynecol. Surv., *26*:739, 1971.

159. Schroeder, J. S., and Harrison, D. C.: Repeated cardioversion during pregnancy. Treatment of refractory paroxysmal atrial tachycardia during three successive pregnancies. Am. J. Cardiol., *27*:445, 1971.

160. Schwartz, D. B., and Schamroth, L.: The effect of pregnancy on the frontal plane QRS axis. J. Electrocardiol., *12*:279, 1979.

161. Seitchik, J.: Total body water and total body density of pregnant women. Obstet. Gynecol., *29*:155, 1967.

162. Shaver, P. J., Carrig, T. F., and Baker, W. P.: Postpartum coronary artery dissection. Br. Heart J., *40*:83, 1978.

163. Shaxted, E. J., and Milton, P. J.: Disopyramide in pregnancy: A case report. Curr. Med. Res. Opin., *6*:70, 1979.

164. Shell, W. E., Walton, J. A., Clifford, M. E., and Willis, P. W., III: The familial occurrence of the syndrome of mid-late systolic click and late systolic murmur. Circulation, *39*:327, 1969.

165. Sherman, S., and Hall, B. D.: Warfarin and fetal abnormality. Lancet, *1*:692, 1976.

166. Slaughter, L., Morris, J. E., and Starr, A.: Prosthetic valvular endocarditis: A 12-year review. Circulation, *47*:1319, 1973.

167. Snaith, L., and Szekely, P.: Cardiovascular surgery in relation to pregnancy. *In* Marcus, S. L., and Marcus, C. C. (eds.): Advances in Obstetrics and Gynecology, Vol. I. Baltimore, Williams & Wilkins Co., 1967.

168. Stevenson, R. E., Burton, M., Ferlauto, G. J., and Taylor, H. A.: Hazards of oral anticoagulants during pregnancy. J.A.M.A., *243*:1549, 1980.

169. Stubblefield, P. G.: Pulmonary edema occurring after therapy with dexamethasone and terbutaline for premature labor: A case report. Am. J. Obstet. Gynecol., *132*:341, 1979.

170. Sundsfjord, J. A.: Plasma renin activity and aldosterone excretion during prolonged progesterone administration. Acta Endocrinol., *67*:483, 1971.

171. Swan, D. A., Bell, B., Oakley, C. M., and Goodwin, J.: Analysis of symptomatic course and prognosis and treatment of hypertrophic obstructive cardiomyopathy. Br. Heart J., *33*:671, 1971.

172. Szekely, P., and Snaith, L.: Heart Disease and Pregnancy. Edinburgh, Churchill Livingstone, 1974.

173. Szekely, P., Turner, R., and Snaith, L.: Pregnancy and the changing pattern of rheumatic heart disease. Br. Heart J., *35*:1293, 1973.

174. Tanz, R. D.: Inotropic effects of certain steroids upon heart muscle. Rev. Can. Biol., *22*:147, 1963.

175. Tapia, H. R., Johnson, C. E., and Strong, C. G.: Effect of oral contraceptive therapy on the renin-angiotensin system in normotensive and hypertensive women. Obstet. Gynecol., *41*:643, 1973.

176. Tunstall, M. E.: The effect of propranolol on the onset of breathing at birth. Br. J. Anaesth., *41*:792, 1969.

177. Turner, G. M., Oakley, C. M., and Dixon, H. B.: Management of pregnancy complicated by hypertrophic obstructive cardiomyopathy. Br. Med. J., *4*:281, 1968.

178. Ueland, K., Akamatsu, T. J., and Der Yuen, D.: Maternal cardiovascular dynamics. VIII. Cesarean section under epidural anesthesia incorporating epinephrine. In preparation, 1980.

179. Ueland, K., Akamatsu, T. J., Eng, M., Bonica, J. J., and Hansen, J. M.: Maternal cardiovascular dynamics. VI. Cesarean section under epidural anesthesia without epinephrine. Am. J. Obstet. Gynecol., *114*:775, 1972.

180. Ueland, K., Gills, R. E., and Hansen, J. M.: Maternal cardiovascular dynamics. I. Cesarean section under subarachnoid block anesthesia. Am. J. Obstet. Gynecol., *100*:42, 1968.

181. Ueland, K., and Hansen, J. M.: Maternal cardiovascular dynamics. III. Labor and delivery under local and caudal analgesia. Am. J. Obstet. Gynecol., *103*:8, 1969.

182. Ueland, K., Hansen, J., Eng, M., Kalappa, R., and Parer, J. T.: Maternal cardiovascular hemodynamics. V. Cesarean section under thiopental, nitrous oxide, and succinylocholine anesthesia. Am. J. Obstet. Gynecol., *108*:615, 1970.

183. Ueland, K., and Metcalfe, J.: Acute rheumatic fever in pregnancy. Am. J. Obstet. Gynecol., *95*:586, 1966.

184. Ueland, K., Novy, M. J., and Metcalfe, J.: Cardiorespiratory responses to pregnancy and exercise in normal women and patients with heart disease. Am. J. Obstet. Gynecol., *115*:4, 1973.

185. Ueland, K., Novy, M. J., Peterson, E. N., and Metcalfe, J.: Maternal cardiovascular dynamics. IV. The influence of gestational age on the maternal cardiovascular response to posture and exercise. Am. J. Obstet. Gynecol., *104*:856, 1969.

186. Ueland, K., and Parer, J. T.: Effects of estrogens on the cardiovascular system of the ewe. Am. J. Obstet. Gynecol., *96*:400, 1966.

187. Walters, W. A. W., and Lim, Y. L.: Cardiovascular dynamics in women receiving oral contraceptive therapy. Lancet, *2*:879, 1969.

188. Weaver, J. B., and Pearson, J. F.: Influence of digitalis on time of onset and duration of labor in women with cardiac disease. Br. Med. J., *3*:519, 1973.

189. Werkö, L., Lagerlöf, H., Bucht, H., and Holmgren, A.: Circulatory changes in pregnancy. Acta Med. Scand., *239* (Suppl.):263, 1950 (abstract).

190. Wilson, M. G., Lim, W. N., and Birch, A. M.: The decline of rheumatic fever. Recurrence rates of rheumatic fever among 782 children for twenty-one consecutive calendar years, (1936–1956). J. Chronic. Dis., *7*:183, 1958.

191. Wilson, W. R., Danielson, G. K., Giulani, E. R., Washington, J. A., II, Jaumin, P. M., and Geraci, J. E.: Valve replacement in patients with active infective endocarditis. Circulation, *58*:585, 1978.

192. Wood, J. E.: The cardiovascular effects of oral contraceptives. Mod. Concepts Cardiovasc. Dis., *41*:37, 1972.

John G. Kelton, M.D.
Jack Hirsh, M.D.

7

VENOUS THROMBOEMBOLIC DISORDERS

Pulmonary embolism is a major cause of morbidity and death during the childbearing period. A maternal mortality survey completed in England and Wales over the 5 year period ending 1966 reported a total of 221 maternal deaths due to pulmonary embolism,[4] a mortality second only to that of abortion. An understanding of venous thromboembolic disorders is particularly important to the obstetrician, because unlike some of the other causes of death in pregnancy, many thromboembolic events can be prevented. In this chapter the incidence, pathogenesis, diagnosis, and treatment of venous thromboembolism in pregnancy and the postpartum period will be considered.

PATHOGENESIS OF VENOUS THROMBOEMBOLISM IN PREGNANCY

Our understanding of the pathogenesis of venous thrombosis has not increased greatly in the 150 years since Virchow's suggestion that three factors — alteration in the composition of the blood, alterations in flow, and vessel wall damage — predispose to venous thrombosis. Changes in all three of these components occur in pregnancy and may contribute to the increased incidence of venous thromboembolism in the puerperium.

Venous thrombi are intravascular deposits consisting predominantly of fibrin and red cells with a variable platelet and leukocyte component. The formation of venous thrombi reflects an imbalance between thrombogenic stimuli and a variety of protective mechanisms. The factors that predispose to venous thrombosis are activation of blood coagulation, vascular damage, and stasis. The protective mechanisms are the inactivation of activated coagulation factors by circulating inhibitors, clearance of activated coagu-

lation factors by the liver, and dissolution of fibrin by a variety of fibrinolytic enzymes derived from plasma, endothelial cells, and circulating leukocytes.

Venous thrombi can be produced experimentally by a combination of stasis and increased blood coagulability, by stasis and vessel wall damage, or by the sole effects of either a marked increase in blood coagulability or severe vessel wall damage. In all of these circumstances, thrombosis is augmented if the fibrinolytic system is inhibited or defective. Stasis predisposes to thrombosis by impairing the clearance of activated coagulation factors, which increase in concentration locally through the autocatalytic activity of the coagulation system.

During pregnancy and in the immediate postpartum period, changes occur in the blood coagulation system, in the fibrinolytic system, in venous flow, and in the vessel wall.

Factors Predisposing to Thrombosis in Pregnancy

The final step in blood coagulation is the conversion of the soluble protein fibrinogen to an insoluble fibrin gel. The coagulation proteins circulate in very low concentrations (micrograms) as proenzymes, which are converted to active enzymes in a sequence that is progressively amplified as it proceeds down the coagulation cascade. The blood coagulation process can be activated through either the intrinsic pathway or the extrinsic pathway (Fig. 7–1). Intrinsic pathway activation occurs when blood comes in contact with a nonendothelialized surface. This triggers the activation of Factor XII, which results in the sequential activation of Factor XI, Factor IX, and Factor X. The activation of Factor X requires Factor VIII, platelet phospho-

169

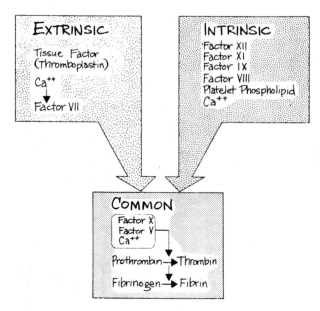

FIGURE 7–1. A simplified version of the coagulation cascade.

lipid, and calcium. The extrinsic pathway is activated when blood is exposed to a phospholipoprotein known as tissue thromboplastin. Tissue thromboplastin combines with and activates Factor VII, which in turn activates Factor X, bypassing a number of time-consuming steps in the intrinsic coagulation pathway. The extrinsic pathway is activated in vivo by exposure of blood to the injured vessel wall or to extravascular substances released into the blood stream during tissue injury.

The intrinsic and extrinsic pathways meet at a common point at the activation of Factor X, and beyond this point blood coagulation continues along a common pathway. Activated Factor X in the presence of calcium, phospholipid, and Factor V converts prothrombin to thrombin, which in turn converts fibrinogen into fibrin monomer and small polypeptide fragments known as fibrinopeptides A and B. The fibrin monomer polymerizes to fibrin polymers, which circulate as soluble complexes and precipitate as insoluble fibrin when they reach a critical size.

Alterations in the levels of several coagulation factors occur during pregnancy. The plasma fibrinogen level increases by approximately 50 per cent.[17] Factors VIII and XII are also consistently elevated in an uncomplicated pregnancy.[76] Factor XI is frequently decreased during pregnancy, and the level of Factor XIII may be decreased by as much as 50 per cent.[22, 77, 81]

Several observations indicate that the blood coagulation system is activated during pregnancy. The most compelling are the increased levels of fibrinopeptide A (the peptide cleaved from fibrinogen by the action of thrombin)[45] and the increased concentrations of circulating fibrin

monomer complexes.[35, 72] There is also evidence in experimental animals that fibrinogen turnover is increased during pregnancy.[75] An increased ratio of Factor VIII antigen to Factor VIII coagulation activity has also been proposed as evidence of increased thrombin generation during pregnancy.[102] However, this finding is not specific for thrombin formation and could be caused by synthesis of Factor VIII antigen devoid of coagulant activity.

There are two possible sites for the activation of blood coagulation during normal pregnancy. The first is the systemic circulation, producing a "hypercoagulable" state. The second (and more likely) is the placental circulation, where the thrombin generation and fibrin formation are localized and therefore unlikely to lead to an increase in systemic blood coagulability.

Observations in program animals and in humans indicate that coagulation is activated during placental separation. Marked activation of coagulation in uterine vein blood during placental separation has been observed.[17] Evidence supporting the activation of blood coagulation during parturition is also provided by the sharp increase in fibrinopeptide A plasma levels and in circulating fibrin monomer complexes at the time of delivery.

Activated blood coagulation factors are inactivated by circulating inhibitors and are cleared by the liver and reticuloendothelial system. Fibrin that has deposited in the vessels is lysed by the fibrinolytic system.

The activated blood coagulation factors are serine proteases, which are inhibited by a number of naturally occurring protease inhibitors. One of the most important of these is antithrombin III, also known as heparin cofactor. The level of antithrombin III is decreased in pregnancy,[49, 112] and there are several reports of a major pulmonary embolism (sometimes fatal) occurring in pregnancy as the first manifestation of an inherited antithrombin III deficiency.[112]

The basic reaction of the fibrinolytic system is the conversion of the proenzyme plasminogen to the active proteolytic enzyme plasmin. This reaction is mediated by plasminogen activators. Plasmin hydrolyzes fibrin, fibrinogen, and Factor VIII. Plasminogen activators are derived from endothelial cells and other tissues. Like the coagulation system, the activity of the fibrinolytic system is modulated by inhibitors that inhibit both the conversion of plasminogen to plasmin and the proteolytic effect of plasmin on fibrinogen or fibrin. The main inhibitor of plasmin is alpha-2-antiplasmin, which rapidly inactivates plasmin when it forms in plasma. Excess plasmin is inactivated by other proteolytic inhibitors, but if the inhibitory system is overwhelmed, during the course of thrombolytic therapy for example, then other coagulation proteins (including fibrinogen) are hydrolyzed. When fibrin is formed, both plasminogen and plasminogen activator are adsorbed to the fibrin. The plasmin molecules formed in close proximity to fibrin are only slowly inactivated by antiplasmin, and fibrinolysis can proceed despite relatively low levels of plasma fibrinolytic activity.

Several changes in the fibrinolytic system occur in pregnancy. Both an increase and a decrease in total fibrinolytic activity have been reported.[35, 45] There are reports that the level of plasminogen activator is decreased during pregnancy but rapidly becomes normal after delivery. The level of fibrin-fibrinogen degradation products is elevated in normal pregnancy, but it is uncertain whether this reflects lysis of intravascular fibrin (for example, in the placenta) or an increase in systemic fibrinolytic activity.[35] It is reported that fibrinolytic activity is decreased in the third trimester and rapidly returns to normal following delivery of the placenta; it has been suggested that the placenta synthesizes a substance that inhibits fibrinolysis,[5] but the nature of this process has not been defined.

Vessel Damage. The normal intact endothelium is nonthrombogenic and reacts neither with platelets nor with blood coagulation proteins. Various reasons have been proposed to explain this nonreactivity, including electrostatic repulsion by the negative charge on the endothelial surface of the cells; the synthesis by endothelial cells of prostacyclin, a prostaglandin that inhibits platelet aggregation; and the presence on the surface of the endothelial cells of a heparin-like material. When a vessel is damaged, there is exposure of subendothelial layers, which react both with platelets and with the blood coagulation system.

The vessel wall remains intact during pregnancy, but local damage to pelvic veins can occur during delivery, particularly if it is complicated or if it is by cesarean section. Traumatic damage is likely to be an important predisposing cause to venous thrombosis in the early postpartum period.

Blood Flow. Venous stasis predisposes to thrombosis in a number of ways. It prevents clearance of activated coagulation factors by the liver and the mixing of activated coagulation factors with their inhibitors. Venous return from the limbs is greatly enhanced by contraction of calf muscles, which act as venous pumps and propel blood from the deep veins of the calf. During recumbency, the soleal sinuses are dependent and are dilated with blood. Venous stasis also occurs when there is impairment of venous return, by a gravid uterus or as a result of venous dilation, for example.

Several changes occur during pregnancy and parturition that predispose to venous stasis. Venous blood flow decreases as pregnancy progresses.[20] Plethysmographic studies indicate that venous dilation occurs during pregnancy, probably as a result of the effect of estrogens on smooth muscle cells in the veins.[39a] This estrogenic effect may also be responsible for the formation of varicose veins during pregnancy. As the uterus grows it compresses the external iliac vein, a process that can lead to significant venous obstruction in the last trimester. The pelvic veins also become markedly dilated during pregnancy, and this could predispose to pelvic vein thrombosis. During prolonged and complicated deliveries or during cesarean section, venous stasis occurs as a result of immobilization of the lower limbs, and by the pressure exerted by the fetal head on the pelvic veins.[109] Venous tone returns to normal 8 to 12 weeks post partum.[33, 70]

INCIDENCE AND DIAGNOSIS OF VENOUS THROMBOEMBOLIC DISORDERS IN PREGNANCY AND THE PUERPERIUM

The precise incidence of venous thromboembolic disorders complicating pregnancy is unknown, because in the majority of studies the incidence is based on clinical examination. It is now well accepted that the clinical diagnosis of venous thrombosis lacks sensitivity and specificity. As many as 50 per cent of patients clinically suspected of having deep venous thrombosis do not have thrombosis.[51] Some of them have other conditions, such as a ruptured tendon or a torn muscle, that could be complicated by anticoagulant treatment. The majority of deep vein thrombi are entirely asymptomatic, and studies using clinical criteria to diagnose venous thromboembolism are of limited value. Maneuvers such as Homan's sign are of historical interest only. Perhaps the only definitive clinical sign of a deep venous thrombosis occurs when a proximal thrombosis produces sufficient venous obstruction to cause leg swelling, pain, and cyanosis. This uncommon condition is termed phlegmasia cerulea dolens.

The accurate clinical diagnosis of pulmonary embolism is also difficult, since other conditions complicating the postpartum period, including atelectasis, can mimic pulmonary emboli. Pulmonary emboli, like venous thrombi, are often silent.

Incidence of Superficial Thrombophlebitis

Superficial thrombophlebitis is the most common venous thromboembolic disorder of pregnancy. In a retrospective survey reviewing 32,337 pregnancies, it was found that superficial thrombophlebitis occurred once in 622 pregnancies prior to delivery and once in 95 pregnancies after delivery.[2] Superficial thrombophlebitis is increased in patients with pre-existing varicose veins but not in patients whose infants are delivered by cesarean section or who have obstetric complications.[1]

Incidence of Deep Vein Thrombosis

Historically, pregnancy and the puerperium have been regarded as high risk conditions for the development of venous thromboembolic disease.[21, 53] However, since the diagnosis was made clinically in most studies, the reported incidences may not be accurate. ^{125}I-fibrinogen leg scanning studies have shown that as many as 3 per cent of patients undergoing normal delivery develop venous thrombi.[36] However, fibrinogen leg scanning may lead to underestimations of the frequency of venous thrombosis occurring during parturition, since some thrombi could arise in proximal leg or pelvic veins and therefore would not be detected by leg scanning.

The incidence of clinically diagnosed deep vein thrombosis is virtually identical in the preg-

nant or nonpregnant patient prior to delivery, with an estimated incidence of approximately 0.007 case per month.[26] In contrast, the postpartum incidence rises dramatically to an average of 10.4 cases per 1000 deliveries. Postpartum thrombophlebitis occurs more frequently in patients who have had a traumatic or complicated delivery or are delivered by cesarean section.[32, 43, 55]

Incidence of Pulmonary Embolism

Various investigators have reported that the incidence of clinically diagnosed nonfatal pulmonary embolism in pregnancy and the puerperium ranges from 0.5 to 12 per 1000 deliveries.[2, 32, 74, 79, 103] There has been one study in which sensitive diagnostic techniques were used to diagnose pulmonary emboli in pregnant patients.[74] Patients were investigated with isotopic perfusion lung scans and pulmonary angiography, and pulmonary emboli complicated 1 in 750 pregnancies.

Mortality figures from England and Wales indicate that death from pulmonary embolism follows 1 in 1500 to 2500 deliveries by cesarean section.[4]

Diagnosis of Superficial Vein Thrombophlebitis

Superficial vein thrombophlebitis is clinically obvious and is characterized by an erythematous superficial vein, which is usually accompanied by pain and tenderness along its distribution.

Diagnosis of Deep Vein Thrombosis in the Nonpregnant Patient

The majority of patients with venous thrombosis have no clinical manifestations. When symptoms or signs of venous thrombosis occur, they are caused by obstruction to venous outflow, by inflammation of the vessel wall or perivascular tissue, by a combination of these two factors, or by embolization of the thrombus into the pulmonary circulation. The common clinical symptoms and signs of venous thrombosis are pain, tenderness, and swelling of the legs. It should be emphasized that these are highly nonspecific, and while they may lead the clinician to suspect venous thrombosis,[10] they should not be used to make a definitive diagnosis or as a basis for therapeutic decisions.

DIAGNOSTIC TESTS FOR DEEP VEIN THROMBOSIS

The available objective tests that have been adequately evaluated are venography, plethysmography, Doppler ultrasound, and ^{125}I-fibrinogen leg scanning.

Venography. Venography is the most definitive method available for diagnosing venous thrombosis.[47] If adequately performed and interpreted, it can be used to either confirm or exclude the diagnosis in patients with clinically suspected venous thrombosis. The external iliac veins and the common iliac veins are not always well visualized by ascending venography, so that femoral venography may occasionally be required to exclude isolated external or common iliac vein thrombosis. The internal iliac veins and their tributaries are not visualized by standard venographic techniques.

Venography is an invasive procedure, which is performed by injecting radiopaque contrast medium into a superficial vein in the dorsum of the foot. The dye opacifies the venous system, and thrombi are identified as persistent intraluminal filling defects, which are constant in all films and are seen in a number of projections. Other venographic abnormalities, such as nonfilling of the segment of the deep venous system or nonfilling of the entire deep venous system above the knee, may be caused by technical artifacts, particularly if the dye is injected proximally into the dorsal foot vein. The nonfilling may then be incorrectly interpreted as being caused by a thrombus. Misinterpreting an inadequate venogram (usually in the direction of a falsely positive diagnosis of venous thrombosis) is a serious and common problem with the increasing use of venography in centers whose staff members are inexperienced in this technique. Venography has several disadvantages. The radiopaque contrast medium damages endothelial cells, and pain can follow the injection of contrast medium. Venography can induce clinically significant phlebitis in a small percentage of patients (1 to 2 per cent), probably as a result of the endothelial damage that it produces. The risk of postvenographic phlebitis can be reduced if the leg is elevated after the procedure is completed and the radiopaque dye washed out with an infusion of 150 to 250 ml of saline.

Impedance Plethysmography (IPG). Plethysmography, a noninvasive method, detects volume changes in the leg. Impedance plethysmography is sensitive and specific for thrombosis of the popliteal, femoral, and iliac veins (proximal veins), but it is relatively insensitive to calf vein thrombosis.[52] The method is based on the principle that blood volume changes in the calf produced by inflation and deflation of the pneumatic thigh cuff result in changes in electrical resistance (impedance). These changes are reduced in patients with proximal vein thrombosis.

Occlusive cuff impedance plethysmography is performed with the patient supine and the leg slightly elevated in a relaxed position. A pneumatic cuff is applied to the midthigh and inflated to occlude venous return. The cuff is then rapidly deflated, and the change in electrical resistance (impedance) resulting from alterations in the blood volume distal to the cuff are detected by circumferential cuff electrodes. Venous outflow obstruction (which most frequently is caused by venous thrombosis) produces characteristic changes. In patients with clinically suspected venous thrombosis, a positive IPG result can be used to make therapeutic decisions in the absence of conditions that cause falsely positive results. A normal result essentially excludes a diagnosis of an occlusive proximal vein thrombosis but does not exclude calf vein thrombosis. Falsely positive results may occur with disorders that interfere with arterial inflow or venous outflow. These include severe congestive cardiac failure, constrictive pericarditis, severe arterial insufficiency, hypotension, and external compression of veins (particularly the external iliac vein by a pelvic mass). Falsely positive results may also occur if the technician performs the test incorrectly or the patient is not relaxed.

Doppler Ultrasonography. Like impedance plethysmography, Doppler ultrasound examination is sensitive to proximal vein thrombosis but relatively insensitive to calf vein thrombosis. Its major drawbacks are that its interpretation is subjective and it requires considerable skill and experience to perform reliably.[10] However, in skilled hands it is as sensitive to proximal vein thrombosis as is impedance plethysmography.

The Doppler ultrasound examination is performed with the patient lying in bed in the semiupright position. The examining probe is placed over the common femoral, superficial femoral, popliteal, or tibial vein. A beam of ultrasound is directed percutaneously at the underlying vein, where it is reflected from blood cells. If the blood is stationary, the frequency of the reflected beam is identical with that of the incident beam and no sound is recorded. On the other hand, if the blood is moving, then the incident beam is reflected at a changed frequency (Doppler shift), which is proportional to the velocity of flow. This difference in frequency between the incident and reflected ultrasound beam is amplified into an audible signal or flow sound. An experienced operator can detect and localize the site of venous obstruction in the proximal venous system by listening to the patterns of sound produced by normal respiration and by various maneuvers that augment and arrest blood flow.

[125]I-fibrinogen Leg Scanning. ^{125}I-fibrinogen leg scanning detects calf vein thrombi and thrombi in the distal half of the thigh in which fibrin is actively accreting.[52] The test is performed by intravenous injection of ^{125}I-fibrinogen into the patient. The patient's legs are scanned with a hand-held probe, and if the radioactive fibrinogen is incorporated into a thrombus, it is detected by an increase in surface radioactivity. Falsely positive results occur when scanning is performed over a hematoma, a wound, or an area of inflammation. In the absence of these conditions, leg scanning is both sensitive and specific for acute calf and lower thigh vein thrombosis. Leg scanning should not be used as the only diagnostic test in patients with clinically suspected venous thrombosis, because it fails to detect femoral or iliac vein thrombi and there may be a delay before enough fibrinogen accumulates in the thrombus to make the test positive. Such a delay is unacceptable in patients with proximal vein thrombosis. However, ^{125}I-fibrinogen leg scanning is a very valuable diagnostic test when used to complement impedance plethysmography in patients with clinically suspected venous thrombosis.

Diagnosis of Venous Thrombosis During Pregnancy

The diagnosis of venous thrombosis in pregnancy is difficult because its clinical features are even less specific in pregnant than in nonpregnant women, and there are limitations to both the performance and interpretation of the objective tests. The nonspecificity of the clinical diagnosis of deep vein thrombosis is augmented in pregnancy by a number of factors, including (1) venous dilation due to the effect of estrogens; (2) superficial thrombophlebitis in varicosities, which often develop during pregnancy; and (3) compression of the iliac veins by the gravid uterus.

The use of objective diagnostic tests for venous thrombosis is complicated in pregnancy because standard ascending venography exposes the fetus to the potential risk of the radiation; ^{125}I-fibrinogen leg scanning is contraindicated because ^{125}I-fibrinogen crosses the placenta; and impedance plethysmography may lose diagnostic specificity in the latter half of the third trimester of pregnancy. These potential difficulties can be overcome in most patients by the use of impedance plethysmography in combination with limited venography. A negative IPG result has the same high negative predictive value in the pregnant as in the nonpregnant patient. Therefore, a negative test result in a patient effectively rules out a diagnosis of proximal vein thrombosis, but it does not exclude a calf vein thrombosis. When a negative result is obtained with the IPG, the patient can either be followed up by serial impedance plethysmography to detect an extending calf vein thrombus or investigated by performance of a limited venogram. If the IPG result is positive in the first or second trimester or in the first half of the third trimester, the diagnosis of venous thrombosis is made and the patient treated for venous thrombosis. However, a positive IPG result obtained in the latter part of the third trimester must be interpreted with caution, because it could be caused by external venous compression by the pregnant uterus, and further investigation with venography should be done. If the venogram is negative and the impedance plethysmograph remains positive despite positioning of the patient to minimize external iliac compression, then the clinician is faced with two options. Either the patient is treated as having venous thrombosis, or a standard venogram is performed with visualization of the common femoral, external, and common iliac veins.

Should a venogram be required during pregnancy, the fetus must be shielded from x-rays by a lead-lined apron covering the patient's abdomen. An ascending venogram is then performed in the standard manner to obtain visualization of calf veins, popliteal veins, and superficial femoral veins. This examination can be performed with minimal risk to the fetus.

Most deep vein thrombi occur in the puerperium. If the patient is not breast-feeding, a combination of radiolabeled fibrinogen leg scanning (to detect calf vein thrombi) with IPG or Doppler ultrasound (to detect proximal thrombi) is the diagnostic approach of choice. Until there is adequate information on the diagnostic specificity of a positive IPG or ultrasound result in the postpartum patient, venography should be performed to confirm the diagnosis.

Diagnosis of Pulmonary Embolism

The clinical diagnosis of pulmonary embolism is nonspecific and insensitive — nonspecific because many conditions produce similar clinical manifestations, and insensitive because many pulmonary emboli are clinically silent. Pulmonary embolism may present in a variety of ways, depending on the size, number, or location of the emboli and on the underlying condition of the patient. The clinical manifestations of pulmonary embolism can be characterized by (1) transient dyspnea and tachypnea with no other associated clinical manifestations; (2) the syndrome of pulmonary infarction or congestive atelectasis, which includes pleuritic chest pain, hemoptysis, pleural effusion, and pulmonary infiltrate on chest x-ray; (3) right-sided heart failure associated with severe dyspnea and tachypnea; (4) cardiovascular collapse with hypotension, syncope, and coma; and (5) various less common and less specific symptom complexes, including confusion or coma, pyrexia, wheezing, resistant heart failure, and unexplained arrhythmia.

The syndromes of acute right heart failure and of cardiovascular collapse are caused by major pulmonary embolism or multiple small emboli that obstruct more than 60 per cent of the pulmonary vasculature. The clinical syndromes of transient dyspnea and pulmonary infarction may be caused by either large or small pulmonary emboli.

The most common symptoms of pulmonary embolism include dyspnea and tachypnea, pain (which may be either pleuritic or central substernal), hemoptysis, syncope, cyanosis, and hypotension. The cardiac manifestations and chest signs of pulmonary infarction include pleural effusion, localized rales, elevated jugular venous pressure with a prominent A wave, right ventricular heave, accentuated pulmonary second sound, and gallop rhythm.

Pulmonary embolism is usually associated with venous thrombosis. If the embolus is small there are usually no clinical manifestations, but if it is large there are usually symptoms. Most clinically significant emboli arise from thrombi in the proximal veins of the leg, but occasionally they may arise from pelvic or calf veins.

DIAGNOSTIC TESTS FOR PULMONARY EMBOLISM

The available objective tests include chest x-ray, perfusion lung scan, ventilation scan, and pulmonary angiography.

Chest X-ray. The chest radiograph may be normal; more frequently it shows nonspecific abnormalities. Chest x-rays are necessary for the proper interpretation of perfusion lung scanning and may show characteristic features of conditions that simulate pulmonary embolism, pneumothorax or pulmonary edema, for example.

Perfusion Lung Scan. The perfusion lung scan detects areas of reduced blood flow and is a valuable test in the investigation of patients clinically suspected of having pulmonary embolism. A normal lung scan effectively excludes the diagnosis of pulmonary embolism.[18] However, an abnormal lung scan cannot be taken as evidence of pulmonary embolism, since many pulmonary disorders are associated with impaired pulmonary perfusion. The test is performed by intravenous injection of the gamma-emitting isotope [99]technetium, which is coupled to macro-aggregates of human albumin. These macro-aggregates have a particle size of approximately 20 microns and lodge in the pulmonary capillaries. The distribution of radioactivity in the lungs is measured by scanning the patient's chest with a gamma camera.

Ventilation Scan. The ventilation scan increases the specificity of the perfusion scan by excluding pulmonary disorders in which the reduction in perfusion is a result of impaired ventilation. Perfusion defects associated with matching ventilation abnormalities are unlikely to be caused by pulmonary embolism, while large perfusion defects (particularly if they are multiple) associated with normal ventilation are usually caused by pulmonary embolism.

During the ventilation scan,[133] xenon is inhaled and exhaled by the patient while the gamma camera records its distribution within the lungs. The patient breathes from a closed circuit spirometer for 5 minutes in order to equilibrate the radioactive xenon, and then the patient breathes room air for 5 minutes while the xenon washes out of the lungs. Imaging with a gamma camera is recorded during the initial breath, during equilibration, and during and after washout. There is no need to perform the ventilation scan if the perfusion scan is normal.

Pulmonary Angiography. Pulmonary angiography is considered the most definitive method for diagnosing pulmonary embolism.[18] Its accuracy has been improved in recent years by performance of selective pulmonary arterial catheterization and by the use of magnification techniques. A diagnosis of pulmonary embolism is made if there is a constant intraluminal filling defect present or if sharp cutoffs can be seen in vessels greater than 2.5 mm in diameter. Other abnormalities such as oligemia, vessel pruning, and loss of filling of small vessels are nonspecific and may occur in other pulmonary disorders.

Other Tests. Other tests used in the past to diagnose pulmonary embolism, such as the diagnostic triad of increased lactate dehydrogenase, normal serum aspartate aminotransferase, and increased bilirubin,[105] lack sensitivity and specificity and are not clinically useful.[99] Similarly, the measurement of arterial blood gases, which was initially reported to be promising,[99] has subsequently been demonstrated to be nonspecific and relatively insensitive.[15]

Diagnosis of Pulmonary Embolism in Pregnancy

All of the available tests for diagnosing pulmonary embolism carry with them the potential hazard of fetal irradiation. However, since the diagnosis of pulmonary embolism has serious implications, the potential risks of these diagnostic tests must be weighed against the risks of not treating a pulmonary embolism when it is present or of treating patients with anticoagulants when their clinical symptoms or signs are not caused by pulmonary embolism. If a chest x-ray, pulmonary angiogram, or venogram is performed, the fetus should be shielded from radiation by a lead-lined apron covering the patient's abdomen. Perfusion and ventilation scanning expose the fetus to minimal irradiation, and these investigations should be performed initially. Since technetium can cross the placenta and is potentially fetotoxic, lung scanning should be avoided in the first trimester if at all possible. The combination of impedance plethysmography and limited venography is a useful approach, since venous thrombosis is frequently associated with pulmonary embolism and a decision can be made to treat the patient for pulmonary embolism if a positive diagnosis of venous thrombosis is made. However, negative tests for venous thrombosis cannot be used to rule out pulmonary embolism in patients who present with clinically suspected pulmonary embolism.

If the clinical features, chest x-ray, and electrocardiogram are compatible with pulmonary embolism, further investigations are required. The chest x-ray is helpful in demonstrating conditions that may simulate a pulmonary embolism, including pneumothorax, a fractured rib, and mitral stenosis. If the chest x-ray is normal or nondiagnostic, a six-view perfusion lung scan should be performed. If the perfusion scan is technically adequate and normal, a diagnosis of pulmonary embolism can be excluded and no further investigation is required. However, an abnormal perfusion lung scan requires further investigation. Two approaches can be used: (1) perform a ventilation scan; (2) investigate the patient for evidence of leg vein thrombosis. If facilities are available, a ventilation scan should be performed, since the results obtained can be used to either confirm or exclude a diagnosis of pulmonary embolism in many patients. Larger perfusion abnormalities that are normal on chest x-ray and involve either a single lobe or multiple segments that ventilate normally are highly predictive for pulmonary embolism and can be considered diagnostic. Small subsegmental perfusion defects with matching abnormalities on the ventilation scan are unlikely to be caused by pulmonary embolism. When this pattern of lung scan abnormality is present, a diagnosis of pulmonary embolism can be excluded without further investigation.

Between these two extremes of very high and very low probability for pulmonary embolism, there are many abnormal lung scan patterns that require further investigation. A combination of impedance plethysmography and venography can be used, as described previously. If the results of these tests are diagnostic of venous thrombosis, then the patient can be treated as having pulmonary embolism. If they are negative, then a decision has to be made to either perform a pulmonary angiogram or make a treatment decision based on the clinical findings.

Diagnosis of Venous Thromboembolism in the Puerperium

With the exception of ^{125}I-fibrinogen leg scanning, which should not be used in the nursing mother, the approach to the diagnosis of venous thromboembolism in the puerperium is identical to that in the nonpregnant patient.

The patient can be investigated either by ascending venography or by noninvasive tests. If the IPG or Doppler ultrasound is normal and the patient is not nursing, she should be injected with ^{125}I-fibrinogen and scanned for 3 days to exclude the possibility of calf vein thrombosis. Alternatively, the patient can be followed up by serial impedance plethysmography, and if this remains normal a diagnosis of clinically significant proximal venous thrombosis can be excluded. Positive results with Doppler ultrasound, impedance plethysmography, or leg scanning should be confirmed by venography, since the specificity of this finding in the puerperium has not been adequately established. The approach to pulmonary embolism during the puerperium is similar to that in the nonpregnant patient.

TREATMENT OF VENOUS THROMBOEMBOLIC DISORDERS IN PREGNANCY

The decision to treat a patient is made after balancing the risks of no treatment, (i.e., the natural history of the disorder) against the risks associated with treatment.

Natural History of Superficial Vein Thrombophlebitis

Superficial phlebitis can develop spontaneously or can follow minor trauma to the vein such as that occurring with intravenous injection. Uncomplicated superficial phlebitis usually resolves spontaneously in 1 to 2 weeks and should not be overtreated. Bed rest, elevation of the limb, application of local heat, and mild analgesics are adequate for many patients. Patients who do not respond to local measures can be given anti-inflammatory agents.

Natural History of Deep Vein Thrombosis

The fate of venous thrombi is determined by the balance between factors that promote the formation of the thrombus and those that lead to its removal. Thrombi may extend, undergo lysis, or embolize. Extension of thrombosis is more likely to occur if the original thrombogenic stimulus persists, if there is marked endothelial damage, of if stasis occurs as a consequence of the original thrombus. Complete spontaneous lysis of large thrombi is relatively uncommon,[85] and even when patients are treated with heparin to limit further thrombus formation, complete lysis occurs in less than 20 per cent of cases.

The results of one randomized study and a number of unrandomized surveys indicate that untreated venous thrombi or pulmonary emboli in nonpregnant patients have a high mortality rate, ranging from 18 to 32 per cent.[9, 11, 13, 63, 110] Since the majority of these studies were performed in postoperative patients and in medical patients with other associated illnesses, their applicability to an otherwise healthy patient can be questioned. There have been several retrospective studies on the natural history of untreated venous thromboembolism in pregnancy. In one, the outcome in 297 pregnant women with antepartum venous thrombosis was reported. One hundred and sixty-three were not given anticoagulant therapy, and 26 (16 per cent) developed a complicating pulmonary embolus, which was lethal in 21 of these patients for an overall mortality of 12.8 per cent. One hundred and thirty-four patients were treated with anticoagulant therapy, and only one death occurred in this group (mortality 0.7 per cent).[103] Another report described 22 pregnant women who developed venous thrombosis. Thirteen were treated with anticoagulants and all recovered, while 9 were untreated and 2 subsequently had emboli.[107] In another series of 172 cases of venous thromboembolism in pregnancy and the puerperium, none of the 13 patients who were treated with anticoagulants died, while 7 of 21 untreated patients with pulmonary embolism died.[101] The results of these studies should be interpreted with caution because they are retrospective and therefore subject to several potential biases. For example, it is possible that the more severely ill patients with bleeding complications or infections may not have been treated with anticoagulants, and they may have been at greater risk of dying of pulmonary embolism. Despite this, the clinical outcome in untreated patients with venous thrombosis in pregnancy is consistent with the results obtained in nonpregnant patients and indicates that patients with venous thromboembolism have an unacceptably high mortality rate if they are untreated.

Natural History of Pulmonary Embolism

Most clinically detectable pulmonary emboli are associated with, and probably arise from, thrombi in the deep venous system of the leg and pelvis. The pathophysiologic effects of pulmonary emboli relate to their effect on lung tissue, on gas exchange, and on right heart function. The consequences of pulmonary emboli are influenced by several factors, including the size of the embolus and its location in the pulmonary circulation, the condition of the patient's cardiorespiratory reserve, and the rate of lysis of the pulmonary embolus. Most pulmonary emboli in hospitalized patients are small and clinically unimportant. Small emboli produce clinical symptoms or signs only if they are multiple or recurrent, if the patient's cardiorespiratory system is compromised by other disease, or if they obstruct a peripheral pulmonary artery and produce atelectasis or pulmonary infarction. Larger pulmonary emboli may also be asymptomatic but frequently produce clinical manifestations because they compromise gas exchange, are associated with pulmonary infarction or congested atelectasis, or produce hemodynamic changes that interfere with right heart function. If the cardiorespiratory status of the patient is compromised, even relatively small pulmonary emboli may produce a critical rise in pulmonary vascular resistance that can result in right heart failure. In addition, these patients are more likely to develop atelectasis or pulmonary infarction because the oxygen supply to the pulmonary parenchyma may be compromised.

In most cases, pulmonary emboli undergo rapid lysis and are markedly reduced in size weeks or months after the embolic event. Impaired resolution may occur in patients with very large emboli or in patients with chronic heart or lung disease, possibly because local fibrinolytic activity is impaired. Most patients, including those with impaired resolution, suffer no long-term consequences from pulmonary embolism. However, a minority of patients with impaired resolution develop chronic thromboembolic pulmonary hypertension.

Treatment of Venous Thromboembolism

The main objectives of treating venous thromboembolism are (1) to prevent death from pulmonary embolism, (2) to prevent the postphlebitic syndrome, (3) to prevent morbidity from the acute event, and (4) to achieve these objectives with the minimum of side effects and costs. A number of different approaches are available but none are free from side effects, and since the patient must be hospitalized, they are expensive. It is therefore important to insure that the diagnosis of venous thromboembolism is confirmed by objective tests before treatment is begun. The available therapeutic approaches are directed at removing the obstruction by mechanical or enzymatic means, preventing its extension by inhibiting blood coagulation, or preventing pulmonary emboli by interrupting the vena cava.

Although removing the thromboembolic obstruction is clearly the most desirable on theoretical grounds, for various reasons this procedure is almost never done and most patients are treated with anticoagulants. This treatment is highly effective and prevents death from pulmonary embolism in over 95 per cent of patients. Heparin may also prevent the postphlebitic syndrome in patients with calf vein thrombosis by limiting propagation of thrombi into the proximal veins. Heparin is less effective in preventing the postphlebitic syndrome in patients who have proximal vein thrombosis at presentation. Total lysis is infrequent with heparin therapy.[85, 88] Instead, the thrombus usually becomes recanalized and eventually produces valvular incompetence, which in turn leads to venous hypertension and the postphlebitic syndrome. Most patients with

pulmonary embolism, including those with major embolism, recover completely if treated with heparin. However, a few remain unresponsive to conservative measures and die shortly after the embolic event unless the pulmonary embolic obstruction can be rapidly removed by either pulmonary embolectomy or thrombolytic therapy. The correct application of these latter techniques requires considerable experience and clinical judgment, since both are often associated with complications.

Mode of Action of Anticoagulants

Heparin is a negatively charged polysaccharide with an average molecular weight of 16,000 daltons (range 3000 to 57,000). It exerts its anticoagulant effect in the presence of a plasma cofactor, antithrombin III.[90] Antithrombin III is an alpha$_2$ globulin that inhibits the activated clotting Factors IX_a, X_a, XI_a, XII_a and thrombin by binding their active serine residues. Heparin markedly accelerates this interaction between the activated clotting factors and antithrombin III by binding to the antithrombin III molecule.[69]

Heparin is not absorbed orally and must be given parenterally. The anticoagulant effect of heparin is immediate, and it is cleared from the plasma with a half-life of 60 minutes.

Heparin is the drug of choice for the treatment of acute venous thromboembolism. However, its clinical use is related to several unresolved issues. They are reviewed in detail elsewhere[58] and will not be discussed here. The major side effect of heparin is bleeding, which occurs more frequently in elderly patients, patients with an underlying hemostatic disorder, and patients who have recently sustained trauma or surgery. When these high risk patients are excluded from analysis, heparin therapy is associated with a 5 per cent incidence of major bleeding. Several studies have demonstrated a relationship between the risk of bleeding and the dose of heparin.[12, 62, 80, 82] Others have reported a lower incidence of bleeding when heparin is given by continuous infusion than when it is given by intermittent injection.[38, 92, 106] It should be noted, however, that in studies reporting a lower incidence of bleeding with continuous intravenous heparin, patients received a lower 24 hour dose of heparin than those who received intermittent heparin. The differences in the incidence of bleeding, therefore, could be related to the total dose of heparin used rather than to the method of administration.

Opinions differ as to whether heparin therapy should be monitored using an in vitro laboratory

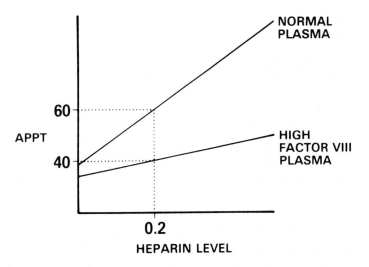

FIGURE 7–2. The relationship between the prolongation of the activated partial thromboplastin time, APTT (in seconds), and a therapeutic concentration of heparin (0.2 unit per ml). The upper line illustrates the heparin-induced prolongation of the APTT with normal plasma, and the lower line represents the APTT prolongation of plasma with a high concentration of Factor VIII.

test. Most authorities recommend that heparin should be monitored to insure that sufficient amounts are administered to prevent thrombus extension. A number of coagulation tests can be used to monitor heparin therapy, including coagulation time, activated partial thromboplastin time (APTT), thrombin clotting time, and heparin assay. The APTT is the test most commonly used to monitor heparin therapy; however, the reagents and instruments used to perform it vary from one laboratory to another, and the results may not be interchangeable.[83] Several APTT systems do not show a linear relationship between the heparin level and the APTT over the therapeutic range, and they should not be used for monitoring heparin therapy.[94, 100] The effect of heparin on the APTT is influenced by several variables (Fig. 7–2), one of which is the level of Factor VIII. Factor VIII increases during pregnancy, and the pretreatment of APTT is shortened. More importantly, a high Factor VIII level can interfere with the prolongation of the APTT by heparin,[28, 39] so that if the dose of heparin is adjusted to prolong patient APTT to twice that of the normal control, a very high dose of heparin may be required (Fig. 7–2). This problem can be overcome by using either the thrombin clotting time or heparin levels to monitor the dose of heparin.[58]

Recommended Method of Administering Heparin in Therapeutic Doses

Heparin should be administered by continuous intravenous infusion in a dose that maintains an in vitro test level equivalent to that caused by 0.2 to 0.4 units of heparin per ml. Usually, this corresponds to an APTT of approximately one and a half to two times the patient's pretreatment APTT value. Unless a hemostatic disorder is

suspected, a preheparin "coagulation screen" is unnecessary. Patients with venous thrombosis should have the monitoring test performed 6 to 8 hours after initiation of treatment and then daily to ensure adequate treatment. In patients with pulmonary embolism, adequate levels of heparin should be achieved as quickly as possible to prevent recurrence and to limit intrapulmonary extension of the embolus. These patients may be resistant to standard doses of heparin, so it may be necessary to perform monitoring tests more frequently during the initial period of treatment.

The average patient requires a bolus injection of 70 units of heparin per kilogram followed by a dose of 300 to 400 units per kilogram over a 24 hour period. Heparin is administered by continuous infusion by suspending 20,000 units of heparin in 500 ml of 5 per cent dextrose in water. It is then administered either by continuous pump or by a graduated cylinder. When the cylinder is used, it is inserted directly into the intravenous bag and filled to provide a 4 hour dose. This avoids the possibility of a sudden infusion of large amounts of heparin. If heparin is diluted to provide a concentration of 20,000 units in 500 ml suspending fluid, the volume of fluid in milliliters infused per hour times 1000 is equal to the total 24 hour dose of heparin. For example, 25 ml per hour is equivalent to a dose of 25,000 units per 24 hours. The average patient requires between 22,000 and 28,000 units of heparin per 24 hours.

Resistance to Heparin

The pregnant patient may have apparent resistance to heparin if the heparin effect is monitored by calculating a ratio of the postheparin APTT level with that obtained using a normal control.

For reasons just discussed, and illustrated in Figure 7–2, these patients may have a short pretreatment APTT because of high Factor VIII levels, so that the post-treatment APTT may not be a true reflection of the anticoagulant effect of heparin. The problem of apparent heparin resistance can be overcome by using the patient's own pretreatment APTT as the baseline in determining the desired post-treatment APTT (i.e., two times the pretreatment APTT). Alternatively, a heparin assay or thrombin clotting time can be performed and the patient maintained at a heparin level of 0.2 to 0.4 units per ml.

Less commonly, true heparin resistance occurs in patients with major pulmonary embolism because the heparin is rapidly cleared from the circulation.[48, 97] Differentiation between apparent and real heparin resistance is important. If the resistance is apparent, an increased heparin dose could lead to bleeding. If the resistance is real, the patient requires more heparin to achieve an adequate antithrombotic effect. Differentiation between these two possible mechanisms of "heparin resistance" is possible by obtaining a thrombin clotting time or measuring the heparin level.

Complications of Heparin Therapy

The complications include hemorrhage, thrombocytopenia, and osteoporosis.

Hemorrhagic Complications. Major hemorrhage is the most serious complication of heparin therapy. It occurs in more than 10 per cent of high risk patients but usually occurs in less than 5 per cent of low risk patients receiving therapeutic doses of heparin. Bleeding can follow procedures such as paracentesis, arterial punctures, and vascular cutdowns, and these should be avoided if possible in patients receiving heparin therapy.

The management of bleeding depends upon its severity. In all cases, the APTT, prothrombin time, and platelet count should be assessed immediately. If the APTT is within the therapeutic range but the prothrombin time is prolonged, a complicating vitamin K deficiency is likely, and the patient should be treated with subcutaneous or intravenous vitamin K. The platelet count should be determined, since heparin can be associated with the development of thrombocytopenia. In many patients who bleed during heparin therapy, it is possible to continue treatment with a lower dose of heparin and to treat the patient with blood transfusion and local measures to control bleeding. If the APTT is markedly prolonged, treatment should be stopped for 1 to 2 hours until the heparin effect has worn off and bleeding has stopped. Treatment is then reinstituted at a lower dosage. On the other hand, if bleeding is life-threatening (e.g., retroperitoneal, cerebral, or into a deep wound), treatment should be stopped and the effect of heparin reversed with protamine sulfate. This positively charged substance combines with and inactivates heparin. The appropriate neutralizing dose depends upon the amount of heparin given, its route of administration, and the time that it was given. When bleeding occurs within minutes of intravenous heparin injection, a full neutralizing dose (1 mg of protamine for 100 units of heparin) should be administered. If bleeding occurs 60 minutes after heparin injection, only 50 per cent of this dose is required, and if it occurs after 2 hours, only 25 per cent is required. Hypotensive reactions can follow the rapid intravenous injection of protamine sulfate, and it should be administered slowly over 20 to 30 minutes. Once the heparin effect is reversed, alternative therapy must be considered. If treatment has only recently been initiated, venal caval interruption is indicated to prevent pulmonary emboli. If the patient has received heparin for several weeks, therapy can be discontinued and the patient followed up closely.

Heparin-Associated Thrombocytopenia. Heparin-associated thrombocytopenia (HAT) is a recently recognized complication of heparin therapy.[16] Thrombocytopenia may occur alone or may occasionally be associated with arterial thrombosis.[57] It may occur after intravenous or subcutaneous administration of heparin and usually appears approximately one week after the beginning of treatment.[59] Heparin-associated thrombocytopenia is relatively common, while heparin-associated thrombocytopenia with associated arterial thrombosis is rare. The reported incidence of HAT varies from less than 5 per cent to more than 30 per cent.[18, 86] One group of investigators reported that it is more common in patients receiving heparin of bovine origin than of porcine origin, but this has not been observed in other studies.[14, 29]

The pathogenesis of heparin-associated thrombocytopenia is uncertain. There is some evidence that the thrombocytopenia is caused by immune mechanisms; however, it is unlike a typical drug immune thrombocytopenia because the thrombocytopenia can resolve while the patient continues to receive heparin. Furthermore, if the patient is rechallenged with heparin after the thrombocytopenia has resolved, it may not recur.[60] The management of heparin-associated thrombocytopenia is uncertain. It is generally recommended that heparin should be stopped and the patient be treated with alternative therapy such as inferior venal caval interruption of oral anticoagulant therapy.[58] However, if the thrombocytopenia is mild, the heparin may be continued with frequent monitoring of the platelet count, since the thrombocytopenia often resolves spontaneously.

Heparin-Induced Osteoporosis. A major concern in patients receiving long-term treatment with heparin is heparin-induced osteoporosis.[54, 91] Heparin may cause osteoporosis by complexing with calcium ions or by augmenting the effect of parathormone on bone reabsorption. The exact incidence of this syndrome is uncertain, since it is difficult to diagnose osteoporosis objectively. It has been reported to occur in six of ten patients treated with subcutaneous heparin in doses of 15,000 to 30,000 units per day for over 6 months.[42] Recently, a patient was described who developed this complication while receiving 10,000 units of heparin subcutaneously twice daily.[108]

Risks to the Fetus of Administering Heparin and Oral Anticoagulants During Pregnancy. Heparin does not cross the placenta, does not enter the fetal circulation,[34] and therefore would not be expected to produce fetal complications. It has been suggested that maternal treatment with heparin is associated with significant risks to the fetus — a conclusion based on reports of a high incidence of stillbirth or prematurity in others treated with heparin.[44] However, review of the indications for the heparin therapy in these patients indicates that much of the fetal loss occurred in mothers who were receiving heparin for pre-eclampsia or toxemia, conditions that are known to be associated with a high rate of fetal loss. Three mothers died while receiving heparin, but only one death was due to bleeding complications. The other two died of thrombotic complications. Critical analysis of the literature yields no good evidence that heparin therapy is associated with increased fetal loss during pregnancy.

Oral anticoagulants cross the placenta and can cause fetal malformations if administered in the first trimester. They can also cause fetal hemorrhage during delivery if treatment is continued throughout pregnancy.[46, 64, 87] Oral anticoagulants are contraindicated during the first trimester of pregnancy because they can induce a syndrome, termed warfarin embryopathy, which is manifested as nasal hypoplasia and skeletal abnormalities.[24, 95] More recently, a second fetal complication of maternal warfarin therapy has

been described. It is characterized by multiple central nervous system abnormalities, including dorsal midline dysplasia, abnormalities of the ventricular system, and optic atrophy.[44] These abnormalities have been reported to occur in the infants of mothers treated with oral anticoagulants at any time during pregnancy. Oral anticoagulants are therefore contraindicated at all times during pregnancy.

Use of Anticoagulants in the Nursing Mother. Heparin is not secreted into breast milk and can be safely administered to the nursing mother. The literature on the safety of oral anticoagulants in nursing mothers is confusing. Based on one case report,[27] it has been suggested that phenindione enters the breast milk. Ethyl biscoumacetate was also detected in breast milk, although in one study no adverse effects occurred in 22 breast-fed infants of mothers receiving this drug. Warfarin is a weakly acidic drug and is highly ionized. It is also very strongly protein bound and therefore does not enter the breast milk. Warfarin in the plasma and breast milk of 13 nursing mothers has been measured; no warfarin was detected in their breast milk or in the plasma of their infants.[68]

Use of Anticoagulants for Treatment of Venous Thrombosis and Pulmonary Embolism

Heparin is the treatment of choice in patients with venous thromboembolic disease because it is relatively safe and effective. Heparin is usually administered for a period of 7 to 10 days, the dose being monitored as has been described. In the nonpregnant patient, heparin therapy is followed by treatment with oral anticoagulants for a period of 6 to 12 weeks. The oral anticoagulant treatment is begun 4 or 5 days before heparin is stopped, since there is a delay before the antithrombotic effect of oral anticoagulants is achieved.[31] A "loading dose" is not used. In the average patient, 10 mg warfarin daily for 2 days is administered. Beginning on the second day, the prothrombin time (PT) should be monitored daily and the dose of warfarin adjusted to give a prothrombin time of one and a half to two times the control prothrombin time.

In patients who are at increased risk of bleeding, or when oral anticoagulant control is difficult, inconvenient, or contraindicated (for example in pregnancy), moderate doses of subcutaneous heparin can be used instead of oral anticoagulants.[98] They can usually be administered by the patient and are particularly valuable in the pregnant patient. Moderate dose subcutaneous heparin is as effective as oral anticoagulants and is associated with less bleeding,[50] but the treatment is expensive.

Treatment of Acute Venous Thromboembolism in Pregnancy

Patients who develop acute venous thrombosis or pulmonary embolism in pregnancy should be treated by continuous intravenous infusion of heparin for 10 to 14 days and then by subcutaneous heparin in moderate doses. As detailed previously, the usual dose of intravenous heparin is 22,000 to 28,000 units per 24 hours. The usual "moderate" dose of subcutaneous heparin is 10,000 units twice a day. This dose should be individualized for each patient by adjusting it so that the heparin level is 0.2 to 0.3 units per ml 6 hours after injection. When the patient is admitted to hospital for delivery, heparin therapy should be stopped. Following delivery, it should be restarted, then continued for 1 week or longer if the patient remains immobilized. Patients who develop venous thrombosis in the last trimester of pregnancy should have moderate dose subcutaneous heparin continued for 3 months after the acute thromboembolic event.

If the patient develops a venous thrombosis in the first trimester or early in the second trimester, she should be treated with moderate doses of subcutaneous heparin for 3 months after an acute event and then treated with low dose heparin (5000 units twice a day) for the duration of the pregnancy. The heparin should be discontinued when labor begins and then restarted at a moderate dose several hours after delivery.

Treatment of Venous Thrombosis and Pulmonary Embolism in the Postpartum Period

Patients who develop venous thromboembolism in the postpartum period should be treated in the same manner as the nonpregnant patient, that is, administration of heparin for 7 to 10 days followed by oral anticoagulants for a period of 6 weeks to 3 months. Warfarin, 5 to 10 mg daily, should be given 5 days after the beginning of heparin therapy and the prothrombin time maintained at one and a half to two times control level. Heparin is then discontinued and the patient maintained on warfarin. Many drugs interact with oral anticoagulants,[89, 96] and they should be avoided during warfarin therapy.

If bleeding occurs during oral anticoagulant therapy, treatment should be stopped and vitamin K administered. If the prothrombin time is markedly prolonged and bleeding is potentially life-threatening, then fresh frozen plasma or Factor II, VII, IX, and X concentrate should be administered. The subsequent management of the patient is influenced by the specific time during the course of anticoagulant therapy that the bleeding occurs. If bleeding occurs toward the end of the course of anticoagulant therapy (more than 6 weeks after starting treatment), then anticoagulants can be terminated. If bleeding occurs early in the course of anticoagulant therapy, then moderate dose subcutaneous heparin should be used, since it has a lower risk of bleeding.[50]

Management of Patients with a Previous History of Venous Thromboembolism

The optimal management of a patient with a previous history of venous thrombosis during subsequent pregnancies is difficult to define, because the risk of recurrent thrombosis in subsequent pregnancies is unknown and the risk of osteoporosis developing in later life in these patients treated with long-term heparin is unknown. Patients with a past history of a documented deep vein thrombosis or pulmonary embolism that occurred in the antepartum period should be treated with low dose heparin in subsequent pregnancies. These patients would be exposed to the same risk (pregnancy) that precipitated the initial episode of thrombosis. The low dose heparin should continue for 1 to 2 weeks following delivery, since that is a high risk period.

The management of patients with a history of a previous postpartum venous thromboembolic event unrelated to pregnancy or in the puerperium is less certain.[8] The clinician has two options. If objective tests were not used to confirm the previous thromboembolic event, bilateral ascending venography should be performed. If the result of venography is normal, a baseline impedance plethysmography should be performed and the patient allowed to proceed throughout pregnancy without anticoagulant prophylaxis. Following delivery, subcutaneous heparin prophylaxis should be administered for 1 to 2 weeks. If the venogram shows evidence of extensive previous thrombosis, or if objective evidence confirms the previous episode of venous thrombosis, the clinician may elect either to treat the patient prophylactically throughout pregnancy using low dose subcutaneous heparin (5000 units twice a day) or to follow up the patient with serial impedance plethysmography at monthly intervals.

SEPTIC PELVIC THROMBOPHLEBITIS

Thrombosed pelvic veins are occasionally observed incidentally during surgery, but the incidence of pelvic vein thrombosis is unknown and the significance uncertain, largely because there is no reliable objective test for diagnosing this disorder. The clinical syndrome of pelvic thrombophlebitis cannot be distinguished from other forms of pelvic inflammatory disease. One group of clinicians has suggested that suppurative pelvic vein thrombosis should be suspected if a fever does not resolve despite treatment with broad-spectrum antibiotics;[93] however, the reliability of these criteria is difficult to validate.

Patients with suspected pelvic thrombophlebitis are often ill with recurrent spiking fevers and complain of abdominal pain and tenderness.[78] Results of pelvic examination may be normal or there may be pelvic tenderness. It has been reported that approximately one third of patients have palpable thrombosed parametrial veins.[19] The first sign of pelvic thrombophlebitis may be the presence of septic pulmonary emboli. The chest x-ray in these patients may reveal a variety of abnormalities, including small multiple infiltrates, but often it is normal. In most studies, blood cultures are positive in 20 to 40 per cent of patients, the most common infecting organism being *Streptococcus*. This may represent an underestimate of the total incidence of positive blood cultures, since the culturing techniques used in the earlier reports may not have detected anaerobic bacteria.[71]

Management of Suspected Suppurative Pelvic Thrombophlebitis

In the preantibiotic era, the clinical condition known as suppurative pelvic thrombophlebitis had a mortality rate of 50 per cent.[73] The more recent reports (in the antibiotic era) have indicated a drop in the mortality rate to 10 per cent.[19, 56]

If suppurative pelvic thrombophlebitis is suspected, the patient's condition should be investigated by a series of at least three blood cultures for both aerobic and anaerobic organisms, and treatment with broad-spectrum antibiotics should be commenced. An impedance plethysmogram and chest x-ray should be performed, and if the impedance plethysmogram is positive, the diagnosis of thrombosis involving the external iliac system should be confirmed by venography. Ventilation and perfusion lung scans should be performed because a pattern showing high probability of pulmonary embolism is useful in making management decisions. Any objective evidence of venous thromboembolism is an indication for the immediate administration of heparin. Surgical interruption of the pelvic vena cava is seldom required.

The management of patients without evidence of thrombosis who fail to respond to antibiotics is controversial. Various approaches have been recommended, including heparin therapy, pelvic vein ligation and inferior vena caval interruption, hysterectomy, and drainage of pelvic abscess. None of these have been formally evaluated.

Pelvic surgery should be considered if a pelvic abscess is suspected on clinical grounds, but pelvic vein ligation or vena caval interruption should be considered only if patients have proven pulmonary emboli that have recurred despite adequate anticoagulant therapy.

CEREBRAL VENOUS THROMBOSIS

Cerebral venous thrombosis is an uncommon but serious complication of pregnancy and the puerperium. Spontaneously occurring cerebral venous thrombosis must be differentiated from that secondary to trauma or to a septic process in the ear, face, or paranasal sinus. Difficulty in diagnosing this condition may account for the considerable variation in the estimated incidence, which ranges from 1 in 2000 to 3000 deliveries[67] to 1 in 600,000 deliveries.[23]

Typically, patients with cerebral venous thrombosis have a sudden onset of severe headache, which may precede other objective neurologic signs by several days. The majority of patients also have vomiting and seizures. Other common signs include focal neurologic signs (often hemiplegia) and an altered state of consciousness ranging from mild confusion to coma.[3] The differential diagnosis includes space-occupying lesions, cerebral hemorrhage, cerebral embolism, and subarachnoid hemorrhage. Space-occupying lesions and cerebral embolism can usually be diagnosed by brain scan. The nausea, vomiting, and seizures that often accompany cerebral venous thrombosis may incorrectly be attributed to pre-eclampsia and toxemia, but unlike toxemia, cerebral venous thrombosis is not accompanied by hypertension. The definitive diagnosis can be made by angiographic examination of the cerebral vessels.[7, 41, 104] It is possible that computerized axial tomographic examination of the brain will prove a useful technique for diagnosing this disorder.

The management of cerebral venous thrombosis remains uncertain. All patients should be treated supportively with antiseizure medication and agents such as corticosteroids or mannitol to decrease intracranial pressure. The patients should not be dehydrated, because dehydration can precipitate this disorder.[7] Some clinicians advocate anticoagulant therapy,[6, 30, 65, 104] but others have reported hemorrhage following heparin therapy.[25, 37] Anticoagulant therapy should be considered if the diagnosis is certain and if other disorders that could be worsened by anticoagulants (such as cerebral hemorrhage) are excluded.

Patients who recover from cerebral venous thrombosis should not receive oral contraceptives because these agents have been associated with the development of this disorder.[6, 25, 30, 84] Further pregnancies are not contraindicated,[66, 67] but it is not known if subcutaneous heparin should be administered prophylactically during pregnancy or the puerperium.

References

1. Aaro, L. A., Johnson, T. R., and Juergens, J. L.: Acute superficial venous thrombophlebitis associated with pregnancy. Am. J. Obstet. Gynecol., 97:514, 1967.
2. Aaro, L. A., and Juergens, J. L.: Thrombophlebitis associated with pregnancy. Am J. Obstet. Gynecol., 109:1128, 1971.
3. Amias, A. G.: Cerebral vascular disease in pregnancy. J. Obstet. Gynaecol. Br. Commonw., 77:312, 1970.
4. Arthure, H.: Maternal deaths from pulmonary embolism. J. Obstet. Gynaecol. Br. Commonw., 75:1309, 1968.
5. Astedt, B.: Fibrinolytic activity of veins in the puerperium. Acta Obstet. Gynecol. Scand., 51:325, 1972.
6. Atkinson, E. A., Fairburn, B., and Heathfield, K. W. G.: Intracranial venous thrombosis as a complication of oral contraceptives. Lancet, 1:914, 1970.
7. Averback, P.: Primary cerebral venous thrombosis in young adults: The diverse manifestations of an underrecognized disease. Ann. Neurol., 3:81, 1978.
8. Badaracco, M. A., and Vessey, M. P.: Recurrence of venous thromboembolic disease and use of oral contraceptives. Br. Med. J., 1:215, 1974.
9. Barker, N. W., Nygaard, K. K., Walters, W. W., et al.: A statistical study of postoperative venous thrombosis and pulmonary embolism. III. Time of occurrence during the postoperative period. Proc. Staff Meet. Mayo Clin., 16:17, 1941.
10. Barnes, R. W., Wu, K. K., and Hoak, J. C.: Fallibility of the clinical diagnosis of venous thrombosis. J.A.M.A., 234:605, 1975.
11. Barritt, D. W., and Jordan, S. C.: Anticoagulant drugs in the treatment of pulmonary embolism. Lancet, 1:1309, 1960.
12. Basu, D., Gallus, A., Hirsh, J., and Cade, J.: A prospective study of the value of monitoring heparin treatment with the activated partial thromboplastin time. N. Engl. J. Med., 287:324, 1972.
13. Bauer, G.: Clinical exeriences of a surgeon in the use of heparin. Am. J. Cardiol., 14:29, 1964.
14. Bell, W. R., and Royall, R. M.: Heparin-associated thrombocytopenia: A comparison of three heparin preparations. N. Engl. J. Med., 303:902, 1980.
15. Bell, W. R., Simin, T. L., and Demets, D. L.: The clinical features of submassive and massive pulmonary embolism. Am. J. Med., 62:355, 1977.
16. Bell, W. R., Tomasulo, P. A., Alving, B. M., and Duffy, T. P.: Thrombocytopenia occurring during the administration of heparin: A prospective study in 52 patients. Ann. Intern. Med., 85:155, 1976.
17. Bonnar, J., McNicol, G. P., and Douglas, A. S. Coagulation and fibrinolytic mechanisms during and after normal childbirth. Br. Med. J., 2:200, 1970.
18. Cheely, R., McCartney, W. H., Perry, J. R., Delany, D. J., Bustad, L., Wynia, V. H., and Griggs, R. T.: The Role of noninvasive tests versus pulmonary angiography in the diagnosis of pulmonary embolism. Am. J. Med., 70:17, 1981.
19. Collins, G. C.: Suppurative pelvic thrombophlebitis. Am. J. Obstet. Gynecol., 108:681, 1970.
20. Coon, W. W.: Epidemiology of venous thromboembolism. Ann. Surg., 186(2):149, 1977.
21. Coon, W. W., Willis, P. W., III, and Keller, J. B.: Venous thromboembolism and other venous disease in the Tecumseh Community Health Study. Circulation, 158:839, 1973.
22. Coopland, A., Alkjaersig, N., and Fletcher, A. P.: Reduction in plasma factor XIII (fibrin stabilizing factor) concentration during pregnancy. J. Lab. Clin. Med., 73:144, 1969.
23. Cross, J. N., Castro, P. O., and Jennett, W. B.: Cerebral strokes associated with pregnancy and the puerperium. Br. Med. J., 3:214, 1968.
24. DiSaia, P. J.: Pregnancy and delivery of a patient with a Starr-Edwards mitral valve prosthesis. Report of a case. Obstet. Gynecol., 28:469, 1966.
25. Dinder, F., and Platts, M. E.: Intracranial venous thrombosis complicating oral contraception. Can. Med. Assoc. J., 111:545, 1974.
26. Drill, V. A., and Calhoun, D. W.: Oral contraceptives and thromboembolic disease. J.A.M.A., 206:77, 1968.
27. Eckstein, H. B., and Jack, B.: Breast feeding and anticoagulant therapy. Lancet, 1:672, 1970.
28. Edson, J. R., Krivit, W., and White, J. G.: Kaolin partial thromboplastin time: High levels of procoagulants producing short clotting times or masking deficiencies of other procoagulants or low concentrations of anticoagulants. J. Lab. Clin. Med., 70:463, 1967.
29. Eika, C., Godal, H. C., Laake, K., and Hamborg, T.: Low incidence of thrombocytopenia during treatment with hog mucosa and beef lung heparin. Scand. J. Haematol., 25:19, 1980.
30. Fairburn, B.: Intracranial venous sinus thrombosis complicating oral contraception: Treatment by anticoagulant drugs. Br. Med. J., 2:647, 1973.
31. Fenech, A., Winter, J. H., and Douglas, A. S.: Individualisation of oral anticoagulant therapy. Drugs, 18:48, 1979.
32. Finnerty, J. J., and MacKay, B. R.: Antepartum thrombophlebitis and pulmonary embolism. Obstet. Gynecol., 19:405, 1962.
33. Flessa, H. C., Glueck, H. I., and Dritschilo, A.: Thromboembolic disorders in pregnancy: Pathophysiology, diagnosis and treatment with emphasis on heparin. Clin. Obstet. Gynecol., 17:195, 1974.
34. Flessa, H. C., Kapstrom, A. B., Glueck, H. I., and Will, J. J.: Placental transport of heparin. Am. J. Obstet. Gynecol., 93:570, 1965.
35. Fletcher, A. P., Alkjaersig, N. K., and Burstein, R.: The influence of pregnancy upon blood coagulation and plasma fibrinolytic enzyme function. Am. J. Obstet. Gynecol., 134:743, 1979.
36. Friend, J. R., and Kakkar, V. V.: The diagnosis of deep vein thrombosis in the puerperium. J. Obstet. Gynaecol. Br. Commonw., 77:820, 1970.
37. Gettelfinger, D. M., and Kokmen, E.: Superior sagittal sinus thrombosis. Arch. Neurol., 34:2, 1977.
38. Glazier, R. L., and Crowell, E. B.: Randomized prospective trial of continuous vs. intermittent heparin therapy. J.A.M.A., 236:1365, 1976.
39. Glynn, M. F. X.: Heparin monitoring and thrombosis. Am. Soc. Clin. Pathol., 71:397, 1979.
39a. Goodrich, S. M., and Wood, J. E.: Peripheral venous dis-

tensibility and velocity of venous blood flow during pregnancy or during oral contraceptive therapy. Am. J. Obstet. Gynecol. *90*:740, 1964.

40. Gowers, W. R.: A Manual of Diseases of the Nervous System. London, Churchill, 1888, p. 116.

41. Greitz, T., and Link, H.: Aseptic thrombosis of intracranial sinuses. Radiol. Clin. Biol., *35*:111, 1966.

42. Griffith, G. C., Nichols, G., Asher, J. D. et al.: Heparin osteoporosis. J.A.M.A., *193*:85, 1965.

43. Gurll, N., Helfand, Z., Salzman, E. F., and Silen, W.: Peripheral venous thrombophlebitis during pregnancy. Am. J. Surg., *121*:449, 1971.

44. Hall, J. G., Pauli, R. M., and Wilson, K. M.: Maternal and fetal sequelae of anticoagulation during pregnancy. Am. J. Med., *68*:122, 1980.

45. Hathaway, W. E., and Bonnar, J.: Perinatal Coagulation. New York, Grune & Stratton Inc., 1978, pp. 27–52.

46. Hirsh, J., Cade, J. F., and Gallus, A. S.: Fetal effects of coumadin administered during pregnancy. Blood, *36*:623, 1970.

47. Hirsh, J., and Hull, R.: Comparative value of tests for the diagnosis of venous thrombosis. World J. Surg., *2*:27, 1978.

48. Hirsh, J., VanAken W. G., Gallus, A. S., Dollery C. T., Cade, J. F., and Yung, W. L.: Heparin kinetics in venous thrombosis and pulmonary embolism. Circulation, *53*:691, 1976.

49. Howie, P. W., Evans, K., Forbes, C. D., and Prentice, C. R.: The effects of stilboestrol and quinestrol upon coagulation and fibrinolysis during the puerperium. Br. J. Obstet. Gynaecol., *82*:968, 1975.

50. Hull, R., Delmore, T., Genton, E., Hirsh, J., Gent, M., Sackett, D., McLoughlin, D., and Armstrong, P.: Warfarin sodium versus low-dose heparin in the long-term treatment of venous thrombosis. N. Engl. J. Med., *301*:855, 1979.

51. Hull, R., Hirsh, J., Sackett, D. L., Powers, P., Turpie, A. G. G., and Walker, I.: Combined use of leg scanning and impedance plethysmography in suspected venous thrombosis. An alternative to venography. N. Engl. J. Med., *296*:1497, 1977.

52. Hull, R., Hirsh, J., Sackett, D. L., Taylor, D. W., Carter, C., Turpie, A. G. G., Zielinsky, A., Powers, P., and Gent., M.: Replacement of venography in suspected venous thrombosis by impedance plethysmography and ¹²⁵I-fibrinogen leg scanning. Ann. Intern. Med., *94*:12, 1981.

52a. Illingworth, R.: Ethyl biscoumacetate (Tromexan) in human milk. J. Obstet. Gynaec. Br. Empire *66*:487, 1959.

53. Inman, W. H. W., and Vessey, M. P.: Investigation of deaths from pulmonary, coronary, and cerebral thrombosis and embolism in women of childbearing age. Br. Med. J., *2*:193, 1968.

54. Jaffe, M. D., and Willis, P. W.: Multiple fractures involved with long-term sodium heparin therapy. J.A.M.A., *193*:158, 1960.

55. Jeffcoate, T. N. A., and Tindall, V. R.: Venous thrombosis and embolism in obstetrics and gynecology. Aust. N. Z. J. Obstet. Gynaecol., *5*:114, 1965.

56. Josey, W. E., and Cook, C. C.: Septic pelvic thrombophlebitis. Report of 17 patients treated with heparin. Obstet. Gynecol., *35*:891, 1970.

57. Kapsch, D. N., Adelstein, E. H., Rhodes, R., and Silver, D.: Heparin-induced thrombocytopenia, thrombosis and hemorrhage. Surgery, *86*:148, 1979.

58. Kelton, J. G., and Hirsh, J.: Bleeding associated with antithrombotic therapy. Semin. Hematol., *17*:259, 1980.

59. Kelton, J. G., and Powers, P.: Heparin associated thrombocytopenia: An immune disorder. *In* Lundblad, R. (ed.): The Chemistry and Biology of Heparin. Amsterdam, Elsevier, 1980.

60. Kelton, J. G., Powers, P. J., Turpie, A. G., and Carter, C. J.: Heparin associated thrombocytopenia is not a typical drug induced thrombocytopenia. Clin. Res., *29*:339A, 1981.

61. Kendall, D.: Thrombosis of intracranial veins. Brain, *71*:386, 1948.

62. Kernohan, R. J., and Todd, C.: Heparin therapy in thromboembolic disease. Lancet, *1*:621, 1966.

63. Kistner, R. L., Ball, J. J., Nordyke, R. A., et al.: Incidence of pulmonary embolism in the course of thrombophlebitis of the lower extremities. Am. J. Surg., *124*:169, 1972.

64. Kraus, A. P., Perlow, S., and Singer, K.: Danger of dicumarol treatment in pregnancy. J.A.M.A., *139*:758, 1949.

65. Krayenbuhl, H. A.: Cerebral venous and sinus thrombosis. Clin. Neurosurg., *14*:1, 1966.

66. Lemmi, H., and Little, S. C.: Occlusion of intracranial venous structures. A consideration of the clinical and electroencephalographic findings. Arch. Neurol., *3*:252, 1960.

67. Lorincz, A. B., and Moore, R. Y.: Puerperal cerebral venous thrombosis. Am. J. Obstet. Gynecol., *83*:311, 1962.

68. L'e Orme, M., Lewis, P. J., De Swiet, M., Serlin, M. J., Sibeon, R., Baty, J. D., and Breckenridge, A. M.: May mothers given warfarin breast-feed their infants? Br. Med. J., *1*:1564, 1977.

69. Machovich, R., and Aranyi, P.: Effect of heparin on thrombin inactivation by antithrombin-III. Biochem. J., *173*:869, 1978.

70. McCausland, A. M., Hyman, C., Winsor, T., and Trotter, A. D.: Venous distensibility during pregnancy. Am. J. Obstet. Gynecol., *81*:472, 1961.

71. McElin, T. W., LaPata, R. E., Westenfelder, G. O., and Hohf, R. P.: Postpartum ovarian vein thrombophlebitis and microaerophilic streptococcal sepsis. Obstet. Gynecol., *35*:632, 1970.

72. McKillop, C., Howie, P. W., Forbes, C. O., et al.: Soluble fibrinogen-fibrin complexes in pre-eclampsia. Lancet, *1*:56, 1976.

73. Miller, C. J.: Ligation or excision of pelvic veins in the treatment of puerperal pyaemia. Surg. Gynecol. Obstet., *25*:431, 1917.

74. Moore, J. G., O'Leary, J. A., and Johnson, P. M.: The changing impact of pulmonary thromboembolism in obstetrics. Am. J. Obstet. Gynecol., *97*:507, 1967.

75. Muller-Berghaus, G., Moeller, R. M., and Mahn, I.: Fibrinogen turnover in pregnant rabbits. Am. J. Obstet. Gynecol., *131*:655, 1978.

76. Nilsson, I. M., and Kullander, S.: Coagulation and fibrinolytic studies during pregnancy. Acta. Obstet. Gynecol. Scand., *46*:273, 1967.

77. Nossel, H. L., Lanzkowsky, P., Levy, S., Mibashan, R. S., and Hansen, J. D. L.: A study of coagulation factor levels in women during labour and in their newborn infants. Thromb. Diath. Haemorrh., *16*:185, 1966.

78. O'Lane, J. M., and Lebherz, T. B.: Puerperal ovarian thrombophlebitis. Obstet. Gynecol., *26*:676, 1965.

79. O'Leary, J. A., Moore, J. G., and Johnson, P. M.: Detection of postpartum pulmonary emboli by lung scan. Obstet. Gynecol., *30*:721, 1967.

80. O'Sullivan, E. F., Hirsh, J., McCarthy, R. A., and de Gruchy, C.: Heparin in the treatment of venous thromboembolic disease. Administration, control and results. Med. J. Aust., *2*:153, 1968.

81. Phillips, L. L., Rosano, L., and Skrodelis, V.: Changes in factor XI (plasma thromboplastin antecedent) levels during pregnancy. Am. J. Obstet. Gynecol., *116*:1114, 1973.

82. Pitney, W. R., Pettit, J. E., and Armstrong, L.: Control of heparin therapy. Br. Med. J., *4*:139, 1970.

83. Poller, L., Thomson, J. M., and Yee, K. F.: Heparin and partial thromboplastin time: An international survey. Br. J. Haematol., *44*:161, 1980.

84. Poltera, A. A.: The pathology of intracranial venous thrombosis in oral contraception. J. Pathol., *106*:209, 1972.

85. Porter, J. M., Seaman, A. J., Common, H. H., Rosch, J., Eidemiller, L. R., and Calhoun, A. D.: Comparison of heparin and streptokinase in the treatment of venous thrombosis. Am. Surg., *41*:511, 1975.

86. Powers, P. J., Cuthbert, D., and Hirsh, J.: Thrombocytopenia found uncommonly during heparin therapy. J.A.M.A., *241*:2396, 1979.

87. Quick, A. M.: Experimentally induced changes in the prothrombin level of the blood. III. Prothrombin concentration of newborn pups of a mother given dicumarol before parturition. J. Biol. Chem., *164*:371, 1946.

88. Robertson, B. R., Nilsson, I. M., and Nylander, G.: Thrombolytic effect of streptokinase as evaluated by phlebography of deep venous thrombi of the leg. Acta. Chir. Scand., *136*:173, 1970.

89. Robinson, D. S., and Sylvester, D.: Interaction of commonly prescribed drugs and warfarin. Ann. Intern. Med., *72*:853, 1970.

90. Rosenberg, R. D.: Actions and interactions of antithrombin and heparin. N. Engl. J. Med., *292*:146, 1975.

91. Sackler, J. P., and Liu, L.: Case reports, heparin-induced osteoporosis. Br. J. Radiol., *46*:548, 1973.

92. Salzman, E. W., Deykin, D., Shapiro, R. M., and Rosenberg, R.: Management of heparin therapy. Controlled prospective trial. N. Engl. J. Med., *292*:1046, 1975.

93. Schulman, H., and Zatuchni, G.: Pelvic thrombophlebitis in the puerperal and postoperative gynecologic patient. Am. J. Obstet. Gynecol., *90*:1293, 1964.

94. Shapiro, G. A., Huntzinger, S. W., and Wilson, J. E.: Variation among commercial activated partial thromboplastin time reagents in response to heparin. Am. J. Clin. Pathol., *67*:477, 1977.

95. Shaul, W. L., and Hall, J. G.: Multiple congenital anomalies associated with oral anticoagulants. Am. J. Obstet. Gynecol., 127:191, 1977.
96. Sigell, L. T., and Flessa, H. C.: Drug interactions with anticoagulants. J.A.M.A., 214:2035, 1970.
97. Simon, T. L., Hyers, T. M., Gaston, J. P., and Harker, L. A.: Heparin pharmacokinetics: Increased requirements in pulmonary embolism. Br. J. Haematol., 39:111, 1978.
98. Spearing, G., Fraser, I., Turner, G., and Dixon, G.: Long-term self-administered subcutaneous heparin in pregnancy. Br. Med. J., 1:1457, 1978.
99. Szucs, M. M., Brooks, H. L., Grossman, W., Banas, J. S. Jr., Meister, S. G., Dexter, L., and Dalen, J. E.: Diagnostic sensitivity of laboratory findings in acute pulmonary embolism. Ann. Intern. Med., 74:161, 1971.
100. Ts'ao, C-H., Galluzzo, T. S., Lo, R., and Peterson, K. G.: Whole blood clotting time, activated partial thromboplastin time, and whole blood recalcification time as heparin monitoring tests. Am. J. Clin. Pathol., 71:17, 1979.
101. Ullery, J. C.: Thromboembolic disease complicating pregnancy and the puerperium. Am. J. Obstet. Gynecol., 68:1243, 1954.
102. van Royen, E. A., and ten Cate, J. W.: Antigen/biological activity ratio for factor VIII in late pregnancy. Lancet, 2:449, 1973.
103. Villasanta, U.: Thromboembolic disease in pregnancy. Am. J. Obstet. Gynecol., 93:142, 1965.
104. Vines, F. S., and Davis, D. O.: Clinical radiological correlation in cerebral venous occlusive disease. Radiology, 98:9, 1971.
105. Wacker, W. E., Rosenthal, M., Snodgrass, P. J., and Amadore, E.: A triad for the diagnosis of pulmonary embolism and infarction. J.A.M.A., 178:8, 1961.
106. Wilson, J. R., and Lampman, J.: Heparin therapy: A randomized prospective study. Am. Heart J., 97:155, 1979.
107. Wingfield, J. G.: Anticoagulation for antenatal thromboembolic disease. J. Obstet. Gynaecol. Br. Commonw., 76:518, 1969.
108. Wise, P. H., and Hall, A. J.: Heparin-induced osteopenia in pregnancy. Br. Med. J., 2:110, 1980.
109. Wright, H. P., Osborn, S. B., and Edmonds, D. G.: Changes in the rate of flow of venous blood in the leg during pregnancy, measured with radioactive sodium. Surg. Gynecol. Obstet., 90:481, 1950.
110. Zilliacus, H.: II. History of thrombo-embolic disease. 1. Etiology and pathogenesis. Acta Med. Scand., 171:1, 1946.
111. Zucker, M. L., Gomperts, E. D., and Marcus, R. G.: Prophylactic and therapeutic use of anticoagulants in inherited antithrombin-III deficiency. S. Afr. Med. J., 50:1743, 1976.

Gerard N. Burrow, M.D.

8

THYROID DISEASES

THYROID FUNCTION DURING PREGNANCY

Hormonal changes and metabolic demands during pregnancy result in complex changes in thyroid function. Furthermore, pregnancy outcome may be profoundly altered by abnormal thyroid function. Changes that occur in the various parameters of thyroid function are mainly due to increased thyroxine-binding globulin, which is induced by increased estrogen production during pregnancy. Although the normal pregnant woman is considered to be euthyroid, there is also an increase in the basal metabolic rate, radioactive iodine thyroid uptake, and thyroid gland size.

Thyroid disease is much more common in women than in men and is not rare during pregnancy. Clinically, the diagnosis of thyroid dysfunction in the pregnant woman can be difficult, and thyroid function tests may offer little help. Once a diagnostic decision has been reached, therapy is complicated by the presence of the fetus. Pharmacologic therapy that is beneficial to the mother may be harmful to the fetus. An understanding of the normal physiologic processes of the thyroid gland during pregnancy will be very helpful in understanding pathologic processes during gestation.

Goiter

The histologic picture of the thyroid gland during pregnancy is that of the active formation and secretion of thyroid hormone. Characteristically, the gland has large follicles with abundant, well-stained colloid and frequent vacuolization. Papillary infolding indicative of follicular hyperplasia may be seen, and the impression is reinforced by finding columnar follicular cells.[168]

The prevalence of goiter during pregnancy varies with the geographic area studied. In a study done in Scotland, 70 per cent of pregnant women were diagnosed as having a goiter in contrast with 38 per cent of nonpregnant women.[33] Goiter was considered to be present if the glands were both palpable and visible. Previous pregnancies did not appear to affect this incidence, since goiters were found in 39 per cent of nulliparous women and 35 per cent of nonpregnant parous women. These investigators repeated the study in Iceland under the same experimental conditions but noted no increase in goiter during pregnancy.[34] Goiter was found in 19 per cent of nonpregnant and 23 per cent of pregnant Icelandic women. A multiple observer design, blind study done in the United States on 49 pairs of pregnant and nonpregnant women also failed to show any increase in goiter during pregnancy.[107]

Increased Iodine Excretion During Pregnancy. The differences between these studies have been attributed to differences in the dietary iodine content, which is low in Scotland but high in Iceland and the United States. An early and sustained rise in the renal clearance of iodine has been considered to be the major factor in the decreased plasma inorganic iodine concentration in pregnancy.[1] The increased glomerular filtration rate during pregnancy results in an increased renal loss of iodine, beginning early in pregnancy. The thyroid gland compensates by enlarging and increasing the plasma clearance of iodine to produce sufficient thyroid hormone to maintain the euthyroid state.

Whether goiter ensues depends on the ability of the thyroid gland to compensate, which in turn depends on the concentration of the plasma inorganic iodide. Iodine deficiency goiter is unlikely to occur at a plasma iodine concentration above 0.08 μg per 100 ml.[2] In most Europeans, the plasma inorganic iodine concentration ranges from 0.10 to 0.15 μg per 100 ml and during pregnancy may fall below 0.08 μg per 100 ml.[103] In residents of North America and Iceland, on the other hand, the plasma inorganic iodine is about 0.30 μg per 100 ml. Even if this value is halved during pregnancy, it remains above 0.08 μg per 100 ml. An iodine balance study done in the United States revealed no difference between pregnant and nonpregnant women.[44a] The pregnant woman in North America also has an increased renal clearance of iodine, but ample dietary intake prevents excess iodine loss. Iodized salt should be sufficient to supply an adequate intake of 250 μg of iodine needed during pregnancy, and the iodine in most prenatal vitamin supplements ensures an adequate intake. In areas of marginal iodine intake, e.g., 50 μg per day, supplementary iodine (160 μg per day) given to pregnant women reduced neonatal goiter from 33 to 7 per cent.[181] An excessive iodine intake because of unusual dietary practices, e.g., greater than 2000 μg daily, may cause difficulties for both mother and child and will be subsequently discussed.

Radioiodine Thyroid Uptake

The decreased plasma inorganic iodine concentration during pregnancy results in a smaller iodine pool and an increased thyroid clearance of iodine. Since the thyroid radioiodine uptake depends on the size of the iodine pool in addition to thyroid-stimulating activity, the thyroid radioiodine uptake is elevated in pregnancy.

Specific problems occur with the use of radioisotopes in the pregnant woman, because possible radiation effects on the fetus must be considered. Whether radiation effects depend on a threshold dose is not clear, and all radiation to the fetus should be regarded as harmful.[165]

However, when pregnant women have been studied, the radioactive iodine thyroid uptake has been increased. Three of five women had an elevated radioactive iodine thyroid uptake at 12 weeks of pregnancy.[76] Urinary excretion of administered radioactive iodine is an indirect measure of thyroid uptake. In 22 women in the third trimester, the mean urinary excretion of radioiodine was in the range between normal and thyrotoxic values.[138] However, with this method, maternal thyroid uptake cannot be distinguished from fetal uptake. In one study, the short-lived isotope ^{132}I was administered to 25 pregnant women and the two-hour thyroid uptake measured at 12, 24, and 36 weeks of gestation as well as 1 and 6 weeks post partum.[76] The thyroid uptakes during pregnancy and at least 1 week post partum were significantly elevated compared with both nonpregnant values and those at 6 weeks post partum.

Two pregnant patients also had a triiodothyronine suppression test with this isotope, and thyroid uptake was suppressed to the same extent as in four nonpregnant women. The same worker also compared the effect of a single injection of TSH in three pregnant and three nonpregnant women with a similar response found in both groups. The uptake doubled 22 hours after the administration of TSH and returned to normal on the third day.

Basal Metabolic Rate

Thyroid function was originally monitored by the basal metabolic rate (BMR), and studies indicated that the BMR was elevated in pregnant women.[130] The BMR began to increase during the fourth month of pregnancy and continued to rise slowly until the eighth month. There was a 15 to 20 per cent increase, the largest occurring in patients who had had the lowest BMR when they were not pregnant. Under scrupulously basal conditions, it was demonstrated that the uterus and its contents could account for 70 to 80 per cent of the rise in oxygen consumption above nonpregnant values. Increased maternal work accounted for the rest.[25a]

Although clinical tests continue to be introduced for the appraisal of thyroid function, a true BMR is still a good indicator of overall thyroid function. However, even in experienced hands the BMR correlates with the final clinical appraisal in only about one half of the patients. The major reason is the difficulty in separating basal from total metabolism, which includes increases in oxygen consumption from digestive and muscular activity. Only the true basal metabolism is a measure of thyroid activity. Most errors in the interpretation of the BMR are due to a failure to recognize this distinction.

Thyroxine-Binding Globulin

The other major change in thyroid function during pregnancy is a rise in thyroxine-binding globulin concentrations to about twice normal values. The increased estrogens in pregnancy induce thyroxine-binding globulin and cause a fall in thyroxine-binding pre-albumin capacity.[66, 148] About 85 per cent of thyroid hormone is transported in serum-bound thyroxine-binding globulin (TBG), and 15 per cent by thyroxine-binding prealbumin (TBPA). The maximum binding capacity of these proteins can be determined by the addition of saturating concentrations of thyroxine. TBG has a normal binding capacity that ranges from 19 to 30 μg per 100 ml of thyroxine and increases to 40 to 60 μg per 100 ml of thyroxine during pregnancy. TBG concentration can also be measured directly by radioimmunoassay and has a normal range of 12.5 $\pm$ 0.75 mg per

1 which increases to 24.9 ± 1.08 mg per 1 during pregnancy.[19] The maximum binding capacity for TBPA has been determined to be 219 to 393 μg thyroxine per 100 ml.[140] Although TBPA has a greater binding capacity for thyroxine, TBG has a greater affinity and actually binds more thyroxine in vivo. Thyroxine binds more tightly to TBG than does triiodothyronine. This difference in affinity of TBG for thyroxine and triiodothyronine is the basis for the resin triiodothyronine uptake. The role of the increased TBG in pregnancy has also been studied by examining pregnant patients with partial or total TBG deficiency.[136, 148] Although there was no increase or only a minimal increase in TBG during pregnancy, no significant changes in thyroid function occurred. Serum thyroxine does not increase unless there is an increase in TBG. Conversely, there must be adequate amounts of thyroid hormone produced to maintain normal thyroid function in the presence of increased binding. In one study, the administration of estrogen to euthyroid patients resulted in an increase in the serum protein–bound iodine concentration; however, no increase was noted in hypothyroid patients receiving inadequate thyroid hormone replacement even though estrogens resulted in an increase in thyroxine-binding capacity.[48]

Although hazardous, the temptation to speculate on the reason for estrogen induction of TBG is overwhelming. A number of hepatic proteins are induced during pregnancy, including cortisol-binding globulin, ceruloplasmin, and the blood clotting factors I, VII, and IX. Perhaps the increased estrogens during pregnancy switch on a genome that results in the increase in certain clotting factors and incidentally in an increase in TBG.

Thyroxine Production During Pregnancy

After free thyroid hormones enter the cell, they exert their effect, perhaps by binding to nuclear receptors and initiating new protein synthesis. Thyroid hormone is subsequently degraded, and this degradation can be measured with radio-isotope-labeled thyroxine. In the steady state, thyroxine degradation is a measure of thyroid hormone production. Serum thyroxine has an approximate volume of distribution of 10 liters. With a normal serum thyroxine of 8 μg per 100 ml, the entire thyroidal pool of thyroxine is approximately 800 μg T_4. Thyroxine disappears from the serum of a euthyroid nonpregnant adult with a half-life of 6 to 8 days, which results in a fractional turnover of about 10 per cent per day.

Therefore, about 10 per cent of the extrathyroidal pool of T_4, or about 80 μg, turns over per day. In a steady state, 80 μg of T_4 is produced daily.

One study showed a decrease in the fractional rate of thyroxine turnover when thyroxine-binding globulin capacity was increased by estrogen administration.[41] The authors suggested that thyroxine binding by TBG exerted a rate-limiting effect upon the peripheral metabolism of thyroid hormone. However, the absolute rate of thyroid hormone disposal was unchanged, because the total serum thyroxine concentration increased. In another study, net thyroxine turnover and presumably thyroid hormone requirements were unchanged in normal human pregnancy.[40] Net thyroxine turnover was 90 μg per day in the nonpregnant women and 97 μg per day in the pregnant women. The two values were identical when expressed as the daily turnover per square meter of body surface. These findings are for one period in pregnancy, but because of necessary restrictions on the use of radioisotopes in pregnant women, further data will not be available. Increased thyroxine turnover has been reported during pregnancy in monkeys.[170]

Most of the studies of thyroid hormone turnover in pregnancy have concerned thyroxine, because until recently, triiodothyronine was considered to be relatively unimportant in thyroid hormone economy. However, triiodothyronine is now known to be the major thyroid hormone. The weaker binding affinity of TBG for triiodothyronine leads to a greater volume of distribution and a more rapid turnover. Triiodothyronine has been estimated to have an extrathyroidal distribution space of approximately 40 liters with a fractional turnover rate of 70 per cent per day. The T_3 extrathyroidal pool approximates 45 μg. Therefore, T_3 turnover would approximate 33 μg per day. Since T_3 is three or four times as potent as T_4 on a weight basis, the metabolic effects of triiodothyronine would at least equal those of thyroxine.

Laboratory Tests of Thyroid Function

The increase in thyroxine-binding globulin results in changes in the laboratory parameters of thyroid function. These changes are important to understand because diagnostic and therapeutic decisions are based on the interpretation of these laboratory tests. Before the radioimmunoassay for TBG was developed, determination of thyroxine-binding capacity was technically difficult. Therefore, an indirect measure of thyroxine-

RIA for TBG.

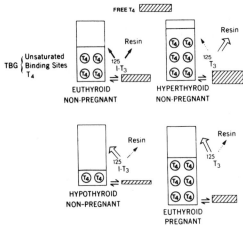

FIGURE 8–1. Resin triiodothyronine uptake. The clear area represents the unsaturated binding sites on TBG. In a hypothyroid nonpregnant woman there is less bound thyroid hormone and more available binding sites. Conversely, in hyperthyroidism there are fewer unsaturated binding sites, and more $^{125}I\text{-}T_3$ binds to the resin. In the pregnant woman the increase in TBG results in an increase in bound thyroid hormone, but there are also an increased number of unsaturated binding sites compared with the nonpregnant state, and less $^{125}I\text{-}T_3$ binds to the resin.

binding capacity was, and still is, obtained with the resin T_3 uptake (RT_3U) test[177] (Fig. 8–1). With the increase in TBG during pregnancy, there is a marked increase in the number of thyroxine-binding sites. Even though more thyroid hormone is bound, the number of unsaturated binding sites still exceeds normal nonpregnant levels. As a consequence, the RT_3U tends to be in the hypothyroid range during pregnancy. The exact values depend on the particular test used. The combination of an elevated serum thyroxine and an RT_3U in the hypothyroid range is characteristic of pregnancy. However, any condition that increases thyroid-binding protein capacity may result in similar changes.

Serum T_4 and T_3. Serum thyroxine and triiodothyronine concentrations are now determined directly by radioimmunoassay. These determinations measure the total thyroxine or triiodothyronine content in the serum and therefore are elevated during pregnancy because of the increased thyroid hormone binding (Fig. 8–2). The serum T_4 and T_3 concentrations are significantly elevated early in pregnancy and remain elevated throughout gestation.[78, 141] The values return to normal shortly after delivery.[187] Although triiodothyronine may play a dominant role in thyroid hormone economy, changes in the serum thyroxine concentration are for the most part mimicked by changes in serum triiodothyronine. Therefore, a serum thyroxine determination usually will suffice as an indicator of thyroid function during pregnancy. Since the total thyroxine concentration is being determined, this should be accompanied by some measure of thyroxine-binding capacity such as RT_3U.

Free Thyroid Hormone. Although the bound thyroxine and triiodothyronine are increased, the free or unbound thyroid hormones have been found within the normal range. Although there is disagreement,[90] two recent studies have reported elevated values for both free T_4 and free T_3 (Fig. 8–3).[78, 187] In the larger study the elevated levels were not above the normal range of the nonpregnant female controls, and this was borne out by a third study.[141] Urinary thyroid hormone levels correlate closely with circulating free thyroid hormone concentrations.[28] The increase in free thyroid hormone concentration could result from changes in peripheral metabolism or increased

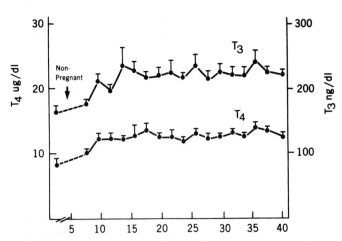

WEEK OF PREGNANCY

FIGURE 8–2. Serum T_4 and T_3 concentrations during pregnancy. Nonpregnant control values are at left. Values are based on samples obtained from 339 women; each point represents mean ± S.E.M. (Modified from Harada et al.: J. Clin. Endocrinol. Metab., *48*:793, 1979.)

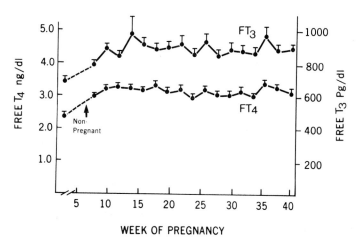

FIGURE 8–3. Serum free T_4 and free T_3 concentrations during pregnancy. Nonpregnant control values are at left. Values are based on samples obtained from 339 women; each point represents mean ± S.E.M. (Modified from Harada et al.: J. Clin. Endocrinol. Metab., *48*:793, 1979.)

secretion of thyroid hormone. As mentioned previously, there are no data clearly relating the slightly elevated free thyroid hormone concentrations with altered metabolic effects of thyroid hormones.

The absolute concentration of free T_4 and T_3 is determined with tracer amounts of ^{125}I-T_4 and equilibrium dialysis of the patient's serum. A per cent of dialyzable fraction is found and, when multiplied by the serum thyroxine determination, yields the free thyroxine concentration. The free thyroxine concentration is the only direct method of estimating thyroid function that compensated for changes in the TBG capacity, but the procedure is technically difficult. Recently another method of determining the free thyroxine concentration, utilizing the kinetics of binding to ligands such as glass beads, has been developed.[185] The determination is relatively easy to perform and will probably supplant the more cumbersome and technically difficult equilibrium dialysis method. However, in some of the procedures the values are not accurate in the presence of large amounts of thyroid-binding protein, like those present during pregnancy.[185]

To compensate for the effect of increased thyroxine binding on the serum thyroxine, a derived value, the free thyroxine index has been obtained. Derived from the determination of the serum thyroxine and the RT_3U, the free thyroxine index gives an indirect approximation of the absolute free thyroid hormone concentration. However, like some of the nonequilibrium dialysis methods, the test may not provide a true index of free T_4 concentration.[19, 163a] This may be due to the failure of the resin T_3 uptake test to determine TBG capacity accurately. Whatever the cause, the free thyroxine index is not directly proportional to the free thyroxine concentration, and the two tests should not be used interchangeably in the pregnant woman.

Hypothalamic-Pituitary-Thyroid Axis

Thyroid hormone secretion is dependent on TSH, and TSH secretion in turn is dependent on the circulating thyroid hormone concentration. Thyroid function is therefore an example of the classic negative feedback mechanism. The level of thyroid hormone — particularly pituitary triiodothyronine, which shuts off TSH — is determined by thyrotropin-releasing hormone, a tri-peptide, L-pyroglutamyl-L-histidyl-L-prolineamide. This hypothalamic releasing hormone determines the set point at which circulating thyroid hormone suppresses TSH secretion of the pituitary.

There are conflicting reports about the responsiveness of the hypothalamic-pituitary-thyroid axis during pregnancy. Two pregnant women given 80 μg of T_3 for 1 week had depression of the thyroidal ^{131}I uptake similar to that in nonpregnant controls.[145] The increase in ^{131}I uptake with TSH was also similar in pregnant and in nonpregnant women. Pregnant women in the second and third trimester were suppressed with 75 to 125 μg T_3 daily for 7 days. Thyroid uptakes were suppressed to the same extent as in nonpregnant women.[180] Serum protein-bound iodine values fell more than 1.0 μg per 100 ml at all time periods studied, but more triiodothyronine was needed to lower the serum PBI concentration in the latter months of pregnancy. Some patients did not respond regardless of the dose of triiodothyronine. One group found that only one of five pregnant women who received 150 to 200 μg T_3 daily had a serum PBI determination consistent with complete suppression.[150] The ^{131}I thyroidal uptake appears to be normally responsive to thyroid hormone suppression during pregnancy, but the serum PBI concentration is not. Part of this apparent lack of responsiveness may be due to the increase in TBG during pregnancy.

We administered TRH to patients in different stages of pregnancy who were to undergo therapeutic abortion.[25] Women between 16 and 20 weeks of pregnancy had an increased TSH response to TRH compared with patients in the 6th to 12th weeks of pregnancy. This increase appeared to be due to estrogens, since nonpregnant women on oral contraceptive steroids also had a greater response to TRH. Other workers, however, have not found an increased TSH response to TRH in pregnant women.[93a, 175, 188] The failure to find an increase in the TSH response to TRH might be due to iodine deficiency,[108] although the mechanism is not clear. TRH crosses the placenta and stimulates the fetal pituitary in animal studies.[36, 101] TRH activity was found in the human placenta,[159] and lower levels of thyrotropin-releasing hormone degrading activity were found in both cord and maternal sera compared with sera from euthyroid nonpregnant adults.[134] These data all suggest that TRH may play a role in the modulation of thyroid function during pregnancy. However, fetal pituitary TSH secretion appears to be controlled independently of both the maternal and the fetal hypothalamus.

Thyroid-Stimulating Activity. TSH concentrations during pregnancy have been reported to be within normal limits[55] or slightly increased during the early trimesters.[115a, 150a] These conflicting results are attributable in part to lack of sensitivity of particular assays. Recent work suggests that serum TSH concentrations are not increased during pregnancy and in fact are decreased during the early weeks of gestation (Fig. 8–3).[78, 187]

Three thyroid stimulators have been reported in normal pregnancy: normal pituitary TSH (hTSH), chorionic TSH (hCT), and chorionic gonadotropin (hCG). In patients with hydatidiform mole and choriocarcinoma, markedly elevated levels of hCG may result in hyperthyroidism.[83, 93]

Material with thyrotropic activity has been extracted from some human placentas (hCT).[81a] Bioassayable thyrotropin in the serum of pregnant women, as well as hCT activity in the placenta, has been found.[80b] With improved assays, the levels of hCT have been found to be quite low. Only one third of the samples in one report contained more than 0.25 μU per ml of activity.[78] With improved techniques it has also

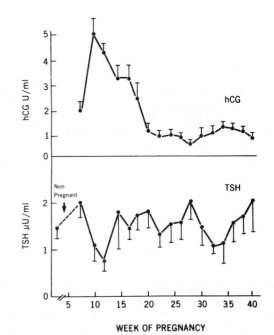

FIGURE 8–4. Serum hTSH and hCG concentrations during pregnancy. Nonpregnant control values are at left. Values are based on samples obtained from 339 women; each point represents mean ± SEM. (Modified from Harada et al.: J. Clin. Endocrinol. Metab., *48*:793, 1979.)

been impossible to recover significant hCT activity from the placenta.[77] hCT does not appear to play a significant role in the modulation of thyroid function during pregnancy.

On the other hand, hCG has an activity in the TSH bioassay of 0.2 μU TSH per U hCG.[78] Based on this activity, hCG concentrations in early pregnancy would be equivalent to 3 to 10 μU TSH per ml. The concentrations of TSH activity are high enough to stimulate thyroid function mildly. The slight decrease in serum TSH concentrations might be explained by the increase in hCG[78, 187] (Fig. 8–4). However, recent studies have suggested that pure hCG may not have intrinsic thyrotropic activity.[7]

FETAL THYROID FUNCTION

The fetal thyroid gland must reach a certain stage of development before thyroid hormone is produced. Any thyroid hormone necessary for fetal development before that stage is reached must be supplied by the maternal thyroid.

Ontogenesis of Thyroid Function

No organic iodine is present in the fetal thyroid gland before 10 weeks.[159a] By 11 to 12 weeks of gestation, the fetal thyroid attains maturity with the ability to produce iodotyrosines and iodothyronines. When radioactive iodine was administered to women immediately prior to termination of pregnancy, the fetus was found to concentrate iodine at about 12 to 14 weeks.[30, 50, 81] Serum TSH is detectable in fetal serum as early as 10 weeks[71] but remains relatively low until 20 weeks of gestation, when it increases over the next 10 weeks to 15 μU per ml and then falls until it is about 7 μU per ml.[139] Fetal serum T_4 concentrations progressively increase in response to the TGH rise after midgestation, increasing from 2 to 3 μg per 100 ml at 10 weeks to 5 to 10 μg per 100 ml at 30 weeks. A similar progressive increment in serum free thyroxine also occurs.[55] These data suggest that fetal pituitary control of thyroid function must exist as early as 12 weeks of gestation and 1 month of postnatal life. The ability of anencephalic fetuses to synthesize iodotyrosines has been taken as evidence that TSH is not necessary. However, careful studies suggest that in these fetuses pituitary tissue is usually present but the hypothalamus is absent; in fact, it was demonstrated that anencephalic fetuses had a hyperresponse of TSH to thyrotropin-releasing hormone.[80b]

Requirements for Fetal Thyroid Hormone. Whether the fetus requires its own thyroid hormone or whether the hormone can be supplied by the mother is unresolved. Fetal access to maternal thyroid hormone is suggested by athyreotic infants who are normal or only mildly retarded at birth. However, maternal thyroid hormone probably cannot completely replace fetal thyroid production, and most athyreotic infants do show a lack of thyroid hormone. The role of maternal thyroid hormone in early fetal development remains unknown, but it does not appear to be necessary during the latter part of pregnancy.[164]

Amniotic Fluid

The increased frequency of amniocentesis in pregnant women has led to an interest in thyroid hormone concentrations in amniotic fluid. Thyroid-stimulating hormone has been difficult to detect in amniotic fluid.[31] During the first half of pregnancy, amniotic fluid thyroxine concentrations increase progressively, reaching peak concentrations at 25 to 30 weeks (Fig. 8–5).[9a, 100] Amniotic fluid triiodothyronine concentrations are low during early pregnancy and increase slowly. During the last half of pregnancy, amniotic fluid thyroxine concentrations decrease

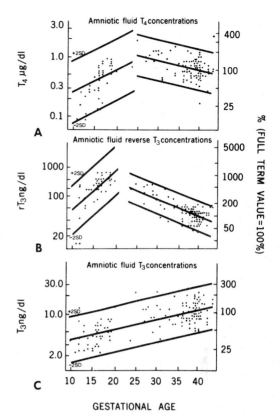

FIGURE 8–5. Amniotic fluid T_4, T_3, and reverse T_3 concentrations during pregnancy. *A,* Amniotic fluid T_4 concentrations. The vertical axis on the left is a logarithmic scale of standard concentrations and the one on the right is the percentage of the term mean value ± 2 SD calculated from the regression lines, which are also plotted. *B,* Amniotic fluid reverse T_3 concentrations plotted in the same manner. *C,* Amniotic fluid T_3 concentrations plotted in the same manner. (From Klein et al.: Am. J. Obstet. Gynecol.,*136*:626, 1980. Reprinted with permission.)

while amniotic fluid triiodothyronine continues to increase. Most of the triiodothyronines (3,5,3'-triiodothyronine) are formed from monodeiodination of the outer ring. Deiodination of the inner ring produces 3,3',5'-triiodothyronine, or reverse T_3 (rT_3), which has minimal biological activity. In the fetus thyroxine is predominantly metabolized to rT_3, perhaps because of immaturity of the enzyme systems.[31] Reverse T_3 concentrations are markedly increased in the amniotic fluid, reaching peak levels at 17 to 20 weeks. This pattern of change in amniotic fluid thyroid hormones is compatible with an increase in 5'-iodothyronine monodeiodinase activity in the fetal compartment.

Whether amniotic fluid thyroid hormone concentrations reflect the fetal compartment is of particular interest. The suggestion has been made that amniotic fluid iodothyronine concentrations

TABLE 8–1 THYROID FUNCTION TESTS IN MATERNAL AND CORD BLOOD AT TERM

Test	Maternal	Cord
Serum thyroxine (μg/100 ml)	10.0–16.0	6.0–13.0
Free thyroxine (ng/100 ml)	2.5–3.5	1.5–3.0
Serum triiodothyronine (ng/100 ml)	150–250	40–60
Reverse triiodothyronine (ng/100 ml)	35–65	80–360
Resin T_3 uptake (per cent)	10	10–15
TBG (μg/100 ml)	40–50	10–16
Serum TSH (μU/ml)	0–6	0–20

Absolute values for these tests may vary according to the method used, but the relation between maternal and cord values should remain constant.

can be used for the prenatal diagnosis of fetal thyroid abnormalities[31, 85] A normal amniotic fluid rT_3 concentration was found in a fetus whose mother had inadvertently received a therapeutic dose of ^{131}I at 10 to 11 weeks gestation. The infant was treated with thyroxine injected into the amniotic fluid and was euthyroid at birth.[108] Furthermore, the amniotic fluid rT_3 concentration rose after the T_4 injection. However, amniotic fluid concentrations have been found to be high in a hypothyroid child and low in a normal infant.[105] TRH also has been found in amniotic fluid.[126]

Neonatal Thyroid Function

Serum T_3 values in cord serum are low, and reverse T_3 concentrations are elevated (Table 8–1). Immediately following birth there is a sharp rise in the serum TSH concentration caused by increased pituitary secretion of TSH.[58] TRH degrading activity is absent in the newborn but appears after three days.[8] This acute surge in TSH may be mediated by TRH secretion, which has been reported to be elevated in newborns.[111] Neonatal serum TSH concentration increases minutes after birth from a mean of 7.5 μU per ml to a peak of 30 μU per ml within 3 hours (Fig. 8–6).[171] In response to TSH stimulation, there is a sharp increase in total and free serum thyroxine concentrations. Serum triiodothyronine also increases dramatically, but this rise is at least in part TSH-independent.[154] Neonatal tissues rapidly acquire an increased capacity to monodeiodinate T_4 to T_3, which contributes importantly to the early rise in serum T_3 concentration and the fall in serum reverse T_3 concentrations. The capacity of neonatal tissues to monodeiodinate T_4 to T_3 is reflected in the progressively changing serum T_3/T_4, rT_3/T_4 ratios between 30 weeks gestation and the first postnatal month.[54]

Neonatal radioactive iodine thyroid uptake is elevated as early as 10 hours postpartum. Thyroid uptake reaches a peak by the second day and drops to adult normal limits by the fifth day post partum.[57] The plasma inorganic iodine and iodine pool are increased, as is the absolute amount of iodide taken up by the thyroid gland.[146] The factors responsible for this stimulation of iodide transport are unknown but probably involve more than stimulation of the hypothalamic-pituitary-thyroid axis.

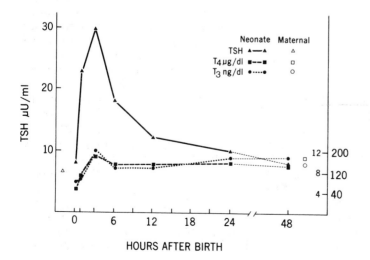

FIGURE 8–6. Serum TSH, T_4, and T_3 concentrations during the first 48 hours in the neonate. (Modified from Stubbe et al.: Horm. Metab. Res., *10*:58, 1978.)

TABLE 8–2 PLACENTAL TRANSFER AND FETAL THYROID FUNCTION

Placental transfer without difficulty
  Iodides
  Thioamides
  Thyroid-stimulating immunoglobulins
  TRH

No transfer
  TSH

Minimal transfer
  T_3
  T_4

PLACENTAL TRANSFER

Any effect of maternal thyroid hormone on the fetus must depend on placental transfer. In fact there are a number of agents that may affect fetal thyroid function depending upon whether or not they are transferred across the placental barrier (Table 8–2).

Transfer of Thyroid Hormone

Pregnant women at term were administered ^{131}I-T_3 or T_4, and the ratio of radioactivity in maternal and fetal sera was determined at the time of delivery.[73a] Both hormones were transferred slowly, but ^{131}I-T_3 appeared to be transferred at a faster rate. Similar observations were made of women who had received the isotopes between the 11th and 26th weeks of pregnancy prior to therapeutic abortion. In another study, 13 pregnant women were given infusions of 500 to 8000 μg of L-thyroxine at term, and the serum PBI and RT_3U were determined in maternal and cord blood.[56] Neonatal serum BEI values increased progressively with increasing amounts of maternal hormone and increasing diffusion time, but the values did not approach those of maternal sera. The placenta again appeared to be relatively impermeable to thyroxine, at least at term, and placental impermeability persisted despite progressive saturation of maternal TBG and a presumed increase in maternal free thyroxine concentrations.

Triiodothyronine was administered to pregnant women for 4 to 6 weeks before delivery and serum thyroxine determined in maternal and cord sera.[150] Transfer of triiodothyronine across the placenta would be expected to decrease fetal TSH with a resulting decrease in serum T_4 values. In five of eight infants born to mothers who had received 300 μg T_3 daily, which is approximately three times the normal dose, serum T_4 values were low. In the other three children, however, values were comparable with control values. Little decrease in cord blood T_4 was noted in infants whose mothers received 150 to 200 μg T_3 daily. The need to administer large doses of triiodothyronine in order to suppress cord blood T_4 again appeared to reflect placental impermeability. In a similar study, the serum T_3 concentration was determined directly in maternal and cord blood.[44] Cord serum T_3 concentrations were elevated in those infants who had a decrease in serum T_4, but again there was evidence of minimal placental transfer.

Available evidence suggests that triiodothyronine and thyroxine cross the placenta but do so with difficulty. Placental transfer of thyroid hormone may also change with duration of pregnancy and aging of the placenta. Triiodothyronine appears to cross more easily than thyroxine; however, fetal serum triiodothyronine concentrations are normally low. The available evidence suggests that thyroid hormone transfer across the placenta is such that administration of physiologic amounts of thyroid hormone to the mother is not helpful in elevating the fetal serum thyroid hormone concentration.

Animal studies have indicated that it may be possible to modify the structure of the thyroid hormone molecule to increase placental transfer. A nonhalogenated thyroid hormone analog, dimethyl-isopropyl thyronine (DIMIT), was found by us to be 20 times as effective as thyroxine in preventing fetal rat goiter without inducing maternal thyrotoxicosis.[32] Placental transfer depends on molecular weight, protein binding, and lipid solubility,[9] and DIMIT is smaller, binds less tightly, and is more lipid soluble than thyroxine. Whether DIMIT has any role in the treatment of hypothyroidism in utero is not clear. The data raise the possibility that the thyroid hormone molecule can be altered to improve transfer across the placenta.

MATERNAL HYPOTHYROIDISM

Hypothyroidism is relatively uncommon in the pregnant patient.[63] This low incidence of hypothyroidism during pregnancy, coupled with the widely held belief that fertility and thyroid function are closely related, is probably responsible for statements that hypothyroid women are infertile.[147]

"The relationship of the thyroid gland to the sex organs is the most ancient and classical interrelation of the function of the glands of internal secretion. Known to the ancients and a subject of daily gossip, it was passed down through the ages."[110]

In one study, 7 of 10 myxedematous women were anovulatory.[68]

Because of this reported association with infertility as well as the absence of definitive therapy, thyroid hormone has been administered to euthyroid infertile women. Desiccated thyroid hormone or placebo was given to 339 euthyroid women with either infertility or menstrual disorders; 75 infertile women eventually received thyroid hormone and 50 received placebo. The authors concluded that thyroid hormone appeared to have no definite benefit.[26] We have treated 20 women who had no identifiable causes of infertility with a combination of thyroxine and triiodothyronine or placebo in a randomized double-blind study. Two of 6 women who received thyroid hormone became pregnant, while 6 of the 14 women who had received placebo also became pregnant. Controlled studies offer no support for the use of thyroid hormone for infertility in euthyroid women.

Pregnancy Outcome in Hypothyroidism

Animal data suggest that mild or moderate hypothyroidism has a minimal effect on fertility, although hypothyroid animals do have difficulty maintaining pregnancy.[91a] This was confirmed in a study of 244 pregnant hypothyroid women in whom the rate of stillbirth was double that in controls.[137] Other workers studied a group of children whose mothers had proved or suspected thyroid disorders during pregnancy. The outcome of six of seven pregnancies in women with clinically suspected hypothyroidism and low BEI values was poor. In addition to a spontaneous abortion and a stillbirth, one child was born with congenital defects and three children had undifferentiated developmental retardation at 8 months of age. Only two of the mothers had received even inadequate thyroid hormone replacement during pregnancy. Although there was no firm evidence that these women were actually hypothyroid, an attenuated rise in the serum BEI concentration was associated with a poor pregnancy outcome.

One group monitored thyroid function in women during pregnancy and subsequently obtained developmental data on the children born to these mothers.[119] About 4 per cent of pregnancies were classified as "hypothyroxinemic" based on two low thyroid hormone values relative to normal pregnancy values or one low value in conjunction with clinical hypothyroidism, previous reproductive failure, or thyroidectomy. Of the 135 pregnancies in which the diagnosis of "hypothyroxinemia" was made, 81 per cent of infants examined 8 months post partum whose mothers had received adequate thyroid hormone replacement were classified as normal. In comparison, only 46 per cent of infants whose mothers had received inadequate replacement were classified as normal. In a 7 year followup study, the progeny of inadequately treated "hypothyroxinemic" women had lower psychologic scores.[118] There was no compelling clinical evidence that these patients were actually hypothyroid, and perhaps their socioeconomic situation might have played a role in the poor outcome. The premise that there may be significant numbers of women with subclinical hypothyroidism that only becomes apparent during pregnancy should be viewed with caution.

Thyroid Function and Spontaneous Abortion. Since hypothyroid women experience increased fetal loss, serum thyroid hormone determinations were done in women who aborted; these were found to be low.[116] Low values were not found, however, in patients who had induced abortions.[60] Followup studies indicated that patients with low thyroid hormone values who aborted were euthyroid and presumably had not been hypothyroid during pregnancy.[112] The data suggested that the low serum thyroid values were secondary to the abortion rather than the cause. Presumably, fetal death resulted in decreased estrogen production with a concomitant decrease in TBG and serum thyroid hormone concentration.

The balance of evidence suggests that the great majority of women with early spontaneous abortions have normal thyroid function. Since the low serum thyroxine merely reflects the decreased estrogen production and TBG, there is no reason to suppose that thyroid hormone would be helpful in these situations.[135] However, hypothyroidism does occur during pregnancy, and decreased thyroid function should be considered in pregnant women with low serum thyroxine concentrations. In one study of 31 women who had previously had at least one spontaneous abortion, half of the women had some evidence of diminished thyroid reserve as determined by TSH responsiveness.[133]

Pregnancy in Hypothyroid Women. Myxedematous patients have been reported to carry their pregnancies to term successfully (Fig. 8–7).[84, 94, 104, 125] Any thyroid hormone necessary for fetal growth before the second trimester must therapy. Idiopathic hypothyroidism is a more insidious cause of decreased thyroid function and is related to Hashimoto's disease. An interesting association has been noted in that mothers of children with Down's syndrome have sometimes been found to have high titers of thyroid antibodies.[52] The reason suggested is that maternal thyroid autoimmunity predisposes to aneuploidy in the child and plays a major role in the birth of children with Down's syndrome in younger mothers. Hashimoto's disease is more common in patients with diabetes mellitus; in one study of 100 diabetic women, 20 per cent of Class D and F diabetics also had Hashimoto's disease.[163]

Regardless of the cause, hypothyroid patients may complain of cold intolerance, constipation, cool dry skin, coarse hair, inability to concentrate, and irritability. However, euthyroid pregnant women may also complain of the same symptoms, which makes the clinical diagnosis difficult. Paresthesia is an early symptom in about 75 per cent of patients with hypothyroidism and may be helpful in the diagnosis. A pregnant woman is unlikely to present with gross myxedema, and the obvious signs, including a low body temperature, periorbital edema, large tongue, and hoarse voice, are the exception rather than the rule. The patient may feel more fatigued than she felt during previous pregnancies and may complain of coarse hair and dry skin. Delayed deep tendon reflexes would be very helpful in making the diagnosis. Postpartum amenorrhea and galactorrhea associated with hyperprolactinemia may be indicative of hypothyroidism.[95, 173a]

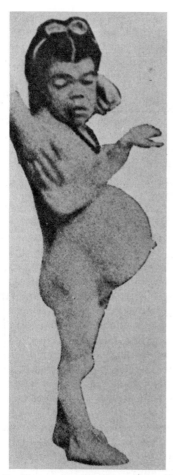

FIGURE 8–7. Pregnant cretin. (From Osler, W.: Sporadic cretinism in America. Transactions of the Congress of American Physicians and Surgeons, 1897. Reprinted with permission.)

come from the maternal side. In severely hypothyroid mothers this hormone would be lacking. Although the offspring have not been subjected to extensive developmantal testing, they have been reported as normal.[147] Whether maternal thyroid hormone is absolutely necessary for fetal development is not clear; certainly, it is desirable. The suggestion has been made that fetal-maternal transfer of thyroxine may occur under these circumstances. In one patient the BMR increased from −40 per cent to −4 per cent with a subsequent decrease again to −28 per cent after delivery of a euthyroid baby.[18] However, such changes are probably due to the pregnancy.

Diagnosis of Hypothyroidism

Hypothyroidism is most commonly iatrogenic following either surgery or radioactive iodine

TABLE 8–3 INITIAL THYROID FUNCTION TESTS IN NINE PREGNANT HYPOTHYROID WOMEN

	Normal, Nonpregnant Range	Mean Pregnant, Hypothyroid
Serum T_4 μg/100 ml	4.5–13.2	2.2
Serum T_3 ng/100 ml	100–200	84
RT_3U	0.88–1.19	.61
TSH μU/ml	0–5	40

Pregnant hypothyroid values represent mean of initial values from nine hypothyroid women presenting between 8 and 30 weeks of gestation. (From Montoro et al., Ann. Intern. Med., *94*:31, 1981)

The most sensitive indicator of primary hypothyroidism is an elevated serum TSH determination in association with a low serum thyroxine concentration. Because of the elevated TBG in pregnancy, the serum thyroxine determination may not be as low as would be expected. The RT_3U is not very helpful because the increased unsaturated binding sites are difficult to quantitate. Representative thyroid function test results are shown in Table 8–3. Thyroid antibodies may provide supporting evidence for hypothyroidism, particularly in the absence of a past history of surgery or radioactive iodine therapy. Elevated serum cholesterol and carotene concentrations occur in hypothyroidism but are not helpful in the diagnosis. During normal pregnancy, serum cholesterol concentration may increase 60 per cent above prepregnancy values.

Therapy of Hypothyroidism During Pregnancy

Once the diagnosis of hypothyroidism has been made in the pregnant woman, full replacement doses of L-thyroxine should be given immediately, regardless of the degree of thyroid function. Although L-triiodothyronine may cross the placenta with greater facility than L-thyroxine, serum T_3 concentrations in the mother rise to thyrotoxic values, and normal fetal serum T_3 concentrations are very low. In the young pregnant woman without other complications, therapy can be begun rapidly even if the patient experiences some initial discomfort. One reasonable schedule is 0.15 mg of L-thyroxine daily for 3 weeks and then readjustment of the dose depending on the thyroid function test results. Thyroxine need only be given once a day because of the long half-life. With adequate treatment, the serum TSH concentration should decrease to values below 6 μU per ml, and the serum T_4 concentration should increase to normal values for pregnancy. If the values do not return to normal, the dose of L-thyroxine should be increased by 0.05 mg increments. In the study illustrated by Table 8–3, the dose of L-thyroxine administered ranged from 0.15 mg to 0.30 mg daily.[125]

Pregnant Women Receiving Thyroid Hormone. The number of women in whom hypothyroidism is diagnosed during pregnancy is small. More commonly, pregnant women are receiving thyroid hormone when first seen, and the initial diagnosis of hypothyroidism may have been obscure. Either thyroid hormone therapy can be stopped for 5 to 6 weeks and the patient reevaluated, or full doses of thyroid hormone can be given for the rest of the pregnancy. Since hypothyroidism, if present, would represent a risk to the continuation of the pregnancy, the latter course seems wiser because the possibility of several weeks of decreased thyroid function is obviated. To be sure the pregnant woman is receiving adequate thyroid hormone, full replacement doses must be given. During the postpartum period, thyroid hormone can be discontinued and thyroid function evaluated 5 to 6 weeks later. Normal thyroid function may be suppressed for a number of weeks after prolonged thyroid hormone therapy.

In recent years the recommended replacement dose of L-thyroxine has decreased from 0.3 mg to about 0.15 mg daily, based on the amount of thyroxine necessary to suppress the elevated serum TSH concentration.[167] With the increase in thyroxine bound to TBG during pregnancy, the woman may require more L-thyroxine during that time. In order for the serum thyroxine to increase, there must be an adequate amount of circulating thyroid hormone. In subjects receiving inadequate thyroid hormone replacement, no increase in the serum thyroid hormone iodine concentration occurred despite an increase in thyroxine-binding capacity.[48] If a hypothyroid woman received 0.15 mg or 0.2 mg of L-thyroxine daily before pregnancy, the dose during pregnancy may be increased to 0.2 or 0.25 mg daily. Serum thyroxine concentrations should be monitored during pregnancy.

Postpartum Hypothyroidism

Physiologic and immunologic changes associated with pregnancy ameliorate autoimmune thyroiditis during gestation. In the postpartum period the autoimmune thyroiditis may intensify; transient thyrotoxicosis may develop, followed by transient hypothyroidism.[4, 63] The patients studied often had a previous history of goiter with the development of thyroid enlargement 1 to 4 months post partum. When they were examined carefully, a period of transient thyrotoxicosis was observed, followed by hypothyroidism with spontaneous recovery in 90 per cent of cases at 5 to 10 months post partum. High titers of antithyroid microsomal antibodies were present, and usually a small goiter persisted. Women with a previous episode of postpartum hypothyroidism tended to develop similar episodes with the same severity of hypothyroidism in subsequent pregnancies.

Although usually transient, the hypothyroidism may last for several months, and it is reasonable to treat the patient as though she had classic hypothyroidism. After 3 months of therapy, the administration of thyroid hormone can be stopped and thyroid function re-evaluated.

NEONATAL HYPOTHYROIDISM

Thyroid hormone deficiency during the fetal and neonatal period results in generalized developmental retardation.[82] Both the severity of thyroid hormone deficiency and the time of onset during development play an important role in the degree and potential reversibility of the ensuing brain damage. Hypothyroidism beginning after the age of 2 years appears to exert little if any irreversible effects on mental development. The earlier hypothyroidism occurs during fetal development, the more likely it is that severe retardation will occur.

With the availability of exogenous thyroid hormone therapy, the possibility of reversing mental retardation in cretinous children appeared reasonable. Osler, in 1897, stated: "Not the magic wand of Prospero or the brave kiss of the daughters of Hippocrates ever effected such a change as that which we are now enabled to make in these unfortunate victims doomed heretofore to live in hopeless imbecility, an unspeakable affliction to their parents and their relatives."[142]

Unfortunately, mere availability is not sufficient; for thyroid hormone therapy to be effective it must be started early in life. If hypothyroidism is diagnosed and treated before 3 months of age, four fifths of affected children will have an IQ above 90. Unfortunately, the early clinical diagnosis of congenital hypothyroidism is difficult.[42] Since early diagnosis and treatment of congenital hypothyroidism is important, yet early clinical diagnosis so difficult, the solution is to screen all newborns for congenital hypothyroidism.[21]

Etiology and Incidence

Neonatal thyroid screening programs have provided a great deal of information on the etiology and incidence of congenital hypothyroidism. Congenital hypothyroidism occurs once in about 4000 births. The various causes of congenital hypothyroidism are outlined in Table 8–4. Primary hypothyroidism is most common, about two thirds of children having ectopic thyroids, one third having thyroid agenesis, and a few having dyshormonogenesis.[39] In developing countries where goiter is endemic, the incidence of congenital hypothyroidism may be as common as 14 per cent of births.[49]

TABLE 8–4 ETIOLOGY AND INCIDENCE OF CONGENITAL HYPOTHYROIDISM

Primary hypothyroidism	*Incidence*
Thyroid dysgenesis	1 in 4,000
Inborn errors of thyroid function	1 in 30,000
Drug-induced	1 in 10,000
Endemic hypothyroidism	1 in 7
Secondary and tertiary hypothyroidism	1 in 60,000

Thyroid Dysgenesis. The cause of thyroid dysgenesis is unknown, but there seems to be a hereditary predisposition. Although the term athyreotic cretinism has been used, some thyroid tissue is usually present.[109] Although it has been postulated that thyrocytotoxic factors are transferred across the placenta, most workers believe that thyroid antibodies that do cross the placenta represent a reaction to thyroid injury rather than a primary event. However, transplacental transfer of a thyrosuppressive factor has been observed in one family.[67, 172]

Inborn Errors of Thyroid Function. Approximately one child in 30,000 is born with an inborn error in thyroid function that can result in goitrous cretinism. Usually these children do not have significant thyroid enlargement at birth, but the goiter develops subsequently.[15] These defects in thyroid hormone biosynthesis are inherited as an autosomal recessive trait with a biochemical defect to correspond to each step in hormone biosynthesis. A family history of goitrous cretinism should alert the physician to this possibility in the neonate.

Drug-Induced Hypothyroidism. A number of compounds ingested by the mother may adversely affect fetal thyroid function. Data from the neonatal thyroid screening programs suggest that transient hypothyroidism may occur in 1 in 10,000 births.

An important cause of neonatal goiter and hypothyroidism is maternal iodide ingestion during pregnancy. Although this has been most commonly reported in women receiving large doses of iodides for chronic lung disease, goiters may occur with the maternal ingestion of as little as 12 mg of iodide daily.[27] The large amount of iodides in the radiopaque dyes used for amniography may result in transient neonatal hypothyroidism.[10, 153] Maternal ingestion of iodides appears to produce a relatively greater enlargement of the fetal thyroid, and the goiters may be large and obstructive (Fig. 8–8).[61] The major problem encountered is maintenance of an adequate airway. With a huge goiter, surgery may be necessary. The hypothyroidism is usually transient, but mental retardation has occurred.

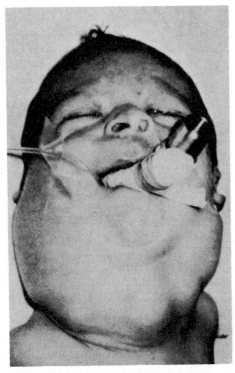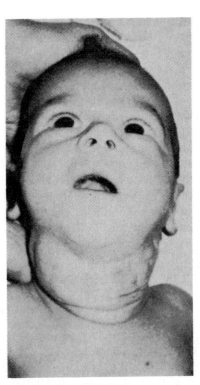

FIGURE 8–8. Iodide-induced neonatal goiter. Left, appearance on the first day of life. Right, appearance at 2 months of age. (From Senior and Chernoff: Pediatrics, 47:510, 1971. Reprinted with permission.)

In contrast to iodides, children who have been exposed to PTU in utero may be born with a small goiter and transient hypothyroidism. Based on screening data, perhaps one infant in 100 who is exposed to PTU in utero will develop transient hypothyroidism.

Diagnosis

During the first weeks of life when the diagnosis is crucial, clinical features of hypothyroidism are so uncommon that the diagnosis is rarely suspected. The clinical features of neonatal hypothyroidism are variable and include prolonged gestation with large size at birth, feeding and respiratory difficulties, constipation, abdominal distention with vomiting, and protracted icterus. Hypothermia, cyanosis, a large posterior fontanel, umbilical hernia, and rough dry skin have commonly been found.[97, 106, 162]

Cretinism may be mistaken for Down's syndrome, because both diseases are characterized by short stature and mental retardation. Howev-

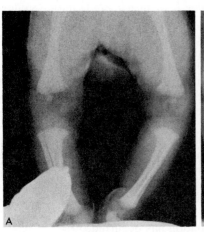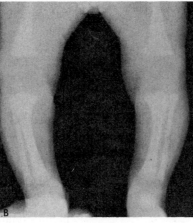

FIGURE 8–9. Distal femoral epiphyses appear in x-ray of normal infant (A) but are absent in a cretin (B). (From Beierwaltes: Hosp. Pract., 3:31, 1968. Reprinted with permission.)

er, the child with Down's syndrome is more active and has specific stigmata. Cretinism may also be confused with the Beckwith-Wiedemann syndrome, which includes umbilical hernia and macroglossia.[53]

A low serum thyroxine (<4 μg per 100 ml) in combination with a very high TSH (>80 μU per 100 ml) is diagnostic of hypothyroidism. Infants with borderline T_4 (4 to 7 μg per 100 ml) or borderline TSH (20 to 80 μU per 100 ml) or both detected in a screening program will require further assessment. Reverse T_3 determinations add little to the diagnosis of neonatal hypothyroidism.[64, 96] X-rays for bone age estimation may be helpful, because the low osteoblastic activity is reflected in a slow rate of skeletal gravity and maturation. In the neonate the lack of ossification of the distal femoral epiphysis on the proximal tibial epiphysis suggests thyroid hormone deficiency in utero.[113] Epiphyseal dysgenesis is commonly seen in the proximal femoral epiphysis but may affect any center of endochondral ossification.[183] The ossification center appears late and at first is not a single center but multiple small centers scattered throughout the epiphysis (Fig. 8–9). These centers eventually coalesce to form a single center with an irregular shape and a stippled appearance.

Therapy of Congenital Hypothyroidism

If thyroid hormone is to be effective, therapy must be started as soon as possible after birth. Early treatment will minimize the degree of mental retardation.[43, 99] In the most complete study, 35 hypothyroid infants were compared by the Griffiths Developmental Test with 37 normal children having comparable socioeconomic characteristics for age and sex.[43] The results indicated that at 12 and 18 months, early treatment of hypothyroidism resulted in a mean IQ above 100. There were no statistically significant differences between the two groups in any of the scores at age 12 months. However, at age 18 months there was a significant decrease in the global quotient in the hypothyroid infants compared with normal control infants. No hypothyroid child had a quotient below 85. Whether these results indicate the first signs of minimal brain damage remains to be determined.

When an infant with possible hypothyroidism is identified by the screening program, a complete evaluation including a thyroid scan should be done. Infants with residual thyroid tissue, no signs or symptoms of hypothyroidism, and a normal bone age and serum T_3 concentration have an excellent prognosis for normal development. Infants without visible thyroid tissue, with detectable signs of bone age retardation, and with low serum T_4 and T_3 concentrations have a more guarded prognosis for entirely normal development, even with early treatment.

The preferred therapeutic approach is the prompt institution of oral L-thyroxine at an initial dose of 50 μg per day. Readjustment of the thyroxine dose on the basis of clinical signs and symptoms and thyroid function tests should be done within the first 4 weeks of therapy. Too much thyroid hormone is equally undesirable for the developing brain.[16] In doubtful cases, when transient hypothyroidism has not been excluded, cessation of therapy and reassessment of thyroid function after the age of 1 to 3 years may be desirable.

In Utero Therapy. Because of the possibility that irreversible central nervous system damage may occur before birth in congenital hypothyroidism, there has been interest in intrauterine treatment of fetal hypothyroidism. As previously discussed, the intrauterine diagnosis of hypothyroidism is difficult.[100, 105] In one instance, intramuscular T_4 was administered to the fetus because the mother had radioablation of the thyroid in the 13th week of pregnancy.[176] The last dose of T_4 was given 2 weeks before delivery. At birth, cord blood T_4 determination was undetectable and the TSH determination was 340 μU per ml. Transabdominal transuterine injections of 120 μg of L-thyroxine were given into the fetal buttock at 2 week intervals. The dose of thyroxine was inadequate, but the calculated dose of 500 μg could not be given intramuscularly.

The fetus effectively absorbs L-thyroxine from amniotic fluid, which would obviate the problems of fetal intramuscular injections.[98] This approach was tried in a woman who inadvertently had received 150 mc of ^{131}I during week 10 to 11 of pregnancy.[108] Because of the potential risks of fetal hypothyroidism, an amniocentesis with an injection of 500 μg of thyroxine was performed weekly from week 33 until delivery. The concentration of T_4 in the cord serum was in the hypothyroid range, and the TSH concentration was low. However, the infant was not hypothyroid. Although the authors suggested that the amniotic fluid reverse T_3 concentration might be useful in the intrauterine diagnosis of hypothyroidism, this has not been substantiated.[105] In addition, it was necessary to follow up the infant for possible results of exposure to large amounts of thyroxine. At present both the intrauterine diagnosis and the therapy of congenital hypothyroidism are difficult.

MATERNAL THYROTOXICOSIS

Thyrotoxicosis occurs in about 2 of every 1000 pregnancies.[137] Seventy-five women with hyperthyroidism were identified in this prenatal research study, and, while the relatively small numbers preclude definitive statements, hyperthyroidism during pregnancy appeared to be associated with a slight increase in the neonatal mortality rate and a significant increase in the frequency of delivery of low birthweight infants. There is no evidence that pregnancy makes the thyrotoxicosis more difficult to control. In fact, perhaps related to the immunology of pregnancy, hyperthyroidism tends to be more easily controlled during pregnancy, whereas relapses tend to occur post partum.

Convincing evidence is lacking that fertility is impaired in mild to moderate hyperthyroidism, and there is disagreement whether fetal mortality is increased once pregnancy is established. Early workers thought that there was a hazard to the fetus proportional to the degree of hyperthyroidism.[131] However, the fetal loss of 8.4 per cent from 57 thyrotoxic pregnancies compared favorably with a total fetal loss of 17.2 per cent in a group of normal euthyroid women. The women in this study had received treatment for their hyperthyroidism, and there are no available data for untreated thyrotoxicosis during pregnancy. The balance of available evidence suggests that mild to moderate thyrotoxicosis is not inimical to the continuation of the pregnancy. An increased incidence of toxemia has been reported in thyrotoxic pregnancies, but the studies were not well controlled, and this correlation appears doubtful.[123, 174] Down's syndrome has also been reported to occur more frequently in the offspring of thyrotoxic mothers, but again, the studies were not well controlled.[132]

Etiology

Although there are a variety of possible causes of hyperthyroidism in pregnant women, including trophoblastic tumors and hydatidiform mole, toxic diffuse goiter (Graves' disease) and toxic nodular goiter (Plummer's disease) are of major importance. Plummer's disease is much less common during the childbearing years, since it arises in long-standing nodular goiter. Graves' disease is the most common form of hyperthyroidism occurring in conjunction with pregnancy.

Patients with Graves' disease have tended to undergo remission during pregnancy and exacerbation in the postpartum period. Recent studies on the immunology of pregnancy have provided possible explanations for these observations. Pregnancy has been described as a successful allograft of foreign tissue, and maternal immunologic inertness has been postulated as the mechanism for protecting the fetal allograft.[11] Both humoral and cell-mediated immunity have been reported to be depressed during normal pregnancy. Thyroid antibodies have been observed to decrease during pregnancy in Graves' disease.[3, 6] The amelioration of Graves' disease during pregnancy with exacerbation after delivery is thought to be due to these immunologic changes. The disappearance of immunosuppression at delivery and a transient enhancement of the immune reaction may be responsible for the transient recurrence of hyperthyroidism occurring after delivery in patients with Graves' disease.[4, 5, 64]

Diagnosis of Hyperthyroidism in Pregnancy

The clinical diagnosis of thyrotoxicosis in the pregnant woman may be difficult. The euthyroid woman may have a number of hyperdynamic symptoms and signs, including an increase in cardiac output with systolic flow murmurs and tachycardia, skin warmth, and heat intolerance. Diagnostic difficulties are further compounded because the usual diagnostic laboratory tests of thyrotoxicosis may easily give rise to suspicion but are confirmed only with difficulty. Signs of hyperthyroidism such as weight loss may be obscured by the weight gain of pregnancy. The presence of the eye changes of Graves' disease or pretibial myxedema may be helpful but do not necessarily indicate thyrotoxicosis. A resting pulse above 100 is helpful, and if the pulse fails to slow during a Valsalva maneuver, thyrotoxicosis becomes more likely. The presence of onycholysis, or separation of the distal nail from the nailbed, may also be helpful in making the clinical diagnosis of thyrotoxicosis.

Although the serum thyroxine concentration is elevated in normal pregnancy, values above 15 μg per 100 ml are suggestive of hyperthyroidism. The exact cutoff value depends on the particular assay. Provided that the patient does not have TBG deficiency, an RT_3U in the euthyroid range during pregnancy is also suggestive of thyrotoxicosis. These two determinations can be combined mathematically to obtain a free thyroxine index that makes a comparison of thyroxine to thyroxine-binding protein in a single value. Unfortunately, because of the elevated TBG during pregnancy, the free thyroxine index is not an accurate measure of the actual free thyroxine concentration.[163a] The newer nonequilibrium dialysis methods for the estimation of free thyroxine may be helpful, although some of them are also affected by changes in TBG.[185] If the patient is clearly thyrotoxic clinically but has normal values for serum thyroxine, the possibility of T_3 toxicosis should be considered.[179]

Hydatidiform mole may produce enough hCG to stimulate the thyroid and produce thyrotoxicosis.[83] For reasons that are not totally clear, such patients may have few clinical signs of thyrotoxicosis despite elevated thyroid function tests.[62]

Thioamide Therapy

Since radioactive iodine therapy is contraindicated during pregnancy, treatment involves a choice between antithyroid drugs and surgery.[144] There are arguments for and against both forms of treatment, and, in the final analysis, the individual decision depends on the physicians' treatment bias and recent past experience. Even if the decision is made to operate, the thyrotoxicosis must first be controlled by antithyroid drug therapy.

The mainstay of antithyroid drug therapy involves thioamides, which inhibit thyroid hormone synthesis by blocking iodination of the tyrosine molecule. Since these drugs block the synthesis but not the release of thyroid hormone, a clinical response to thioamides does not occur until the thyroid hormone stored in the colloid is utilized. Therefore, the time required to achieve control of the thyrotoxicosis will depend on the amount of colloid stored in the thyroid gland. Commonly, the patient will notice some clinical improvement after the first week of therapy and may approach euthyroidism after 4 to 6 weeks of therapy. Both propylthiouracil and methimazole have a short duration of action. Although most patients can probably be maintained on a single daily dose,[73] some women may require the thioamides every 8 hours or even more frequently for adequate control of the thyrotoxicosis.

Propylthiouracil (PTU) and methimazole (Tapazole) have been used interchangeably without evidence that one or the other has definite therapeutic advantages. However, propylthiouracil has the advantage of blocking the conversion of T_4 to T_3 in addition to inhibiting thyroid hormone synthesis. Furthermore, there is some evidence that methimazole therapy may be associated with aplasia cutis in the offspring[127] (Fig. 8–10). For these reasons, propylthiouracil is the drug of choice in the therapy of thyrotoxicosis in pregnancy.

PTU Dose. Once the diagnosis of hyperthyroidism has been made, the patient should be given PTU, 100 to 150 mg every 8 hours. After control of thyrotoxicosis has been achieved, as determined by an improvement in symptoms and signs as well as a fall in serum thyroxine, the dose of PTU should be decreased to 50 mg four times a day. If the patient remains euthyroid, the PTU could be decreased to 150 mg per day and then after three weeks to 50 mg twice a day. Serial serum T_4 determinations obtained monthly may be helpful in monitoring the course of the disease. The serum thyroxine concentrations may increase before clinical signs of thyrotoxicosis recur. Pregnant women with thyrotoxicosis should be maintained on as low a dose of PTU as possible, preferably under 100 mg daily.[22]

If thyrotoxicosis recurs, the PTU should again be increased to 300 mg per day. As mentioned earlier in the chapter, a recurrence is particularly likely post partum, and PTU could be increased to 300 mg daily at that time. If control of thyrotoxi-

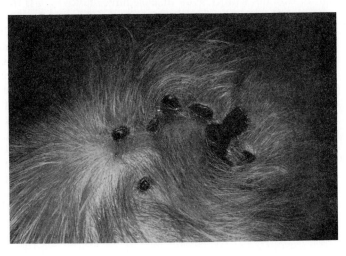

FIGURE 8–10. Aplasia cutis in a child whose mother had received methimazole. (From Burrow et al.: Yale J. Biol. Med. 51:13, 1978. Reprinted with permission.)

Mother   Placenta   Fetus

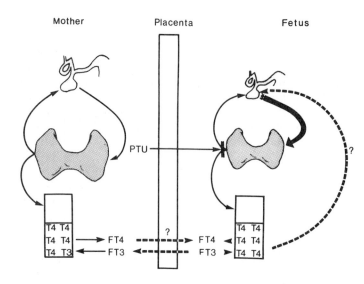

FIGURE 8–11.   Effect of PTU on fetal thyroid function.

cosis in the pregnant woman is not achieved on this treatment schedule. the PTU should be increased to 600 mg daily and given more frequently, e.g., every 4 to 6 hours. Rarely will it be necessary to give more than 600 mg PTU daily.

Complications of PTU Therapy. The most common complications of thioamide therapy include a mild, occasionally purpuric skin rash, pruritus, drug fever, and nausea, which occur in about 2 per cent of patients taking PTU. These minor side effects tend to occur during the first 4 weeks of therapy. If a drug reaction occurs with PTU, therapy may be continued with methimazole. However, the development of agranulocytosis requires that thioamide drug therapy be stopped immediately. Agranulocytosis usually occurs after 4 to 8 weeks of therapy in about 0.3 per cent of the treated population but leads to a fatal outcome in less than 1 in 10,000 treated patients. A leukocyte count should be obtained before thioamide therapy, since about 10 per cent of patients with Graves' disease have leukopenia. Weekly monitoring of the patient's leukocyte count during therapy is probably not helpful, because the white blood cell count may fall precipitously over several days.

Effect on the Fetus. The major concern with the use of PTU during pregnancy is the development of fetal goiter and hypothyroidism.[30a] Propylthiouracil crosses the placenta without difficulty[120] and blocks the fetal thyroid gland (Fig. 8–11). When the concentration of the fetal serum thyroid hormone decreases, stimulation of the thyroid gland by TSH might result in goiter formation.[22, 151] This effect may not depend solely on the amount of PTU. Many women have given birth to normal children even after receiving large amounts of antithyroid drugs during pregnancy.

Four out of 400,000 children screened in the Quebec neonatal thyroid screening program had transient hypothyroidism due to PTU. The number of mothers receiving antithyroid drugs was unknown, but a crude estimate suggests that only 1 to 5 per cent of children exposed to PTU develop transient hypothyroidism. Under ordinary circumstances, sufficient maternal thyroid hormone may cross the placenta to prevent fetal goiter.

Since a decrease in fetal thyroid hormone concentration may cause neonatal goiter, maternal thyroid hormone supplementation has been suggested.[157a] However, the added hormone may increase the dosage of PTU that is needed to control the thyrotoxicosis.[69, 88, 90, 102, 144] Certainly every effort should be made to avoid maternal hypothyroidism during pregancy. Propylthiouracil should be decreased or discontinued, and thyroid hormone should be administered if hypothyroidism is even suspected.

If the pregnant thyrotoxic woman on antithyroid medication can be followed at monthly intervals with laboratory determinations of thyroid function, then thyroid hormone supplementation is probably unnecessary. If she cannot be followed closely, then thyroid hormone supplementation may ensure against the development of maternal hypothyroidism. Certainly, an attempt should be made to treat the pregnant thyrotoxic woman with the lowest possible dose of antithyroid medication.[103a] Pregnant women tolerate mild degrees of hyperthyroidism without great difficulty, and it would be better to err by giving too small a dose of antithyroid medication rather than too large. Finally, if early diagnosis and treatment of neonatal hypothyroidism prevent the sequelae of in utero hypothyroidism, then these affected children can be successfully treated after birth.

Breast-Feeding by a Mother Receiving PTU. Another possible effect on the infant may occur after delivery when a lactating mother receives thioamides. Because these agents were once thought to be concentrated in breast milk, breast-feeding was discouraged.[184] Recently, however, studies have indicated that thioamides reach breast milk in a considerably lower concentration than previously thought. PTU concentrations are lower than methimazole; the amount of PTU excreted in the breast milk was 0.025 per cent of the administered dose.[92] These authors studied one child who was breast-fed for 5 months during which the mother received 200 to 300 mg of PTU daily. The infant was calculated to have received only about 0.15 mg of PTU daily, and no changes occurred in thyroid function tests. They concluded that mothers on PTU could breast-feed with close supervision. Even though the dose of PTU is probably low, it seems unwise to subject the child to even this minimal risk unless there are compelling reasons.

Possible Long-Term Effects. Unlike iodide-induced goiter, the neonatal goiter associated with PTU therapy is not large and obstructing. Although cretinism has been reported in the offspring of women treated with thioamides, there is no conclusive evidence that it was caused by the drugs. A more difficult question is whether children who were exposed to thioamides in utero attain full intellectual development. To study this problem we compared 18 children exposed to PTU in utero with 17 nonexposed siblings.[20] The children ranged in age from 2 to 12 years, and there were no important differences in their physical or mental characteristics. Thyroid function tests were normal in both groups, and there was no evidence of abnormal physical development or delayed bone growth. Physiologic testing revealed no marked differences between the groups, either in overall intellectual development or in patterning of various mental skills.

The small size of the sample precluded definite conclusions, but, in a subsequent study, intelligence tests administered to 28 children who had been exposed to propylthiouracil in utero and 32 nonexposed siblings also showed no important differences between the groups.[23] Similar data were reported for 25 children aged 3 to 13 years who were exposed in utero to carbimazole, which is metabolized to methimazole.[121] These results indicate that with careful attention, thioamides can be given to pregnant women without interfering with the subsequent intellectual development in the offspring.

Propranolol

Because the pregnant woman treated with PTU must be followed up very carefully, there has been interest in alternative therapy, particularly with the beta blocking agent propranolol.[17] However, the pharmacologic actions of propranolol on the fetus and neonate have been associated with small placenta, intrauterine growth retardation, impaired responses to anoxic stress, and postnatal bradycardia and hypoglycemia.[65, 75, 149] These observations indicate that propranolol should not be the primary agent for long-term treatment of hyperthyroidism during pregnancy. Whether a selective β_1-blocker has a role in chronic therapy remains to be determined. In 101 hypertensive women, fetal growth retardation was lower with metoprolol (12 vs 16 per cent).[157]

For rapid control of thyrotoxicosis, the combination of propranolol, 40 mg every 6 hours, with iodides, which block the release of thyroid hormone, will usually result in marked improvement within 2 to 7 days. Iodides act by inhibiting the secretion of thyroid hormone and acutely inhibiting the uptake of iodide into the thyroid. Unfortunately, iodides cause similar effects on the fetal thyroid gland in doses as low as 12 mg daily. Five drops of Lugol's solution twice a day, which is equivalent to a total of 100 mg of iodide, may be added to the therapeutic regimen for no more than a week or so. Once control of the thyrotoxicosis has been achieved, the patient may undergo subtotal thyroidectomy, but the anesthesiologist should be made aware that the patient has received propranolol.

Surgery

If a subtotal thyroidectomy is to be performed, surgery is often delayed until after the first trimester. The rationale for this delay is that the spontaneous abortion rate is highest during the first trimester and surgery during this period might increase the risk of abortion. However, thyroid surgery probably need not be avoided during the first trimester if indicated. The argument against subtotal thyroidectomy for the treatment of the pregnant woman with thyrotoxicosis is twofold. First, there is a finite surgical risk, which is probably higher than that of fatal complications of medical therapy.[16a] Second, the surgical complications of hypoparathyroidism and recurrent laryngeal nerve paralysis are disabling and difficult to treat. Although uncommon, they do occur, and, as fewer thyroidectomies are done because of medical therapy, the complication rate rises.

In one study of 12 thyrotoxic women treated with subtotal thyroidectomy, all the patients were first controlled with PTU and a brief course of iodides.[173] Three women were operated upon during the first trimester, 7 in the second, and 2 early in the last trimester. Seven women received thyroid hormone postoperatively. Of the 12 patients, 9 were delivered of normal children weighing more than 2500 grams. One patient had a spontaneous abortion 12 hours postoperatively, one intrauterine death occurred at 20 weeks; and one infant was premature. There was a total pregnancy wastage of 16 per cent for this group compared with 33 per cent in the medically treated group. The spontaneous abortion rate was 3.5 per cent in the surgically treated group and 11.5 per cent in the women receiving antithyroid medication. When the difference in spontaneous abortion was eliminated, the overall fetal salvage was similar.

The difficulty with these studies is that patients must be controlled medically before they can undergo surgery. The spontaneous abortion rate is higher during early pregnancy and may be labeled a "medical failure" when the patient aborts during preoperative preparation.[79] In a study in which subtotal thyroidectomy had been planned after control was achieved with antithyroid drugs, only seven patients were actually operated upon for various reasons.[186] With one exception the more severe cases were treated medically. In spite of this, 70 per cent of women treated with medical therapy had a successful pregnancy outcome, while 28 per cent of surgically treated women were in the same category. Other workers have found that subtotal thyroidectomy after appropriate preparation resulted in no surgical complications.[47] If the patient is to have surgery, she should be observed carefully for signs of hypothyroidism postoperatively. At the first chemical signs of hypothyroidism, the pregnant woman should be started on a regimen of 0.2 mg of L-thyroxine.[13]

Since surgical complications do occur, and since the majority of patients who receive propylthiouracil have uncomplicated pregnancies, medical therapy seems to be the preferred treatment of hyperthyroidism during pregnancy. Subtotal thyroidectomy should probably be reserved for antithyroid drug hypersensitivity, poor compliance, and the rare instance in which the drugs are ineffective.[90]

Thyroid Storm

The major risk to the pregnant woman with thyrotoxicosis is the development of thyroid storm. This uncommon but frightening complication occurs as a life-endangering augmentation of the signs and symptoms of hyperthyroidism. Thyroid storm is more likely to occur when there is some precipitating factor such as labor, cesarean section, or infection.[74] The pregnant woman may present with a fever as high as 106°F, marked tachycardia, prostration, and severe dehydration, a course ending fatally in up to 25 per cent of cases despite good medical management. Thyroid storm is more commonly seen in patients in whom the diagnosis of hyperthyroidism has not been recognized, but it also occurs in inadequately treated patients.

Precipitating factors should be alleviated if possible and specific therapy should include (1) propranolol, 40 mg by mouth every 6 hours to control the beta-adrenergic activity. If necessary, the drug can be given intravenously in doses of 1.0 to 2.0 mg. (2) Sodium iodide, 1 gm intravenously to block the secretion of thyroid hormone. (3) Lithium, 300 mg three times a day, also to block thyroid hormone secretion. (4) PTU, 1200 mg orally in divided doses to block the formation of thyroid hormone and the deiodination of T_4 to T_3. (5) Dexamethasone, 8 mg a day to further block the deiodination of T_4 to T_3. (6) Five liters of fluids to replace severe fluid losses. (7) Hypothermia for malignant hyperpyrexia.[89] If hyperthyroidism is considered in the pregnant woman and adequate therapy initiated, this frightening complication of thyrotoxicosis should be virtually eliminated.

Inadvertent Administration of [131]I During Pregnancy

As mentioned previously, radioactive iodine is absolutely contraindicated during pregnancy. However, occasionally patients not known to be pregnant at the time are given a dose of radioactive iodine. Although all women in the childbearing age should have a pregnancy test before receiving therapeutic doses of radiation, this is not always done.

Maternal Irradiation. During a radioisotope thyroid uptake, both mother and fetus are exposed to radiation. The amount of radiation that the mother receives is insignificant in terms of a radiation dose to the thyroid or ovaries. However, a treatment dose of ^{131}I for hyperthyroidism is 1000 times the dose required for an uptake study. Hyperthyroidism is the only common nonmalignant disease for which patients receive significant amounts of ionizing radiation. Although the incidence of leukemia and thyroid malignancy is not increased in thyrotoxic patients receiving radioactive iodine,[155] subsequent effects of the gonadal dose are less certain.[156] The radiation dose to the maternal and fetal thyroid as well as to the gonads has been estimated.[76] In a similar study a patient was estimated to receive a total body dose of 0.51 rad per mc.[179a] Therefore, a thyrotoxic patient receiving a therapeutic dose of 10 mc of ^{131}I would receive a total body dose of about 5 rads. There are five sources of radiation to the gonads: beta radiation from blood flowing through the gonads and gamma radiation from the thyroid, extrathyroidal tissue, bladder, and colon. The mean gonadal dose has been estimated at about 0.3 to 0.45 rad per mc of [131]I.[152, 179a] Whether this radiation dose is sufficient to cause genetic effects is not clear. Persistent chromosomal abnormalities have been found in the white blood cells of patients who had received 5 mc of ^{131}I for the treatment of thyrotoxicosis. There is no reason to suppose that similar changes do not also occur in gonadal chromosomes.

Fetal Irradiation. The fetal thyroid begins to concentrate iodine at about the 10th to 12th week of gestation and has an avidity for iodine 20 to 50 times that of the maternal thyroid. As a consequence, any dose of radioiodine will be more concentrated per gram of thyroid tissue in the fetus than in the mother. Congenital hypothyroidism has been reported in offspring of mothers who received therapeutic doses of radioiodine.[129] A thyrotoxic mother who inadvertently received 14.5 mc of ^{131}I at the end of the first trimester was estimated to have received a dose of 20,000 rads to her thyroid, while the fetus received an estimated dose of 250,000 rads to the thyroid with resulting hypothyroidism.

Not only is the fetal thyroid gland more avid for iodine, fetal tissues in general are more radiosensitive. Studies have demonstrated a causal relationship between prenatal irradiation and the subsequent development of malignant disease, with indications that the risk is related to both the dose and the time of exposure.[114, 166] Microcephaly has also been noted in children who were heavily irradiated in utero.[68a] Children who were in utero at the time of the atomic bombing of Hiroshima and Nagasaki have been studied intensively. Radiation in utero resulted in increased fetal and infant mortality and a higher prevalence of microcephaly and mental retardation. Microcephaly was most common when the child was irradiated between 7 and 15 weeks of gestation. Children exposed to ionizing radiation in utero also lagged behind nonexposed peers during adolescence in several aspects of growth and development.[22] These findings suggested that subtle defects that are not easy to detect may occur because of radiation. Most of the long-term effects occurred with whole body radiation above 50 rads. Whether there is a threshold effect for radiation damage or whether the damage is linear is important, since the whole body radiation dose to the fetus from a therapeutic dose of ^{131}I for thyrotoxicosis is well below 50 rads. At least some of the effects may be linear, and all radiation should be regarded as harmful.

Therapeutic Considerations

If a woman is subsequently found to be pregnant after a radioactive iodine uptake, nothing further need be done. Although radiation is absolutely contraindicated in the pregnant woman, the amount received during a diagnostic thyroid study is not sufficient to cause concern. However, in a pregnant woman who has inadvertently received a therapeutic dose of ^{131}I for hyperthyroidism, the question of termination of the pregnancy arises. This situation tends to occur early in pregnancy when the fetal thyroid is not trapping iodine. The relatively low fetal whole body irradiation is probably not sufficient to justify pregnancy termination. If the fetal thyroid is trapping iodine, hypothyroidism is a risk. However, the neonatal thyroid screening program is predicated on the supposition that prompt postnatal thyroid hormone therapy prevents the sequelae of in utero hypothyroidism.

If a pregnant woman with thyrotoxicosis is given a therapeutic dose of ^{131}I and this is discovered within a week of administration, she might be treated with propylthiouracil, 300 mg daily for 7 days, to block the recycling of the ^{131}I in the fetal gland. Iodides would dilute the uptake pool but would also inhibit the release of radioactivity. By 10 days after treatment, more than 90 per cent of the dose of ^{131}I has been delivered, and such treatment would not be helpful. The mother will be thyrotoxic and will have to be treated, which will also complicate fetal thyroid function. Regardless of possible preventive measures, the condition of the infant should be carefully evaluated for hypothyroidism at birth and immediate treatment begun if indicated.

Long-Term Management of Thyrotoxicosis. The long-term management of a young thyrotoxic patient who is planning subsequent pregnancies represents a difficult therapeutic decision. A medical remission in this age group is unlikely, and therapy during the subsequent pregnancies will probably be indicated. A full 2 year course of PTU therapy seems indicated — possibly a second course, if necessary. If the patient is still thyrotoxic, then active consideration should be given to radioactive iodine therapy. Long-term antithyroid drug therapy in such a situation may be undesirable.[127] Despite the attendant risks, subtotal thyroidectomy also deserves active consideration in this situation.

NEONATAL THYROTOXICOSIS

Approximately 1 per cent of pregnant women with a history of Graves' disease give birth to infants with neonatal thyrotoxicosis.[128] Although the mothers themselves were not necessarily thyrotoxic during pregnancy, virtually all of them had some clinical or laboratory manifestations of Graves' disease. The neonatal thyrotoxicosis was transient, usually lasting 2 to 3 months or less. Hyperthyroidism has been a most frequent problem in the infant; eye changes of Graves' disease have not always been present. Neonatal thyrotoxicosis is not a benign condition and has been associated with a mortality rate of 16 per cent.[86] Perhaps the most serious, long-term complication in surviving infants is premature craniosynostosis that might result in inadequate cerebral development.[124]

Etiology

Neonatal thyrotoxicosis is most likely due to the placental transfer of a thyroid-stimulating immunoglobulin from the mother with Graves' disease to the fetus. This concept was based on the finding of LATS in maternal and cord serum and the decline of LATS activity in fetal serum as the neonatal thyrotoxicosis resolved.[122, 128] After great initial enthusiasm, the inability to detect LATS in the sera of many hyperthyroid patients raised questions whether it was the etiologic agent.[86, 87]

However, it was found that LATS-protector was much more commonly detected than LATS[128] (Fig. 8–12). Serum LATS-protector was 20 units per ml or higher in 11 of 12 mothers who gave birth to thyrotoxic infants. With two exceptions, infants born live to mothers with LATS-protector levels of more than 20 units per ml were thyrotoxic. Cases of neonatal thyrotoxicosis have also been observed in which the LATS assay was negative but the presence of thyroid-stimulating immunoglobulin was confirmed. The evidence suggests that neonatal thyrotoxicosis is caused by the 7S immunoglobulin, and failure to detect elevated levels is a reflection of the particular assay used. The equal sex incidence in neonatal thyrotoxicosis also favors the concept of placental transfer of the etiologic agent when compared with the female-to-male ratio of 3 or 4:1 for Graves' disease. The duration of neonatal thyrotoxicosis appears to be a function of the initial neonatal serum concentration of the thyroid-stimulating immunoglobulin and the rate of degradation. The half-life of the antibody in the

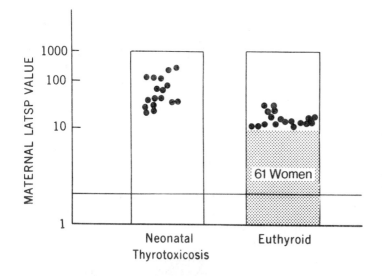

FIGURE 8–12. Maternal serum concentrations of LATS protector in 93 pregnant women with Graves' disease. Sixty-one euthyroid women with LATS-P values of less than 10 are represented by the dotted area. (Modified from Munro et al.: Br. J. Obstet. Gynaecol., *85*:837, 1978.)

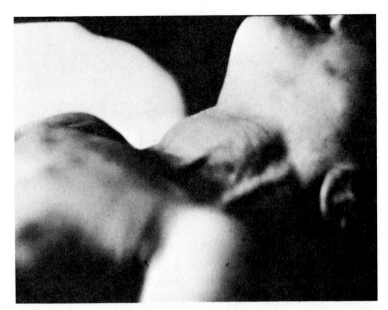

FIGURE 8–13. Neonatal thyrotoxicosis.

serum of the thyrotoxic neonate, based on studies with LATS-protector, is between 4 and 10 days.[115, 127a]

The question has been raised whether neonatal thyrotoxicosis is transient.[86, 87] A number of children have been described in whom the hyperthyroidism persisted beyond 1 year of age. These patients, particularly females, appear to inherit congenital Graves' disease as an autosomal dominant trait. Certainly, the majority of patients with neonatal thyrotoxicosis appear to have the disease only transiently.

Diagnosis

The diagnosis of neonatal thyrotoxicosis can usually be made on the basis of the total clinical picture (Fig. 8–13). If the mother has Graves' disease, then the possibility of neonatal thyrotoxicosis should be carefully considered. The presence of goiter, exophthalmos, and tachycardia in a hyperirritable infant with an elevated serum thyroxine is sufficient to enable the diagnosis to be made with a reasonable degree of certainty.[159] Infants with neonatal thyrotoxicosis have also presented with other signs, such as cardiac failure, hepatosplenomegaly, jaundice, and thrombocytopenia.[46] Such patients can be detected in the population screening programs for neonatal hypothyroidism if the T_4 radioimmunoassay is used.[178] The diagnosis would be greatly strengthened by a positive assay for thyroid-stimulating immunoglobulin. A high titer is diagnostic in the infant and virtually predictive in the mother. Unfortunately, this assay is only readily available in research laboratories.

Although a history of Graves' disease is the rule, the mother may not have active thyrotoxicosis and may be euthyroid or hypothyroid. Another problem in the diagnosis of neonatal thyrotoxicosis may occur in children exposed to antithyroid drugs in utero. These children may not be thyrotoxic at birth but may develop the disease subsequently.[127] Presumably, the antithyroid drugs block the clinical expression of thyrotoxicosis in the neonate so that it may not become evident until after the child has left the hospital.[182] The neonatal narcotic withdrawal syndrome could be confused with neonatal thyrotoxicosis with irritability and tremulousness, and the serum thyroxine may also be elevated.[91]

Therapy

If neonatal thyrotoxicosis is mild, no specific antithyroid therapy is necessary because the disease is self-limited. Otherwise, the infant can be treated with Lugol's solution, one drop (8 mg iodine) three times a day, and propranolol, 2 mg per kg per day.[80, 161] Propylthiouracil, 10 mg every 8 hours, can also be added but is perhaps better reserved for children whose condition cannot be controlled with iodides or propranolol. Patients with neonatal thyrotoxicosis who have died have usually been premature and have had severe hyperthyroidism accompanied by congestive heart failure. However, most children recover without incident. The majority of infants who require treatment do so for 3 to 6 weeks, depending upon the serum titer of thyroid-stimulating immunoglobulin. Some children with neonatal thyrotoxicosis have been considered to be prema-

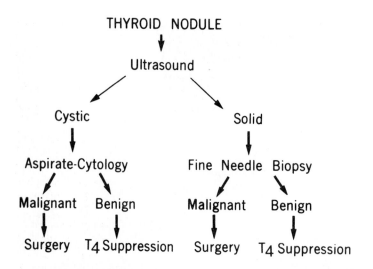

THYROID NODULE

Ultrasound

Cystic · Solid

Aspirate-Cytology · Fine Needle Biopsy

Malignant · Benign · Malignant · Benign

Surgery · T4 Suppression · Surgery · T4 Suppression

FIGURE 8–14. Management of a solitary thyroid nodule during pregnancy.

ture because of low birth weight. However, these children may actually have accelerated maturity on the basis of bone age, the low birth weight being secondary to the thyrotoxicosis.[51]

THYROID NODULE AND THYROID CARCINOMA

The presence of nontoxic diffuse goiter in response to relative iodine deficiency during pregnancy has been discussed earlier in the chapter. A more difficult problem concerns the pregnant woman who is discovered to have a solitary thyroid nodule.

Management of the Thyroid Nodule

Our study reported 26 women who had been operated upon for a clinically solitary nodule that had arisen during, or was affected by, pregnancy.[35] At surgery most of the nodules represented nontoxic nodular goiter, but there were nine true adenomas. Parity seemed to have no influence on the development of thyroid nodules.

Evaluation of the solitary thyroid nodule during pregnancy is limited because the radioisotope thyroid scan is contraindicated. However, it is possible to obtain ultrasound evaluation of the nodule to determine whether it is solid or cystic and to follow that procedure by a fine needle aspiration biopsy of the nodule (Fig. 8–14). If the biopsy does not reveal suspicious cells, then the thyroid should be suppressed with 0.2 mg of L-thyroxine for the duration of the pregnancy.

Following delivery the thyroid nodule should be re-evaluated. If the biopsy is suggestive of malignancy, then surgery is indicated even though the patient is pregnant.

Management of Thyroid Carcinoma

Pregnancy apparently has no effect on the natural history of thyroid carcinoma, nor does thyroid carcinoma have any significant effect on the pregnancy. In one study of 60 women who had thyroid carcinoma in association with pregnancy, 38 women had been treated and were free of disease for 2 to 15 years before becoming pregnant.[153a] The second group in that study included 22 women with consistent thyroid carcinoma who were pregnant one to five times in this condition. Two therapeutic abortions were performed, one because of extensive metastases and one because of radioiodine therapy. In another study, 70 women with thyroid carcinoma who became pregnant were compared with 109 women with thyroid carcinoma who did not.[83a] There was no significant difference in the overall recurrence rate between the two groups, and the authors concluded that pregnancy subsequent to the diagnosis of thyroid carcinoma had no effect on the course of the disease.

The diagnosis of carcinoma during pregnancy is not an absolute indication for terminating the pregnancy, nor is pregnancy a contraindication to necessary thyroid surgery. Radioactive iodine therapy should be withheld until after delivery but is rarely indicated.

References

1. Aboul-Khair, S. A., Crooks, J., Turnbull, A. C., and Hytten, F. E.: The physiological changes in thyroid function during pregnancy. Clin. Sci., 27:195, 1964.
2. Alexander, W. D., Koutras, D. A., Crooks, J., Buchanan, W. W., MacDonald, E. M., Richmond, M. H., and Wayne, E. J.: Quantitative studies of iodine metabolism in thyroid disease. Q. J. Med., 31:281, 1962.
3. Amino, N., Kuro, R., Tanizawa, O., Tanaka, F., Hayashi, C.,

Kotani, K., Kawashima, M., Miyai, K., and Kumahara, Y.: Changes of serum anti-thyroid antibodies during and after pregnancy in autoimmune thyroid diseases. Clin. Exp. Immunol., *31*:30, 1978.

4. Amino, N., Miyai, K., Kuro, R., Tanizawa, O., Azukizawa, M., Takai, S., Tanaka, F., Nishi, K., Kawashima, M., and Kumahara, Y.: Transient postpartum hypothyroidism: Fourteen cases with autoimmune thyroiditis. Ann. Intern. Med., *87*:155, 1977.

5. Amino, N., Miyai, K., Yamamoto, T., Kuro, R., Tanaka, F., Tanizawa, O., and Kumahara, Y.: Transient recurrence of hyperthyroidism after delivery in Graves' disease. J. Clin. Endocrinol. Metab., *44*:130, 1977.

6. Amino, N., Tanizawa, O., Miyai, K., Tanaka, F., Hayashi, C., Kawashima, M., and Ichihara, K.: Changes of serum immunoglobulins IgG, IgA, IgM, and IgE during pregnancy. Obstet. Gynecol., *52*:415, 1978.

7. Amir, S. M., Sullivan, R. C., and Ingbar, S. H.: In vitro responses to crude and purified hCG in human thyroid membranes. J. Clin. Endocrinol. Metab., *51*:51, 1980.

8. Aratan-Spire, S., and Czernichow, P.: Thyrotropin-releasing hormone-degrading activity of neonatal human plasma. J. Clin. Endocrinol. Metab., *50*:88, 1980.

9. Asling, J., and Way, E. L.: Placental transfer of drugs. In La Du, B. N., Mandel, H. G., and Way, E. L. (Eds.): Fundamentals of Drug Metabolism and Drug Disposition, pp. 88–105. Baltimore, The Williams & Wilkins Co., 1971.

9a. Bashmore, B. A., Reed, A., Morley, J. E., Carlson, H., and Hershman, J. M.: Thyrotropin-releasing hormone and thyroid hormones in amniotic fluid. J. Clin. Endocrinol. Metab., *134*:581, 1979.

10. Becroft, D. M. O., Smeeton, W. M. I., and Stewart, J. H.: Fetal thyroid hyperplasia, rhesus isoimmunisation, and amniography. Arch. Dis. Child., *55*:213, 1980.

11. Beer, A. E., and Billingham, R. E.: Immunobiology of mammalian reproduction. Adv. Immunol., *14*:1, 1971.

12. Beierwaltes, W. H.: Hosp. Pract., *3*:31, 1968.

13. Bell, G. O., and Hall, J.: Hyperthyroidism and pregnancy. Med. Clin. North Am., *44*:363, 1960.

14. Black, J. A.: Neonatal goitre and mental deficiency. The role of iodides taken during pregnancy. Arch. Dis. Child., *38*:526, 1963.

15. Bongiovanni, A. M., Eberlein, W. R., Thomas, P. Z., and Anderson, W. B.: Sporadic goiter of the newborn. J. Clin. Endocrinol. Metab., *16*:146, 1956.

16. Brasel, J. A., and Boyd, D. B.: Influence of thyroid hormone on fetal brain growth and development. In Fisher, D. A., and Burrow, G. N. (Eds.): Perinatal Thyroid Physiology and Disease, pp. 59–71. New York, Raven Press, 1975.

16a. Brodsky, J. B., Cohen, E. N., Brown, B. W. Jr., Wu, M. L., and Whitcher, C.: Surgery during pregnancy and fetal outcome. Am. J. Obstet. Gynecol., *138*:115, 1980.

17. Bullock, J. L., Harris, R. E., and Young, R.: Treatment of thyrotoxicosis during pregnancy with propranolol. Am. J. Obstet. Gynecol., *121*:242, 1975.

18. Burk, K., and Kerr, A., Jr.: Pregnancy in a patient with myxedema. Am. J. Obstet. Gynecol., *68*:1623, 1954.

19. Burr, W. A., Ramsden, D. B., Evans, S. E., Hogan, T., and Hoffenberg, R.: Concentration of thyroxine-binding globulin: Value of direct assay. Br. Med. J., *1*:485, 1977.

20. Burrow, G. N., Bartsocas, C., Klatskin, E. H., and Grunt, J. A.: Children exposed in utero to propylthiouracil. Am. J. Dis. Child., *116*:161, 1968.

21. Burrow, G. N., and Dussault, J. H. (Eds.): Neonatal Thyroid Screening. New York, Raven Press, 1980.

22. Burrow, G. N., Hamilton, H. B., and Hrubec, Z.: Study of adolescents exposed in utero to the atomic bomb, Nagasaki, Japan. II. Growth and development. J.A.M.A., *192*:357, 1965.

23. Burrow, G. N., Klatskin, E. H., and Genel, M.: Intellectual development in children whose mothers received propylthiouracil during pregnancy. Yale J. Biol. Med., *51*:151, 1978.

24. Burrow, G. N., Mutjtaba, Q., LiVolsi, V., and Cornog, J.: The incidence of carcinoma in solitary "cold" thyroid nodules. Yale J. Biol. Med., *51*:13, 1978.

25. Burrow, G. N., Polackwich, R., and Donabedian, R.: The hypothalamic-pituitary-thyroid axis in normal pregnancy. In Fisher, D. A., and Burrow, G. N. (Eds.): Perinatal Thyroid Physiology and Disease, pp. 1–10. New York, Raven Press, 1975.

25a. Burwell, C. S.: Circulating adjustments to pregnancy. Bull. Johns Hopkins Hosp., *95*:115, 1954.

26. Buxton, C. L., and Herrmann, W. L.: Effect of thyroid therapy on menstrual disorders and sterility. J.A.M.A., *155*:1035, 1954.

27. Carswell, F., Kerr, M. M., and Hutchison, J. H.: Congenital goitre and hypothyroidism produced by maternal ingestion of iodides. Lancet, *1*:1241, 1970.

28. Chan, V., Paraskevaides, C. A., and Hale, J. F.: Assessment of thyroid function during pregnancy. Br. J. Obstet. Gynaecol., *82*:137, 1975.

29. Chandler, J. W., Blizzard, R. M., Hung, W., and Kyle, M.: Thyroid antibodies passing to fetus. N. Engl. J. Med., *278*:1153, 1968.

30. Chapman, E. M., Corner, G. W., Jr., Robinson, D., and Evans, R. D.: The collection of radioactive iodine by the human fetal thyroid. J. Clin. Endocrinol. Metab., *8*:717, 1948.

30a. Cheron, R. G., Kaplan, M. G., Larsen, P. R., Selenkow, H. A., and Crigler, J. F. Jr.: Neonatal thyroid function after propyl thiouracil therapy for maternal Graves' disease. N. Engl. J. Med., *304*:525, 1981.

31. Chopra, I. J., and Crandall, B. F.: Thyroid hormones and thyrotropin in amniotic fluid. N. Engl. J. Med., *293*:740, 1975.

32. Comite, F., Burrow, G. N., Jorgensen, E. C.: Thyroid hormone analogs and fetal goiter. J. Clin. Endocrinol. Metab., *102*:1670, 1978.

33. Crooks, J., Aboul-Khair, S. A., Turnbull, A. C., and Hytten, F. E.: The incidence of goiter during pregnancy. Lancet, *2*:334, 1964.

34. Crooks, J., Tulloch, M. I., Turnbull, A. C., Davidsson, D., Skulason, T., and Snaedel, G.: Comparative incidence of goitre in pregnancy in Iceland and Scotland. Lancet, *2*:625, 1967.

35. Cunningham, M. P., and Slaughter, D. P.: Surgical treatment of disease of the thyroid gland in pregnancy. Surg. Gynecol. Obstet., *131*:486, 1970.

36. D'Angelo, S. A., and Wall, N. R.: Maternal fetal endocrine interrelations: Effects of synthetic thyrotropin releasing hormone (TRH) on the fetal-pituitary-thyroid system of the rat. Neuroendocrinology, *9*:197, 1972.

37. Dawood, M. Y., Ylikorkala, O., Trivedi, D., and Fuchs, F.: Oxytocin in maternal circulation and amniotic fluid during pregnancy. J. Clin. Endocrinol. Metab., *49*:429, 1979.

38. Dekaban, A., and Baird, R.: The outcome of pregnancy in diabetic women. I. Fetal wastage, mortality and morbidity in the offspring of diabetic and normal control mothers. J. Pediatr., *55*:563, 1959.

39. Delange, F., Beckers, C., Hofer, R., Konig, M. P., Monaco, F., and Varrone, S.: Progress report on neonatal screening for congenital hypothyroidism in Europe. In Burrow, G. N., and Dussault, J. H. (Eds.): Neonatal Thyroid Screening, pp. 107–131. New York, Raven Press, 1980.

40. Dowling, J. T., Appleton, W. G., and Nicoloff, J. T.: Thyroxine turnover during human pregnancy. J. Clin. Endocrinol. Metab., *27*:1749, 1967.

41. Dowling,. J. T., Freinkel, N., and Ingbar, S. H.: The effect of estrogens upon the peripheral metabolism of thyroxine. J. Clin. Invest., *39*:1119, 1960.

42. Dussault, J. H., Coulombe, P., and Laberge, C., et al.: Preliminary report on a mass screening program for neonatal hypothyroidism. J. Pediatr., *86*:670, 1975.

43. Dussault, J. H., Letarte, J., Glorieux, J., Morissette, J., and Guyda, H.: Psychological development of hypothyroid infants at age 12 and 18 months: Experience after neonatal screening. In Burrow, G. N., and Dussault, J. H. (Eds.): Neonatal Thyroid Screening, pp. 271–276. New York, Raven Press, 1980.

44. Dussault, J., Row, V. V., Lickrish, G., and Volpe, R.: Studies of serum triiodothyronine concentration in maternal and cord blood: Transfer of triiodothyronine across the human placenta. J. Clin. Endocrinol. Metab., *29*:595, 1969.

44a. Dworkin, H. J., Jacquez, J. A., and Beierwaltes, W. H.: Relationship of iodine ingestion to iodine excretion in pregnancy. J. Clin. Endocrinol. Metab., *26*:1329, 1966.

45. Echt, C. R., and Doss, J. F.: Myxedema in pregnancy. Obstet. Gynecol., *22*:615, 1963.

46. Elsas, L. J., Whittemore, R., and Burrow, G. N.: Maternal and neonatal Graves' disease. J.A.M.A., *200*:250, 1967.

47. Emslander, R. F., Weeks, R. E., and Malkasian, G. D., Jr.: Hyperthyroidism and pregnancy. Med. Clin. North Am., *58*:835, 1974.

48. Engbring, N. H., and Engstrom, W. W.: Effects of estrogen and testosterone on circulating thyroid hormone. J. Clin. Endocrinol. Metab., *19*:783, 1959.

49. Ermans, A. M., Bourdoux, P., Lagasse, R., Delange, F., and

Thilly, C.: Congenital hypothyroidism in developing countries. *In* Burrow, G. N., and Dussault, J. H. (Eds.): Neonatal Thyroid Screening, pp. 61–73. New York, Raven Press, 1980.

50. Evans, T. C., Kretzchmar, R. M., Hodges, R. E., and Song, C. W.: Radioiodine uptake studies of the human fetal thyroid. J. Nucl. Med., *8*:157, 1967.

51. Farrehi, C.: Accelerated maturity in fetal thyrotoxicosis. Clin. Pediatr., *7*:134, 1968.

52. Fialkow, P. J.: Autoimmunity and chromosomal aberrations. Am. J. Hum. Genet., *18*:93, 1966.

53. Fillippi, G., and McKusick, V. A.: The Beckwith-Wiedemann syndrome. Medicine, *49*:279, 1970.

54. Fisher, D. A.: Thyroid function in the premature infant. Am. J. Dis. Child., *131*:842, 1977.

55. Fisher, D. A., Hobel, C. J., Gazara, R., and Pierce, C. A.: Thyroid function in the preterm fetus. Pediatrics, *46*:208, 1970.

56. Fisher, D. A., Lehman, H., and Lackey, C.: Placental transport of thyroxine. J. Clin. Endocrinol. Metab., *24*:393, 1964.

57. Fisher, D. A., Oddie, T. H., and Burroughs, J. C.: Thyroidal radioiodine uptake rate measurement in infants. Am. J. Dis. Child., *103*:738, 1962.

58. Fisher, D. A., and Odell, W. D.: Acute release of thyrotropin in the newborn. J. Clin. Invest., *48*:1670, 1969.

59. Fisher, W. D., Voorhess, M. L., and Gardner, L. I.: Congenital hypothyroidism in infant following maternal I¹³¹ therapy. J. Pediatr., *62*:132, 1963.

60. Friis, T., and Secher, E.: Protein-bound iodine of serum in induced abortion and at delivery. Acta Endocrinol., *18*:428, 1955.

61. Galina, M. P., Arnet, M. L., and Einhorn, A.: Iodides during pregnancy. N. Engl. J. Med., *267*:1124, 1962.

62. Galton, V. A., Ingbar, S. H., Jimenez-Fonseca, J., and Hershman, J. M.: Alterations in thyroid hormone economy in patients with hydatidiform mole. J. Clin. Invest., *50*:1345, 1971.

63. Ginsberg, J., and Walfish, P. G.: Post-partum transient thyrotoxicosis with painless thyroiditis. Lancet, *1*:1125, 1977.

64. Ginsberg, J., Walfish, P., and Chopra, J. J.: Cord blood reverse T₃ in normal, premature euthyroid and hypothyroid newborns. J. Endocrinol. Invest., *1*:73, 1978.

65. Gladstone, G. R., Hordof, A., and Gersony, W. M.: Propranolol administration during pregnancy: Effects on the fetus. J. Pediatr., *86*:962, 1975.

66. Glinoer, D., Gershengorn, M. C., Dubois, A., and Robbins, J.: Stimulation of thyroxine-binding globulin synthesis by isolated rhesus monkey hepatocytes in vivo β-estradiol administration. Endocrinology, *100*:807, 1977.

67. Goldsmith, R. E., McAdams, A. J., Larsen, P. R., MacKenzie, M., and Hess, E. V.: Familial autoimmune thyroiditis: Maternal-fetal relationship and the role of generalized autoimmunity. J. Clin. Endocrinol. Metab., *37*:265, 1973.

68. Goldsmith, R. E., Sturgis, S. H., Lerman, J., and Stanbury, J. B.: The menstrual pattern in thyroid disease. J. Clin. Endocrinol., *12*:846, 1952.

68a. Goldstein, L., and Murphy, D. P.: Etiology of the ill-health in children born after maternal pelvic irradiation. II. Defective children born after postconception pelvic irradiation. Am. J. Roentgenol., *22*:322, 1929.

69. Goluboff, L. G., Sisson, J. C., and Hamburger, J. I.: Hyperthyroidism associated with pregnancy. Obstet. Gynecol., *44*:107, 1974.

70. Green, H. G., Gareis, F. J., Shepard, T. H., and Kelley, V. C.: Cretinism associated with maternal sodium iodide I 131 therapy during pregnancy. Am. J. Dis. Child., *122*:247, 1971.

71. Greenberg, A. H., Czernichow, P., Reba, R. C., Tyson, J., and Blizzard, R. M.: Observations on the maturation of thyroid function in early fetal life. J. Clin. Invest., *49*:1790, 1970.

72. Greenman, G. W., Gabrielson, M. O., Howard-Flanders, J., and Wessel, M. A.: Thyroid dysfunction in pregnancy. Fetal loss and follow-up evaluation of surviving infants. N. Engl. J. Med., *267*:426, 1962.

73. Greer, M. A., Meihoff, W. C., and Studer, H.: Treatment of hyperthyroidism with a single daily dose of propylthiouracil. N. Engl. J. Med., *272*:888, 1965.

73a. Grumbach, M. M., and Werner, S. C.: Transfer of thyroid hormone across the human placenta at term. J. Clin. Endocrinol. Metab., *16*:1392, 1956.

74. Guenter, K. E., and Friedland, G. A.: Thyroid storm and placenta previa in a primigravida. Obstet. Gynecol., *26*:403, 1965.

75. Habib, A., and McCarthy, J. S.: Effects on the neonate of propranolol administered during pregnancy. J. Pediatr., *91*:808, 1977.

76. Halnan, K. E.: The radioiodine uptake of the human thyroid in pregnancy. Clin. Sci., *17*:281, 1958.

77. Harada, A., and Hershman, J. M.: Extraction of human chorionic thyrotropin (hCT) from term placentas: Failure to recover thyrotropic activity. J. Clin. Endocrinol. Metab., *47*:681, 1978.

78. Harada, A., Hershman, J. M., Reed, A. W., Braunstein, G. D., Dignam, W. J., Derzko, C., Friedman, S., Jewelewicz, R., and Pekary, A. E.: Comparison of thyroid stimulators and thyroid hormone concentrations in the sera of pregnant women. J. Clin. Endocrinol. Metab., *48*:793, 1979.

79. Hawe, P., and Francis, H. H.: Pregnancy and thyrotoxicosis. Br. Med. J., *2*:817, 1962.

80. Hayek, A., and Brooks, M.: Neonatal hyperthyroidism following intrauterine hypothyroidism. J. Pediatr., *87*:446, 1975.

80a. Hayek, A., Driscoll, S. G., and Warshaw, J. B.: Endocrine studies in anencephaly. J. Clin. Invest., *52*:1636, 1973.

80b. Hennen, C., Pierce, J. G., and Freychet, P.: Human chorionic thyrotropin: Further characterization and study of its secretion during pregnancy. J. Clin. Endocrinol. Metab., *29*:581, 1969.

81. Hershman, J. M., and Hershman, F. K.: Development of the thyroid control system. *In* Stanbury, J. B., and Kroc, R. L. (Eds.): Human Development and the Thyroid Gland: Relation to Endemic Cretinism. Proceedings, Symposium on Endemic Cretinism, Kroc Foundation. New York, Plenum Press, 1972.

81a. Hershman, J. M., and Starnes, W. R.: Extraction and characterization of a thyrotropic material from the human placenta. J. Clin. Invest., *48*:923, 1969.

82. Hetzel, B. S., and Hay, I. D.: Thyroid function, iodine nutrition and fetal brain development. Clin. Endocrinol., *11*:445, 1979.

83. Higgins, H. P., Hershman, J. M., Kenimer, J. G., Patillo, R. A., Bayley, T. A., and Walfish, P.: The thyrotoxicosis of hydatidiform mole. Ann. Intern. Med., *83*:307, 1975.

83a. Hill, C. S., Jr., Clark, R. L., and Wolf, M.: The effect of subsequent pregnancy on patients with thyroid carcinoma. Surg. Gynecol. Obstet., *122*:1219, 1966.

84. Hodges, R. E., Hamilton, H. E., and Keettel, W. C.: Pregnancy in myxedema. Arch. Intern. Med., *90*:863, 1952.

85. Hollingsworth, D. R., and Austin, E.: Thyroxine derivatives in amniotic fluid. Fetal outcome in three patients with thyroid problems. J. Pediatr., *79*:923, 1971.

86. Hollingsworth, D. R., and Mabry, C. C.: Congenital Graves' disease. Four familial cases with long-term follow-up and perspective. Am. J. Dis. Child., *130*:148, 1976.

87. Hollingsworth, D. R., Mabry, C. C., and Eckerd, J. M.: Hereditary aspects of Graves' disease in infancy and childhood. J. Pediatr., *81*:446, 1972.

88. Ibbertson, H. K., Seddon, R. J., and Croxson, M. S.: Fetal hypothyroidism complicating medical treatment of thyrotoxicosis in pregnancy. Clin. Endocrinol., *4*:521, 1975.

89. Ingbar, S. H.: Management of emergencies. IX. Thyrotoxic storm. N. Engl. J. Med., *274*:1252, 1966.

90. Innerfield, R., and Hollander, C. S.: Thyroidal complications of pregnancy. Med. Clin. North Am., *61*:67, 1977.

91. Jhaveri, R. C., Glass, L., Evans, H. E., Dube, S. K., Rosenfeld, W., Khan, F., Salazar, J. D., and Chandavasu, O.: Effects of methadone on thyroid function in mother, fetus, and newborn. Pediatrics, *65*:557, 1980.

91a. Jones, G., Delfs, E., and Foote, E. C.: The effect of thiouracil hypothyroidism on reproduction in the rat. Endocrinology, *38*:337, 1946.

92. Kampmann, J. P., Hansen, J. M., Johansen, K., and Helweg, J.: Propylthiouracil in human milk. Lancet, *1*:736, 1980.

93. Kannan, V., Sinha, M. D., Devi, P. K., and Pastogi, G. K.: Plasma thyrotropin and its response to thyrotropin releasing hormone in pregnancy. Obstet. Gynecol., *42*:547, 1973.

93a. Kenimer, J. C., Hershman, J. M., and Higgins, H. P.: The thyrotropin in hydatidiform moles is human chorionic gonadotropin. J. Clin. Endocrinol. Metab., *40*:482, 1975.

94. Kennedy, A. L., and Montgomery, D. A. D.: Hypothyroidism in pregnancy. Br. J. Obstet. Gynaecol., *85*:225, 1978.

95. Kinch, R. A., Plunkett, E. R., and Devlin, M. C.: Postpartum amenorrhea — galactorrhea of hypothyroidism. Am. J. Obstet. Gynecol., *105*:766, 1969.

96. Klein, A. H., Foley, T. P., Bernard, B., Ho, R. S., and Fisher, D. A.: Cord blood reverse T₃ in congenital hypothyroidism. J. Clin. Endocrinol. Metab., *46*:336, 1978.

97. Klein, A. H., Foley, T. P., Jr., Larsen, P. R., Agustin, A. V.,

and Hopwood, N. J.: Neonatal thyroid function in congenital hypothyroidism. J. Pediatr., 89:545, 1976.

98. Klein, A. H., Hobel, C. J., Sack, J., and Fisher, D. A.: Effect of intraamniotic fluid thyroxine injection on fetal serum and amniotic fluid iodothyronine concentrations. J. Clin. Endocrinol. Metab., 47:1034, 1978.

99. Klein, A. H., Meltzer, S., and Kenny, F. M.: Improved prognosis in congenital hypothyroidism treated before age three months. J. Pediatr., 81:912, 1972.

100. Klein, A. H., Murphy, B. E. P., Artal, R., Oddie, T. H., and Fisher, D. A.: Amniotic fluid thyroid hormone concentrations during human gestation. Am. J. Obstet. Gynecol., 136:626, 1980.

101. Kojima, A., and Hershman, J. M.: Effects of thyrotropin-releasing hormone (TRH) in maternal, fetal and newborn rats. Endocrinology, 94:1133, 1974.

102. Komins, J. I., Snyder, P. J., and Schwarz, R. H.: Hyperthyroidism in pregnancy. Obstet. Gynecol. Surv., 30:527, 1975.

103. Koutras, D. A., Pharmakoitis, A. D., Koliopoulos, N., Tsoukalos, J., Souvatzoglou, A., and Stontouris, J.: The plasma inorganic iodine and the pituitary thyroid axis in pregnancy. J. Endocrinol. Invest., 1:227, 1978.

103a. Lamberg, B. A., Ikonen, E., Teramo, K., Wägar, G., Österlund, K., Mäkinen, T., and Pekonen, F.: Treatment of hyperthyroidism with antithyroid agents and changes in thyrotropin and thyroxine in the newborn. Acta Endocrinol., 97:186, 1981.

104. Lachelin, G. C.: Myxedema and pregnancy: A case report. J. Obstet. Gynaecol. Br. Commonw., 77:77, 1970.

105. Landau, H., Sack, J., Frucht, H., Palti, Z., Hochner-Celnikier, D., and Rosenmann, A.: Amniotic fluid 3,3′,5′-triiodothyronine in the detection of congenital hypothyroidism. J. Clin. Endocrinol. Metab., 50:799, 1980.

106. Letarte, J., Guyda, H., and Dussault, J. H.: Clinical, biochemical, and radiological features of neonatal hypothyroid infants. In Burrow, G. N., and Dussault, J. H. (Eds.): Neonatal Thyroid Screening, pp. 225–236. New York, Raven Press, 1980.

107. Levy, R. P., Newman, D. M., Rejali, L. S., and Barford, D. A. G.: The myth of goiter in pregnancy. Am. J. Obstet. Gynecol., 137:701, 1980.

108. Lightner, E. S., Fismer, D. A., Giles, H., and Woolfenden, J.: Intra-amniotic injection of thyroxine (T4) to a human fetus. Am. J. Obstet. Gynecol., 127:487, 1977.

109. Little, G., Meador, C. K., Cunningham, R., and Pittman, J. A.: "Cryptothyroidism," the major cause of sporadic "athyreotic" cretinism. J. Clin. Endocrinol. Metab., 25:1529, 1965.

110. Litzenberg, J. C.: The relation of basal metabolism to sterility. Am. J. Obstet. Gynecol., 12:706, 1926.

111. Lombardi, G., Lupoli, G, Scopacasa, F., Panza, R., and Minozzi, M.: Plasma immunoreactive thyrotropin releasing hormone (TRH) values in normal newborns. J. Endocrinol. Invest., 1:69, 1978.

112. Lum, J., and Man, E. B.: Serum butanol-extractable iodines in abortions. Yale J. Biol. Med., 28:105, 1955.

113. Lusted, L. B., and Pickering, D. E.: The hypothyroid infant and child — the role of roentgen evaluation in therapy. Radiology, 66:708, 1956.

114. MacMahon, B.: Prenatal x-ray exposure and childhood cancer. J. Natl. Cancer Inst., 28:1173, 1962.

115. Maisey, M. N., and Stimmler, L.: The role of long acting thyroid stimulator in neonatal thyrotoxicosis. Clin. Endocrinol., 1:81, 1972.

115a. Malgasian, G. D., and Mayberry, W. E.: Serum total and free thyroxine in normal and pregnant women, neonates and women receiving progestogens. Am. J. Obstet. Gynecol., 108:1234, 1971.

116. Man, E. B., Heinemann, M., Johnson, C. E., Leary, D. C., and Peters, J. P.: The precipitable iodine of serum in normal pregnancy and its relation to abortions. J. Clin. Invest., 30:137, 1951.

117. Man, E. B., Holden, R. H., and Jones, W. S.: Thyroid function in human pregnancy. VII. Development and retardation of four year old progeny of euthyroid and hypothyroxinemic women. Am. J. Obstet. Gynecol., 109:12, 1971.

118. Man, E. B., Jones, W. S., Holden, R. H., and Mellits, E. D.: Thyroid function in human pregnancy. VIII. Retardation of progeny aged 7 years; relationships to maternal age and maternal thyroid function. Am. J. Obstet. Gynecol., 111:905, 1971.

119. Man, E. B., Reid, W. A., Hellegirs, A. E., and Jones, W. S.: Thyroid function in human pregnancy. III. Serum thyroxine-binding prealbumin (TBPA) and thyroxine binding globulin

(TBG) of pregnant women aged 14 through 43 years. Am. J. Obstet. Gynecol., 103:338, 1969.

120. Marchant, B., Brownlie, B. E. W., Hart, D. M., Horton, P. W., and Alexander, W. D.: The placental transfer of propylthiouracil, methimazole and carbimazole. J. Clin. Endocrinol. Metab., 45:1187, 1977.

121. McCarroll, A. M., Hutchinson, M., McAuley, R., and Montgomery, D. A. D.: Long-term assessment of children exposed in utero to carbimazole. Arch. Dis. Child., 51:532, 1976.

122. McKenzie, J. M., and Zakarija, M.: Pathogenesis of neonatal Graves' disease. J. Endocrinol. Invest., 2:182, 1978.

123. McLaughlin, C. W., Jr., and McGoogan, L. S.: Hyperthyroidism complicating pregnancy. Am. J. Obstet. Gynecol., 45:591, 1943.

124. Menking, M., Wiebel, J., Schmid, W. U., Schmidt, W. T., Ebel, K. D., and Ritter, R.: Premature craniosynostosis associated with hyperthyroidism in 4 children with reference to 5 further cases in the literature. Monatsschr. Kinderheilkd., 120:106, 1972.

125. Montoro, M. N., Collea, J. A., Frasier, S. N., and Mestman, J. H.: Successful outcome of pregnancy in women with hypothyroidism. Ann. Intern. Med., 94:31, 1981.

126. Morley, J. E., Bashore, R. A., Reed, A., Carlson, H. E., and Hershman, J. M.: Thyrotropin-releasing hormone and thyroid hormones in amniotic fluid. Am. J. Obstet. Gynecol., 134:581, 1979.

127. Mujtaba, Q., and Burrow, G. N.: Treatment of hyperthyroidism in pregnancy with propylthiouracil and methimazole. Obstet. Gynecol., 46:282, 1975.

127a. Munro, D. S., Cooke, I. D., Dirmikis, S. M., Humphries, H., James, V., Lee, D., Milner, R. D. G., and Stewart, C. R.: Neonatal thyrotoxicosis. Q. J. Med., 45:689, 1976.

128. Munro, D. S., Dirmikis, S. M., Humphries, H., Smith, T., and Broadhead, G. D.: The role of thyroid stimulating immunoglobulins of Graves' disease in neonatal thyrotoxicosis. Br. J. Obstet. Gynaecol., 85:837, 1978.

129. Murray, I. P. C.: The current status of radioactive iodine. Practitioner, 199:696, 1967.

130. Mussey, R. D.: The thyroid gland and pregnancy. Am. J. Obstet. Gynecol., 36:529, 1938.

131. Mussey, R. D.: Hyperthyroidism complicating pregnancy. Mayo Clin. Proc., 14:205, 1939.

132. Myers, C. R.: An application of the control group method to the problem of the etiology of mongolism. Proc. Am. Assoc. Mental Def., 62:142, 1938.

133. Naumoff, N., and Shook, D. M.: Abortion and low thyroid reserve. Int. J. Fertil., 8:811, 1963.

134. Neary, J. T., Nakamura, C., Davies, I. J., Soodak, M., and Maloof, F.: Lower levels of thyrotropin-releasing hormone–degrading activity in human cord and in maternal sera than in the serum of euthyroid, nonpregnant adults. J. Clin. Invest., 62:1, 1978.

135. Nicoloff, J. T., Nicoloff, R., and Dowling, J. T.: Evaluation of vaginal smear, serum gonadotropin, protein-bound iodine, and thyroxine-binding as measures of placental adequacy. J. Clin. Invest., 41:1998, 1962.

136. Nikolai, T. F., and Seal, U. S.: X-chromosome linked familial decrease in thyroxine-binding globulin activity. J. Clin. Endocrinol. Metab., 26:835, 1966.

137. Niswander, K. R., Gordon, M., and Berendes, H. W.: The Women and Their Pregnancies. Philadelphia, W. B. Saunders Co., 1972.

138. Noble, M. J. D., and Rowlands, S.: Utilization of radio-iodine during pregnancy. J. Obstet. Gynaecol. Br. Emp., 60:892, 1953.

139. Oddie, T. H., Fisher, D. A., Bernard, B., and Lam, R. W.: Thyroid function at birth in infants of 30 to 45 weeks' gestation. J. Pediatr., 90:803, 1977.

140. Oppenheimer, J. H., Squef, R., Surks, M. I., and Hauer, H.: Binding of thyroxine by serum proteins evaluated by equilibrium dialysis and electrophoretic techniques. Alteration in nonthyroidal illness. J. Clin. Invest., 42:1769, 1963.

141. Osathanondh, R., Tulchinsky, D., and Chopra, I. J.: Total and free thyroxine and triiodothyronine in normal and complicated pregnancy. J. Clin. Endocrinol. Metab., 42:98, 1976.

142. Osler, W.: Sporadic cretinism in America. Trans. Cong. Am. Physicians Surg., 4:169, 1897.

143. Packard, G. B., Williams, E. T., and Wheelock, S. E.: Congenital obstructing goiter. Surgery, 48:422, 1960.

144. Pekonen, F., and Lamberg, B.-A.: Thyrotoxicosis during pregnancy. Ann. Chir. Gynaecol., 67:165, 1978.
145. Pochin, E. E.: The iodine uptake of the human thyroid throughout the menstrual cycle and in pregnancy. Clin. Sci., 11:441, 1952.
146. Ponchon, G., Beckers, C., and DeVisscher, M.: Iodide kinetic studies in newborns and infants. J. Clin. Endocrinol. Metab., 26:1392, 1966.
147. Potter, J. D.: Hypothyroidism and reproductive failure. Surg. Gynecol. Obstet., 150:251, 1980.
148. Premachandra, B. N., Gossain, V. V., and Perlstein, I. B.: Effect of pregnancy on thyroxine binding globulin (TBG) in partial TBG deficiency. Am. J. Med. Sci., 274:189, 1977.
149. Pruyn, S. C., Phelan, J. P., and Buchanan, G. C.: Long-term propranolol therapy in pregnancy: Maternal and fetal outcome. Am. J. Obstet. Gynecol., 135:485, 1979.
150. Raiti, S., Holsman, G. B., Scott, R. L., and Blizzard, R. M.: Evidence for the placental transfer of triiodothyronine in human beings. N. Engl. J. Med., 277:456, 1967.
150a. Rastogi, G. K., Sawhney, R. C., Sinha, M. K., Thomas, Z., and Devi, P. K.: Serum and urinary levels of thyroid hormones and normal pregnancy. Obstet. Gynecol. 44:176, 1974.
151. Refetoff, S., Ochi, Y., Selenkow, H. A., and Rosenfield, R. L.: Neonatal hypothyroidism and goiter in one infant of each of two sets of twins due to maternal therapy with antithyroid drugs. J. Pediatr., 85:241, 1974.
152. Robertson, J. S., and Gorman, C. A.: Gonadal radiation dose and its genetic significance in radioiodine therapy of hyperthyroidism. J. Nucl. Med., 17:826, 1976.
153. Rodesch, F., Camus, M., Ermans, A. M., Dodion, J., and Delange, F.: Adverse effect of amniofetography on fetal thyroid function. Am. J. Obstet. Gynecol., 126:723, 1976.
153a. Rosvoll, R. V., and Winship, T.: Thyroid carcinoma and pregnancy. Surg. Gynecol. Obstet., 121:1039, 1965.
154. Sack, J., Beaudry, M., DeLamater, P. V., Oh, W., and Fisher, D. A.: Umbilical cord cutting triggers hypertriiodothyroninemia and nonshivering thermogenesis in the newborn lamb. Pediatr. Res., 10:169, 1976.
155. Saenger, E. L., Thoma, G. E., and Tompkins, E. A.: Incidence of leukemia following treatment of hyperthyroidism. J.A.M.A., 205:855, 1968.
156. Safa, A. M., Schumacher, O. P., and Rodriguez-Antunez, A.: Long-term follow-up results in children and adolescents treated with radioactive iodine (131I) for hyperthyroidism. N. Engl. J. Med., 292:167, 1975.
157. Sandstrom, B.: Antihypertensive treatment with the adrenergic beta-receptor blocker metoprolol during pregnancy. Gynecol. Invest., 9:195, 1978.
157a. Selenkow, H. A.: Antithyroid-thyroid therapy of thyrotoxicosis during pregnancy. Obstet. Gynecol., 40:117, 1972.
158. Senior, B., and Chernoff, H. L.: Iodide goiter in the newborn. Pediatrics, 47:510, 1971.
159. Shambaugh, G., III Kubek, M., and Wilber, J. F.: Thyrotropin-releasing hormone activity in the human placenta. J. Clin. Endocrinol. Metab., 48:483, 1979.
159a. Shepard, T. H.: Onset of function in the human fetal thyroid: Biochemical and radioautographic studies from organ culture. J. Clin. Endocrinol. Metab., 27:945, 1967.
160. Smallridge, R. C., Wartofsky, L., Chopra, I. J., Marinelli, P. V., Broughton, R. E., Dimond, R. C., and Burman, K. D.: Neonatal thyrotoxicosis: Alterations in serum concentrations of LATS-protector, T4, T3, reverse T3 and 3,3'T2. J. Pediatr., 93:118, 1978.
161. Smith, C. S., and Howard, N. J.: Propranolol in treatment of neonatal thyrotoxicosis. J. Pediatr., 83:1046, 1973.
162. Smith, D. W., Klein, A. M., Henderson, J. R., and Myrianthopoulos, N. C.: Congenital hypothyroidism — signs and symptoms in the newborn period. J. Pediatr., 87:958, 1975.
163. Soler, N. G., and Nicholson, H.: Diabetes and thyroid disease during pregnancy. Obstet. Gynecol., 54:318, 1979.
163a. Souma, J. A., Niejadlik, D. C., Cottrell, S., and Rankel, S.: Comparison of thyroid function in each trimester of pregnancy with the use of triiodothyronine uptake, thyroxine iodine, free thyroxine and free thyroxine index. Am. J. Obstet. Gynecol., 116:905, 1973.
164. Stanbury, J. B.: Cretinism and the fetal-maternal relationship. In Stanbury, J. B., and Kroc, R. L. (Eds.): Human Development and the Thyroid Gland: Relation to Endemic Cretinism. Proceedings, Symposium on Endemic Cretinism, Kroc Foundation. New York, Plenum Press, 1972.

165. Sternberg, J.: Irradiation and radiocontamination during pregnancy. Am. J. Obstet. Gynecol., 108:490, 1970.
166. Stewart, A., Webb, J., and Hewitt, D.: A survey of childhood malignancies. Br. Med. J., 1:1495, 1958.
167. Stock, J. M., Surks, M. I., and Oppenheimer, J. H.: Replacement dosage of L-thyroxine in hypothyroidism. N. Engl. J. Med., 290:529, 1974.
168. Stoffer, R. P., Koeneke, I. A., Chesky, V. E., and Hellwig, C. A.: The thyroid in pregnancy. Am. J. Obstet. Gynecol., 74:300, 1957.
169. Stoffer, S. S., and Hamburger J. I.: Inadvertent 131I therapy for hyperthyroidism in the first trimester of pregnancy. J. Nucl. Med., 17:146, 1976.
170. Stolte, L., Kock, H., van Kessel, H., and Kock, L.: Thyroxine utilization in non-pregnant, steroid-induced pseudopregnant, and pregnant monkeys. Acta Endocrinol., 52:383, 1966.
171. Stubbe, P., Gatz, J., Heidemann, P., Muhlen, A., and Hesch, R.: Thyroxine-binding globulin, triiodothyronine, thyroxine and thyrotropin in newborn infants and children. Horm. Metab. Res., 10:58, 1978.
172. Sutherland, J. M., Esselborn, V. M., Burket, R. L., Skillman, T. B., and Benson, J. T.: Familial nongoitrous cretinism apparently due to maternal antithyroid antibody. Report of a family. N. Engl. J. Med., 263:336, 1960.
173. Talbert, L. M., Thomas, C. G., Jr., Holt, W. A., and Rankin, P.: Hyperthyroidism during pregnancy. Obstet. Gynecol., 36:779, 1970.
173a. Thorner, M. O.: Prolactin. Clin. Endocrinol. Metab., 6:201, 1977.
174. Ueda, Y., Hayaski, K., Kishimoto, Y., and Mizusawa, S.: Sexual function in women with diseases of the thyroid gland. J. Jap. Obstet. Gynecol. Soc., 11:48, 1964.
175. Vandalem, J. L., Pirens, G., Hennen, G., and Gaspard, U.: Thyroliberin and gonadoliberin tests during pregnancy and the puerperium. Acta Endocrinol., 86:695, 1977.
176. Van Herle, A. J., Young, R. T., Fisher, D. A., Uller, R. P., and Brinkman, C. R., III.: Intra-uterine treatment of a hypothyroid fetus. J. Clin. Endocrinol. Metab., 40:474, 1975.
177. Visscher, P. D.: T3-131I binding capacity of serum proteins. Am. J. Obstet. Gynecol., 86:829, 1963.
178. Walker, P., Dussault, J. H., Hart, I. R., Langelier, P., and Szots, F.: Thyrotoxicosis detected in a mass-screening program for neonatal hypothyroidism: Demonstration of placental transfer of an immunoglobulin with marked lipolytic activity. J. Pediatr., 91:400, 1977.
179. Wallace, E. Z., and Gandhi, V. S.: Triiodothyronine thyrotoxicosis in pregnancy. Am. J. Obstet. Gynecol., 130:106, 1978.
179a. Weijer, D. L., Duggan, H. E., and Scott, D. B.: Total body radiation and dose to the gonads from the therapeutic use of iodine131. J. Can. Assoc. Radiol., 11:50, 1960.
180. Werner, S. C.: The effect of triiodothyronine administration on the elevated protein-bound iodine level in human pregnancy. Am. J. Obstet. Gynecol., 75:1193, 1958.
181. Wespi-Eggenberger, H. J.: Untersuchungen über das Vorkommen und die Verhuntung des Neugeborenenkropfes im Einzugsgebeit. Schweiz. Med. Wschr., 78:130, 1948.
182. Wilkin, T. J., Kenyon, E., and Isles, T. E.: The behaviour of thyroid hormones in an infant with untreated neonatal thyrotoxicosis. Clin. Endocrinol., 7:227, 1977.
183. Wilkins, L.: Epiphysial dysgenesis associated with hypothyroidism. Am. J. Dis. Child., 61:13, 1941.
184. Williams, R. H., Kay, G. A., and Jandorf, B. J.: Thiouracil. Its absorption, distribution, and excretion. J. Clin. Invest., 23:613, 1944.
185. Witherspoon, L. R., Shuler, S. E., Garcia, M. M., and Zollinger, L. A.: An assessment of methods for the estimation of free thyroxine. J. Nucl. Med., 21:529, 1980.
186. Worley, R. J., and Crosby, W. M.: Hyperthyroidism during pregnancy. Am. J. Obstet. Gynecol., 119:150, 1974.
187. Yamamoto, T., Amino, N., Tanizawa, O., Koi, K., Ichihara, K., Azukizawa, M., and Miyai, K.: Longitudinal study of serum thyroid hormones, chorionic gonadotrophin and thyrotropin during and after normal pregnancy. Clin. Endocrinol., 10:459, 1979.
188. Ylikorkala, O., Kivinen, S., and Reinila, M. I.: Serial prolactin and thyrotropin responses to thyrotropin-releasing hormone throughout normal human pregnancy. J. Clin. Endocrinol. Metab., 48:288, 1979.

Gerard N. Burrow, M.D.

9

PITUITARY, ADRENAL, AND PARATHYROID DISORDERS

THE PITUITARY GLAND

Pituitary integrity is necessary for conception, and pregnancy is uncommon in women with pituitary abnormalities. During the course of pregnancy the anterior lobe of the pituitary may double or triple in size because of an increase in prolactin-secreting cells.[15] The pituitary may enlarge during apparently normal pregnancy to the degree that it impinges upon the optic chiasm and causes bitemporal hemianopsia.[30] Whether this phenomenon occurs in a completely normal pituitary gland is a subject for dispute; the possibility exists that these patients have small, clinically undetected prolactinomas. However, with the rapid postpartum regression of pituitary size, visual fields usually return to normal by the tenth postpartum day.

Physiologic changes occur in the pituitary in addition to the anatomic changes. Pituitary gonadotropin levels are low,[21] presumably because of increased concentrations of circulating estrogens. There is a reduced growth hormone response to both hypoglycemia and arginine during the third trimester.[44] Whether this decreased growth hormone release occurs because of increased human placental lactogen or progesterone is not clear.[6, 42] Although conflicting results have been reported, we found an increased TSH response to TRH during the second half of the pregnancy.[7, 45] In contrast, ACTH secretion is apparently diminished, as is indicated by the metyrapone test.[4] Both the TSH and the ACTH effects may be due, at least in part, to the increased concentration of circulating estrogens. Finally, the serum prolactin concentration is markedly elevated during pregnancy.[43]

These changes in pituitary hormones make evaluation of pituitary function in pregnancy difficult. Serum FSH and LH concentrations are low during normal pregnancy. Serum growth concentrations can be determined only with difficulty during the first two trimesters of pregnancy. Stimulation of growth hormone secretion by hypoglycemia is undesirable in pregnancy, and arginine infusion is probably the best choice. For screening purposes, a plasma growth hormone can be obtained 60 to 90 minutes after nocturnal sleep, or samples can be obtained 20 minutes after vigorous exercise. Plasma concentrations greater than 5 ng per ml make further testing unnecessary. A low serum TSH concentration in conjunction with low serum thyroxine determinations indicates hypothyroidism at the pituitary or hypothalamic level. If necessary, TRH could be used to differentiate pituitary or secondary hypothyroidism from hypothalamic or tertiary hypothyroidism. Although the response in normal pregnancy is decreased, metyrapone can be used to test the pituitary-adrenal axis. However, neither TSH nor metyrapone is recommended for use in pregnant women.

Pituitary Tumors in Pregnant Women

Increasing numbers of pregnancies are being reported in patients with prolactinomas as a consequence of the use of bromocriptine for ovulation induction.[41] This is a calculated risk, and it should be made clear to the women that pituitary tumors are probably estrogen dependent with a potential risk of enlargement during pregnancy. The exact degree of risk is unclear, and such women have usually carried uneventful pregnancies to term.[22, 38] Interestingly, these tumors have been reported to have become smaller after pregnancy.[8a]

At the present time most workers would agree that a woman with a prolactin-secretin macroadenoma should not conceive unless the tumor has been treated surgically. Radiation treatment

215

to limit subsequent tumor expansion during pregnancy has been suggested.[41] Whether this has a role in the treatment of women with microadenomas remains to be determined.

As soon as pregnancy is confirmed in a patient with a prolactin-secretin microadenoma who is receiving bromocriptine, the drug should be stopped. During pregnancy the patient should be followed up closely with monthly visual field examinations by Goldman perimetry. Sellar tomography and CT scans should be done at any time during pregnancy if visual field changes, headaches, blurred vision, or funduscopic changes occur. If visual field defects due to tumor enlargement arise during pregnancy, bromocriptine may be reinstituted with successful reversal of the visual field defects.[5] Transsphenoidal hypophysectomy is also effective.[38] If the patient is close to term, the pregnancy may be terminated by induction of labor or cesarean section. Immediately post partum, bromocriptine therapy should be reinstituted in all patients so affected. If the pregnant woman has undergone previous transsphenoidal hypophysectomy, she should be followed up with frequent visual field examinations throughout pregnancy to be sure there is no recurrence.

Acromegaly. Acromegaly may also occur during pregnancy. Although amenorrhea is common in women with acromegaly, pregnancy does occur.[1, 14] Six normal pregnancies occurred in 19 young women with acromegaly who had continued to menstruate. Despite other soft tissue changes in acromegaly, no major changes occur in the genital tract that would complicate delivery. Occasionally pregnant women may have some new edematous thickening of features that might be mistaken for acromegaly.

Lymphocytic Hypophysitis. There have been several case reports of women with apparent pituitary tumors who were found to have lymphocytic hypophysitis on biopsy. In about half the cases the disease was detected in the postpartum period, and in two cases the onset was during gestation.[2] The cause may be related to changes in autoimmunity during pregnancy and the postpartum period with resulting inflammation and hypopituitarism.

Sheehan's Syndrome

Before clinical manifestations of pituitary hypofunction become evident, about three quarters of the entire pituitary must be destroyed. In the adult female, postpartum pituitary necrosis or Sheehan's syndrome is the most common cause of anterior pituitary insufficiency.[37] The cause of the syndrome is not clear, but it is a sequel to acute ischemic necrosis of the pituitary subsequent to blood loss during delivery.[27] Sheehan's syndrome may be related to the pituitary hypertrophy, which makes the gland more sensitive to an inadequate blood supply. The syndrome is distinctly uncommon with other conditions associated with shock and vascular collapse. Furthermore, there is no direct correlation between the severity of the hemorrhage and the occurrence of Sheehan's syndrome.[17]

Course of Sheehan's Syndrome. Classically, the clinical appearance of pituitary deficiency has been considered to follow a pattern of consecutive loss of gonadotropins, growth hormone, TSH, and ACTH. This orderly loss of pituitary function would make Sheehan's syndrome a problem for long-term medical followup but would preclude further pregnancies. However, only rarely does the functional impairment in spontaneous hypopituitarism approach that which occurs with a large tumor. Only half of 25 women with Sheehan's syndrome developed amenorrhea and did not lactate.[13] The other half menstruated and lactated to varying degrees. A woman who had only scanty menses for 16 years after a massive postpartum hemorrhage had three uneventful pregnancies during this time.[29] During the fourth pregnancy she had evidence of decreased thyroid and adrenal function, and evaluation of pituitary function after delivery revealed decreased levels of TSH, ACTH, and growth hormone. Other patients with Sheehan's syndrome have also developed impaired anterior pituitary function following a subsequent uncomplicated pregnancy.[20] Hypoglycemia may occur during pregnancy because of a combination of ACTH and growth hormone deficiency superimposed on the tendency of the pregnant woman toward hypoglycemia.[39]

Failure of lactation and rapid breast involution are the earliest postpartum signs of hypopituitarism in patients with Sheehan's syndrome. These women fail to regain strength and vigor after delivery and are often treated for postpartum depression. Menses are scanty or absent. Fatigue and cold intolerance are common complaints, and the patients may present with frank myxedema. On examination the skin is pale and waxy. Axillary and pubic hair is sparse; virtually none remains after several years of marked hypopituitarism. The decrease in melanin pigmentation in the skin also affects the areolae of the breasts.

Differential Diagnosis. Pituitary necrosis

may also occur in pregnant diabetics.[12, 35] Nineteen cases of hypopituitarism in diabetic females have been reported, and eight occurred during pregnancy.[12] Characteristically, a deep midline headache developed during the third trimester, lasted several days, and was followed by a decrease in insulin requirements. The affected women were not necessarily long-standing diabetics. In three of seven patients the condition was associated with maternal death.

In the postpartum period Sheehan's syndrome must be separated from other causes of amenorrhea. Perhaps the commonest cause of postpartum amenorrhea in association with galactorrhea (Chiari-Frommel syndrome) is prolactinoma. However, the symptom complex can also occur in association with hypothyroidism.[26] The failure of menstrual periods to return within 4 to 6 months after delivery in a non–breast-feeding mother is a matter of concern and should be investigated at least with serum prolactin and serum thyroxine determinations.

Treatment. Treatment of pituitary hypofunction diagnosed during pregnancy involves replacement of adrenal corticosteroids and thyroid hormone.[23] Unlike Addison's disease, there is usually a sufficient quantity of aldosterone produced in the absence of ACTH, and mineralocorticoid replacement is not necessary.

The question of growth hormone replacement is of interest, particularly in view of the fact that with cloning procedures, abundant clinical supplies of human growth hormone will become available. Sexually ateliotic dwarfs have no growth hormone, nor may their offspring in utero. In such cases, not only is the birth weight normal, but so is the birth length. The speculation has been made that perhaps human placental lactogen takes over the role of growth hormone.[42]

In addition to the management of pituitary function during pregnancy, long-term medical followup should be provided for any patient who has significant intrapartum bleeding. In an attempt to determine whether there were significant numbers of women without overt Sheehan's syndrome but compromised pituitary function following intrapartum bleeding, we studied 13 women.[25] Complete evaluation of anterior pituitary function with hypothalamic-releasing hormones failed to reveal any patients with decreased function, although one patient was found to have a prolactinoma. The results of this study suggest that there are not large numbers of women with subclinical pituitary hypofunction following intrapartum hemorrhage.

Diabetes Insipidus

Changes occur in posterior pituitary function as well as in anterior pituitary function during pregnancy. The plasma concentration of neurophysin is elevated during pregnancy, apparently because of the increased estrogen concentrations.[32, 34] Neurophysins are present in the neurohypophysis in association with the peptide hormones oxytocin and vasopressin and are thought to act as intraneuronal carrier proteins for these hormones. Any condition that causes damage to the neurohypophyseal system may result in inadequate secretion of vasopressin with resulting diabetes insipidus.

Clinical Picture. Most cases of diabetes insipidus belong to the symptomatic group of patients with a history of trauma or tumor that has damaged the hypothalamic-hypophyseal region. About a third of all patients with diabetes insipidus have an idiopathic type for which no definite etiology can be found. The hereditary form, inherited as an autosomal dominant trait, is rare, accounting for less than 1 per cent of patients with diabetes insipidus.

The main symptoms in typical diabetes insipidus are polyuria and polydipsia. The specific gravity of the urine is less than 1.005. The diagnosis is made by water deprivation with increasing serum osmolality in the face of low urine osmolalities and a return toward normal values after the administration of vasopressin.[3] This has to be done very cautiously in a pregnant woman.

Diabetes Insipidus and Pregnancy. Diabetes insipidus is of particular interest during pregnancy because of the relation to the other neurohypophyseal hormone, oxytocin.[11] Observation of a diabetes insipidus patient in labor who had uterine atony that did not respond to exogenous pituitrin suggested the possible importance of this relationship.[28] Subsequent reports have not substantiated the presence of inadequate labor in women with diabetes insipidus.[16, 18, 31] One study has suggested that oxytocin and vasopressin are released independently in pregnant women. Changes in uterine activity and urine osmolality were used as indicators of oxytocin or vasopressin release in a group of women in late pregnancy or early puerperium. Direct measurement of oxytocin in a pregnant woman with diabetes insipidus demonstrated a surge of plasma oxytocin during labor.[36]

Patients with diabetes insipidus have no impairment in fertility, and pregnancy is not affected adversely by the disease. Although vasopressin may cause uterine contractions, there have been no consistent reports of abortion or premature labor.[19] Two patients have been reported in whom the symptoms of diabetes insipidus appeared during pregnancy and disappeared after parturition.[24]

Treatment. The standard treatment for diabetes insipidus has been parenteral vasopressin. However, great variability in the requirement for vasopressin has occurred during pregnancy.[10, 31] Recently L-deamino-8-d-arginine vasopressin (DDAVP), a synthetic analogue, has replaced vasopressin as the drug of choice.[33] DDAVP can be given intranasally and is reliable, and patients do not develop tolerance. The drug has been successfully used in pregnant women.[8] Certainly, the drug is more desirable than chlorpropamide, which has been used in patients with partial diabetes insipidus.

THE ADRENAL GLAND

Evaluation of the condition of a pregnant woman with suspected adrenal pathology may be very difficult because of the gestational changes in adrenal function. Adrenal corticosteroid therapy in the pregnant woman, if indicated, is complicated because of possible effects on the fetus. In order to understand the changes in adrenal function during pregnancy, a clear understanding of adrenal function in the nonpregnant woman is necessary.

Normal Adrenal Function

Maintenance of normal adrenal function depends on continual glucocorticoid secretion, which is accomplished by intermittent release of cortisol with apparent diurnal variation.

Regulation of Glucocorticoid Release. Patients who are stressed require increased quantities of the corticosteroids. However, if too much steroid is delivered to the tissues, the effects may be harmful, as in Cushing's disease. Diurnal variation in cortisol secretion characterized by higher concentrations in the early morning and lower concentrations in the evening is due to similar variations in ACTH release, which in turn are presumably secondary to variations in corticotropin-releasing factor (CRF) from the hypothalamus. Diurnal variation of ACTH does not follow a smooth curve. Rather, there is episodic release of ACTH and stimulation of corticosteroid secretion. Stress results in increased release of ACTH, presumably mediated through the central nervous system and CRF.

The pathway of cortisol synthesis in the adrenal is of importance, because defects in synthesis may occur through a congenital or acquired block in the steroid pathway (Fig. 9–1). The side chain of cholesterol is cleaved to form pregnenolone, which is transformed into progesterone, the immediate precursor of all active adrenocortical hormones. A series of stepwise hydroxylations then takes place in the 17, 21, and 11 positions, resulting in the formation of cortisol and aldosterone. Androgens are formed from 17-hydroxylated precursors and in turn are precursors for the estrogens.

Tests of Adrenal Function. Adrenal corticosteroids are excreted almost quantitatively in the urine after conjugation and metabolism. Measurement of the 24 hour excretion of adrenal steroids gives an integrated measure of daily corticosteroid production, which is important because of the diurnal variation. Much of the cortisol produced can be measured in the urine, as 17-hydroxycorticosteroids (17-OHCS) by the Porter-Silber reaction (Fig. 9–2). The determination is not specific, however, and determination of the urinary free cortisol by radioimmunoassay is desirable, if the latter is available. The plasma cortisol concentration can be determined by any of several procedures, including fluorescent competitive protein binding and radioimmunoassay methods. The radioimmunoassay may be highly specific and sensitive and is relatively simple.

The value of these tests is greatly enhanced if physiologic manipulations are performed that help to separate normal from pathologic conditions. Dexamethasone, 0.5 mg every 6 hours, inhibits ACTH secretion and results in a decrease in plasma cortisol concentration and urinary 17-OHCS in normal persons. Patients with adrenal hyperplasia but not autonomous adrenal adenomas will usually be suppressed with 2 mg of dexamethasone every 6 hours. A rapid dexamethasone screening test can be done by administration of 1 mg of dexamethasone at 11 PM. A plasma cortisol determination the next morning should be less than 10 μg per 100 ml.

The pituitary-adrenal axis may be evaluated by the administration of metyrapone, which inhibits 11B-hydroxylation in the adrenal gland (see Fig. 9–1). Alternatively, hypoglycemia can be induced by insulin, which results in increased ACTH release and a rise in the plasma cortisol. The ability of the adrenal to respond can be tested with synthetic corticotropin (Cortrosyn). A rapid screening test can be performed by obtaining a base-line plasma cortisol and administering 0.25 mg of Cortrosyn intramuscularly. The plasma cortisol determination is repeated an

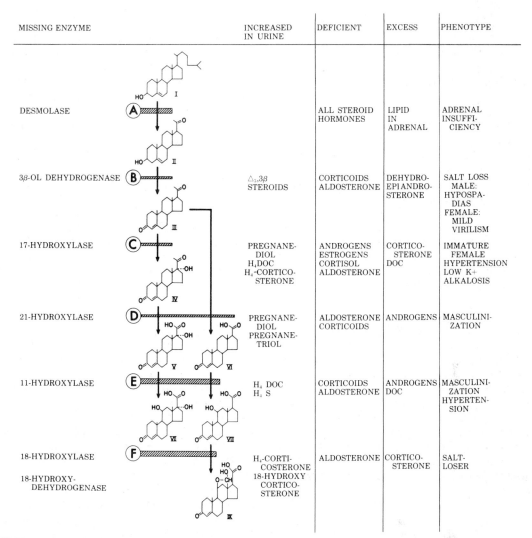

MISSING ENZYME		INCREASED IN URINE	DEFICIENT	EXCESS	PHENOTYPE
DESMOLASE	(A)		ALL STEROID HORMONES	LIPID IN ADRENAL	ADRENAL INSUFFI- CIENCY
3β-OL DEHYDROGENASE	(B)	Δ₅,3β STEROIDS	CORTICOIDS ALDOSTERONE	DEHYDRO- EPIANDRO- STERONE	SALT LOSS MALE: HYPOSPA- DIAS FEMALE: MILD VIRILISM
17-HYDROXYLASE	(C)	PREGNANE- DIOL H₂DOC H₄-CORTICO- STERONE	ANDROGENS ESTROGENS CORTISOL ALDOSTERONE	CORTICO- STERONE DOC	IMMATURE FEMALE HYPERTENSION LOW K+ ALKALOSIS
21-HYDROXYLASE	(D)	PREGNANE- DIOL PREGNANE- TRIOL	ALDOSTERONE CORTICOIDS	ANDROGENS	MASCULINI- ZATION
11-HYDROXYLASE	(E)	H₄ DOC H₄ S	CORTICOIDS ALDOSTERONE	ANDROGENS DOC	MASCULINI- ZATION HYPERTEN- SION
18-HYDROXYLASE 18-HYDROXY- DEHYDROGENASE	(F)	H₄-CORTI- COSTERONE 18-HYDROXY CORTICO- STERONE	ALDOSTERONE	CORTICO- STERONE	SALT- LOSER

FIGURE 9–1. Steroid pathway for cortisol synthesis and possible metabolic blocks (From Bondy, P. K., and Rosenberg, L. E.: Metabolic Control and Disease, 8th ed. Philadelphia, W. B. Saunders Co., 1980, p. 1480.)

REACTION	17-HYDROXY- CORTICOIDS	17-KETOGENIC STEROIDS				17-KETOSTEROIDS	
REQUIRES							
INCLUDES	CORTISOL CORTISONE TETRAHYDRO- CORTISOL TETRAHYDRO- CORTISONE and their 3β-OH, Δ⁵ counterparts	17-HYDROXY- CORTICOIDS	CORTOLS CORTOLONES	17-HYDROXY- PROGESTERONE + 21-DEOXYCORTISOL	PREGNANETRIOL	DEHYDROEPI- ANDROSTERONE ANDROSTERONE ETIOCHOLANOLONE (Androgen derivatives)	11β-HYDROXYANDROSTER- ONE 11β-HYDROXYETIOCHOLAN- OLONE 3α,11β-HYDROXYANDROS- TENE-17-ONE 3α-UREIDO, 11β-HYDROXY- ANDROSTADIENE, 17-ONE 11β-HYDROXY 3,5 ANDROS- TADIENE, 17-ONE (Derivatives of cortisol.

FIGURE 9–2. Steroids measured by various urinary determinations. (From Bondy, P. K., and Rosenberg, L. E.: Metabolic Control and Disease, 8th ed. Philadelphia, W. B. Saunders Co., 1980, p. 1452.)

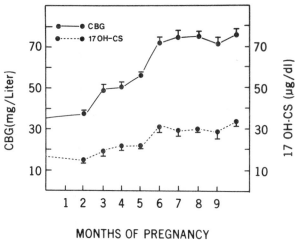

FIGURE 9–3. Cortisol-binding globulin concentration during pregnancy. (From Doe et al.: J. Clin. Endocrinol. Metab., 24:1029, 1964. Copyright 1964 The Endocrine Society. Reprinted with permission.)

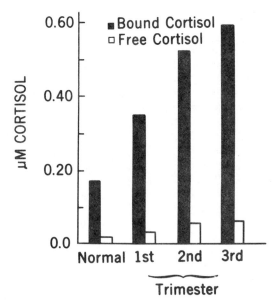

FIGURE 9–4. Free and bound cortisol concentrations during pregnancy. (From Rosenthal et al.: J. Clin. Endocrinol. Metab., 29:352, 1969. Copyright 1969 The Endocrine Society. Reprinted with permission.)

hour later, and there should be at least a doubling of the plasma cortisol value.

Adrenal Function During Pregnancy

Although the weight of the adrenal glands does not increase significantly during pregnancy, an increase in the thickness of the zona fasciculata was observed in 24 women who died suddenly during pregnancy or in the immediate postpartum period.[100]

Corticosteroid-Binding Globulin. Plasma cortisol concentrations rise progressively during pregnancy and reach a plateau that is above the upper limits of normal during the second trimester. A large part of this increase is due to a rise in corticosteroid-binding globulin concentration (CBG) during pregnancy.[95] Biologically active unconjugated cortisol circulates in plasma bound to CBG, which is an alpha-globulin. Progesterone also binds to CBG in the serum.

During pregnancy the mean CBG concentration rose from 33 mg per liter in 16 normal females to a plateau of 70 mg per liter in the second trimester (Fig. 9–3). In another study of 253 pregnant women, CBG capacity increased from 24 μg cortisol per 100 ml in normal nonpregnant females to a mean peak of 45 μg cortisol per 100 ml at 28 to 31 weeks of gestation (values expressed as μg cortisol bound per 100 ml).[59] This increase in CBG can be mimicked by estrogen administration to nonpregnant women. In normal women who received 200 mg ethinyl estradiol for 2 weeks, the mean CBG concentration rose from 38 mg per liter to 99 mg per liter with a concomitant increase in the mean morning plasma cortisol concentration from 19 to 51 μg per 100 ml.[60]

Cortisol. Cortisol bound to CBG does not enter the cell, but rather it is the free plasma cortisol that is metabolically active. In contrast to thyroid hormone, free plasma cortisol concentrations are also clearly elevated in pregnancy (Fig. 9–4).[57, 80] During pregnancy, free cortisol concentrations are increased in both the morning

TABLE 9–1 FREE AND BOUND CORTISOL CONCENTRATIONS

	CBG *mg/l*	Plasma 17-OHCS *μg/100 ml*		Free 17-OHCS *μg/100 ml*	
		9 AM	9 PM	9 AM	9 PM
Nonpregnant female	39	19	7.4	1.4	0.4
Estrogen treated female	99	51	19	2.3	0.6
Pregnancy	80	43	24	2.6	1.0

(From Doe, R., Dickinson, P., Zinneman, H. H., and Seal, U. S.: J. Clin. Endocrinol. Metab., 29:757, 1980.)

and the evening[57, 60] (Table 9–1). The elevated free cortisol concentrations approach those found in Cushing's syndrome. Although the free plasma cortisol is elevated, diurnal variation is qualitatively similar to that in nonpregnant women.[80] Estrogen administration, in contrast, causes an increase in free cortisol in the morning but not in the evening. Plasma aldosterone concentrations are also increased.[96] Urinary free cortisol concentrations increase during pregnancy concomitant with the increase in plasma free cortisol values.[54] The increase in the urinary free cortisol is due to the increased excretion of cortisol during the evening.[79]

The half-life of plasma cortisol is prolonged in the pregnant woman.[56, 76] Estrogen administration to nonpregnant women also results in a prolonged half-life for plasma cortisol.[77, 85] The increase in CBG may allow less cortisol to be extracted by the liver, with a consequent prolongation of the half-life of cortisol. Another possibility is that the prolongation of the half-life of plasma cortisol is an indication that the liver has an impaired ability to metabolize plasma cortisol in the pregnant woman.[92]

The cortisol production rate is more than twice as high during pregnancy than in the nongravid state.[80] Presumably, the small amount of cortisol secreted by the fetus contributes little to the maternal level, since the gradient would favor transfer of cortisol from mother to fetus. The combination of increased cortisol production and delayed plasma clearance would explain the increase in free cortisol concentration during pregnancy.

The urinary excretion of cortisol metabolites as measured by 17-OHCS is decreased during pregnancy. Thirteen pregnant women had a mean urinary 17-OHCS excretion of 2 mg per 24 hours, which was significantly lower than the mean nonpregnant value of 3.4 mg for 24 hours.[77] Similar decreases in urinary 17-OHCS excretion also occur after estrogen administration.[65] The decreased urinary 17-OHCS excretion is due to a decrease in the excretion of the tetrahydro metabolites of cortisol,[58, 73] which may be partially due to the formation of 6B-hydroxy compounds that are not measured in the 17-OHCS assay.

Despite apparent decreased urinary 17-OHCS excretion, the adrenal gland appears to be more responsive to ACTH during pregnancy with a greater rise in plasma cortisol concentration for a given dose of ACTH[9a, 58, 68] (Fig. 9–5). Although the adrenal appears more responsive, the pituitary-adrenal axis is less responsive to metyrapone. The rise in 17-OHCS following metyrapone administration is decreased in normal

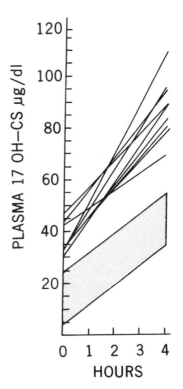

FIGURE 9–5. Plasma 17-OH-corticosteroid response to ACTH in pregnancy. Solid lines represent nine pregnant women tested with 25 U ACTH over four hours during the third trimester of pregnancy. Shaded area represents normal response of nonpregnant women. (From Jailer et al.: Am. J. Obstet. Gynecol., 78:1, 1959. Reprinted with permission.)

pregnancy,[50, 53] and similar results occur in nonpregnant women given estrogens.[75]

Fetal Contribution to Maternal Adrenal Function. The fetal adrenal grows rapidly and by the fourth month of gestation is larger than the fetal kidney.[99] About 80 per cent of this large gland is made up by the fetal zone, which is extremely active in steroid metabolism. By parturition, the fetal adrenal has decreased to half the size of the kidney and continues its rapid involution. The fetal adrenal provides the placenta with precursors for the synthesis of estrogens and progesterone. Marked increases in the urinary excretion of corticosteroid and 11-deoxycorticosteroid sulfates occur in pregnant women at term, and this has been interpreted as indirect evidence that the steroid sulfates originate from the fetus.[69] Studies with radioactive cortisol suggest that maternal cortisol must cross the placenta at least at term.[76] However, ACTH does not cross the placenta or does so poorly.[46]

Adrenal State During Pregnancy. CBG and plasma cortisol concentrations increase in the pregnant woman. Free cortisol concentrations also increase, which raises the question whether adrenal function is truly increased during pregnancy. Pregnant women have a urinary amino acid pattern similar to that of patients receiving pharmacologic doses of cortisol. Increased adrenal function in pregnancy could contribute to striae gravidarum, impaired carbohydrate tolerance, hypertension, fluid retention, and amelioration of the inflammatory process. However, it is not actually the free cortisol that determines steroid action, but the steroid bound to nuclear receptors. Progesterone concentrations in pregnancy are high enough to compete with cortisol for intracellular binding sites. The elevated cortisol concentrations during pregnancy may reflect diminished intracellular cortisol binding in the hypothalamus and pituitary.[49] Whether adrenal function in pregnancy is actually increased at the cellular level must remain cloaked in rhetoric.

Adrenocortical Insufficiency

Insufficient adrenal corticosteroids, whether as a result of primary obstruction of the adrenals, insufficient ACTH secretion from the pituitary, or inadequate steroid replacement, can result in an acute state with life-threatening collapse or a chronic process with numerous ill-defined signs and symptoms.

Chronic Adrenal Insufficiency. Adrenocortical insufficiency appearing during pregnancy for the first time may be difficult to diagnose, both from the clinical and the laboratory presentations. This is especially true during the period of development of the disease when the patient may have adequate steroids for daily living but cannot cope with stress. Pregnant patients in whom the diagnosis of adrenocortical insufficiency has been established may need to have their steroid replacement therapy regulated to meet the changing demands of gestation.

The systemic effects of insufficient mineralocorticoids are expressed by a reduced ability to retain sodium and excrete potassium. Along with the decrease in extracellular electrolytes, glucocorticoid deficiency results in decreased renal perfusion and cardiac output. As a result of these factors, intravascular volume decreases, and with poor vascular tone, vascular collapse ultimately ensues. The systemic effects of insufficient glucocorticoids include a tendency toward gastrointestinal disturbances, difficulty in maintaining fasting blood glucose levels, and spontaneous hypoglycemia.[93] Because of the decreased cortisol concentration, there is a loss of ACTH

feedback control, and the pituitary responds by excreting excessive amounts of ACTH and melanocyte-stimulating hormone (MSH). The nausea and vomiting, the increased pigmentation, and the tendency toward fasting hypoglycemia in the normal pregnant woman may confuse the diagnosis of Addison's disease during pregnancy and at the same time potentiate the clinical signs of adrenal insufficiency. Addison's disease may also occur as part of a syndrome of multiple end-organ failure, which further confuses the diagnosis.[87]

Diagnosis During Pregnancy. The signs and symptoms of Addison's disease in pregnancy are the same as in the nonpregnant state. Weakness, fatigue, increased pigmentation, weight loss, anorexia, hypoglycemia, and nervousness, occur in both conditions. Asthenia, marked pigmentation, intensified gastrointestinal symptoms, and weight loss are particularly common presenting complaints in pregnancy, and unfortunately, the normal pregnant woman may present with these signs and symptoms. However, weight loss and persistent nausea and vomiting should alert the physician. In a review of 39 cases of Addison's disease occurring in pregnancy, seven patients were diagnosed for the first time after they developed adrenal crisis during the puerperium.[52] In each instance, fatigue, increased pigmentation, and nausea and vomiting had been attributed to the pregnancy. Patients with untreated Addison's disease tended to tolerate pregnancy without difficulty but to develop difficulties in the puerperium. Twelve out of 22 patients with adrenocortical insufficiency who carried their pregnancies to term developed adrenal crisis post partum. This tendency to develop adrenal crisis post partum is probably related to the diuresis and dehydration that may follow delivery.

The laboratory diagnosis of adrenal insufficiency during pregnancy is made more difficult by the increased CBG. Plasma cortisol concentrations may be within the normal nonpregnant range. The diagnosis of Addison's disease rests on the lack of rise in the plasma cortisol concentration after Cortrosyn infusions. Although urinary 17 OHCS excretion is decreased during pregnancy, the values should increase after Cortrosyn stimulation if adrenal function is intact.

Acute Adrenal Insufficiency. In contrast to the relatively indolent course of chronic adrenal insufficiency, acute adrenal insufficiency, or addisonian crisis, is a true medical emergency. Anorexia rapidly progresses to nausea and vomiting, diarrhea, and abdominal pain. Shortly after the onset of vomiting, the blood pressure may plummet and the patient may appear to be in severe shock. Fever is usually present.

A patient with suspected addisonian crisis should be treated without waiting for the laboratory results. After plasma cortisol determinations have been obtained, the patient should be treated with cortisol and fluids. Cortisol hemisuccinate (Solu-Cortef), 200 mg, should be given as a bolus intravenously, and fluid replacement with isotonic saline should be instituted. The first liter, which should be given over about 30 minutes, should also contain 50 gm of glucose to obviate hypoglycemic attacks. In addition, each liter of fluid should contain 100 mg of cortisol hemisuccinate. The addisonian crisis may require 5 or 6 liters for hydration, and thus the patient may receive as much as 600 mg of cortisol. This much cortisol has sufficient mineralocorticoid activity, and no extra mineralocorticoid is necessary. Within 24 hours it is usually possible to switch to intramuscular cortisol hemisuccinate, 25 mg every 6 hours.

Maintenance of the Pregnant Woman with Addison's Disease. For the pregnant woman with Addison's disease, adequate adrenal replacement is cortisone acetate, 25 mg in the morning and 12.5 mg at night, with 0.05 or 0.10 mg 9-alpha-fluoro-hydrocortisone daily. Prednisone, 5 mg in the morning and 2.5 mg in the evening, is less expensive for prolonged maintenance. However, the decreased mineralocorticoid activity of prednisone makes the 9-alpha-fluoro-hydrocortisone more necessary. Hypertension or edema may necessitate reduction of the mineralocorticoid. Although induction of labor would allow the patient with Addison's disease to be optimally maintained on steroid replacement, the great majority of patients can be allowed to have spontaneous delivery. During labor the woman should be maintained in a good state of hydration with normal saline and given 25 mg of cortisol hemisuccinate every 6 hours. At the delivery or if labor is prolonged, 100 mg of cortisol may be given intravenously over several hours. Following delivery the patient should continue to receive parenteral steroids and fluids for several days in order to avoid a postpartum adrenal crisis.

Offspring of mothers receiving steroids for Addison's disease have been reported to have a tendency toward low birth weights, which have been attributed to fetal hypoglycemia.[83] However, in most instances corticosteroid treatment of the newborn is not thought to be indicated, although blood glucose determinations at frequent intervals are recommended. Cortisol, 2 mg per kg every 8 hours, and 10 per cent glucose given intravenously are adequate for the rare infant who develops temporary decreased adrenal responsiveness secondary to maternal steroid therapy.

Cushing's Syndrome

Excess circulating glucocorticoids result in Cushing's syndrome, characterized by a variety of metabolic abnormalities that may be caused by adrenal hyperplasia, adrenal adenomas, or exogenous corticosteroid therapy.

Adrenocortical hyperplasia develops as a result of excessive ACTH stimulation, presumably caused by a pituitary adenoma.[98] The increased production of glucocorticoid is manifested by obesity, easy bruisability, weakness, glucose intolerance, osteoporosis, and emotional disturbances. Increased mineralocorticoid activity results in hypertension, and increased androgens result in hirsutism and acne. The increased steroid production also results in polycystic ovaries — about a third of women with early Cushing's syndrome have amenorrhea, and another 20 per cent have menstrual irregularities. Eventually two thirds of affected women may have amenorrhea.[63] However, some women continue to have normal menses and may become pregnant.

The classic features of Cushing's syndrome include a round face with full cheeks (moon face) and increased fat deposition over the upper dorsal vertebrae (buffalo hump) and in the supraclavicular bursae. Striae are present, which may be undistinguishable from those seen in pregnancy or may be broader and purple in color. Tinea versicolor is common.

Diagnosis in Pregnancy. The diagnosis of Cushing's syndrome in pregnancy is made more difficult because weight gain, hypertension, striae, edema, and increased pigmentation may occur in normal pregnancy. However, increased hirsutism and acne are particularly common in pregnant women with Cushing's syndrome (Fig. 9–6). A partial explanation for this increased androgenic component may be the increased incidence of adrenal adenomas in pregnant women. Seven of ten pregnant women with Cushing's syndrome had adrenal adenomas.[71] The combination of excess androgens with the increased cortisol in these patients may prevent the increase in protein catabolism but result in more hirsutism and acne. Whether the increase in adrenal adenomas in these women simply reflects a selective process in fertility is not clear.

The laboratory diagnosis of Cushing's syndrome in pregnancy is complicated by the changes in adrenal function in normal pregnancy.

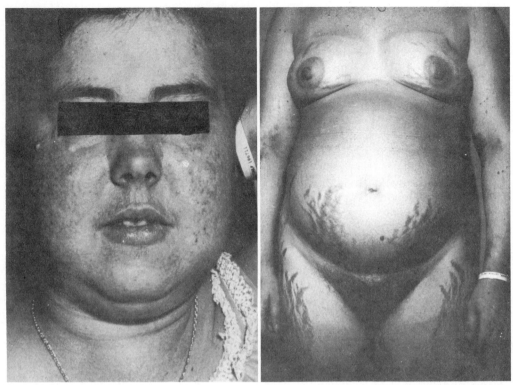

FIGURE 9–6. Cushing's syndrome in pregnancy. (From Grimes et al.: Obstet. Gynecol., *42*:550, 1973. Reprinted with permission.)

Patients with Cushing's syndrome typically have elevated plasma cortisol concentrations without diurnal variation. Urinary steroid excretion is elevated and not suppressed by 2 mg of dexamethasone daily. In normal pregnancy the plasma cortisol is also elevated, with diminished diurnal variation and an exaggerated response to Cortrosyn. Consequently, the diagnosis of Cushing's syndrome during pregnancy depends on the dexamethasone suppression test. Since the diagnosis depends on suppression, a complete dexamethasone suppression test should be performed in suspected cases with both plasma and urinary steroid determinations. With the high incidence of adrenal adenomas, a significant percentage of these women may not suppress adrenal steroid production with "high dose" (8 mg) dexamethasone suppression.[66]

Cushing's syndrome may appear during pregnancy and, if untreated, disappear with delivery and recur with a subsequent pregnancy[55, 72, 84, 101] (Tables 9–2 and 9–3). Whether the increased adrenal stimulation during pregnancy is sufficient to make subclinical Cushing's syndrome apparent is not clear. In the two patients in whom the Cushing's syndrome disappeared after delivery only to recur with another pregnancy,

adrenal adenomas were found at surgery. Although the clinical evidence of Cushing's syndrome disappeared, several of these women continued to have abnormal dexamethasone suppression test results. These observations sug-

TABLE 9–2 PLASMA 11-OHCS LEVELS DURING ADRENAL SUPPRESSION IN A PREGNANT PATIENT WITH CUSHING'S SYNDROME WHICH DISAPPEARED POST PARTUM

Medication	11-OHCS $\mu g/100\ ml$
Base line: AM	44
PM	41
After dexamethasone, 1.0 mg prior evening	47
Dexamethasone, 0.5 mg every 6 hr, 8 days	40
Dexamethasone, 2.0 mg every 6 hr, 8 days	45
2 weeks after D & C	22
After dexamethasone, 1.0 mg prior evening	22
Dexamethasone, 0.5 mg every 6 hr, 8 days	11
Dexamethasone, 2.0 mg every 6 hr, 8 days	7
5 months after D & C: AM	18
PM	8
After dexamethasone, 1.0 mg prior evening	5

Source: Wieland, R., Schaffer, M., and Glove, R.: Obstet. Gynecol., *38*:841, 1971.

TABLE 9–3 URINARY STEROID LEVELS DURING ADRENAL SUPPRESSION IN A PREGNANT PATIENT WITH CUSHING'S SYNDROME WHICH DISAPPEARED POST PARTUM

Medication	17-KS *mg/24 hr*	17-OHCS *mg/24 hr*	11-OHCS *μg/24 hr*
Base line	31.5	75.9	
Dexamethasone, 0.5 mg every 6 hr, 8 days	34.2	135.5	
2.0 mg every 6 hr, 8 days	42.6	115.7	7566
2 weeks after D & C	4.5	17.4	528
Dexamethasone, 0.5 mg every 6 hr, 8 days	3.0	24.2	234
2.0 mg every 6 hr, 8 days	1.3	9.5	133
5 months after D & C	3.0	7.0	65
Dexamethasone, 0.5 mg every 6 hr, 8 days	2.6	3.0	84
2.0 mg every 6 hr, 8 days		3.3	99
HCG, 4000 U per day, 4 days	6.1	17.4	350
6 months after D & C		8.7	72
HCG, 2000 U*	5.6	10.9	102
TIW, 2 wks	4.4	8.9	78
9 months after D & C	4.2	8.5	
Days 19 and 20 of sequential estrogen-progestogen	3.2	6.2	

*Samples obtained on Days 12 and 13.
(From Wieland, R., Schaffer, M., and Glove, R.: Obstet. Gynecol., *38*:841, 1971.)

gest that these women should be followed up carefully after delivery, since they may well have an underlying adrenal pathologic condition.

Course and Therapy. Not only is pregnancy unusual in Cushing's syndrome, but there is an increased fetal loss during pregnancy. Four of 16 pregnancies associated with Cushing's syndrome resulted in spontaneous abortion, and another 4 resulted in stillbirths.[71] Of the 8 pregnancies that resulted in live births, premature labor occurred in every instance between the 32nd and 37th weeks of pregnancy. The same authors described a premature infant, born at 30 weeks to a mother with Cushing's syndrome, who required steroid therapy for apparent adrenal insufficiency. Two similar offspring were stillborn and had a marked decrease in adrenal size.

Cushing's syndrome during pregnancy clearly represents a real risk to the fetus and should be treated if diagnosed during pregnancy. Cushing's syndrome with bilateral adrenal hyperplasia appears to be most likely due to small pituitary adenomas.[98] If so, therapy would be a transsphenoidal hypophysectomy, which could be done during pregnancy. Two successful pregnancies occurring after cyproheptadine therapy have been reported.[24a] However, the incidence of adrenal tumor, including adrenal carcinoma, in pregnant women with Cushing's syndrome makes it mandatory to rule out this possibility. Failure to suppress with the "high dose" dexamethasone is good indirect evidence. In the nonpregnant patient the abdominal CT scan has been very helpful in identifying adrenal tumors.

In the pregnant woman up to 20 weeks the fetus would receive approximately 100 mR, a dose comparable with that received from a single abdominal radiograph; after 20 weeks the dose would be higher because of direct exposure. If the index of suspicion is high that the Cushing's syndrome is due to an adrenal tumor, then surgery is the treatment of choice. Following treatment, the pregnancy may continue normally. A normal infant weighing 2600 grams was born to a mother with Nelson's syndrome who had been treated with pituitary radiation and partial adrenalectomy and O,P'-DDD.[74]

Congenital Adrenal Hyperplasia

Congenital adrenal hyperplasia is an inherited enzymatic defect of steroid biosynthesis that interfers with the production of normal amounts of cortisol. Defective enzyme activity may occur at each step in the pathway of cortisol biosynthesis (see Fig. 9–1). Approximately 95 per cent of all patients with congenital adrenal hyperplasia have a deficiency of the 21-hydroxylase enzyme necessary for the conversion of 17-hydroxyprogesterone to 11-desoxycortisol, the immediate precursor of cortisol. The decreased cortisol results in increased ACTH secretion and adrenal hyperplasia. The disease may not manifest itself at birth and may not be recognizable until adolescence or later (postnatal adrenal hyperplasia).

The relative or absolute deficiency in specific enzymatic activity results in decreased cortisol formation and an increase in ACTH secretion. The resulting hyperplastic adrenal glands may secrete sufficient cortisol to maintain life in conjunction with an overproduction of other adrenal steroids. These other steroids, including androgens, cause the characteristic clinical abnormalities. Patients with untreated congenital adrenal hyperplasia have low-normal or decreased plasma cortisol values and excrete increased amounts of 17-ketosteroids and abnormal steroid intermediates.

Excessive amounts of androgens in utero result in masculinization.[48] In the female fetus, masculinization results in clitoral enlargement and fusion of the labia, so that there is difficulty differentiating the infant from a male. In the male fetus exposed to androgens in utero, the major abnormality is premature enlargement of the phallus.

Course in Pregnancy. Pregnancy is rare in inadequately treated women. In a study of adequately treated women under the age 20 years, 10 of 18 were able to conceive.[70] Infertility and menstrual irregularities may be due to ovarian inactivity as a result of the inhibition of pituitary gonadotropins by adrenal androgens and estrogens, or possibly by a direct peripheral influence on the ovary. The state of the ovaries varies with the age of the patient. In infancy the ovaries are normal, but by late adolescence there are numerous primordial follicles with sparse stroma and no sign of luteinization. As the patients with adrenal hyperplasia become older, the ovaries may become cystic, resembling those of the Stein-Leventhal syndrome.

Of the approximately 20 infants born to mothers with congenital or postnatal adrenal hyperplasia, 15 were female.[78, 97] Only 4 of the patients were delivered vaginally. The major indication for cesarean section has been a congenitally narrow birth canal or cephalopelvic disproportion due to a contracted pelvis. Spontaneous abortion occurs with high frequency (20 per cent) in adrenal hyperplasia. Most of these patients have been treated with adrenocorticosteroids during pregnancy. If the steroid dosage is correct, the pregnancy should be normal in all other respects, although maternal hypertension is common. With adequate steroid replacement, neither congenital abnormality nor adrenal insufficiency has been noted in the offspring.

The usual maintenance dose of 37.5 mg cortisone or 7.5 mg prednisone need not be altered during pregnancy. Although the urinary excretion of 17-ketosteroids does not change appreciably during pregnancy, there is a peak of pregnanetriol excretion (3.4 to 9.3 mg per 24 hours) during the last trimester because of placental production. Therefore, increases in pregnanetriol excretion may not mean that the maintenance steroid dosage is inadequate. The patient with adrenal hyperplasia should be carefully studied to determine whether cesarean section is indicated. Steroid coverage should be provided during delivery.[88] There is evidence that the fetal pituitary-adrenal axis may play an important role in the initiation of labor. Pregnancies tend to be prolonged in patients whose offspring have adrenal hypoplasia.[89] However, no differences in length of gestation have been noted in patients whose offspring have congenital adrenal hyperplasia.[88]

Prenatal Diagnosis. Since congenital adrenal hyperplasia is inherited as an autosomal recessive trait, parents of affected children have a 25 per cent risk of having another affected child, and a treated woman has a 1:100 to 1:200 chance of producing affected infants. The gene responsible for 21-hydroxylase deficiency appears to be closely linked to the HLA-B locus.[62] This relationship can also be used to indicate the risk of congenital adrenal hyperplasia in the fetus by HLA typing of amniotic cells in high risk families.[86] Although feasible, the test is complex and time-consuming. Determination of the 17-OH-progesterone content in amniotic fluid appears to be a simple, effective way to make the diagnosis of congenital adrenal hyperplasia in utero.[67] The 17-OH-progesterone concentration determined by radioimmunoassay in amniotic fluid was more than three times the mean value determined in pregnancies of comparable gestation with normal outcome. A rare form of congenital adrenal hyperplasia, 11-B-hydroxylase deficiency, has also been successfully diagnosed in utero by determining the 11-deoxycortisol concentration in amniotic fluid.[91, 94]

Long-Term Therapy with Pharmacologic Doses of Steroid

Patients with a variety of disease processes may be given pharmacologic doses of glucocorticoids as part of long-term therapy. When these patients become pregnant they present special problems because they are receiving pharmacologic rather than maintenance doses of glucocorticoids. Cleft palate in the offspring of mice given cortisone has been reported.[64] Cleft palate associated with the antenatal administration of pharmacologic doses of glucocorticoid has been reported in the human fetus. To produce a cleft palate, an effective dose of steroid is necessary before the closure of the palatal process, which is usually complete by the 12th week of gestation.

A review of the world literature in 1960, of 260 pregnancies in which the women had received pharmacologic doses of glucocorticoids, showed that two infants were born with cleft palates and that both had been exposed to steroids before the 14th week of gestation.[51] The problem of cleft palate appears small but real.

In addition to the cleft palate, one infant in the same review presented with adrenal insufficiency, which lasted 3 days. Adrenal insufficiency secondary to maternal steroid ingestion must be very rare, although one case of adrenal hemorrhage in the offspring of a patient receiving large doses of steroids during pregnancy has been reported.[82] The introduction of treatment with high doses of corticosteroids during pregnancy to prevent the respiratory distress syndrome has created a patient group in which the fetus is intentionally exposed.[81]

Pregnant patients receiving steroids should also receive steroid coverage during delivery. It is important to realize that patients receiving large doses of steroids may have a withdrawal syndrome characterized by weakness and fever if there is an abrupt change to maintenance steroid therapy.[47] Therefore, pharmacologic doses of steroids may be necessary throughout labor and delivery. These high doses of steroid may also interfere with wound healing, but this may be unavoidable.

THE PARATHYROID GLANDS

The normal nonpregnant woman requires about 0.5 gm of calcium daily to maintain normal calcium balance. In contrast, the pregnant woman requires 1.5 to 2 gm of calcium daily during the last half of pregnancy to maintain calcium balance. The fetus requires a total of 25 to 30 gm of calcium, mostly during the second half of pregnancy. This is achieved by an increase in maternal 1,25 dihydroxy vitamin D levels and an increase in the intestinal absorption of calcium.[117, 121b] Under normal circumstances calcium balance in pregnancy is easily maintained by a normal diet, and osteomalacia in the pregnant woman occurs only under unusual social circumstances.[128] The custom of providing calcium supplements to the pregnant women ensures an adequate intake.[102]

Evaluation of Parathyroid Function

The serum calcium concentration is the key determination in evaluating parathyroid function. The concentration of serum calcium by the most accurate method, atomic absorption flame photometry, ranges from 9 to 10.5 mg per 100 ml. About 40 per cent of the total serum calcium is bound to plasma proteins, primarily albumin. The ionized fraction of serum calcium is considered to be the metabolically active fraction. With a decrease in the serum protein concentrations the total serum calcium concentration decreases, but the ionized calcium fraction remains unchanged. An estimation of the normal serum calcium concentration can be obtained despite decreased serum protein concentration because 1 gm albumin binds 0.8 mg calcium. The urinary excretion of calcium can also be measured but can be difficult to interpret because of dietary variation.

In contrast to the serum calcium concentration, the serum phosphorus concentration varies with age, diet, and hormonal status. However, the renal excretion of phosphorus is commonly used in tests of parathyroid function. Inorganic phosphorus is filtered through the glomerulus and largely resorbed in the proximal tubule. Phosphate resorption is inhibited by parathyroid hormone. In normal nonpregnant women, tubular resorption of phosphate (TRP) ranges from 82 to 97 per cent of the filtered load, while patients with hyperparathyroidism have a TRP of less than 82 per cent. The availability of the parathyroid hormone radioimmunoassay is helpful but has not consistently separated normal from pathologic parathyroid states. Parathyroid hormone increases urinary cyclic AMP, and this has been used as a measure of parathyroid hormone.

Parathyroid Function in Normal Pregnancy

The total serum calcium concentration begins to fall during the second or third month of gestation and reaches a nadir between the 28th and 32nd weeks (Fig. 9–7).[127] This decrease in serum calcium has been attributed to the dilutional hypoalbuminemia of pregnancy without alterations in the protein binding of calcium.[121a] The serum ionized calcium concentration remains almost unchanged during pregnancy. Thus, maternal serum ionic calcium concentration is important in normal perinatal calcium homeostasis.[131] Calcium ions are transferred from mother to fetus against a concentration gradient, a process that presumably reflects active transport by the placenta. Despite the hypocalcemia and diversion of calcium to the fetus, the urinary excretion of calcium is increased in normal pregnant women because of increased glomerular filtration.[116] Even with the increase in glomerular filtration, there is no change in tubu-

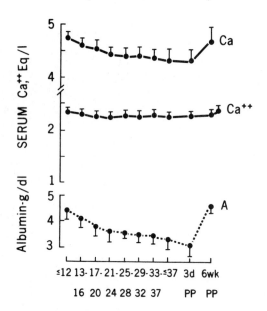

DURATION OF PREGNANCY (WEEKS)

FIGURE 9–7. Serum calcium, ionized calcium, and albumin concentrations during pregnancy. (From Pitkin et al.: Am. J. Obstet. Gynecol., *133*:781, 1979. Reprinted with permission.)

lar reabsorption of phosphate during pregnancy. In patients not receiving calcium supplementation, the urinary excretion of calcium decreases between early gestation and the month prior to term.[115]

The occurrence of maternal parathyroid hyperplasia during normal pregnancy suggests increased hormone production. Serum parathyroid hormone values rise progressively throughout pregnancy[127] (Fig. 9–8), but there is no correlation between the total serum calcium concentration and serum parathyroid hormone concentrations. However, normal serum parathyroid hormone concentrations during the last trimester have been reported.[119] No differences were found between maternal and cord blood at term.[122a] Serum calcitonin concentrations have also been found to be elevated during pregnancy in some but not all studies.[119, 130] Calcitonin may be of importance during pregnancy in inhibiting parathyroid hormone–induced bone resorption and in conserving skeletal calcium.[134]

Significant changes in the secretion, absorption, and turnover in calcium occur well in advance of fetal skeletal mineralization.[117] High doses of estrogen and progesterone failed to reproduce the changes in calcium metabolism observed in pregnancy. The biologically active form of vitamin D, 1,25 dihydroxy vitamin D, is also elevated at term in pregnant women.[132a] Increased production of 1,25 dihydroxy vitamin D

would be consistent with a need for increased calcium retention. The increased calcium drain to the fetus could create a hypocalcemic tendency in the mother with increased parathyroid hormone production.[125] Hypocalcemia and an increase in parathyroid hormone are physiologic signals for increased 1,25 dihydroxy vitamin D production.[122b] The elevated prolactin concentrations in pregnancy might also have a role in the stimulation of 1,25 dihydroxy vitamin D production.

Hyperparathyroidism

The continued secretion of excess parathyroid hormone results in a chronic disease characterized by an elevated serum calcium associated with generalized muscular weakness and a variety of other nonspecific findings. The diagnosis may be suspected immediately, or the symptoms and signs may be so vague that diagnosis is extremely difficult. In about half the cases, hyperparathyroidism is caused by a single parathyroid adenoma and this rate is even higher in pregnancy.[121] These adenomas have been considered to be autonomous because hormone is secreted despite an elevated serum calcium. However, with the availability of the parathyroid hormone radioimmunoassay, the adenomas ap-

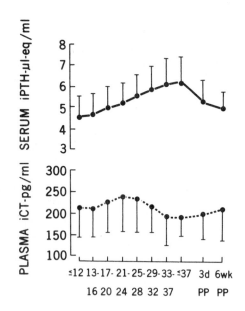

DURATION OF PREGNANCY (WEEKS)

FIGURE 9–8. Serum parathyroid hormone and calcitonin concentrations during pregnancy. (From Pitkin et al.: Am. J. Obstet. Gynecol., *133*:781, 1979. Reprinted with permission.)

pear to respond to the serum calcium level but at a higher set point. Hyperparathyroidism is rare before puberty and is two to three times more common in females than in males. In addition to the usual findings in hyperparathyroidism, there are specific problems in pregnancy with the fetus, which is exposed to high levels of serum calcium. Some women with hyperparathyroidism have more pronounced nausea and vomiting during a pregnancy.[123a]

The increased parathyroid hormone causes phosphaturia and a fall in serum phosphate concentration. With prolonged PTH secretion there is an increase in bone resorption and an elevation of the serum calcium. Parathyroid hormone actually causes decreased excretion of calcium. However, hypercalciuria occurs when the serum calcium is elevated because of a limited ability of the kidney to reabsorb calcium. The hypercalciuria is associated with an alkaline urine, and hyperphosphaturia leads to the formation of renal calculi and nephrocalcinosis. The hypercalcemia may lead to a loss of renal concentrating ability, which, in conjunction with an increased osmotic load, causes polyuria and polydipsia. The increased bone resorption may lead to thinning of the bony trabeculae with fractures or, in its most advanced form, to osteitis fibrosa cystica.

The decrease in total serum calcium concentration during pregnancy makes the diagnosis of hyperparathyroidism more difficult. In pregnant patients with hyperparathyroidism, serum calcium levels ranged from 9.5 to 20.6 mg per 100 ml; 27 of 30 patients had a serum calcium value greater than 12 mg per 100 ml.[121] However, the diagnosis will be missed in some pregnant patients if the usual value of 10.6 mg per 100 ml in nonpregnant patients is taken as the upper limit of normal. Other tests of parathyroid function, such as serum phosphate and tubular resorption of phosphatate, may be helpful, but serum calcium concentration remains the best single test.

Effect on the Fetus. The effect of maternal hyperparathyroidism on the fetus is detrimental, with high fetal morbidity and variable mortality. One group reviewed reports of 37 pregnancies in untreated hyperparathyroid patients and noted 5 spontaneous abortions, 5 stillbirths, and 4 neonatal deaths; 18 offspring developed neonatal tetany.[121] In another study analyzing 15 pregnancies, in 13 women with hyperparathyroidism during pregnancy, complications occurred in 80 per cent of cases.[108] Spontaneous abortions and neonatal deaths occurred in 20 per cent. Fertility does not appear to be reduced in hyperparathyroid patients, and labor and delivery have been

reported to be normal, although low birth weights have been observed.[135]

Over half the pregnant patients with hyperparathyroidism had offspring with neonatal tetany, and this should be an important although retrospective diagnostic clue. Calcium crosses the placenta by active transport, and the fetal serum calcium is 1 to 2 mg per 100 ml higher than maternal calcium levels. Parathyroid hormone does not apparently cross the placenta. Presumably, transplacental passage of elevated maternal ionized calcium suppresses the fetal parathyroid. In addition, the neonate has immature kidneys and parathyroid glands at birth. In a series of 250 normal mothers observed during pregnancy, subclinical hypocalcemia was common in newborns at about the sixth day of life.[136] Neonatal tetany may become manifest about 5 to 14 days post partum, probably because of a limited ability to handle the increased phosphorus of cow's milk. The serum calcium is lowered still further, and tetany ensues. Hypomagnesemia may occur in conjunction with the neonatal hypocalcemia.[110] The tetany is usually transient, and complete recovery often occurs without treatment. One woman with asymptomatic hyperparathyroidism had eight children, four of whom developed neonatal tetany with hypocalcemia.[120] Interestingly, the nontetanic neonates had been given a low phosphorus milk product. An unsuccessful attempt has been made to transplant the mother's resected parathyroid adenoma into the hypoparathyroid offspring.[106]

Treatment. The high fetal and neonatal morbidity and the variable mortality rate indicate the need for surgery when the diagnosis of hyperparathyroidism is made in the pregnant woman.[111] When surgery is contraindicated, in selected cases therapy with oral phosphate may be an effective alternate treatment until surgery can be safely performed. Termination of the pregnancy is not indicated except for selected patients with advanced renal insufficiency when maternal risk is increased and there is a poor fetal prognosis. The neonate's condition should be carefully evaluated and he should be followed up after delivery. Prophylactic calcium administration might be important to prevent neonatal tetany. A large number of patients are not suspected of having hyperparathyroidism during the pregnancy. One potentially lethal complication is the development of hyperparathyroid crisis during the postpartum period because of bed rest and dehydration[132] (Fig. 9–9).

Whether patients with minimal elevations of serum calcium and no evidence of complications such as renal calcinosis should be treated medi-

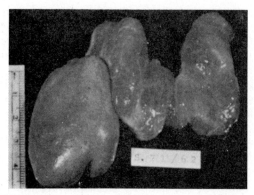

FIGURE 9–9. Parathyroid adenoma opposite inferior pole of right lobe of thyroid gland. (From Schenker and Kallner: Obstet. Gynecol., 25:705, 1965. Reprinted with permission.)

cally during the pregnancy is equivocal. Avoiding surgery during pregnancy would spare the fetus unnecessary stress. However, despite an asymptomatic maternal state, neonatal tetany may occur, and surgery is probably indicated in most cases of primary hyperparathyroidism during pregnancy.

Hypoparathyroidism

The normal maintenance of calcium balance depends heavily on adequate parathyroid hormone, and significant hypocalcemia occurs in the absence of this hormone. Hypoparathyroidism is characterized by tetany, seizures, weakness, fatigue, and psychiatric aberrations. The most common cause of hypoparathyroidism is iatrogenic, when parathyroid glands are inadvertently removed or their blood supply compromised during thyroid surgery. Idiopathic hypoparathyroidism may be an autoimmune disorder, but the possibility of recessive inheritance has also been raised. Hypoparathyroidism needs to be distinguished from pseudohypoparathyroidism, in which the parathyroids are normal but the end-organs do not respond to the hormone.

Diagnosis. Cessation of parathyroid hormone leads to a decrease in the serum calcium concentration and a rise in the serum phosphate concentration. Urinary calcium and phosphate excretion are both decreased. The major signs and symptoms of hypoparathyroidism are directly attributable to the decreased level of serum ionized calcium, which causes increased neuromuscular excitability. Tetany is the most prominent feature of this increased excitability. Numbness and tingling of the extremities, cramps, and carpopedal spasm may be followed in rare instances by laryngeal stridor and generalized convulsions.

Tetany can be induced either by alkalosis, which increases calcium binding, or by a decrease in the total serum calcium concentration with a proportionate decrease in the ionized calcium concentration. The absolute value of the ionized calcium at which tetany will occur depends on the rate of change of calcium concentration. A rapid fall, as in alkalosis, leads to the development of tetany at a calcium concentration that is usually high enough to prevent overt tetany in chronic hypocalcemia.

Hypoparathyroidism in Pregnancy. Hypoparathyroidism in pregnancy is complicated both by the response of the fetus to the low serum ionized calcium and by the increased need for calcium during the pregnancy. One group studied eight women with hypoparathyroidism during pregnancy and concluded that treated hypoparathyroidism had no deleterious effect on pregnancy or on the newborn.[116] However, the calcium depletion that occurs during pregnancy may make hypoparathyroidism clinically evident.[109] Offspring of mothers with untreated hypoparathyroidism may develop neonatal hyperparathyroidism.[105] Patients with both iatrogenic and idiopathic hypoparathyroidism have given birth to hyperparathyroid infants. The disease is self-limiting in the offspring, and x-ray evidence of osteitis fibrosa cystica at birth disappears within 4 months. One hypoparathyroid mother who had undergone thyroidectomy gave birth to twins, who died in the newborn period from hyaline membrane disease and intracranial hemorrhage.[122] At autopsy both infants had parathyroid hyperplasia and osteitis fibrosa (Fig. 9–10). The hyperparathyroidism is thought to be secondary and to represent a physiologic response to the low maternal calcium. Hypercalcemia in these children is uncommon because, presumably, the parathyroid hyperplasia and bone resorption are a physiologic response to the low maternal serum calcium. Since idiopathic hypoparathyroidism is an inherited disease, the offspring may also be hypoparathyroid. A mother with idiopathic hypoparathyroidism had a child with hyperparathyroidism, but her second child had congenital hypoparathyroidism.[114]

Although tetany occurring during pregnancy is most likely due to alkalosis, hypoparathyroidism should be considered, particularly in a patient who has previously undergone thyroid surgery. Latent tetany may be elicited by tapping over the facial nerve in front of the ear, causing a twitch of the upper lip (Chvostek's sign). This may be positive in 10 per cent of normal adults. Trous-

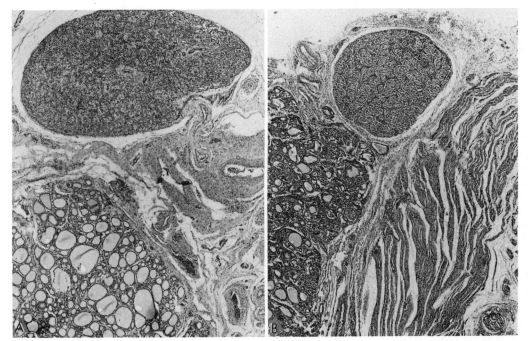

FIGURE 9–10. Parathyroid hyperplasia secondary to low maternal calcium (A) compared with normal parathyroid gland (B). (From Landing and Kamashita: J. Pediatr., 77:842, 1970. Reprinted with permission.)

seau's sign can be used to roughly quantitate the latent tetany. Carpopedal spasm is induced by inflating the sphygmomanometer above the systolic pressure. This constriction should be maintained for 3 minutes before the test is considered negative; the length of time necessary to induce carpopedal spasm can be monitored.

Therapy. The pregnant hypoparathyroid patient is much more apt to be receiving vitamin D and calcium therapy already, and it does not appear to be necessary to alter this therapy during pregnancy. Fifteen women with 27 pregnancies were studied; they received 100,000 IU vitamin D daily and calcium supplementation. Normal serum calcium was maintained throughout pregnancy. All the pregnancies resulted in live births.[113] The question has been raised whether maternal vitamin D therapy might result in cardiovascular abnormalities in the offspring.[133] However, in the group just mentioned, no evidence was found of cardiovascular abnormalities or craniofacial abnormalities associated with infantile hypercalcemia in the children, who were examined from 6 weeks to 16 years of age. It was thought that the serum calcium level, not the amount of vitamin D, was important in producing these abnormalities.[113] Moreover, a patient receiving extremely high doses of 1,25 dihydroxy vitamin D gave birth to a normal child despite evidence that the vitamin D had entered the fetal circulation.[123] The net tubular reabsorp-

tion of calcium is significantly lowered in patients with treated hypoparathyroidism.[116] The renal threshold for calcium is low because of the lack of parathyroid hormone. Because of the low renal threshold and the increased glomerular filtration during pregnancy, urinary calcium excretion is markedly increased at normal levels of serum calcium when these hypoparathyroid patients are treated with vitamin D.

Two patients have been reported with postthyroidectomy hypoparathyroidism who were treated during pregnancy with normal maintenance doses of calcium and vitamin D without difficulty.[137] However, in the immediate postpartum period, serum calcium levels rose to 12 to 15 mg per 100 ml and persisted at an elevated level for 3 months despite normal or reduced vitamin D and calcium therapy. The findings suggest that treated hypoparathyroid patients should be carefully followed up during the immediate postpartum period. These patients should also be watched carefully during labor, since hyperventilation might lead to alkalosis and tetany.[104] During labor and delivery, calcium gluconate infusion can be used to maintain a normal serum calcium level.[124] The pregnant hypoparathyroid patient requires 2 gm elemental calcium a day, which is equivalent to 24 gm calcium gluconate or 8 gm calcium lactate. The dose of vitamin D may be omitted during labor if the patient is not taking oral fluids.

Breast feeding by a hypoparathyroid mother is undesirable. Human milk contains about 400 mg calcium per liter, and adequate supplementation to meet this loss is difficult in the hypopara- thyroid patient. Furthermore, there is evidence that large amounts of 25-hydroxycholecalciferol appear in the milk of mothers receiving vitamin D therapy for hypoparathyroidism.[112]

References

PITUITARY GLAND

1. Abelove, W. A., Rupp, J. J., and Paschkis, K. E.: Acromegaly and pregnancy. J. Clin. Endocrinol. Metab., *14*:32, 1954.
2. Asa, S. L., Bilbao, J. M., Kovacs, K., Josse, R. E., and Kreines, K.: Lymphocytic hypophysitis of pregnancy resulting in hypopituitarism: A distinct clinicopathologic entity. Ann. Intern. Med., *95*:166, 1981.
3. Barlow, E. D., and De Wardener, H. E.: Compulsive water drinking. Q. J. Med., *28*:235, 1959.
4. Beck, P., Eaton, C. J., Young, I. S., and Kupperman, H. S.: Metyrapone response in pregnancy. Am. J. Obstet. Gynecol., *100*:327, 1968.
5. Bergh, T., Nillius, S. J., and Wide, L.: Clinical course and outcome of pregnancies in amenorrhoeic women with hyperprolactinaemia and pituitary tumours. Br. Med. J., *1*:875, 1978.
6. Bhatia, S. K., Moore, D., and Kalkhoff, R. K.: Progesterone suppression of the plasma growth hormone response. J. Clin. Endocrinol. Metab., *35*:364, 1972.
7. Burrow, G. N., Polackwich, R., and Donabedian, R.: The hypothalamic-pituitary-thyroid axis in normal pregnancy. *In* Fisher, D. A., and Burrow, G. N. (eds.): Perinatal Thyroid Physiology and Disease, pp. 1–10. New York, Raven Press, 1975.
8. Burrow, G. N., Wassenar, W., Robertson, G. L., and Sehl, H.: DDAVP treatment of diabetes insipidus during pregnancy and the post partum period. Acta Endocrinol., *97*:23, 1981.
8a. Campagnoli, C., Belforte, L., Massara, F., Peris, C., and Molinatti, C. M.: Partial remission of hyperprolactinemic amenorrhea after bromocriptine-induced pregnancy. J. Endocrinol. Invest., *4*:85, 1981.
9. Campbell, J. W.: Diabetes insipidus and complicated pregnancy. J.A.M.A., *243*:1744, 1980.
9a. Carr, B. R., Parker, C. R. Jr., Madden, J. D., MacDonald, P. C., and Porter, J. C.: Maternal plasma adrenocorticotropin and cortisol relations throughout human pregnancy. Am. J. Obstet. Gynecol., *139*:416, 1981.
10. Chau, S. S., Fitzpatrick, R. J., and Jamieson, B.: Diabetes insipidus and parturition. J. Obstet. Gynaecol. Br. Commonw., *76*:444, 1969.
11. Dawood, M. Y., Ylikorkala, O., Trivedi, D., and Fuchs, F.: Oxytocin in maternal circulation and amniotic fluid during pregnancy. J. Clin. Endocrinol. Metab., *49*:429, 1979.
12. Dorfman, S. G., Dillaplain, R. P., and Gambrell, R. D., Jr.: Antepartum pituitary infarction. Obstet. Gynecol., *53*(Suppl.):21S, 1979.
13. Drury, M. I., and Keelan, D. M.: Sheehan's syndrome. J. Obstet. Gynaecol. Br. Commonw., *73*:802, 1966.
14. Finkler, R. S.: Acromegaly and pregnancy. Case report. J. Clin. Endocrinol. Metab., *14*:1245, 1954.
15. Goluboff, L. G., and Ezrin, C.: Effect of pregnancy on the somatotroph and the prolactin cell of the human adenohypophysis. J. Clin. Endocrinol. Metab., *29*:1533, 1969.
16. Gordon, G., and Bradford, W. P.: Pregnancy in patient with diabetes insipidus following induction of ovulation with clomiphene. J. Obstet. Gynaecol. Br. Commonw., *77*:467, 1970.
17. Hall, M. R. P.: The incidence of anterior pituitary deficiency following postpartum haemorrhage: Cases reviewed from the Oxfordshire and Buckinghamshire area. Proc. R. Soc. Med., *55*:468, 1962.
18. Hendricks, C. H.: The neurohypophysis in pregnancy. Obstet. Gynecol. Surv., *9*:323, 1954.
19. Hime, M. C., and Richardson, J. A.: Diabetes insipidus and pregnancy. Obstet. Gynecol. Surv., *33*:375, 1978.
20. Jackson, I. M. D., Whyte, W. G., and Garrey, M. M.: Pituitary function following uncomplicated pregnancy in Sheehan's syndrome. J. Clin. Endocrinol. Metab., *29*:315, 1969.
21. Jeppsson, S., Rannevik, G., Liedholm, P., and Thorell, J. I.: Basal and LRH-stimulated secretion of FSH during early pregnancy. Am. J. Obstet. Gynecol., *127*:32, 1977.
22. Jewelewicz, R., and Vande Wiele, R. L.: Clinical course and outcome of pregnancy in twenty-five patients with pituitary microadenomas. Am. J. Obstet. Gynecol., *136*:339, 1980.
23. Jorgensen, P. I., Sele, V., Buus, O., and Damkjaer, M.: Detailed hormonal studies during and after pregnancy in a previously hypophysectomized patient. Acta Endocrinol., *73*:117, 1973.
24. Jouppila, P., and Vuopala, U.: Diabetes insipidus and pregnancy. Ann. Chir. Gynaecol., *60*:57, 1971.
24a. Kasperlik-Zaluska, A., Migdalska, B., and Hartwig, W.: Two pregnancies in a woman with Cushing's syndrome treated with cyproheptadine. Br. J. Obstet. Gynecol., *87*:1171, 1980.
25. Kayne, R. D., and Burrow, G. N.: Anterior pituitary function in women with postpartum hemorrhage. Yale J. Biol. Med., *51*:143, 1978.
26. Kinch, R. A., Plunkett, E. R., and Devlin, M. C.: Postpartum amenorrhea — galactorrhea of hypothyroidism. Am. J. Obstet. Gynecol., *105*:766, 1969.
27. Kovacs, K.: Necrosis of anterior pituitary in humans. Neuroendocrinology, *4*:170, 1969.
28. Maranon, G.: Diabetes insipidus and uterine atony: A case observed over a period of 26 years. Br. Med. J., *2*:769, 1947.
29. Martin, J. E., MacDonald, P. C., and Kaplan, N. M.: Successful pregnancy in a patient with Sheehan's syndrome. N. Engl. J. Med., *282*:425, 1970.
30. Pearce, H. M.: Physiologic bitemporal hemianopsia in pregnancy. Obstet. Gynecol., *22*:612, 1963.
31. Pico, I., and Greenblatt, P. B.: Diabetes insipidus and pregnancy. Fertil. Steril., *20*:385, 1969.
32. Robinson, A. G.: Elevation of plasma neurophysin in women on oral contraceptives. J. Clin. Invest., *54*:209, 1974.
33. Robinson, A. G.: DDAVP in the treatment of central diabetes insipidus. N. Engl. J. Med., *294*:507, 1976.
34. Robinson, A. G., Archer, D. F., and Tolstoi, L. F.: Neurophysin in women during oxytocin-related events. J. Clin. Endocrinol. Metab., *37*:645, 1973.
35. Schalch, D. S., and Burday, S. Z.: Antepartum pituitary insufficiency in diabetes mellitus. Ann. Intern. Med., *74*:357, 1971.
36. Sende, P., Pantelakis, N., Suzuki, K., and Bashore, R.: Plasma oxytocin determinations in pregnancy with diabetes insipidus. Obstet. Gynecol., *48*(Suppl.):38S, 1976.
37. Sheehan, H. L.: The frequency of post-partum hypopituitarism. J. Obstet. Gynaecol. Br. Commonw., *72*:103, 1965.
38. Shewchuk, A. B., Adamson, G. D., Lessard, P., and Ezrin, C.: The effect of pregnancy on suspected pituitary adenomas after conservative management of ovulation defects associated with galactorrhea. Am. J. Obstet. Gynecol., *136*:659, 1980.
39. Smallridge, R. C., Corrigan, D. F., Thomason, A. M., and Blue, P. W.: Hypoglycemia in pregnancy. Arch. Intern. Med., *140*:564, 1980.
40. Thorner, M. O.: Prolactin. Clin. Endocrinol. Metab., *6*:201, 1977.
41. Thorner, M. O., Edwards, C. R. W., Charlesworth, M., Dacie, J. E., Moult, P. J. A., Rees, L. H., Jones, A. E., and Besser, G. M.: Pregnancy in patients presenting with hyperprolactinaemia. Br. Med. J., *2*:771, 1979.
42. Tyson, J. E., Barnes, A. C., McKusick, V. A., Scott, C. L., and Jones, G. S.: Obstetric and gynecologic considerations of dwarfism. Am. J. Obstet. Gynecol., *108*:688, 1970.
43. Tyson, J. E., Hwang, P., Guyda, H., and Friesen, H. G.: Studies of prolactin secretion in human pregnancy. Am. J. Obstet. Gynecol., *113*:14, 1972.
44. Tyson, J. E., Rabinowitz, D., Merimee, T. J., and Friesen, H.: Response of plasma insulin and human growth hormone to arginine in pregnant and postpartum females. Am. J. Obstet. Gynecol., *103*:313, 1969.
45. Ylikorkala, O., Kivinen, S., and Reinila, M.: Serial prolactin and

thyrotropin responses to thyrotropin-releasing hormone throughout normal human pregnancy. J. Clin. Endocrinol. Metab., 48:288, 1979.

ADRENAL GLAND

46. Allen, J. P., Cook, D. M., Kendall, J. W., and McGilvra, R.: Maternal-fetal ACTH relationship in man. J. Clin. Endocrinol. Metab., 37:230, 1973.
47. Amatruda, T. T., Jr., Jurst, M. M., and D'Esopo, N. D.: Certain endocrine and metabolic facets of steroid withdrawal syndrome. J. Clin. Endocrinol. Metab., 25:1207, 1965.
48. Bacon, G. E., and Kelch, R. P.: Congenital adrenal hyperplasia due to 21 hydroxylase deficiency: A review of current knowledge. J. Endocrinol. Invest., 2:93, 1979.
49. Baxter, J. D., and Forsham, P. H.: Tissue effects of glucocorticoids. Am. J. Med., 53:573, 1972.
50. Beck, P., Eaton, C. J., Young, I. S., and Kupperman, H. S.: Metyrapone response in pregnancy. Am. J. Obstet. Gynecol., 100:327, 1968.
51. Bongiovanni, A. M., and McPadden, A. J.: Steroids during pregnancy and possible fetal consequences. Fertil. Steril., 1:181, 1960.
52. Brent, F.: Addison's disease and pregnancy. Am. J. Surg., 79:645, 1950.
53. Brownie, A. C., and Sprunt, J. G.: Metopirone in the assessment of pituitary-adrenal function. Lancet, 1:773, 1962.
54. Burke, C. W., and Roulet, F.: Increased exposure of tissues to cortisol in late pregnancy. Br. Med. J., 1:657, 1970.
55. Calodney, L., Eaton, R. P., Black, W., and Cohn, F.: Exacerbation of Cushing's disease during pregnancy: Report of a case. J. Clin. Endocrinol. Metab., 36:81, 1973.
56. Christy, N. P., Wallace, E. Z., Gordon, W. E. L., and Jailer, J. W.: On the rate of hydrocortisone clearance from plasma in pregnant women and in patients with Laennec's cirrhosis. J. Clin. Invest., 38:299, 1959.
57. Clerico, A., Del Chicca, M. G., Ghione, S., and Materazzi, F.: Progressively elevated levels of biologically active (free) cortisol during pregnancy by a direct radioimmunological assay of cortisol in an equilibrium dialysis system. J. Endocrinological Invest., 3:185, 1980.
58. Cohen, M., Steifel, M., Reddy, W. J., and Laidlaw, J. C.: The secretion and disposition of cortisol during pregnancy. J. Clin. Endocrinol. Metab., 18:1076, 1958.
59. DeMoor, P., Steeno, O., Brosens, I., and Hendrikx, A.: Data on transcortin activity in human plasma as studied by gel filtration. J. Clin. Endocrinol. Metab., 26:71, 1966.
60. Doe, R. P., Dickinson, P., Zinneman, H. H., and Seal, U. S.: Elevated nonprotein-bound cortisol (NPC) in pregnancy, during estrogen administration and in carcinoma of the prostate. J. Clin. Endocrinol. Metab., 29:757, 1969.
61. Doe, R. P., Fernandez, R., and Seal, U. S.: Measurement of corticosteroid-binding globulin in man. J. Clin. Endocrinol. Metab., 24:1029, 1964.
62. Dupont, B., Smithwick, E. M., Oberfield, S. E., Lee, T. D., and Levine, L. S.: Close genetic linkage between HLA and congenital adrenal hyperplasia (21-hydroxylase deficiency). Lancet, 2:1309, 1977.
63. Eisenstein, A. B., Karsh, R., and Gall, I.: Occurrence of pregnancy in Cushing's syndrome. J. Clin. Endocrinol. Metab., 23:971, 1963.
64. Fraser, F. C., and Fainstat, T. D.: Production of congenital defects in the offspring of pregnant mice treated with cortisone. Pediatrics, 8:527, 1951.
65. Grant, S. D., Pavlatos, F. C., and Forsham, P. H.: Effects of estrogen therapy on cortisol metabolism. J. Clin. Endocrinol. Metab., 25:1057, 1965.
66. Grimes, E. M., Fayez, J. A., and Miller, G. L.: Cushing's syndrome and pregnancy. Obstet. Gynecol., 42:550, 1973.
67. Hughes, I. A., and Laurence, K. M.: Antenatal diagnosis of congenital adrenal hyperplasia. Lancet, 2:7, 1979.
68. Jailer, J. W., Christy, N. P., Longson, D., Wallace, E. Z., and Gordon, W. E. L.: Further observations on adrenal cortical function during pregnancy. Am. J. Obstet. Gynecol., 78:1, 1959.
69. Klein, G. P., Kertesz, J. P., Chan, S. K., and Giroud, C. J. P.: Urinary excretion of corticosteroid C-21 sulfates during human pregnancy. J. Clin. Endocrinol. Metab., 32:333, 1971.
70. Klingensmith, G. J., Garcia, S. C., Jones, H. W., Jr., Migeon, C.

J., and Blizzard, R. M.: Glucocorticoid treatment of girls with congenital adrenal hyperplasia: Effects on height, sexual maturation, and fertility. J. Pediatr., 90:996, 1977.
71. Kreines, K., and DeVaux, W. D.: Neonatal adrenal insufficiency associated with maternal Cushing's syndrome. Pediatrics, 47:516, 1971.
72. Kreines, K., Perin, E., and Salzer, R.: Pregnancy in Cushing's syndrome. J. Clin. Endocrinol. Metab., 24:75, 1964.
73. Layne, D. S., Meyer, C. J., Vaishwanar, P. S., and Pincus, G.: The secretion and metabolism of cortisol and aldosterone in normal and in steroid treated women. J. Clin. Endocrinol. Metab., 22:107, 1962.
74. Leiba, S., Kaufman, H., Winkelsberg, G., and Bahary, C. M.: Pregnancy in a case of Nelson's syndrome. Acta Obstet. Gynecol. Scand., 57:373, 1978.
75. Mestman, J. H., and Nelson, D. H.: Inhibition by estrogen administration of adrenal-pituitary response to methopyrapone. J. Clin. Invest., 42:1529, 1963.
76. Migeon, C. J., Bertrand, J., and Wall, P. E.: Physiological disposition of 4–C14 cortisol during late pregnancy. J. Clin. Invest., 36:1350, 1957.
77. Migeon, C. J., Kenny, F. M., and Taylor, F. H.: Cortisol production rate. VIII. Pregnancy. J. Clin. Endocrinol. Metab., 28:661, 1968.
78. Mori, N., and Miyakawa, I.: Congenital adrenogenital syndrome and successful pregnancy. Obstet. Gynecol., 35:394, 1970.
79. Murphy, B. E. P.: Clinical evaluation of urinary cortisol determinations by competitive protein-binding radioassay. J. Clin. Endocrinol. Metab., 28:343, 1968.
80. Nolten, W. E., Lindheimer, M. D., Rueckert, P. A., Oparil, S., and Ehrlich, E. N.: Diurnal patterns and regulation of cortisol secretion in pregnancy. J. Clin. Endocrinol. Metab., 51:466, 1980.
81. Ohrlander, S., Gennser, G., Batra, S., and Lebech, P.: Effect of betamethasone administration on estrone, estradiol-17B, and progesterone in maternal plasma and amniotic fluid. Obstet. Gynecol., 49:148, 1977.
82. Oppenheimer, E. H.: Lesions in the adrenals of an infant following maternal corticosteroid therapy. Bull. Johns Hopkins Hosp., 114:146, 1964.
83. Osler, M.: Addison's disease and pregnancy. Acta Endocrinol., 41:67, 1962.
84. Parra, A., and Cruz-Krohn, J.: Intercurrent Cushing's syndrome and pregnancy. Am. J. Med., 40:961, 1966.
85. Peterson, R. E., Nokes, G., Chen, P. S., Jr., and Black, R. L.: Estrogen and adrenocortical function in man. J. Clin. Endocrinol. Metab., 20:495, 1960.
86. Pollack, M. S., Levine, L. S., Pang, S., Owens, R. P., Nitowsky, H. M., Maurer, D., New, M. I., Duchon, M., Merkatz, I. R., Sachs, G., and Dupont, B.: Prenatal diagnosis of congenital adrenal hyperplasia (21-hydroxylase deficiency) by HLA typing. Lancet, 1:1107, 1979.
87. Poonai, A., Jelercic, F., and Pop-Lazic, B.: Pregnancy with diabetes mellitus, Addison's disease, and hypothyroidism. Obstet. Gynecol., 49(Suppl.):86S, 1977.
88. Price, H. V., Cone, B. A., and Keogh, M.: Length of gestation in congenital adrenal hyperplasia. J. Obstet. Gynaecol. Br. Commonw., 78:430, 1971.
89. Roberts, G., and Cawdery, J. E.: Congenital adrenal hypoplasia. J. Obstet. Gynaecol. Br. Commonw., 77:654, 1970.
90. Rosenthal, H. E., Slaunwhite, W. R., Jr., and Sandberg, A. A.: Transcortin: A corticosteroid-binding protein of plasma. X. Cortisol and progesterone interplay and unbound levels of these steroids in pregnancy. J. Clin. Endocrinol. Metab., 29:352, 1969.
91. Rosler, A., Leiberman, E., Rosenmann, A., Ben-Uzilio, R., and Weidenfeld, J.: Prenatal diagnosis of 11B-hydroxylase deficiency congenital adrenal hyperplasia. J. Clin. Endocrinol. Metab., 49:546, 1979.
92. Sandberg, A. A., and Slaunwhite, W. R., Jr.: Physical state of adrenal cortical hormones in plasma. In Christy, N. P. (ed.): The Human Adrenal Cortex, pp. 69–86. New York, Harper & Row, 1971.
93. Satterfield, R. G., and Williamson, H. O.: Isolated ACTH deficiency and pregnancy. Obstet. Gynecol., 48:693, 1976.
94. Schumert, Z., Rosenmann, A., Landau, H., and Rosler, A.: 11-deoxycortisol in amniotic fluid: Prenatal diagnosis of congenital adrenal hyperplasia due to 11 β-hydroxylase deficiency. Clin. Endocrinol., 12:257, 1980.

95. Slaunwhite, W. R., Jr., and Sandberg, A. A.: Transcortin: A corticosteroid-binding protein of plasma. J. Clin. Invest., 38:384, 1959.
96. Smeaton, T. C., Andersen, G. J., and Fulton, I. S.: Study of aldosterone levels in plasma during pregnancy. J. Clin. Endocrinol. Metab., 44:1, 1977.
97. Speroff, L.: The adrenogenital syndrome and its obstetrical aspects: A review of the literature and case report. Obstet. Gynecol. Surv., 20:185, 1965.
98. Tyrrell, J. B., Brooks, R. M., Fitzgerald, P. A., Cofoid, P. B., Forsham, P. H., and Wilson, C. B.: Cushing's disease. Selective trans-sphenoidal resection of pituitary microadenomas. N. Engl. J. Med., 298:753, 1978.
99. Villee, D. B.: Development of endocrine function in the human placenta and fetus. N. Engl. J. Med., 281:533, 1969.
100. Whiteley, H. J., and Stoner, H. B.: The effect of pregnancy on the human adrenal cortex. J. Endocrinol., 14:325, 1957.
101. Wieland, R. G., Shaffer, M. B., Jr., and Glove, R. P.: Cushing's syndrome complicating pregnancy. A case report. Obstet. Gynecol., 38:841, 1971.

PARATHYROIDS

102. Ashe, J. R., Schofield, F. A., and Gram, M. R.: The retention of calcium, iron, phosphorus, and magnesium during pregnancy: The adequacy of prenatal diets with and without supplementation. Am. J. Clin. Nutr., 32:286, 1979.
103. Bodansky, M., and Duff, V. B.: Regulation of the level of calcium in the serum during pregnancy. J.A.M.A., 112:223, 1939.
104. Bolen, J. W.: Hypoparathyroidism in pregnancy. Am. J. Obstet. Gynecol., 117:178, 1973.
105. Bronsky, D., Weisbery, M. G., Gross, M. C., and Barron, J. J.: Hyperparathyroidism and acute postpartum pancreatitis with neonatal tetany in the child. Am. J. Med. Sci., 260:160, 1970.
106. Bruce, J., and Strong, J. A.: Maternal hyperparathyroidism and parathyroid deficiency in the child. Q. J. Med., 24:307, 1955.
107. Cushard, W. G., Jr., Creditor, M. A., Canterbury, J. M., and Reiss, E.: Physiologic hyperparathyroidism in pregnancy. J. Clin. Endocrinol. Metab., 34:767, 1972.
108. Delmonico, F. L., Neer, R. M., Cosimi, A. B., Barnes, A. B., and Russell, P. S.: Hyperparathyroidism during pregnancy. Am. J. Surg., 131:328, 1976.
109. DeYcaza, M. M., and Stinebaugh, B. J.: Idiopathic hypoparathyroidism with hyperthyroidism. South. Med. J., 65:246, 1972.
110. Ertel, N. H., Reiss, J. S., and Spergel, G.: Hypomagnesemia in neonatal tetany associated with hyperparathyroidism. N. Engl. J. Med., 280:260, 1969.
111. Gaeke, R. F., Kaplan, E. L., Lindheimer, M. D., Coe, F., and Shen, K.-L.: Maternal primary hyperparathyroidism of pregnancy. J.A.M.A., 238:508, 1977.
112. Goldberg, L. D.: Transmission of a vitamin-D metabolite in breast milk. Lancet, 2:1258, 1972.
113. Goodenay, L. S., and Gordon, G. S.: No risk from vitamin D in pregnancy. Ann. Intern. Med., 75:807, 1971.
114. Gorodischer, R., Aceto, T., Jr., and Terplan, K.: Congenital familial hypoparathyroidism and fetal undermineralization. Am. J. Dis. Child., 119:74, 1970.
115. Goss, D. A.: Renal conservation of calcium during pregnancy. Obstet. Gynecol., 20:199, 1962.
116. Graham, W. P., Gordon, G. S., Loken, H. F., Blum, A., and Halden, A.: Effect of pregnancy and of the menstrual cycle on hypoparathyroidism. J. Clin. Endocrinol. Metab., 24:512, 1964.
117. Heany, R. P., and Skillman, T. G.: Calcium metabolism in normal human pregnancy. J. Clin. Endocrinol. Metab., 33:661, 1971.
118. Hillman, L. S., and Haddad, J. G.: Human perinatal vitamin D metabolism. I. 25-hydroxyvitamin D in maternal and cord blood. J. Pediatr., 84:742, 1974.
119. Hillman, L. S., Slatopolsky, E., and Haddad, J. G.: Perinatal vitamin D metabolism. IV. Maternal and cord serum 24,25-dihydroxyvitamin D concentrations. J. Clin. Endocrinol. Metab., 47:1073, 1978.
120. Hutchin, P., and Kessner, D. M.: Neonatal tetany. Diagnostic lead to hypoparathyroidism in the mother. Ann. Intern. Med., 61:1109, 1964.
121. Johnstone, R. E., II, Kreindler, T., and Johnstone, R. E.: Hyperparathyroidism during pregnancy. Obstet. Gynecol., 40:580, 1972.
121a. Kerr, C., Loken, H. F., Glendening, M. B., Gordon, G. S., and Page, E. W.: Calcium and phosphorous dynamics in pregnancy. Am. J. Obstet. Gynecol., 83:2, 1962.
121b. Kumar, R., Cohen, W. R., Silva, P., and Epstein, F. H.: Elevated 1.25 dihydroxy vitamin D levels in normal human pregnancy and lactation. J. Clin. Invest., 63:342, 1979.
122. Landing, B. H., and Kamashita, S.: Congenital hyperparathyroidism secondary to maternal hypoparathyroidism. J. Pediatr., 77:842, 1970.
122a. Lequin, R. M., Hackeng, W. H. L., and Schopman, W.: A radioimmunoassay for parathyroid hormone in man. II. Measurement of parathyroid concentrations in human plasma by means of radioimmunoassay for bovine hormone. Acta Endocrinol., 63:655, 1970.
122b. Lowe, W., and Lester, G. E.: Vitamin D and pregnancy: the maternal fetal metabolism of vitamin D. Endocr. Rev., 2:264, 1981.
123. Marx, S. J., Swart, E. G., Jr., Hamstra, A. J., and DeLuca, H. F.: Normal intrauterine development of the fetus of a woman receiving extraordinarily high doses of 1,25-dihydroxyvitamin D_3. J. Clin. Endocrinol. Metab., 51:1138, 1980.
123a. McGeown, M. G., and Field, C. M. B.: Asyptomatic hyperparathyroidism. Lancet, 2:1268, 1960.
124. O'Leary, J. A., Klainer, L. M., and Neuwirth, R. S.: The management of hypoparathyroidism in pregnancy. Am. J. Obstet. Gynecol., 94:1103, 1966.
125. Pitkin, R. M.: Calcium metabolism in pregnancy: A review. Am. J. Obstet. Gynecol., 121:724, 1975.
126. Pitkin, R. M., and Gebhardt, M. P.: Serum calcium concentrations in human pregnancy. Am. J. Obstet. Gynecol., 127:775, 1977.
127. Pitkin, R. M., Reynolds, W. A., Williams, G. A., and Hargis, G. K.: Calcium metabolism in normal pregnancy: A longitudinal study. Am. J. Obstet. Gynecol., 133:781, 1979.
128. Rab, S. M., and Baseer, A.: Occult osteomalacia amongst healthy and pregnant women in Pakistan. Lancet, 2:1211, 1976.
129. Samaan, N. A., Anderson, G. D., and Adam-Mayne, M. E.: Immunoreactive calcitonin in the mother, neonate, child, and adult. Am. J. Obstet. Gynecol., 121:622, 1975.
130. Samaan, N. A., Hill, C. S., Jr., Beceiro, J. R., and Schultz, P. N.: Immunoreactive calcitonin in medullary carcinoma of the thyroid and in maternal and cord serum. J. Lab. Clin. Med., 81:671, 1973.
131. Schauberger, C. W., and Pitkin, R. M.: Maternal-perinatal calcium relationships. Obstet. Gynecol., 53:74, 1979.
132. Schenker, J. G., and Kallner, B.: Fatal postpartum hyperparathyroid crisis due to primary chief cell hyperplasia of parathyroids. Obstet. Gynecol., 25:705, 1965.
132a. Steichen, J. J., Tsang, R. C., Gratton, T. L., Hamstra, A., and DeLuca, H. F.: Vitamin D homeostasis in the perinatal period. N. Engl. J. Med., 302:315, 1980.
133. Taussig, H. B.: Possible injury to the cardiovascular system from vitamin D. Ann. Intern. Med., 65:1195, 1966.
134. Taylor, T. G., Lewis, P. E., and Balderstone, O.: Role of calcitonin in protecting the skeleton during pregnancy and lactation. J. Endocinrol., 66:297, 1975.
135. Wagner, G., Transbol, I., and Melchior, J. C.: Hyperparathyroidism and pregnancy. Acta Endocrinol., 47:549, 1964.
136. Watney, P. J. M., Chance, G. W., Scott, P., and Thompson, J. M.: Maternal factors in neonatal hypocalcaemia: A study in three ethnic groups. Br. Med. J., 2:432, 1971.
137. Wright, A. D., Joplin, G. F., and Dixon, H. G.: Post-partum hypercalcaemia in treated hypoparathyroidism. Br. Med. J., 1:23, 1969.

Thomas F. Ferris, M.D.

10

RENAL DISEASES

Because pregnancy is occasionally associated with toxemia, a disease manifesting hypertension, proteinuria, and edema, the presence of underlying renal disease in a pregnant woman has been viewed with alarm. However, with the greater understanding of the natural history and diverse pathology of chronic renal diseases, this attitude is no longer justified. Most women with renal disease can, with proper medical supervision, have uneventful pregnancies without adverse affects on their underlying renal disease or their ultimate prognosis. This chapter will cover the changes in renal physiology occurring with pregnancy and the effect of pregnancy on preexisting renal disease.

PHYSIOLOGIC CHANGES DURING PREGNANCY

Renal Blood Flow — Renal Function in Pregnancy

A striking increase in renal blood flow occurs early in pregnancy. In one woman studied prior to conception, renal plasma flow increased 45 per cent by the ninth week of pregnancy.[114] A review of the four published studies of the serial changes in renal plasma flow, utilizing PAH clearance, throughout pregnancy reveals a mean renal plasma flow of 809 ± ml per min in the first trimester, 695 ± ml per min the last 10 weeks of pregnancy, and 482 ± ml per min following delivery.[3, 27, 32, 114] Although it has been suggested that the measurements obtained with the patient in the supine position in late pregnancy caused a spurious reduction in renal plasma flow because compression of the inferior vena cava by the uterus,[15, 90] two studies have been unable to demonstrate such positional effects.[31, 114] Thus, it seems that the reduction in renal plasma flow in late pregnancy is real.

The cause of the rise in renal blood flow during pregnancy is not clear. Although an increase in cardiac output of approximately 40 per cent occurs as early as the first trimester, blood flow to all regional beds does not increase uniformly; no increase in cerebral or hepatic blood flow has been detected in pregnancy. A decrease in renal vascular resistance accounts in large measure for the increase in renal blood flow. Filtration fraction, the percentage of renal plasma flow filtered by the glomeruli, decreases in early pregnancy, reflecting a fall in postglomerular efferent arteriolar resistance. One can calculate the change in renal vascular resistance occurring with pregnancy from the published data on renal plasma flow during and after pregnancy. Assuming a blood pressure of 120/80 (MAP 93 mm Hg) and a hematocrit of 40, renal blood flow (renal plasma flow 482 × 1.4) is 675 ml per min after pregnancy, and renal resistance (MAP/renal blood flow), 0.138 mm Hg per ml. Assuming during pregnancy a blood pressure of 100/70 (MAP 80 mm Hg) and a hematocrit of 30, renal blood flow (809 × 1.3) is 1052 ml per min in the first trimester and renal resistance .076 mm Hg per ml, approximately half that in nonpregnant women. The cause of the decrease in renal vascular resistance is unclear, but recent observations that urinary excretion of PGE_2 and 6-keto-$PGF_{1\alpha}$, the major metabolite of PGI_2, is elevated in pregnancy might be of significance.[6, 69] Infusions of PGE_2 and PGI_2 into the renal circulation decrease renal vascular resistance with an increase in renal blood flow, whereas prostaglandin-inhibiting drugs, such as indomethacin or aspirin, may reduce renal blood flow in certain experimental and clinical circumstances.[126] Whether an increase in prostaglandin synthesis during pregnancy is the cause of the low renal resistance is not known.

A modest increase in renal blood flow occurs with the administration of human growth hormone.[103] Although growth hormone levels are normal during pregnancy, human placental lactogen, which is immunologically and chemically similar to human growth hormone, increases as early as the sixth week of gestation. Whether placental lactogen has an effect similar to that of growth hormone is not known. Placental lactogen increases with a hydatidiform mole and

235

choriocarcinoma, but no increase in renal blood flow has been documented in these clinical circumstances. It does not appear to be a major factor in the increase in renal blood flow that occurs during normal pregnancy.

Glomerular Filtration Rate

Homer Smith has stated, "A pregnant woman is a very interesting phenomenon. I do not know of any other way to increase glomerular filtration rate by 50 per cent or better for prolonged periods."[115] The increase in glomerular filtration, like the increase in renal blood flow, occurs early in pregnancy. In a study of eight women, creatinine clearance was found to be significantly increased within 4 weeks of the last menstrual period.[23] As shown by inulin clearance, the glomerular filtration rate (GFR) rose from 96 ± ml per min in nonpregnant women to 143 ± ml per min in the first trimester of pregnancy and re-

mained at this level throughout the remainder of the pregnancy. The increase in GFR occurs in spite of a fall in filtration fraction, which is 0.20 in nonpregnant women, 0.18 in the first 30 weeks of pregnancy, and 0.22 in the last 10 weeks of pregnancy. The increase in GFR in pregnancy is probably due to the increase in glomerular plasma flow that must occur. The rise in filtration fraction in late pregnancy may have multiple causes, including efferent arteriolar constriction as well as a fall in plasma oncotic pressure.[96] Serum protein concentration falls approximately 1 gram per 100 ml in late pregnancy, which diminishes plasma oncotic pressure by approximately 7 mm Hg; this tends to increase filtration fraction by increasing the proportion of glomerular plasma flow that is filtered. Glomerular filtration depends upon the balance between glomerular hydrostatic pressure minus plasma oncotic pressure, and a fall in plasma oncotic pressure increases glomerular filtration. The increase in glomerular filtration rate in pregnancy is reflect-

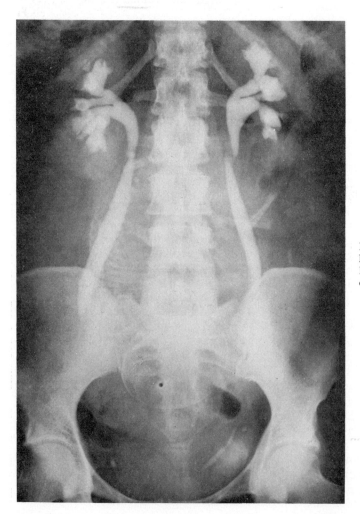

FIGURE 10–1. An IVP in a pregnant woman in her 38th week of gestation. Note the physiologic hydronephrosis with ureteral dilation greater on the right side.

ed by the low blood urea nitrogen, 8.7 ± 1.5 mg per 100 ml, and serum creatinine, 0.46 ± 0.6 mg per 100 ml in pregnant women compared with nonpregnant values of 13 ± 3 mg per 100 ml and 0.67 ± 0.17 mg per 100 ml, respectively.

ANATOMIC CHANGES OF THE URINARY TRACT DURING PREGNANCY

From early pregnancy through the puerperium, the renal collecting system is dilated, which produces the so-called physiologic hydronephrosis of pregnancy (Fig. 10–1). The right ureter tends to dilate more than the left in late pregnancy, which may indicate some element of obstruction from the uterine enlargement. There is evidence in animals that hydronephrosis is induced by estrogen and progesterone administration and in women taking oral contraceptives.[46] A similar smooth muscle atony of the stomach and gallbladder also occurs with pregnancy.[11] Since the dilation persists for up to 12 weeks post partum,[35] obstruction does not appear to be a major causative factor. Comparisons of pyelographic studies done in the immediate puerperium and repeated 6 months later reveal that renal length increases approximately 1 cm during pregnancy. This enlargement is probably a reflection of the increase in renal vascular volume and blood flow occurring with pregnancy.

The increase in urinary tract volume in pregnancy is probably the major cause of the increased incidence of acute pyelonephritis during pregnancy in women with asymptomatic bacteriuria. Nonpregnant rats given diethylstilbestrol manifest similar dilation and are more susceptible to pyelonephritis.[2]

RENAL TUBULAR FUNCTION IN PREGNANCY

Sodium Absorption

Pregnancy is the most striking example in humans of the need for renal glomerular-tubular balance if extraordinary losses of sodium are to be prevented. The increase in GFR during pregnancy necessitates an equal increase in sodium reabsorption by the renal tubules. The magnitude of this increase in tubular reabsorption can be assessed by calculating the increase in sodium reabsorption necessitated by a 50 per cent increase in GFR. Assuming a sodium concentration of 140 mEq per l in glomerular filtrate and a

GFR of 100 ml per min, the daily filtered sodium equals 20,160 mEq sodium. An increase in GFR to 150 ml per min would increase daily sodium filtration to 30,240 mEq; in other words, the renal tubules must reabsorb 10,080 mEq sodium more than in the nonpregnant state if sodium wasting is not to occur. Since the normal intake of sodium is approximately 150 to 200 mEq per day, the renal tubules reabsorb approximately 99.5 per cent of the filtered sodium.

This concept of glomerular-tubular balance, which is essential to maintenance of extracellular volume, has been a subject of intensive research effort. The peritubular capillary oncotic and hydrostatic pressures are important factors in controlling proximal tubular sodium reabsorption, but other factors are undoubtedly important as well, since approximately 30 per cent of filtered sodium is reabsorbed in more distal segments of the nephron.

In spite of this extraordinary increase in filtered sodium with pregnancy, there is no evidence that pregnant women do not conserve sodium normally. Sodium balance is attained in third trimester pregnant women receiving a 10 mEq sodium intake as readily as in nonpregnant women, and urinary sodium falls as rapidly as in nonpregnant women (Fig. 10–2).[6] Plasma aldosterone is approximately two and a half times higher in pregnant women on a low sodium intake, but whether this is a major factor in the capacity of the pregnant woman to maintain

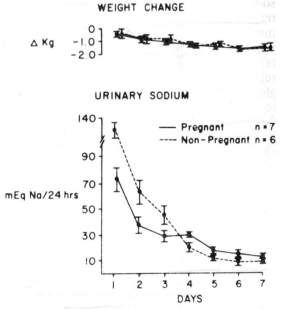

FIGURE 10–2. Serial weight change and urinary sodium excretion on a 10 mEq Na intake in seven pregnant and six nonpregnant women. (From Bay and Ferris: Hypertension, 1:410, 1979. Reprinted with permission.)

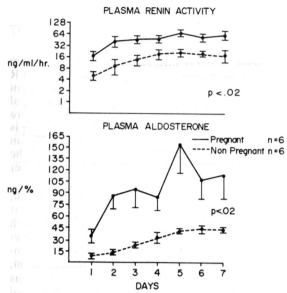

PLASMA RENIN ACTIVITY

ng/ml/hr.

p < .02

PLASMA ALDOSTERONE

ng/%

——Pregnant n=6
----Non Pregnant n=6

p<.02

DAYS

FIGURE 10–3. Plasma renin and aldosterone in pregnant and nonpregnant women on a 10 mEq Na intake for 7 days. (From Bay and Ferris: Hypertension, 1:410, 1979. Reprinted with permission.)

sodium balance on a low sodium intake is not clear (Fig. 10–3). Women with Addison's disease maintain sodium balance during pregnancy without an increase in mineralocorticoid dosage. Since aldosterone does not have an effect on the proximal tubule, where approximately two thirds of the increase in filtered sodium is reabsorbed, other factors are of obvious importance.

When pregnant women receive a 300 mEq sodium intake, plasma aldosterone and plasma renin do not decrease to the same extent as in nonpregnant women (see Figure 1–1, page 3) but urinary sodium excretion increases to equal intake. Pregnancy, like so many clinical states, represents an example of the failure of change in glomerular filtration rate or aldosterone secretion to explain change in sodium excretion. Other factors, simplistically termed "third factor" but probably representing many hormonal and physiologic factors not yet understood, maintain sodium balance in both nonpregnant and pregnant humans.

Glucose Reabsorption

Although the increase in glomerular filtration rate does not compromise the pregnant woman's ability to maintain sodium balance, pregnancy is frequently associated with glucosuria, which is due to the inability of some women to increase glucose reabsorption parallel with the increase in glucose filtration. A reduction in the renal thresh-

hold for glucose in pregnancy has been observed: 155 ± 17 mg per 100 ml compared with 194 ± 6 mg per 100 ml in nonpregnant women.[16] Since the tubular maximum for glucose transport (TM_G), a measure of the capacity of the tubules to reabsorb glucose in a given time, was the same in pregnant and control women, that worker believed the reduced threshold was due to the increase in filtered glucose. Although it is now known that the concept of TM_G is an oversimplification, since many factors affect glucose transport in the proximal tubule, the concept provides comparison of the changes in glucose reabsorption in pregnant women who develop glucosuria. In 29 pregnant women, 16 without glucosuria and 13 with glucosuria, GFR was the same in both groups but TM_G was significantly lower in pregnant women with glucosuria (310 ± 18 mg per min) compared with those without glucosuria (378 ± 18 mg per min) or in a nonpregnant control group (366 ± 16 mg per min).[127] There is a normal increase in TM_G with increase in GFR, but pregnancy displaces the slope of the regression line of TM_G on GFR to the right, and pregnant women with glucosuria have an even greater reduction in TM_G relative to GFR (Fig. 10–4). Since the increase in filtered load of glucose is not associated with as great an increase in glucose reabsorption as occurs in nonpregnant women with increased GFR, all pregnant women have a propensity to develop glucosuria. In a comparison of the renal handling of glucose in

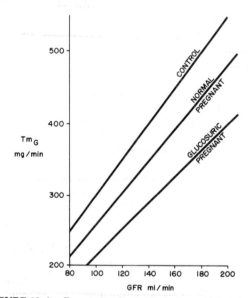

FIGURE 10–4. Regression lines of maximum tubular glucose absorption (TM_G) on GFR in nonpregnant control subjects, pregnant women without glucosuria, and pregnant women with glucosuria. (Adapted from Welsh and Sims, 1960.)

late pregnancy and 8 to 12 weeks after delivery, the reabsorption of glucose was shown to be decreased in all pregnant women compared with postpartum values.[26] However, women with glucosuria had the lowest fractional glucose reabsorption both during and after pregnancy. In women who had glucosuria greater than 150 mg per day during pregnancy, the disappearance of glucosuria post partum was due to diminished filtration of glucose as GFR returned to nonpregnant levels. Women with greater glucosuria demonstrated diminished reabsorption of glucose during and after pregnancy. These studies confirm earlier findings[127] that glucosuria in pregnancy is due to an increase in filtered glucose in women who have a diminished capacity for glucose reabsorption in the nonpregnant state.

Micropuncture studies have demonstrated that the distal tubule reabsorbs glucose and that glucose reabsorption is reduced at that site in pregnant rats.[8] Hormonal changes occurring with pregnancy seem to be the most likely cause of these changes in reabsorption of glucose, but no convincing evidence that estrogen or progesterone alters the tubular reabsorption of glucose has been provided.

Amino Acid Reabsorption

In addition to glucosuria, aminoaciduria occurs during pregnancy. Excretion of many amino acids is increased, with corresponding reduction in plasma amino acid levels.[17, 123] In the case of histidine, the percentage of reabsorbed filtered amino acid is actually decreased. An increase in urinary histidine was first proposed as a test for pregnancy in 1929 and serves as the basis for one commercial test for detection of pregnancy. Interestingly, cortisone administration causes a pattern of aminoaciduria similar to pregnancy, and the aminoaciduria of pregnancy has been interpreted as indicating an increased cortisol effect upon the renal tubules.[134] Glycine, histidine, threonine, serine, and alanine excretion increase early in pregnancy, and by term the urinary loss of these amino acids can be substantial. In one study, up to 20 per cent of the filtered glycine and histidine was excreted daily in some pregnant women,[54] which indicates a decrease in the reabsorptive capacity for these two amino acids. There is not a uniform increase in excretion of amino acids during pregnancy; for instance, excretion of glutamic acid or methionine does not increase at any time during pregnancy.

Uric Acid

Uric acid, the end product of purine metabolism, is freely filtered by the glomerulus and actively reabsorbed in the proximal tubule. The urate clearance, which is approximately 10 per cent of the creatinine clearance, is the net result of reabsorption of filtered urate and secretion of urate into the tubule at a site distal to the reabsorption site. Men and women excrete between 500 and 800 mg of urate daily in the urine, and there is no evidence that this is increased during pregnancy. There is, however, an increase in urate clearance in pregnancy; the mean serum urate in pregnancy is 3 ± 0.17 mg per 100 ml compared with 4.2 ± 1.2 mg per 100 ml in nonpregnant women. The estimation of the contribution of glomerular filtration, tubular secretion, and reabsorption to urate clearance has been difficult to determine and has depended upon inferences made in humans based upon changes in urate clearance following the administration of pyrazinamide, a drug known to inhibit urate secretion.[117] Since these studies suggest that urinary urate largely represents the effect of tubular secretion, the rise in urate clearance in pregnancy might be the result of the increase in renal plasma flow with delivery of greater amounts of urate to the tubular secretory site. As pregnancy progresses, serum uric acid concentration gradually rises, so that by late pregnancy the serum urate is similar to that in nonpregnant women. The decrease in urate clearance may be the result of the decrease in renal plasma flow and increase in filtration fraction occurring in late pregnancy. It has been demonstrated that urate clearance is decreased by a decrease in renal plasma flow with an increase in filtration fraction induced by either angiotensin or norepinephrine infusions.[37] The decrease in urate clearance during maintenance of GFR was thought to be the result of diminished postglomerular blood flow. A similar change in renal hemodynamics occurs with volume depletion, and hyperuricemia occurs with salt depletion, as is seen following the use of diuretics.

The characteristic decrease in urate clearance that occurs with the development of toxemia may be due to decrease in renal plasma flow. Essential hypertension is associated with hyperuricemia accompanied by reduced renal plasma flow and elevated filtration fraction, but the changes in toxemia are not clear. Studies of renal blood flow depend upon para-aminohippuric acid (PAH) clearance, which are unreliable during the conditions of low urine flow present in the published studies of renal hemodynamics with toxemia.

Toxemia, like other hypertensive states, is associated with diminished plasma volume and hemoconcentration, and this fact as well as other changes in the renal circulation induced by hypertension undoubtedly play a role in the diminished urate clearance. Saline loading in normotensive pregnant women in the third trimester does not increase fractional urate clearance, but this does not clarify what occurs to reduce urate clearance with toxemia. Urate clearance is decreased by organic acids such as lactate or ketoacids, but no consistent elevation in either has been noted in toxemia.[34, 44, 47]

ACID-BASE BALANCE IN PREGNANCY

Pregnancy is associated with a compensated respiratory alkalosis, which begins early in pregnancy and continues to term.[70] Arterial Pco_2 decreases from 40 mm Hg to approximately 30 mm Hg during gestation, pregnant women having an arterial pH of 7.44 compared with the normal value of 7.4. The alkalosis is thought to be due to the effect of elevated progesterone in causing hyperventilation.[74] Pregnant women are thus more prone to develop severe acidosis with either ketoacidosis or lactic acidosis in pregnancy, since their total buffering capacity is reduced because of the low bicarbonate. Mean plasma bicarbonate decreases to 18 to 20 mEq per l compared with 24 to 28 mEq per l in nonpregnant women. There is no defect in acid excretion by the kidney in pregnancy; studies have demonstrated normal excretion of both titratable acid and ammonium following ammonium chloride loading.[4]

URINARY CONCENTRATION AND DILUTION IN PREGNANCY

Pregnant women are capable of attaining normal maximal and minimal urinary osmolality. In a study of 75 normotensive pregnant women, maximum osmolality after water deprivation averaged 900 mOsm per kg of water, a figure not different from that in nonpregnant women.[57] Thus, in spite of increased renal blood flow and decreased renal vascular resistance, there is no evidence that papillary osmolality is reduced. Since urinary PGE_2 is elevated in pregnancy, the normal capacity for urine concentration is interesting. PGE_2 is known to antagonize the effect of antidiuretic hormone in causing water move-

ment across the collecting tubule. The failure to demonstrate a defect in maximum urine concentration in spite of increased renal synthesis of PGE_2 is similar to other conditions in which there is an increase in PGE_2 excretion but no prostaglandin-dependent defect in concentrating ability.[101] Minimal urine osmolality following a water load is also unimpaired in pregnancy; the urinary osmolalities are between 25 and 88 mOsm per kg, a value similar to that in nonpregnant women.[71]

In spite of the normal ability to dilute the urine in pregnancy, serum sodium falls approximately 5 mEq per l during late pregnancy with a fall in serum tonicity of approximately 10 mOsm per kg H_2O.[75] Studies in pregnant rats have demonstrated a similar fall in tonicity with a resetting of ADH release to maintain lower serum osmolality.[33] Thus, increased ADH secretion is probably one factor in maintaining hypotonicity during pregnancy, but in the Brattleboro rat, which is unable to synthesize ADH, hyponatremia also occurs during pregnancy because of increased water intake. Pregnant women demonstrate increased thirst during pregnancy; 24 hour urine volumes are approximately 25 per cent greater than in nonpregnant women. Since angiotensin is known to increase thirst in other clinical situations,[40] elevated angiotensin in pregnancy may be a factor in the increased water intake.

RENAL DISEASES AND PREGNANCY

In the past there has been great reluctance on the part of physicians to allow pregnancy in women with underlying renal disease. However, convincing data have now been accumulated to demonstrate that pregnancy does not have an adverse effect upon underlying renal disease. With control of blood pressure, a woman with chronic renal disease has an excellent chance for a successful pregnancy. Table 10–1 represents a compilation of several series of pregnant women with underlying renal disease reported from 1956 through 1969. These studies were retrospective, and most did not examine the effect of pregnancy on the underlying renal disease. However, in the total reported group of 365 patients having 424 deliveries, the fetal loss was 18 per cent. When the women were grouped into those with proteinuria alone and those with proteinuria plus hypertension, there were 176 deliveries in the proteinuric group, with a fetal loss of 7 per cent, and an incidence of toxemia of 16 per cent. In women with hypertension and proteinuria there were 123 deliveries, with a fetal loss of 45 per cent and an incidence of toxemia, defined as an increase in

TABLE 10–1 PREGNANCY AND CHRONIC RENAL DISEASE

	Patients	Deliveries	Fetal Loss _Per Cent_	Toxemia _Per Cent_
Combined series[58,62,78,92,117,129,131]	365	424	18	
Proteinuria alone		176	7	16
Proteinuria + hypertension		123	45	50
Katz et al.[60]	89	121	4.1	25

arterial blood pressure, greater than 50 per cent. These observations are compared with the recent study of renal disease and pregnancy by Katz et al., who prospectively evaluated the effect of 121 pregnancies in 89 women with renal disease.[60] Fetal loss was only 4.1 per cent, and hypertension occurred in 25 per cent of these pregnancies. The fetal loss of 4.1 per cent in Katz's series compares with an overall 1.2 per cent fetal loss in the United States. Although all the women had underlying renal disease, manifested by proteinuria, all had normal renal function with serum creatinine levels of less than 1.4 mg per 100 ml before the pregnancy. Since renal function was measured before, during, and after pregnancy, the study represents the first opportunity to document in a large group of women the effect of pregnancy upon underlying renal disease. Although renal function decreased in 16 per cent of the pregnancies, the decrease was usually mild, and reversal occurred in every case following delivery. The worsening of renal function in these women probably represented superimposed toxemia. Proteinuria increased in over half of the women and was greater than 3 gm per day in 39 of the 57 pregnancies. However, only five of these women had proteinuria greater than 3 gm per day post partum. Women were followed up from 3 months to 23 years after the pregnancy, and only five went on to develop chronic renal failure. In none did the authors feel that pregnancy was a factor in the ultimate outcome of the disease. The serum creatinine and urea decreased in half of the women during the pregnancy. In women with diminished glomerular filtration rate prior to pregnancy, an increase occurred during pregnancy that returned to the prepregnant level post partum. Figure 10–5 shows 2 hour inulin clearance in 16 women with renal disease studied before, during, and after pregnancy. It is remarkable that increases in GFR occur with underlying renal disease during pregnancy. Even in women with more compromised renal function and serum creatinine between 3 and 4 mg per 100 ml, an increase in glomerular filtration may occur.

The observations by Katz are different from

the report of Kincaid-Smith that in 12 patients with chronic diffuse glomerulonephritis and azotemia, all but one had higher BUN levels after the pregnancy.[62] Two of Kincaid-Smith's patients died of renal failure within months of pregnancy, two required dialysis or transplantation, and one died 3 years after the pregnancy. Toxemia appeared as early as the 14th week of pregnancy in some of her patients. Since the decrease in glomerular filtration rate in the Katz series occurred in only 16 per cent of the women and was transient in all, the patients reported by Kincaid-Smith probably had deteriorating renal function prior to the pregnancy. In Mackay's series of 38 women with chronic glomerulonephritis and hypertension but normal renal function at the start of pregnancy, 50 per cent showed deterioration of renal function during pregnancy, but information is not provided concerning postpartum renal function.[76] In all series of patients, fetal mortality is higher than in pregnant women without renal disease, ranging from 4 per cent

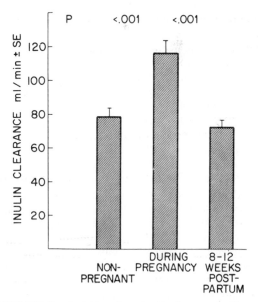

FIGURE 10–5. Serial two-hour inulin clearance in 19 pregnancies of 16 women with renal disease before, during, and after pregnancy. (From Katz et al.: Kidney Int., _18_:192, 1980. Reprinted with permission.)

when proteinuria is the only manifestation to 45 per cent when hypertension and proteinuria are present.

In women with the nephrotic syndrome, defined as proteinuria, hypoproteinemia, and edema, the risk created by pregnancy does not appear greater than in those with chronic glomerulonephritis without the nephrotic syndrome.[117] Lipoid nephrosis, in which minimal changes are found in the glomeruli by light microscopy, is a rare cause of the nephrotic syndrome in adults. Patients with lipoid nephrosis usually have uncomplicated pregnancies, although there is a higher incidence of prematurity. Birth weight correlates best with serum albumin levels, and severe hypoproteinemia often results in prematurity. Lipoid nephrosis usually responds to steroid therapy, and women have had normal pregnancies and deliveries while receiving steroid therapy for the nephrotic syndrome.

The most frequent cause of the nephrotic syndrome in adults is either membranous or membranoproliferative glomerulonephritis. In a series of 22 women with the nephrotic syndrome and either membranous or membranoproliferative glomerulonephritis, there were 35 pregnancies with 33 live births.[117] In the 5 patients treated with steroids throughout the pregnancy there were 8 successful pregnancies. Followup study of these patients from 1 to 20 years after pregnancy revealed 3 deaths from renal disease. The authors believed these deaths were due to the natural history of the disease, since there was no evidence that pregnancy had exerted a deleterious effect upon the renal disease. These workers did not note a difference in the incidence of toxemia in membranous or membranoproliferative glomerulonephritis, but it is this author's impression that membranoproliferative glomerulonephritis is more often associated with toxemia during pregnancy. A rise in blood pressure of 20 mm Hg or more occurred in 12 of the 22 nephrotic women who were normotensive at the start of the pregnancy. Of the 8 women who were hypertensive at the start of the pregnancy, 2 showed a severe increase in blood pressure at the 16th week, and pregnancy was terminated; 3 others showed a significant rise toward term. An inordinate number of premature infants were born to hypertensive mothers. When the nephrotic syndrome is associated with azotemia, a successful pregnancy is not likely. Infection, particularly of the urinary tract, may be a problem during pregnancy in nephrotic patients because of associated hypogammaglobulinemia.

Some workers have believed that patients with the nephrotic syndrome were more apt to develop thromboembolism during pregnancy, particularly in the puerperium, and have advocated routine use of anticoagulants post partum;[78, 107] but this complication has not appeared prominently in other reports. However, with peripheral edema, hyperlipidemia, and other factors in pregnancy predisposing to clotting, nephrotic patients may be at greater risk for thromboembolic phenomena and should be observed carefully in the postpartum period. Renal vein thrombosis has occurred during pregnancy in women with the nephrotic syndrome, resulting in worsening of renal function.[99, 100]

A rare form of nephrosis is the "nephrotic syndrome of pregnancy," in which proteinuria develops during pregnancy, disappears after delivery, and recurs with subsequent pregnancies.[107] The possibility of a sensitizing antigen, either a fetal or a placental protein, resulting in immune-complex deposits in glomeruli has been postulated, but no studies of the glomeruli in this rare disease have been described. It is possible that the increase in protein excretion during pregnancy noted in patients with underlying renal disease but minimal proteinuria was the cause of the nephrotic syndrome in this patient.

Diagnosis of Renal Disease During Pregnancy

The diagnosis of renal disease can usually be made by the physician on the basis of clinical history, physical examination, and urinalysis. Examination of the urine is the single most valuable procedure in the recognition and differential diagnosis of renal disease. Since urine can be concentrated or dilute depending on the hydration of the patient, and 24 hour urinary excretion of protein, cells, and casts is constant, any urinalysis showing a specific gravity of less than 1.020 can be misleading. Although proteinuria, cylindruria, hematuria, or pyuria in a dilute urine is significant, absence of those conditions does not exclude renal disease. It is thus essential that a concentrated urine (the first voided urine in the morning is usually concentrated) be examined when the presence of renal disease is being established. There is no doubt that an examination of the urine done casually or by an inexperienced person is the most common cause of failure to detect renal disease.

Proteinuria. Proteinuria is an important sign of renal disease, and significant proteinuria points to changes in glomerular basement membrane permeability to plasma proteins. Protein excretion is abnormal when the total daily excretion exceeds 150 mg, but with pregnancy, daily protein excretion may reach 250 mg.[122] Although trace quantities of protein can normally be present in concentrated urine, concentration alone never results in proteinuria exceeding 10 to 20 mg per 100 ml. Presently, the most commonly used method for detection of urinary protein is based upon a color-producing reaction between albumin and paper strips impregnated with tetra-bromphenol blue dye. This reaction is specific for albumin and will not detect globulin in urine. This test is so sensitive that frequent trace reactions occur in patients who subsequently prove to have less than 150 mg protein in a 24 hour urine collection. Adding approximately 7.5 ml salicylic acid (3 gm per 100 ml) to 2.5 ml urine results in turbidity in the presence of significant proteinuria. This is a reliable semiquantitative measurement, which gives a reaction with proteins other than albumin, but false positive results can occur with several substances, including x-ray contrast media and tolbutamide. If both the dip stick and sulfosalicyclic acid tests give positive reaction, a 24 hour urine specimen should be obtained to document total protein excretion.

The extent to which serum proteins normally penetrate the glomerular basement membrane in human beings is not clear. In the dog, micropuncture of the proximal tubule has revealed protein concentrations of 2 to 8 mg per 100 ml in about one half of the animals.[28] If the human glomerular filtrate contained 1 mg protein per 100 ml, approximately 1.8 gm protein would be filtered daily. There is good evidence in the rat that tubular reabsorption of filtered protein occurs. The fact that GFR can be increased 50 per cent in normal pregnancy without causing proteinuria indicates either that tubular reabsorption of protein increases with pregnancy or that the glomerulus is more impermeable to plasma protein in human beings than it is in animals.

Heavy proteinuria (more than 2 gm daily) is caused by renal diseases that primarily affect the glomerulus. These diseases include acute and chronic glomerulonephritis, intercapillary glomerulosclerosis, systemic lupus erythematosus, membranous glomerulonephritis, lipoid nephrosis, and renal venous congestion. Moderate proteinuria, between 150 mg and 2 gm daily, is more apt to be present with chronic interstitial nephritis or nephrosclerosis.

The microscopic examination of the urine sediment provides a great deal of information concerning the nature of the renal disease and aids in differentiating the various renal disorders resulting in proteinuria. Cells in the urine sediment arise from either desquamation of tubular cells lining the urinary tract or entrance of cells into the urinary tract in response to inflammation and infection. Tubular epithelial cells are seen in all forms of renal disease but particularly in tubular necrosis and nephrotoxic nephritis. In the nephrotic syndrome, tubular epithelial cells filled with lipid give the typical "Maltese cross" appearance under polarized light. With renal disease, increased numbers of red and white blood cells are found in the urine. These cells may be added at any site in the urine's passage through the nephron or collecting system. Only when these cells form casts can one be certain that they come from the kidney and not from the pelvis, bladder, or urethra. Casts are cylindric masses of cells that form in the nephron, and the width of the cast indicates where it was formed. Most casts are formed in the distal nephron. Cellular casts are formed when cells agglutinate because of precipitation of protein. The precipitation of protein is abetted by an acid pH and low urine flow rate, conditions that are more apt to be present with the first voided specimen of the morning. Tamm-Horsfall mucoprotein is the matrix material in hyaline and granular casts and is secreted by cells of the distal nephron. It is readily precipitated in an acid urine with high concentrations of solute, which probably accounts for the absence of casts in dilute or alkaline urines. Although a few red and white blood cells can be seen in normal urine, they are not sufficient to cause cast formation. Red blood cells usually have the characteristic rusty or reddish-brown appearance of hemoglobin; this distinguishes them from other casts, which are colorless.

Normal Sediment. The mean excretion rate of red blood cells is approximately 300,000 cells per day in normal adults. This number rarely gives more than 1 red blood cell per high-power field in the spun urinary sediment. Microscopic hematuria can be increased by severe exercise, kidney trauma, and acute febrile illness. The mean rate of excretion of white blood cells is 600,000 to 1,000,000 cells daily. This results in approximately 2 white blood cells per high-power field in men. In women there may be up to 5 white blood cells per high-power field. Whether the increased number of white blood cells in women would be present on a catheter sample is unclear, since epithelial cells from the mucosal surfaces of the vulva and vagina are indistinguishable from white blood cells in the urine. Normal adults may excrete from 5000 to 10,000 casts per 24 hours. Thus, a rare hyaline cast (no more than 1 every 15 to 20 high-power fields) may be found in normal urine, and these can be increased in situations that can cause functional proteinuria, i.e., exercise, fever, and posture. However, a granular or cellular cast should always be viewed with suspicion.

Urinary Sediment in Renal Disease. Hematuria is so frequently caused by extrarenal bleeding from the genitourinary tract that one must determine whether red blood cell casts are present. Finding them locates the bleeding in the kidney and indicates that there is inflammation and injury, usually in the glomerulus. The causes of hematuria run the gamut of glomerulonephritides, including acute and subacute glomerulonephritis, systemic lupus erythematosus, periarteritis, focal glomerulonephritis, and malignant hypertension. It is of note that in pre-eclampsia, in which a definite lesion of the glomerulus has been demonstrated, proteinuria occurs usually without hematuria. The presence of microscopic hematuria with casts in a toxemic patient suggests underlying renal disease. However, when thrombocytopenia occurs with toxemia, hematuria may be significant.

Pyuria may be seen in any renal disease but when pronounced usually indicates the presence of infection. White blood cells, casts, and pyuria can, however, be present in the absence of infection in response to inflammation of either the glomerulus or the interstitium of the kidney. Thus, it is not unusual in acute glomerulonephritis to find leukocytes and leukocyte casts because of the polymorphonuclear inflammation in the glomeruli. Similarly, in chronic interstitial nephritis increased numbers of white blood cells are seen in the urine in the absence of bacteriuria. Indeed, by inducing fever one can produce pyuria frequently in patients with chronic inflammation of the renal interstitium. This has been utilized by some to diagnose chronic interstitial nephritis by infusing bacterial pyrogen and quantitating the pyuria obtained. Like hematuria, pyuria in the absence of leukocyte casts can be found whenever infection is present in the genitourinary tract. The presence of leukocyte casts indicates infection or inflammation in the renal parenchyma. In the past, diagnostic significance was placed on the appearance and staining properties of leukocytes in the urine. Leukocytes arising from infections in the kidney were thought to have characteristic pale and swollen cytoplasm ("glitter cells"), and they demonstrated brownian movement in the cytoplasm. It now appears more likely that these cells are caused by hypotonicity or other changes in urinary composition and do not necessarily imply the presence of infection. A quantitative urine culture with more than 100,000 organisms per ml of urine is necessary to document the presence of infection in suspected cases of pyelonephritis.

In the absence of a quantitative urine culture, the presence of bacteriuria on microscopic examination in a drop of unspun urine usually indicates significant bacteriuria (greater than 100,000 organisms per ml). Since pyelonephritis is a disease of the kidney caused by bacterial infection, it is illogical to make that diagnosis unless significant bacteriuria is documented. Many nonbacterial renal diseases involving the interstitium can present with pyuria and leukocyte casts. The inflammatory response of the interstitium can be immunologic, nephrotoxic, or vascular.

Clinical History. Although chronic renal disease is usually an insidious and asymptomatic process, there are clues frequently in the history. Previous hematuria, described as cola- or wine-colored urine, is sometimes uncovered. Enuresis beyond the age of 6 sometimes indicates polyuria, particularly if it is followed by subsequent nocturia. Although polyuria may reflect inability to concentrate urine, nocturia can be caused by loss of the normal diurnal variation in urine flow. Normal persons have reduced urine output at night, whereas patients with either renal disease or hypertension show no diurnal variation in urine flow. Polyuria may be accompanied by symptoms of excessive fluid intake, particularly in renal diseases affecting the renal medulla. Symptoms of urinary tract infection — dysuria, foul-smelling urine, urgency — must be searched for. Although a history of urinary tract infection in sexually active women is not unusual, urinary infection before the age of sexual activity may indicate underlying renal disease, possibly obstructive. The examiner should ask whether proteinuria or albuminuria has been detected at any time as well as whether hypertension was noted at physical examination. The family history is important in determining whether hypertension, diabetes, gout, or renal disease is present. Hypertension, gout, and diabetes are associated with early vascular disease, and nephrosclerosis can precede the development of overt hypertension in some families.

Laboratory Studies. After a careful urinalysis, base-line studies of renal function in patients with abnormal results should include a serum creatinine, BUN, and uric acid. In patients with heavy proteinuria, serum protein and cholesterol should be determined. The BUN and serum creatinine must be interpreted in light of the knowledge that it is only after a 60 to 70 per cent reduction in GFR that these levels rise above the "normal" values. As one can see from Figure

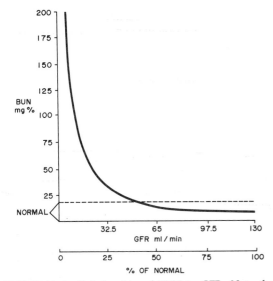

FIGURE 10–6. Relationship of BUN to GFR. Note that BUN remains within the normal range until GFR is approximately 40 per cent normal. The hyperbolic curve then causes a precipitous change in BUN with slight change in GFR.

10–6, a rise in BUN and creatinine is barely detectable with changes in GFR from 125 to 50 ml per minute, but thereafter there is a sharp rise in BUN and creatinine with relatively slight change in GFR. Once creatinine and BUN have become elevated, one can expect precipitous changes in both with slight reductions in GFR or with changes in protein intake that increase urea production. In addition to increased protein intake, BUN is affected by catabolism of protein, such as that occurring during infection, surgical stress, steroid administration, and extravasation of blood into various body compartments. Since serum creatinine, a metabolic by-product of muscle metabolism, is unaffected by changes in protein intake or catabolism, its serum level reflects only GFR and creatinine synthesis, which is dependent upon muscle mass. When renal disease exists without elevation in BUN or serum creatinine, a 24 hour creatinine clearance is needed to determine GFR. Creatinine clearance is an accurate guide to GFR and can be followed serially throughout pregnancy. A creatinine clearance involves collecting a 24 hour urine specimen and determining the serum creatinine the day of the collection. It is important to standardize the timing of the urine collections so that each 24 hour collection is similar. The patient discards the first voided specimen the first morning and collects each subsequent urine specimen, including the first of the following morning. The most frequent error in creatinine

clearance is incomplete collection of the 24 hour urine sample. Creatinine clearance is calculated thus:

$$\frac{\text{Urine creatinine concentration (mg per 100 ml)} \times}{\text{Plasma creatinine (mg per 100 ml)} \times}$$
$$\frac{\text{24 hour urine volume (ml)}}{\text{1440 (minutes per day)}}$$

For example,

$$\frac{90 \text{ mg per 100 ml} \times 1500 \text{ ml}}{1.2 \text{ mg per 100 ml} \times 1440} = 78.1 \text{ ml per minute}$$

A base-line serum urate determination is important in early pregnancy since a rise in serum urate points to the development of pre-eclampsia. Elevated urate in the face of normal BUN and creatinine is sometimes indicative of diseases affecting tubular function, i.e., nephrosclerosis or interstitial nephritis. Excretion of urate, like that of other organic acids, is dependent upon tubular secretion, and tubular function may be disproportionately affected in nonglomerular diseases.

Radiologic Studies. Abdominal x-rays are avoided during pregnancy because of the radiation risk to the fetus. However, with careful shielding of the lower pelvis and with image intensification techniques, renal x-ray can be obtained when necessary. Seldom, however, is an intravenous pyelogram needed in the diagnosis of parenchymal renal disease. Proteinuria and microscopic hematuria are indicative of chronic glomerulonephritis, and a renal echogram may be used to estimate renal size. The creatinine clearance is the measure of function; there frequently is little correlation between kidney size and function, particularly with rapidly progressive glomerulonephritis. Chronic interstitial nephritis or nephrosclerosis results in renal scarring that gives the kidney an irregular surface, with distortion and clubbing of the renal calyces and pelvis. However, the diagnosis of pyelonephritis is made by demonstration of urinary tract infection and not by nonspecific radiologic findings, which can be the result of many noninfectious diseases.

Renal colic from stones is uncommon in pregnancy, occurring in less than 1 in 1000 pregnancies, but when symptoms suggest a renal stone, a renal echogram is indicated. Gross hematuria without significant proteinuria is an indication for an intravenous pyelogram, since tumors or cysts can present in this way.

The radiologic evaluation of a pregnant woman for hypertension should be deferred until the postpartum period unless the clinical history strongly suggests a pheochromocytoma. Pheochromocytomas are associated with high mortality during pregnancy and must be removed surgically. All other hypertensive states should be treated with drug therapy and the hypertensive evaluation postponed until after delivery. This topic is covered in more detail in Chapter 1, Toxemia and Hypertension.

Renal Biopsy. The understanding of renal disease in both pregnant and nonpregnant patients has been greatly increased as a result of the use of renal biopsy and the study of these biopsy specimens by electron microscopy, special histochemical staining, and immunofluorescent techniques. Renal biopsies performed during pregnancy have demonstrated the renal pathology of pre-eclampsia. However, there is an increased risk with renal biopsy during pregnancy, particularly in the hypertensive patient. Both perirenal hematoma and gross hematuria are more frequent following renal biopsy, and surgical intervention for postbiopsy bleeding was reported in 2 of 90 pregnant patients in contrast to none of 450 nonobstetric patients by the same investigators.[105] One patient died following surgery for a perirenal hematoma. The increase in risk is probably related to the technical difficulties in performing a biopsy in a pregnant patient, the increase in renal blood flow, and the hypertension that is usually present in the pregnant patient undergoing a renal biopsy. Because of these risks, renal biopsy should not be performed during pregnancy unless the potential benefit to the patient's care warrants the risk.

Orthostatic Proteinuria. Orthostatic or postural proteinuria is a clinical syndrome in which proteinuria is present during ambulation or standing but is absent when the patient is recumbent. The relationship of orthostatic proteinuria to underlying renal disease is uncertain. Although it was originally thought to be a benign condition in young adults, studies utilizing renal biopsy in patients with orthostatic proteinuria revealed that 8 per cent had unequivocal evidence of well-defined renal disease and 45 per cent had subtle but definite alterations of glomerular structure.[97] The clinical significance of these findings is not clear, since the subtle and focal changes of the glomeruli might be reflections of the proteinuria and not pathognomonic of glomerular disease. In followup studies of 531 patients with orthostatic proteinuria for an average of 6 years, 18 per cent had developed constant proteinuria and 14 per cent had diastolic hypertension. In another 10 year followup of young men with orthostatic proteinuria, approximately

50 per cent continued to have proteinuria, but none showed evidence of renal disease or hypertension; half of the patients no longer demonstrated proteinuria.[97] It will be of interest to determine whether any of the patients with persistent orthostatic proteinuria for 10 years demonstrate clearing of the proteinuria in subsequent followup examinations.

Orthostatic proteinuria has been thought to be caused by an unusual sensitivity in some individuals to the reduction in renal blood flow and the rise in filtration fraction that occur during standing. It has been reported in 5 per cent of pregnant women, but there is no evidence that pregnancy is associated with increased risk in these women. Since patients with underlying renal disease can demonstrate an increase in proteinuria with standing, it is important to document the absence of proteinuria with the patient supine and, during late pregnancy, lying on her side. The presence of systemic disease, such as hypertension or diabetes mellitus, should be excluded, and a careful examination of the urinary sediment must be done. Base-line BUN and serum creatinine values should be obtained.

Acute Glomerulonephritis

Acute glomerulonephritis is a rare complication during pregnancy. Twenty patients have been reported in the literature, and the calculated incidence of the disease is approximately 1 in every 40,000 pregnancies.[81] In most pregnant patients developing acute glomerulonephritis, fetal loss occurs, although successful pregnancies have been reported.[53] In two of three women reported by Wilson with acute glomerulonephritis, the condition rapidly progressed after pregnancy, but this experience is not usual. Most women recover normal renal function post partum.[131] The treatment of the condition is similar to that for the nonpregnant patient: careful control of blood pressure and fluid balance. Blood pressure must be maintained in the normotensive range by use of appropriate antihypertensive agents and salt restriction. This is particularly important if congestive heart failure or evidence of hypertensive encephalopathy is present. After the blood pressure has been controlled, correction of the expanded extracellular volume, a prominent factor in the hypertension of acute glomerulonephritis, should be accomplished if possible. The edema of acute glomerulonephritis, like toxemia, can be clinically subtle, since it primarily involves areas (i.e., periorbital area, hands) with low tissue turgor pressure. Pitting edema of the legs usually indicates congestive heart failure with elevation of venous pressure. No intravenous solutions containing sodium should be administered until blood pressure and edema are controlled. If the patient can eat, the salt intake should be restricted to 500 mg daily. If the daily urine volume is below 1000 ml, potassium restriction to 40 mEq daily is necessary, and serum potassium must be carefully monitored. Although therapeutic abortion has been advocated when acute glomerulonephritis occurs during pregnancy, there seems little reason to evacuate the uterus if blood pressure and fluid balance are controlled. Of 15 patients with acute glomerulonephritis reported in the literature in whom blood pressure was recorded, 7 had diastolic pressures above 110 mm Hg. Six of these patients had either a fetal death or a termination of the pregnancy. In the 8 patients with diastolic pressures below 100 mm Hg, 6 had successful pregnancies with living infants.[81] No evidence of renal disease was noted in the babies, possibly indicating that the soluble antigen-antibody complexes causing the glomerulonephritis are too large to cross the placental circulation or that fetal glomeruli do not react similarly to soluble immune complexes. When infants develop acute glomerulonephritis in the first year of life, the juxtamedullary glomeruli are predominantly involved, and they are the most mature.

There is no evidence that acute glomerulonephritis improves following delivery, but if superimposed pre-eclampsia is suspected, delivery of the fetus is indicated. This is a difficult clinical differentiation; however, if blood pressure is controlled and renal function does not deteriorate, continuation of the pregnancy seems a reasonable course. In early pregnancy an attack of acute glomerulonephritis may resolve, and the remainder of the pregnancy may be uneventful. Each situation must be evaluated individually, attention being directed to the clinical status of the patient, the risk of the abortion, and the patient's attitude toward the pregnancy.

Acute glomerulonephritis during the last trimester may be difficult to differentiate from pre-eclampsia, but the presence of microscopic hematuria with red blood cell casts, low serum complement, and a rising antistreptolysin O (ASO) titer point to acute post-streptococcal glomerulonephritis. Since many cases of acute glomerulonephritis in adults are nonstreptococcal, one must not rely upon the ASO titer except as an indication of streptococcal involvement. This would be one of the rare circumstances in which a renal biopsy is justified in pregnancy to differentiate between the two conditions.

There is no increased risk of pregnancy in women with a preceding history of acute glomerulonephritis in whom activity of the disease has cleared, as demonstrated by a negative urinalysis at the time of pregnancy. One study suggested an increase in perinatal mortality in women having children within 3 years of acute glomerulonephritis,[92] but this has not been confirmed by others.[58] Since normal urine after acute glomerulonephritis has been described in patients in whom renal biopsy has demonstrated persistent activity of the disease, patients with a history of glomerulonephritis should be followed closely during pregnancy so that any change in blood pressure or appearance of proteinuria is quickly detected.

Focal glomerulitis is of particular interest because it represents a relatively common cause of hematuria and minimal proteinuria in young adults.[38, 65] In childhood this disease has been called recurrent benign hematuria.[5] Although microscopic hematuria, frequently associated with episodes of gross hematuria, is prominent, the disease can usually be differentiated from diffuse glomerulonephritis by the minimal proteinuria, which is usually under 500 mg per 24 hours. Rarely, patients have sufficient proteinuria to cause the nephrotic syndrome. Blood pressure and glomerular filtration rate are characteristically normal. The glomerular lesions consist of focal segmental capillary hypercellularity or sclerosis and mesangial thickening due to increase in mesangial cells and matrix. IgA, IgG, and complement are frequently demonstrated in the mesangial areas of the glomeruli. The prognosis in these patients is excellent, and only rarely does progressive renal failure occur. In the author's experience, pregnancy in women with focal glomerulonephritis is not associated with a greater risk of pre-eclampsia or fetal mortality.

Systemic Lupus Erythematosus

Because systemic lupus erythematosus (SLE) occurs frequently in young women, the effect of pregnancy in women with underlying lupus nephropathy is clinically an important issue. A 1962 report suggested that exacerbation of SLE was three times greater in the first 20 weeks of pregnancy and eight times greater in the immediate postpartum period.[43] No evidence of exacerbation of the disease from the 20th to the 40th week of pregnancy was reported in this study. However, more recent studies do not support these findings. The best study of lupus nephropathy was published by Hayslett and Lynn and represents data obtained on 65 pregnancies in 47 patients with lupus nephropathy reported from 13 centers.[50] Renal biopsy was obtained in 77 per cent of these patients, so the patients have proven lupus nephropathy. Information on renal function and activity of the SLE was recorded before, during, and after the pregnancy. In nine pregnancies the SLE occurred for the first time either during the pregnancy or immediately post partum, whereas in the remaining 56 pregnancies the onset of SLE occurred before gestation. In a comparison of the clinical activity of the lupus during and after pregnancy, the clinical course was not adversely influenced by the pregnancy in 65 per cent of the pregnancies. Thirty-nine per cent had an exacerbation, either a relapse or a worsening of the disease activity, during gestation or in the immediate postpartum period. Exacerbation was more common during the pregnancy than immediately following delivery. It was found that the activity of the lupus in the 6 month interval before conception was an important indicator of relapse during the pregnancy; thus, in 31 pregnancies in which there was no evidence of disease activity within 6 months of conception, the remission was sustained in 21 throughout the pregnancy. However, in 10 pregnancies with evidence of disease activity 6 months before conception, an exacerbation occurred during gestation in 6 and post partum in 4. Eighty-eight per cent of these women with SLE had live births, and the prematurity rate did not exceed the rate of 8.2 per cent recorded in a population of healthy subjects. There were three spontaneous abortions in women with quiescent lupus, making the likelihood of a successful outcome in these patients 92 per cent. In women with sustained remission throughout pregnancy, evidence of lupus nephropathy was present in 20 of the 21 cases; two patients had nephrotic syndrome and one had renal insufficiency. In the 10 pregnancies that were characterized by exacerbation during pregnancy or in the immediate postpartum period, evidence of renal disease prior to the pregnancy was present in 8. The relapse of the SLE involved activation of the renal disease in all but 1 woman; renal insufficiency occurred in 3 cases and the nephrotic syndrome in 3. Hypertension was present in most of these exacerbations, so superimposed toxemia in some patients probably occurred. There were no patient deaths in this series. In 8 women followed up for more than 3 months post partum, there was a complete or partial reversal of the exacerbation. This is similar to the findings of Katz in women with chronic glomerulonephritis. The major findings of the Hayslett study are these: (1) if there is evidence of clinical remission of the SLE for at least 6 months prior to conception, the outlook for a live birth is reduced only slightly below the rate expected in the normal population, and (2) in the 30 per cent of cases in which there was an exacerbation of the lupus, significant morbidity occurred in only 10 per cent, and in most patients there was reversal of the exacerbation following delivery.

In the 25 pregnancies in which activity of the SLE was evident in the 6 month interval before conception, clinical manifestations of the disease remained unchanged in 10 (40 per cent), improved in 3 (12 per cent), and worsened in 12 (48 per cent) during pregnancy or in the postpartum period. The incidence of live births in this group of pregnancies was 64 per cent after exclusion of those in which a therapeutic abortion was performed. There were 2 fetal deaths in the 12 women with renewed activity of the lupus during pregnancy, 1 stillbirth, and 1 abortion at 24 weeks. The onset of lupus during pregnancy caused significant maternal morbidity: a fetal loss of approximately 35 per cent. It was not believed, however, that the subsequent course of the lupus was different. Five of 9 of these patients had subsequent uncomplicated pregnancies.

When proteinuria preceded the pregnancy, an increase in proteinuria occurred frequently with pregnancy. It did not necessarily indicate an exacerbation of the lupus and usually subsided after delivery. Thus, the increased proteinuria with lupus nephropathy is similar to other forms of chronic glomerulonephritis in which the hemodynamic effects of pregnancy on glomerular filtration rate may increase protein excretion.

Sixteen pregnancies in Hayslett's series were in women with the nephrotic syndrome. When these women were classified on the basis of serum creatinine level, nine of ten with a level of 1.5 ml per 100 ml or less had full term live births, and only two of five with a level greater than 1.5 mg per 100 ml had a successful outcome. If all women with lupus nephropathy were grouped on the basis of serum creatinine level, fetal loss was 50 per cent when the serum creatinine was greater than 1.5 mg per ml. However, in the four women with live births in this group, the serum creatinine was 4 mg per 100 ml or higher in three. Thus, even with severe renal insufficiency from lupus nephropathy a successful pregnancy is possible.

There was no evidence that either glucocorticoids or cytotoxic agents induced developmental anomalies in the offspring. This is similar to results obtained in women becoming pregnant following renal homografts (vide infra). Although there is evidence in laboratory animals that steroids can cause fetal abnormalities such as cleft palate and harelip, there are no reports of such changes in human pregnancy. Some studies have linked glucocorticoids with reduced fetal growth,[126] but this has not been observed by others.[134] Appropriate treatment with either prednisone or cytotoxic agents in doses needed to suppress clinical activity of SLE should not be withheld from women who become pregnant. However, since the 5 year survival rate of patients with SLE treated between the years 1968 and 1978 was 93 per cent, compared with a 70 per cent survival between 1957 and 1968 when treatment with high dose steroids was more popular, high dose glucocorticoid therapy with or without cytotoxic drugs is now avoided unless it is needed to suppress clinical evidence of disease activity. This also improves the quality of life for patients with SLE by preventing superimposition of Cushing's disease.

Glucocorticoids and immunosuppressant therapy can cause a reduction in thymic size with lymphocytopenia and reduced plasma cortisol in the neonate. However, cortisol secretion rate and the response to ACTH in most neonates born to mothers treated with glucocorticoids are normal.[88] The fetus may be protected from excess prednisolone and hydrocortisone by the presence in placenta of 11 beta-dehydrogenase, which oxidizes glucocorticoids to the inactive 11-ketoform.[9] Dexamethasone and betamethasone undergo limited metabolism by 11-beta dehydrogenase, so theoretically these glucocorticoids have greater potential in harming the fetus than does prednisone.

In the UCLA series, 39 patients with known lupus nephropathy had 52 pregnancies.[39] When serum creatinine was less than 1 mg per 100 ml and proteinuria less than 1 gm per day, in 30 of 38 pregnancies there was no change in renal function, in 5 there was transient deterioration, and in only 3 did persistent deterioration occur. In the 14 pregnancies in 13 patients with more extensive renal involvement, i.e., proteinuria from 1 to 3 grams per day and creatinine clearance 50 to 80 ml per min, in 5 there was no deterioration in renal function, in 2 there was transient deterioration in renal function, and in 2 there was persistent deterioration. Of the 52 pregnancies, 37 resulted in full term births, 4 in spontaneous abortions, and 11 in therapeutic abortions. In only 5 pregnant patients (9.6 per cent) did renal function deteriorate and remain suppressed during the 3 to 12 month followup period.

Although other studies involving small numbers of patients have suggested permanent renal damage occurred frequently during pregnancy in women with lupus nephropathy,[7, 10] the combined reports of all the reported studies do not support such a conclusion. If one combines the 114 pregnancies reported in these studies, only 15 patients had permanent deterioration in renal function during pregnancy. Also, when an abortion was performed in the first trimester, there was no evidence that a deleterious effect on renal function occurred, in contrast to an early report where severe exacerbation of SLE following therapeutic abortion was described.[30]

Pregnancy Following Renal Transplantation

With the increased numbers of women receiving renal transplantation, the potential for them to have children is increasing. About 1 of every 50 women of childbearing age with a functional renal transplant become pregnant. In men following renal transplantation, impotence remains a problem in 22 to 43 per cent.[68] Despite this incidence of impotence in some men, many male transplant recipients have been parents. In the largest series, reported from Colorado, of female transplant recipients who have become pregnant there were 37 women who had 56 pregnancies.[87] Seven had therapeutic abortions because the patient did not desire the pregnancy, 1 had a spontaneous abortion, and 24 had live births with a fetal survival of 90 per cent. The incidence of toxemia in these women was 25 per cent, and 1 patient demonstrated evidence of deterioration of renal function during the pregnancy that persisted in the postpartum period. Although in 4 of 56 pregnancies there was deterioration of renal function thought to be attributable to pregnancy, a comparison of creatinine clearance before, during, and after the pregnancy revealed no significant difference. The creatinine clearance was 72 ± 4 before, 75 ± 4 during, and 72 ± 4 after pregnancy in these 37 patients. Three of the 4 in whom there was deterioration of the renal function during pregnancy had impaired function before conception. The authors recommended termination of the gestation if deterioration of renal function occurs during the pregnancy; this was necessary in 5 patients. In the 15 patients developing toxemia during pregnancy, 10 developed toxemia superimposed on preexisting hypertension, whereas in 5 the toxemia occurred in previously normotensive women. Four children born to female patients had congenital abnormalities. Whether these anomalies were related to the immunosuppressive agents is unclear.

Vaginal delivery was thought possible in all of these patients, although in nine a cesarian section was performed because of avascular necrosis of both hips with impaired abduction, cephalopelvic disproportion, or fetal distress. All women were given supplemental corticosteroid therapy from the onset of parturition, 100 mg hydrocortisone intravenously every 8 hours for 24 hours.

Of the 44 infants, 31 had an uncomplicated neonatal course, but 13 had one or more complications. Four had respiratory distress syndrome, 2 had adrenal insufficiency, and two, septicemia.

The recommendation of the Colorado group is that all patients who have completed their families and have no desire for further children should be offered sterilization at the time of transplantation. Those wishing to become parents should be advised to practice contraception for at least 18 months after the renal transplant. Since thromboembolism and hypertension are more common in transplantation patients, oral contraceptive agents are not recommended. Also, because of the potential for infection following the insertion of intrauterine devices, this mode of contraception is discouraged in immunosuppressed patients.

Postpartum Hemolytic Uremic Syndrome

During the immedate postpartum period acute renal failure may occur because of hemorrhagic shock, abruptio placentae, eclampsia, or sepsis. However, as described in 1968, the syndrome of renal failure with typical lesions of thrombotic microangiopathy may occur up to 2 months post partum.[98, 124] In the 10 years since, 49 cases have been reported under various terms: malignant nephrosclerosis in women post partum,[104] postpartum renal failure with microangiopathic hemolytic anemia,[73] postpartum hemolytic uremic syndrome,[108] and idiopathic postpartum renal failure.[119] A review of 49 published cases revealed a symptom-free interval lasting up to 2 months in nearly all the cases.[108] Symptoms preceding the onset of renal failure included vomiting, diarrhea, or an influenza-like illness. When oliguria occurred, hematuria and proteinuria were most often found. Thirty-six of the 49 patients had an associated severe microangiopathic hemolytic anemia with anisocytosis and schizocytosis. Frequent findings were indirect hyperbilirubinemia, hemoglobinemia, reticulocytosis, and thrombocytopenia. Some patients had disseminated intravascular coagulation, evidenced by reduction in clotting factors. Although the initial reports emphasized the invariably fatal outcome of the disease, this is not a uniform finding. In 49 reported cases, death has occurred in 30, a fatality rate of 61 per cent. Terminal renal failure occurred in 8 patients maintained on dialysis, in 2 of whom malignant hypertension, requiring bilateral nephrectomy, was necessary. In the other 11 cases, slow improvement in renal function occurred for as long as 1½ years from the onset of the symptoms. Complete recovery occurred in only 5 patients (9.5 per cent).

Neurologic signs and symptoms are less common than in childhood hemolytic-uremic syndrome, although convulsions were noted in 14 of the 49 cases. In 27 of 52 published cases heparin has been administered. Eleven of these patients died (40.8 per cent), four went into terminal renal failure (14.8 per cent), and twelve had partial or complete improvement in renal function (44.4 per cent). In 25 untreated cases, nineteen died (75 per cent), three went into terminal renal failure (12 per cent), and three had partial or complete improvement in renal function (12 per cent). Although this suggests that the prognosis is improved by anticoagulant therapy, there are no convincing studies on this matter.

The characteristic pathologic lesion is thickening of the glomerular capillary wall due to endothelial cell swelling and the appearance of a widened subendothelial space containing mucinous material, which gives a double contoured effect. Capillary thrombi are seen in about half the cases. Vascular changes in the arterioles are constant, involvement of the intralobular arteries being more frequent than in childhood hemolytic uremic syndrome (Fig. 10–7). The most constant finding by electron microscopy is the subendothelial space in glomeruli and blood vessels. When biopsy specimens are obtained late in the disease, the features of malignant nephrosclerosis are most prominent. Immunofluorescent studies were done in 12 cases and showed fibrinogen in the mesangium, glomerular capillary wall, and arterioles. C3 deposits were commonly found, but C1q and C4 were usually absent.

It appears that disseminated intravascular coagulation is not the starting point in the pathogenesis of the disease, but rather local renal intravascular coagulation, possibly due to endothelial cell damage. Because of the emerging evidence that endothelial cell PGI$_2$ synthesis is increased in late pregnancy[69] and reduced in the umbilical arteries of patients with toxemia,[13, 118] it is intriguing to speculate that the intrarenal vascular occlusions are due to an aberration in renal endothelial cell PGI$_2$ synthesis in the postpartum period.

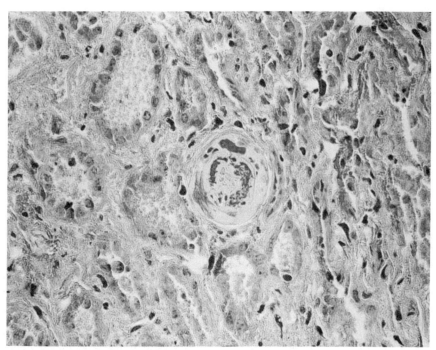

FIGURE 10–7. Postpartum renal failure. Intimal hyperplasia and organization of fibrin deposit in renal artery. (Courtesy of Dr. R. Luke.)

The reason that the hemolytic uremic syndrome seems to have a better prognosis in children is that in adults the medium-sized vessels of the kidney are more often involved. Unlike the case in children, extrarenal manifestations of vascular occlusions are uncommon in postpartum renal failure. Fibrinolytic therapy, administration of antiplatelet drugs, plasmaphoresis, and plasma infusion have all been advocated. No convincing evidence of a beneficial effect with these treatment modalities has been presented, however.

It is interesting to note other diseases with multisystem involvement, occurring either during or immediately after pregnancy, that might have intravascular clotting as a common basis. Acute fatty liver of pregnancy,[49, 82] postpartum myocardiopathy,[12] and postpartum necrosis of the anterior pituitary[112] all could be manifestations of small vessel thrombosis occurring either during or immediately after pregnancy.

Acute Renal Failure in Pregnancy

Because the major cause of acute renal failure during pregnancy was formerly septic abortion, the incidence has decreased since the liberalization of abortion laws. In France the percentage of cases of acute renal failure during pregnancy has fallen from 40 per cent of all patients with acute renal failure in 1966 to 4.5 per cent of patients with acute renal failure in 1978.[45] Although the mortality rate from acute renal failure in pregnancy is lower than in the nonpregnant state, probably because of the younger age of pregnant patients, acute renal failure in pregnancy bears a greater risk of development of renal cortical necrosis and consequent chronic renal failure. Among 38 cases of bilateral renal cortical necrosis, 26 (68 per cent) were of obstetric origin, and the incidence in pregnant women who develop acute renal failure ranges from 27 to 33 per cent. A 21 per cent incidence of bilateral renal cortical necrosis following postpartum renal failure has been reported.[63] The incidence seems higher with abruptio placentae or intrauterine death and prolonged retention of the fetus. In contrast, only 2 per cent of pregnant women dying of toxemia were found to have cortical necrosis at post mortem.[72] Although toxemia is often stated to be a setting in which bilateral renal cortical necrosis occurs, cortical necrosis is less apt to happen in that condition than with other obstetric complications. Bilateral cortical necrosis should be suspected in any pregnant woman with acute renal failure, particularly when it develops before the 30th week of gestation and when the oliguric or anuric phase is longer than 10 days. Even with cortical necrosis, renal function may improve slowly with time and has been documented to improve for up to 3 years after the onset of the disease.[63]

In addition to the decrease in number of criminal abortions, improvement in the management of obstetric complications has also contributed to the lowered incidence of acute renal failure. In a series of 154 women with eclampsia, only 1 developed acute renal failure.[89] In 57 cases of acute renal failure during pregnancy from the Hopital Necker in Paris, 13 were associated with abruptio placentae, 12 with severe toxemia, 6 with acute pyelonephritis, and the remainder with miscellaneous conditions occurring during pregnancy.[45] Acute renal failure is more apt to occur in pregnant women who are hypertensive or have signs of pre-eclampsia. In one series, as many as 62 per cent of patients developing acute renal failure had toxemia; in another, 33 per cent had toxemia.[45, 60] However, the likelihood of the development of acute renal failure with toxemia is low. In the largest series of women dying following eclampsia, only 3 of 33 had pathologic evidence of acute tubular necrosis.[72] When acute renal failure develops in toxemia, it does so more often in older multiparous women in whom underlying nephrosclerosis is more apt to be present.

The incidence of acute renal failure with acute fatty liver of pregnancy is high. Although maternal mortality (as high as 75 per cent in most series) is usually the result of hepatic rather than of renal failure, tubular necrosis with glomerular thrombi has been found at autopsy.[56] In one series segmental occlusions of the capillary lumen by fibrin material were present in 50 per cent of the glomeruli.[82] This suggests that acute fatty liver is associated with a hemolytic syndrome in which both the liver and the kidneys have fibrin deposits. Jaundice is present in approximately 33 per cent of pregnant women developing acute renal failure.

Hemodialysis During Pregnancy

There have now been several reports of patients with chronic renal failure who become pregnant and require hemodialysis during the pregnancy, in some instances because of either acute renal failure or drug overdose. Fifteen pregnant women with chronic renal disease requiring dialysis have been reported; the babies of two were normal and those of two were born dead. The remaining infants were premature, weighing under 2000 grams;[39] most of them did well despite the low birth weight.

Hypotension and vaginal bleeding, but no other complications, have been reported to occur during hemodialysis in the pregnant woman. Because of low peripheral vascular resistance in pregnancy, ultrafiltration with dialysis needs to be carefully monitored to prevent hypotension. Because pregnant women are prone to develop hypoglycemia, particularly when fasting, glucose-containing dialysates have been recommended. Low dose heparin, with maintenance of the activated clotting time at less than 2 minutes, should be administered. One group noted the removal of progesterone by hemodialysis and questioned whether premature contractions or labor might be caused by depletion of progesterone.[55] This report suggested parenteral progesterone administration during hemodialysis in the pregnant patient.

With the chronic respiratory alkalosis of pregnancy, the use of a bicarbonate rather than an acetate-containing bath is probably preferable. Bicarbonate may fall substantially in early hemodialysis with the use of an acetate bath because of the movement of bicarbonate into the dialysate.

Renal Tuberculosis

In the three published series of pregnant women with a history of renal tuberculosis there was no increased risk of toxemia or perinatal mortality, provided that renal function and blood pressure were normal.[74, 83, 103] If azotemia is present, pregnancy is contraindicated, and any worsening of renal tuberculosis during pregnancy in spite of antituberculosis therapy is indication for termination of the pregnancy. Hypertension, if present, should be treated with antihypertensive drugs throughout the pregnancy.

Polycystic Kidney Disease

Because the average age for the onset of symptoms and signs of polycystic renal disease is 41, women with undiagnosed or asymptomatic polycystic kidney disease are usually past childbearing age when clinical manifestations of the disease appear. In large retrospective studies, no risk of pregnancy was demonstrable in women with polycystic kidney disease without hypertension or azotemia.[22, 67] As with other renal diseases, when hypertension or azotemia precedes the pregnancy, the incidence of pre-eclampsia and perinatal mortality is increased. In one series of 11 pregnant patients with polycystic kidney disease there were 20 deliveries with 3 fetal deaths.[67] The deaths occurred in women with either hypertension or azotemia.

Since polycystic kidney disease is transmitted as an autosomal dominant trait with high penetrance, the incidence of the disease in large families is 50 per cent. Thus, couples may wish to limit family size or adopt children when they are aware of the presence of the disease. Approximately 20 per cent of patients with polycystic kidney disease have intracranial aneurysms, which may pose a problem during pregnancy and delivery.

Diabetic Nephropathy

Some degree of renal disease is probably present in all diabetic patients of childbearing age if the diabetes appeared before the age of 10. Fanconi et al. reported that of 87 juvenile diabetics, all had nephropathy within 16 years of the onset of the disease,[36] whereas Dolger found hypertension, proteinuria, and retinopathy in 50 per cent of juvenile diabetics within 13 years of onset.[29] Although renal failure is rarely the cause of death when diabetes appears in adulthood, it is the most common cause when diabetes appears in early childhood. Glomerulosclerosis, both diffuse and nodular, is the characteristic feature of diabetic nephropathy, but vascular disease of both the large and the small arteries of the kidney is prominent. The renal vascular changes include atheromatous changes in large arteries, hyalinization of the intima and media of arterioles, and thickening of the basement membrane with proliferation of mesangial material and cells in glomeruli. Vascular disease of the kidneys can cause severe scarring of the renal interstitium and changes that are indistinguishable from those of chronic pyelonephritis. Although hypertension is usually associated with diabetic nephropathy, vascular changes can occur in diabetics without hypertension. The increased incidence of hypertension in the diabetic population is, in all likelihood, due to renal vascular changes.

Nodular glomerulosclerosis was described by Kimmelstiel and Wilson as the specific renal lesion of diabetes.[61] Although the nodular lesion is virtually pathognomonic of the disease, the clinical features of diabetic nephropathy — heavy proteinuria, azotemia, and hypertension — are due to diffuse involvement of the glomeruli. Diffuse glomerulosclerosis consists of thickening of the intercapillary regions of the glomeruli, the mesangium, with basement membrane–like material.[21] This basement membrane-like matrix can become compacted into homogeneous masses characteristic of the Kimmelstiel-Wilson nodule. Glomerulosclerosis is part of a wide-spread angiopathy that involves small vessels throughout the body. In addition to basement membrane thickening, there is a tendency of the retinal vessels to develop aneurysms, which frequently become filled with hyaline material. Since retinal and renal angiopathy usually coincide, significant proteinuria from diabetic nephropathy is almost invariably associated with capillary aneurysms, exudates, and retinal arteriolosclerosis. The absence of diabetic retinopathy in a diabetic patient with the nephrotic syndrome indicates that glomerulosclerosis is quite unlikely to be the cause.

It is not clear whether acute pyelonephritis is more frequent in diabetic patients. One worker found the incidence of bacteriuria to be significantly higher in diabetic women,[122] but another group reported no significant difference between diabetic and nondiabetic patients of either sex in the incidence of bacteriuria.[86] Studies from the Joslin Clinic revealed a 15 per cent incidence of bacteriuria in 65 pregnant juvenile diabetics, and an incidence of 18 per cent was found in nonpregnant diabetics at the Boston City Hospital.[79] Since 30 per cent of untreated pregnant women with bacteriuria develop acute pyelonephritis during pregnancy, the potential danger of gram-negative infection is present in approximately 6 per cent of pregnant diabetics. Physicians caring for diabetics should eradicate bacteriuria because diabetic ketoacidosis can be readily precipitated by acute pyelonephritis, particularly during pregnancy. If eradication is not possible, continuous urinary antisepsis is warranted.

The course of diabetic nephropathy during pregnancy is similar to that of other renal diseases. There is no evidence that the renal disease is worsened. Although therapeutic abortion has been advocated when diabetic nephropathy precedes pregnancy, studies at the Joslin Clinic[132] and by Sims[113] have demonstrated that diabetics can have normal pregnancies with good chance for fetal survival. The experience at the Joslin Clinic is particularly helpful, because 24 hour urine collections for creatinine clearance were obtained from 209 diabetic pregnant women. Using the six categories (A through F) of diabetes, based on the severity of the disease, in 6 women with only a positive glucose tolerance test (class A) the mean GFR was 109 + 32 ml per minute per 1.73 square meters of body surface area during pregnancy. These women had uneventful pregnancies with viable infants. In class B (onset of diabetes after age 20, present for 0 to

9 years without evidence of vascular disease) there were 35 patients with a mean GFR of 92 + 33 ml per minute per 1.73 square meters. Five patients had spontaneous abortions, but 26 live babies were delivered, resulting in a fetal survival rate of 87 per cent. In class C (onset of diabetes between ages 10 and 19 years, present for 10 to 19 years, and no evidence of vascular disease) 36 women had a mean GFR of 97 + 29 ml per minute per 1.73 square meters. Four had spontaneous abortions, but 30 were delivered of live babies, resulting in a fetal survival rate of 94 per cent. In class D (onset of diabetes from age 10, present longer than 20 years, and evidence of vascular disease with retinopathy) there were 73 women with a mean GFR of 89 + 32 ml per minute per 1.73 square meters. Eight had spontaneous abortions, and 52 of the remaining 65 patients had live babies — a fetal survival rate of 71 per cent. In class F (evidence of renal disease with proteinuria greater than 100 mg per 100 ml or a BUN over 20 mg per 100 ml at the start of pregnancy) there were 14 patients with a mean GFR of 57 + 20 ml per minute per 1.73 square meters. There were 4 spontaneous abortions and 1 therapeutic abortion in this group, but 6 of the 9 remaining women had living babies. Serial measurements of GFR were performed in class F patients throughout pregnancy, and there was no significant change during pregnancy, although the GFR increased significantly post partum.

The study by Sims included 8 pregnant patients with diabetes of 8 to 23 years' duration (average, 14 years); 4 had retinopathy, 3 had biopsy-proved intercapillary glomerulosclerosis, and 5 had absent patellar reflexes. GFR (measured by inulin clearance) and renal plasma flow (measured by PAH clearance) increased in all with pregnancy.[113] The increase in GFR and renal plasma flow was indistinguishable from that in the pregnant control group, although there seemed to be a reduction in filtration fraction in diabetics compared with that in normal pregnant women. Even in patients with biopsy-proved glomerulosclerosis, GFR and renal plasma flow rose during pregnancy.

It is possible that the Joslin Clinic patients had lower initial GFR and did not demonstrate a rise in GFR during pregnancy because they were given maintenance doses of 25 to 100 mg hydrochlorothiazide throughout pregnancy.

In another series there were 40 pregnant women in class D and 2 in class F.[64] The infant survival for these women was 55 per cent, and 16 per cent of the women developed toxemia. There were no maternal deaths and no evidence that renal disease worsened during pregnancy. Although the chance for a successful pregnancy diminishes with the extent of diabetic complications, renal involvement per se does not appear to be the factor deciding the outcome of the pregnancy.

It was of interest that BUN was significantly higher in diabetic patients than in control subjects with similar GFR. Although catabolism of protein by the diabetic might be a factor in causing this effect, the higher BUN could also be related to the greater reduction in GFR and renal blood flow that occurs in the diabetic patient during standing. This inordinate decrease in renal blood flow in the diabetic has been attributed to impaired vasomotor reflexes because of autonomic neuropathy. Such a defect might induce inordinate ADH release with standing, which, by concentrating the urine, disproportionately reduces urea clearance.

Renal Calculi

Although ureteral and renal pelvis dilation predisposes to stasis and infection, renal calculi are relatively rare during pregnancy. The incidence of approximately 1 in 1150 pregnant women is about the same as in nonpregnant women.[19, 41] Although uncommon, calculi represent the most common cause of pain requiring hospitalization for diagnosis and treatment during pregnancy. Of the 93 women in one series, 63 required surgical intervention during pregnancy, and in 5 a therapeutic abortion was deemed necessary.[41] In another series, 10 of 19 pregnant women with symptoms of renal calculi spontaneously passed the stones. In an analysis of 78 women with nephrolithiases, no adverse effects occurred during pregnancy other than an increase in urinary tract infections.[19] Pregnancy did not alter the activity or severity of renal calculi. Idiopathic hypercalciuria accounted for 42 per cent of these cases of calculi; idiopathic lithiasis was the diagnosis in 20 per cent. Although intestinal absorption of calcium increases greatly during pregnancy, urinary calcium rarely exceeds 250 mg daily.[51]

Treatment for renal calculi during pregnancy is similar to that of the nonpregnant patient. There is no need to perform surgical exploration for a stone unless it is causing acute obstruction of a ureter. Even in such cases, unless infection is present, transient obstruction of urine flow will not permanently impair renal function. In one series of 20 stone episodes during pregnancy, none required surgical intervention.[19] Dilation of the ureters during pregnancy may allow passage of the stone. In all patients with renal stones, the cause should be investigated. Serum calcium and phosphorus should be evaluated to exclude hyperparathyroidism, and a serum urate determination is indicated.

Recurrent urinary tract infection with a urease-containing organism causes alkalinization of the urine, predisposing to precipitation of calcium phosphate. This type of infection is a common cause of staghorn calculi. The treatment consists of long-term urinary antisepsis and forced diuresis to maintain hypotonicity of the urine. Surgery for staghorn calculi is rarely indicated, and nephrectomy should not be performed unless recurrent sepsis with pyelonephritis is present. If urinary tract infection is the cause of a staghorn calculus, recurrent stone formation is likely, and renal insufficiency from chronic pyelonephritis may occur. Thus, preservation of renal mass is essential in prolonging life or avoiding dialysis.

The milk-alkali syndrome as a cause of nephrocalcinosis can be diagnosed by taking a careful history with regard to ingestion of extraordinary amounts of milk and absorbable alkali, such as sodium bicarbonate and other antacids, to control symptoms of peptic ulcer. Renal tubular acidosis of the distal type and medullary sponge kidney may present with nephrocalcinosis and stones. Such patients have had uneventful pregnancies.

Cystinuria is a rare cause of renal stones, often staghorn calculi, and it can now be treated with D-penicillamine. One woman had a successful pregnancy during penicillamine therapy for control of cystinuria, and the stone dissolved during the pregnancy as a result of therapy.[20]

The diagnosis of a renal stone is sometimes difficult during pregnancy, and less than 50 per cent of the patients in one series had microscopic hematuria.[48] It seems reasonable to perform an intravenous pyelogram in all pregnant women with (1) a history suggestive of a renal stone, (2) acute symptoms of infection and a previous history of a renal calculus, or (3) recurrent urinary tract infection during pregnancy. The danger to the fetus from radiation is minimal if shielding and image-intensification procedures are followed.

COUNSELING THE PREGNANT PATIENT WITH RENAL DISEASE

The decision concerning pregnancy is extremely difficult for the women with renal disease and for her family. This is particularly true at present, since the prognosis of chronic renal disease is quite changed because of the availability of hemodialysis and transplantation. Many women with chronic renal disease may wish to attempt to have children prior to transplantation with the consequent risks of immunosuppressive therapy on fetal development. Thus, in counseling women and their families it is imperative for the physician to keep in mind that the decision must be made by the patient and her family after complete and thorough presentation of the best medical opinion. The physician must be willing to accept the patient's decision to bear some risk in an attempt to have a successful pregnancy, as well as accept her wish if she desires termination of a pregnancy. The woman with renal disease who wishes to become pregnant places a great deal of responsibility upon the physician, and this frequently affects the medical opinion. However, with the availability of antihypertensive agents and diuretics, the dangers of pregnancy to the mother should be minimal if the physician has confidence in the treatment of hypertension and renal disease. It must be emphasized to the patient, however, that fetal mortality is increased. If the patient accepts the need for frequent neonatal visits and the potential risk of taking antihypertensive medication throughout pregnancy, there is no reason not to allow a woman to become pregnant. It is fortunate that renal disease with hypertension and azotemia impairs fertility, since it is in this group that the potential problems of pregnancy are greater.

The patient must be willing to accept the need for continued close observation during pregnancy, at least every 3 weeks before the 28th week and weekly thereafter. Thus, the pregnancy becomes the mutual responsibility of both physician and patient.

References

1. Alexander, E. A., Churchill, S., and Bengele, H. H.: Renal hemodynamics and volume homestasis during pregnancy in the rat. Kidney Int., *18*:173, 1980.
2. Andriole, V. T., and Cohn, G. L.: The effect of diethylstilbestrol on the susceptibility of rats to hematogenous pyelonephritis. J. Clin. Invest., *43*:1136, 1964.
3. Assali, N. S., Dignam, W. J., and Dasgupta, K.: Renal function in human pregnancy: Effects of venous pooling on renal hemo-

dynamics and water, electrolyte, and aldosterone excretion during normal gestation. J. Lab. Clin. Med., *54*:394, 1959.

4. Assali, N. S., Herzig, D., and Singh, B. P.: Renal responses to ammonium chloride acidosis in normal and toxemic pregnancies. J. Appl. Physiol., *7*:367, 1955.

5. Ayoub, E. M., and Vernier, R. L.: Benign recurrent hematuria. Am. J. Dis. Child., *109*:217, 1965.

6. Bay, W. H., and Ferris, T. F.: Factors controlling plasma renin and aldosterone during pregnancy. Hypertension, *1*:410, 1979.

7. Bear, R.: Pregnancy and lupus nephritis: A detailed report of six cases with a review of the literature. Obstet. Gynecol., *47*:715, 1976.

8. Bishop, J. H. V., and Green, R.: Effects of pregnancy on glucose handling by distal segments of the rat nephron. J. Physiol., *289*:98P, 1978.

9. Blanford, A. T., and Murphy, B. E.: In vitro metabolism of prednisone, dexamethasone, betamethasone, and cortisol by the human placenta. Am. J. Obstet. Gynecol., *127*:264, 1977.

10. Boedlaert, J., Morel-Maroger, L., Mery, J. P.: Renal insufficiency in lupus nephritis. Adv. Nephrol., *4*:249, 1974.

11. Braverman, D. Z., Johnson, J. G., and Kern, F.: Effects of pregnancy and contraceptive steroids on gallbladder function. N. Engl. J. Med., *302*:362, 1980.

12. Burch, G. E., Giles, T. D., and Tsui, C. Y.: Postpartal cardiomyopathy, Cardiovasc. Clin., *4*:270, 1972.

13. Carreras, L. O., Defreyn, G., VanHoutte E., Verhylen, J., and VanAssche, A.: Pratacyclin and pre-eclampsia, Lancet *1*:442–1981.

14. Chesley, L. C.: Hypertension in pregnancy: Definitions, familial factor, and remote prognosis.

15. Chesley, L. C., and Sloan, D. M.: The effect of posture on renal function in late pregnancy. Am. J. Obstet. Gynecol., *89*:754, 1964.

16. Christensen, P. J.: Tubular reabsorption of glucose during pregnancy. Scand. J. Clin. Lab. Invest., *10*:364, 1958.

17. Christensen, P. J., Date, J. W., Schonheyder, F., and Volqvartz, K.: Amino acids in blood plasma and urine during pregnancy. Scand. J. Clin. Lab. Invest., *9*:43, 1957.

18. Chugh, K. S., Singhal, P. C., Sharma, B. K., Pal, Y., Mathew, M. T., Dhall, K., and Datta, B. N.: Acute renal failure of obstetric origin. Obstet. Gynecol., *48*:642, 1976.

19. Coe, F. L., Parks, J. H., and Lindheimer, M. D.: Nephrolithiasis during pregnancy. N. Engl. J. Med., *302*:362, 1980.

20. Crawhall, J. C., and Thompson, C. J.: Cystinuria: Effect of D-penicillamine on plasma and urinary cystine concentration. Science, *147*:1459, 1965.

21. Dach, S., Churg, J., Mautner, W., and Grishman, E.: Diabetic nephropathy. Am. J. Pathol., *44*:155, 1964.

22. Dalgaard, O. Z.: Polycystic disease of the kidneys. In Strauss, M. B., and Walt, L. G. (eds.): Diseases of the Kidney, 2nd ed. Boston, Little, Brown & Co., 1971, p. 1223.

23. Davidson, J. M.: Changes in renal function and other aspects of homeostasis in early pregnancy. J. Obstet. Gynaecol. Br. Commonw., *81*:1003, 1974.

24. Davison, J. M., and Dunlop, W.: Renal hemodynamics and tubular function in normal human pregnancy. Kidney Int., *18*:152, 1980.

25. Davison, J. M., and Hytten, F. E.: Renal handling of glucose in pregnancy. In Sutherland, H. W., and Stowers, J. M. (eds.): Proceedings, Symposium on Carbohydrate Metabolism in Pregnancy and the Newborn. London, Churchill Livingstone, 1974, p. 2.

26. Davison, J. M., and Hytten, F. E.: The effect of pregnancy on the renal handling of glucose. Br. J. Obstet. Gynaecol., *82*:374, 1975.

27. DeAlvarez, R. R.: Renal glomerulotubular mechanisms during normal pregnancy: I. Glomerular filtration rate, renal plasma flow and creatinine clearance. Am. J. Obstet. Gynecol., *75*:931, 1958.

28. Dirks, J. H., Clapp, R. R., and Berliner, R. W.: The protein concentration in the proximal tubule of the dog. J. Clin. Invest., *43*:916, 1964.

29. Dolger, H.: Clinical evaluation of vascular damage in diabetes mellitus. J.A.M.A., *134*:1289, 1947.

30. Donaldson, L. B., and DeAlvarez, R. R.: Further observation on lupus erythematosus associated with pregnancy. Am. J. Obstet. Gynecol., *83*:1461, 1962.

31. Dunlop, L.: Investigations into the influence of posture on renal plasma flow and glomerular filtration rate during late pregnancy. Br. J. Obstet. Gynaecol., *83*:17, 1976.

32. Dunlop, L.: Renal physiology in pregnancy. Postgrad. Med. J., *55*:329, 1979.

33. Durr, J. A., Stamoutsos, B. A., and Lindheimer, M. D.: Plasma osmolality in pregnant rats in the absence of vasopressin. J. Clin. Invest. (In press.)

34. Fadel, H. E., Northrop, G., and Misenhimer, H. R.: Hyperuricemia in pre-eclampsia. A reappraisal. Am. J. Obstet. Gynecol., *125*:640, 1976.

35. Fainstat, T.: Ureteral dilation in pregnancy: A review. Obstet. Gynecol. Surv., *18*:845, 1963.

36. Fanconi, G., Botstny, A., and Kousmine, C.: Hephropathic bein kindlichen diabetes mellitus. Helv. Paediatr. Acta, *3*:341, 1948.

37. Ferris, T. F., and Gorden, P.: Effect of angiotensin and norepinephrine upon urate clearances in man. Am. J. Med., *44*:359, 1968.

38. Ferris, T. F., Gorden, P., Kashgarian, M., and Epstein, F. H.: Recurrent hematuria and focal nephritis. N. Engl. J. Med., *276*:770, 1967.

39. Fine, L. G., Barnett, E. V., Danovitch, G. M., Nissenson, A. R., Connolly, M. E., Lieb, S. M., and Barrett, C. T.: Systemic lupus erythematosus in pregnancy. Ann. Intern. Med., *94*:667, 1981.

40. Fitzsimons, J. T.: The physiological basis of thirst. Kidney Int., *10*:3, 1976.

41. Folger, G. K.: Abdominal pain and pregnancy with particular reference to urinary calculi. Obstet. Gynecol., *5*:513, 1955.

42. Gant, N. F., Worley, R. J., Everett, R. B., and MacDonald, P. C.: Control of vascular responsiveness during human pregnancy. Kidney Int., *18*:253, 1980.

43. Garsenstein, M., Pollak, V. E., and Kark, R. M.: Systemic lupus erythematosus and pregnancy. N. Engl. J. Med., *267*:165, 1962.

44. Goldfinger, S., Klinenberg, J. R., and Seegmiller, J. E.: Renal retention of uric acid induced by infusion of betahydroxybutyrate and acetoacetate. N. Engl. J. Med., *272*:351, 1965.

45. Grunfeld, J. P., Ganaval, D., and Bournerias, F.: Acute renal failure in pregnancy. Kidney Int., *18*:179, 1980.

46. Guyer, P. B., and Delany, D.: Urinary tract dilation and oral contraceptives. Br. Med. J., *4*:488, 1970.

47. Handler, J. S.: The role of lactic acid in the reduced excretion of uric acid in toxemia of pregnancy. J. Clin. Invest., *39*:1526, 1960.

48. Harris, R. E., and Dunnihoo, D. R.: The incidence and significance of urinary calculi during pregnancy. Am. J. Obstet. Gynecol., *99*:237, 1967.

49. Hatfield, A. K., Stein, J. H., Greenberger, N. J., Abernathy, R. W., and Ferris, T. F.: Idiopathic acute fatty liver of pregnancy. Am. J. Dig. Dis., *17*:167, 1972.

50. Hayslett, J. P., and Lynn, R. I.: Effect of pregnancy in patients with lupus nephropathy. Kidney Int., *18*:207, 1980.

51. Heany, R. P., and Skillman, T. G.: Calcium metabolism in normal human pregnancy. J. Clin. Endocrinol. Metab., *33*:661, 1971.

52. Holzbach, R. T.: Jaundice in pregnancy. Am. J. Med., *61*:367, 1976.

53. Hughes, J.: Acute glomerulonephritis during pregnancy. Br. J. Clin. Pract., *19*:583, 1965.

54. Hytten, F. E., and Cheyne, G. A.: The aminoaciduria of pregnancy. J. Obstet. Gynaecol. Br. Commonw., *79*:424, 1972.

55. Johnson, T. R., Jr., Lorenz, R. P., Menon, K. M. J., and Nolan, G. H.: Successful outcome of a pregnancy requiring dialysis: Effects on serum progesterone and estrogens. J. Reprod. Med., *22*:217, 1979.

56. Kahil, M. E., Fred, H. L., Brown, H., and Davis, J. S.: Acute fatty liver of pregnancy. Arch. Intern. Med., *113*:63, 1964.

57. Kaitz, A. L.: Urinary concentrating ability in pregnant women with asymptomatic bacteriuria. J. Clin. Invest., *49*:1331, 1961.

58. Kaplan, A. L., Smith, J. P., and Tillman, A. J. B.: Healed acute and chronic nephritis in pregnancy. Am. J. Obstet. Gynecol., *83*:1519, 1962.

59. Katz, A. I., Davison, J. M., Hayslett, J. P., Singson, E., and Lindheimer, M. D.: Pregnancy in women with kidney disease. Kidney Int., *18*:192, 1980.

60. Kennedy, A. C., Burton, J. A., Luke, R. G., Briggs, J. D., Lindsay, R. M., Allison, M. E. M., Edward, N., and Dargie, H. J.: Factors affecting the prognosis in acute renal failure. Q. J. Med., *42*:73, 1973.

61. Kimmelstiel, P., and Wilson, C.: Intercapillary lesions in the glomeruli of the kidney. Am. J. Pathol., *12*:83, 1936.

62. Kincaid-Smith, P., and Fairley, K. F.: Kidney disease and pregnancy. Med. J. Aust., *2*:1155, 1967.

63. Kleinknecht, D., Grunfeld, J. P., Cia Gomez, P., Moreau, J. F., and Garcia-Torres, R.: Diagnostic procedures and long-term prognosis in bilateral renal cortical necrosis. Kidney Int., *4*:390, 1973.

64. Knowles, H. C., Guest, G. M., Lampe, J., Kessler, M., and Skillman, T. G.: The course of juvenile diabetes treated with unmeasured diet. Diabetes, *14*:239, 1965.

65. Labovitz, E. D., Steinmuller, S. R., Henderson, L. W., McCurdy, D. K., and Goldberg, J.: "Benign" hematuria with focal glomerulitis in adults. Ann. Intern. Med., *77*:723, 1972.

66. Lancet, J., and Fisher, I. L.: The value of blood uric acid levels in toxemia of pregnancy. J. Obstet. Gynaecol. Br. Emp., *63*:115, 1956.

67. Landesman, R., and Scheer, L.: Congenital polycystic kidney disease in pregnancy. Obstet. Gynecol., *8*:673, 1956.

68. Levy, N. B.: Sexual adjustment to maintenance hemodialysis and renal transplantation: National survey by questionnaire, preliminary report. Trans. Am. Soc. Artif. Intern. Organs, *19*:138, 1973.

69. Lewis, P. J., Boylan, P., Friedman, L. A., Nensby, C. N., and Dowing, I.: Prostacyclin in pregnancy. Br. Med. J., *280*:1581, 1980.

70. Lim, V. S., Katz, A. I., and Lindheimer, M. D.: Acid-base metabolism in pregnancy. Am. J. Physiol., *231*:1764, 1976.

71. Lindheimer, M. D., and Weston, P. V.: Effect of hypotonic expansion on sodium, water, and urea excretion in late pregnancy: The influence of posture on these results. J. Clin. Invest., *48*:947, 1969.

72. Lopez-Llera, M., and Linares, G. R.: Factors that influence maternal mortality in eclampsia. *In* Lindheimer, M. D., Katz, A. I., Zuspan, F. P. (eds.): Hypertension in pregnancy. New York, John Wiley and Sons, 1975, p. 41.

73. Luke, R. G., Siegel, R. R., Talbert, W., and Holland, H.: Heparin treatment for postpartum renal failure with microangiopathic hemolytic anemia. Lancet, *2*:750, 1970.

74. Lyons, H. A., and Antonio, R.: The sensitivity of the respiratory center in pregnancy and after the administration of progesterone. Trans. Assoc. Am. Physicians, *72*:173, 1959.

75. MacDonald, H. N., and Good, W.: The effect of parity on plasma sodium, potassium, chloride and osmolality levels during pregnancy. J. Obstet. Gynaecol. Br. Commonw., *79*:441, 1972.

76. Mackay, E. V.: Pregnancy and renal disease. Aust. N.Z.J. Obstet. Gynaecol., *3*:21, 1963.

77. Macquet, P., and Patoir, G.: Tuberculose urinaive et grossesse. J. Urol. Med. Chiv., *62*:690, 1956.

78. Marcus, S. L.: The nephrotic syndrome during pregnancy. Obstet. Gynecol. Surv., 18:511, 1963.

79. McCartney, C. P.: Renal morphology and function among patients with pre-eclampsia and gravidas with essential hypertension. Clin. Obstet. Gynecol., *11*:596, 1968.

80. Morrin, P. A. F., Handa, S. P., Valberg, L. S., Bencosme, S. A., Kipkie, G. F., and Wyllie, J. C.: Acute renal failure in association with fatty liver in pregnancy: Recovery after fourteen days of complete anuria. Am. J. Med., *42*:844, 1967.

81. Nadler, N., Salinas-Madrigal, L., Charles, A. G., and Pollak, V. E.: Acute glomerulonephritis during late pregnancy. Obstet. Gynecol., *34*:277, 1969.

82. Nash, D. T., and Tomaszewicz, T.: Acute yellow atrophy of liver in pregnancy. N.Y. State J. Med., *71*:458, 1971.

83. Nersisian, R. K.: The course of pregnancy in patients with renal tuberculosis. Akush. Ginekol., *41*:31, 1965.

84. Nolten, W. E., and Ehrlich, E. N.: Sodium and mineralocorticoids in normal pregnancy. Kidney Int., *18*:162, 1980.

85. Norden, C. W., and Kass, E. H.: Bacteriuria of pregnancy: A critical appraisal. Ann. Rev. Med., *19*:431, 1968.

86. O'Sullivan, D. J., Fitzgerald, M. G., Mynell, J. J., and Malins, J. M.: Urinary tract infections: A comparative study in the diabetic and general populations. Br. Med. J., *5228*:786, 1961.

87. Penn, I., Makowski, E. L., and Harris, P.: Parenthood following renal transplantation. Kidney Int., *18*:221, 1980.

88. Price, H. B., Salaman, J. R., Laurence, K. M., and Langmaid, H.: Immunosuppressive drugs and the foetus. Transplantation, *21*:294, 1976.

89. Pritchard, J. A.: Management of pre-eclampsia and eclampsia. Kidney Int., *18*:259, 1980.

90. Pritchard, J. A., Barnes, A. C., and Bright, R. H.: The effect of the supine position on renal function in the near-term pregnant woman. J. Clin. Invest., *34*:777, 1955.

91. Pritchard, J. A., and Pritchard, S. A.: Standardized treatment of 154 cases of eclampsia. Am. J. Obstet. Gynecol., *123*:543, 1975.

92. Rauramo, L., Kasanen, A., Elfving, K., and Salmi, H.: Fertility, pregnancy and labour in women with a history of nephritis or pyelonephritis. Acta. Obstet. Gynecol. Scand., *41*:357, 1963.

93. Redman, C. W. G.: Treatment of hypertension in pregnancy. Kidney Int., *18*:267, 1980.

94. Redman, C. W. G., Beilin, L. J., Bonnar, J., and Wilkinson, R. H.: Plasma urate measurement in predicting fetal death in hypertensive pregnancy. Lancet, *1*:1370, 1976.

95. Remuzzi, G., Zoja, D., Marchesi, D., Schreppeti, A., Mecca, G., Misiani, R., Donati, M. G., and DeSaetons, G.: Plasmatic regulation of vascular prostacyclin in pregnancy. Br. Med. J., *282*:512, 1981.

96. Robertson, E. G.: Increased erythrocyte fragility in association with osmotic changes in pregnancy serum. J. Reprod. Fertil., *16*:323, 1968.

97. Robinson, R. R.: Idiopathic proteinuria. Ann. Intern. Med., *71*:1019, 1969.

98. Robson, J. S., Martin, A. M., and Burkley, V. A.: Irreversible postpartum renal failure: A new syndrome. Q. J. Med., *37*:423, 1968.

99. Rosenmann, E., Kanter, A., Bacani, R. A., Pirani, C. L., and Pollak, V. E.: Fatal late postpartum intravascular coagulation with acute renal failure. Am. J. Med. Sci., *257*:259, 1969.

100. Rosenmann, E., Pollak, V. E., and Pirani, D. L.: Renal vein thrombosis in the adult: A clinical and pathologic study based on renal biopsies. Medicine, *47*:269, 1968.

101. Rutecki, G. W., Cox, J. W., Robertson, G. W., Francisco, L. L., and Ferris, T. F.: Urinary consent rating ability and ADH responsiveness in the K-depleted dog. J. Lab. Clin. Med. (In press.)

102. Sala, N. L., and Rubi, R. A.: Ureteral function in pregnant women. V. Incidence of vesicoureteral reflux and its effect upon ureteral contractility. Am. J. Obstet. Gynecol., *112*:871, 1972.

103. Schaefer, G., Douglas, R. G., and Dreishpoon, I. H.: Extrapulmonary tuberculosis and pregnancy. Am. J. Obstet. Gynecol., *67*:605, 1954.

104. Scheer, R. L., and Jones, D. B.: Malignant nephrosclerosis in women postpartum. A note on micro-angiopathic hemolytic anemia. J.A.M.A., *299*:600, 1967.

105. Schewitz, L. J., Friedman, I. A., and Pollak, V. E.: Bleeding after renal biopsy in pregnancy. Obstet. Gynecol., *26*:295, 1965.

106. Schreiner, G. E.: Nephrotic syndrome. *In* Strauss, M. B., and Welt, L. G. (eds.): Diseases of the Kidney. Boston, Little, Brown & Co., 1971, p. 572.

107. Seftel, H. C., and Schewitz, L. J.: The nephrotic syndrome in pregnancy. J. Obstet. Gynaecol. Br. Emp., *64*:862, 1957.

108. Segonds, A., Louradour, N., Suc, J. M., and Orfila, C.: Postpartum hemolytic uremic syndrome: A study of three cases with a review of the literature. Clin. Nephrol., *12*:229, 1979.

109. Seitchek, J.: Observations on the renal tubular reabsorption of uric acid. I. Normal pregnancy and abnormal pregnancy with and without pre-eclampsia. Am. J. Obstet. Gynecol., *65*:981, 1953.

110. Sheehan, H. L.: Renal morphology in pre-eclampsia. Kidney Int., *18*:241, 1980.

111. Sheehan, J. L.: Neurological complications of pregnancy. Proc. R. Soc. Med., *32*:584, 1939.

112. Sims, E. A. H.: The kidney in pregnancy complicated by diabetes mellitus. Clin. Obstet. Gynecol., *5*:462, 1962.

113. Sims, E. A. H., and Krantz, K. E.: Serial studies of renal function during pregnancy and the puerperium in normal women. J. Clin. Invest., *37*:1764, 1958.

114. Smith, H.: Summary interpretation of observations of renal

hemodynamics in pre-eclampsia. *In* Fomon, S. J. (ed.): Report of First Ross Obstetric Research Conference. Ross Laboratories, Ohio, 1956, p. 75.

115. Smith, K., Browne, J. C. M., Shackman, R., and Wrong, O. M.: Acute renal failure of obstetric origin: An analysis of 70 patients. Lancet, *2*:351, 1965.

116. Steele, T. H., and Rieselbach, R. E.: Renal urate excretion in normal man. Nephron, *14*:21, 1975.

117. Studd, J. W. W., and Blainey, J. D.: Pregnancy and the nephrotic syndrome. Br. Med. J., *1*:276, 1969.

118. Stuart, J. J., Clark, D. A., Sundeji, S. G., Yambo, T., Allen, J. B., Elrod, H., and Slott, J. H.: Decreased prostacyclin production: A characteristic of chronic placental insufficiency syndromes. Lancet, *2*:1126, 1981.

119. Sun, N. C. J., Johnson, W. J., Sung, D. T. W., and Woods, J. E.: Idiopathic postpartum renal failure. Review and case report of a successful renal transplantation. Mayo Clin. Proc., *59*:395, 1975.

120. Thompson, A. L., Durrett, R. R., and Robinson, R. R.: Fixed and reproducible orthostatic proteinuria: Results of a 10 year follow-up evaluation. Ann. Intern. Med., *73*:235, 1970.

121. Toback, F. G., Hall, P. W., and Lindheimer, M. D.: Effect of posture on urinary protein patterns in nonpregnant, pregnant, and toxemic women. Obstet. Gynecol., *35*:765, 1970.

122. Vejlsgaard, R.: Bacteriuria in patients with diabetes mellitus. *In* Kass, E. H. (ed.): Progress in Pyelonephritis. Philadelphia, F. A. Davis, 1965, p. 478.

123. Wallraff, E. B., Brodie, E. C., and Borden, A. L.: Urinary excretion of amino acids in pregnancy. J. Clin. Invest., *29*:1542, 1950.

124. Wagoner, R. D., Holley, K. E., and Johnson, W. R.: Acceler-

ated nephrosclerosis and postpartum acute renal failure in normotensive patients. Ann. Intern. Med., *69*:237, 1968.

125. Walshe, J. J., and Venuto, R. C.: Acute oliguric renal failure induced by indomethacin: Possible Mechanisms. Ann. Intern. Med., *91*:47, 1979.

126. Warrell, W. W., and Taylor, R.: Outcome for the foetus of mothers receiving prednisolone during pregnancy. Lancet, *1*:117, 1968.

127. Welsh, G. W., Sims, E. A. H.: The mechanisms of renal glucosuria in pregnancy. Diabetes, *9*:363, 1960.

128. Weinman, E. J., Eknoyan, G., and Suki, W. N.: The influence of extracellular fluid volume on the tubular reabsorption of uric acid. J. Clin. Invest., *55*:283, 1975.

129. Werko, L., and Bucht, H.: Glomerular filtration rate and renal blood flow in patients with chronic diffuse glomerulonephritis during pregnancy. Acta. Med. Scand., *153*:166, 1956.

130. Williams, G. G., et al.: Vesicoureteric reflux in patients with bacteriuria in pregnancy. Lancet, *2*:1202, 1968.

131. Wilson, C.: *In* Morris, N., and Browne, J. D. M. (eds.): Nontoxemic hypertension in pregnancy. Boston, Little, Brown & Co., 1958.

132. Younger, D., Rees, S. B., and White, P.: Quoted by Sims, E. A.: The kidney in pregnancy complicated by diabetes mellitus. Clin. Obstet. Gynecol., *5*:469, 1962.

133. Zinneman, H. H., Seal, U. S., and Doe, R. P.: Urinary amino acids in pregnancy, following progesterone and estrogen. J. Clin. Endocrinol. Metab., *27*:397, 1967.

134. Zurier, R. B., Argyros, T. G., Urman, J. D., Warren, J., and Rothfield, N. F.: Systemic lupus erythematosus management during pregnancy. Obstet. Gynecol., *51*:178, 1978.

John W. Dobbins, M.D.
Howard M. Spiro, M.D.

11

GASTROINTESTINAL COMPLICATIONS

Pregnancy has many effects on the gastrointestinal tract, from altering lower esophageal sphincteric function to decreasing colonic motility, which can lead to clinical problems, such as reflux esophagitis, or set the stage for the development of future problems, such as gallstone formation. Moreover, pregnancy may make the diagnosis of gastrointestinal disorders more difficult. For example, nausea and vomiting is common in pregnant women but also occurs with many gastrointestinal disorders. Another example is acute appendicitis, which is the major nonobstetric cause for laparotomy in pregnancy.[11] Despite modern technology, the diagnosis of appendicitis is still made primarily by history and physical examination, i.e., chills, fever, nausea, vomiting, right lower quadrant pain and tenderness, and rebound tenderness. The enlarging uterus, however, shifts the appendix to the right upper quadrant and changes the classic signs; the tenderness and guarding of appendicitis seem less pronounced in the pregnant woman than in the nonpregnant one.[1] Nausea, vomiting, and right *upper* quadrant tenderness with little guarding could mean acute cholecystitis, acute pancreatitis, or even peptic ulcer disease, conditions that the physician would prefer to treat medically if possible. Appendicitis, however, still demands operation as soon as possible, because delay may lead to rupture and greatly increase the risk to the fetus.[11] The reader can readily appreciate the dilemma produced by the uterus shifting the usual landmarks. When in doubt, the surgeon must operate, as the risk of a negative laparotomy for the fetus is slight,[18] whereas the danger from pus in the peritoneum is great. The surgeon must "look and see, not wait and see."[1]

Fortunately for patient and physician, the usual gastrointestinal complications of pregnancy rarely require operation. To manage these complications successfully when they do arise,

however, the physician must be aware of the physiologic, anatomic, and clinical alterations induced by pregnancy.

NAUSEA AND VOMITING OF PREGNANCY

Nausea and vomiting in the first 14 to 16 weeks of pregnancy is common, affecting 50 to 60 per cent of pregnant women. It is usually mild, consisting of no more than morning nausea and occasional vomiting, and is not accompanied by any evidence of disturbed nutrition. Although its cause is unknown, the most commonly held theory relates it to the levels of gonadotropic hormones.[24]

Hyperemesis gravidarum, or pernicious vomiting of pregnancy, is severe, persistent vomiting in early pregnancy resulting in fluid and electrolyte disturbances and nutritional deficiency. Fortunately, it is relatively rare, with an average incidence of 3.5 per 1000 deliveries. Hyperemesis rarely persists into the second half of pregnancy and does not result in toxemia, spontaneous abortion, or an abnormal infant.[5] The cause of hyperemesis is unknown, but psychologic theories abound.[5, 24]

Nausea and vomiting of pregnancy must, of course, be distinguished from nausea and vomiting from a more important cause. Therefore, a careful history and physical examination as well as appropriate laboratory tests are in order for every patient with vomiting that is (1) severe or protracted; (2) in the latter half of pregnancy; or (3) associated with weight loss, abdominal pain, fever, or specific localizing symptoms — dysuria, epigastric pain, or the like. Only when no disease process can be found should severe vomiting be ascribed to pregnancy or hyperemesis gravidarum.

Mild nausea and vomiting of early pregnancy

259

can be treated optimistically with assurance that the symptoms are temporary. Small feedings, avoidance of symptom-provoking foods, and the occasional use of such antiemetics as meclizine or prochlorperazine, which have no apparent teratogenic potential, are helpful. Hyperemesis gravidarum, which must be treated with hospitalization, intravenous fluid and electrolyte replacement, and psychotherapy, is beyond the scope of this discussion.

REFLUX ESOPHAGITIS

Reflux esophagitis may be defined as inflammation of the distal esophagus, usually from reflux of acid gastric juice. Its typical symptom is heartburn, a burning or hot sensation located substernally with occasional radiation to the back of the throat. Heartburn typically occurs postprandially, but also on lying down, bending over, or lifting heavy objects. Orange juice faithfully produces heartburn in many susceptible persons, and sometimes aspirin or alcohol does the same. Heartburn is typically relieved by antacids, though frequently only temporarily. It may be accompanied by "water-brash," the regurgitation of gastric contents into the mouth. Esophageal stricture may result from prolonged reflux esophagitis or even the vomiting of pregnancy; remotely, other more serious complications ensue.

Status in Pregnancy

Heartburn is a frequent complaint during pregnancy, especially during the third trimester.[13, 16] Of 563 pregnant women interviewed during and after pregnancy, 203 developed heartburn. No heartburn was reported in the first two months; the per cent of women noting heartburn for the first time increased from 7.4 in the third month to 20.7 in the seventh month and declined to 14.4 in the ninth month.[13] When heartburn occurred early in pregnancy, it was usually not related to meals or position; nausea and vomiting were common, and antacids afforded little relief. In contrast, heartburn that began later in pregnancy was more persistent, related to meals and position, associated with water brash, and relieved by antacids; nausea and vomiting were rare. In 10 per cent of the women with heartburn, it developed during the first 4 months and disappeared in the fifth and sixth months, only to reappear during the third trimester. When this occurred, the type of heartburn in early and late

pregnancy was as already described. Spontaneous relief of heartburn was noted by 45 per cent of affected women in the last few weeks of pregnancy. After delivery, 98 per cent had no heartburn. Rarely, esophageal stricture results from the vomiting of pregnancy.[23]

Pathophysiology

Since heartburn usually disappears after delivery, it is presumably related to some physiologic alterations during pregnancy. Overwhelming evidence suggests that the cause of heartburn is the reflux of hydrochloric acid into the esophagus, although reflux of bile acids can also cause heartburn.

Explanations for the heartburn of pregnancy have included (1) increased intrabdominal pressure from the enlarging uterus, (2) delayed gastric emptying secondary to the mass of the uterus, (3) development of a hiatus hernia, (4) alterations of anatomical structures surrounding the lower esophageal sphincter (LES), and (5) decreased LES pressure. Little evidence supports the first four proposals, in large part because appropriate studies in pregnant women are very difficult. Indeed, relatively few studies have documented acid reflux and esophagitis in pregnant women.[3, 7]

Most investigations have focused on the role of the LES as a factor in the heartburn of pregnancy. A decrease in the LES pressure during pregnancy was first noted in 1961 by use of a nonperfused catheter method; in 20 per cent of pregnant women with heartburn, LES pressure was decreased.[15] These early findings were confirmed by later investigators using the more sensitive perfused catheter technique.[7, 12, 21] Measurement of LES pressures in four pregnant women at 12, 24, and 36 weeks of gestation and at 1 to 4 weeks after delivery showed that the LES pressure fell successively during pregnancy but returned to normal after delivery (Fig. 11–1). LES pressure was only slightly lower than normal at 12 and 24 weeks but was profoundly depressed at 36 weeks. There was no accompanying change in basal gastric pH, basal and peak gastric acid output, or serum gastrin levels. As expected, serum estrone, estradiol, and progesterone levels increased progressively during pregnancy; the implication was that the decreasing LES pressure was related to increasing estrogen and progesterone levels. This suggestion, which might have been regarded with skepticism as overinterpretation of parallel events, is strengthened by evidence that LES pressure

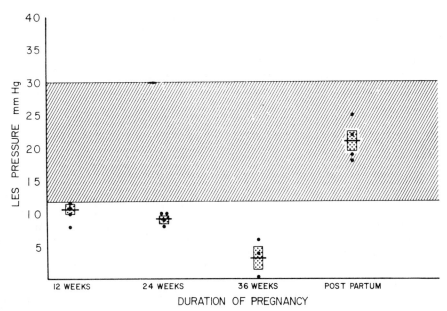

FIGURE 11–1. Measurement of lower esophageal pressures during pregnancy. (Reprinted by permission of the publisher from Van Thiel et al.: Heartburn of pregnancy. Gastroenterology, 72:667, 1977. Copyright by The American Gastroenterological Association.)

decreased in seven women taking sequential oral contraceptives.[22] LES pressure remained unchanged when women took ethinylestradiol but decreased when they were taking both ethinylestradiol and the progestation agent dimethisterone (Fig. 11–2). There were no concomitant changes in gastric acidity or serum gastrin levels. Of course, the increase in serum estrogens and progesterone, along with the decrease in LES pressure, does not prove a causal relationship, but

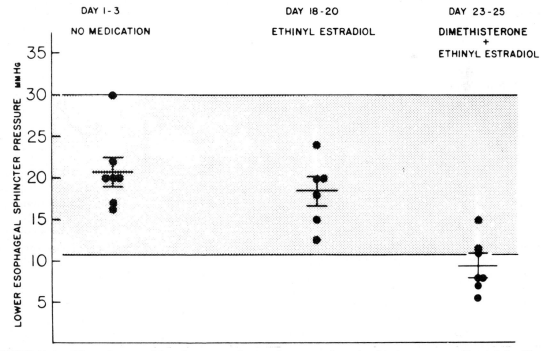

FIGURE 11–2. Effect of sequential oral contraceptives on lower esophageal sphincter pressure. (Reprinted with permission from Van Thiel, et al.: Gastroenterology, 71:233, 1976. Copyright by The American Gastroenterological Association.)

other evidence suggests that these hormones may be important. Progesterone is a smooth muscle relaxant,[9] and its administration depresses LES pressure in the opossum.[19] Such studies make it seem likely that estrogens alone do not decrease LES pressure; whether progesterone alone has any effect is uncertain, since estrogens have been given before or during all studies of progesterone administration to date.

In a study of eight women about to undergo abortion during early pregnancy at 14 to 19 weeks of gestation, LES pressure was normal, but its response to physiologic stimuli such as a protein meal or to pharmacologic stimuli such as pentagastrin, edrophonium, and methacholine injection was depressed.[6] The LES responses returned to normal after pregnancy was terminated. Estrogen and progesterone levels were elevated before the abortion, but serum gastrin levels were normal. Functional abnormalities in the LES, therefore, can be detected early in pregnancy, further implicating its dysfunction in the heartburn of pregnancy.

Several investigators have described increased intragastric pressure during the third trimester.[7, 12, 20] Ordinarily, any increase in intra-abdominal pressure leads to a reflex increase in LES pressure that equals the rise in intra-abdominal pressure, to maintain the pressure differential between stomach and LES that provides the barrier against reflux. In pregnancy, however, the following sequence of events may take place: (1) LES sphincter dysfunction develops early in pregnancy as the result of hormonal changes; most women remain asymptomatic, however, because increased intra-abdominal pressure does not rise until later; (2) Once intra-abdominal pressure rises, the already weakened LES is unable to respond adequately; and (3) acid reflux develops. The decreased frequency of heartburn during the last few weeks of pregnancy may be the result of the descent of the uterus, leading to decreased intragastric pressure. In support of this overall hypothesized sequence is the observation that the response of the LES to abdominal compression was depressed in early as well as in late pregnancy.[21] Not all investigators, however, have recorded an increased intragastric pressure late in pregnancy, and the postulated sequence of events does not take into account the decrease in LES pressure noted in nonpregnant women receiving oral contraceptives.

Further, although LES dysfunction is widely accepted as a prerequisite for reflux esophagitis, many patients with reflux esophagitis have normal LES pressures. Even more important, LES pressure as measured manometrically may not remain constant with time. When LES pressures are measured continuously overnight in normal subjects, they frequently decrease to low levels and acid reflux occurs.[4, 10] If the same phenomenon occurs in the pregnant women, as seems likely, then increased intra-abdominal pressure or delayed gastric emptying could lead to acid reflux whenever the LES pressure decreases transiently.

Decreased propulsive activity in the distal third of the esophagus has also been noted during pregnancy.[15, 20] This abnormality may lead to decreased clearing of acid from the esophagus once reflux has occurred. Needless to say, additional observations are needed to clarify the importance of factors other than LES dysfunction in the heartburn of pregnancy.

Diagnosis

Reflux esophagitis during pregnancy can be recognized from its symptoms. Clearly, all radiologic and radioactive diagnostic studies should be avoided unless absolutely necessary, the physician taking comfort from the fact that duodenal ulcer exacerbations are extremely rare in pregnancy and symptomatic treatment is usually all that is needed for heartburn of pregnancy. Women with reflux symptoms should undergo diagnostic measures such as pH monitoring *only* if the physician believes that a treatable condition will be discovered. It is almost never necessary to operate or otherwise intervene for heartburn of pregnancy.

Treatment

The standard measures utilized for reflux esophagitis are appropriate for pregnant women. These include (1) elevating the head of the bed about 4 inches on bed blocks, (2) avoiding large meals, especially snacks, just before going to bed, and (3) taking liquid antacids for symptomatic relief. Other measures that have proved quite successful for reflux esophagitis should not be used in pregnant women at present. These include cimetidine and metoclopramide. An H_2 receptor antagonist, cimetidine is a very potent inhibitor of basal and stimulated acid secretion and is therefore effective for the symptomatic relief of heartburn in men and in nonpregnant women.[2] There has been no reported experience with cimetidine during pregnancy; however, since it crosses the placental barrier and affects the H_2 receptors on T cells, the heart, and the brain, cimetidine should be avoided in pregnancy, even though teratogenic studies so far have revealed no adverse effects.

Metoclopramide, a dopamine antagonist, has three properties that make it potentially useful in the treatment of heartburn of pregnancy. It (1) is an antiemetic, (2) increases LES pressure, and (3) stimulates gastric emptying.[14] Currently not approved for such uses in the United States, metoclopramide has been used in Europe in pregnant women as an antiemetic and in the treatment of reflux esophagitis. A single injection of metoclopramide increased LES pressure in about 50 per cent of pregnant women, but the symptomatic response to prolonged oral administration was said to be much better.[8] A major problem with metoclopramide, however, is its high incidence of neurologic, extrapyramidal, and psychologic side effects and its induction of galactorrhea and increased serum prolactin levels.[17] The clinician in the United States will not wish to use this drug for the heartburn of pregnancy, at least until there have been further studies of its side effects. Clinicians outside the United States, where metoclopramide is more freely available, are advised to refrain from giving it to pregnant women without more evidence.

PEPTIC ULCER

"Peptic ulcer" usually refers to duodenal or gastric ulcer, but the clinician concerned with the pregnant woman should remember that the spectrum of acid-peptic disease encompasses everything from reflux esophagitis through gastritis and duodenitis to the jejunal ulcers of gastrinoma and even the ileal ulcers of Meckel's diverticulum. Here we will be concerned only with gastric and duodenal ulcer in pregnancy, as the other lesions are covered elsewhere in this chapter or are so rare in pregnancy as to deserve no extended attention.

It is important to remember that an ulcer is distinguished from an erosion by the fact that an ulcer extends below the muscularis mucosae; therefore after it heals, it leaves a scar. The erosions of gastritis or duodenitis, on the other hand, are superficial, heal without a trace, and may therefore be considered transitory.

The most common complaint of patients with gastric or duodenal ulcer is epigastric pain, often described as discomfort, acid feeling, burning, or indigestion. Classically, the pain is temporally related to eating; that is, it occurs before meals and is relieved by food, only to recur 30 minutes to 1 hour postprandially. This sequence of events parallels gastric acidity, food acting as a buffer. Antacids usually relieve this pain; if not, the physician should consider the possibility of a penetrating ulcer or another diagnosis. Nausea and vomiting immediately after eating in the patient with a duodenal ulcer should arouse suspicion of a pyloric channel ulcer with irritability and spasm, whereas nausea and vomiting several hours after eating should suggest gastric outlet obstruction. Weight loss is uncommon in duodenal ulcer but occurs in about one third of patients with gastric ulcer. As already suggested, poor response to medical therapy suggests a penetrating ulcer.

Status in Pregnancy

Pregnancy has a protective effect against the development of a peptic ulcer and also against the symptoms. Onset of ulcer disease during pregnancy is very unusual; indeed, when a woman with an established ulcer becomes pregnant, her symptoms usually improve. In a retrospective study conducted nearly 30 years ago, 400 women with documented peptic ulcer who had had a total of 313 pregnancies were interviewed. Forty-five per cent reported that they were symptom-free during pregnancy, 43 per cent reported that they were better, and only 12 per cent had no change or worsening of their symptoms.[26] Four per cent had to be admitted to the hospital with increasing symptoms, usually near term and frequently with other complications of pregnancy. No subsequent studies have refuted these observations based on patient recall; indeed, the notion that pregnancy relieves the woman with peptic ulcer is generally accepted. Such evidence, slight as it is, makes it reasonable to conclude that during pregnancy symptoms of peptic ulcer decrease in most women. The women in that study commented that they enjoyed pregnancy for the relief of gastric symptoms that it provided.

Not only does pregnancy protect against exacerbations of ulcer disease, but it also seems to militate against complications such as bleeding, perforation, and obstruction. The complications of peptic ulcer disease are so rare during pregnancy that they are reported in the literature when they occur. For example, it is an old clinical aphorism that gastrointestinal bleeding during pregnancy should not suggest duodenal ulcer but, instead, either pseudoxanthoma elasticum or Marfan's syndrome!

Pathophysiology

Peptic ulcer results from an imbalance between aggressive and defensive factors, of which the two apparently most important are (1) acid-pepsin secretion and (2) mucosal resistance.

Unfortunately, almost no attention has been paid to mucosal resistance, a feature that may prove to be particularly pertinent in the pregnant woman. Gastrin, and no doubt other hormones, is trophic to the gastric mucosa in animals, and trophic factors originating in placenta or fetus may conceivably prove to protect the mother's gastric mucosa, but these conjectures have not been examined. No studies of gastric mucosal resistance in the pregnant woman or animal have come to our attention.

Decreased mucosal resistance has been well documented in patients with gastric ulcer, to some extent as a result of the reflux of bile acids and pancreatic enzymes into the stomach from the duodenum. The increased prevalence of gastritis and gastric ulcers in chronic aspirin users and abusers appears to be the result of decreased mucosal resistance brought about by aspirin.[42] Aspirin is a prostaglandin synthetase inhibitor; other prostaglandin synthetase inhibitors, such as the nonsteroidal anti-inflammatory agents, can also cause gastritis.[34] Since prostaglandins exert a protective benefit on the gastric mucosa by mechanisms yet to be elucidated that have come to be known as "cytoprotection,"[39] the relationship of prostaglandin levels in the pregnant woman to the decreased prevalence of peptic ulcer disease in pregnancy deserves investigation. Undoubtedly, much remains to be learned about mucosal resistance in the normal man or woman as well as in the pregnant woman.

Whereas decreased mucosal resistance clearly plays an important role in gastric ulcer, acid hypersecretion may be more important in the genesis of duodenal ulcer. Acid secretion is necessary for both types of ulceration, however, and the rarity of an ulcer in the stomach without acid has led to the dictum "No acid, no ulcer."

Patients with duodenal ulcer tend to have the following characteristics: (1) basal and stimulated acid secretion is greater than normal; (2) the number of parietal cells in the gastric mucosa is increased above normal; (3) postprandial serum gastrin levels are modestly elevated and there is increased sensitivity to gastrin; (4) the so-called "feedback inhibition" of acid secretion by acid in the stomach is impaired; and (5) there is a more rapid emptying of liquids, but not solids, from the stomach.[30] Whether gastric emptying, apparently more rapid in duodenal ulcer patients than in normals, is also affected by the general slowing of the gastrointestinal tract in the pregnant woman is unknown. Conceivably, reduced gastric emptying could contribute to the remarkably infrequent occurrence of duodenal ulcer during pregnancy, as a direct inhibitory effect of progesterone on human gastric muscle has been demonstrated in vitro.[33]

Gastric secretion has only rarely been studied in the pregnant woman, and even more rarely in the pregnant woman with a duodenal ulcer. What studies there are have suggested that gastric secretion diminishes little or not at all during pregnancy. In one woman with an active duodenal ulcer, basal acid secretion decreased during the second half of pregnancy but returned rapidly to normal on the first postpartum day and remained normal during the period of observation, to the 48th day of the postpartum period.[43] Other studies of normal women have found either no change in gastric acid during pregnancy or a slight decrease.[27, 36, 45] The matter may be regarded as uncertain.

Attempts to assess gastric secretion have utilized indirect measures, like serum pepsinogen levels, that have been shown to be correlated with maximal gastric acid secretion.[41] Serum pepsinogen I, from the fundus of the stomach, is elevated in about one half of patients with peptic ulcer.[40] In normal women, values do not change significantly during pregnancy, which suggests that gastric acid secretion remains unchanged during that period.[31, 46]

Men and women have different levels of gastric secretion and a different prevalence of peptic ulcer, matters germane to any consideration of ulcer during pregnancy. Duodenal ulcer and gastric ulcer are about twice as common in men as in women, although this difference may be decreasing.[29] The reasons for the lesser susceptibility of women to duodenal ulcer are not apparent; acid secretion is greater in men than in women more as a result of their larger size than for any other reason. Some studies have suggested that estrogens have a protective effect; they ameliorate the symptoms of duodenal ulcer and promote radiographic healing, but in men exogenous estrogens have very little effect on acid secretion.[28, 32, 37, 44]

The older literature reported that women had the onset of duodenal ulcer more frequently after the menopause, although women, like men, have a decreasing incidence of peptic ulcer as they get older.[26] Thus, estrogens appear to exert some protective effect other than the decrease in gastric acid secretion, perhaps by altering mucosal resistance.

Plasma histaminase levels increase dramatically during pregnancy, presumably as a result of production by the placenta.[27] Such increased amounts of histaminase could lead to increased destruction of histamine at the level of the parietal cells and in this way to decreased acid production. In rats, pregnancy protected against the development of histamine-produced ulcers but did not affect ulcers produced by other mechanisms.

Diagnosis

Usually, the physician treating the pregnant woman with heartburn or indigestion will think of reflux esophagitis and "the heartburn of pregnancy." Ordinarily relying on symptomatic management, he will feel that diagnosis is neither necessary nor useful. In the very rare woman with a history of previous duodenal ulcer, the recurrence of symptoms alone is sufficient to establish the diagnosis. On the even rarer occasion when a diagnosis is deemed necessary in a woman without a previous history, panendoscopy offers the appropriate diagnostic approach. The new flexible endoscopes, particularly the pediatric endoscope, are sufficiently thin that the procedure is comfortable for the mother and without danger to the fetus, as it can be carried out without premedication. At panendoscopy, the clinician will see the ulcer crater in the stomach or duodenum.

Barium studies are clearly to be avoided except as a last resort because of the possible hazards to the fetus; radiologic studies should be performed only after considerable attention to the risks, benefits, and expected change in therapeutic plan. Neither gastric analysis, nor serum pepsinogen levels, nor other diagnostic maneuvers sometimes helpful in the nonpregnant woman are useful enough in establishing the diagnosis of peptic ulcer disease to be warranted in the pregnant woman. The stools should obviously be checked for blood.

Rarely, a gastric ulcer is found during pregnancy or is recognized before pregnancy. There is certainly not enough experience to suggest a firm plan; there have been several reports of gastric ulcer in pregnant women that turned out to be gastric carcinoma or lymphoma. It makes sense, therefore, to consider performing endoscopy and biopsy in the rare woman in whom a gastric ulcer is found by whatever means.

Treatment

Although therapy for peptic ulcer now centers on the H_2 blockers that speed the healing of duodenal ulcer, they should not be used in the pregnant woman, at least until much more experience suggests that they are harmless to the fetus.[47] Carbenoxolone has not proved effective in the United States and is therefore unavailable to the clinicians; sucralfate, currently undergoing testing and apparently not absorbed, may prove to be a useful drug in the pregnant woman with peptic ulcer, but its indications will have to await further testing and experience.

Therapy for peptic ulcer in the pregnant woman should therefore be based on symptom relief and particularly on dietary manipulation and antacids.[38] The pregnant woman should avoid any foods that provoke symptoms and should probably avoid coffee, tea, and alcohol if she is not already doing so. From a physiologic standpoint, it makes sense for the woman to avoid bedtime snacks, not only because they may stimulate nocturnal acid secretion but also because of the tendency to gastroesophageal reflux during middle and late pregnancy.

Small amounts of antacids make sense for the pregnant woman with a suspected duodenal ulcer because acid levels are low and therapeutic objectives usually limited. Although considerable attention has been given to the promotion of ulcer healing by large amounts of high potency antacids 1 and 3 hours after meals and at bedtime, 7 times a day, it seems more judicious to give smaller amounts of antacids less frequently to the pregnant woman. If relief of symptoms quickly follows, the clinician can be assured that the effectiveness of such small amounts of antacid in promoting ulcer healing is probably high. To be sure, proponents of vigorous antacid therapy in the nonpregnant patient have tried to eliminate all acid secretion, but reduction of acid to the point at which mucosal healing can occur on its own is enough in the pregnant woman. Indeed, evidence from cimetidine trials suggests that restoring acid levels to normal is all that is necessary in the nonpregnant patient and that it is unnecessary to eradicate acid completely.

In this spirit, then, we recommend that the pregnant woman with symptoms of duodenal ulcer take 15 ml of antacid 1 hour after meals and again at bedtime. If this gives relief of symptoms, the physician should be satisfied. If symptoms persist, however, then an increase in the amount of antacids to 30 ml of Mylanta II, Gelusil II, or Maalox Plus can be tried as often as seven times a day or 1 and 3 hours after meals and at bedtime. Such large amounts of antacid cause diarrhea in 30 per cent of nonpregnant patients, but the constipated pregnant woman may find an increase in the frequency of her bowel movements a bonus[38]!

The amount of aluminum or other constituents absorbed from antacids and their potential effects on the fetus are unknown. Moreover, the possibility of phosphorus depletion in the patient taking large amounts of aluminum-containing antacid should be kept in mind. This is rare enough, however, so that even in the pregnant woman there is no need to monitor serum phosphorus levels. Although calcium-containing antacids are currently condemned for most patients because calcium stimulates acid secretion, they may well have a useful place in providing calcium supplementation for the pregnant woman. The clinician must keep in mind that antacids can interfere with the absorption of a number of drugs.[25, 35]

Because an ulcer ordinarily takes about 4 to 6 weeks to heal, it makes sense to give regular antacid therapy for at least that length of time. The clinician treating a pregnant woman, however, should use common sense. In the unlikely event that a peptic ulcer in a pregnant woman proves intractable, the therapeutic program should be individualized. Indeed, we have not seen such intractability except with extreme marital and social tension. In that rare event, it is appropriate to admit the woman to the hospital in order to remove her from whatever tensions may be producing exacerbations at home. The help of a gastroenterologist should be searched for, rather than instructions from a textbook. If necessary, a nasogastric tube can be passed to withdraw any acid from the stomach and to determine whether this procedure gives relief. The possibility that the pain is not the result of an ulcer deserves consideration. Other causes of intractability should be considered, but we will not here recite the litany of gastric cancer, pancreatic cancer, and the rest. Presumably, cimetidine will be considered in such circumstances, but as already noted, it is a new drug, and although animal studies show no teratogenic effects, it should be avoided in pregnancy unless there seem to be no alternatives. It is of interest that cimetidine has "antiandrogen effects" in that it produces gynecomastia, galactorrhea, decreased sperm count, and increased testosterone levels, all of which suggest that some of the beneficial effects of cimetidine could be related to its antiandrogen effects. This question should be answered by the studies of some of the new H_2 antagonists that are apparently devoid of such effects.

The complications of peptic ulcer during pregnancy should be treated in the usual fashion, although, as already suggested, they are so rare as to deserve no extended discussion. Recurrent gastrointestinal bleeding or obstruction will call for the usual diagnostic and therapeutic measures. Surgical intervention should not be postponed when it seems in order.

CHOLELITHIASIS AND BILIARY TRACT DISEASE

Frequently asymptomatic, gallstones may go undetected throughout life. They may lead to biliary colic or cholecystitis when they obstruct the cystic duct or to jaundice, cholangitis, and pancreatitis when they pass into the common bile duct. Biliary colic is visceral pain of short duration, usually lasting 2 to 3 hours, that results from transient obstruction of the cystic duct. It is steady rather than intermittent, despite its name, and it usually occurs an hour or two after the evening meal. Biliary pain commonly is felt in the epigastrium or right upper quadrant, although rarely it may be felt in the left upper quadrant, precordium, or lower abdomen. The pain may radiate to the angle of the scapula in the back or directly between the shoulder blades, particularly when a common duct stone is present. Nausea and vomiting may accompany the pain, but vomiting only very rarely relieves it; vomiting is rarely protracted except in the presence of pancreatitis or common duct obstruction. Cystic duct obstruction that progresses to inflammation of the gallbladder leads to fever, leukocytosis, and signs of inflammation in the right upper quadrant.

Status in Pregnancy

Fortunately, acute cholecystitis and other complications of gallstones requiring surgical intervention are rare in pregnancy.[63] In one review of 175,000 pregnancies, only 11 cholecystectomies had been performed;[71] of 1884 cholecystectomies in women aged 16 to 45, only 6 (0.3 per cent) were in pregnant women.[66] Assuming two pregnancies in a 30 year time span, these women were pregnant 5 per cent of the time, suggesting that pregnancy decreased the incidence of cholecystectomy! Such statistical manipulation presumably is not valid, since women ordinarily have babies in their twenties and undergo cholecystectomy in their thirties or forties. Still, it is not unreasonable to postulate that the sluggish gallbadder of pregnancy makes the occurrence of cystic duct obstruction unlikely. There are many reports of recurrence of biliary colic after delivery and a seemingly high incidence of cholecystectomy in the year after delivery.[71] Furthermore, when acute cholecystitis requiring operation occurs during pregnancy, it is most common during the first trimester when gallbladder contractions are still normal.[66] Gallstones are also an uncommon cause of jaundice in pregnancy, accounting for only 7 per cent of cases, hepatitis and cholestasis being the most common causes.[63]

Pathophysiology

Gallstones are more common in women than in men in areas where cholesterol gallstones are prevalent.[52] The increased risk of cholelithiasis begins at the menarche and ends at the menopause, a relationship that strongly suggests that the sex hormones are involved in gallstone formation. Since estrogen and progesterone levels are further increased during pregnancy, there is reason to believe that pregnancy increases the already greater risk of gallstones in women. During the past 15 years, a considerable amount has been learned about how gallstones form, much of which proves the pathophysiologic basis of the adage "female, fat, forty, and fertile." There is good reason, then, for the physician caring for pregnant women to be aware of biliary tract physiology as it is currently understood.

There are two types of gallstones: cholesterol stones, composed almost exclusively of cholesterol, and pigment stones, composed primarily of calcium bilirubinate. Since cholesterol stones are far more common than pigment stones, particularly in pregnant women, we will focus primarily on the mechanism of cholesterol stone formation. Moreover, the frequency of pigment stone does not seem to be increased in women, even if they have been pregnant or are fat, although one report suggests that women with hemolytic disorders are more likely than men to develop pigment stones.[65]

Gallstone formation is divided into three events: (1) formation of bile supersaturated with cholesterol, (2) nucleation and crystallization of cholesterol to begin stone formation, and (3) growth of the crystal to clinically detectable size. Most recent investigations have been directed toward the first event, saturation, but the latter two steps are beginning to receive more study.

For the physician interested in pregnancy, however, the role of cholesterol deserves the most attention. Cholesterol in the body is mainly eliminated by being secreted into the bile. Because cholesterol is very insoluble in water,

however, it must be incorporated into soluble micelles with bile acids and phospholipids. Bile that has solubilized all the cholesterol it can is said to be "saturated"; theoretically, any excess cholesterol will precipitate out of solution as cholesterol crystals and lead to gallstone formation. In reality, however, normal bile frequently is supersatured with cholesterol, and yet the cholesterol does not precipitate out of solution, or does so very slowly, in this so-called *metastable zone*. When supersaturation is increased sufficiently, however, cholesterol crystals form; this is called the *labile zone*. Apparently, the normal liver frequently secretes bile supersaturated with cholesterol without the formation of crystals or stones; thus, other factors are clearly important in stone formation. By the same token, however, gallstones will not form if bile is not supersaturated with cholesterol, regardless of other factors.

Supersaturation of bile tends to occur whenever there is a high rate of cholesterol secretion or a low rate of bile acid secretion. Bile is relatively more saturated with cholesterol at lower rates of bile acid secretion.[72] Moreover, dilute bile is less capable of holding cholesterol in solution than is concentrated bile.[56] An increased rate of cholesterol secretion occurs in obesity,[51, 69] in conformity with the oft-quoted quartet. A high calorie diet, even in the absence of obesity, increases cholesterol secretion into the bile,[51, 68] but whether the increased caloric intake and relative "obesity" of pregnancy increase biliary cholesterol secretion has not been determined.

A low rate of bile acid secretion uncommonly but classically occurs in persons who have undergone massive ileal resection, usually for Crohn's disease. Such an anatomic rearrangement results in a decreased bile acid pool size, because bile acids cannot be absorbed from the normal ileal site and instead pass out into the colon and are lost to the body. If the liver cannot increase synthesis sufficiently, the bile acid pool decreases in size until synthesis matches fecal losses. Such decreased pool size leads to reduction in the rate at which bile acids are secreted into the bile so that the bile becomes more saturated with cholesterol.

Evidence seems conclusive that either endogenous or exogenous estrogens or progestins increase the risk of gallstone formation, largely by increasing biliary cholesterol saturation. Women have a smaller total bile acid and chenodeoxycholic acid pool than men; this is important, because the amount of cholesterol saturation in the bile is inversely related to the chenodeoxycholic acid pool size.[49] In this regard, the development of lithogenic bile during puberty in Pima Indians is pertinent.[53] Pima Indians are highly susceptible to the formation of cholesterol gallstones and have served as a model that has been extended to the general population. Before puberty, cholesterol saturation of bile is no greater in Pima Indians than in normal white adults. With the onset of puberty, however, cholesterol saturation increases sharply in both Pima men and women but is 15 per cent higher in women when adjusted for age. In the Pima Indians, bile cholesterol saturation is related to obesity, as already noted, and to urinary estrogen excretion in both men and women. In Pima men, total bile acid pool size increases with age, but this does not happen in women; chenodeoxycholic acid pool size in women actually decreases with age to some extent. Only 13 per cent of girls and no boy under the age of 13 had bile saturated with cholesterol in the labile zone; whereas over the age of 19, 71 per cent of women but only 29 per cent of men had cholesterol supersaturation in the labile zone. This finding correlates remarkably with the ultimate 70 per cent prevalence of cholelithiasis in Pima women.

The bile acid pool size increases, while biliary cholesterol saturation decreases, in premenopausal women after oophorectomy.[48] Estrogen use for any reason — oral contraception, postmenopausal replacement, or therapeutically in men — has been associated with gallstone formation.[52] Oral contraceptive use increases biliary cholesterol saturation and decreases the proportion of chenodeoxycholic acid in the bile acid pool.[50] Chenodeoxycholic acid therapy dissolves gallstones primarily by decreasing biliary cholesterol secretion.[57]

Those observations make it appear that either estrogens or progestins or both, endogenous or exogenous, increase the risk of gallstone formation by increasing biliary cholesterol saturation. The increase in cholesterol saturation results from (1) a decrease in the total bile acid pool size in general and a decrease in the chenodeoxycholic acid pool size in particular and (2) an increased secretion of biliary cholesterol. The mechanism for the decreased bile acid pool size remains unknown, but the increased secretion of cholesterol appears to be secondary to the decreased amount of chenodeoxycholic acid. Such increased cholesterol secretion in the bile is enhanced by obesity. In Pima women, the prevalence of lithogenic bile rises in the teens, a parallel rise in the prevalence of gallstones occurs about 10 years later, and gallbladder disease — at least as determined by nonvisualization of the gallbladder — peaks around age 40 (Fig. 11–3). Thus, scientific investigation has provided insight into three fourths of the adage.

Whether pregnancy adds an additional risk is controversial. In baboons, pregnancy is accompanied by a decrease in bile acid pool size, a decrease in the relative proportion of chenodeoxycholic acid, and an increase in biliary cholesterol saturation.[59] Data regarding the effect of pregnancy on human bile composition, however, are scanty and inconsistent.[52] Considering the additional risk of gallstones with oral contraceptive use, which in essence induces a state of pseudopregnancy, the physician can reasonably assume that (1) pregnancy increases the risk of gallstones by increasing biliary cholesterol saturation and (2) multiple pregnancies have an additive effect on risk.

Even though it has not been established with certainty that pregnancy alters the physical chemistry of biliary lipids, it is certain that pregnancy affects gallbladder function.[55] In

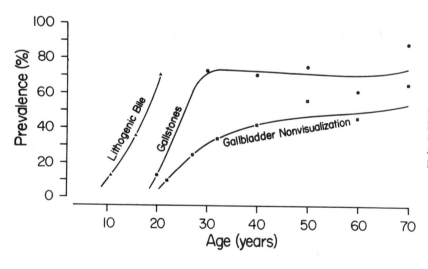

FIGURE 11–3. Development of lithogenic bile in Pima Indians. (From Bennion: N. Engl. J. Med., 300:876, 1979. Reprinted with permission.)

women who have been pregnant for 14 or more weeks, ultrasound studies have shown that (1) fasting gallbladder volume is twice as large as normal, (2) the rate of gallbladder emptying is significantly slower, (3) the maximum per cent emptied is lower than normal, and therefore (4) the residual gallbladder volume is twice as great as in control nonpregnant women. Interestingly enough, women taking oral contraceptives have normal gallbladder function.[55]

As has been already emphasized, dilute bile is less capable of solubilizing cholesterol than is concentrated bile. Thus, when the normal gallbladder concentrates bile by removing water from it, it increases micelle formation and the solubilization of cholesterol. Estrogen and pregnancy seem to inhibit fluid transport by the gallbladder, at least as shown by in vitro study of the guinea pig, in which 17 β-estradiol inhibits fluid transport.[62] This phenomenon may be related to the inhibition of the sodium pump enzyme, sodium-potassium ATPase.[58, 67] This process results in a large gallbladder in the fasting patient, testimony to the fact that the concentrating ability of the gallbladder diminishes during pregnancy, and therefore its ability to solubilize cholesterol is less than normal.

The diminished ability of the gallbladder to contract during pregnancy is not unexpected, since progesterone is a general inhibitor of smooth muscle function. Progesterone also inhibits cholecystokinin-induced gallbladder contraction in animals,[70] and cholecystokinin is probably the major stimulus for gallbladder contraction after a meal. Impaired gallbladder contraction and the resulting increase in gallbladder residual volume may increase the risk of gallstone formation by causing sequestration of cholesterol crystals, the final stage in the growth of gallstones.[64] These latter two hypotheses are largely unproved, however. On the other hand, it could be argued that the "sluggish" gallbladder of pregnancy actually serves a protective function by sequestering bile acids in the gallbladder. Making bile acids unavailable to the general bile acid pool would result in less "feedback inhibition," thus increasing bile acid synthesis, secretion, and pool size, events that decrease cholesterol saturation.[61]

Diagnosis

Since at least 50 per cent of gallstones cause no symptoms, there is no reason to search for them in the asymptomatic woman. Only if the pregnant women develops biliary colic, jaundice, pancreatitis, or other potential complications of gallstones should diagnostic procedures be undertaken. The differential diagnosis of jaundice and pregnancy is considered elsewhere; however, recurrent intrahepatic cholestasis, viral hepatitis, and acute fatty liver of pregnancy are all disorders that must enter into consideration.

Ultrasonography has greatly simplified the diagnosis of cholelithiasis in pregnancy. Indeed, because of its speed, safety, and accuracy, ultrasonography has replaced oral cholecystography in most medical centers. Correct performance and interpretation of sonograms require considerable skill, however, and this factor must be weighed in the evaluation of the patient considered to have one of the complications of cholelithiasis. Ultrasonography in skilled hands is also quite accurate at distinguishing extrahepatic from intrahepatic biliary obstruction in the jaundiced patient, but only rarely will it detect stones in the common bile duct.

As pregnancy progresses, the appendix is displaced to the right upper quadrant, and in late pregnancy it may be difficult to distinguish between acute cholecystitis and acute appendicitis or between acute pancreatitis and acute cholecystitis. In such patients, intravenous cholangiography or the radionuclide HIDA scans are very useful in determining whether cystic duct obstruction is present. Both techniques, however, involve radiation, thus posing a risk to the fetus, and should be used only when surgery is being seriously contemplated. Currently HIDA is the most common of the technetium scans and has proved as accurate as the intravenous cholangiogram in demonstrating cystic duct obstruction, without the potential allergic reaction that intravenous cholangiography entails. HIDA scans have the future advantage of displaying the common duct at bilirubin levels as high as 8 mg per 100 ml; some of the new agents being developed may show the duct when the levels of bilirubin are even higher.

Treatment

Asymptomatic gallstones discovered incidentally during pregnancy by ultrasound or abdominal film can be ignored on the supposition that they will not cause any trouble, particularly in a sluggish gallbladder, which is less likely to propel them into the cystic duct. The asymptomatic woman with gallstones contemplating pregnancy can be advised that it is unlikely that she will develop biliary colic during pregnancy, but it is prudent to advise prophylactic cholecystectomy in such a young woman, who has a long life ahead of her. These are matters for individual judgment, however. Asymptomatic stones should be removed in diabetic women because of the increased morbidity and mortality of acute cholecystitis in such patients.

Although chenodeoxycholic acid and ursodesoxycholic acid dissolve gallstones by decreasing biliary cholesterol secretion, these agents are not yet available for general use in the United States and their effect in pregnant women is completely unknown. For the time being, therefore, physicians will have to rely upon symptomatic treatment and, when necessary, upon operative therapy for gallstones and the complications they produce.

The pregnant woman who develops biliary colic should be treated symptomatically, since the attacks usually subside within a few hours. Subsequent attacks during pregnancy should be treated expectantly if at all possible, but operation may sometimes be necessary. In any case the pregnant woman who develops biliary colic should be advised to undergo cholecystectomy after the conclusion of her pregnancy.

Acute cholecystitis during pregnancy may also be treated medically in the hope that it will respond to nasogastric suction, antibiotics, and intravenous hydration; operation should ordinarily be postponed until after delivery. If acute cholecystitis does not resolve with medical management, however, or if ascending cholangitis or persistent pancreatitis develops, then operation must be performed without delay. As a general rule, operation should be performed early for an acute condition of the abdomen during pregnancy, as delay is associated with increased mortality for mother and fetus.[63] Fetal mortality is less than 5 per cent after cholecystectomy, especially in the second and third trimester, but approaches 60 per cent when pancreatitis secondary to biliary tract disease is left untreated.[66]

PANCREATITIS AND PREGNANCY

The syndromes "pancreatitis of pregnancy" and "postpartum pancreatitis" have turned out to be a simple association with gallstones and not a metabolically predetermined event, as was originally suggested. Pancreatitis in pregnancy is related to gallstones in more than two thirds of women and may also, of course, be related to the biliary stasis of pregnancy already commented upon.[60, 73]

Pathophysiology

Pancreatitis generally has two origins. By far the commonest in the female population is that which results from a gallstone passing down the common duct and impacting briefly at the ampulla. Then, it leads to a short-lived attack of pancreatitis, which ordinarily lasts no more than 24 to 48 hours. Such pancreatitis is known as "large duct pancreatitis." The other form of pancreatitis, which is less common among women, is "small duct pancreatitis." This is usually the result of excessive use of alcohol for many years but at times may be the result of such drugs as the birth control pill, chlorothiazide, and even steroids. Alcohol produces pancreatitis by metabolic events, and such pancreatitis may usually be thought of as chronic rather than as an acute remediable event. Estrogens in the birth control pill are likely to cause pancreatitis in women with type IV hyperlipemia because they remarkably increase the level of lipids in the serum, usually by a direct effect on the liver.

Diagnosis

For practical purposes, the clinician should think of acute pancreatitis whenever the pregnant woman has acute cholecystitis or biliary colic. Severe epigastric pain associated with prolonged nausea and vomiting, and particularly with any development of jaundice or pain in the back, should be an important clinical clue. As already pointed out, physical examination of the pregnant woman may not be very helpful or may be misleading. Therefore, the diagnosis should be approached in the usual manner, with determinations of serum amylase and lipase and with ultrasound evaluation. All radiologic studies should be avoided just as in biliary tract disorders.

Treatment

The therapy for the patient with acute pancreatitis during pregnancy should consist of nasogastric suction, maintenance of normal fluid and electrolyte balance with intravenous fluids, and pain relief, usually by means of narcotic analgesics (intramuscular Demerol). Antibiotics should be used only if pancreatic abscess is suspected or if there is concomitant ascending cholangitis. Ordinarily, pancreatitis subsides within a day or two, if it is related to biliary tract disease.

Pancreatitis that lasts more than 48 hours should always raise the question of associated alcoholism or some other cause and may well need operation — matters of importance but not to be discussed further here.

Rarely, stenosis of the sphincter of Oddi or pancreatic cancer will turn up during pregnancy as a cause of pancreatitis, purely by chance.[54]

INFLAMMATORY BOWEL DISEASE

The incidence and prevalence of inflammatory bowel disease (IBD) has risen spectacularly over the past 30 years. As women of childbearing years are in the age group most likely to develop inflammatory disease, concern has grown for the effect of IBD on fertility, on the course of pregnancy, and on the fetus. There has been a generally pessimistic but entirely unjustified view that pregnancy may worsen the course of inflammatory bowel disease. In this section we emphasize that the course of inflammatory bowel disease in pregnant young women does not differ from that in nonpregnant women of the same age except insofar as (1) drugs are used much less frequently in pregnant women, (2) mechanical complications of the enlarged uterus interfere with recognition of acute complications, and (3) the justifiable fear of radiation precludes many of the studies usually required for diagnosis.

Definitions. In the 1980s the old rigid classifications of regional enteritis, ulcerative colitis, and granulomatous or Crohn's colitis have yielded to a recognition that these disorders constitute a spectrum that is best considered inflammatory bowel disease. Regional enteritis occupies one end of that spectrum and ulcerative proctitis the other. In the patient with a hose-like narrowing of the terminal ileum and the typical radiologic involvement of a short segment of terminal ileum, it is easy to make a diagnosis of regional enteritis, even if thoughts of tuberculosis or lymphoma briefly cross the mind of the clinician who is looking for rare causes. Similarly, in the young person with proctitis involving the distal 10 cm of the rectum, the rest of the sigmoid appearing normal to fiberoptic scrutiny, the diagnosis is clearly ulcerative proctitis. In these circumstances, the past few years have seen the necessity for excluding a host of infectious disorders. Still, the point applicable to the care of the pregnant woman is that more than 25 per cent of the time the practicing physician will not be able to get a definitive answer to the question of just which disorder the young woman patient has.

For that reason, the term inflammatory bowel disease has achieved wide popularity, the more specific categories being reserved for patients with classic manifestations and course. As a general rule, therapy is almost exactly the same for all three disorders, but the prognosis for the patient with clear-cut Crohn's colitis is rather gloomy after operation. These are matters that can be looked at in appropriate sources.

Status in Pregnancy

Women with ulcerative colitis become pregnant at about the same rate as healthy women,[89] but the same does not hold true for women with Crohn's disease.[88] The reported studies leave it unclear whether women with colonic disease are less likely to be able to become pregnant than women with disease of the small bowel only.[78, 80, 81] A general impression is left that women with ulcerative colitis may become pregnant when they are otherwise healthy. However, in women with Crohn's colitis, local complications such as tubo-ovarian abscess, perineal fistula, and the chronic ill health of that disorder sometimes preclude fertility.[88] As already noted, figures are hard to come by because of the varying definitions of infertility, the varying lengths of the followup by which the nonpregnant woman is defined as infertile or subfertile, and the surprising lack of statistics on the male partner. In any case, it is not unfair to conclude that at least half of the women with ulcerative colitis can become pregnant and that a figure only slightly less holds for the "average" woman with Crohn's disease of any variety.

No studies have examined the fertility of men with inflammatory bowel disease. Sulfasalazine, a drug commonly used in the management of the ambulatory patient with IBD, may diminish fertility in the male,[83, 87] but nothing is known about its effect in women.

Effect of IBD on Pregnancy. There has been a prevailing impression that during pregnancy patients with IBD fare less well than other women. This is not borne out, however, by careful study of the course of the disease in women of *equal age*, whether pregnant or not.[78, 79, 89] In this regard, it is important to disregard all studies of the course of inflammatory bowel disease in pregnant women before the 1950s to 1960s, since up to that time steroid therapy, the mainstay of treatment, and even sulfasalazine were not widely used. Generally speaking, over the past 20 to 30 years the incidence of ulcerative colitis, which tends to have a more spectacular downhill course, has diminished while the incidence of Crohn's disease, which is characterized by a more indolent but less dramatic series of events, has increased. In going over reports it is not always easy to be sure that the clinicians have been able to make the careful distinctions that, as we have already pointed out, are so difficult. In any event, women with ulcerative colitis who become pregnant have an abortion rate no greater than that of normal women of the same age.[79, 89] They have about the same prospects of having a normal child unless they become ill enough to require operation during pregnancy, in which case they run a greater than normal risk.

Somewhat greater pessimism has rightly attended reports of the effects of Crohn's disease on pregnancy. Higher abortion rates, ranging from 10 to 25 per cent are reported in patients with Crohn's disease, but overall the fetus that is carried to term has no greater risk of stillbirth, prematurity, or congenital deformity.[88]

At present, then, physicians caring for the pregnant woman or for the woman who wishes to become pregnant should rethink their usually somewhat pessimistic advice to women with inflammatory bowel disease. Generally, the inclination to counsel patients to conceive only when the disease is quiescent and when they are not taking medication, and when they have not been taking medication for some months if possible, seems reasonable.[89] That is not always possible, however, and the clinician should probably advise the woman to have her inflammatory bowel disease controlled, whether by operation or by medication, before embarking on pregnancy. But in general there is little evidence that IBD under good control, or even active disease, adversely affects either the course of pregnancy or the product of pregnancy. Complications that may develop are more difficult to recognize and to treat, however.

Effect of Pregnancy on IBD. The general impression that pregnancy has an adverse effect on ileitis and colitis is not true, but it is an extremely hardy belief. It stems from the initial case reports that described complications of ulcerative colitis during pregnancy,[76] studies done before the use of steroids,[74] and the failure of early studies to include a control group.[77] When such factors are accounted for, it turns out that pregnant women with ulcerative colitis fare about as well during pregnancy as other young women.[79, 89] There seems no evidence that women aged 15 to 45 years with ulcerative colitis have any different course regardless of whether they are pregnant. It is important for the physi-

cian taking care of the woman in childbearing years to keep in mind the fact that, regardless of pregnancy, there is about a 50-50 chance of any patient's developing recurrent disease during any given year. Similarly, it may be accepted that pregnancy generally has little adverse effect on the course of Crohn's disease.[78, 80] Relapses occur, but they generally do not cause serious trouble and are readily controlled.

Speculation as to why some patients with inflammatory bowel disease do badly and why certain periods of pregnancy tend to have more exacerbations and remissions center on variations in endogenous cortisol levels.[79] No firm evidence emerges, however. Part of the problem in evaluating what happens to the woman with inflammatory bowel disease during pregnancy comes from varying definitions of improvement or recurrence. A little reflection suggests how difficult they are to analyze: The woman who wants a baby very badly may have a different reaction to recurrent symptoms of inflammatory bowel disease than a woman who only tolerates the pregnancy. Surely the woman who finds pregnancy disagreeable will react much more intensely to any diarrhea or abdominal pain that she develops. These are matters difficult to analyze, and unfortunately no reported studies have taken such emotional factors into account.

Overall, then, we may summarize the effects of IBD on pregnancy by stating that (1) about half of women with known ulcerative colitis at conception may have a flareup of symptoms during pregnancy; (2) women with quiescent disease do somewhat better than women with active disease, but probably no differently from nonpregnant women of similar age; (3) recurrences tend to be most frequent during the first trimester and during the postpartum period and give the highest mortality and morbidity rate; (4) women who first develop ulcerative colitis during pregnancy or in the postpartum period run a somewhat greater risk; (5) overall, about half the patients may have a relapse during the postpartum period but not at a different rate from the relapse rate in women who have not been pregnant.[88]

There is no way to predict from a preceding pregnancy how a woman will do in the next pregnancy.[84, 88] In other words, successive pregnancies tend to have different effects on inflammatory bowel disease and the physician cannot guarantee what that effect will be. The physician has no firm ground for advising a second pregnancy, or a third one for that matter, or for advising against it. The decision, as in so many matters, should be left to the woman and to her partner.

Complications of IBD During Pregnancy. The complications of IBD are no more frequent during pregnancy than at any other time, but they are much harder to recognize and to treat. Minor problems such as diarrhea or lower abdominal cramps clearly arising from the colon usually need little investigation. Sigmoidoscopy can be performed if necessary without extra hazard, but dietary manipulation, as discussed later, is ordinarily all that is necessary.

In the woman who develops more severe abdominal pain, the problem becomes more complicated. Ordinarily the physician caring for a patient with IBD, particularly one who is taking steroids, orders abdominal x-ray films to check on the possibility of obstruction or perforation. In the pregnant woman, however, fear of radiation to the fetus, particularly during the first trimester, usually precludes most radiologic studies except in great emergency. Fortunately, ultrasound has proved helpful in excluding the possibility of a confined perforation in the patient with Crohn's disease. Obviously, x-ray films may be necessary, but the need must be tempered by concern for risks of the fetus and by the severity of the abdominal pain.

If the clinician thinks it probable that a catastrophe such as a perforation has occurred, then abdominal x-ray films must be made. In these circumstances it is useful to give the woman a small amount of Hypaque or barium to drink before a single upright plain film is made; it is wise to wait 10 minutes or so after the radiopaque agent has been taken before making the film. It is useful also to remember that large amounts of Hypaque may produce osmotic diarrhea. As already noted, ultrasound is harmless, so far as is currently known, and is helpful. It may be necessary to perform barium studies.

Treatment

As already noted, the standard management of an exacerbation of IBD of any variety centers on dietary control and the use of steroids. In the ordinary patient with inflammatory bowel disease it is customary to give 20 to 40 mg of prednisone in the early morning and decrease the dose as the patient improves. In the pregnant woman, however, it is well known that corticosteroids cross the placenta,[75] and therefore there has been considerable concern about the effect of steroids given for inflammatory bowel disease during pregnancy. In general, the bulk of human data suggests that steroids, when used to treat a variety of conditions including IBD, pose little risk to the human fetus.[85, 88]

Sulfasalazine is a valuable drug in the management of patients with inflammatory bowel disease of any variety. It is broken down by bacterial action in the gut into 5-aminosalicylate and sulfapyridine. Current views of its mechanism of action suggest that sulfasalazine inhibits prostaglandin synthesis. Its use in dosages varying from 2 grams to 12 grams a day has become common. Again, such drugs should not be used in a pregnant woman unless absolutely necessary, particularly in view of the reported congenital abnormalities in women taking certain other sulfonamide drugs.[86] If the drug is to be taken during pregnancy, the dose should be as small as possible, and the woman should take folic acid daily, particularly as sulfasalazine inhibits the transfer of folate across the intestinal mucosa.

We emphasize, however, that nothing is known about the effect of sulfasalazine in the pregnant woman. If sulfasalazine is to be used, it is probably wise *not* to use it in the last trimester of pregnancy because sulfonamides displace bilirubin from plasma protein and may cause kernicterus. Two recent studies, however, suggest that this may be only a theoretical risk and that there is no greater incidence of kernicterus in infants born to mothers treated with sulfsalazine.[85, 89] Although nothing is known about the safety of sulfasalazine during breast-feeding, it has been concluded that sulfasalazine can be safely given to nursing mothers, a conclusion that should be accepted only with reservations at present.[82]

Other, more experimental drugs, including azathiaprine or 6-mercaptopurine, should be avoided in treatment of the pregnant woman. These drugs cause fetal abnormalities and, as they only have a much-debated, experimental place in the therapy of inflammatory bowel disease generally, they have no place in the management of the pregnant woman with inflammatory bowel disease. Hydrocortisone enemas may be given as necessary, in approximately the same spirit as steroids are given, but the clinician should recall that they are absorbed and their local effect is great but that they have a general metabolic influence.

Codeine, Lomotil, and Imodium are useful drugs in the management of diarrhea. While we regard them as harmless, as with all other drugs their judicious use in pregnancy must be gauged by other considerations. Presumably, they are less likely to cause harm in the latter half of pregnancy.

In summary then, the management of inflammatory bowel disease in the pregnant woman is complicated. If diarrhea is the major complaint, then dietary control, omitting lactose, fruits, and vegetables as necessary, is in order. If the pregnant woman is to go on a restricted diet, omitting milk, ice cream, and American and cottage cheese, then the likelihood of calcium deficiency is not very great as long as she eats other cheeses and fortified bread. If a lactose-free diet is used, however, then calcium supplementation, as in the form of Oscal three times a day, is certainly in order. The use of such constipating agents as Pepto-Bismol, Amphojel, or Metamucil, all of which are presumably not absorbed in significant amounts, is preferable to the use of other drugs. For example, several tablespoons of Pepto-Bismol or Metamucil two or three times a day in a glass of water is quite effective in the management of diarrhea. The use of codeine, Lomotil, or Imodium must be guided by obstetric considerations. If prednisone is used, it should be used for the specific indications of weight loss, anorexia, and partial intestinal obstruction, and not simply for diarrhea; its use may be necessary for persistent bleeding as well. It should be used in the smallest possible doses, but if larger amounts are necessary, the clinician should not automatically assume that the fetus has been irreparably damaged. Generally, the foregoing comments about sulfasalazine suggest caution in its use, particularly in the last few months of pregnancy. However, the human data regarding its use during pregnancy are reassuring.[85, 89]

Finally, it should be clear from this discussion that the management of a woman with inflammatory bowel disease who becomes pregnant is a matter not so much for textbooks as for careful collaboration between the physician, the gynecologist, the internist, the gastroenterologist, and possibly the surgeon.

DISORDERED BOWEL FUNCTION

Constipation is a frequent complaint in Western society, although there are very few studies of this lowly phenomenon in the literature. Objective criteria for constipation include (1) a change in the usual bowel habits of the patient, (2) discomfort because the stools are difficult to pass or are too hard, or their passage produces pain, (3) incomplete evacuation, and (4) infrequent evacuation. The discomfort is usually a painful sensation of fullness in the rectum or left lower quadrant; other less well-defined symptoms, including bloating, excessive flatus, anorexia, malaise, and the like, are legion.[95] Constipation increases in frequency as pregnancy progresses, but happily it is self-limited.

Status in Pregnancy

The incidence of constipation is almost universally said to be increased in pregnancy, but there are few clinical studies of the phenomenon. In a study of 1000 postpartum Jewish and Arabic Israelis, constipation requiring laxative treatment was rare, in only 1.5 per cent of women studied; only 10 per cent reported decreased bowel frequency.[94] Whether this surprising report can be extrapolated to women in Western culture seems doubtful.

Pathophysiology

The pathophysiology of constipation is as poorly understood in pregnancy as it is in the general population. Aside from a few rare neuromuscular disorders such as Hirschsprung's disease, or other forms of obvious obstruction, very little is known about the mechanisms resulting in constipation. Currently popular is the idea that the responsible mechanisms include specific slow-wave electrical discharges in the myoelectric apparatus, but most often constipation seems to be a variation of normal bowel function.

Slow transit of fecal contents through the colon is widely believed to be important in the genesis of constipation. Some investigators determine the colonic transit time of radiopaque markers in their evaluation of refractory constipation,[95, 96] whereas others look for "slow waves."

It is possible that no neuromuscular abnormality exists in most patients who become constipated after the first decade of life but that their diet is just deficient in fiber. Increasing the amounts of dietary fiber decreases colonic transit time in constipated subjects. Constipation from birth or in the first decade of life strongly suggests neuromuscular disorder.

The constipation of pregnancy has not been studied, and therefore we can only speculate about its mechanisms. As stated earlier, progesterone is a smooth muscle relaxant with an inhibitory effect on human colonic musculature.[93] The increasing progesterone levels of pregnancy may slow colonic transport and result in constipation. On the other hand, constipation has not been reported with the use of oral contraceptives, something which suggests that other factors are involved in the constipation of pregnancy. Another major factor frequently cited is the pressure of the enlarged fetus on the rectum, in essence creating a mechanical obstruction. Hemorrhoids are also quite common during pregnancy and may contribute to constipation to the extent that defecation is delayed or inhibited by the pain.

Diagnosis

In women without a prior history of constipation, the diagnosis can be made by history alone. If there is rectal pain, then external hemorrhoids should be excluded and a digital exam and anoscopy should be done to rule out internal hemorrhoids and a rectal fissure. Other diagnostic procedures such as sigmoidoscopy, colonoscopy, and barium enema are indicated *only* if there is evidence of serious colonic obstruction threatening the health of the mother. Unless blood is present in or on the stool, the development of constipation during pregnancy may be considered normal and does not require further investigation. Occasionally, the physician may wish to rule out hypercalcemia and hypothyroidism, which can cause constipation. Since heartburn is so frequent in pregnancy, it is wise to ask about the intake of aluminum and calcium antacids, whose overuse can cause constipation.

Treatment

Any disorder contributing to constipation, such as hemorrhoids or hypothyroidism, should be treated, and constipating antacids should be eliminated. The treatment of uncomplicated constipation depends upon increased dietary fiber together with increased fluid intake; this combination increases stool weight and decreases colonic transit time.[90, 91, 92] Dietary fiber can be increased easily by increasing the intake of fruits, vegetables, and grains such as bran. The patient should be instructed to eat at least three servings of fruit and three of vegetables each day and to drink eight to ten glasses of water. If this is not effective, then bulk agents such as Metamucil or Konsyl can be added. Therapy can begin with one teaspoon twice daily, increasing as needed up to one tablespoonful three to four times daily.

Exercise has been advocated in the treatment of constipation, though the only evidence to support this is the observation that constipation is frequent in hospitalized patients at bed rest. A large breakfast, followed by a visit to the toilet regardless of whether the urge is present, has also been advocated in order to "retrain" the colon.

Dietary therapy including the use of bran and bulk agents will be successful in most patients. This approach should be tried for at least six weeks before being considered ineffective. A few patients will require laxatives or enemas, but the use of these agents should be avoided unless there is no response to a high fiber diet. Milk of magnesia, magnesium citrate, or dioctyl sodium sulfosuccinate (Colace) also relieves severe constipation. Likewise, a tap water enema (500 to 1000 cc) or Fleets enema may prove helpful. Laxatives and enemas should be used only sporadically to relieve severe constipation, not on a regular basis to prevent constipation. Chronic habitual laxative use, especially of senna or cascara, may lead to damage to colonic neurons that may impair motility and induce megacolon, resulting presumably in even more severe constipation.

References

NAUSEA AND VOMITING, REFLUX ESOPHAGITIS

1. Acute appendicitis in pregnancy (editorial). Br. Med. J., *4*:668, 1975.
2. Behar, J., Brand, D. L., Brown, E. C., Castell, D. O., Cohen, S., Crossley, R. J., Pope, C. E., and Winanis, C. S.: Cimetidine in the treatment of symptomatic gastroesophageal reflux. Gastroenterology, *74*:441, 1978.
3. Castro, L. de P.: Reflux esophagitis as the cause of heartburn in pregnancy. Am. J. Obstet. Gynecol., *98*:1, 1967.
4. Dent, J., Dodds, W. J., Friedman, R. H., Seikiguchi, T., Hogan, W. J., Arndorter, R. C., and Petrie, D. J.: Mechanism of gastroesophageal reflux in recumbent asymptomatic human subject. J. Clin. Invest., *65*:256, 1980.
5. Feldman, M., and Fordtran, J. S.: Vomiting. *In* Sleisinger, M. H., and Fordtran, J. S. (eds.): Gastrointestinal Disease, 2nd ed. Philadelphia, W. B. Saunders Co., 1978.
6. Fisher, R. S., Roberts, G. S., Grabowski, C. J., et al.: Altered lower esophageal sphincter function during early pregnancy. Gastroenterology, *74*:1233, 1978.
7. Hey, V. M. F., Cowley, D. S., Ganguli, P. C., Skinner, L. D., Ostick, D. G., and Sharp, D. S.: Gastro-esophageal reflux in late pregnancy. Anesthesia, *32*:372, 1977.
8. Hey, V. M. F., and Ostick, D. G.: Metoclopramide and the gastro-oesophageal sphincter: A study in pregnant women with heartburn. Anesthesia, *33*:462, 1978.
9. Hytten, F. E., and Leitch, I.: The Physiology of Human Pregnancy, 2nd ed. Philadelphia, F. A. Davis Co., 1971.
10. Johnson, L. F., and Demeester, T. R.: Twenty four hour pH monitoring of the distal esophagus. Am. J. Gastroenterol. *62*:325, 1974.
11. Kammerer, W. S.: Nonobstetric Surgery During Pregnancy. Med. Clin. North Am., *63*:1157, 1979.
12. Lind, J. F., Smith, A. M., McIver, D. K., et al.: Heartburn in pregnancy — a monometric study. Can. Med. Assoc. J., *98*:571, 1968.

13. Marchand, P.: The gastroesophageal sphincter and the mechanism of regurgitation. Br. J. Surg., 42:504, 1955.
14. McCallum, R. W., Ippoliti, A. F., Cooney, C., and Sturdevant, R. A. L.: A controlled trial of metoclopramide in symptomatic gastroesophageal reflux. N. Engl. J. Med., 296:354, 1977.
15. Nagler, R., and Spiro, H. M.: Heartburn in late pregnancy. Manometric studies of esophageal motor function. J. Clin. Invest., 40:954, 1961.
16. Nagler, R., and Spiro, H. M.: Heartburn in pregnancy. Am. J. Dig. Dis., 7:648, 1962.
17. Pinder, R. M., Brogden, R. D., Sawyer, P. R., et al.: Metoclopramine: A review of its pharmacological properties and clinical use. Drugs, 12:81, 1976.
18. Saunder, P., and Milton, P. J. D.: Laparotomy during pregnancy: An assessment of diagnostic accuracy and wastage. Br. Med. J., 3:165, 1973.
19. Schulze, K., and Christensen, J.: Lower sphincter of the opossum esophagus in pseudopregnancy. Gastroenterology, 73:1082, 1977.
20. Ulmsten, U., and Sundstrom, G.: Esophageal manometry in pregnant and non-pregnant women. Am. J. Obstet. Gynecol., 132:260, 1978.
21. Van Thiel, D. H., Galvaler, J. S., Joshi, S. N., et al.: Heartburn of pregnancy. Gastroenterology, 72:666, 1977.
22. Van Thiel, D. H., Gavaler, J. S., and Stremple, J.: Lower esophageal sphincter pressure in women using sequential oral contraceptives. Gastroenterology, 71:232, 1976.
23. Vinson, P. P.: Esophageal stricture following the vomiting of pregnancy. Surg. Gynecol. Obstet., 33:412, 1921.
24. Winship, D. H.: Gastrointestinal diseases. In Burrow, G. N., and Ferris, T. F. (eds.): Medical Complications During Pregnancy, 1st ed. Philadelphia, W. B. Saunders Co., 1975.

PEPTIC ULCER

25. Brown, D. D., and Juhl, R. P.: Decreased bioavailability of digoxin due to antacids and kaolin-pectin. N. Engl. J. Med., 259:1034, 1976.
26. Clark, D. H.: Peptic ulcer in women. Br. Med. J., 1:1254, 1953.
27. Clark, D. H., and Tankel, H. I.: Gastric acid and plasma-histaminase during pregnancy. Lancet, 2:886, 1954.
28. Doll, R., Hill, I. D., and Hutton, C. F.: Treatment of gastric ulcer with carbenoxolone sodium and estrogens. Gut, 6:19, 1965.
29. Elashoff, J. D., and Grossman, M. I.: Trends in hospital admissions and death rates for peptic ulcer in the United States from 1970 to 1978. Gastroenterology, 78:280, 1980.
30. Grossman, M. I.: Abnormalities of acid secretion in patients with duodenal ulcer. Gastroenterology, 75:524, 1978.
31. Gryboski, W. A., and Spiro, H. M.: The effect of pregnancy on gastric secretion. N. Engl. J. Med., 255:1131, 1965.
32. Kaufmann, H. J., and Spiro, H. M.: Estrogens and gastric secretion. Gastroenterology, 54:913, 1968.
33. Kumar, D.: In vitro inhibitory effect of progesterone on extrauterine human smooth muscle. Am. J. Obstet. Gynecol., 84:1300, 1962.
34. Lanza, F. L., Royer, G. L., Nelson, R. S., Chen, T. T., Seckman, C. E., and Rack, M. E.: The effects of ibuprofen, indomethacin, aspirin, naproxen and placebo on the gastric mucosa of normal volunteers. Dig. Dis. Sci., 24:823, 1979.
35. Littman, A., and Pine, B. H.: Antacids and anticholinergic drugs. Ann. Intern. Med., 82:544, 1975.
36. Murray, F. A., Erskine, J. P., and Fielding, J.: Gastric secretion in pregnancy. J. Obstet. Gynaecol. Br. Emp., 64:373, 1957.
37. Parbhoo, S. P., and Johnston, I. D. A.: Effects of estrogens on gastric secretion in patients with duodenal ulcer. Gut, 7:612, 1966.
38. Peterson, W. L., Sturdevant, R. A. L., Frankle, H. D., et al.: Healing of duodenal ulcers with an antacid regimen. N. Engl. J. Med., 297:341, 1977.
39. Robert, A.: Cytoprotection by prostaglandins. Gastroenterology, 77:761, 1979.
40. Rotter, J. I., Jones, J. Q., Samloff, I. M., Richardson, C. T., Gursky, J. M., Walsh, J. H., and Rimoin, D. L.: Duodenal ulcer disease associated with elevated serum pepsinogen I. N. Engl. J. Med., 300:63, 1979.
41. Samloff, I. M., Secrist, D. M., and Passaro, E.: A study of the relationship between serum group I pepsinogen levels and gastric acid secretion. Gastroenterology, 69:1196, 1975.
42. Silvoso, G. R., Ivey K. J., Butt, J. H., Lockard, D. O., Holt, S. D., Sisk, C., Baskin, W. N., Mackercher, P. A., and Hewett, J.: Incidence of gastric lesions in patients with rheumatic disease on chronic aspirin therapy. Ann. Intern. Med., 91:517, 1979.
43. Spiro, H. M., Schwartz, R. D., and Pilot, M. L.: Peptic ulcer in pregnancy. Am. J. Dig. Dis., 4:289, 1959.
44. Truelove, S. C.: Stilboesterol, phenobarbitone and diet in chronic duodenal ulcer. Br. Med. J., 2:559, 1960.
45. Van Thiel, D. H., Gavaler, J. S., Joshi, S. N., et al.: Heartburn of pregnancy. Gastroenterology, 72:666, 1977.
46. Waldum, H. L., Straume, B. K., and Lundgren, R.: Serum group I pepsinogens during pregnancy. Scand. J. Gastroenterol., 15:61, 1980.
47. Wastell, C., and Lanie, P. (eds.): Cimetidine: The Westminster Hospital Symposium 1978. Edinburgh, London, and New York, Churchill Livingstone, 1978.

CHOLELITHIASIS, BILIARY TRACT DISEASE, PANCREATITIS

48. Bennion, L. J.: Changes in bile lipids accompanying oophorectomy in a premenopausal woman. N. Engl. J. Med., 297:709, 1977.
49. Bennion, L. J., Drobyn, E., Knowler, W. C. et al.: Sex differences in the size of bile acid pools. Metabolism, 27:961, 1978.
50. Bennion, L. J., Ginsberg, R. L., Garnick, M. B. et al.: Effects of oral contraceptives on the gallbladder bile in normal women. N. Engl. J. Med., 294:189, 1976.
51. Bennion, L. J., and Grundy, S. M.: Effects of obesity and caloric intake on biliary lipid metabolism in man. J. Clin. Invest., 56:996, 1975.
52. Bennion, L. J., and Grundy, S. M.: Risk factors for the development of cholelithiasis in man. N. Engl. J. Med., 299:116, 1978.
53. Bennion, L. J., Knowler, W. C., Mott, D. M., Spagnola, A. M., and Bennett, P. H.: Development of lithogenic bile during puberty in Pima Indians. N. Engl. J. Med., 300:873, 1979.
54. Boyle, J., and McLeod, M.: Pancreatic cancer presenting as pancreatitis of pregnancy. Am. J. Gastroenterol., 70:371, 1978.
55. Braverman, D. Z., Johnson, M. L., and Kern, F.: Effects of pregnancy and contraceptive steroids on gallbladder function. N. Engl. J. Med., 302:363, 1980.
56. Carey, M. C., and Small, D. M.: The physical chemistry of cholesterol solubility in bile: Relationship to gallstone formation and dissolution in man. J. Clin. Invest., 61:998, 1978.
57. Danzinger, R. G., Hoffmann, A. F., Thistle, J. L., and Schoenfield, L. J.: Effect of oral chenodeoxycholic acid on bile acid kinetics and biliary lipid composition in women with cholelithiasis. J. Clin. Invest., 52:2809, 1973.
58. Davis, R. A., Kern, F., Showalter, R., Sutherland, E., Sinesky, M., and Simon, F. R.: Alterations on hepatic Na^+, K^+-ATPase and bile flow by estrogen: Effects on liver surface membrane structure and function. Proc. Natl. Acad. Sci. USA, 75:4130, 1978.
59. Deitrick, J. E., McSherry, C. K., Javitt, N. B., et al.: Bile salt kinetics in the pregnant baboon: A new model for the study of gallbladder function. Gastroenterology, 65:536, 1973.
60. Dreiling, D., Bordalo, O., Rosenber, V., et al.: Pregnancy and pancreatitis. Am. J. Gastroenterol., 64:23, 1975.
61. Duane, W. C., and Hanson, K. C.: Role of gallbladder emptying and small bowel transit in regulation of bile acid pool size in man. J. Lab. Clin. Med., 92:858, 1978.
62. France, V. M., Menon, A., Reay, S. R., and Richardson, P. S.: The effect of 17 β-oestradiol on fluid transport in the in vitro guinea-pig gallbladder. J. Physiol. (Lond)., 286:67, 1977 (abstract).
63. Kammerer, W. S.: Nonobstetric surgery during pregnancy. Med. Clin. North Am., 63:1157, 1979.
64. LaMorte, W. N., Schoetz, D. J., Birkett, D. H., and Williams, L. F.: The role of the gallbladder in the pathogenesis of cholesterol gallstones. Gastroenterology, 77:580, 1979.
65. McCall, I. W., Desai, P., Serjeant, B. E., and Serjeant, G. R.: Cholelithiasis in Jamaican patients with homozygous sickle cell disease. Am. J. Hematol., 3:15, 1977.
66. Printen, K. J., and Ott, R. A.: Cholecystectomy during pregnancy. Am. Surg., 44:432, 1978.
67. Reyes, H., and Kern, F.: Effect of pregnancy on bile flow and biliary lipids in the hamster. Gastroenterology, 76:144, 1979.
68. Sarles, H., Crotte, C., Gerolami, A., et al.: The influence of

caloric intake and of dietary protein on the bile lipids. Scand. J. Gastroenterol., 6:189, 1971.

69. Shaffer, E. A., and Small, D. M.: Biliary lipid secretion in cholesterol gallstone disease: The effect of cholecystectomy and obesity. J. Clin. Invest., 59:828, 1977.

70. Smith, J. J., Pomarance, M. M., and Ivy, A. C.: The influence of pregnancy and sex hormones on gallbladder motility in the guinea pig. Am. J. Physiol., 132:129, 1941.

71. Sparkman, R. S.: Gallstones in young women. Ann. Surg., 145:813, 1957.

72. Wagner, C. I., Trotman, B. W., and Soloway, R. D.: Kinetic analysis of biliary lipid secretion in man and dog. J. Clin. Invest., 57:473, 1976.

73. Wilkinson, E.: Acute pancreatitis in pregnancy. Obstet. Gynecol. Surv., 28:281, 1973.

INFLAMMATORY BOWEL DISEASE

74. Abramson, D., Jankelson, I. R., and Milner, L. R.: Pregnancy in idiopathic ulcerative colitis. Am. J. Obstet. Gynecol., 61:121, 1951.

75. Ballard, P. L., Granberg, P., and Ballard, R.: Glucocorticoid level in maternal and cord sperm after prenatal betamethasone therapy to prevent respiratory distress syndrome. J. Clin. Invest., 56:1548, 1978.

76. Barnes, C. S., and Hayes, H. M.: Ulcerative colitis complicating pregnancy and the puerperium. Am. J. Obstet. Gynecol., 22:907, 1931.

77. Crohn, B. B., Varnis, H., et al.: Ulcerative colitis and pregnancy. Gastroenterology, 30:391, 1956.

78. DeDombal, F. T., Burton, I. L., and Goligher, J. C.: Crohn's disease and pregnancy. Br. Med. J., 3:550, 1972.

79. DeDombal, F. T., Watts, J. M., Watkinson, G., and Goligher, J. C.: Ulcerative colitis and pregnancy. Lancet, 2:599, 1965.

80. Fielding, J. F., and Cooke, W. T.: Pregnancy and Crohn's Disease. Br. Med. J., 2:76, 1970.

81. Homan, W. P., and Thorbjarnarson, B.: Crohn's disease and pregnancy. Arch Surg., 111:545, 1976.

82. Jarnerot, G., and Into-Malmberg, M. B.: Sulfasalazine treatment during breast feeding. Scand. J. Gastroenterol., 14:869, 1979.

83. Levi, A. J., Fisher, A. M., et al.: Male infertility due to sulfa-salazine. Lancet, 2:276, 1979.

84. MacDougall, I.: Ulcerative colitis and pregnancy. Lancet, 2:641, 1956.

85. Mogadam, M., Dobbins, W. O., Korelitz, B. I., and Ahmed S. W.: Pregnancy in inflammatory bowel disease: Effect of sulfa-salazine and corticosteroids on fetal outcome. Gastroenterology, 80:72, 1981.

86. Physicians' Desk Reference, 34th ed. Oradell, N. J., Medical Economics Co., 1980, pp. 1379–80.

87. Toth, A.: Male infertility due to sulfasalazine. Lancet, 2:904, 1979.

88. Vender, R. J., and Spiro, H. M.: Inflammatory bowel disease and pregnancy: A review of the literature. J. Clin. Gastroenterol. (in press).

89. Willoughby, C. P., and Truelove, S. C.: Ulcerative colitis and pregnancy. Gut, 21:469, 1980.

DISORDERED BOWEL FUNCTION

90. Brodribb, J., Condon, R. E., Cowles, V., and DeCosse, J. J.: Influence of dietary fiber on transit time, fecal composition and myoelectrical activity of the primate right colon. Dig. Dis. Sci., 25:260, 1980.

91. Burkitt, D. P., Walter, A. R. P., and Painter, N. S.: Effect of dietary fiber on stools and transition times, and its role in the causation of disease. Lancet, 2:1408, 1972.

92. Cumming, J. H., Jenkins, D. J. A., and Wiggins, H. S.: Measurement of mean transit time of dietary residue through the human gut. Gut, 17:210, 1976.

93. Kuman, D.: In vitro inhibitory effect of progesterone on extra-uterine human smooth musculature. Am. J. Obstet. Gynecol., 84:1300, 1962.

94. Levy, N., Lemberg, E., and Sharf, M.: Bowel habit in pregnancy. Digestion, 4:216, 1971.

95. Martelli, H., Devroede, G., Arhan, P., and Dugay, C.: Mechanisms of idiopathic constipations: Outlet obstruction. Gastroenterology, 75:623, 1978.

96. Martelli, H., Devroede, G., Arhan, P., Dugay, C., Dornic, C., and Faverdin, C.: Some parameters of large bowel motility in normal man. Gastroenterology, 75:612, 1978.

12

Harold J. Fallon, M.D.

LIVER DISEASES

The effects of pregnancy on normal liver function are substantial. Although these changes are reversible, they often confront the physician with difficulty in distinguishing those patients with liver disease. This is especially important because of the improved treatment of patients with chronic liver diseases, resulting in more frequent pregnancies in this group.

Most of the common forms of acute and chronic liver diseases occur during pregnancy and often present special difficulties in diagnosis and management. In addition, there is a group of liver disorders relatively unique to pregnancy, which also must be identified and managed appropriately. The implications of these various disorders for the fetus and the mother are diverse and mandate precision in diagnosis.

The changes in liver function related to pregnancy will be reviewed initially, followed by a description of the major forms of liver disease specifically associated with pregnancy. The common liver diseases that complicate pregnancy will then be described and a practical approach to the patient with liver abnormalities proposed.

THE EFFECTS OF PREGNANCY ON THE LIVER

Anatomic Changes

A substantial increase in liver weight occurs during pregnancy in the experimental animal, but a corresponding enlargement in the human has not been documented. Although liver size is difficult to estimate clinically, especially in late pregnancy when displacement is caused by uterine enlargement, a review of autopsy records of women dying during pregnancy failed to show any substantial increase in liver weight in comparison with a nonpregnant control group.[24] Therefore, it seems unlikely that pregnancy causes enlargement of the human liver, and the latter size is strong evidence for the presence of liver disease.

Minor histologic changes have been reported in human liver during pregnancy. In a series of liver biopsies reported in 1945, variations in size and shape of the hepatocytes, occasional lympocytic infiltrations in the portal area, and variable increases in glycogen and fat were noted.[57] These minimal findings are nonspecific and may be seen in apparently healthy nonpregnant women. Administration of estrogens or oral contraceptives is also unaccompanied by significant histologic or electron microscopic alterations except in patients who develop obvious clinical and laboratory evidence of cholestasis in response to these agents.

Physiology

Hepatic blood flow is maintained in pregnancy despite marked changes in the cardiovascular system. An increase in plasma and blood volume of 50 per cent or more and a rise in cardiac output of up to 50 per cent occur during pregnancy. These changes are maximum at the beginning of the third trimester. Nevertheless, hepatic blood flow is unaltered, resulting in a decline in the proportion of cardiac output delivered to the liver of approximately 35 per cent.[46] The relative decrease in hepatic blood flow may contribute to the reduction in clearance of various compounds from blood, especially during the latter half of pregnancy.

Liver Function in Pregnancy

Protein Metabolism. Significant changes occur in the synthesis, catabolism, and serum concentration of various plasma proteins during pregnancy. Virtually all serum proteins known to be synthesized in liver are affected by pregnancy or by the administration of estrogens to nonpreg-

278

nant females. The total serum protein concentration declines approximately 20 per cent in mid-pregnancy, an effect largely attributed to the substantial decline in serum albumin. There is a small increase in the alpha and beta globulin fractions and a slight decline in gamma globulin. A portion of the decrease in serum albumin may be attributed to simple dilution caused by the increase in total blood volume, although an increase in albumin catabolism without a compensating increase in synthesis has also been described in pregnancy.[52] Dilution cannot explain the variable changes in the several globulin fractions, and their mechanism remains unexplained. The hepatic parenchymal cell is not the site of globulin biosynthesis, and therefore other tissues are probably involved in the serum globulin alterations during pregnancy.

A significant rise in serum fibrinogen regularly accompanies pregnancy. Experimental evidence suggests that this is a consequence of increased fibrinogen synthesis.[99] Similarly, administration of estrogens or combined estrogen and progestin preparations to human beings induces a rise in serum fibrinogen levels. Other coagulation protein, including factors VII, VIII, IX, and X, may be increased in pregnancy or following estrogen treatment. The prothrombin time is normal in pregnancy, but fibronolytic activity is slightly reduced.

Several other serum proteins synthesized in liver are altered in pregnancy. Ceruloplasmin levels gradually increase, reaching a maximum at term.[106a] Estrogens stimulate a similar increase in serum ceruloplasmin concentrations. In some pregnant patients with Wilson's disease, the level of ceruloplasmin has been reported to increase to nearly normal values.[125] In such patients, pregnancy is often associated with improvement in the symptoms of Wilson's disease and a reduction in the requirement for therapy.[26] However, this may be a result of distribution of copper to the fetus rather than a consequence of a rise in the serum ceruloplasmin level in such patients.

Transferrin levels are increased in the last trimester but are not affected by estrogen administration. An increase in serum binding capacity for thyroxin, vitamin D, folate, corticosteroid, and testosterone also occurs in pregnancy, affecting the serum concentration of these hormones. These changes are attributed to increased levels of specific binding proteins and have been reported following estrogen administration to nonpregnant women. Serum haptoglobin levels are decreased following estrogen administration, possibly accounting for the higher concentration of haptoglobin in males. Pregnancy does not alter haptoglobin concentration.

Bilirubin. A slight rise in serum bilirubin has been reported in a small number (approximately 5 per cent) of otherwise normal pregnancies. However, other studies have failed to document significant bilirubin elevation in the absence of specific cause during normal pregnancy.[46] Therefore, an increased serum bilirubin in pregnancy should be considered evidence for the presence of liver or hematologic disease.

Pregnanediol and 5β-pregnane-3α,20β-diol are competitive inhibitors of glucuronyltransferase in vitro. Excretion of the latter hormone in human milk has been associated with hyperbilirubinemia in infants. However, the significance of such compounds in clinical jaundice in the mother during pregnancy has not been proved. There is evidence that elevated maternal unconjugated bilirubin, from whatever cause, may be transferred to the fetus.[76]

Sulfobromophthalein. Significant changes in sulfobromophthalein (BSP) metabolism occur in normal pregnancy.[24] Although BSP retention in serum 45 minutes after intravenous administration is usually within the normal range, both uptake and excretion are altered. The relative storage capacity for BSP is increased twofold in the latter half of pregnancy, but maximal tubular excretory rate (Tm) into bile is decreased 27 per cent. It is likely that these changes in BSP excretion are mediated by hormonal events in late pregnancy and are quickly reversible following delivery. Increased plasma binding of BSP in pregnancy has also been noted, although the mechanism of this change and its relationship to the alterations in BSP metabolism are unknown. There is evidence that the BSP removal rate is more rapid in the presence of hypoalbuminemia,[45] a common alteration in pregnancy.

Serum Enzymes. Total serum alkaline phosphatase is regularly elevated during pregnancy. The rise is modest during the first half of pregnancy but accelerates rapidly in the third trimester, reaching a peak of nearly two to four times normal at term. The source of the elevation in alkaline phosphatase appears to be the placenta, as established by differential inhibition studies, gel electrophoresis, heat stability determination, and immunochemical techniques. The portion of total serum alkaline phosphatase derived from placenta increases from less than 10 per cent in the first month of pregnancy to over 50 per cent at the time of delivery. The placental phosphatase decreases rapidly after delivery, reaching normal levels about 20 days post partum.[147] A pattern of decreasing placental alkaline phosphatase during the last trimester has been associated with fetal death in utero.[128]

The serum alkaline phosphatase may be increased in nonpregnant females by administration of estradiol or estriol in amounts corresponding to those found during pregnancy.[85] It is obvious that the phosphatase under these conditions is not of placental origin and is probably derived from the liver. The major sources of serum alkaline phosphatase in normal persons are liver, bone, and intestine.[65, 94] Liver alkaline phosphatase production is stimulated by a variety of injuries to the canalicular membrane, including mechanical bile duct obstruction and intrahepatic cholestasis. Estrogens may produce the latter type of injury.[122] This possibility is supported by observations that serum 5'-nucleotidase, a more specific indicator of canalicular membrane disturbance, is also increased in some women receiving estrogens.[71, 72]

The serum gamma-glutamyl-transpeptidase (GGPT) is an enzyme that is regularly elevated in cholestasis and hepatocellular injury. It is increased during the third trimester of pregnancy and is not useful as an indicator of liver injury during this time.[21] Serum lactic dehydrogenase and ornithine transcarbamylase are also increased near term.

In contrast to these serum enzyme changes, it is noteworthy that serum glutamic oxaloacetic transaminase (ASP or SGOT) and serum glutamic pyruvic transaminase (ALT or SGPT) are only slightly altered by normal pregnancy. Although both may rise near term, the increase is usually within the normal range.[109] Therefore, these two serum enzyme determinations are especially useful as sensitive indications of liver or other organ damage during pregnancy.

Serum Lipids. A substantial increase in the serum concentration of the major lipid classes occurs during pregnancy and is most marked at term.[130] Inhibition of postheparin esterase activity and lipoprotein lipase occurs in late pregnancy with a rapid return to normal following delivery.[36] These effects may be attributable to estrogenic compounds, which are known to reduce lipoprotein lipase activity in nonpregnant females. In addition, there is evidence that estrogens accelerate hepatic triglyceride biosynthesis.

Although the elevation in serum triglyceride may be quantitatively the most marked, the rise in serum cholesterol may cause the greatest confusion in the differential diagnosis of suspected liver disease. The upper limit of normal for cholesterol during the last trimester of pregnancy is approximately double the normal limit for

nonpregnant women of the same age. Therefore, hypercholesterolemia cannot be taken as evidence of cholestasis during pregnancy. The changes in serum lipid constituents are a consequence of corresponding increases in low density lipoproteins and very low density lipoproteins.

Porphyrins. There are minor changes in porphyrin metabolism during pregnancy.[70] Total urine coproporphyrin excretion may be increased slightly, but there is a marked decrease in urinary excretion of the coproporphyrin III isomer and a relative increase in the coproporphyrin I isomer. Porphobilinogen excretion is normal, but δ-aminolevulinic acid excretion is increased in about one half of women with normal pregnancies.

A summary of the major biochemical changes in liver function during pregnancy is shown in Table 12–1.

Effects of Female Sex Hormones on Liver Function

Several authors have reviewed the effects of the anabolic steroids, estrogens, progestins, and oral contraceptives on liver structure and function.[4, 122] Each of these classes of agents has significant and somewhat different effects on the liver. However, their role in mediating the physi-

TABLE 12–1 LIVER FUNCTION TESTS IN NORMAL PREGNANCY

Test	Effects	Period of Maximum Change *Trimester*
Albumin	↓ 20 per cent	second
γ-globulin	nl to sl ↓	third
α-globulin	sl ↑	third
β-globulin	sl ↑	third
Fibrinogen	↑ 50 per cent	second
Ceruloplasmin	↑	third
Transferrin	↑	third
Bilirubin	nl to sl ↑	third
BSP	nl to sl ↑	third
Alkaline phosphatase	2- to 4-fold ↑	third
Lactic dehydrogenase	sl ↑	third
SGOT	nl	—
SGPT	nl	—
GGTP	↑	third
Cholesterol	2-fold ↑	third

nl — normal
sl — slight
↑ — increase
↓ — decrease

ologic and biochemical alterations associated with normal pregnancy or in mediating the liver diseases specifically related to pregnancy is not clear.

Many of these natural and synthetic hormones produce variable degrees of cholestasis. Cholestasis is defined as centrilobular bile stasis associated with dilation of the canaliculi and loss of the normal microvillus structure of the canaliculus as seen by electron microscopy. The biochemical changes of cholestasis are extremely variable but usually include increases in the serum level of alkaline phosphatase, 5'-nucleotidase, GGTP, bile acids, and occasionally bilirubin. In addition, disturbances in the biliary clearance of such compounds as BSP are common.

The anabolic steroids most likely to cause significant cholestasis are those containing a methyl or ethyl group in the C-17 position. Virtually all these agents cause BSP retention, primarily as a result of defective BSP transport into bile. The relative storage capacity for this compound remains normal. Many of these compounds cause a small rise in SGOT (ASP) without histologic evidence of hepatocellular injury and apparently unrelated to the degree of BSP retention. Much less commonly, alkaline phosphatase, lactic dehydrogenase, and serum bilirubin may be elevated. Intrahepatic cholestasis with anatomic changes limited to the canalicular membrane and sparing most of the intracellular organelles is characteristic of this class of drugs.

Progesterone, in contrast, causes proliferation of the smooth endoplasmic reticulum and an increase in cytochrome P450 in rats. The rise in mixed function oxidase activity is preceded by an increase in δ-aminolevulinic acid synthetase and corresponds to a similar effect of such drugs as phenobarbital. The progestins have no effect on BSP metabolism, and cholestasis is not produced.

Estrogens and drugs with estrogenic activity may produce cholestasis, occasional hepatocellular necrosis, and a decreased clearance of bilirubin. In contrast to the progestational agents, the estrogens increase hepatic rough endoplasmic reticulum and accelerate the associated synthesis of proteins. The estrogens frequently elevate serum alkaline phosphatase activity and decrease the Tm for BSP transport into bile. Bile flow may also be reduced, and the maximum bilirubin secretion rate is impaired.

The possible role of hormones in the production of cholestatic jaundice of pregnancy and other forms of liver injury in pregnancy is considered later.

LIVER DISEASES OF PREGNANCY

Cholestasis of Pregnancy

This disorder has been called recurrent jaundice of pregnancy, cholestatic jaundice of pregnancy, jaundice of late pregnancy, hepatosis of pregnancy, and intrahepatic cholestasis of pregnancy. The syndrome originally described consisted of pruritus and mild jaundice appearing in Swedish women during the last trimester of pregnancy.[136] Subsequently, the disease has been recognized in various parts of the world, in different racial groups, and in the absence of clinical jaundice. However, the frequency may be higher among Scandinavian and Chilean women, in whom cholestasis complicates as many as 2.4 per cent of pregnancies.[97] There is apparent hereditary predisposition to this syndrome in Sweden, since 18 to 44 per cent of affected women give a history of relatives with similar symptoms during pregnancy.[40, 47]

Jaundice and Pruritus. The subsequent course of the original reported cases has shown that 15 of the 27 multiparous women with cholestasis of pregnancy have had jaundice or pruritus during subsequent pregnancies, and 3 women during several pregnancies.[40, 101] Therefore, the syndrome is not always recurrent. Other reports have described the onset of cholestasis before the last trimester in 25 per cent of patients and rarely in early pregnancy.[40, 46, 101] Since there are no clinical or biochemical features that distinguish these cases appearing early in pregnancy or in a single pregnancy, the term cholestatic jaundice of pregnancy has been preferred by many authors. However, it is evident that many patients with this disorder present with pruritus and chemical evidence of cholestasis but without jaundice.[62] The general term cholestasis of pregnancy most accurately reflects the diversity of this syndrome.

Characteristically, the disorder is heralded by the onset of pruritus at the beginning of the third trimester. Pruritus remains the dominant and most disturbing feature of cholestasis of pregnancy. The symptom may become very severe if untreated and may involve the trunk and the extremities, including the palms and the soles of the feet. Insomnia, fatigue, and mental disturbance often accompany the pruritus. In many cases, the pruritus is followed in 1 to 2 weeks by the onset of mild jaundice, dark urine, and light colored stools.

The duration of the syndrome varies from 1 to 33 weeks, depending on the time of onset. Both the pruritus and jaundice begin to clear shortly after delivery, although pruritus is usually the first symptom to remit completely, most often within 24 hours. Throughout the duration of the syndrome, the patient generally feels well, and there is no fever, anorexia, nausea, vomiting, diarrhea, or arthralgia. Abdominal pain is usually absent, although some patients complain of vague right upper quadrant discomfort. However, there is a significantly increased incidence of emesis in early pregnancy among patients with cholestasis of pregnancy, suggesting that the underlying metabolic abnormality exists throughout pregnancy.[62] Physical examination is unremarkable except for evidence of scratching. In one series, an increased prior history of gall bladder disease and drug reactions was observed in patients with cholestasis of pregnancy.

The syndrome may recur during each subsequent pregnancy, or it may appear only once or in some, but not all, pregnancies. Furthermore, pruritus may be the only manifestation in one pregnancy, but both pruritus and jaundice may appear in others.[40] The explanation for this variation in presentation is unknown.

Histologic Features. The histologic appearance of the liver is characteristic of simple cholestasis. The centrilobular canaliculi are dilated and many contain bile plugs. There is mild Kupffer cell proliferation, and often PAS-positive granules are seen in macrophages. There are no hepatocellular changes, and the portal areas are entirely normal. Electron microscopy of the liver shows swelling, distortion, and atrophy of the canalicular microvilli.[3, 47] In some areas, the parenchymal cells have enlarged and irregular mitochondria. The histologic and other changes seen under electron microscopy do not seem to be progressive during the pregnancy, and repeat liver biopsy taken some months after delivery no longer reveals any abnormalities.[3]

There is no apparent correlation between the severity of the pathologic findings and the clinical symptoms of the disorder.

Biochemical Changes. The biochemical changes noted are those of cholestasis and are outlined in Table 12–2. The serum alkaline phosphatase increases to values significantly higher than those observed during normal pregnancy. Values seven to ten times normal are not unusual. In contrast to the other biochemical changes, the rise in serum alkaline phosphatase may persist or further increase after delivery. Serum 5'-nucleotidase levels are also increased in cholestasis of pregnancy, indicating that the rise in alkaline phosphatase in this syndrome is more likely of hepatic than of placental origin. The rise in alkaline phosphatase is entirely of placental origin in normal pregnancy.

The serum bilirubin is elevated in many patients, but the increase is usually less than 5 mg per 100 ml and is virtually never above 10 mg per 100 ml. The bilirubin is almost entirely of the direct-reacting fraction, and consequently bilirubinuria occurs. Urobilinogen is never absent from the urine and is either normal or moderately increased in amount. The serum protein changes noted in normal pregnancy — i.e., a decrease in albumin and γ-globulin, a slight rise in α_1- and α_2-globulins, and a greater rise in β-globulin — are somewhat exaggerated but not qualitatively different.[38] Prothrombin time is usually normal except when jaundice appears early in pregnancy and malabsorption of fat-soluble vitamins occurs. The prothrombin time responds quickly to parenteral administration of vitamin K in this latter group.

The serum transaminases may be normal, as in uncomplicated pregnancy, or moderately increased. Values of SGOT or SGPT are usually

TABLE 12–2 CHOLESTASIS OF PREGNANCY

Clinical Features	Biochemical Changes	
Pruritus	Alkaline phosphatase	7- to 10-fold ↑
Jaundice*	5'-Nucleotidase	2-fold ↑
	Bilirubin (total)	nl to 5 mg per 100 ml
No anorexia or malaise	SGOT	< 250 units
Emesis first trimester*	BSP	10–25 per cent retention
Last trimester onset*	Prothrombin time	nl to 2-fold ↑
Recurrent*	Serum bile acids	10-to 100-fold
Familial*	Cholesterol	2- to 4-fold ↑
	Triglyceride	nl to 2-fold↑

*These clinical features are not invariably present.
nl — normal
sl — slight
↑ — increase
↓ — decrease

less than 250 Sigma units, although occasional values up to 1000 units have been reported. The latter situation is clearly unusual and may cause confusion with viral hepatitis. Diagnosis in such cases would depend upon immunologic markers of acute viral hepatitis or liver biopsy.

Serum lipids are commonly altered but are substantially elevated only in those with severe disease.[47, 62, 131] The large variation in serum cholesterol in the last trimester of normal pregnancy often precludes any interpretation of hypercholesterolemia in this syndrome. Lipoprotein-X, usually associated with cholestasis of any cause, is frequently raised in cholestasis of pregnancy.

BSP retention is always observed. Usually the retention at 45 minutes varies between 10 and 25 per cent, considerably higher than the minimal elevation reported occasionally in normal pregnancy. A depression in BSP storage capacity and Tm is observed in patients manifesting pruritus alone as well as in those with both jaundice and pruritus. This provides support for the suggestion that jaundice is but one facet of the syndrome and need not always be present. The changes in BSP metabolism quickly revert to normal after delivery.

Serum bile acid levels are regularly increased in cholestasis of pregnancy.[33, 82a] Increases range from 10- to 100-fold, and there is a rise in serum cholic acid as well as in chenodeoxycholic and deoxycholic acids. Presumably, the major symptom of this disease, pruritus, is related to the deposition of bile acids in the skin. Therapy aimed at lowering serum and tissue bile acid levels is often successful in correcting the pruritus.

Coproporphyrin excretion is increased in this syndrome, but the excretion of coproporphyrin III isomer is markedly decreased.[70] δ-Aminolevulinic acid excretion is increased above that observed in normal pregnancy.

The mechanism of cholestasis is not entirely clear, although several lines of evidence suggest an unusual sensitivity to the rise in estrogenic hormones during pregnancy. Estriol metabolism has been studied in patients with cholestasis of pregnancy, and abnormalities in the excretion of estriol metabolites have been observed. Urinary estriol glucuronide is depressed, and the sulfate conjugate is increased. Biliary excretion of estriol is also markedly diminished. These changes may be a reflection of the cholestasis and a reduced biliary excretion of estrogen rather than contributors to the pathogenesis of the disorder. However, the frequent observation that patients with this syndrome may develop similar clinical symptoms and biochemical changes following administration of oral contraceptives strongly incriminates female sex hormones in the development of the cholestasis.[71, 72, 137] As noted earlier, some of these hormones may cause abnormalities of biliary excretion in normal and nonpregnant women. Despite these observations, not all patients with cholestasis are susceptible to recurrence when estrogens are administered after delivery,[97] and the precise relationship of the cholestasis to such hormones remains obscure.

Diagnosis. The most common disorders that are confused with cholestasis of pregnancy are cholestatic viral hepatitis, cholestatic drug reaction, primary biliary cirrhosis, biliary tract disease, and acute fatty liver of pregnancy. Diagnosis is based on the clinical history, laboratory findings, abdominal ultrasonography, and, when necessary, the histologic findings at liver biopsy.

Laboratory studies may be useful in diagnosis because serum transaminase levels are usually much higher in viral hepatitis, and elevations in immunoglobulin (IgM) and mitochondrial antibodies are characteristic of primary biliary cirrhosis. In many reviews, cholestasis of pregnancy has been reported as the second most common cause of jaundice pregnancy. In one series, it accounted for more than 50 per cent of the cases of liver abnormality in the last trimester.[46] The disease bears no relationship to benign recurrent cholestasis, which may appear in males and females and is not worsened by pregnancy.

Effects on the Mother. The major effects of cholestasis of pregnancy on the mother are those related to the discomfort of the pruritus, the occasional occurrence of coagulation abnormalities related to impaired Vitamin K absorption, and difficulty in distinguishing this syndrome from other cases of cholestasis. Maternal mortality and spontaneous abortion are not increased by cholestasis of pregnancy. In one series postpartum hemorrhage was most frequent, presumably as a result of vitamin K deficiency. Recognition of the characteristic features of the syndrome is important in distinguishing this form of cholestasis from other common conditions, including biliary tract disease, cholestatic drug reactions, cholestatic viral hepatitis, and primary biliary cirrhosis.

Effects on the Fetus. Several reviews have reported an increased incidence of prematurity and fetal death in patients with cholestasis of pregnancy.[40, 47, 124] The incidence of premature labor varied from 33 to 87 per cent, and the fetal mortality ranged from 6 to 40 per cent. However, another series does not record an increase in either prematurity or fetal mortality.[62] Most likely the severity of the syndrome and the health of the mother affect the incidence of these complications.

Treatment. Therapy is directed at lowering serum and skin bile acid levels and thereby alleviating the pruritus. This can usually be achieved with cholestyramine resin given daily in three doses of 4 gm each as a liquid suspension. The pruritus usually is relieved promptly but recurs in 1 to 2 days if the drug is discontinued. Cholestyramine should not be given in conjunction with other medications because of the nonspecific anion-binding capacity of the resin. Side effects are minimal at this dose, but mild nausea, anorexia, bloating, or constipation may occur. Steatorrhea and malabsorption of fat-soluble vitamins do not customarily appear unless doses over 20 to 30 gm per day are given. Nonetheless, prothrombin time should be monitored because of the possible effects of cholestasis itself on vitamin K absorption. Parenteral vitamin K therapy should be given near term in mothers with steatorrhea and prolonged prothrombin time. No other form of therapy is indicated in these patients, and induction of labor is not recommended.[47] It is advisable for women with this syndrome to avoid oral contraceptives, unless they are aware of the possibility of recurrence.

Acute Fatty Liver of Pregnancy

This rare and often fatal liver disease was first associated with pregnancy by Sheehan in 1940. Over 60 cases have been reported with an overall mortality rate of approximately 85 per cent. The incidence appears higher in first pregnancies, but it has been reported after multiple pregnancies and at all ages in the childbearing period.

Clinical Course. The disease begins abruptly, usually in the 36th to 40th week of pregnancy. A few cases have been reported as early as 30 weeks, and the onset of symptoms may be delayed until after delivery.[47] Severe and persistent vomiting is usually followed by abdominal pain and then jaundice.[82a, 115] Tachycardia is common, and about one half of patients develop significant fever. Many patients present with features suggestive of pre-eclampsia, including hypertension and proteinuria. Disseminated intravascular coagulation also has been reported in these patients. Somnolence, followed by coma, often appears 1 to 2 weeks after onset but may occur as early as the third day or may be delayed for a month or more. Survivors usually begin to im-

prove shortly after the birth of a dead fetus; however, fetal survival is possible.[146] It is of interest that survivors may be delivered of normal infants in subsequent entirely uncomplicated pregnancies.[15]

Histologic Changes. The histologic findings are characteristic and consist of marked fatty infiltration of the hepatocytes, often with relative sparing of the periportal areas and absence of necrosis or inflammatory cell infiltration (Fig. 12–1). The portal triad is unaffected, but bile plugs are often seen in the central areas.[32, 46] Several authors have reported cases of acute fatty liver of pregnancy presenting with this histologic picture but with massive or submassive pericentral necrosis as well.[26, 63] It is not certain whether the spectrum of this disease occasionally includes necrosis or whether some additional process such as hypotension, passive congestion, or drug reaction has occurred during the course of illness in these patients. Such cases might also represent the coincidence of acute fatty liver of pregnancy with subacute hepatic necrosis due to viral hepatitis, although there is no evidence to support this possibility. In one patient who survived the disease, repeat liver biopsy at several intervals after the onset of illness showed remarkably rapid removal of the fat beginning at the periphery of the lobule.[32] The liver biopsy was normal 37 days after the onset of liver failure. Electron microscopy shows mild cystic changes in the smooth endoplasmic reticulum and mitochondrial alterations.[139]

A number of other organ systems have shown histologic changes, often associated with clinical manifestations. The pancreas, central nervous system, bone marrow, and proximal tubule of the kidney may be involved with vacuolar changes.[32, 48, 84, 108, 145] Acute renal failure, disseminated intravascular coagulation, or acute hemorrhagic pancreatitis may be the immediate cause of death or may be a contributing factor. Since many patients with this disorder are eclamptic, the histologic features of eclampsia may be superimposed on the fatty changes. The term acute fatty liver of pregnancy merely describes the most obvious pathologic finding in this disorder, and certainly it is to be preferred to the erroneous designation acute yellow atrophy. The cause of the syndrome remains unexplained at present. Several authors have noted certain similarities between fatty liver of pregnancy and Reye's syndrome, which appears most often in childhood.[14] However, differences in ultrastructure, serum amino acid levels, and enzymatic changes in the liver distinguish the two syndromes.[139]

Laboratory Values. The laboratory changes in acute fatty liver are extremely variable. Most patients develop jaundice, but the bilirubin elevation is usually below 10 mg per 100 ml. Rarely, values above 25 mg per 100 ml have been recorded. The alkaline phosphatase level is elevated above that of normal pregnancy, and the SGOT is most often increased in the range of 300 to 500

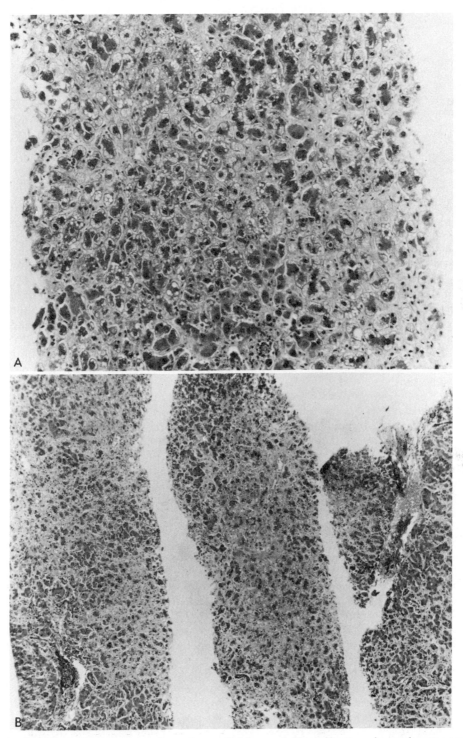

FIGURE 12–1. Fatty liver of pregnancy as shown by needle biopsy. *A,* The infiltration of many hepatocytes with small droplets of fat is well shown. These droplets stained positively with a Sudan stain for lipid. *B,* The predominance of the infiltration in pericentral areas is shown. There is relative sparing of the peripheral and periportal areas of the lobule. (Courtesy of Dr. G. Klatskin.)

TABLE 12–3   ACUTE FATTY LIVER OF PREGNANCY

Clinical Features	Biochemical Changes	
Abrupt onset	Bilirubin	< 10 mg per 100 ml
Vomiting	Alkaline phosphatase	sl ↑
Abdominal pain	SGOT	300–500 units
Jaundice	Prothrombin time	2- to 5-fold ↑
Fever, coma*	Leukocytes	20,000–30,000 cells per cu mm
Pre-eclampsia*	Serum glucose	↓
36th–40th weeks	Arterial ammonia	↑
Bleeding*	Serum amino acids	↓

*Indicates clinical findings that are most variable.
nl — normal
sl — slight
↑ — increase
↓ — decrease

units per ml. The prothrombin time is markedly prolonged (usually greater than 25 seconds), and polymorphonuclear leukocytosis with counts of 20,000 to 30,000 cells per cu mm is common. In contrast to the hyperaminoacidemia reported in hepatic encephalopathy due to cirrhosis or fulminant hepatitis, generalized hypoaminoacidemia is reported in fatty liver of pregnancy.[139] Severe hypoglycemia[14] and marked elevation in arterial ammonia contribute to the deep coma. Shock, acidosis, and renal failure may also influence the neurologic state. The clinical and laboratory findings in this syndrome are listed in Table 12–3.

Effects on Mother and Fetus. The maternal mortality rate is extremely high and varies between 65 and 90 per cent. Infant mortality is only slightly less because many infants are delivered promptly by cesarean section. There are no long-term effects on either mother or infant if they survive the acute disease.

Treatment. Correct diagnosis in this setting is essential to appropriate therapy. Although laboratory findings are suggestive, liver biopsy, when possible, is definitive. The use of fresh frozen plasma may permit biopsy in cases with coagulopathy.

Since survival is possible, careful attention to the details of medical care is imperative. Maintenance of a normal serum glucose level and correction of electrolyte imbalance take precedence. Airway should be maintained, hypertension managed, gastrointestinal hemorrhage controlled with blood transfusions, and clotting abnormalities corrected with fresh frozen plasma. Most authors recommend immediate delivery of the fetus by cesarean section as soon as the essential functions in the mother are restored, because of the rapid clinical deterioration that frequently accompanies spontaneous vaginal delivery. Too few cases have been reported to establish the effectiveness of these recommendations, but in view of the potential complete reversibility of the syndrome,[15, 32, 108] aggressive efforts to support vital functions seem indicated.

Tetracycline-Induced Fatty Liver of Pregnancy. This entity was first described in 1963,[110] although cases may have appeared earlier. A histologic picture and clinical course identical with that of acute fatty liver of pregnancy has been associated with intravenous administration of excessive doses of tetracycline (2.4 to 4.0 gm per day). All the initial patients died in coma within 5 to 13 days. The typical pericentral fatty changes, and an absence of hepatocellular necrosis or inflammatory exudate within the liver, were noted at autopsy. In subsequent reports, both pancreatitis and renal failure have been associated with tetracycline-induced fatty liver.[107] Tetracycline is known to inhibit hepatic protein synthesis and results in fat deposition in the liver. It is possible that this effect is exaggerated during pregnancy.

In contrast to the usual cases of acute fatty liver of pregnancy, the fatty liver associated with tetracycline administration in large intravenous doses may occur in nonpregnant women as well.[27, 92] In such cases, 1 to 3 gm tetracycline were given intravenously and the patients developed fatty infiltration of the liver, pancreatitis, and necrosis of the proximal renal tubule. The changes in liver chemistries, amylase, and urea nitrogen resembled those reported in pregnant women with fatty liver.

Since the clinical symptoms, laboratory changes, and course of this disorder are identical to those of acute fatty liver of pregnancy, the recommendations regarding therapy are the same. Obviously, this disorder is preventable if tetracycline is administered in appropriate oral doses or if alternative antibiotics are given.

PRE-ECLAMPSIA AND ECLAMPSIA

The liver may be involved in eclampsia or pre-eclampsia as a part of the generalized vascular disorder. The incidence of liver function changes in eclampsia has been estimated as less than 50 per cent, and marked functional change is usually associated with severe or fatal disease.[46, 56] However, liver injury seems more common if disseminated intravascular coagulation accompanies the eclampsia or pre-eclampsia.[69, 78] The true incidence of this complication is not clear, but it may be frequently overlooked. In addition to biochemical changes in liver function, hepatic rupture, hemorrhage, and death may occur.[18, 19, 82]

Typically, a patient in the last trimester presents with onset of hypertension and proteinuria. Nausea and vomiting occur as well as moderate to severe epigastric pain. Occasionally, frank jaundice may appear.

The physical findings in these patients include those common to pre-eclampsia and eclampsia, but in addition, tender hepatomegaly is common. Splenomegaly, ascites, and peripheral signs of chronic liver disease do not occur. The coma and convulsions of eclampsia should not be confused with hepatic encephalopathy, which has not been reported with eclampsia.

The liver function changes associated with pre-eclampsia and eclampsia consist of an elevation in alkaline phosphatase and a rise in SGOT, which may be modest but in some cases reaches more than 1000 IU/ml. The extent of these functional changes usually parallels the clinical course, and a rapid fall is indicative of a good prognosis. Bilirubin elevation occurs in about 10 per cent of patients with eclampsia and is usually mild (<6 mg per ml).[78] In patients with jaundice, hemolysis has been considered a major contributing factor. The hemolysis is often accompanied by disseminated intravascular coagulation under these conditions. Therefore, the presence of jaundice is an indication for appropriate diagnostic studies of these two complications.

The histologic changes in the liver resemble those reported for other tissues in eclampsia. They are very different from those of fulminant hepatitis or fatty liver of pregnancy. Fibrin thrombi are seen in the hepatic sinusoids, occasionally associated with surrounding focal necrosis of liver cells. Hemorrhagic necrosis may

appear in severe or fatal cases and probably predisposes to the hepatic hemorrhage or rupture occasionally reported in eclampsia. Inflammatory exudate is absent, but when shock occurs, massive centrilobular necrosis may be found at autopsy.

Treatment of the disorder must be directed at the pre-eclampsia and eclampsia rather than the often mild and freely reversible hepatic lesion. In the more severe cases complicated by disseminated intravascular coagulation, prompt delivery is recommended. Reversal of hypertension, proteinuria, and liver derangement usually begins 12 to 24 hours after delivery. It is important to monitor any eclamptic patient carefully for evidence of hepatic hemorrhage, a serious but potentially correctable complication.

Hepatic Rupture and Hematoma

As noted in the section on eclampsia, hepatic rupture during pregnancy commonly occurs in the setting of hypertension and proteinuria[12,86] and often with frank toxemia. The patients almost regularly complain of severe epigastric or right upper quadrant pain, and they present abruptly with unexplained shock. Rupture usually occurs in the last trimester or shortly after delivery and is accompanied by hemoperitoneum. In some cases, abdominal trauma or convulsions have been considered as contributing factors, but this is not uniform. Disseminated intravascular coagulation has recently been recognized in approximately 10 per cent of eclamptic patients, and it is postulated that this complication contributes to hematoma formation and rupture. Subcapsular hematoma without rupture has also been recognized in this setting and is presumed to be a direct precursor of rupture.

The clinical findings of rupture include shock, oliguria, fever, and leukocytosis. Abdominal ultrasound often defines an intrahepatic hematoma in these patients. Diagnosis of rupture is confirmed by peritoneal aspiration of blood, and immediate surgical intervention is indicated to preserve maternal life. Although elevations in alkaline phosphatase, bilirubin, and SGOT are common in patients with hepatic rupture, they are not specific. However, when these chemical changes are associated with disseminated intravascular coagulation in a patient with pre-eclampsia and eclampsia, the patient is at risk of hepatic rupture.

Treatment consists of surgical control of bleeding by local packing, resection, or hepatic artery ligation. Survival is recorded when prompt diagnosis is made and appropriate cardiovascular support and surgical correction are provided.[43, 80]

OTHER DISORDERS OF PREGNANCY AFFECTING THE LIVER

Hyperemesis Gravidarum

This disorder, occurring in the first trimester, is rarely accompanied by jaundice, although serum bilirubin elevation has been described in 10 per cent of patients. Urine urobilinogen may be increased, and SGOT is occasionally elevated. The association of such findings with anorexia and vomiting may suggest viral hepatitis, but the characteristic functional and histologic liver changes of viral hepatitis are absent.

Pyelonephritis

Pyelonephritis is not uncommon in pregnancy, and if it is untreated or is associated with toxemia, changes in liver function may occur.[132] Jaundice is rare, and the liver abnormalities respond when the infection is controlled by the proper use of antibiotics. It is important to recognize that some of the therapeutic agents used in treating urinary tract infections may also cause liver function changes.

Cholelithiasis

Although it was formerly thought that cholelithiasis and cholecystitis were common during pregnancy, recent evidence does not support this view.[56, 66, 101, 102, 124] However, pregnancy may contribute to the future development of gallstones, as is indicated by a review of 219 women with gallstones.[42] Diagnosis of cholelithiasis or cholecystitis in pregnancy is complicated by the anatomic changes created by the enlarged uterus and by the frequent abnormalities in liver function tests in pregnancy, which may mimic the findings of extrahepatic cholestasis. Abdominal ultrasound is the procedure of choice in diagnosis because it offers no known hazard to mother or infant.

LIVER DISEASE DURING PREGNANCY

Most of the common forms of liver disease occur during pregnancy, although the diagnosis, clinical course, and therapy of these diseases may be altered. The major diseases of the liver will be reviewed, special emphasis being placed on features relevant to pregnancy, including effects on the fetus.

Viral Hepatitis

Rapid progress in research on viral hepatitis has occurred since the seminal discovery of hepatitis B antigen by Blumberg in 1963. Because viral hepatitis remains the most common cause of jaundice during pregnancy, an understanding of the clinical and epidemiologic advances in this field is essential for those caring for women during pregnancy. It is now known that there are at least three distinct forms of viral hepatitis. Some of the characteristics of these viruses are shown in Table 12–4. Although the clinical illnesses produced by these agents may be similar, considerations regarding complications, transmission, and risk to fetus or neonate are quite different. Therefore, each type of hepatitis will be considered independently.

Viral Hepatitis A. This common disease is of worldwide distribution but occurs more frequently in impoverished populations or lower socioeconomic groups because of poor hygienic conditions. It is a disease of childhood and adolescence in such groups but more commonly affects adults in the developed nations of western Europe and North America. Evidence of prior infection with hepatitis A as measured by the presence of antibody increases with age in the United States and exceeds 65 per cent in some urban populations.

Characteristically, the disease is transmitted by fecal-oral spread from patients during the incubation or early prodromal period. Shedding of virus in the feces begins approximately 2 weeks before symptoms occur and persists for 1 to 2 weeks after the onset of illness. Therefore, precaution in handling stool is indicated only during this early phase of the disease. Viremia occurs for a short period, and blood is infectious during this time. Chronic viremia has not been demonstrated. Contaminated food and water may transmit hepatitis A, shellfish being one of the more common sources.

The clinical illness is inseparable from other types of hepatitis and includes a vague "flu-like" onset with fatigue, weakness, nausea, and loss of appetite during the prodromal phase. More seriously ill patients present with vomiting, abdominal pain, myalgia, pruritus, and fever. In the majority of patients icterus does not occur, and

TABLE 12-4 FORMS OF VIRAL HEPATITIS

Characteristics	Hepatitis A	Hepatitis B	Non A, Non B
Earlier terminology	Infectious hepatitis	Serum hepatitis	Unrecognized
Virus type	RNA	DNA	Unknown
Virus size	27 nm	42 nm	Unknown
Incubation period	15–50 days	30–180 days	30–160 days
Transmission	Fecal-oral	Parenteral or body fluids	Parenteral, close contacts
Vertical transmission to fetus	Rare	Common	Probable
Diagnosis	HA antibody IgM and IgG types	$HB_s Ag$, $HB_c Ab$ $HB_s Ab$, $HB_e Ag$	by exclusion
Maximum infectivity	Prodrome	Prodrome or $HB_s Ag$ carriers	Probably prodrome
Carrier state	None	5–10 per cent	More than 10 per cent
Acute clinical forms	Asymptomatic to fulminant	Asymptomatic to fulminant	Asymptomatic to fulminant
Chronic clinical forms	None	Chronic persistent hepatitis Chronic active hepatitis	Chronic persistent hepatitis Chronic active hepatitis

the diagnosis may be overlooked in such patients. Verification of the disease by appearance of hepatitis A antibody is now possible. In the early recovery phase, the antibody is of the I_gM type, but several months later it is predominantly I_gG. Therefore, acute infection in the presence or absence of icterus and physical findings of liver disease can be accurately determined by these immunologic tests.

Characteristic liver function changes include marked elevation in SGOT (ASP) and SGPT (ALT) to levels of 1000 to 2000. In some, cholestasis occurs with a marked rise in levels of alkaline phosphatase, serum cholesterol, and bilirubin, often accompanied by pruritus and light stools. Differentiation from extrahepatic obstruction may be difficult in such patients but is suggested by the usual absence of marked elevation in SGOT and SGPT in biliary obstruction and the normal ultrasonography of the biliary tree in viral hepatitis.

The symptomatic phase of hepatitis A usually lasts 10 to 15 days, and the patients then enter a gradual recovery phase. Rarely, fulminant hepatitis has been attributed to hepatitis A virus, although no chronic illness or carrier state is reported.

Pregnancy does not alter either the course or the management of patients with hepatitis A. Rest and a nutritious diet as tolerated are recommended. For those with severe anorexia or with nausea and vomiting, admission to the hospital for fluid therapy is occasionally required. No specific drug treatment is indicated.

The effect of hepatitis A on pregnancy is probably minimal. There are reports of prematurity when the disease occurs in the latter part of pregnancy; however, there is no evidence that hepatitis A causes birth defects in infants.[50]

Hepatitis A may be prevented in close household contacts by the administration of immune serum globulin. This precaution has been suggested in the rare situation in which infants are born to mothers during the infectious period of hepatitis A. However, recent information indicates that the risk of transmission to the infant under these conditions is very small.[137a] If hepatitis A occurs early in pregnancy, the disease is not transmitted to the fetus.

Viral Hepatitis B. Although this disease bears many clinical similarities to hepatitis A, hepatitis B may be more serious because of the development of chronic clinical sequelae and the frequency of the chronic carrier state. The disease is of worldwide distribution but is endemic in certain areas, especially Africa and Asia, where it has been implicated in the extremely high incidence of hepatoma. Hepatitis B is now defined by the presence of various immunologic markers as shown in Table 12–5.

TABLE 12-5 HEPATITIS B TERMINOLOGY

Hepatitis B virus	Dane particle
Hepatitis B core antigen	$HB_c Ag$
Hepatitis B core antibody	$HB_c Ab$
Hepatitis B surface antigen	$HB_s Ag$
Hepatitis B surface antibody	$HB_s Ab$
Hepatitis "e" antigen	$HB_e Ag$
Hepatitis "e" antibody	$HB_e Ab$
Hyperimmune serum globulin	HBIG

In the United States, the frequency of hepatitis B is highest among drug abusers, health care personnel, male homosexuals, and patients repeatedly treated with blood products, e.g., hemophiliacs. It accounts for about one third of sporadic cases of hepatitis in the general population.[81]

In contrast to hepatitis A, this disease is transmitted primarily by exposure to infected blood or blood products and probably by semen, vaginal secretions, and saliva as well. Other bodily fluids contain the hepatitis B surface antigen (HB_sAg) but are not clearly implicated in transmission. In contrast to hepatitis A, feces are not contaminated with intact infectious particles. Shortly after transmission of the intact hepatitis B virus (called the Dane particle), hepatic infection occurs. The viral genome is incorporated into the nucleus, and production of the viral core is initiated within the nucleus and of the viral coat, in the cytoplasm. These two separate materials are assembled and secreted from the cell in infectious form. Usually the viral coat material is produced in great excess and is detectable in serum as HB_sAg. This 17–25 nm material is noninfectious but is extremely useful as a marker of hepatitis B infection, appearing in serum 10 to 14 days before clinical symptoms are manifest. The Dane particle (intact hepatitis B virus) also appears during this period, but neither the intact Dane particle nor the core antigen is of clinical use at present in defining acute infection. However, the "e" antigen (HB_eAg), which is closely related to the intact viral particle, is usually present during this early phase. It is frequently used as an indirect measure of the presence of complete virus particles and therefore of the infectious state. The HB_eAg usually clears 6 to 8 weeks after the onset of the symptoms of hepatitis. Its persistence beyond 3 months is often associated with some form of chronic hepatitis.

HB_cAb appears about the time of maximum clinical symptoms and persists for many years after infection. HB_sAb appears late in the recovery phase of hepatitis B and persists for years.

The clinical symptoms of hepatitis B are very similar to those of hepatitis A, except that the prodrome and early infectious period may be much more prolonged and insidious. The onset is often accompanied by arthralgia, frank arthritis, and skin rash. Glomerulonephritis has been reported in children and young adults with this disease.

It was proposed earlier that acute hepatitis B in pregnancy was associated with a much higher risk of fulminant hepatitis and death. While this seems to be true for populations in areas with extreme protein malnutrition in Africa, Asia, and the Middle East, it does not seem to be valid for western populations.[47] There is no evidence in the United States that pregnancy predisposes to fulminant viral hepatitis or massive hepatic necrosis due to hepatitis B.[50]

The disease is diagnosed by clinical and laboratory features and is confirmed by characteristic immunologic changes (Fig. 12–2). Considerable variability exists in this pattern, and all of the immunologic markers may be present simultaneously in some cases. Failure of HB_sAg to clear and HB_sAb to appear is characteristic of the carrier state seen in some 10 per cent of patients with this disease. Approximately half the carriers will show evidence of chronic persistent or chronic active hepatitis. The latter is associated with the development of postnecrotic cirrhosis and hepatoma and has a substantial mortality rate. However, an increasing number of patients with chronic active hepatitis are well enough to conceive; they present such clinical problems as hepatic failure, bleeding varices, prematurity, and the potential for vertical transmission of hepatitis B to the newborn.[141]

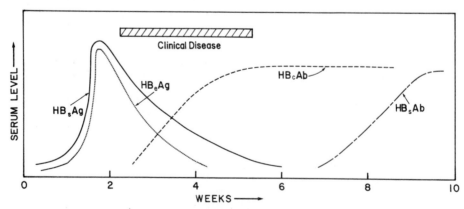

FIGURE 12–2. Immunologic changes in hepatitis B.

TABLE 12–6 MANAGEMENT OF TYPICAL VIRAL HEPATITIS IN PREGNANCY

Establish type by immunologic test
Institute appropriate isolation and precautions
Determine need for contact prophylaxis with serum globulin preparations
Activity — determined by tolerance
Diet — patient preference, parenteral if necessary
Antiemetics — phenothiazines may be used
Corticosteroids — not indicated

Management of acute hepatitis B in pregnancy is the same as for other patients and should include rest (strict bed rest is not essential), adequate fluids, and a nutritious diet, as shown in Table 12–6. Protein content of the diet must be restricted if signs or symptoms of hepatic encephalopathy occur. Precautions with the patient's blood or serum are critical during the infectious period in such patients, but stool and urine are not considered highly infectious to family or health care personnel. The most contagious period is usually past by the time patients seek medical advice.

The effect of acute hepatitis B on pregnancy is not substantial if the infection occurs during the first or second trimester. However, disease in the third trimester has been associated, in some studies, with an increased risk of prematurity and therefore fetal mortality.[2, 50, 67, 120] Moreover, transmission of hepatitis infection to the infant is extremely common (estimated at 65 per cent) when infection occurs in the third trimester regardless of racial, nutritional, or socioeconomic status.[59]

The appearance of HB_sAg and the increase in transaminase in the infant are usually at day 40 to 100 of life. This suggests that transmission occurs at the time of birth, possibly by fetal ingestion of contaminated blood or vaginal secretions.[8] However, a few infants are HB_sAg positive from birth onward, indicating transplacental transmission of hepatitis virus. Infection as a consequence of breast feeding or close contact after birth is probably of much less significance.[74]

Although most affected infants are asymptomatic, some develop acute hepatitis, fulminant disease, and cirrhosis and do not survive. Others become chronic carriers of the virus with the attendant risks of infection to others and of late development of hepatoma.[111]

A much more common clinical problem is the vertical transmission of hepatitis B infection from mothers who are chronic carriers of the HB_sAg (Table 12–7). The frequency of HB_sAg carriers varies dramatically among population groups and is usually 1 per cent or less in western countries but may be 30 to 40 per cent in Asia or Africa. Moreover, the risk of transmission is also widely different and varies from 65 to 70 per cent in Asia to nearly zero in Scandinavia and approximately 15 per cent in the United States.[28, 74, 116]

TABLE 12–7 VERTICAL TRANSMISSION OF HEPATITIS

MATERNAL INFECTION	Hepatitis A ACUTE INFECTION	Hepatitis B ACUTE INFECTION	CARRIER STATE
Transmission Risk to Infant	Rare	1st and 2nd trimester: < 10 per cent 3rd trimester: ≅ 65 per cent	HB_eAg positive: 75–95 per cent HB_eAg negative: < 5 per cent HB_eAb positive: < 5 per cent
Infant Disease	Rare clinical hepatitis (at 14–30 days of age) No carriers	Usually mild hepatitis, rarely severe hepatitis (at 30–120 days of age) Commonly become carriers	May have severe or fatal hepatitis (at 30–120 days of age) Commonly become carriers Cirrhosis or hepatoma late complications (10–20 years later)
Prophylaxis for Infant	ISG — only for infant of mother with acute infection HBIG — no	ISG — no HBIG — useful	ISG — no HBIG — useful

Although several factors may account for these variations, recent studies have shown that the "e" antigen (HB$_e$Ag) status of the mother is the most important.[83, 87, 88] HB$_e$Ag is closely related to the number of circulating Dane particles and is an excellent marker of infectivity in other clinical settings. Recently, a more sensitive radioimmunoassay for HB$_e$Ag has been used to study vertical transmission of hepatitis B. HB$_s$Ag mothers who are also HB$_e$Ag positive have a high risk of transmitting the disease to their infants, estimated at 95 per cent in one report.[126] Those who are HB$_e$Ag negative and HB$_e$Ab positive do not transmit infection. Therefore, this additional marker is exceedingly important in assessing the risk of infection to an infant of a mother who is an HB$_s$Ag carrier. This is true regardless of the status of liver injury in the mother. Although many HB$_s$Ag carriers have no significant liver findings, approximately half have chronic persistent or chronic active hepatitis (vide infra). The same mechanisms of transmission seem to occur in HB$_s$Ag carrier mothers as in the less common situation of acute hepatitis in the third trimester, and evidence of infection in the infant is usually delayed until 2 to 3 months of age.

It is obvious that any attempts at prevention of disease in the newborn infants of mothers who are carriers or have acute hepatitis in the third trimester must be initiated at birth. Unfortunately, cesarean section has not proved useful in the prevention of vertical transmission of hepatitis B.[8] For newborn infants in either setting, nasogastric aspiration at birth is recommended to remove secretions. In addition, there is evidence that neonatal infection may be prevented or at least delayed if hyperimmune serum (HBIG, 0.5 ml per kg) is given immediately at birth or during the first 48 hours and at monthly intervals (0.16 ml per kg) for 6 months.[30, 60, 98] This regimen is currently recommended for infants born of mothers with third trimester acute hepatitis B regardless of "e" antigen status and for infants of mothers who are HB$_s$Ag positive and HB$_e$Ag positive.

However, there is a report of repetitive transmission of fatal hepatitis B to the infant of a HB$_s$Ag positive mother who was "e" antigen negative.[30] Although this may be explained by an insensitive test for HB$_e$Ag, HBIG should be used in subsequent pregnancies if transmission has occurred previously.

Non A, Non B Hepatitis. Recognition that additional forms of hepatitis exist quickly followed the development of immunologic markers of hepatitis A and B. Although specific markers for the additional hepatitis type(s) have not become widely available, it is clear that the vast majority of patients with postransfusional hepatitis have non A, non B type.[138] A substantial portion of sporadic hepatitis (30 to 40 per cent) is also attributed to non A, non B hepatitis in the United States. The incubation period is long and there is high risk of transmission by the parental route and between sexual partners.

The clinical illness in the pregnant woman is treated in the same manner as other forms of hepatitis. Virtually nothing is now known about the mode and frequency of transmission from mother to infant of this type of hepatitis because of the absence of appropriate markers. However, similarity to hepatitis B is anticipated, based on epidemiologic data. In the absence of precise information, no recommendation for the use of immune globulin to prevent newborn infection can be made. The clinical illness is treated in the same manner as other forms of hepatitis during pregnancy.

ATYPICAL FORMS OF HEPATITIS

Fulminant Hepatitis. A small percentage of patients with hepatitis, regardless of type, may present with fulminant hepatitis. This is defined as an acute serious disease with encephalopathy, marked aberrations in coagulation factors, and often renal failure. The mortality is approximately 80 per cent. The pathologic lesion in the liver may consist of massive hepatocellular necrosis in which virtually every hepatocyte is necrotic or abnormal, or submassive necrosis in which multilobular collapse and "bridging" necrosis alternate with areas of substantial hepatocyte preservations. Data suggest that the former is almost uniformly fatal, whereas some patients with the milder lesion survive. Although such a catastrophic illness will hardly escape the attention of patient and physician, the important aspects of differentiating this disease from acute fatty liver of pregnancy may be difficult in patients during the third trimester. Most often, the transaminase and bilirubin elevations are higher in fulminant hepatitis, but overlap may occur. The presence of immunologic markers of acute hepatitis B, or rarely of A, is helpful; however non A, non B hepatitis cannot be distinguished from fatty liver by current techniques. Liver biopsy is definitive but often difficult to obtain because of attendant coagulopathy.

Rapid delivery of the fetus is clearly indicated in fatty liver of pregnancy and may be desirable in fulminant hepatitis to spare the life of the infant.[113] Therefore, this course of action is reasonable for both diseases when the diagnosis is in doubt. Restriction of protein intake, the use of lactulose, prompt treatment of gastrointestinal bleeding, and supplementation of clotting factors with fresh frozen plasma and platelets are imperative if patients are to be provided opportunity for survival. It is important to note that medical personnel and newborn infants are at no special risk by contact with patients with the fulminant form of the disease, since these patients have already passed the most infectious phase of the disease.

Prolonged or Relapsing Viral Hepatitis. In some patients, the course of acute viral hepatitis may be prolonged for 4 to 12 months.[138] The clinical features, laboratory findings, and course are not different from those of typical viral hepatitis of any type, yet the recovery phase is protracted. It may be difficult to separate this group of patients clinically from those with subacute (bridging) hepatic necrosis or chronic active hepatitis. Since therapeutic intervention may be indicated in the latter, liver biopsy is indicated. Needle biopsy is safe during pregnancy, provided the patient is cooperative and the results of coagulation studies are acceptable. No specific therapy is indicated for prolonged hepatitis, and management of the newborn is dependent upon the immunologic studies described earlier.

Relapsing hepatitis refers to a form of the illness in which repetitive episodes of acute hepatitis occur after apparent full recovery. It is important, as in prolonged hepatitis, to differentiate this disease from the more pernicious forms of hepatitis, and this can be done with assurance only by liver biopsy. Management is as described for typical acute hepatitis.

Subacute (Bridging) Hepatic Necrosis. An estimated 10 to 15 per cent of patients with hepatitis B, or non A, non B hepatitis, will present with a prolonged and occasionally severe illness but without severe encephalopathy. Compared with patients having typical viral hepatitis, these patients have more profound hypoprothrombinemia and hypoalbuminemia. Liver biopsy is necessary to confirm the presence of subacute hepatic necrosis or multilobular collapse. Although the eventual outcome in young patients with this clinical and histologic form of hepatitis is often that of complete recovery, some develop chronic active hepatitis as a sequel to their disease. There is no clear evidence that corticosteroids can alter this latter transition, and their use cannot be recommended.

A diagnosis of chronic active hepatitis following an acute episode of subacute (bridging) hepatic necrosis is not made until the disease has been present for at least 3 months and histologic study of the liver reveals the characteristic fibrotic and inflammatory characteristics of this disease. If the initial disease occurs early in pregnancy, it is possible for patients to develop chronic acute hepatitis well before delivery.

Chronic Active Hepatitis. Chronic active hepatitis is a clinical-pathologic entity that is best defined by the histologic findings on liver biopsy. Increased fibrous tissue extends from portal areas, often in a "bridging" manner, and is accompanied by focal and periportal necrosis and extensive inflammatory exudate consisting predominantly of lymphocytes, plasma cells, and mononuclear elements. Cirrhosis of the postnecrotic type is frequently found. The clinical manifestations are extremely varied; the disease may be nearly asymptomatic or may result in persistent fatigue, anorexia, weight loss, and debility. Evidence of portal hypertension (splenomegaly, ascites, superficial abdominal venous distention) is common, although the liver is usually small or only modestly enlarged. All of the signs, symptoms, and laboratory changes characteristic of cirrhosis may be seen, and in some patients, rashes, arthralgia, myalgia, and pruritus are prominent.

Several studies have shown that therapy with corticosteroids or corticosteroids and azathioprine reduces morbidity and mortality in established chronic active hepatitis.[25, 121] However, it is less certain that the subset of patients in whom the disease is a consequence of hepatitis B infection will benefit from such immunosuppressive treatment. Therefore, specific therapy in this latter group should be avoided during pregnancy unless severe or life-threatening clinical deterioration occurs. In this uncommon circumstance or in severe chronic active hepatitis without evidence of hepatitis B infection, prednisone alone should be used because no serious adverse effects on pregnancy or the fetus are recorded. Azathioprine and other immunosuppressive agents are usually contraindicated in pregnancy because of their teratogenic effects.

The effect of chronic active hepatitis on the course of pregnancy is variable.[13, 22, 141] If the patient has cirrhosis and chronic active hepatitis, early termination and perinatal mortality are clearly increased.[22] There is also an increased risk to the mother of esophageal bleeding, anemia, and toxemia. In one series, maternal complications occurred in 42 per cent of patients. The relative reduction in hepatic blood flow and the increase in intravascular volume in pregnancy may account for reports of reduced hepatic function and increased risk of esophageal bleeding. Nonetheless, a patient with milder disease may proceed safely through pregnancy and be delivered of a normal infant. Careful observation of the mother during the pregnancy should include monthly measurement of liver function and control of weight gain and blood pressure.

In those patients with HB_sAg negative chronic active hepatitis, the frequency of pregnancy is reduced but is no longer uncommon because of the generally favorable response of this disease to therapy with prednisone.[127] However, the risk of complications is high, with increased toxemia and urinary tract infection. Overall fetal mortality is estimated at about one third, largely attributable to prematurity and low birth rate. In most patients, prednisone has been continued throughout pregnancy without adverse effect on mother or fetus. Azathioprine may be teratogenic in animals and, until further information in humans is available, should be avoided in patients planning pregnancy. In patients whose condition is well controlled by prednisone therapy, the risk of variceal bleeding is not high, in contrast to early reports of untreated patients with a variety of forms of cirrhosis.[127]

Chronic Persistent Hepatitis. In this disease, a persistent, predominantly periportal, inflammatory reaction occurs, with only minimal hepatocellular injury. Often the disease persists for 4 to 6 years. It is frequently associated with HB_sAg. Treatment is not recommended because of the generally benign nature of this form of chronic hepatitis.

Pregnancy has been reported in such patients, and the prenatal and postnatal course was entirely uneventful.[58] There was no worsening of liver function or clinical status. Normal full-term deliveries were recorded in each case. It is likely that chronic persistent hepatitis presents no hazard to the mother and none to the fetus except for the risk of hepatitis B transmission in those mothers who are HB_sAg and HB_eAg positive.

Drug Reactions

Liver manifestations of drug reactions can be divided into two general classes: those which predominantly cause cholestasis and those which produce widespread hepatocellular injury. Some agents produce a mixed reaction. Although any of the drugs associated with hepatic injury in nonpregnant patients also may cause reactions during pregnancy, several agents are of special importance because of their frequent use in the treatment of complications. These include the antiemetic agents, especially chlorpromazine

and structurally related compounds; the antibiotics, especially tetracyclines and the sulfonamides; and tranquilizers or antidepressants. The various hormonal preparations associated with cholestasis or other forms of hepatic injury have been discussed previously. Other commonly used agents that may cause hepatocellular injury include alpha-methyldopa, isoniazid, acetaminophen, cimetidine, and penicillin.

Diagnosis of hepatic injury related to drugs is difficult because liver function changes are variable and nonspecific, and even liver biopsy may be inconclusive. Improvement with cessation of the drug or recurrence when treatment is resumed is the most convincing evidence.

There are no special risks of hepatocellular or cholestatic drug reactions during pregnancy, with the exception of intravenous tetracycline. However, confusion in diagnosis may cause difficulties in management. Cessation of treatment or substitution with a drug of different chemical structure usually results in clinical improvement, although recovery may be slow (many weeks). The effects of drugs on fetal development are independent of their potential for causing hepatocellular or cholestatic reactions.

Cirrhosis and Pregnancy

Pregnancy in patients with cirrhosis is unusual but is no longer considered rare.[55, 95, 141] Cirrhosis often leads to amenorrhea and infertility. However, the advent of therapy for certain forms of cirrhosis has resulted in an increasing number of young women of childbearing age who improve sufficiently to conceive and to survive pregnancy.

Natural History. The natural history of 95 pregnancies in 78 patients with cirrhosis or chronic active hepatitis has been described.[55] The majority of these patients had postnecrotic cirrhosis, although a few were diagnosed as having Laennec's cirrhosis, primary biliary cirrhosis, or chronic active hepatitis. In two thirds of the cases, there was no significant change in liver function during pregnancy. In the remaining patients, a deterioration of liver function appeared, and in some, jaundice occurred. Two patients improved during the pregnancy. Of 23 patients with demonstrated esophageal varices, 18 had gastrointestinal bleeding during the pregnancy. Six of the nine deaths in the series were a result of variceal bleeding. Several patients underwent successful portal decompressive surgical procedures during pregnancy. No adverse effects on the mother or fetus from these proce-

TABLE 12–8 CIRRHOSIS AND PREGNANCY

Outcome	Per Cent
Early termination (< 20 weeks)	18
Prematurity (21–37 weeks)	20
Vaginal delivery	85
Perinatal mortality	18
Maternal complication	42

dures were reported. The survival of the fetus was affected by the presence of maternal cirrhosis. There were 10 stillbirths, 7 abortions, and 61 live births among the 78 patients with cirrhosis.

The results of another study are shown in Table 12–8. In this group, 70 per cent of patients had postnecrotic cirrhosis or chronic active hepatitis; 20 per cent, primary biliary cirrhosis; and 10 per cent, Laennec's cirrhosis. The incidence of premature delivery and fetal mortality was high. The maternal complications included anemia, toxemia, postpartum hemorrhage, and bleeding from esophageal varices. The latter occurred in 20 per cent of patients and was associated with maternal death in approximately one third of patients.

These studies indicate that pregnancy may occur in cirrhotic women and may result in a normal, healthy infant. The risk of complications, including deterioration in liver function and hemorrhage from varices, is high in the mother. Variceal hemorrhage accounts for most of the maternal deaths in cirrhotic patients. Prematurity and infant mortality are also increased. These risks, in themselves, are not sufficiently high to be considered absolute indications for interruption of the pregnancy. However, in patients with cirrhosis and varices, the mother should be aware of the high risk of bleeding.

Problems in Therapy. Therapy for certain chronic liver diseases presents specific problems during pregnancy. The effectiveness of corticosteroid or combined corticosteroid and azathioprine therapy in the treatment of severe chronic active hepatitis with cirrhosis has been established in several controlled studies.[25, 121] Corticosteroids are less effective in HB_sAg positive chronic hepatitis, and one report suggests they may be harmful in this disease.

The many undesirable side effects of long-term corticosteroid therapy may appear during pregnancy and complicate management. In addition, there is a potential higher risk of congenital deformities in infants born to mothers on such therapy.[141] Nonetheless, serious deterioration in liver function during pregnancy in patients with cirrhosis may present a still greater risk to both mother and fetus. Therapy with the minimum effective dose of corticosteroid is desirable. The dose necessary to control the disease varies, and in some patients, alternate day therapy is adequate. Azathioprine is not known to be teratogenic in the rat,[134] but it may be in other species.[106] There is little experience with the use of this drug in human pregnancy, although at least one report describes the successful delivery of a normal infant to a mother given 50 mg per day of azathioprine daily and prednisone for 4 months of her pregnancy.[34] The drug should probably be used in pregnancy only when the liver disease cannot be adequately controlled with corticosteroid therapy. Neither agent is known to be effective in any form of chronic liver disease except chronic active hepatitis.

Portal Hypertension

The presence of severe portal hypertension with esophageal varices is associated with a high risk of hemorrhage during pregnancy. Patients previously treated with portacaval shunt for varices have become pregnant. Twenty-one pregnancies in 17 patients with portacaval shunts prior to pregnancy resulted in 17 live births, 2 neonatal deaths, 1 stillbirth, and 1 abortion. No maternal deaths were recorded. Therefore, the presence of a portacaval shunt is not a contraindication to pregnancy and does not contribute an additional risk to that of the chronic liver disease alone.[100, 142]

The potential hazard of pregnancy to noncirrhotic patients with portal hypertension who have not had a prior shunt procedure is indicated by a report of two patients with extrahepatic portal hypertension.[49] Both patients had had multiple episodes of hematemesis, which were controlled by transthoracic ligation of varices. During pregnancy, both patients bled, presumably because of increased portal hypertension resulting from the pregnancy. It is apparent that the risk of variceal hemorrhage is increased during pregnancy, regardless of the cause of the portal hypertension.

The use of sclerotherapy for bleeding varices during pregnancy may provide a safe alternative to portacaval anastomosis. Controlled trials have suggested efficacy in nonpregnant patients, and such treatment seems reasonable for the pregnant patient with varices.

Other Hepatic Disorders Occurring During Pregnancy

Wilson's Disease. Wilson's disease is a rare disorder characterized by cirrhosis, neurologic abnormalities, the Kayser-Fleischer corneal ring, and, less commonly, hematologic and renal dysfunction. Pregnancy has been reported rarely in affected women.[31, 49, 142] The advent of effective therapy for this disease has increased the possibility of pregnancy but has also raised the question of fetal injury produced by penicillamine.[142] If therapy with pencillamine is begun early in the disease, considerable improvement in all the manifestations of Wilson's disease results. The secondary amenorrhea is often corrected, and since many patients are in the childbearing period, pregnancies have ensued.[49] However, abortion has been reported in patients treated with penicillamine, indicating the need for caution in the use of this drug during pregnancy. It is possible that abortion results from reduction in tissue copper or cystine depletion affecting fetal collagen formation. It may be possible to reduce penicillamine dosage or to discontinue the agent entirely in pregnancy because of the favorable effect of pregnancy on this disease. This phenomenon has been attributed to an increase in serum ceruloplasmin levels in pregnancy,[31] but this interpretation is open to question, since it is known that estrogens also increase the serum ceruloplasmin levels in nonpregnant women with Wilson's disease without improving clinical aspects of the disorder. If penicillamine is discontinued in the pregnant woman with Wilson's disease, she must be followed up closely for evidence of hepatic or neurologic deterioration. The drug should be reinstituted promptly following delivery.[39]

Sickle Cell Disease. Liver disease, primarily of a cholestatic type, has been reported in patients with sickle cell (SS) disease.[105] The disorder is associated with marked sickling of cells in the hepatic sinusoids and prominent swelling of the Kupffer cells, which are often seen engulfing the abnormal red blood cells. The process is exaggerated during sickle cell crisis and has been associated with pregnancy as well. Marked jaundice, elevation in alkaline phosphatase, and a moderate increase in SGOT occur. The process subsides after delivery, and some authors recommend induction of labor in such patients.[46] The possible association of sickle cell trait (SA) with infarction of the liver during pregnancy has been noted.[123]

Cholelithiasis. The incidence of cholelithiasis is greater in females than in males and pregnancy has been implicated as a major factor in this predominance. In one large series of young women with cholelithiasis, 89 of 219 patients developed symptoms during pregnancy and 67 developed symptoms within 6 months after delivery.[42] Seventy-five per cent of the women with cholelithiasis had been pregnant. Unfortunately, the incidence of pregnancy in a control population of women of the same age was not recorded, and some studies do not support the concept that cholelithiasis is more common in women who have previously been pregnant.[103] Furthermore, cholelithiasis is not a common cause of jaundice during pregnancy.[46, 101, 124] In one review of this subject, it was found to be the cause of jaundice in only 5.9 per cent of pregnant women.[46] Such a finding does not exclude a contributing role of pregnancy in the future development of cholelithiasis. Pregnancy may be too brief for the gallstones to become clinically evident. It is also possible that some factor related to pregnancy reduces the chance of cystic or common duct obstruction, and therefore, gallstones formed during pregnancy are not clinically evident until after delivery. Whatever the explanations for these various observations, it is clear that cholelithiasis is not a major factor in the differential diagnosis of jaundice of pregnancy.

Budd-Chiari Syndrome. Budd-Chiari syndrome, or hepatic vein occlusion, is an uncommon disease that has been associated with both pregnancy and the use of oral contraceptives.[51, 68] The disease may be of sudden onset, usually involving the major hepatic veins, and may result in death within several weeks to months. Alternatively, it may be more insidious, involve smaller intralobular veins, and be associated with prolonged survival. Unfortunately, it is the former type that has been most often recorded in association with pregnancy.[68] Symptoms may appear near term or, more commonly, within hours or days after delivery. Most authors have attributed the occurrence to the hypercoagulable state in pregnancy, although the precise mechanism is uncertain. However, the association of Budd-Chiari syndrome with oral contraceptive use does suggest a possible hormonal mechanism in both circumstances.

Most often, pain in the upper abdomen is rapidly followed by abdominal distention and development of ascites. Fever, vomiting, and jaundice may occur but are not constant. The ascitic fluid often shows a high protein content (about 50 per cent of cases). The results of coagulation studies are usually normal, and variable minor changes in liver function test results are reported.

Liver biopsy reveals a characteristic centrilobular zonal congestion with hemorrhage and necrosis. Usually sclerosis of the central vein radicle is not seen, although veno-occlusive disease has been reported in pregnancy.[51] Wedged hepatic vein pressures are elevated and roentgenologic studies most often show blockage of the main hepatic veins, often with collateral circulation. In addition, inferior vena caval obstruction may occur. Hepatic scintigraphy often shows an unusual pattern with hypertrophy and increased uptake in the caudate lobe, which has auxiliary drainage into the vena cava. The course of such patients is usually that of rapid deterioration manifested by portal hypertension, bleeding varices, severe ascites, and hepatic failure. Anticoagulants have not generally been useful, and direct surgical removal of the block is rarely successful. Side to side portacaval shunts have improved portal hypertension and ascites and are recommended for those with stable liver function. Since this complication usually occurs after delivery, there are no direct effects on the fetus.

Hepatic Rupture. Pregnancy has been associated with rupture of the liver.[12, 86] Although most of the 91 reported cases have been accompanied by pre-eclampsia or eclampsia,[18, 19] hepatic rupture in pregnancy has been reported in the absence of these diseases.[6, 93] Rupture of the liver in eclampsia is probably related to the sinusoidal fibrin deposits, infarction of liver parenchyma, and subsequent intrahepatic hemorrhage.

A similar sequence has been reported in nonpregnant women during oral contraceptive therapy, suggesting a possible hormonal factor in the pathogenesis. Initially, an unruptured subcapsular hematoma accumulates and under various conditions may then rupture freely into the peritoneum. Trauma, convulsions, and normal delivery have all been incriminated in rupture of the subcapsular hemorrhage. Thirty-seven of the 45 cases reported up to 1972 were multigravidas.[93] The risk is highest in the third trimester or soon after delivery, and the incidence is greater in older patients (ages 35 to 45). The symptoms include sudden onset of severe right upper quadrant or epigastric pain with tenderness to palpation in both upper quadrants. Pain may be referred to the back or the right shoulder. Shock, coma, and death promptly ensue unless the diagnosis is suspected and laparotomy performed.

The diagnosis, once suspected, is usually established by peritoneal tap revealing hemoperitoneum. In cases of unruptured subcapsular hematoma, ultrasonography may be useful. In cases of rupture, immediate surgery offers the best opportunity for survival. Hepatic artery ligation has been recommended for prompt control of bleeding.[80] Partial hepatectomy is suggested by others or may be necessary in addition to ligation. Despite prompt blood replacement and surgical intervention, maternal mortality remains extremely high (60 to 80 per cent). Early diagnosis and control of hemorrhage are essential to survival.

In patients with unruptured subcapsular hematoma, prompt cesarean section is recommended to avoid the trauma of vaginal delivery. It is important to control the accompanying pre-eclampsia or eclampsia to avoid convulsions. In one series, all infants born to mothers with hepatic rupture died. However, survival is recorded when cesarean section is performed.[86] The overall fetal mortality is estimated at 60 per cent.

An Approach to the Diagnosis of Liver Disease in Pregnancy

Symptoms. The appearance of jaundice is most often the first indication of liver disorder in pregnancy. However, it is important for the physician to be aware that significant liver disease may be present in the absence of overt jaundice. Symptoms such as vague gastrointestinal complaints, fatigue, pruritus, abdominal pain, edema, and fever may be the earliest manifestations of liver dysfunction. Unless an obvious explanation exists for such complaints, careful physical examination and performance of liver function tests are indicated to evaluate the possibility of liver disease.

Physical Examination. The physical examination should include a careful search for icterus, spider angiomas, and palmar erythema. The latter two are extremely common in uncomplicated pregnancy, appearing in approximately two thirds of normal pregnancies. However, if prominent in early pregnancy, they are more suggestive of antecedent liver disease. Estimation of liver size in late pregnancy is difficult, but in early pregnancy measurement by percussion or direct palpation is useful in estimating liver size. Similarly, enlargement of the spleen may be exceedingly useful in directing attention to the possibility of long-standing liver disease with secondary portal hypertension. The relative size and consistency of the two organs is of assistance to the experienced clinician in suggesting various diagnostic possibilities. Other physical findings include evidence of ascites, edema, abdominal venous distention, and abdominal bruits or rubs.

Initial Laboratory Studies. Liver function studies for initial diagnostic purposes should

TABLE 12–9 MAJOR CAUSES OF LIVER FUNCTION ABNORMALITIES IN PREGNANCY

First Trimester	Second Trimester	Third Trimester
Infectious hepatitis Hyperemesis gravidarum Drug reaction	Normal pregnancy Infectious hepatitis Gallstones Cirrhosis Pyelonephritis	Normal pregnancy Cholestasis of pregnancy Infectious hepatitis Eclampsia, pre-eclampsia Gallstones Cirrhosis Fatty liver of pregnancy Pyelonephritis

include measurements of the major synthetic and excretory functions of the liver. Most often, these include determination of serum total protein, albumin, and globulin; direct and total bilirubin; alkaline phosphatase or 5'-nucleotidase; SGOT and SGPT; cholesterol; and prothrombin time. More specific immunologic tests are not usually useful as screening tests. If the physical findings or liver function test results suggest the possibility of liver disease, various clinical disorders must be considered and distinguished.

Stage of Pregnancy.   The stage of pregnancy in which liver disease first becomes clinically evident can often assist in delineating the major diagnostic possibilities. Certain diseases may be manifest in all three trimesters; however, others are much more likely to appear in early or late pregnancy.

The most common causes of major liver dysfunction in each trimester are indicated in Table 12–9. The incidence varies in different series and in various parts of the world; however, it is apparent that the number of disorders to be considered is greatest in the third trimester. This is also the period in which maximum abnormalities in liver function tests occur during normal pregnancy, hence complicating diagnosis in those with milder illness. It is not surprising that episodes of anicteric hepatitis or mild cholestasis are frequently overlooked during the last trimester. Nevertheless, the importance of correct diagnosis is perhaps greatest during this stage of pregnancy because of the possible value of induced labor to the health and survival of mother and infant.

Clinical Course of Disease.   The clinical course is the most useful in deciding among these various possibilities. For example, the abrupt onset of abdominal pain, encephalopathy, bleeding, and labor should suggest fatty liver of pregnancy, fulminant hepatitis, or eclampsia (with or without hepatic rupture). Each is a serious life-threatening illness and is an indication for provision of an adequate airway, maintenance of normal blood pressure, and replacement of coagulation factors by intravenous infusion of fresh plasma or a suitable substitute. When vital signs have become stabilized, delivery of the infant is indicated in patients with fatty liver of pregnancy or fulminant hepatitis. Immediate surgery is nec-

TABLE 12–10 DIAGNOSIS OF LIVER DISEASE IN THIRD TRIMESTER

Condition	Histology	Albumin Per Cent	SGOT*	Bilirubin*	Alkaline Phosphatase
Normal pregnancy	Normal	↓ 20	nl	sl ↑	2-fold ↑
Infectious hepatitis	Typical	↓ 20–40	500–1000	1–5 mg per 100 ml	2- to 3-fold ↑
Cholestasis of pregnancy	Cholestasis	↓ 20	nl	1–5 mg per 100 ml	10-fold ↑
Eclampsia	Sinusoidal fibrin	↓ 20	100–1000	sl ↑	2- to 3-fold ↑
Gallstone	Cholestasis	↓ 20	nl to sl ↑	variable	3- to 10-fold ↑
Cirrhosis and chronic active hepatitis	Cirrhosis	↓ 20–40	50–150	1–5 mg per 100 ml ↑	3-fold ↑
Fatty liver of pregnancy	Steatosis	↓ 40	300–500	1–10 mg per 100 ml	3-fold ↑
Pyelonephritis	Portal inflammation	↓ 20	100–300	sl ↑	3-fold ↑

*These values indicate the usual range for each condition.
nl — normal
sl — slight
↑ — increase
↓ — decrease

essary in hepatic rupture complicating eclampsia or pre-eclampsia. Final proof of diagnosis may require liver biopsy following stabilization of the clinical status. The clinical setting for most of the other disorders is considerably different and has been described. Awareness of the typical clinical presentation and course will often permit a reasonable presumptive diagnosis and should identify quickly those patients requiring immediate obstetric or surgical intervention.

Further Evaluation of the Liver. The usual liver function changes for major forms of liver disease that occur in the third trimester are indicated in Table 12–10. None of these changes are diagnostic, and there is considerable overlap in the range of abnormalities. These studies are often useful in helping to suggest the clinical diagnosis and are more important in evaluating the adequacy of treatment. In many cases, the course of the changes is important; for example, rapid improvement is seen following delivery in the eclamptic patient, but this is not the case in patients with infectious hepatitis.

When the diagnosis is equivocal and specific therapy is indicated, as in chronic active hepatitis, liver biopsy is the only means of establishing diagnosis. Under such circumstances, liver biopsy is indicated despite the greater technical difficulties related to displacement of the liver by the enlarged uterus.

References

1. Abide, J. K.: Liver function in pregnancy utilizing sulfobromophthalein. Obstet. Gynecol., 27:544, 1966.
2. Adams, R. H., and Combes, B.: Viral hepatitis during pregnancy. J.A.M.A., 192:95, 1965.
3. Adlercreutz, H., Svanborg, A., and Anberg, A.: Recurrent jaundice in pregnancy. I. A clinical and ultrastructural study. Am. J. Med., 42:335, 1967.
4. Adlercreutz, H., and Tenhunen, R.: Some aspects of the interaction between natural and synthetic female sex hormones and the liver. Am. J. Med., 49:630, 1970.
5. Aickin, D. R., and Campbell, D. G.: Anomalous amniotic fluid bilirubin after hepatitis in an Rh immunized patient. Obstet. Gynecol., 37:687, 1971.
6. Albukerk, J. N.: Wilson's disease and pregnancy. A case report. Fertil. Steril., 24:494, 1973.
7. Arora, B.: Infective hepatitis and pregnancy in Bristol. J. Obstet. Gynaecol. Br. Commonw., 74:763, 1967.
8. Beasley, R. P., and Stevens, C. E.: Vertical transmission of HBV and interruption with globulin. *In* Vyas, G. N., et al. (eds.): Viral Hepatitis. Philadelphia, Franklin Institute Press, 1978, p. 333.
9. Beecham, J. B., Braun, T. E., Clapp, J. F., and Lucey, J. F.: Intrauterine diagnosis of fetal liver dysfunction. Obstet. Gynecol., 41:556, 1973.
10. Bennett, N. M., Forbes, J. A., Lucas, C. R., and Kucers, A.: Infective hepatitis and pregnancy: Analysis of liver function test results. Med. J. Aust., 2:974, 1967.
11. Bernstein, L. M., Siegel, E. R., Koff, R. S., Merritt, A. D., and Goldstein, C. M.: The hepatitis knowledge base. Ann. Intern. Med., 93:169, 1980.
12. Bis, K. A., and Waxman, B.: Rupture of the liver associated with pregnancy: A review of the literature and report of 2 cases. Obstet. Gynecol., 31:763, 1976.
13. Borhanmanesh, F., and Haghighi, P.: Pregnancy in patients with cirrhosis of the liver. Obstet. Gynecol., 36:315, 1970.
14. Breen, K. J., Perkins, K. W., Mistilis, S. P., and Shearman, R.: Idiopathic acute fatty liver of pregnancy. Gut, 11:822, 1970.
15. Breen, K. J., Perkins, K. W., Schenker, S., Dunkerley, R. C., and Moore, H. C.: Uncomplicated subsequent pregnancy after idiopathic fatty liver of pregnancy. Obstet. Gynecol., 40:813, 1972.
16. Brown, D. F., Porta, E. A., and Reder, J.: Idiopathic jaundice of pregnancy. Arch. Intern. Med., 111:592, 1963.
17. Burston, G. R.: Fetal malformations associated with maternal infective hepatitis. Practitioner, 197:664, 1966.
18. Call, M., and Lorentzen, D.: Rupture of the liver in pregnancy. Obstet. Gynecol., 25:468, 1965.
19. Castaneda, H., Garcia-Romero, H., and Canto, M.: Hepatic hemorrhage in toxemia of pregnancy. Am. J. Obstet. Gynecol., 107:578, 1970.
20. Center for Disease Control, U.S. Public Health Service: Isolation Techniques for Use in Hospitals. Washington, D.C., U.S. Government Printing Office, 1970.
21. Cerutti, R., Ferrari, S., Grella, P., Castelli, G. P., and Rizzotti, P.: Behavior of serum enzymes in pregnancy. Clin. Exp. Obstet. Gynecol., 3:22, 1976.
22. Cheng, Y. S.: Pregnancy in liver cirrhosis and/or portal hypertension. Am. J. Obstet. Gynecol., 128:812, 1977.
23. Clinich, J., and Tindall, V. R.: Effect of oestrogens and progestogens on liver function in the puerperium. Br. Med. J., 1:602, 1969.
24. Combes, B., Shibata, J., Adams, R., Mitchell, B. O., and Trammell, V.: Alterations in sulfobromophthalein sodium-removal mechanisms from blood during normal pregnancy. J. Clin. Invest., 42:1431, 1963.
25. Cook, G. C., Mulligan, R., and Sherlock, S.: Controlled prospective trial of corticosteroid therapy in active chronic hepatitis. Q. J. Med., 40:159, 1971.
26. Czernobilsky, B., and Bergnes, M. A.: Acute fatty metamorphosis of the liver in pregnancy with associated liver cell necrosis. Obstet. Gynecol., 26:792, 1965.
27. Damjanov, I., Arnold, R., and Faour, M.: Tetracycline toxicity in a nonpregnant woman. J.A.M.A., 204:934, 1968.
28. Derson, A., Boxall, E. H., Tarlow, M. J., and Flewett, T. H.: Transmission of HB$_s$Ag from mother to infant in four ethnic groups. Br. Med. J., 1:949, 1978.
29. DiZoglio, J. D., and Cardillo, E.: The Dubin-Johnson syndrome and pregnancy. Obstet. Gynecol., 42:560, 1973.
30. Dosik, H., and Jhaveri, R.: Prevention of neonatal hepatitis B infection by high-dose hepatitis B immune globulin. N. Engl. J. Med., 298:602, 1978.
31. Dreifuss, F. E., and McKinney, W. M.: Wilson's disease (hepatolenticular degeneration) and pregnancy. J.A.M.A., 195:960, 1966.
32. Duma, R. J., Dowling, E. A., Alexander, H. C., Sibrans, D., and Dempsey, H.: Acute fatty liver of pregnancy. Ann. Intern. Med., 63:851, 1965.
33. Engstrom, J., Hellstrom, J., Posse, N., and Sjovall, J.: Recurrent cholestasis of pregnancy. Treatment with cholestyramine of one case with an unusually early onset. Acta Obstet. Gynecol. Scand., 49:29, 1970.
34. Erkman, J., and Blythe, J. G.: Azathioprine therapy complicated by pregnancy. Obstet. Gynecol., 40:708, 1972.
35. Extrahepatic manifestations of serum hepatitis (editorial). Lancet, 2:805, 1971.
36. Fabian, E., Stork, A., Kucerova, L., and Sonarova, J.: Plasma levels of free fatty acids, lipoprotein lipase, and postheparin esterase in pregnancy. Am. J. Obstet. Gynecol., 100:904, 1968.
37. Flewett, T. H., Parker, G. F., Philip, W. M.: Acute hepatitis due to herpes simplex virus in an adult. J. Clin. Pathol., 22:60, 1969.
38. Forkman, B., Ganrot, P. O., Gennser, G., and Rannevik, G.: Plasma protein pattern in recurrent cholestasis of pregnancy. Scand. J. Clin. Lab. Invest., 29(Suppl. 124):89, 1972.
39. Fukuda, K., Ishii, A., Matsue, Y., Funaki, K., Hoshiai, H., and Maeda, S.: Pregnancy and delivery in penicillamine treated

patients with Wilson's disease. Tohoku J. Exp. Med., *123*:279, 1977.

40. Furhoff, A. K., and Hellstrom, K.: Jaundice in pregnancy. A follow-up study of the series of women originally reported by L. Thorling. I. The pregnancies. Acta Med. Scand., *193*:259, 1973.

41. Galbert, M. W., and Gardner, A. E.: The anesthetic and obstetric management of the parturient with acute hepatitis. Anesth. Anal., *51*:549, 1972.

42. Glenn, F., and McSherry, C. K.: Gallstones and pregnancy among 300 young women treated by cholecystectomy. Surg. Gynecol. Obstet., *127*:1067, 1968.

43. Golan, A., and White, R. G.: Spontaneous rupture of the liver associated with pregnancy. S. Afr. Med. J., *56*:133, 1979.

44. Goyette, R. E., Donowho, E. M., Hieger, L. R., and Plunkett, G. D.: Fulminant herpesvirus hominis hepatitis during pregnancy. Obstet. Gynecol., *43*:191, 1974.

45. Grausz, H., and Schmid, R.: Reciprocal relation between plasma albumin level and hepatic sulfobromophthalein removal. N. Engl. J. Med., *284*:1403, 1971.

46. Haemmerli, U. P.: Jaundice during pregnancy with special emphasis on recurrent jaundice during pregnancy and its differential diagnosis. Acta Med. Scand. (Suppl.) *444*:1, 1967.

47. Haemmerli, U. P.: Jaundice during pregnancy. *In* Schiff, L. (ed.): Diseases of the Liver. Philadelphia, J. B. Lippincott Co., 1972, pp. 1023–1036.

48. Hatfield, A. K., Stein, J. H., Greenberger, N. J., Abernethy, R. W., and Ferris, T. F.: Idiopathic acute fatty liver of pregnancy. Death from extrahepatic manifestations. Am. J. Dig. Dis., *17*:167, 1972.

49. Hermann, R. E., and Esselstyn, C. G.: The potential hazard of pregnancy in extrahepatic portal hypertension. Arch. Surg., *95*:956, 1967.

50. Hieber, J. P., Dalton, D., Shorey, J., and Combes, B.: Hepatitis and pregnancy. J. Pediatr., *91*:545, 1977.

51. Hodkinson, H. J., McKibbin, J. K., Ou Tim, L., Segal, F., and Giraud, R. M. A.: Postpartum veno-occlusive disease treated with ascitic fluid reinfusion. S. Afr. Med. J., *54*:366, 1978.

52. Hoffenberg, R.: Control of albumin degradation in vivo and in the perfused liver. *In* Rothschild, M. A., and Waldman, T. (eds.): Plasma Protein Metabolism. New York, Academic Press, 1970, p. 239.

53. Holden, T. E., and Sherline, D. M.: Hepatitis and hepatic failure in pregnancy. Obstet. Gynecol., *40*:586, 1972.

54. Hsia, D. Y., Taylor, R., and Gellis, S.: Long-term follow up study on infectious hepatitis during pregnancy. J. Pediatr., *41*:13, 1952.

55. Huchzermeyer, H.: Pregnancy in patients with liver cirrhosis and chronic hepatitis. Acta Hepatosplenol. (Stuttg.), *18*:294, 1971.

56. Hurwitz, M. D.: Jaundice in pregnancy: A 10-year study and review. S. Afr. Med. J., *44*:219, 1972.

57. Ingerslev, M., and Teilum, G.: Biopsy studies on the liver in pregnancy. II. Liver biopsy on normal pregnant women. Acta Obstet. Gynecol. Scand., *25*:352, 1945.

58. Infeld, D. S., Borkowf, H. I., and Varma, R. R.: Chronic-persistent hepatitis and pregnancy. Gastroenterology, *77*:524, 1979.

59. Isenberg, J. N.: The infant and hepatitis B virus infection. Adv. Pediatr., *24*:455, 1977.

60. Iwarson, S., Norkrans, G., Hermodsson, S., and Nordenfelt, E.: Passive-active immunization in a neonate treated with repeated doses of high-titred hepatitis B immune globulin. Scand. J. Infect. Dis., *11*:167, 1979.

61. Johnson, P., Samsioe, G., and Gustafson, A.: Studies in cholestasis of pregnancy with special reference to lipids and lipoproteins. Acta Obstet. Gynecol. Scand. (Suppl.), *27*:1, 1973.

62. Johnson, P., Samsioe, G., Gustafson, A.: Studies in cholestasis of pregnancy with special reference to clinical aspects and liver function tests. Acta Obstet. Gynecol. Scand. (Suppl.), *54*:77, 1975.

63. Joske, R. A., McCully, D. J., and Mastaglia, F. L.: Acute fatty liver of pregnancy. Gut, *9*:489, 1968.

64. Kahil, M. E., Fred, H. L., Brown, H., and Davis, J. S.: Acute fatty liver of pregnancy. Arch Intern. Med., *113*:63, 1964.

65. Kaplan, M. M.: Alkaline phosphatase. Gastroenterology, *62*:452, 1972.

66. Kater, R. M., and Mistilis, S. P.: Obstetric cholestasis and pruritus of pregnancy. Med. J. Aust., *1*:638, 1967.

67. Keys, T. F., Sever, J. L., Hewitt, W. L., and Gitnick, G. L.: Hepatitis-associated antigen in selected mothers and newborn infants. J. Pediatr., *80*:650, 1972.

68. Khuroo, M. S., and Datta, D. V.: Budd-Chiari syndrome following pregnancy. Am. J. Med., *68*:113, 1980.

69. Killam, A. P., Dillard, S. H., Patton, R. C., and Pederson, P. R.: Pregnancy-induced hypertension complicated by acute liver disease and disseminated intravascular coagulation. Am. J. Obstet. Gynecol., *123*:823, 1975.

70. Koskelo, P., and Toivonen, I.: Urinary excretion of coproporphyrin isomeric 1 and 3 and delta aminolaevulinic acid in normal pregnancy and obstetric hepatosis. Acta Obstet. Gynecol. Scand., *47*:292, 1968.

71. Kreek, M. J., Sleisenger, M. H., and Jeffries, G. H.: Recurrent cholestatic jaundice of pregnancy with demonstrated estrogen sensitivity. Am. J. Med., *43*:795, 1967.

72. Kreek, M. J., Weser, E., Sleisenger, M. H., and Jeffries, G. H.: Idiopathic cholestasis of pregnancy. The response to challenge with the synthetic estrogen, ethinyl estradiol. N. Engl. J. Med., *277*:1391, 1967.

73. Kunelis, C. T., Peters, J. L., and Edmondson, H. A.: Fatty liver of pregnancy and its relationship to tetracycline therapy. Am. J. Med., *38*:359, 1965.

74. Lee, A. K. Y., Ip, H. M. H., and Wong, V. C. W.: Mechanisms of maternal-fetal transmission of hepatitis B virus. J. Infect. Dis., *138*:668, 1978.

75. Liebhart, M., and Wojcicka, J.: Microscopic patterns of placenta in cases of pregnancy complicated by intrahepatic cholestasis (idiopathic jaundice). Pol. Med. J., *11*:1589, 1970.

76. Lipsitz, P. J., Flaxman, L. M., Tartow, L. R., and Malek, B. K.: Maternal hyperbilirubinemia and the newborn. Am. J. Dis. Child., *126*:525, 1973.

77. Lomas, J., Boardman, R. H., and Markowe, M.: Complications of chlorpromazine therapy in 800 mental hospital patients. Lancet, *1*:1144, 1955.

78. Long, R. G., Scheuer, P. J., and Sherlock, S.: Pre-eclampsia presenting with deep jaundice. J. Clin. Pathol., *30*:212, 1977.

79. Mainwarring, R. L., and Bruekner, C. G.: Fibrinogen-transmitted hepatitis. A controlled study. J.A.M.A., *195*:437, 1966.

80. Mays, E. T., Conti, S., Fallahzadeh, H., and Rosenblatt, M.: Hepatic artery ligation. Surgery, *86*:536, 1979.

81. Mihas, A. A., and Conrad, M. E.: Hepatitis B antigen and the liver. J. Med. *57*:129, 1978.

82. Miller, F. G.: Hepatic hemorrhage due to eclampsia. Can. Med. Assoc. J., *106*:964, 1972.

82a. Mistilis, S. P.: Liver disease in pregnancy, with particular emphasis on the cholestatic syndromes. Austr. Ann. Med., *17*:248, 1968.

83. Mollica, F., Musumeci, S., Rucolo, S., and Mattina, T.: A prospective study of 18 infants of chronic HB$_s$Ag mothers. Arch. Dis. Child., *54*:750, 1979.

84. Morrin, P. A. F., Handa, S. P., Valberg, L. S., Bencosme, S. A., Kipkie, G. F., and Wyllie, J. C.: Acute renal failure in association with fatty liver of pregnancy. Am. J. Med., *42*:844, 1967.

85. Mueller, M. N., and Kappas, A.: Estrogen pharmacology. I. The influence of estradiol and estriol on hepatic disposal of sulfobromophthalein (BSP) in man. J. Clin. Invest., *43*:1905, 1964.

86. Nelson, E. W., Archibald, L., and Albo, D.: Spontaneous hepatic rupture in pregnancy. Am. J. Surgery, *134*:817, 1977.

87. Okada, K., Kamiyama, I., Inomata, M., Imai, M., Miyakawa, Y., and Maymi, M.: e Antigen and anti-e in the serum of asymptomatic carrier mothers as indicators of positive and negative transmission of hepatitis B virus to their infants. N. Engl. J. Med., *294*:746, 1976.

88. Papaevangelou, G., and Hoofnagle, J. H.: Transmission of hepatitis B virus infection by asymptomatic chronic Hb$_s$Ag carrier mothers. J. Pediatr., *63*:602, 1979.

89. Parbhoo, S. P., Owens, D., Scheuer, P. J., and Sherlock, S.: Acute fatty liver of pregnancy. Gut, *13*:319, 1972.

90. Parker, M. L.: Infectious hepatitis in pregnancy. Med. J. Aust., *2*:967, 1967.

91. Peltokallio, V., and Peltokallio, P.: Tuberculous hepatitis with jaundice in pregnancy. Acta Obstet. Gynecol. Scand., *46*:1, 1967.

92. Peters, R. L., Edmondson, H. A., Mikkelsen, W. P., and Tatter, D.: Tetracycline-induced fatty liver in nonpregnant patients. Am. J. Surg., *113*:622, 1967.

93. Portnuff, J., and Ballon, S.: Hepatic rupture in pregnancy. Am. J. Obstet. Gynecol., *114*:1102, 1972.
94. Posen, S.: Alkaline phosphatase. Ann. Intern. Med., *67*:183, 1967.
95. Powell, D.: Pregnancy in active chronic hepatitis on immunosuppressive therapy. Postgrad. Med. J., *45*:292, 1969.
96. Prout, B. J., and Marks, V.: Infective hepatitis and acquired hypogammaglobulinaemia during pregnancy with complete recovery. Postgrad. Med. J., *43*:492, 1967.
97. Rannevik, G., Jeppsson, S., and Kullander, S.: Effect of oral contraceptives on the liver in women with recurrent cholestasis (hepatosis) during previous pregnancies. J. Obstet. Gynaecol. Br. Commonw., *79*:1128, 1972.
98. Reesink, H. W., Brongers, E. E. R., Schut, T. L., Benschop, J. K., and Brummelhuis, H. G. J.: Prevention of chronic HB$_s$AG carrier state in infants of HB$_s$AG-positive mothers by hepatitis B immunoglobulin. Lancet, *2*:436, 1979.
99. Regoeczi, E., and Hobbs, K. B.: Fibrinogen turnover in pregnancy. Scand. J. Haematol., *6*:175, 1969.
100. Reisman, T. M., and O'Leary, J. A.: Portacaval shunt performed during pregnancy. A case report. Obstet. Gynecol., *37*:253, 1971.
101. Rencoret, R., and Aste, H.: Jaundice during pregnancy. Med. J. Aust., *1*:167, 1973.
102. Richards, R. L., Willocks, J., and Dow, T. G.: Jaundice in pregnancy. Scot. Med. J., *15*:52, 1970.
103. Robertson, H. E., and Dochat, G. R.: Pregnancy and gallstones: A collective review. Int. Abstr. Surg., *78*:193, 1944.
104. Robinson, W. S., Clayton, D. A., and Greenman, R. L.: DNA of a human hepatitis B virus candidate. J. Virol., *14*:384, 1974.
105. Rosenblate, H. J., Eisenstein, R., and Holmes, A. W.: The liver in sickle cell anemia. Arch. Pathol., *90*:235, 1970.
106. Rosenkrantz, J. G., Githens, J. H., Cox, S. M., and Kellum, D. L.: Azathioprine (Imuran) and pregnancy. Am. J. Obstet. Gynecol., *97*:387, 1957.
106a. Sass-Kortsak, A.: Copper metabolism. Adv. Clin. Chem., *8*:1, 1965.
107. Schiffer, M. A.: Fatty liver associated with administration of tetracycline in pregnant and nonpregnant women. Am. J. Obstet. Gynecol., *96*:326, 1966.
108. Schiffer, M. A., and Dunn, I.: Jaundice with hepatorenal failure associated with pregnancy or gynecologic procedures. Obstet. Gynecol., *39*:241, 1972.
109. Scholtes, G.: Liver function and liver diseases during pregnancy. J. Perinat. Med., *7*:55, 1979.
110. Schultz, J. C., Adamson, J. S., Workman, W. W., and Norman, T. D.: Fatal liver disease after intravenous administration of tetracycline in high dosage. N. Engl. J. Med., *269*:999, 1963.
111. Schweitzer, I. L., Dunn, A. E. G., Peters, R. L., and Spears, R. L.: Viral hepatitis B in neonates and infants. Am. J. Med., *55*:762, 1973.
112. Schweitzer, I. L., Mosley, J. W., Ashcaval, M., Edwards, V. M., and Overby, L. B.: Factors influencing neonatal infection by hepatitis B virus. Gastroenterology, *65*:277, 1973.
113. Shabot, J. M., Jaynes, C., Little, H. M., Alperin, J. B., and Snyder, N.: Viral hepatitis in pregnancy with disseminated intravascular coagulation and hypoglycemia. South. Med. J., *71*:479, 1978.
114. Sheehan, H. L.: The pathology of acute yellow atrophy and delayed chloroform poisoning. J. Obstet. Gynaecol. Br. Commonw., *47*:49, 1940.
115. Sherlock, S.: Jaundice in pregnancy. Br. Med. Bull., *24*:39, 1968.
116. Shiraki, K., Yoshihara, N., Kawana, T., Yasui, H., and Sakurai, M.: Hepatitis B surface antigen and chronic hepatitis in infants born to asymptomatic carrier mothers. Am. J. Dis. Child., *131*:644, 1977.
117. Simcock, M. J., and Forster, F. M.: Pregnancy is cholestatic. Med. J. Aust., *2*:971, 1967.
118. Skinhoj, P., Olesen, H., Cohn, J., and Mikkelsen, M.: Hepatitis-associated antigen in pregnant women. Acta Pathol. Microbiol. Scand., *80*:362, 1972.
119. Skinhoj, P., Sardemann, H., Cohn, J., Mikkelsen, M., and Olesen, H.: Hepatitis associated antigen (HAA) in pregnant women and their newborn infants. Am. J. Dis. Child., *123*:380, 1972.
120. Smithwick, E. M., Pascual, E., and Go, S. C.: Hepatitis-associated antigen: A possible relationship to premature delivery. J. Pediatr., *81*:537, 1972.

121. Soloway, R. D., Summerskill, W. H. J., Baggenstoss, A. H., Geall, M. G., Gitnick, G. L., Elveback, L. R., and Schoenfield, L. J.: Clinical, biochemical and histological remission of severe chronic active liver disease: A controlled study of treatments and early prognosis. Gastroenterology, *63*:820, 1972.
122. Song, C. S., and Kappas, A.: The influence of estrogens, progestins and pregnancy on the liver. Vitam. Horm., *26*:147, 1968.
123. Stähler, E., Stähler, F., and Sturm, G.: Gravidität bei Wilsonscher Kupferstoffwechselstörung. Geburtshilfe Frauenheilkd., *32*:590, 1972.
124. Steel, R., and Parker, M. L.: Jaundice in pregnancy. Med. J. Aust., *1*:461, 1973.
125. Steinlieb, I., and Scheinberg, I. H.: Penicillamine therapy for hepatolenticular degeneration. J.A.M.A., *189*:784, 1965.
126. Stevens, C. E., Neurath, R. A., Beasley, R. P., and Szmuness, W.: HB$_s$Ag and Anti-HB$_c$ detection by radioimmunoassay: Correlation with vertical transmission of hepatitis B virus in Taiwan. J. Med. Virol., *3*:237, 1979.
127. Stevens, M. M., Buckley, J. D., and Mackay, I. R.: Pregnancy in chronic active hepatitis. Q. J. Med., *48*:519, 1979.
128. Sussman, H., Bowman, M., and Lewis, J. L.: Placental alkaline phosphatase in maternal serum during normal and abnormal pregnancy. Nature, *218*:359, 1968.
129. Svanborg, A., and Ohlsson, S.: Recurrent jaundice of pregnancy. Am. J. Med., *27*:40, 1959.
130. Svanborg, A., and Vikrot, O.: Plasma lipid fraction, including individual phospholipids at various stages of pregnancy. Acta Med. Scand., *178*:615, 1965.
131. Svanborg, A., and Vikrot, O.: Plasma lipids in recurrent jaundice of pregnancy. Acta Med. Scand., *181*:83, 1967.
132. Sworn, M. J., and Jones, W. M.: Peripartum hepatic dysfunction and xanthogranulomatous pyelonephritis. Br. J. Urol., *45*:327, 1973.
133. Taylor, J. D.: Liver disease and pregnancy. Med. J. Aust., *1*:15, 1972.
134. Thiersch, J. B.: Effect of 6-(1'-methyl-4'-nitro-5'-imidazolyl)-mercaptopurine and 2-amino-6-(1'-methyl-4'-nitro-5'-imidazolyl)-mercaptopurine on the rat litter in utero. J. Reprod. Fertil., *4*:297, 1962.
135. Tiliacos, M., Tsoulias, A., Aphentoglou, S., Tsantoulas, D., Kokka, E., and Metzantonakis, C.: The Budd-Chiari syndrome in pregnancy. Postgrad. Med. J., *54*:686, 1978.
136. Thorling, L.: Jaundice in pregnancy. A clinical study. Acta Med. Scand. (Suppl.), *302*:131, 1955.
137. Tikkanen, M. J., and Adlercreutz, H.: Recurrent jaundice in pregnancy. III. Quantitative determination of urinary estriol conjugates, including studies in pruritus gravidarum. Am. J. Med., *54*:600, 1973.
137a. Tong, M. J., Thursby, M. et al.: Gastroent. *80*:999, 1981.
138. Wands, J. R.: Viral hepatitis and its effect on pregnancy. Clin. Obstet. Gynecol., *22*:301, 1979.
139. Weber, F. L., Snodgrass, P. J., Powell, D. E., Rao, P., Huffman, S. L., and Brady, P. G.: Abnormalities of hepatic mitochondrial urea-cycle enzyme activities and hepatic ultrastructure in acute fatty liver of pregnancy. J. Lab. Clin. Med., *94*:27, 1979.
140. Werther, J. L., and Korelitz, B. I.: Chlorpromazine jaundice. Am. J. Med., *22*:351, 1957.
141. Whelton, M. J., and Sherlock, S.: Pregnancy in patients with hepatic cirrhosis. Management and outcome. Lancet, *2*:995, 1968.
142. Wilbanks, G. D., and Klinges, K. G.: Pregnancy after portacaval shunt. Report of 2 cases and review of the literature. Obstet. Gynecol., *29*:44, 1967.
143. Wojcicka, J.: Erythrocytic enzymes of phosphorylating glycolysis. The aldolase activity in full blood, erythrocytes and plasma in women with a normal course of gestation and with intrahepatic cholestasis of pregnancy. Pol. Med. J., *11*:1013, 1972.
144. Wojcicka, J., Roszkowski, I., Wichrzycki, A., and Frydrychowska, T.: Acid-base balance in women with jaundice in late pregnancy. Clin. Chim. Acta, *32*:109, 1971.
145. Wood, E. E.: A case of acute fatty liver of pregnancy. J. Obstet. Gynaecol. Br. Commonw., *77*:337, 1970.
146. Woolf, A. J., Johnston, A. W., Stokes, J. F., and Roberton, N. R. C.: Acute liver failure in pregnancy. J. Obstet. Gynaecol. Br. Commonw., *71*:914, 1964.
147. Zuckerman, H.: Serum alkaline phosphatase in pregnancy and puerperium. Obstet. Gynecol., *25*:819, 1965.

13

Vincent T. Andriole, M.D.

BACTERIAL INFECTION

INTRODUCTION

Even though the pregnant woman requires specific and appropriate medical care, pregnancy is not considered a disease state. Nevertheless, certain physiologic changes occur during pregnancy that seem to predispose the expectant mother to specific infections. Other bacterial infections occur that although relatively nonthreatening to the mother, may result in high perinatal morbidity and mortality and thus are of equal importance to the obstetrician. This chapter, therefore, is intended to provide the reader with a practical approach to the recognition of only the most common bacterial infections likely to be encountered in the pregnant patient and to their currently accepted treatment. In addition, the efficacy, kinetics, and toxicity of various antimicrobial agents in pregnancy and on the fetus are reviewed.

URINARY TRACT INFECTIONS DURING PREGNANCY

Urinary tract infections are among the most common infections during pregnancy. Although effective therapy for most bacterial infections has been developed since the advent of antimicrobial agents, considerable controversy still exists over the proper approach to the treatment of urinary tract infections. Nevertheless, the results of some investigations into specific areas of urinary tract infections, particularly during pregnancy, have provided definitive conclusions and now permit the clinician to proceed with a consistent modus operandi in dealing with their diagnosis, treatment, and prevention. However, the major difficulty for the clinician caring for pregnant patients with urinary tract infections is to be able to separate those approaches which are based upon scientific facts from those which represent tradition and are essentially stylistic rather than substantive. Furthermore, the clinician must also learn to use only those methods which are practical, yet reliable, economical, and, of equal importance, readily available to all of his or her pregnant patients with urinary tract infections.

Physiologic Changes

The normal female urinary tract undergoes profound physiologic changes during pregnancy that affect the entire urinary tract. The most obvious is physiologic hydroureter of pregnancy.[13] Dilation of the ureters and renal pelves has been attributed in the past to obstruction of the ureters by the pregnant uterus,[4] to hypertrophy of the longitudinal sheath of muscle bundles at the lower end of the ureter,[18] and to hormonal "imbalance," producing atony of the ureter with resultant diminished peristaltic activity.[32] Careful studies in humans and animals, most made prior to the late thirties, have shown that these changes occur in varying degrees as early as the seventh week of gestation, gradually progress up to term, and rapidly return to normal (in the absence of infection) in one third of women by the seventh postpartum day, in two thirds of women by 1 month, and in almost all women by the second month following delivery.[19]

Dilation of the upper collecting system occurs during pregnancy and extends down to the level of the pelvic brim. During most normal pregnancies, calycine cups lose their tone and no longer fit closely to the renal papillae. The renal pelves and upper ureters, above the pelvic brim, dilate and become elongated and tortuous. This is more common and more marked on the right. The ureter takes a precipitous drop into the pelvic cavity at the pelvic brim, and the angle is sharper on the right. Ureteral peristalsis is reduced after the first 2 months, and in the seventh and eighth months of pregnancy there are no contractions for long periods.[17] However, intraureteric pressures begin to rise again during the last few weeks of gestation. The rate of urine flow is normal during the first two months but decreases

302

as pregnancy advances. Ureteral volume may increase up to 25 times normal. Marked hypertrophy of the longitudinal musculature (Waldeyer's sheath) of the ureter occurs below the pelvic brim as early as the seventh week of gestation and may be important in preventing dilation of the lower third of the ureter. The bladder also undergoes a progressive decrease in tone and an increase in capacity, so that in late pregnancy it may contain double its normal volume (1000 ml) without discomfort.

These changes vary from patient to patient, are more marked on the right, and are more likely to occur in primigravidas or multiparas who have had their pregnancies in rapid succession.[12] Thus, marked physiologic changes begin around the second month of gestation, progress throughout pregnancy, and may persist in some patients, in the absence of infection, for as long as 2 months into the puerperium. Infection may enhance these changes.

Compression of the ureter at the pelvic brim by the enlarging uterus or by hypertrophy of Waldeyer's sheath in the lower third of the ureter has been thought to be a cardinal factor responsible for the hydroureter of pregnancy.[8, 18] Other studies have suggested that increased production of progesterone, gonadotropins, and estrogens during pregnancy are primary etiologic factors and that the pregnant uterus may play an important but clearly secondary role.[13] To investigate the effect of estrogens on these changes, we treated nonpregnant female and male rats (to avoid the possible effect of obstruction from an enlarging uterus) with estrogens and obtained intravenous pyelograms prior to and at intervals during estrogen treatment. Hydroureter and marked increased susceptibility to *Escherichia coli* pyelonephritis were observed in both nonpregnant female and male animals. These observations suggested that the physiologic and anatomic urinary tract changes of pregnancy may well be attributed to "hyperestrogenism" and also provided at least a partial explanation for the increased frequency of acute pyelonephritis in the last trimester of human pregnancy.[3] Similar observations have been described in women taking oral contraceptives,[15, 22] who also have been found to have an increased prevalence of bacteriuria.[31] However, other studies have been unable to show a cause and effect relationship between excess estrogens or progestins and changes in ureteral activity.[6, 21] Regardless of the cause, it is clear that specific physiologic changes occur during pregnancy and provide an opportunity for the development of symptomatic infection of the urinary tract.

Specific Problems in Pregnancy

The presence of asymptomatic bacteriuria in women during pregnancy may lead to acute symptomatic pyelonephritis with its associated serious complications for both mother and fetus. Furthermore, an association between acute pyelonephritis during pregnancy and premature delivery has been well documented in the preantibiotic era, and rates of prematurity in the range of 20 to 50 per cent have been observed.[9]

BACTERIURIA AND PREGNANCY

The prevalence of asymptomatic bacteriuria in *pregnancy* ranges from 4 to 6.9 per cent, is higher in pregnant patients from a lower socioeconomic status, and rises with parity and age.[23] Most women with bacteriuria at the time of delivery have been bacteriuric since the first prenatal visit. Only 1 per cent acquire bacteriuria later in pregnancy and these patients are detected at the initial visit. From 20 to 40 per cent of patients with bacteriuria detected in early pregnancy develop acute pyelonephritis later in pregnancy, whereas this syndrome occurs only rarely in those women whose urine is uninfected in early pregnancy. Thus, the high frequency of symptomatic urinary tract infection in pregnancy is simply an expression of asymptomatic bacteriuria acquired early in life, which, because of the specific changes that take place in the urinary tract during the later stages of pregnancy, permits established bacterial colonization of the urine and consequent invasion of the kidney. On the basis of the present data, it would be incorrect to consider that pregnancy itself is responsible for a major increase in the acquisition of significant bacteriuria except in those patients who undergo catheterization of the bladder. Pregnancy simply sets the stage for the development of symptomatic pyelonephritis in those women with asymptomatic bacteriuria. These episodes of acute pyelonephritis can be prevented in 90 per cent of women by detection and treatment of asymptomatic bacteriuria in the early stages of gestation. However, women whose bacteriuria fails to respond to treatment are at highest risk of developing symptomatic infection. Since *acute symptomatic pyelonephritis* is known to occur in the later stages of pregnancy in women with asymptomatic bacteriuria and has associated serious implications for both mother and fetus, screening by quantitative urine cultures of all pregnant patients at the initial visit and at least one subsequent visit during pregnancy, and treatment of bacteriuria of pregnancy, are warranted.

BACTERIURIA IN NONPREGNANT ADULT WOMEN

The prevalence of bacteriuria in adults has been found to be about 1 to 4 per cent in young nonpregnant women and is known to increase with age and parity to about 10 to 15 per cent in older women, but age seems to be the more important factor. Spontaneous remissions and new infections occur annually at the rate of about 1 per cent of the total female population; new infections often develop in women who have had urinary infections previously. The observation that approximately 4 per cent of young nonpregnant women have bacteriuria and that in 1 per cent of this population the bacteriuria spontaneously clears, while in another 1 per cent new infections develop, means that each year spontaneous remissions occur in about 25 per cent of bacteriuric women and are replaced by an equal number of women who have become infected. This also indicates that the prevalence of bacteriuria remains the same at any given time. Although bacteriuria does not appear to be more common in pregnant than in nonpregnant women, bacteriuria in pregnant women differs from that in nonpregnant ones in two respects. First, bacteriuria during pregnancy rarely remits spontaneously, whereas, as pointed out earlier, in nonpregnant adult women, as well as in school-age girls, spontaneous clearing of bacteriuria is common. Second, acute pyelonephritis appears to be less frequent in the nonpregnant than in the pregnant bacteriuric woman.

The natural history of urinary tract infections, as just described, has evolved from studies that have used the concept of significant bacteriuria as the endpoint without reference to the presence or absence of symptoms of urinary tract disease. It is equally important to look at the clinical problem of urinary tract symptoms in relation to significant bacteriuria in adults. A number of studies have indicated that urinary tract symptoms, particularly dysuria, occur in approximately 20 per cent of women each year, but only half of them seek medical attention. Of those who seek medical attention, one third have the "acute urethral syndrome," whereas two thirds have significant bacteriuria by the traditional criteria of greater than 10^5 bacteria per ml of urine. Of those two thirds with significant bacteriuria, half have bladder bacteriuria and the remaining half have renal parenchymal involvement.[27] However, the physician cannot separate patients with the acute urethral syndrome from those with either bladder or renal bacteriuria on clinical grounds alone. Frequency, burning, and suprapubic pain are found approximately equally in all three groups of patients. Costovertebral angle tenderness and elevated temperature may be present as frequently in patients with the acute urethral syndrome as in patients with renal bacteriuria, and rigors occur in approximately equal numbers of patients with the acute urethral syndrome as in those with bladder bacteriuria, though less frequently than in patients with renal bacteriuria.

The cause of the acute urethral syndrome in women has not been well defined. Recent work has shown that women who seek medical attention for acute dysuria and frequency (after excluding patients with vaginitis) can be divided into four groups, of which three have potentially treatable infections.[30] One group has typical acute cystitis with greater than 10^5 bacteria, usually coliform, per ml of urine on culture, plus pyuria (at least 8 leucocytes per cubic millimeter of midstream urine); a second group has bladder bacteriuria with less than 10^5 bacteria, also usually coliform, per ml of urine and will also have pyuria; a third group has sterile bladder urine but pyuria and *Chlamydia trachomatis* urethritis; and a fourth group has sterile bladder urine, no pyuria, no chlamydial infection, and no recognized cause of the symptoms.

Women with low-count bladder bacteriuria (less than 10^5 bacteria per ml of urine) and pyuria cannot be differentiated clinically, in terms of symptoms and signs, from women with typical bacterial cystitis (greater than 10^5 bacteria per ml of urine) and pyuria. However, women with the urethral syndrome due to chlamydial infection (sterile bladder urine and pyuria) more often have a history of a new sex partner in the month before onset of symptoms, less frequently have a history of symptoms of urinary tract infection in the preceding 2 years, and more often use oral contraceptives than do women with low-count bladder bacteriuria and pyuria.

These findings may help in the diagnosis and treatment of the nonpregnant woman who presents with dysuria and frequent urination (Table 13–1). Vaginitis and gonorrhea should be excluded. A clean-catch, midstream voided urine specimen should be obtained for quantitative culture and for microscopic analysis of uncentrifuged urine for leucocytes and bacteria. Acute bacterial cystitis is likely if bacteria are seen with or without pyuria. If bacteria are not seen but pyuria is present microscopically, the history may help to separate women with the acute urethral syndrome due to low-count bladder bacteriuria from those with chlamydial urethritis. Women with low-count bladder bacteriuria are more likely to have a more sudden onset of symptoms, microscopic hematuria, and suprapubic pain than those with chlamydial infection,

TABLE 13–1 DYSURIA-FREQUENCY WORKUP

1. Exclude vaginitis and gonorrhea
2. Clean-catch urine
   a. Quantitative culture
   b. Microscopic analysis for WBC and bacteria
3. Bacteriuria ± pyuria — cystitis
4. Pyuria without bacteriuria plus
   a. Sudden onset of symptoms
   b. Microscopic hematuria
   c. Suprapubic pain
   Diagnosis — low-count bladder bacteriuria

5. Pyuria without bacteriuria plus
   a. New sex partner
   b. Oral contraceptive use
   c. No history of urinary tract symptoms during the previous 2 years
   Diagnosis — chlamydial infection

and the culture results show low count bacteriuria rather than sterile pyuria. Some women have sterile urine and no pyuria and have no recognizable cause for their symptoms. Women with acute cystitis, low-count bladder bacteriuria, or chlamydial infection can be expected to respond to antimicrobial therapy, whereas those without pyuria, or the few who may have pyuria but without bladder bacteriuria or chlamydial infection, may or may not respond.[2]

Most women with typical acute cystitis respond to a single 3-gram oral dose of amoxicillin or a single oral dose of trimethoprim-sulfamethoxazole (3 double-strength tablets, i.e., trimethoprim 0.48 grams; sulfamethoxazole 2.4 grams). Though it has not yet been proved, most women with low-count bladder bacteriuria also would be expected to respond to single-dose antibiotic therapy. Recent studies suggest that women with the urethral syndrome due to chlamydial infection respond to 100 mg doxycycline by mouth for 10 days.[29] The effectiveness of shorter courses of therapy for chlamydial urethritis remains to be determined.

Single-dose therapy can also be used as a guide to future management of women presenting with clinical cystitis or with low-count bladder bacteriuria. After an initial urine culture has been obtained, single-dose therapy can be tried in all women presenting with a presumptive diagnosis of clinical cystitis. Followup urine cultures can be obtained 3 to 5 days later. Bacteriuria is eliminated in most women with lower urinary tract infection, and no further treatment or investigation should be necessary except for periodic followup urine cultures. Reinfection, should it occur, can be treated similarly with single-dose therapy and the patient can be followed up.

However, single-dose therapy should fail for those patients with renal bacteriuria who relapse symptomatically or culturally or continue to have significant bacteriuria on followup. These patients should then be considered for radiologic investigation as well as for an extended (6 week) course of antimicrobial therapy, which will cure some. Single-dose therapy would be expected to also fail in patients with structural urinary tract abnormalities, and this may help to identify those patients who may require urologic evaluation.[2]

Some women have frequently recurrent reinfections (caused by new bacterial species or new serotypes), which tend to occur in clusters. Effective therapy for these women has not been well established. Although prophylaxis with one half tablet of trimethoprim-sulfamethoxazole (containing 40 mg of trimethoprim and 200 mg of sulfamethoxazole) given three times weekly at bedtime for 6 months reduced recurrent urinary tract infections of the reinfection type in some women, reinfections recurred once prophylaxis was discontinued, and less than 10 per cent remained free of infection during a 6 month followup period.[2]

Diagnosis and Laboratory Methods

Proper technique must be used when urine is collected for culture, since unreliable urine collection results in unreliable cultural data. Single *catheterization* of the bladder to obtain urine for quantitative culture requires less cooperation from the patient than other methods of urine collection and has the advantage of avoiding heavy vaginal contamination of the urine in women. Although these are important considerations, a single catheterization also carries a 4 to 6 per cent risk of introducing infection. Catheterization, therefore, is not justified merely to obtain a urine specimen for diagnostic purposes.

Clean-Catch. The *clean-catch method* has the advantage of decreasing the risk of introducing infection compared with catheterization. A standard technique is used to obtain midstream urine specimens for culture in our female patients. The patient, after washing her hands, straddles a commode facing its back and washes her vulva from front to back, using one stroke with each of three separate sterile gauze sponges (4 by 4 inches) that have been soaked in tincture of green soap, followed by two separate sponges soaked in sterile distilled water that are used as rinses. Benzalkonium solution and soaps containing pHisoHex are not used because of their antibacterial effect on culture results when a small amount gets into the urine. Then two sterile gauze pads are used to spread the labia with the fingers of one hand. The first portion of the voided urine is discarded into the commode; the second portion is collected in a sterile container and cultured immediately or refrigerated until it is cultured.

Suprapubic Bladder Aspiration. This procedure can also be used to collect urine for culture and requires a full bladder. An area 2 to 5 cm above the symphysis pubis in the midline is shaved and cleansed with 70 per cent alcohol. The skin is anesthetized, and a 3.5 inch, sterile, 22 gauge needle attached to a sterile 20 ml syringe is introduced into the skin and quickly plunged through the bladder wall into the bladder cavity. The syringe is used to aspirate 5 ml of urine for culture and 15 ml of urine for routine analysis. The needle is withdrawn and a small strip dressing is placed over the area. Even though suprapubic bladder aspiration has been shown to be quite safe, we have reserved this procedure for special situations.

Culture Methods. A number of methods are currently in use to quantitate bacterial counts in urine. The *pour plate dilution technique* is precise, though impractical in clinical laboratories, yet continues to serve as the reference standard. The more commonly employed practical tests are the standardized *calibrated inoculating loop* and the *streak plate methods.* Reasonably accurate results can be obtained with these techniques for the majority of urine specimens that must be cultured. However, the *dip-slide technique* is currently the best available semiquantitative method and is also recommended for use in office practice. Although available from a number of manufacturers, our experience with Uricult (Orion Laboratories, Helsinki, Finland) dip-slide has been excellent.[2] Modifications of the dip-slide have also been introduced in the form of a *filter paper method* (Testuria), *pipet method* (Culture-Pette), *cup method* (Bacturcult, Speci-test), and *pad culture method* (Microstix). All employ the principle of the dip-slide method and are based on the growth of bacteria on media. The pad culture method also has tetrazolium added to the two medium-containing areas on the strip, and a chemical reagent to detect nitrite added to a third area. Nevertheless, greater accuracy has been observed with the dip-slide technique compared with the pad culture method.[10]

Chemical Methods. Several indirect chemical tests have been used to screen samples for significant bacteriuria. The *Griess test* utilizes a chemical reagent that, in the presence of suffi-

cient numbers of bacteria in the urine, reduces nitrate to nitrite, which can be measured colorimetrically. The *TTC test* requires bacteria that possess dehydrogenase activity to reduce colorless triphenyltetrazolium chloride (TTC) to insoluble red triphenyl-formazan. The *glucose oxidase test* is based on the principle that significant bacteriuria results in a subnormal urinary glucose concentration. The *catalase test* attempts to measure bacterial catalase in urine by a catalase-hydrogen peroxide interaction, but it is not specific enough to exclude the presence of catalase of red and white blood cell and renal cell origin. Although these chemical tests are simple to use and provide more rapid results, their sensitivity and specificity are not comparable to the semiquantitative culture methods, e.g., the dip-slide technique, and they are not recommended.

Other Methods. More recently the reliability of a number of other methods to detect significant bacteriuria has been evaluated. These include the detection of bacterial adenosine triphosphate (ATP) by bioluminescence, electrochemical methods, impedence screening, gas liquid chromatography, coulter counter, limulus lysate endotoxin assay, and xanthine oxidase activity in the urine.[2] These methods have not been well studied, nor are they simple, inexpensive, or readily available. The common practice of examining a drop of uncentrifuged urine microscopically has served as a rapid screening procedure but does not exclude the presence of significant bacteriuria (20 per cent) whenever bacteria are not seen and does not permit bacteriologic identification, so that culture of the urine may be required. Since the dip-slide method is simple, inexpensive, and as accurate as other quantitative methods, and colonies can be subcultured for identification and sensitivity tests, and since it is readily adaptable to busy clinics, physicians' offices, and home self-screening programs, it is currently the most acceptable procedure for the detection of bacteriuria. According to traditional criteria, 100,000 or more colonies per milliliter of urine almost always connotes infection, whereas colony counts of less than 10,000 have been thought to reflect contamination, when the urine has been obtained by either the clean-voided technique or catheterization. Urine obtained by suprapubic bladder aspiration is either sterile or contains significant bacterial growth regardless of the number of colonies present per milliliter of urine. However, the colony count *must be interpreted in the light of the patient's symptoms, time of day, methods of urine collection and quantitation, type of organ-*

sm, purity of the culture, and whether the patient is receiving antimicrobial therapy. In a recent study almost half the women who presented with the "frequency-dysuria syndrome" had a bacterial infection but with fewer than 100,000 bacteria per ml when their urine was collected by suprapubic bladder aspiration, whereas their urine, when obtained by midstream or bladder catheterization, was "negative" on culture by traditional criteria, i.e., greater than 10^5 bacteria per ml of urine.[30] These results suggest that traditional definitions of a "positive" urine culture, as applied to symptomatic women, need to be re-examined, and that cultures with less than 10^5 bacteria per ml of urine should not be ignored in women with symptoms of frequency and dysuria.

Localization of the Site of Infection. The ability to consistently differentiate patients with renal parenchymal infection from patients with only bladder bacteriuria would permit us to more accurately evaluate the duration as well as the optimal dose of treatment in an individual patient. A number of methods have been introduced. Some (e.g., *serum antibody titer* to the infecting bacteria, *maximal urinary concentrating ability, urinary enzyme activity,* and *renal biopsy)* are too insensitive to predict the site of infection in individual patients. Others (e.g., *ureteral catheterization* and *bladder washout),* although more accurate and specific, are too cumbersome to use in office practice. Elevated serum *C-reactive protein* (CRP) values and the presence of *antibody-coated bacteria* in the urine sediment (ACB-test) have been suggested as reliable indicators of renal bacteriuria. However, other workers have not been able to confirm these results. Currently, the ACB-test is not available to all clinicians. If the technique can be improved, the sensitivity enhanced, the interpretation standardized, and the limitations clearly defined through future studies, the ACB-test may prove to be a useful method for localizing the site of infection in the urinary tract. The *patterns of response to antimicrobial therapy* have been shown to be significantly different in patients with renal, compared with bladder, bacteriuria. After short course chemotherapy, most patients with renal bacteriuria develop a pattern of recurrence of the *relapse* type, defined as recurrence with the same bacterial species and serologic strain, within 2 weeks of the cessation of therapy, that was present initially. In contrast, most patients with bladder bacteriuria either are cured or develop recurrences with different microorganisms, defined as recurrences of the *reinfection* type. The pattern of response to antimicrobial therapy as a predictor of the site of infection has an overall accuracy of 75 to 80 per cent in women with recurrent bacteriuria. Also, recurrences with the same microorganisms *(relapses)* more than 2 weeks following cessation of short term therapy occur primarily in patients with bladder bacteriuria rather than renal bacteriuria and are more characteristic of reinfection with the same bacterial species from the patient's gastrointestinal tract, urethra, or vagina. Although there are potential disadvantages, the pattern of response to and recurrence after antimicrobial therapy has been of practical value in deciding upon the duration of therapy in selected patients with recurrent infections.[2]

Treatment

Even though there is an understandable concern about the use of antimicrobial agents in pregnancy, there is as yet no way to predict the outcome of bacteriuria in any individual pregnant patient. Therefore, the shortest possible course of antimicrobial agents should be used to minimize the toxicity of these drugs in both mother and fetus. An 8 day course of sulfonamide (sulfisoxazole 1 gm followed by 0.5 gm every 6 hours) is recommended, because approximately 90 per cent of organisms isolated from antenatal patients have been shown to be sensitive and because of their low cost and minimal side effects. This method will cure between 70 and 80 per cent of patients. Similar results have been observed with ampicillin (0.5 gm orally every 8 hours) or nitrofurantoin (100 mg orally two or three times daily). Although it is difficult to recommend any single antimicrobial agent as being more effective than any other, currently up to 20 per cent of *E. coli* isolated from patients seen in office practice may be ampicillin resistant. Treatment failures result from resistance of the infecting organism, failure of the patient to take the medication, or renal parenchymal infection.[35] Followup urine culture studies should be made within a few days after the start of treatment and repeated in patients whose initial culture on treatment is sterile, at periodic intervals throughout pregnancy, and finally at the 6 week postpartum visit. The medication of those patients whose bacteriuria persists (20 to 30 per cent), as determined by the first culture obtained after the start of treatment, may be changed to either ampicillin or nitrofurantoin for 8 days with similar followup cultures. Cures can be expected in more than half of the initial 20 to 30 per cent of patients who do not respond to sulfonamide therapy. Only a few patients fail to respond to sulfonamide followed by ampicillin or nitrofurantoin, and in vitro sensitivity data can be used as a guide to select further therapy. However, the few patients in whom this sequence of treatment fails are not likely to respond to further therapy. These failures occur most commonly in patients with renal parenchymal infection or radiographic abnormalities of the urinary tract.[35] Optimum therapy for this small group of pregnant patients who are not helped by the therapy outlined, or who experience either recurrent infections with the same organism, or repeated reinfections by different organisms is currently unknown. A short course of antimicrobial treatment based on in vitro sensitivity tests, followed immediately by long term prophylaxis with 100 mg of nitrofurantoin each night until term, has been suggested.[35] Patients with documented renal bacteriuria whose infection was difficult to cure during pregnancy should have a complete urologic investigation after the third postpartum month and are more likely to have postpartum bacteriuria and abnormalities, including scars, on postpartum intravenous pyelography. These abnormalities are thought to be a result of childhood infection rather than of infection that occurred during pregnancy.

Those patients who develop acute pyelonephritis of pregnancy should be admitted to the hospital, particularly if bacteremia is suspected and the patient has high fever and chills and may be at risk of developing hypotension. Intravenous antimicrobial therapy is preferred because many of these patients also have nausea, and proper absorption of oral medication may not be optimal. Initially, intravenous ampicillin in a dose of 1 gram every 4 to 6 hours until the patient is afebrile, followed by oral administration for 10 to 14 days, should be adequate unless there is a known history of penicillin allergy or the patient presents with severe or overwhelming sepsis. In the latter circumstance we would add an aminoglycoside, either tobramycin or gentamicin, in a dose of 1.5 mg per kilogram of body weight every 8 hours by intramuscular or intravenous injection until the exact sensitivity of the infecting bacteria is known. Therapy can then be adjusted to a single agent with the least toxicity. Followup therapy for patients who have recovered from acute pyelonephritis is still unsettled. Some workers have observed a high incidence (60 per cent) of recurrent pyelonephritis that required hospital admission in patients who did not receive therapy for the remainder of their pregnancy, whereas this complication occurred in less than 3 per cent of patients who were treated.[16]

Although these patients may require antimicrobial therapy for the duration of pregnancy, confirmatory studies are needed before the necessity for prolonged therapy can be universally accepted.

Effect of Treatment on Mother and Fetus

There are some data on the toxicity of antimicrobial agents used during pregnancy. One group has used sulfonamides for the treatment of bacteriuria of pregnancy for more than 6 years without observing serious toxicity.[35] Sulfonamides were not given to patients with a history of hypersensitivity, nor were they used during the last few weeks of pregnancy because of the possible complications of hyperbilirubinemia and kernicterus. Although this danger has been reported,[11, 24] it may be only theoretical. There is a suggestion that sufficient sulfonamide crosses the placenta to conjugate with enough binding sites to cause dangerous hyperbilirubinemia.[1] Although the use of long-acting sulfonamides has been associated with the development of the Stevens-Johnson syndrome,[5] there is serious question whether an association exists or is only fortuitous.

Ampicillin has essentially the same toxicity as penicillin except for a higher incidence of rash, which may be due to a different mechanism. Gastrointestinal side effects include nausea, vomiting, cramps, and diarrhea. Hypersensitivity reactions consist of rashes, fever, arthralgia, arthritis, eosinophilia, leukopenia, and rarely anaphylaxis. Patients allergic to penicillin are also allergic to ampicillin. Nevertheless, ampicillin does not appear to be harmful to the fetus[33] and is safe for use during pregnancy.

Nitrofurantoin may produce nausea and vomiting, peripheral neuropathy, hemolytic anemia in patients with glucose-6-phosphate dehydrogenase — deficient red blood cells, and hypersensitivity reactions, including allergic pulmonary infiltration with eosinophilia and pleural effusion. Nitrofurantoin passes the placenta[25] but is not harmful to the fetus[26] and is apparently safe for use in pregnancy.

Tetracyclines should not be used in pregnancy. Tetracyclines cross the placenta and when given to pregnant patients, particularly after the fourth month of gestation, may cause yellow discoloration of the deciduous teeth of the child. Their role in the production of hypoplasia of the enamel or defective teeth is disputed. Tetracycline deposition in the bones of infants produces temporary inhibition of bone growth, which is rapidly reversed when the drug is discontinued, and permanent effects on the human skeleton have not been observed. The greatest danger of tetracycline therapy in pregnancy is hepatotoxicity,[20] which is dose-related and occurs particularly with intravenous administration. Symptoms include wide swings of fever, nausea, and vomiting, followed by hyperbilirubinemia and jaundice. In severe cases hematemesis, melena, acidosis, and renal failure occur, followed by coma and terminal hypotension in fatal cases. At autopsy the liver shows extensive fine vacuolar fatty infiltration similar to that first described by Sheehan in 1940 as "idiopathic obstetric acute yellow atrophy."[28]

Trimethoprim-sulfamethoxazole, in standard doses of two tablets twice daily, and trimethoprim alone, in doses of 200 mg twice daily for 7 days, have been shown to be effective (83 per cent) therapy for bacteriuria of pregnancy. Although serious risk of teratogenicity was not observed with either drug, both drugs have been shown to be teratogenic when given to pregnant rats and rabbits. We have avoided the use of either drug in pregnant patients and nursing mothers, even though the risk to the fetus may be minimal but also because trimethoprim is excreted in human milk and may interfere with folic acid metabolism.

Asymptomatic Bacteriuria and Prematurity

The association between acute attacks of pyelonephritis during pregnancy and premature delivery was well documented in the preantibiotic era.[9] Rates of prematurity in the range of 20 to 50 per cent have been observed in pregnant women with symptomatic infections of the urinary tract. In contrast, the relationship of asymptomatic bacteriuria of pregnancy to premature delivery and fetal mortality remains a highly controversial issue, which began in 1959 when an association between asymptomatic bacteriuria and prematurity, and a significant reduction in the rate of premature delivery by the eradication of bacteriuria, were reported.[19a] These observations have been followed by many years of conflicting data, which when summarized suggest that the incidence of prematurity seems to be increased in bacteriuric compared with nonbacteriuric pregnant women, probably more specifically in those bacteriuric women with renal involvement.[7] However, this does not mean that bacteriuria causes prematurity. Furthermore, most studies have failed to show a decreased incidence of prematurity or fetal mortality in women treated for asymptomatic bacteriuria. Therefore, asymptomatic bacteriuria appears to be only a minor factor in the overall problem of prematurity.

POSTPARTUM TREATMENT

Followup studies of patients with bacteriuria of pregnancy have shown a high incidence (approximately 25 per cent) of postpartum bacteriuria. It was suggested that more patients were bacteriuric after delivery if they were not treated during pregnancy,[34] but no significant difference in postpartum bacteriuria between treated and untreated patients was observed.[14] Additional studies showed that patients who responded to chemotherapy were less likely to have radiologic abnormalities, and these abnormalities were less severe than those observed in patients who either had not responded to treatment or had required repeated courses of therapy for bacteriuria of pregnancy.[7, 35] Therefore, patients with bacteriuria of pregnancy should have followup urine cultures after delivery. Patients with recurrent infection or whose infection was difficult to cure during pregnancy should have a complete urologic investigation after the third month post partum.

GROUP B STREPTOCOCCAL DISEASE IN PREGNANCY

The group B beta-hemolytic *Streptococcus* has been known to be pathogenic for man for almost half a century since it was first recognized as a cause of neonatal sepsis by Dunham in 1933. However, group B beta-hemolytic *Streptococcus* had only occasionally been reported as a cause of lethal or life-threatening infection until 1961, when it was found to be a major threat to the fetus and the newborn.[51] During the past decade, the organism has emerged as the predominant pathogen in most newborn nurseries in North America and Western Europe,[44, 45, 53, 56] although it remains an unusual pathogen in other areas of the world.[48, 62] Nevertheless, group B beta-hemolytic *Streptococcus* has been responsible for neonatal sepsis with high morbidity and mortality in the United States and has been the cause of considerable controversy about effective methods of prevention.[57, 62] Since the single most important factor in group B beta-hemolytic *Streptococcus* sepsis in the neonate is the presence of this microorganism in the maternal genital tract at birth, information about the magnitude of this association, as well as its prevention and treatment, are important to the obstetrician.

Disease in the Nonpregnant State

Group B beta-hemolytic streptococci have been isolated from the throat, skin, urine, stool, cervix, vagina, blood, cerebrospinal fluid, joint fluid, exudates, and wounds. These bacteria are commonly found in the genital tract of adult women and in the upper respiratory tract of newborn infants. The gastrointestinal tract is probably the major reservoir of the organism, and it is sexually transmitted. It has been recovered from the urethras of 20 per cent of men seen in a venereal disease clinic[61] and from 63 per cent of asymptomatic sexual partners of women harboring colonies.[54] However, the role of group B beta-hemolytic *Streptococcus* in genital infections in nonpregnant women is still unclear. Group B beta-hemolytic streptococci have been recovered from cervical-vaginal cultures in the absence of clinical signs and symptoms of infections in 5 per cent of patients admitted to a hospital for termination of pregnancy, in 17 per cent of gynecologic patients admitted for elective major surgical procedures,[36] in 18 per cent of healthy college women,[38] and in 36 per cent of sexually active nonpregnant women.[52] The frequency of the recovery of the organism from these women did not appear to be influenced by oral contraceptive use, intrauterine contraceptive devices or infections associated with these devices, sexual practices, history of gonococcal infection, previous pregnancy, race, socioeconomic or marital status, gynecologic symptoms, or antibiotic use. However, vaginal colonization with group B beta-hemolytic streptococci was decreased with increasing age, which suggested that certain, yet undefined local vaginal factors, such as secretory immunoglobulins, pH, and other bacteria, may be important in its elimination from the vagina in older women.[43] Nevertheless, the organism is a potential pathogen and has caused urinary tract and postoperative wound infections.[46]

Diagnosis and Course in Pregnancy

The group B *Streptococcus* has been recovered from the rectum or vagina of 5 to 30 per cent of asymptomatic pregnant women.[62] Most of the information on the prevalence of vaginal colonization with group B *Streptococcus* during pregnancy has been obtained from single observations. However, in a longitudinal 3 year study with repeated observations (4 to 11) of 382 patients followed up through pregnancy, delivery, and the postpartum period, group B streptococci were isolated from the vagina of 15 per cent of these patients at first visit and from 28 per cent of those who had repeated cultures. Of 108 patients with vaginal colonization, 36 per cent were colonized persistently throughout pregnancy, 20 per cent were colonized transiently, and 15 per cent were colonized intermittently. Group B *Streptococcus* carriage was significantly less common in Mexican-Americans, in women 20 years of age or older, and in women in their fourth or subsequent pregnancy.[37] Despite these observations, little is known about the factors responsible for the acquisition of increasing resistance to genital colonization, which seems to occur with advancing age and repeated pregnancy. Also, although there is some question about increased prevalence of vaginal colonization by group B streptococci with advancing gestation,[41] many other studies have failed to demonstrate any difference in prevalence of colonization in any trimester of pregnancy. Instead, there appears to be a relatively constant rate of vaginal colonization throughout pregnancy and immediately following delivery.[37] The fact is that there is a significant correlation between the intrapartum isolation of group B *Streptococcus* from the pregnant patient and the colonization of her newborn with the same serotype during the first week of life.

There are two possible sources of group B beta-hemolytic *Streptococcus,* each of which may lead to colonization of the birth canal. The gastrointestinal tract may be the primary site of colonization with secondary contamination of the genital tract, or colonization of the pregnant patient may occur by her sexual partner. The latter possibility is supported by recovery of the organism from urethral swabs of adult males, by recovery of the same serotypes from genital cultures of pregnant women and their husbands, and by the more frequent recovery of the organism from sexually active than from virginal college women even though a significant correlation between genital colonization and degree of sexual activity has not been demonstrated.[37, 43] Furthermore, intrapartum acquisition may be related to the glycogen-rich mucosa, lactobacillary flora, and acid pH in the normal vagina during pregnancy, which are all highly protective against group A streptococci but are apparently ineffective against endogenous group B streptococci. Regardless of the mechanism of vaginal colonization, vertical transmission from mother to infant during delivery has been documented by means of two epidemiologic markers, i.e., specific cap-

early + Late

5 Serotypes

sular polysaccharide antigens and phage susceptibilities.[40, 63] Similarly, horizontal transmission among infants within a nursery has also been demonstrated, but much less frequently. The key point is that some 50 to 75 per cent of infants delivered from colonized mothers become carriers within 3 days after birth with a serotype identical to that of the mothers. However, invasive disease develops in only 1 to 2 per cent of colonized infants. Thus, the number of neonates who develop group B streptococcal infection is considerably smaller than the number potentially at risk.

Two clinically distinct neonatal infections have been defined and are based on the age at onset. "Early-onset" septicemia presents as a severe, fulminant, multisystemic illness with rapid onset during the first week, most frequently during the first 24 hours of life. Pulmonary involvement is frequent and may be characterized by severe respiratory distress, unexpected apnea, or radiologic evidence of hyaline membrane disease or perinatal pneumonia. Symptoms of septicemia, meningitis, or both may be present, and shock may also occur. Early onset disease is more frequently associated with obstetric complications and has a mortality of approximately 60 per cent. Several factors have been shown to be important in the pathogenesis of early onset infections in the neonate and to increase the risk for disease substantially. These include a high inoculum in the maternal genital tract at the time of delivery, the number of sites from which the streptococci are isolated, a prolonged period between rupture of the membranes and delivery in a colonized mother, premature delivery or low birth weight, low levels of specific humoral antibody directed against B_{III} streptococcal capsular polysaccharide in maternal and infant serum, maternal peripartum infection, septic or traumatic delivery, fetal hypoxia, and infants who are the products of multiple-birth pregnancies.[50, 63] However, early onset disease has also been described in full-term infants in the absence of obstetric complications as well as in infants delivered by cesarean section. Also, intrauterine fetal death due to group B streptococcal infection has occurred despite intact fetal membranes. Nevertheless, the pathogenesis of early onset neonatal infection can best be explained by the acquisition of this organism in utero or during passage through the colonized birth canal. This concept is supported by the fact that the lung is often the primary site of early onset infection, which may be caused by aspiration of infected amniotic fluid. Also, the pathogen may be recovered from several sites, including the skin, nasopharynx, gastric aspirate, meconium, ear, blood, and cerebrospinal fluid of infants with early onset disease. All five serotypes (Ia, Ib, Ic, II, and III) may cause early-onset disease. In contrast, late onset disease occurs after the first week of life (11 days to 12 weeks), is more insidious in onset, is more often associated with meningitis, and occurs more frequently in infants of normal full-term deliveries and in the absence of obstetric complications. The pathogenesis of late onset disease is unclear, and the mortality rate is less than 20 per cent. The organism may have been acquired from the mother, either at delivery or after birth; from other newborns in the nursery; or from nursery personnel. Group B streptococci are recovered infrequently from sites other than blood or CSF, and almost all strains belong to serotype III.[40, 53]

Neonatal disease may also present as any of several focal infections including pneumonia, otitis media, facial or orbital cellulitis, ethmoiditis, conjunctivitis, septic arthritis, osteomyelitis, impetigo, empyema, and bacteremia without signs of sepsis. In the pregnant patient, group B streptococcus may cause chorioamnionitis, septic abortion, or peripartum sepsis.

Laboratory Procedures

Group B *Streptococcus,* or *Streptococcus agalactiae,* produces a mucoid colony with a narrow zone of beta hemolysis on beef heart infusion agar plates enriched with 10 per cent sheep's blood. Genital tract cultures, which are likely to contain several different organisms, are more effectively done on a selective medium containing Todd-Hewitt broth, sheep's blood, nalidixic acid, and gentamycin.[42] Most strains can be differentiated from almost all strains of group A beta-hemolytic streptococci by means of a bacitracin disc pressed onto an agar plate streaked with a heavy inoculum of the test organism. Most group A beta-hemolytic streptococci are inhibited by bacitracin, whereas most strains of group B beta-hemolytic streptococci are resistant, as are some strains of groups G and C streptococci. Therefore, certain other chemical tests are required to differentiate non–group A beta-hemolytic streptococci. The organisms can be further differentiated immunochemically because of their type-specific capsular polysaccharide antigens. Five serotypes have been identified (Types Ia, Ib, Ic, II, and III) and most strains isolated from patients can be identified as one of these types.[64]

Prevention and Treatment

Many studies have attempted to determine an optimal approach to the prevention or treatment of group B streptococcal infection. They have been directed at the pregnant mother, the newborn infant, or both. Three basic plans have been evaluated. The first requires identifying and treating the pregnant carrier with antibiotics to eliminate the organism from the birth canal and thus prevent colonization and subsequent infection of the newborn. The second is based on immunoprophylaxis, wherein antibody-deficient nonpregnant or pregnant women receive either active or passive immunization, respectively. The third involves prophylactic chemotherapy of the newborn in the form of early, single-dose penicillin administration at the time of birth.[42, 57, 63]

Initially, antepartum screening was suggested as a routine component of prenatal care, and carriers were treated with oral antibiotics. Although oral administration of ampicillin to carriers in the third trimester of pregnancy significantly reduced colonization within 3 weeks of completion of therapy, it failed to reduce colonization rates in both mother and child at delivery.[55] Similar results were observed with penicillin.[60] This approach has been unsuccessful because of the difficulty in eliminating the organism from mucosal surfaces, the intermittent nature of colonization, and the possibility of reinfection from asymptomatic but colonized sexual partners. In one study, the administration of penicillin or erythromycin to pregnant women and their spouses daily from 38 weeks of gestation until delivery was successful in reducing the incidence of neonatal colonization and disease.[59] Currently, most workers agree that there is little basis for routine antepartum screening cultures in normal pregnant patients. However, some have suggested that routine antepartum cultures be done at 34 to 36 weeks of gestation and that colonized mothers be treated during labor, but not enough infants were evaluated to determine the effect on rates of neonatal disease.[65] Others have recommended that screening cultures be obtained in that small group of pregnant patients who may be at high risk for infection. Specifically, patients may be candidates for antepartum cultures if they have obstetric histories that are known to be associated with neonatal infection, including premature delivery and low birth weight, a previous newborn with group B streptococcal or undiagnosed sepsis, prolonged rupture of membranes, unexplained stillbirth, postpartum endometritis, or chorioamnionitis.[47]

Although there is little scientific evidence to support the practice of prenatal screening, it has been suggested that pregnant patients at high risk for infection be followed up with quantitative cultures every 4 weeks, beginning at the 24th week of gestation, and those patients found to have a heavy growth be treated with oral penicillin, 500 mg four times daily for 1 week, followed by repeat cultures every 2 weeks until delivery, with re-treatment if recolonization occurs.[47] Furthermore, it is suggested that (1) women with premature rupture of membranes and those in premature labor be cultured on admission; (2) carriers with premature rupture of membranes and who are going to be observed be treated with oral penicillin, and (3) high-risk patients who are known carriers and in labor be treated with ampicillin 500 mg intravenously every 6 hours.[47] Further studies are needed to determine whether any or all of these suggestions have merit. However, based on our current understanding of the epidemiology and pathogenesis of neonatal infection, treatment directed at the high risk newborn at the time of delivery might be a more prudent approach, except of course for those pregnant patients who are at high risk of developing endometritis or chorioamnionitis, i.e., carriers with prolonged premature rupture of membranes.

Immunoprophylaxis is based on the observation that infants with group B streptococcal infections caused by Type III organisms, as well as their mothers, are deficient in Type III specific capsular polysaccharide antibody. Type III accounts for almost all late onset infections and approximately one third of early onset disease. A vaccine has been prepared from the Type III polysaccharide antigen and is immunogenic, and passive immunization of the fetus by means of maternal vaccination has been proposed.[43] However, transfer of maternal antibody may be deficient before 34 weeks of gestation, and the procedure may provide little protection for those most at risk, i.e., premature infants, even if properly timed. Also this vaccine does not provide protection against the other serotypes that account for two thirds of early onset disease.[57] Furthermore, an antigenic cross reaction between serotype III and Type 14 pneumococcal capsular polysaccharide has recently been clarified.[58] Immunization with polyvalent pneumococcal vaccine may transiently boost preexisting titers of Type III antibody but only if the pre-existing Type III antibody titer is above 2 μg per ml.[44] Although further studies may demonstrate a greater role for immunoprophylaxis, currently the prevention of early onset disease by immunizing the mother appears to have specific limitations. Studies of all five capsular polysaccharide vaccines in healthy volunteers and pregnant women must prove to be successful before immunoprophylaxis can be used routinely.

Prevention of group B streptococcal disease through a direct approach to the neonate by administering intramuscular penicillin (50,000 units) at the time of delivery has produced some encouraging results.[57, 63] Specifically, in a prospective randomized study of more than 18,000 infants, a single dose of penicillin given to neonates within 1 hour of delivery significantly decreased infant colonization and disease rates compared with rates observed in untreated control infants. However, the penicillin-treated group had an increased incidence of disease caused by penicillin-resistant organisms during the first year of this study but not during the second year.[63] Although this approach appears promising, further studies are needed to fully define the effect of routine parenteral penicillin at birth on the incidence of disease caused by penicillin-resistant pathogens. Specifically, the use of parenteral penicillin at birth in infants known to be at high risk of early onset disease, (e.g., premature delivery, low birth weight, prolonged rupture of membranes) would be of particular importance in resolving this controversial issue.

SEPTIC ABORTION AND SEPTIC SHOCK

During the decade of the 1960s septic abortion was one of the leading causes of maternal mortality in many states. Our experience with this syndrome during that period clearly indicated that almost all cases of septic abortion seen at the Yale–New Haven Hospital were a result of criminal or nonmedical abortions. Currently, we rarely see patients with this syndrome, because the laws governing abortions have become more liberal and physician-induced abortions to terminate unwanted pregnancies have become readily available to women throughout the United States. In 1978, the fifty states and the District of Columbia reported 1,157,776 legally induced abortions, approximately twice the number of abortions reported in 1972.[84] The national abortion rate was 23 per 1000 women aged 15 to 44 in 1978, and the national abortion ratio was 347 per 1000 live births, or more than one abortion for every three live births. The highest ratios were reported from New York City and the District of Columbia, where more than 1000 abortions oc-

curred per 1000 live births. The risk of maternal death for legal abortion procedures (1972 through 1978) was shown to increase with gestational age. Curettage procedures, the most widely used during the first trimester, had the lowest maternal death rate per 100,000 abortions; dilation and evacuation procedures, used after the twelfth week of gestation, significantly increased the patient's overall risk of dying compared with curettage but was significantly less than the risk from either saline or prostaglandin instillation procedures.[83] The overall maternal death rate for all types of procedures averaged 2.2 per 100,000 abortions. Although the number of legally induced abortions doubled from 1972 through 1978, and septic abortion continues to be a leading cause of maternal mortality, the total number of women dying of septic abortion has decreased by 89.4 per cent from 1969 through 1978.[83]

Current studies suggest that approximately 1 per cent of patients who have had first trimester abortions and 3 per cent of those with midtrimester elective abortions will develop postabortal endometritis (fever, abdominal pain, uterine tenderness, and retained products of conception) and will require hospital admission.[68] The endogenous vaginal bacterial flora (E. coli and other aerobic enteric gram-negative rods, group B beta-hemolytic streptococci, anaerobic streptococci, Bacteroides species, staphylococci, and microaerophilic bacteria) are most often responsible for postabortal endometrial infections, which often may be polymicrobial in cause. Current therapy consists of two key factors: (1) evacuation of the uterus and (2) parenteral antibiotics before, during, and after removal of any necrotic tissue by curettage. Most agree that prompt removal of infected necrotic tissue is the more important therapeutic procedure and should be performed within a few hours after admission to the hospital and *after* the beginning of antibiotic therapy. Numerous antibiotics have been recommended for the regimen of choice, but these variations are more stylistic than substantive. For example, in one study that compared the efficacy of clindamycin with that of penicillin and chloramphenicol in combination, a significantly greater number of complications (tubo-ovarian abscesses several weeks after treatment) was observed in the clindamycin treated group.[69] These investigators concluded that the penicillin-chloramphenicol combination was more effective, probably because of the broader spectrum of antibacterial activity, which may be the key to successful therapy along with evacuation of the uterus. We recommend penicillin or ampicillin plus an aminoglycoside, either tobramycin or gentamicin, for 5 to 7 days, and this regimen has been adequate in most instances. Also, some authors have suggested that prophylactic antibiotic therapy be considered for patients undergoing elective midtrimester abortions.[68] In our own studies with first trimester elective abortion by suction curettage, we observed a high incidence (85 per cent) of transient bacteremia during the abortion procedure or soon after. Bacteremia was intermittent in some and persistent in others; it existed as long as 1 hour after the procedure and was transient in all patients. Bacteremia was caused by normal genital tract flora, predominantly anaerobes, and mixed bacteremia occurred in almost one half of these patients. Our observations (1) suggested that there is some risk of developing bacterial endocarditis during suction abortion in patients with cardiac deformities and (2) provided support for the current practice of antibiotic prophylaxis for abortion patients with cardiac lesions that predispose them to endocarditis.[86]

Although most patients with septic abortions respond favorably to treatment,[81] the *septic shock* syndrome is one of the most serious complications of septic abortion. This syndrome can also occur later in pregnancy in patients with prolonged rupture of the membranes. The syndrome of septic shock as a complication of septic abortion was initially emphasized by Studdiford and Douglas, who described the clinical course and pathologic findings of what they called "placental bacteremia" in seven patients with second trimester septic abortion, all of whom became hypotensive after admission and four of whom died.[92] These patients had a clinical background of attempted induction of abortion, usually in the second trimester. The initial incident was followed by slight vaginal bleeding, often accompanied by leakage of amniotic fluid and lower abdominal pain. Fever and chills occurred after a variable interval, usually after 48 hours, and were followed within 8 to 36 hours by the sudden onset of hypotension unrelated to blood loss. Coliform organisms were recovered from the blood and the placenta of these patients, and a striking placental bacteremia was noted without a significant inflammatory reaction of the decidua or placental tissues.

These observations led the same workers to speculate that bacteria had been introduced into maternal tissues at the time of attempted abortion, where during the next few days they multiplied and because of the nature of the placenta, could be accumulated in huge numbers, ultimately inundating the maternal blood with products of bacterial growth and disintegration. Patients with products of conception in utero seemed to be easily infected, apparently because the products of conception had no perceptible defense mechanism to protect against infection. In fact, the placenta, which at term represents a membrane of 7 square meters in area,[73] appears to serve as a high culture medium, supporting the growth of invading microbes and permitting toxic substances to pass back and forth easily between the fetal and maternal circulations. Consequently, it is not difficult to understand how healthy young women can become so seriously ill so quickly once the placenta and the surrounding tissues become infected.

Gram-negative bacteria are responsible for the majority of these infections, particularly coliform, *Bacteroides,* and *Proteus* species. Gram-positive bacteria, specifically enterococci, staphylococci, anaerobic streptococci, and *Clostridium perfringens,* can be involved, although much less frequently than gram-negative organisms. Although *C. perfringens* has been cultured in 10 to 27 per cent of all septic abortion cases,[91] it is saprophytic in most of these patients. It has been the causative agent in only 0.5 per cent of pregnant patients who develop septic shock,[74] and in these patients early removal of the uterus is essential, combined with high dose intravenous penicillin therapy, 20 million units daily.

Pathophysiology

The pathophysiology of gram-negative bacteremia and its complication, septic shock, has undergone intensive investigation since 1951. However, controversy still exists over the precise mechanisms involved as well as the optimum approach to the therapy of this disease.

Since endotoxin is contained in the cell walls of all gram-negative bacilli and results in chills, fever, hypotension, abnormalities in coagulation, and lethality when given to man or animals, it has been generally assumed that endotoxin per se, when released during either multiplication or destruction of gram-negative bacilli during infection, is the primary pathogenic mechanism responsible for the manifestations of gram-negative bacteremia in humans. However, the chemical mediators epinephrine, norepinephrine, serotonin, 5-hydroxytryptophan, glucocorticoids, histamine, and lysosomal enzymes have also been proposed as responsible mediators for the clinical manifestations of gram-negative bacteremia.[82] Recent studies of host response to endotoxin suggest that endotoxin is not directly toxic but acts through the initiation of a complex series of pathophysiologic events that involve the fibrinolytic, coagulation complement, and kinin systems and their effects on the function of the microcirculation and hemostasis. The precipitating event in this sequence appears to be the activation of Hageman factor (Factor XII) by endotoxin or gram-negative bacilli.[87] Activated Hageman factor in turn can activate the fibrinolytic system as well as the clotting cascade. Intravascular fibrinolysis and concomitant intravascular clotting have been shown to occur in disseminated intravascular coagulation and may occur in gram-negative bacteremia.[79] In addition, gram-negative bacilli, endotoxin, Hageman factor, or antigen-antibody complexes can activate the classic and alternate pathways of the complement system. Complement activation may cause adherence of platelets and leukocytes to each other and to vascular endothelium and may generate chemotactic factors and anaphylatoxin.[76] Anaphylatoxin stimulates smooth muscle contraction, increases vascular permeability, leads to histamine release from mast cells, and is chemotactic for neutrophils. The kinin cascade can also be activated by endotoxin, antigen-antibody complexes, and through an essential intermediate step, by Hageman factor, with the ultimate production of the potent vasoactive substance bradykinin,[78] which can induce increased vascular permeability and leukocyte chemotaxis, marked systemic arteriolar dilation, venoconstriction, and hypotension.[80] Endotoxin can also release lysosomal enzymes capable of producing direct tissue injury, including damage to vascular endothelium and blood vessel walls as well as chemotactic and fibrinolytic activity, histamine release, and fever production.[95] These observations, demonstrating that changes in the kinin, complement, and coagulation systems occur in gram-negative bacteremia and are most marked in those patients who develop hypotension,[82] suggest a causal relationship.

Clinical Features

Classically, gram-negative bacteremia presents with an abrupt onset of chills, fever, prostration, hyperventilation, and occasionally nausea and vomiting. Some degree of hypotension may appear within 30 minutes to a few hours after the initial manifestations of gram-negative bacteremia in some patients with septic abortion.

In others, the clinical features may be much more subtle. In approximately one out of five patients with septic abortion, the disease may pursue a more fulminant course,[92] the onset of chills and fever being followed in 8 to 36 hours by sudden hypotension.

Although it is difficult to define sequential events and a consistent pattern of hemodynamic alterations in patients with bacteremic shock, two distinct clinical syndromes, early phase and late phase, have been described.[93] We have observed similar patterns and have interpreted them as sequential events in the pathogenesis of gram-negative bacteremic shock. Specifically, some patients develop chills, fever, and hypotension but have a warm, dry, flushed skin, full pulse, alert sensorium, neutropenic leukopenia, and hyperventilation with respiratory alkalosis. Initially, these patients usually have decreased peripheral resistance, low central venous pressure, and normal cardiac output, and although high, low, and normal central venous pressures and cardiac outputs have been observed.[96] These patients generally respond to prompt therapy, and their prognosis is excellent.

Some patients progress into a later and more classic clinical syndrome of shock with cold moist skin, weak thready pulse, pallor, cyanosis, mental confusion or obtundation, fall in fever, decreased urinary output, leukocytosis, and occasionally jaundice. In some the shock progresses, and metabolic acidosis, lactic acid accumulation, and a drop in arterial blood pH appear, reflecting inadequate tissue perfusion.[94] Some patients develop the adult respiratory distress syndrome (ARDS) manifested by pulmonary alterations of alveolar hypoventilation with impaired oxygen diffusion and severe hypoxemia. Pulmonary infiltrates that may appear on x-ray histologically consist of pulmonary edema, alveolar thickening, round cell infiltration, and ultimately fibrosis of hyaline membranes and alveolar septa.[70]

Septic shock patients may develop disseminated intravascular coagulation with decreased levels of Factors II, V, and VIII; fibrinogenopenia; thrombocytopenia; and fibrin split products in the serum.[82] These patients have an extremely poor prognosis.

The pathophysiologic events in septic shock are very complex, but the pattern of events in our pregnant patients in general has been one of initially decreased peripheral vascular resistance, increased cardiac output, and low central venous pressure (early phase) followed by a fall in cardiac output, compensatory peripheral arterial vasoconstriction, and in the absence of concomitant blood loss, a rising central venous pressure (late phase).

Management

Optimal treatment of septic abortion and septic shock includes identification of the infecting agent and its susceptibility to antimicrobial agents, prompt parenteral administration of an appropriate antibiotic in adequate doses, drainage of the infected focus either by mechanical or chemical evacuation or in specific situations by surgical removal of the uterus, and maintenance of adequate tissue perfusion by volume replacement and vasoactive amines. Thus, the management of these infections is designed to accomplish two goals — maintenance of adequate tissue perfusion and elimination of the infecting microbial agent.

Cultures

Bacteriologic studies should include aerobic and anaerobic cultures of blood, cervix or purulent cervical discharge, and if possible, uterine cavity. Care must be taken to avoid contaminating the specimen with normal vaginal flora. A Gram stain of cervical or uterine material should be done to attempt to identify the presence of clostridia, which will be meaningful only if these organisms are seen in the purulent discharge or in tissue obtained from the uterus. While clostridial infections are the most impressive and most serious infections in the female genital tract, fortunately they are rare. Other anaerobic organisms, particularly *Bacteroides* species *(B. melaninogenicus* or *B. fragilis* and other *Bacteroides* species), are much more common, as are anaerobic gram-positive cocci, aerobic *E. coli, Proteus, Klebsiella, Streptococcus,* and other bacteria.

Once cultures are obtained, appropriate *parenteral* antibiotic therapy is promptly begun, and then arterial blood pressure and central venous pressure are monitored. A percutaneous radiopaque central venous catheter is inserted, usually through the cephalic but sometimes through the external jugular vein to the superior vena cava and into the right atrium in order to monitor central venous pressure and assess the adequacy of volume replacement. Proper placement of the catheter is confirmed radiologically. On some occasions a Swan-Ganz catheter is inserted to monitor pulmonary wedge pressure in more seriously ill patients or when the routine central venous catheter cannot be properly positioned. The patient's mental status and urine output can be used as a guide for perfusion of vital organs; mental clarity and a urinary output of approximately 50 ml per hour reflect adequate perfusion of the brain and kidneys.

Other Laboratory Studies

Other base-line laboratory studies should also be obtained: typing and cross-matching of whole blood for possible volume replacement, complete blood and platelet counts, prothrombin and partial thromboplastin time and fibrinogen levels, blood urea nitrogen or serum creatinine levels, and serum electrolyte levels. The hematocrit should be repeated every few hours in patients with hypovolemia or hemorrhage.

An abdominal x-ray in the upright position should also be obtained, if possible, to check for free air in the peritoneal cavity as a result of perforation of the bowel or uterus. Arterial blood gases are also obtained in patients in shock in order to monitor the severity of the metabolic acidosis (lactic acidosis) and to provide guidelines for therapy. Severe lactic acidosis has been correlated with a poor prognosis in patients with septic shock. Although treatment of the lactic acidosis does not correct the primary lesion in septic shock, we do attempt to treat it partially with parenteral sodium bicarbonate. Attempts to correct the lactic acidosis rapidly and completely may be hazardous.[89]

Antibiotic Therapy

Once base-line cultures have been obtained, initial parenteral antibiotic therapy should be started promptly. Since the identity and antibiotic sensitivity of the infecting bacteria are rarely known at this time, our *initial* antibiotic therapy is based on the current antibiotic sensitivity patterns of the species of bacteria that statistically are the most likely cause of the infection and is also based on our past experience in treating these infections. We prefer a combination of antibiotics as initial therapy to provide a broad antibacterial spectrum until the infecting agent can be identified and antibiotic sensitivity tests can be performed. This information is usually available within 48 to 72 hours. At that time, the initial combination of antibiotics is altered according to the results of the cultures and antibiotic sensitivity tests, and the single most effective and least toxic antibiotic is selected for further treatment.

Our initial therapy consists of ampicillin in a dose of 1 gm intravenously every 3 to 4 hours (or a cephalosporin, the dose being dependent upon the preparation selected) and an aminoglycoside, either tobramycin or gentamicin in a dose of 1.5 mg per kg intravenously every 8 hours. The daily dose of the aminoglycoside must be decreased appropriately in those patients with compromised renal function. These combinations of antibiotics provide adequate initial antibacterial coverage against most of the infecting pathogens except *Bacteroides fragilis* and *Pseudomonas* species.

B. fragilis are resistant to the aminoglycosides, most cephalosporins, penicillin, and ampicillin in usual doses. The most effective antibiotics in vitro against *B. fragilis* are chloramphenicol, clindamycin, cefoxitin, and carbenicillin in large doses. Any one of these agents is indicated in septic abortion patients when certain clues suggest anaerobic infections. A foul-smelling purulent exudate (although not all anaerobic infections produce a foul odor) or a deep-seated pelvic infection that does not respond to drainage or initial antibiotic therapy is highly suggestive of an anaerobic infection. Chloramphenicol can be given in a loading dose of 1 gm intravenously followed by 500 mg every 4 to 5 hours, as the ester chloramphenicol sodium succinate, which is highly soluble. The ester has no antibacterial activity, but after intravenous administration it is rapidly converted to active chloramphenicol. We use a 10 per cent solution (e.g., 1 gm in 10 ml or 500 mg in 5 ml) for intermittent intravenous injections, and this dose is slowly injected over a period of a few minutes. Rapid intravenous injection does not appear to be dangerous, but patients may complain of an intensely bitter taste. The ester chloramphenicol sodium succinate should not be used intramuscularly, since as much as one third of the ester may not be hydrolyzed to active chloramphenicol when given in this manner.

Two forms of bone marrow depression may occur with chloramphenicol. The rare complication of aplastic anemia with pancytopenia occurs in approximately 1 in 100,000 treated cases and has a mortality rate of approximately 50 per cent. The more common complication of hematopoietic toxicity is manifested by reduced iron utilization for hemoglobin synthesis (rising serum iron level), vacuolation of marrow granulocyte and erythrocyte precursors, leukopenia, thrombocytopenia, and low reticulocyte counts, with a progressive increase in marrow myeloid-erythroid ratio. These changes may occur when plasma levels exceed 25 μg per ml and are usually reversible after cessation of the drug.

Clindamycin is given in a dose of 600 mg intravenously every 6 to 8 hours in a volume of 100 ml of normal saline over a period of approximately 30 minutes. Clindamycin may produce pseudomembranous enterocolitis, which may be fatal. This syndrome occurs shortly after the first week of treatment and presents with crampy abdominal pain and diarrhea in most cases. Clindamycin is not effective against coliforms, *Proteus,* and *Pseudomonas* organisms. In fact, its only role in septic abortion patients may be in treating *B. fragilis* infections, since other *Bacteroides* species are often killed by ampicillin. Also, since many septic abortions are mixed aerobic-anaerobic infections, we do not recommend the use of clindamycin alone as initial therapy and suggest it be combined with an aminoglycoside.

Pseudomonas aeruginosa infections should be treated with a combination of an antipseudomonal penicillin (e.g., carbenicillin or ticarcillin) and an aminoglycoside (tobramycin, gentamicin, or amikacin). These combinations have been shown to be synergistic against most strains of *Pseudomonas* in vitro and in serious *Pseudomonas* infections in animals[66, 67] as well as in preliminary clinical trials in septic abortion patients.[88] Carbenicillin is given intravenously in a dose of 4 to 5 gm every 4 hours (approximately 70 mg per kg) and gentamicin or tobramycin either intramuscularly or intravenously in a dose of 1.5 mg per kg of body weight every 8 hours. Recommended doses for amikacin are either 5 mg per kg every 8 hours or 7.5 mg per kg given every 12 hours. The dose of ticarcillin should be approximately two thirds of that of carbenicillin. The two drugs in the combination should be given at different sites and should not be mixed together in the same solution because of the potential inactivation of the aminoglycoside by carbenicillin or ticarcillin under these conditions.

The management of septic abortion patients with stable blood pressures who are not in acute distress includes obtaining base-line cultures and the laboratory determinations just described, followed immediately by aggressive parenteral antibiotic therapy. Although effective treatment also includes rapid and complete removal of the source of infection by surgical means, attempts to evacuate the uterus by curettage may result in increased risks of postoperative sepsis and hypotension[85] and should be delayed a few hours (3 to 4) while the patient is receiving intensive antibiotic treatment. Some patients may respond to antibiotic treatment but later develop a persistently elevated temperature. These patients should be evaluated for the presence of a tubo-ovarian abscess.

The management of septic abortion patients in shock also includes obtaining base-line cultures and the laboratory determinations previously described as well as instituting parenteral antibiotic therapy and monitoring central venous pressure measurements to determine the adequacy of volume replacement. Our treatment of the hypotensive patient with a low central venous pressure is aimed at expansion of blood volume to restore adequate tissue perfusion. Initially, rapid infusion of isotonic saline, plasma, albumin, or dextran solutions is given, or whole blood if the patient is anemic, and frequent central venous pressure measurements are taken. There is still much debate about the value of colloid versus crystalloid therapy in the treatment of shock.[90] Pragmatic considerations favor crystalloid therapy initially. Volume replacement is continued until the hypotension has been corrected or until central venous pressure rises to 120 mm H_2O. If central venous pressure either is elevated initially or becomes elevated with fluid replacement, and the patient's hypotension persists, we begin administration of a vasoactive amine, either isoproterenol or dopamine. Both agents have a chronotropic effect on the heart, but because of beta-adrenergic activity they can enhance peripheral tissue perfusion. Dopamine causes vasodilation of renal, coronary, and cerebral vessels, and most physicians prefer it over other agents. Initial rates of infusion of dopamine vary from 2 to 5 μg per kg per minute. The rate of infusion can be increased at 15 minute intervals until the systolic blood pressure is 90 to 100 mm Hg and urine output is in the range of 30 to 50 ml per hour. Once a response has been obtained, the infusion rate should be maintained at the lowest level that produces the desired hemodynamic state. Rapid but careful digitalization may be helpful in some cases when cardiac output does not improve after adequate fluid replacement. Oxygen should be administered to patients in shock, and the metabolic acidosis should be partially corrected with parenteral bicarbonate. Oliguria and urea nitrogen retention may complicate septic shock. Initial oliguria may be secondary to decreased effective circulating volume, which may respond to fluid replacement or to replacement followed by a single dose of 12.5 to 25 gm intravenous mannitol in an attempt to achieve a rapid increase in renal blood flow and urinary output and, it is hoped, to prevent further renal damage. If fluid replacement and mannitol fail to induce a satisfactory diuresis, hypoperfusion may persist and renal failure may occur as a result of acute tubular necrosis or, less frequently, bilateral cortical necrosis.

The use of corticosteroids in the treatment of septic shock remains most controversial. Nevertheless, large doses of corticosteroids have been recommended and have been widely used in the treatment of septic shock. The controversy has resulted from the well-known deleterious effects of corticosteroids on mechanisms of host defense against infection and on the lack of suitably controlled clinical studies documenting the effectiveness of corticosteroids in septic shock. In all probability, supraphysiologic doses of corticosteroids given for short periods have no major adverse effects on the course of infections. Corticosteroids may diminish interstitial edema, improve vascular and possibly myocardial responsiveness to catecholamines, and thereby improve tissue perfusion. Consequently, if the septic shock patient fails to respond promptly to fluid replacement and vasoactive substances, we use corticosteroids in doses of 1 gm of hydrocortisone, or an equivalent dose of some other corticosteroid, intravenously and repeat this dose at 4 to 6 hour intervals during the first 24 hours or until the patient responds. We do not use corticosteroids routinely but only in patients who fail to respond to volume replacement and vasoactive drugs.

In addition to corticosteroids, many other pharmacologic agents have been evaluated in animal models and then proposed for use in septic shock. However, no controlled studies in humans support their clinical use. Of these agents, the opiate antagonist naloxone is of interest. Recent studies suggest that stress releases the endogenous opiate beta-endorphin, which if released during septic shock may contribute to hypotension.[77] Studies in animals have shown that naloxone rapidly reverses the hypotension secondary to endotoxin[77] as well as to acute blood loss[75] and, when given prophylactically, blocks the occurrence of shock caused by endotoxin. Obviously, future studies are needed to determine the value of naloxone in humans.

Septic shock, particularly in the obstetric patient, may be associated with disseminated intravascular coagulation (DIC). Therefore, the clotting mechanism must be evaluated periodically with platelet counts, prothrombin and partial thromboplastin times, fibrinogen levels, and the presence of fibrin split products in the serum. The use of heparin in the treatment of disseminated intravascular coagulation is also controversial. Although there is evidence that the coagulopathy can be terminated by heparinization, there is no evidence that anticoagulation prolongs survival.[71, 72] Currently, it appears that absolute control of DIC requires effective removal of the underlying disease state and that anticoagulation results in only temporary beneficial effects. In incomplete septic abortion or fetal death in utero, the development of DIC becomes more likely the longer the products of conception are retained. Removal of the products of conception abolishes disseminated intravascular coagulation, as it does in abruptio placentae, and heparin may be unnecessary. If the hypotensive septicemic patient has bleeding because of the coagulopathy, replacement therapy should consist of transfusions with platelets, cryoprecipitate, and fresh frozen plasma for thrombocytopenia, hypofribrinogenemia, and other coagulation factors, respectively. Although replacement therapy may aggravate the coagulopathy by supplying additional clotting factors, this complication is uncommon if shock and infection are controlled along with the replacement of coagulation factors.[72]

A more radical approach is required in patients who fail to respond to fluid replacement, vasoactive agents, pharmacologic doses of corticosteroid, and intensive antibiotic therapy. We favor abdominal hysterectomy, particularly when the placenta remains attached and is inaccessible or when curettage has produced either a minimal amount of tissue or none and the patient does not improve within 4 to 6 hours. Although uncommon, this high risk category also includes the patient with a large uterus, more than 3 months in gestational size, with extensive spread of infection and with overt evidence of local or generalized peritonitis. The condition of each patient must be evaluated separately, and the decision to intervene surgically must be based on that particular patient's clinical condition and responsiveness to the therapy outlined here.

ANTIMICROBIAL AGENTS IN OBSTETRICS

The appropriate selection of antimicrobial agents in the practice of obstetrics must take into consideration their potential toxicity for the pregnant patient as well as the specific dangers to the fetus created by their passage across the placental barrier. These drugs may create special problems for the pregnant woman that do not exist for other patients. The obstetrician should be fully cognizant of the pharmocokinetics and toxicity of these agents, since antimicrobial

treatment must frequently be begun before the infecting organism has been identified. Consequently, the obstetrician must choose an antimicrobial agent or combination that will be effective against the organism *most likely* to be responsible for the patient's infection but that will not subject the pregnant patient or the fetus to unnecessary risk. The decision, therefore, should be based on a knowledge of the most common infections in obstetric patients, the organisms most likely to be responsible for these infections, the prevailing antimicrobial sensitivity patterns of the organisms, and the potential toxicity of the antimicrobial agents. Similarly, the physician must be aware of antimicrobial agents that are hazardous to the breast-fed newborn, because they appear in the milk of lactating mothers.

In an attempt to provide the reader with a reference guide, available antimicrobial agents have been grouped as follows: those which cross the placental barrier but are not toxic to the mother or fetus and are, therefore, not known to be a problem in pregnancy (Table 13–2); those

TABLE 13–2 ANTIMICROBIAL AGENTS THAT CROSS THE PLACENTAL BARRIER BUT ARE NONTOXIC TO THE FETUS

Penicillin (Greene and Hobby, 1944; Wasz-Hockert et al., 1970)
Ampicillin (Bray et al., 1966; Kraybill et al., 1980; Wasz-Hockert et al., 1970)
Amoxicillin (Kucers and Bennett, 1979)
Methicillin (Depp et al., 1970)
Oxacillin (Prigot et al., 1963)
Cloxacillin (Kucers and Bennett, 1979)
Dicloxacillin (MacAulay et al., 1968; Depp et al., 1970)
Nafcillin (Depp et al., 1970)
Cephalothin (Sheng et al., 1964)
Cephaloridine (Barr and Graham, 1967)
Cephalexin (Creatsas et al., 1980)
Cefazolin (Dekel et al., 1980)
Cephapirin (Creatsas et al., 1980)
Cephradine (Bergogne-Berezin, et al., 1979)
Cefamandole (Berkowitz et al., 1981)
Cefoxitin (Bergogne-Berezin et et al., 1979)
Cefaclor (Berkowitz et al., 1981)
Cefadroxil (Berkowitz et al., 1981)
Cefotaxime (Kafetzis et al., 1980)
Erythromycin (Kiefer et al., 1955; Philipson et al., 1973)
Colistimethate (MacAulay and Charles, 1967)
Isoniazid* (Kucers and Bennett, 1979)
Para-aminosalicylic Acid (Remington and Klein, 1976)
Ethambutol (Kucers and Bennett, 1979)
Amphotericin B† (Author's experience)
Griseofulvin (Rubin and Dvornik, 1965)

---

*Fetal toxicity rare (Varpela, 1964; Monnet, et al., 1967)
†Safety during first trimester not established

which cross the placental barrier and are harmful to the mother, fetus, or both (Table 13–3); those which appear in the milk of lactating mothers and therefore may be harmful to the newborn (Table 13–4); and those for which we have insufficient data about their pharmacokinetic distribution in pregnancy or which are not recommended during pregnancy because of potential toxicity to the fetus (Table 13–5). These tables list reactions of specific toxicity for the pregnant patient, fetus, or newborn and do not include all side effects that have been observed in other patients who have received these drugs and that of course, may also occur in the pregnant woman.

The use of prophylactic antibiotics in pregnant patients with predisposing congenital or acquired cardiovascular disease (rheumatic or other) does not appear warranted during the antepartum course of an uncomplicated pregnancy. The controversial question, however, is whether these patients should receive antibiotic prophylaxis at the onset of labor and during the immediate postpartum period. The incidence of asymptomatic puerperal bacteremia has been reported to be 0.5 and 1.3 per cent in two large groups of

patients (396 and 519 patients, respectively) who were studied at delivery and at various intervals during the immediate postpartum period.[97] The authors of that study question the advisability of using prophylactic antibiotics in patients with heart disease who have an uncomplicated delivery and postpartum course. However, they do not indicate the number of their patients who had predisposing cardiovascular disease nor the incidence of bacteremia in this group of patients. Even though the incidence of asymptomatic bacteremia may be low during the puerperal period, which suggests that the potential risk of developing bacterial endocarditis is small, most agree that pregnant patients with underlying cardiovascular disease that clearly predisposes them to bacterial endocarditis should receive prophylactic procaine penicillin G, 1.2 million units intramuscularly or intravenously, *or* 1 gm ampicillin intramuscularly or intravenously, plus 1 gm streptomycin intramuscularly (or tobramycin or gentamicin 1.5 mg per kg intramuscularly or intravenously) about 1 hour prior to delivery and that this regimen should be repeated at 12 hour intervals for 2 additional doses. Tobramycin or

TABLE 13–3 ANTIMICROBIAL AGENTS THAT CROSS THE PLACENTAL BARRIER AND MAY BE HARMFUL TO MOTHER BECAUSE OF PREGNANCY OR TO FETUS

Drug	Mother*	Fetus
Tetracyclines	Fever, nausea, vomiting, hyperbilirubinemia, jaundice, hematemesis, melena, acidosis, and azotemia (Schultz et al., 1963; Whalley et al., 1964)	Deposited in bones and joints (Kline et al., 1964; Kutscher et al., 1966)
Chloramphenicol	No	Circulatory collapse (Burns et al., 1959)
Streptomycin	No	Ototoxicity, rare (Woltz and Wiley, 1945; Conway and Birt, 1965)
Kanamycin	No	Potential ototoxicity (Kucers and Bennett, 1979)
Gentamycin	No	Potential ototoxicity (Creatsas et al., 1980)
Tobramycin	No	Potential ototoxicity (Kucers and Bennett, 1979)
Amikacin	No	Potential ototoxicity (Kucers and Bennett, 1979)
Carbenicillin	No	†Unknown (Sabath, 1973)
Lincomycin	†	†(Medina et al., 1964)
Clindamycin	†	†(Kucers and Bennett, 1979)
Novobiocin	No	Potential hyperbilirubinemia (Sutherland and Keller, 1961)
Sulfonamides	No	Potential hyperbilirubinemia and kernicterus; hemolysis in G-6-P-D deficiency (Kucers and Bennett, 1979)
Nitrofurantoin	No	Hemolysis in G-6-P-D deficiency (Perry and LeBlanc, 1967; Perry et al., 1967)
Trimethoprim	No	‡(Kucers and Bennett, 1979)
Trimethoprim/Sulfamethoxazole	No	‡(Kucers and Bennett, 1979)
Metronidazole	No	‡(Kucers and Bennett, 1979)
Rifampicin	No	‡(Kucers and Bennett, 1979)
5-Fluorocytosine	No	‡(Kucers and Bennett, 1979)
Ethionamide	No	‡(Kucers and Bennett, 1979)

*Only toxicities exaggerated by the pregnant state are listed.
†Safety not established in pregnancy.
‡High doses may be teratogenic. Not recommended during pregnancy, particularly during first trimester.

TABLE 13–4 ANTIMICROBIAL AGENTS THAT APPEAR IN HUMAN MILK

Drug	Toxic to Newborn
Penicillin G (Greene et al., 1946)	No
Oxacillin (Prigot et al., 1963)	No
Cloxacillin (Sabath, 1973)	No
Erythromycin (Remington and Klein, 1976)	No
Lincomycin (Medina et al., 1964)	No
Dihydrostreptomycin (Remington and Klein, 1976)	No
Chlortetracycline (Guilbeau et al., 1950)	Yes*
Tetracycline (Posner et al., 1954)	Yes*
Chloramphenicol (Burns et al., 1959; Sutherland, 1959)	Gray baby syndrome with circulatory collapse and death*
Novobiocin (Remington and Klein, 1976)	Hyperbilirubinemia*
Oxolinic Acid (Author's experience)	Unknown*
Sulfonamides (Kucers and Bennett, 1979)	Kernicterus, hemolytic anemia (G-6-P-D deficiency)*
Trimethoprim (Kucers and Bennett, 1979)	Interferes with folic acid metabolism*
Trimethoprim/Sulfamethoxazole (Kucers and Bennett, 1979)	Kernicterus*
Cefoxitin (Kucers and Bennett, 1979)	Unknown
Metronidazole (Kucers and Bennett, 1979)	Potentially carcinogenic*
Isoniazid (Kucers and Bennett, 1979)	No
Amantidine (Kucers and Bennett, 1979)	Potentially toxic*

*Should not be used in nursing mothers.

gentamicin should be given at 8 hour intervals. For patients allergic to penicillin, vancomycin (1 gm intravenously) given over 30 minutes to 1 hour plus streptomycin as just described should be given and repeated for 2 additional doses. We believe that bacterial endocarditis is such a serious disease that every effort should be made to prevent its occurrence.

POSTPARTUM INFECTIONS

Puerperal sepsis is sometimes underestimated as a potentially serious postpartum complication. Even though we no longer see epidemics of "childbed fever," postpartum infection continues to be a leading contributor to maternal morbidity and mortality today.

Historically, the streptococcus has been equated with puerperal sepsis, and although Gordon, in 1795,[144] and Holmes, in 1843,[147] were believers in the contagiousness of this disease, person-to-person transmission was not clearly established until the classic studies of Semmelweis were published in 1861.[153] For the most part, some degree of prevention and control of "childbed fever" epidemics was attained with the introduction of antiseptic techniques, isolation procedures, and more recently, antimicrobial drugs. Similarly, the development of specific bacteriologic techniques was responsible for the demonstration that group A beta-hemolytic streptococci were the organisms most frequently isolated from patients with puerperal sepsis, and physicians readily assumed that postpartum sepsis was synonymous with streptococcal infec-

TABLE 13–5 OTHER ANTIMICROBIAL AGENTS — TRANSPLACENTAL PASSAGE AND/OR SAFETY NOT ESTABLISHED IN PREGNANCY

Bacitracin	Nalidixic Acid*‡§	Miconazole*‡
Neomycin	Oxolinic Acid*‡§	Econazole*‡
Cephaloglycin	Cinoxacin*‡§	Ketoconazole†
Polymyxin B	Pyrazinamide†	Idoxuridine†
Vancomycin	Clycloserine	Cytarabine†
Ticarcillin	Capreomycin	Adenine Arabinoside†
Spectinomycin	Viomycin	Amantidine*‡
Methenamine Mandelate	Nystatin	Methisazone†
Pyrimethamine	Pimaricin	

*Not recommended during first trimester
†Not recommended during pregnancy
‡Not recommended during breast feeding
§Not recommended in newborn infants

tion. Recently, however, group A beta-hemolytic streptococci have become less frequent causes of puerperal sepsis, and other bacteria, including other streptococci, have been identified as the more common causative agents. In fact, the organisms involved in postpartum pelvic infections are those normally found in the genital tract of asymptomatic patients and include *E. coli, Klebsiella,* group B beta hemolytic streptococci, enterococci, and a variety of anaerobes, e.g., peptococci, peptostreptococci, and *B. fragilis.* Pathogenic organisms isolated less frequently include group A beta-hemolytic streptococci, *S. aureus*; *P. aeruginosa* and *S. marcescens.* Fortunately, puerperal sepsis caused by bacteria other than group A streptococci is generally less fulminating and is often endogenous in origin, that is, non–hospital acquired. Thus, fulminant puerperal sepsis caused by Group A beta-hemolytic streptococci, as well as its associated high maternal mortality, has been *almost* eliminated as a cause of serious postpartum infection. However, postpartum endometritis, myometritis, bacteremia, septic thrombophlebitis, necrotizing fasciitis, and pelvic abscess still occur frequently and are responsible for the maternal morbidity and mortality caused by postpartum infections.

Factors Predisposing to Postpartum Infections

First, the female genital tract is heavily colonized with potentially pathogenic bacteria. Second, the onset of labor may be associated with frequent internal examinations and internal fetal monitoring devices. Third, vaginal delivery may require manual removal of the placenta, episiotomy, and forceps extraction. Finally, delivery, whether vaginal or by cesarean section, is associated with tissue trauma and blood loss. Thus, potential bacterial contamination of traumatized tissue may set the stage for postpartum uterine infection. Fortunately, such infections occur in only a small percentage of women, probably because of recently recognized factors that appear to aid in their prevention. Specifically, the bacterial flora of the female genital tract changes during pregnancy so that the number of gram-negative aerobic (e.g., *E. coli*) and anaerobic organisms decreases late in pregnancy.[143] Also the antibacterial activity of amniotic fluid increases progressively from the twentieth to the fortieth week of gestation, when it then begins to decrease,[152] and normal pregnant women have elevated white blood cell counts with increased activity during pregnancy, labor, and the early postpartum period.[149] Although these factors are

thought to play a protective role against infection, other factors seem to increase the risk of postpartum infection. Of these, the most critical factor is the route of delivery, i.e., cesarean section is the major predisposing clinical factor for both the frequency and the severity of postpartum pelvic infections.[139] Since cesarean section rates are increasing throughout the country, postpartum infections have become a problem of major significance. A review was recently made of the relative risk of infection complications following cesarean section compared with similar patients following vaginal delivery.[139] Endometritis occurred 5 to 30 times more frequently in patients who were delivered by cesarean section than in similar patients with vaginal deliveries. Similarly, postpartum cesarean section patients experienced septic thrombophlebitis or pelvic abscesses twice as frequently, bacteremia 2 to 10 times more frequently, and death from sepsis 80 times more frequently than comparable patients who had undergone vaginal delivery. In addition to cesarean section, the influence of other factors on the postpartum pelvic infection rate was also reviewed.[139] The risk of developing puerperal infection was lowest 1 to 3 per cent, in patients undergoing uncomplicated vaginal delivery. This risk increased to 3 to 10 per cent in (a) patients with vaginal delivery complicated by prolonged labor, prolonged rupture of membranes, or major trauma, and (b) nonindigent women undergoing *elective* cesarean section. A further increase in the risk of infection (10 to 40 per cent) occurred in (a) indigent women delivered by *elective* cesarean section, (b) indigent women delivered by cesarean section who were in labor with ruptured membranes of less than 6 hours, and (c) nonindigent women with any duration of labor and ruptured membranes who were delivered by cesarean section. The highest risk of postpartum pelvic infection (40 to 85 per cent) occurred in indigent women delivered by cesarean section who required multiple vaginal examinations because of prolonged labor and ruptured membranes of greater than 6 to 12 hours.[139] Thus, the evidence appears to support route of delivery (i.e., cesarean section), presence of labor, rupture of membranes, vaginal examinations, and socioeconomic status as major risk factors that predispose to postpartum pelvic infections. In contrast, the evidence for internal fetal monitoring, manual removal of the placenta, episiotomy, forceps delivery, anemia in the absence of poor nutrition or lower socioeconomic status, obesity (a major risk factor for wound infection), and general anesthesia as major risk factors of and by themselves for postpartum pelvic infections has not been definitively established.[139]

In addition, there has been some concern that classic cesarean sections place the patient at even greater risk of infection in general and severe complications in particular.[154] However, many of these procedures were performed after prolonged rupture of the membranes. In contrast, when classic cesarean sections were performed only in patients with short periods of labor or ruptured membranes, or without either of these predisposing factors, more frequent or more severe postpartum pelvic infections were not encountered.[139]

Clinical Manifestations and Treatment

Puerperal infection usually takes the form of acute endometritis, which may progress to pelvic cellulitis and peritonitis. Symptoms generally do not appear until 3 or more days after delivery. Symptoms appearing earlier or later suggest an infection acquired either before or after labor and delivery. In addition, in infection acquired during delivery, the infectious process is likely to be more virulent the earlier the symptoms of puerperal sepsis appear. Fever, subinvolution, uterine tenderness on abdominal palpation, and vaginal discharge, which may be foul smelling, are the prominent clinical manifestations of puerperal sepsis. A chilly sensation, headache, and malaise may also be present. These symptoms are usually more acute and the patient's condition more toxic, with more pronounced chills and pelvic-abdominal pain, when group A beta-hemolytic streptococci are the causative agents. Furthermore, puerperal beta-hemolytic streptococcal infections may spread along the walls of the cervix, uterus, and vagina, resulting in pelvic cellulitis, peritonitis, or septicemia. Less often an abscess may form in the pelvis and lower abdomen.

Vaginal, uterine, blood, and urine cultures should be obtained before treatment. Often, a Gram stain of material, properly acquired from the uterine cavity before starting antibiotic therapy, may be helpful in identifying the bacteria responsible for the infection. For example, the presence of gram-negative, poorly staining pleomorphic rods suggests infection with Bacteroides species, whereas small gram-positive cocci in chains are likely to be Streptococcus species, gram-positive rods Clostridia species, etc. Frequently, the initial Gram stain suggests polymicrobial infection. Nevertheless, the Gram stain can help the clinician to implement an appropriate therapeutic regimen. Since anaerobes may play a major role in these infections, properly acquired material from the uterine cavity must be submitted for both aerobic and anaerobic cultures.

Antibiotic therapy is often begun for either suspected or obvious infection before bacteriologic identification and antibiotic sensitivity results of cultures are available. Two approaches have been used, both employing combination antibiotic therapy.

One approach is to begin high dose penicillin G (20 million units daily) or ampicillin (1 gram at 4 hour intervals) intravenously combined with an aminoglycoside, either gentamicin or tobramycin (1 to 1.5 mg per kg every 8 hours in patients with normal renal function), the higher dose being given to severely septic patients. A cephalosporin may be substituted for penicillin or ampicillin in patients allergic to penicillin whose history does not include anaphylaxis. These antibiotic combinations are not optimally active against Bacteroides fragilis. Consequently, agents effective against B. fragilis (chloramphenicol, clindamycin, metronidazole, or newer-generation cephalosporins, i.e., cefoxitin, cefotaxime, and moxalactam) are added for women who remain febrile after 48 to 72 hours. This approach is intended to avoid the overuse of the potentially toxic drugs chloramphenicol and clindamycin.

The second approach is to begin therapy with the clindamycin-aminoglycoside (gentamicin or tobramycin) combination. This approach is intended to shorten the clinical course and decrease maternal complications that may occur in women who would remain febrile after 48 to 72 hours of treatment if they had received the penicillin-aminoglycoside combination.

There are equally avid proponents of both approaches, and the "trade-off" is an increased risk of toxicity versus a potentially increased risk of maternal complications. Of course, early treatment for anaerobes, particularly B. fragilis, is indicated whenever infection with this organism is suspected.

Some women who fail to respond to antibiotic therapy may require surgical intervention for drainage of adnexal or pelvic abscesses. A persistent septic course in these patients is often attributed to infection with antibiotic-resistant bacteria, which may result in a delay in diagnosis while the physician adds other antibiotics. In fact, resistant organisms are an infrequent cause of a continued clinically septic course in patients treated with the antibiotic regimens recommended earlier.[148] Prompt diagnosis and localization of the abscess should be attempted, rather than the addition of other antibiotics. We have found ultrasound to be extremely reliable in demonstrating pelvic abscesses, and we use it as a diagnostic tool to support early operative intervention.[155] In our experience, ultrasound accurately diagnosed 32 out of 33 pelvic abscesses and correctly excluded pelvic abscess in 33 out of 34 other patients.[155] Gallium scan, though used frequently, has greater limitations in the postoperative patient (postcesarean section) because of nonspecific inflammation in the operative area. Thus, we feel that failure to respond to appropriate antibiotic therapy, combined with a positive ultrasound for the presence of a fluid-filled mass with highly reflective irregular walls, a rounded contour, and internal echoes suggesting cellular debris contained in pus, is strong evidence in support of surgical intervention.[155]

Septic pelvic thrombophlebitis and *septic pulmonary emboli* were frequently seen at autopsy in patients who died of puerperal sepsis in the preantibiotic era.[145] Although antibiotics have reduced the frequency of this complication of puerperal infection, septic pelvic thrombophlebitis still occurs in about 2 per cent of pelvic infections, presumably as a complication of protracted and extensive pelvic cellulitis that spreads to the major pelvic veins. Anaerobic infections, particularly those caused by *Bacteroides* species, seem to cause septic pelvic thrombophlebitis, and this may be due to the production of heparinase by these organisms.[138] Fortunately, the pulmonary emboli that may occur as a result of septic pelvic thrombophlebitis are small and rarely fatal. Large septic emboli are very uncommon. Nevertheless, septic pelvic thrombophlebitis produces a clinical picture of protracted intermittent fever even though the patient is receiving adequate antibiotic therapy and has no clinical or laboratory evidence of a pelvic abscess. Physical examination may reveal localized lower abdominal or pelvic tenderness, but this tenderness is often minimal and sometimes absent. Consequently, septic pelvic thrombophlebitis should be suspected in patients who remain febrile while receiving adequate antibiotic therapy and who have negative evaluations for a pelvic abscess. A diagnostic trial of a constant intravenous infusion of heparin, in a dose sufficient to achieve a therapeutic range determined by clotting or partial thromboplastin times, should be given.[50, 151] A therapeutic response should occur within 48 hours and may often be dramatic. Treatment should be continued for a minimum of 10 days unless pulmonary emboli have occurred, and then oral anticoagulants can be used for a longer course of treatment. The anticoagulant effect of heparin is thought to be responsible for its therapeutic effect. Ligation of the inferior vena cava and ovarian vein, with possible removal of the infected veins, has been used as the mainstay of therapy[137] but is more often reserved for patients with evidence of embolization despite adequate heparinization. In contrast to septic pelvic thrombophlebitis, ovarian vein thrombophlebitis presents as acute unilateral abdominal pain, usually right-sided and often suggesting acute appendicitis. Fever may or may not be present. Although the diagnosis can be suspected, it can be made only at laparotomy. Ligation and excision of the thrombus with or without heparin therapy, as well as anticoagulation alone, has been successful.

Necrotizing fasciitis, or "synergistic bacterial gangrene," has been described in postpartum patients.[142] Although this complication is rare in the practice of obstetrics, it occurs more commonly after vaginal delivery and episiotomy repair than after cesarean section and has a high mortality. There is rapid progression of edema, necrosis, and gangrene of the skin and adjacent fascia caused by simultaneous infection with aerobes and anaerobes. Early recognition of this condition and prompt and extensive surgical debridement plus high dose broad-spectrum antibiotic therapy are critical.

Extensive paracervical or paravaginal soft tissue infections have been reported following paracervical or pudendal block anesthesia in patients undergoing vaginal delivery.[146] These patients complain of hip pain and difficulty in ambulation early in the postpartum period as well as severe leg pain even with passive movement. These infections are thought to be polymicrobial, and antibiotic therapy should include coverage for anaerobes. Some of these patients may also require surgical drainage.[146]

Toxic-Shock Syndrome. In November 1978, a severe acute disease associated with strains of staphylococci of Phage Group I that produced a unique epidermal toxin was described in seven children.[164] These patients presented with the sudden onset of high fever, headache, confusion, sore throat, vomiting, watery diarrhea, and hypotension. They also developed conjunctival injection, a scarlatiniform rash, subcutaneous edema, acute renal failure, abnormalities in liver function, and desquamation of the hands and feet during convalescence. This illness was named the Toxic-shock syndrome (TSS).[164]

Shortly after this description of toxic-shock syndrome in children, several cases in adults were reported to the Wisconsin Division of Health, and currently more than 600 cases of

TSS have been reported to the Center for Disease Control. These cases have occurred predominantly in young, previously healthy, menstruating women who used tampons (particularly those who used them continuously during menses, and especially the Rely brand tampon) and became ill during the first few days of their menstrual period.[160] In addition to tampon use, another risk factor appears to be vaginal colonization with *Staphylococcus aureus*. In one study this organism has been isolated from 98 per cent of preantibiotic vaginal cultures from women with TSS compared with 7 per cent of control women who had vaginal cultures during their menstrual periods. Although approximately 10 per cent of TSS cases have been reported in postmenopausal women and in males, these patients have usually had a staphylococcal infection of the soft tissue.[160] These observations indicate an etiologic role for *S. aureus* in TSS, and most strains of *S. aureus* isolated have been resistant to penicillin and ampicillin.[162] However, the exact role of the staphylococcus in the pathogenesis of TSS has not been clearly defined. Since bacteremia rarely occurs in TSS, it has been proposed that the widespread systemic effects in this disease have been caused by a staphylococcal toxin. Recent studies have identified both a pyrogenic exotoxin[161] and an enterotoxin-like protein, staphylococcal enterotoxin F (SEF),[158] from strains of *Staphylococcus aureus* isolated from patients with TSS. Furthermore, sera from patients with acute TSS were found to have a lower prevalence of anti-SEF antibodies compared with control sera, which suggests that TSS patients may be more susceptible to the effects of SEF at the onset or in the early phases of their acute illness.[158] However, SEF–anti-SEF complexes were not looked for in this study. Therefore, at least two toxins, a pyrogenic exotoxin and enterotoxin F, have been incriminated as contributing to the clinical picture of the toxic-shock syndrome. Others may be discovered during future studies.

The toxic-shock syndrome typically begins abruptly with fever (frequently above 40° C), vomiting, diarrhea, and sometimes chills and abdominal pain. Hypotension develops within 72 hours or may occur abruptly. A diffuse, blanching, macular, erythematous rash (sunburn-like) develops and may erroneously be attributed to the fever, or to a drug eruption if it later evolves into a discrete macular exantham. Mucous membrane involvement may be prominent, with pharyngeal, conjunctival, or vaginal hyperemia. Sore throat may be a presenting symptom or may occur later in the disease. Diffuse myalgia is frequently present, and the patient may complain of exquisite tenderness of the skin or muscles with touch or movement. Initial laboratory results include leukocytosis with marked shift in immature neutrophils, thrombocytopenia, abnormal urinary sediment and renal and liver function, hyponatremia, hypocalcemia, elevated creatine phosphokinase, hyperamylasemia, and myoglobinuria in some patients. Photophobia, hepatomegaly, paresthesia, arthralgia, joint effusions, pericarditis, vasculitis, adult respiratory distress syndrome, and central nervous system symptoms including seizures have been described.[162] Most patients recover within 7 to 10 days. The rash desquamates within 7 to 14 days, primarily on the palms and soles but also on the face, torso, and tongue. The estimated incidence of the toxic shock syndrome is 6 to 15 cases per 100,000 menstruating women per year, and the mortality rate throughout the country has been 10 to 15 per cent.

TREATMENT. The currently suggested management of suspected TSS in women includes careful vaginal examination with removal of any retained tampon; cultures of vagina, cervix, blood, anterior nose, urine, and stool for *S. aureus* and other organisms *before* initiating antibiotic therapy; and aggressive fluid replacement with parenteral crystalloid solutions. Patients may require 8 to 12 liters per day, because much of this fluid is sequestered in the extravascular space and they may develop peripheral edema. Patients failing to respond promptly should also receive colloid, e.g., plasma, to restore oncotic pressure and a vasoactive amine to maintain adequate tissue perfusion. Patients should also receive beta-lactamase–resistant antistaphylococcal antibotics, because it is difficult to determine clinically which patients with TSS are bacteremic and because beta-lactamase–resistant antistaphylococcal antibiotics decrease the risk of recurrent episodes.[159] Approximately 30 per cent of affected women have had one or more recurrences, usually within a month or two of the initial episode but sometimes as long as a year or more later. For this reason, and even though we are uncertain about the exact role of tampons in the pathogenesis of TSS, women who have had an episode of TSS should be advised to discontinue tampon use at least until *S. aureus* has been eradicated from the vagina. If they and other women choose to use tampons, they probably can reduce the risk of TSS by employing tampons only intermittently during the menstrual period.

The Centers for Disease Control has established a strict clinical case definition, which physicians should use to document the toxic-shock syndrome in their patients.[160] These criteria are as follows:

1. Fever (temperature 38.9 C [102 F]).
2. Rash (diffuse macular erythroderma).
3. Desquamation, 1–2 weeks after onset of illness, particularly of palms and soles.
4. Hypotension (systolic blood pressure ≤90 mm Hg for adults or <5th percentile by age for children <16 years of age, or orthostatic syncope).
5. Involvement of 3 or more of the following organ systems:
   A. Gastrointestinal (vomiting or diarrhea at onset of illness).
   B. Muscular (severe myalgia or creatine phosphokinase level >2 × ULN*).
   C. Mucous membrane (vaginal, oropharyngeal, or conjunctival hyperemia).
   D. Renal (BUN† or Cr‡ ≥2 × ULN or ≥ 5 white blood cells per high power field — in the absence of a urinary tract infection).
   E. Hepatic (total bilirubin, SGOT§, or SGPT‖ ≥ 2 × ULN).
   F. Hematologic (platelets ≥ 100,000/mm³).
   G. Central nervous system (disorientation or alterations in consciousness without focal neurologic signs when fever and hypotension are absent).
6. Negative results on the following tests, if obtained:
   A. Blood, throat, or cerebrospinal fluid cultures.
   B. Serologic tests for Rocky Mountain spotted fever, leptospirosis, or measles.

*Twice upper limits of normal for laboratory.
†Blood urea nitrogen level.
‡Creatinine level.
§Serum glutamic oxaloacetic transaminase level.
‖Serum glutamic pyruvic transaminase level.

TSS is not restricted to menstruating women. In the following case, which was called to my attention by Dr. David Baker, it occurred in this patient during the third day following delivery by cesarean section.

A 27 year old Gravida 2, Para 1 woman was admitted on February 9, 1981, for a repeat cesarean section at the beginning of the 40th week of an uneventful pregnancy. The following morning she was delivered of a 7 lb 8 oz live female infant through a low transverse incision under epidural anesthesia. She had an uneventful course until she began to notice swelling and redness of both hands about 60 hours

postoperatively. Over the next several hours the erythema became generalized, and she became febrile, her temperature being 103° F. At that time, her rash was described as a diffuse, erythematous eruption with "sandpaper" texture, involving her face, trunk, and upper thighs, including her skin folds. She was noted to have circumoral pallor and a white-coated, red-edged tongue. She had a pulse of 130 per min but was not hypotensive, and there was no evidence of wound erythema, induration, or fluctuance. A white blood cell count was 20,300 per cu mm with 85 segmented and 9 band neutrophils, 2 lymphocytes, 1 monocyte, and 3 eosinophils. Cultures of urine, blood, lochia, and pharynx were obtained as well as antistreptolysin O titer and intravenous penicillin G therapy was started.

The following day she continued to be febrile, with a temperature as high as 104° F. The erythematous rash had decreased on her face but retained its "sandpaper" texture elsewhere, and her tongue was now bright red and tender. High dose intravenous penicillin therapy was continued although the blood cultures were negative.

On the morning of February 16, 1981, she was noted to be hypotensive for the first time and her urine output decreased. She continued to have a diffuse erythematous rash and "strawberry tongue" and had a persistent leukocytosis with left shift. Later that morning, because of the development of a wound dehiscence, she was returned to the operating room, where a total abdominal hysterectomy and repair of wound dehiscence were performed under general anesthesia.

Cultures of the abdominal wound and vagina obtained preoperatively as well as intrauterine and peritoneal cultures obtained at surgery all grew a coagulase-positive *Staphylococcus aureus* resistant to penicillin G. All blood cultures remained negative, as did the antistreptolysin O titer.

Additional complications included hyperbilirubinemia (maximum of 4.6 mg per dl on February 18), which returned to normal by February 23, transient rise in serum creatinine to 1.9 mg per 100 ml on February 16, which fell to 1.0 mg per 100 mgl by February 18, and the development of adult respiratory distress syndrome, requiring entubation and respirator support for 2 days and supplemental oxygen for another 2 days before arterial blood gases returned to normal values.

The patient received parenteral antistaphylococcal therapy for 8 days followed by another week of oral dicloxacillin. Prior to discharge, repeat vaginal cultures were negative for staphylococci, and except for desquamation of the skin of the nose and fingertips, the skin had returned to normal. All cultures of the infant were negative for staphylococci throughout her hospital stay.

Although clinicians are constantly challenged by new syndromes, the toxic-shock syndrome probably existed long before it became publicized so recently. In fact, an association between *S. aureus* infection and a diffuse scarlatiniform rash followed by desquamation was reported as far back as 1927.[163] Nevertheless, TSS must be added now to the list of infections that the obstetrician must consider in postpartum patients.

LISTERIA INFECTIONS

Listeriosis, an infectious disease of animals and man, is characterized by a wide range of clinical signs and symptoms. The infection is caused by the bacterium *Listeria monocytogenes,* an opportunistic, motile, aerobic or microaerophilic, hemolytic, gram-positive bacillus. The epidemiology of infections caused by *L. monocytogenes* has not been well defined. Although some evidence suggests that human *Listeria* infections are caused by direct transmission from animal sources (*L. monocytogenes* has been found to infect more than fifty species of animals), the majority of human infections cannot be explained by this mechanism. Circumstantial evidence suggests that certain exogenous factors and environmental pollution may help to explain the worldwide distribution of *Listeria* infection; e.g., this organism survives in large quantities under natural conditions in soil, in the superficial layers of poor silage, on decayed matter, and on wood and other materials. Also, *Listeria* has been cultured frequently from fecal specimens of healthy and sick animals, slaughterhouse workers, and healthy pregnant women. Thus, this organism may be a normal resident of the intestinal tract with the potential to be pathogenic, and soil and feces may be important modes of transmission of *Listeria* infections in animals. In addition, animal-to-animal, animal-to-man, and man-to-man transmission may occur. However, the source of *Listeria* infection in most human cases is not clear, except when transplacental transmission occurs. Even though epidemics have been reported, most cases of human listeriosis are sporadic and occur primarily in newborns, very young infants, and older adults, which suggests that infection with this organism may be associated with deficiencies in host defense mechanisms. Specifically, pregnant women and patients with chronic infectious diseases, diabetes mellitus, alcoholism, diseases of the reticuloendothelial system, and diseases requiring immunosuppressive or corticosteroid therapy are particularly prone to infection with *Listeria*. Also, listeriosis has occurred in a number of hemodialysis patients.

Listeria monocytogenes is well known to produce several clinical syndromes in human beings: listeriosis of pregnancy; disseminated perinatal sepsis (granulomatosis infantiseptica); neonatal or adult meningoencephalitis; sepsis of unknown origin in the neonate or adult; and a variety of focal infections including those of the lymph nodes and skin, purulent conjunctivitis, anterior uveitis, endocarditis, arthritis, osteomyelitis, peritonitis, cholecystitis, and spinal or brain abscess.[167, 170] Excellent reviews of human *Listeria* infections have been published.[167, 169, 170] Consequently, only those infections of concern to the obstetrician will be emphasized here.

Listeriosis During Pregnancy

Infection may occur at any time during pregnancy but more often occurs after the fourth month and particularly during the third trimester. No specific clinical manifestations of maternal listeriosis distinguish it from other complications of pregnancy. Frequently, it presents as an acute but mild febrile illness with chills, fever, malaise, myalgia, headache, and back or flank pain a few days or weeks before abortion or delivery. The syndrome often mimics influenza or pyelonephritis, except that the diagnosis is not supported by examination or culture of the urine, and other laboratory tests are not helpful. These symptoms may subside with or without antibiotic therapy, and the diagnosis can be established only by isolation of *L. monocytogenes* from blood cultures obtained during the illness. However, many cases are probably not detected because blood cultures are often not obtained. In some patients, untreated *Listeria* bacteremia in the mother does not affect the fetus, whereas in others, the infection appears to precipitate labor, which may result in premature delivery of an infected or dead baby.[165] Neonatal infection is presumed to be secondary to maternal bacteremia. The organism must cross the placenta during bacteremia in the mother and infect the placenta, the amniotic fluid, and the fetus. *Listeria* may be recovered from umbilical cord blood, lochia, endometrial tissue obtained by curettage, vaginal mucus, urine, and placental tissue.[169] *Listeria monocytogenes* has been thought to be responsible for 1 to 6 per cent of abortions in western European countries. Although the interval between maternal and fetal infection is still uncertain, abortion or stillbirth has been reported to occur immediately after a febrile illness in a pregnant patient. Two mechanisms have been proposed. Specifically, fetal death may be a result of maternal bacteremia with dissemination to the fetus, or it may be a consequence of reinfection bacteremia in the mother from a previously infected, necrotic placenta.[169] Although the role of *L. monocytogenes* as a cause of repeated abortions is still unclear because definitive data are lacking, a number of studies have provided good circumstantial evidence that such maternal infections may be responsible for recurrent abortions in some women.[169]

Neonatal Listeriosis

Two forms, "early" and "late," of neonatal infection with *L. monocytogenes* have been described. In early onset disease, transplacental transmission of the organism may cause severe disease in the fetus with disseminated abscesses, granuloma, or both in multiple organs, e.g., liver, spleen, brain, lungs, and kidneys. This form of the disease (granulomatosis infantiseptica) is unique for *L. monocytogenes,* appears to be limited to in utero infection, and has a high mortality rate. The infant is usually critically ill at birth and presents primarily with respiratory distress and heart failure. Occasionally a skin eruption consisting of tiny focal cutaneous granulomas and purulent conjunctivitis is present. Cultures of the meconium, amniotic fluid, maternal vagina and lochia, and blood from infant and mother should be obtained, as well as cultures of purulent conjunctival material if present. The laboratory should be alerted that infection with *L. monocytogenes* is suspected so that they will not disregard the preliminary culture results as "diphtheroids" and misinterpret them as contaminants. The infant should be treated immediately on the basis of the presumptive diagnosis. There is some evidence that some cases of early onset neonatal sepsis may be caused by infection acquired during or after birth rather than in utero, perhaps by aspiration of infected amniotic fluid or acquisition of the organism during passage through the birth canal. These neonates become symptomatic after 3 days of age and present with a clinical picture of moderate to severe neonatal sepsis. Although some workers have occasionally observed *L. monocytogenes* as a cause of neonatal sepsis, we have observed only 2 infections with this organism in a series of 359 infants with neonatal sepsis during the years 1966 to 1978.[166]

The more common form ("late" onset) of neonatal listeriosis occurs after the sixth day of life. The infant appears well at birth and then develops either sepsis or, more frequently, central nervous system infection (meningoencephalitis) between 1 and 6 weeks of age. *Listeria* usually cannot be recovered from the mother in late onset disease. Although infection of this type may be acquired during delivery or as a result of low-level maternal bacteremia during the third trimester, postnatal acquisition of this organism may be responsible for "late" onset disease.

Treatment

Penicillin or ampicillin have both been effective therapeutic agents for *Listeria* infections. However, no controlled studies have established a "drug of choice," and there are equally firm opinions about which drug should be used. Both appear to be equally effective. Treatment failures have been reported for both penicillin and ampicillin, and in vitro penicillin resistance has been demonstrated, i.e., the bactericidal level of penicillin may be much greater than the inhibitory level.[170] Aminoglycosides have been shown to act synergistically with penicillin or ampicillin against *L. monocytogenes* in vitro and in experimental infections, although this has not been confirmed clinically and the superiority of combined therapy in human infections is lacking. The appropriate duration of therapy has also not been definitively determined. Although 2 weeks of therapy has proved successful in some patients, relapses have been noted after 2 weeks of therapy, particularly in immunosuppressed patients. We have used a minimum of 2 and preferably 3 weeks of high dose penicillin G (10 to 20 million units) or ampicillin (6 to 9 gm) daily in adults, more severely ill patients receiving the longer course of therapy. Early diagnosis and prompt initiation of treatment appear to be key factors for patient survival.

References

URINARY TRACT INFECTIONS

1. Adamson, K., and Joelsson, J.: The effects of pharmacological agents upon the fetus and newborn. Am. J. Obstet. Gynecol., 96:437, 1966.
2. Andriole, V. T.: Current concepts of urinary tract infections. *In* Weinstein, L., and Fields, B. N. (eds.): Seminars in Infectious Disease, Vol. III. New York, Thieme-Stratton Co., 1980.
3. Andriole, V. T., and Cohn, G. L.: The effect of diethylstilbestrol on the susceptibility of rats to hematogenous pyelonephritis. J. Clin. Invest., 43:1136, 1964.
4. Baker, E. C., and Lewis, J. S.: Comparison of the urinary tract in pregnancy and pelvic tumors. J.A.M.A., 104:812, 1935.
5. Beveridge, J., Harris, M., Wise, G., et al.: Long-acting sulphonamides associated with Stevens-Johnson syndrome. Lancet, 2:593, 1964.

6. Clayton, J. D., and Roberts, J. A.: Radionuclide postpartum evaluation of the urinary tract during anovular therapy. Surg. Gynecol. Obstet., *137*:215, 1973.
7. Condie, A. P., Williams, J. D., Reeves, D. S., et.al.: Complications of bacteriuria in pregnancy. *In* O'Grady, F., and Brumfitt, W. (eds.): Urinary Tract Infection. London, Oxford University Press, 1968, p. 148.
8. Crabtree, E. G., and Prather, G. C.: Clinical aspects of pyelonephritis in pregnancy. N. Engl. J. Med., *202*:357, 1930.
9. Dodds, G. S.: The immediate and remote prognosis of pyelonephritis of pregnancy. J. Obstet. Gynaecol. Br. Emp., *39*:46, 1932.
10. Duerden, B. I., and Moyes, A.: Comparison of laboratory methods in the diagnosis of urinary tract infections. J. Clin. Pathol., *29*:286, 1976.
11. Dunn, P. M.: The possible relationship between the maternal administration of sulphamethoxypyridazine and hyperbilirubinaemia in the newborn. J. Obstet. Gynaecol. Br. Commonw., *71*:128, 1964.
12. Eastman, N. J.: Williams Obstetrics, 11th ed. New York, Appleton-Century-Crofts, 1956.
13. Fainstat, T.: Ureteral dilatation in pregnancy: A review. Obstet. Gynec. Surv., *18*:845, 1963.
14. Gower, P. E., Haswell, B., Sidaway, M. E., et al.: Follow-up of 164 patients with bacteriuria of pregnancy. Lancet, *1*:990, 1968.
15. Guyer, P. B., and Delaney, D.: Urinary tract dilatation and oral contraceptives. Br. Med. J., *4*:588, 1970.
16. Harris, R. E., and Gilstrap, L. C.: Prevention of recurrent pyelonephritis during pregnancy. Obstet. Gynecol., *44*:637, 1974.
17. Hodson, C. J.: Round table discussion: Radiologic changes in the urinary tract associated with pregnancy in relation to the pathogenesis of pyelonephritis. *In* O'Grady, F., and Brumfitt, W. (eds.): Urinary Tract Infection. London, Oxford University Press, 1968, p. 170.
18. Hofbauer, J.: Contribution to the etiology of pyelitis of pregnancy. Bull. Johns Hopkins Hosp., *42*:118, 1928.
19. Hundley, J. M., Siegel, I. A., Hachtel, F. W., et al.: Some physiological and pathological observations on the urinary tract during pregnancy. Surg. Gynecol. Obstet., *66*:360, 1938.
19a. Kass, E.: Bacteriuria and pyelonephritis of pregnancy. Trans. Assoc. Am. Physicians, *72*:257, 1959.
20. Lepper, M. H., Wolfe, C. K., Zimmerman, H. J., et al.: Effect of large doses of aureomycin on human liver. Arch. Intern. Med., *88*:271, 1951.
21. Marchant, D. J.: Effects of pregnancy and progestational agents on the urinary tract. Am. J. Obstet. Gynecol., *112*:487, 1972.
22. Marshall, S., Lyon, R. P., and Minkler, D.: Ureteral dilatation following use of oral contraceptives. J.A.M.A., *198*:782, 1966.
23. Norden, C. W., and Kass, E. H.: Bacteriuria of pregnancy — a critical appraisal. Annu. Rev. Med., *19*:431, 1968.
24. Odell, G. B.: The dissociation of bilirubin from albumin and its clinical implications. J. Pediatr., *55*:268, 1959.
25. Perry, J. E., and LeBlanc, A. L.: Transfer of nitrofurantoin across the human placenta. Tex. Rep. Biol. Med., *25*:265, 1967.
26. Perry, J. E., Toney, J. D., and LeBlanc, A. L.: Effect of nitrofurantoin on the human fetus. Tex. Rep. Biol. Med., *25*:270, 1967.
27. Sanford, J. P.: Urinary tract symptoms and infections. Annu. Rev. Med., *26*:485, 1975.
28. Sheehan, H. L.: The pathology of acute yellow atrophy and delayed chloroform poisoning. J. Obstet. Gynaecol. Br. Commonw., *47*:49, 1940.
29. Stamm, W. E., Running, K., McKevitt, M., Counts, G. W., Turck, M., and Holmes, K. K.: Treatment of the acute urethral syndrome. N. Engl. J. Med., *304*:956, 1981.
30. Stamm, W. E., Wagner, K. F., Amsel, R., Alexander, E. R., Turck, M., Counts, G. W., and Holmes, K. K.: Causes of the acute urethral syndrome in women. N. Engl. J. Med., *303*:409, 1980.
31. Takahashi, M., and Loveland, D. B.: Bacteriuria and oral contraceptives. J.A.M.A., *227*:762, 1974.
32. Traut, H. F., and McLane, C. M.: Physiological changes in the ureter associated with pregnancy. Surg. Gynecol. Obstet., *62*:65, 1936.
33. Wasz-Hockert, O., Nummi, S., Voopala, S., et al.: Transplacental passage of azidocillin, ampicillin, and penicillin G during early and late pregnancy. Acta. Paediatr. Scand. (suppl.), *206*:109, 1970.
34. Whalley, P. J., Martin, F. G., and Peters, P. C.: Significance of asymptomatic bacteriuria detected during pregnancy. J.A.M.A., *193*:879, 1965.
35. Williams, J. D., Reeves, D. S., Condie, A. P., et al.: The treatment of bacteriuria in pregnancy. *In* O'Grady, F., and Brumfitt, W. (eds.): Urinary Tract Infection. London, Oxford University Press, 1968, p. 160.

GROUP B STREPTOCOCCAL DISEASE IN PREGNANCY

36. Amsley, M. S.: Low morbidity in the surgical patient with group B streptococci. Obstet. Gynecol., *50*:428, 1977.
37. Anthony, B. F., Okada, D. M., and Hobel, C. J.: Epidemiology of group B *Streptococcus:* Longitudinal observations during pregnancy. J. Infect. Dis., *137*:524, 1978.
38. Baker, C. J.: Summary of the workshop on perinatal infections due to group B *Streptococcus*. J. Infect. Dis., *136*:137, 1977.
39. Baker, C. J., and Barrett, F. F.: Transmission of group B streptocci among parturient women and their neonates. J. Pediatr., *83*:919, 1973.
40. Baker, C. J., Barrett, F. F., and Gordon, R. C. et al.: Suppurative meningitis due to streptococci of Lancefield group B. A study of 33 infants. J. Pediatr., *82*:724, 1973.
41. Baker, C. J., Barrett, F. F., and Yow, M. D.: The influence of advancing gestation on group B streptococcal colonization in pregnant women. Am. J. Obstet. Gynecol., *122*:820, 1975.
42. Baker, C. J., Clark, D. J., and Barrett, F. F.: Selective broth medium for isolation of group B streptococci. Appl. Microbiol., *26*:884, 1973.
43. Baker, C. J., Goroff, D. K., Alpert, S., et al.: Vaginal colonization with group B *Streptococcus:* A study in college women. J. Infect. Dis., *135*:392, 1977.
44. Baker, C. J., Kasper, D. L., and Edwards, M. S., et al.: Influence of pre-immunization antibody levels on the specificity of the immune response to related polysaccharide antigens. N. Engl. J. Med., *303*:173, 1980.
45. Barton, I. I., Feigin, R. D., and Lins, R.: Group B beta hemolytic streptococcal meningitis in infants. J. Pediatr., *82*:719, 1973.
46. Bayer, A. S., Chow, A. W., Anthony, B. F., et al.: Serious infections in adults due to group B streptococci. Clinical and serotype characterization. Am. J. Med., *61*:498, 1976.
47. Bobitt, J. F., Brown, G. L., and Tull, A. H.: Group B streptococcal neonatal infection: Clinical review of plans for prevention and preliminary report of quantitative antepartum cultures. Obstet. Gynecol., *55*:171S, 1980.
48. Collado, M. del., Kretschmer, R. R., Becker, I., et al.: Colonization of Mexican pregnant women with Group B *Streptococcus*. J. Infect. Dis., *143*:134, 1981.
49. Dunham, E. C.: Septicemia in the newborn. Am. J. Dis. Child, *45*:229, 1933.
50. Edwards, M. S., Jackson, C. F., and Baker, C. J.: Increased risk of Group B streptococcal disease in twins. J.A.M.A., *245*:2044, 1981.
51. Eickhoff, T. C., Klein, J. O., Daly, A. K., et al.: Neonatal sepsis and other infections due to group B beta-hemolytic streptococci. N. Engl. J. Med., *271*:1221, 1964.
52. Finch, R. G., French, G. L., and Phillips, I.: Group B streptococcal neonatal and infant infections. J. Pediatr., *82*:701, 1973.
54. Gardner, S. E., Yow, M. D., Leeds, L. J., et al.: Failure of penicillin to eradicate group B streptococcal colonization in the pregnant woman: A couple study. Am. J. Obstet. Gynecol., *135*:1062, 1979.
55. Hall, R. T., Barnes, W., Krishman, L., et al.: Antibiotic treatment of parturient women colonized with group B streptococci. Am. J. Obstet. Gynecol., *124*:630, 1976.
56. Hey, D. J., Hall, R. I., Burry, V. F., et al.: Neonatal infections caused by group B streptococci. Am. J. Obstet. Gynecol., *116*:43, 1973.
57. Hodes, H. L.: Penicillin prophylaxis and neonatal streptococcal disease. Hosp. Pract., *15*:115, 1980.
58. Kasper, D. L., Baker, C. J., Baltimore, R. S., et al.: Immunodeterminant specificity of human immunity to type III Group B *Streptococcus*. J. Exp. Med., *149*:327, 1979.
59. Merenstein, G. B., Todd, W. A., Brown, G., et al.: Group B β

hemolytic streptococcus: Randomized controlled treatment study at term. Obstet. Gynecol., 55:315, 1980.

60. Paredes, A., Wong, P., and Yow, M. D.: Failure of penicillin to eradicate the carrier state of group B *Streptococcus* in infants. J. Pediatr., 89:191, 1976.

61. Sackel, S. G., Baker, C. J., Kasper, D. L., et al.: Isolation of group B streptococci from men. Presented at the 18th Interscience Conference on Antimicrobial Agents and Chemotherapy, October 1–4, 1978.

62. Siegel, J. D., and McCracken, Jr., G. H.: Sepsis neonatorium. N. Engl. J. Med., 304:642, 1981.

63. Siegel, J. D., McCracken, Jr., G. H., and Threlkeld, N., et al.: Single-dose penicillin prophylaxis against neonatal group B streptococcal infections: A controlled trial in 18,738 newborn infants. N. Engl. J. Med., 303:769, 1980.

64. Wilkinson, H. W., Facklam, R. R., and Wortham, E. C.: Distribution by serological type of group B streptococci isolated from a variety of clinical material over a five-year period (with special reference to neonatal sepsis and meningitis). Infect. Immunol., 8:228, 1973.

65. Yow, M. D., Mason, E. O., Leeds, L. J., et al.: Ampicillin prevents intrapartum transmission of group B streptococcus. J.A.M.A., 241:1245, 1979.

SEPTIC ABORTION AND SEPTIC SHOCK

66. Andriole, V. T.: Synergy of carbenicillin and gentamicin in experimental infection with pseudomonas. J. Infect. Dis. (suppl.), 124:46, 1971.

67. Andriole, V. T.: Antibiotic synergy in experimental infection with pseudomonas. II. The effect of carbenicillin, cephalothin, or cephanone combined with tobramycin or gentamicin. J. Infect. Dis., 129:124, 1974.

68. Burkman, R. T., Atienza, M. F., and King, T. M.: Culture and treatment results in endometritis following elective abortion. Am. J. Obstet. Gynecol., 128:556, 1977.

69. Chow, A. W., Marshall, J. R., and Guze, L. B.: A double-blind comparison of clindamycin with penicillin plus chloramphenicol in treatment of septic abortion. J. Infect. Dis. (suppl.), 135:35, 1977.

70. Connors, A. F., McCaffree, D. R., and Rogers, R. M.: The adult respiratory distress syndrome. Disease-A-Month, 27. Chicago, Yearbook Medical Publishers, 1981, pp. 14–15.

71. Corrigan, J.: Heparin should be used cautiously and selectively. *In* Ingelfinger, F. J., et al. (eds.): Controversy in Internal Medicine II. Philadelphia, W. B. Saunders Co., 1974, p. 623.

72. Corrigan, J. J., Jr.: Heparin therapy in bacterial septicemia. J. Pediatr., 91:695, 1977.

73. Dodds, G. S.: The area of the chorionic villi in the full-term placenta. Anat. Rec., 24:287, 1923.

74. Eaton, C. J., and Peterson, E. P.: Diagnosis and acute management of patients with advanced clostridial sepsis complicating abortion. Am. J. Obstet. Gynecol., 19:1162, 1971.

75. Faden, A. I., Holaday, J. W.: Opiate antagonists: A role in the treatment of hypovolemic shock. Science, 205:317, 1979.

76. Gewurz, H., Shin, H. S., and Mergenhagen, S. E.: Interactions of the complement system with endotoxic lipopolysaccharide: Consumption of each of the six terminal complement components. J. Exp. Med., 128:1049, 1968.

77. Holaday, J. W., Faden, A. I.: Naloxone reversal of endotoxin hypotension suggests role of endorphins in shock. Nature, 275:450, 1978.

78. Kaplan, A. P., and Austen, K. F.: A prealbumin activator of prekallikrein. II. Derivation of activators of prekallikrein from active Hageman factor by digestion with plasmin. J. Exp. Med., 133:696, 1971.

79. Kaplan, A. P., Schreiber, A. D., and Austen, K. F.: Isolation and reaction mechanisms of human plasma plasminogen activator and its precursor. Fed. Proc., 31:624, 1972.

80. Kellermeyer, R. W., and Graham, R. C.: Kinins — possible physiologic and pathologic roles in man. N. Engl. J. Med., 279:754, 1968.

81. Ledger, W. J., and Kriewall, T. J.: The fever index: A quantitative indirect measure of hospital acquired infections in obstetrics and gynecology. Am. J. Obstet. Gynecol., 115:514, 1973.

82. McCabe, W. R.: Gram-negative bacteremia. Adv. Int. Med., 19:135, 1974.

83. Morbidity Mortality Weekly Report, Annual Summary 1979, 28:54, 1980.

84. Morbidity Mortality Weekly Report, Abortion Surveillance — United States, 1978, 30:222, 1981.

85. Neuwirth, R. S., and Friedman, E. A.: Septic abortion. Obstet. Gynecol., 85:24, 1963.

86. Ritvo, R., Monroe, P., and Andriole, V. T.: Transient bacteremia due to suction abortion: Implications for SBE antibiotic prophylaxis. Yale J. Biol. Med., 50:471, 1977.

87. Rodriguez-Erdmann, F.: Studies on the pathogenesis of the generalized Shwartzman reaction. III. Trigger mechanism for the activation of the prothrombin molecule. Thromb. Diath. Haemorrh., 12:471, 1964.

88. Santamarina, B.: Septic abortion and septic shock. *In* Charles, D., and Finland, M. (eds.): Obstretric and Perinatal Infections. Philadelphia, Lea & Febiger, 1973, p. 273.

89. Schwartz, R. H.: Septic abortion. Philadelphia, J. B. Lippincott Co., 1968.

90. Shine, K. I.: Aspects of the Management of Shock. Ann. Intern. Med., 93:723, 1980.

91. Smith, L. P., McLean, A. P. H., and Maughan, G. B.: *Clostridium welchii* septicotoxemia: A review and report of 3 cases. Am. J. Obstet. Gynecol., 110:135, 1971.

92. Studdiford, W. E., and Douglas, G. W.: Placental bacteremia: A significant finding in septic abortion accompanied by vascular collapse. Am. J. Obstet. Gynecol., 71:842, 1956.

93. Waisbren, B. A.: Bacteremia due to gram-negative bacilli other than the salmonella: A clinical and therapeutic study. A.M.A. Arch. Intern. Med., 88:467, 1951.

94. Weil, M. H., and Shubin, H.: Diagnosis and Treatment of Shock. Baltimore, Williams & Wilkins Co., 1967.

95. Weissmann, G.: The role of lysosomes in inflammation and disease. Annu. Rev. Med., 18:97, 1967.

96. Wilson, R. F., Chiscano, A. D., Quadros, E., et al.: Some observations on 132 patients and septic shock. Anesth. Analg., 46:751, 1967.

ANTIMICROBIAL AGENTS IN OBSTETRICS

97. Baker, T. H., and Hubbell, R.: Reappraisal of asymptomatic puerperal bacteremia. Am. J. Obstet. Gynecol., 97:575, 1967.

98. Barr, W., and Graham, R. M.: Placental transmission of cephaloridine. J. Obstet. Gynaecol. Br. Commonw., 74:739, 1967.

99. Belton, E. M., and Jones, R. V.: Hemolytic anemia due to nalidixic acid. Lancet, 2:691, 1965.

100. Bergogne-Berezin, E., Lambert-Zechovsky, N., Rouvillois, J. L.: Study of transplacental transmission of beta-lactam antibiotics. J. Gynecol. Obstet. Biol. Reprod., 8:359, 1979.

101. Berkowitz, R. L., Coustan, D. R., and Mochizuki, T. K., (eds.): Handbook for Prescribing Medications During Pregnancy. Boston, Little, Brown & Co., 1981.

102. Bray, R. E., Boe, R. W., and Johnson, W. L.: Transfer of ampicillin into fetus and amniotic fluid from maternal plasma in late pregnancy. Am. J. Obstet. Gynecol., 96:938, 1966.

103. Burns, L. E., Hodgeman, J. W., and Cass, A. B.: Fatal circulatory collapse in premature infants receiving chloramphenicol. N. Engl. J. Med., 261:1318, 1959.

104. Conway, N., and Birt, B. D.: Streptomycin in pregnancy. Effect on foetal ear. Br. Med. J., 2:260, 1965.

105. Creatsas, G., Pavlatos, M., Lolis, D., et al.: A study of the kinetics of cephapirin and cephalexin in pregnancy. Curr. Med. Res. Opin., 7:43, 1980.

106. Creatsas, G., Pavlatos, M., Lolis, D., et al.: Ampicillin and gentamicin in the treatment of fetal intrauterine infections. J. Perinat. Med., 8:13, 1980.

107. Dekel, A., Elian, I., Gibor, Y., et al.: Transplacental passage of cefazolin in the first trimester of pregnancy. Eur. J. Obstet. Gynaecol. Reprod. Biol., 10:303, 1980.

108. Depp, R., Kind, A. C., Kirby, W. M., et al.: Transplacental passage of methicillin and dicloxacillin into the fetus and amniotic fluid. Am. J. Obstet. Gynecol., 107:1054, 1970.

109. Greene, H. J., Burkhart, B., and Hobby, G. L.: Excretion of penicillin through human milk following parturition. Am. J. Obstet. Gynecol., 51:732, 1946.

110. Greene, H. J., and Hobby, G. L.: Transmission of penicillin through human placenta. Proc. Soc. Exp. Biol. Med., 57:282, 1944.

111. Guilbeau, J. A., Schoenbach, E. B., Schaub, I. G., et al.: Aureomycin in obstetrics: Therapy and prophylaxis. J.A.M.A., 143:520, 1950.

112. Kafetzis, D. A., Lazarides, C. V., Siafas, C. A., et al.: Transfer

of cefotaxime in human milk and from mother to fetus. J. Antimicrob. Chemother., 6:135, 1980.

113. Kiefer, L., Rubin, A., McCoy, J. B., et al.: The placental transfer of erythromycin. Am. J. Obstet. Gynecol., 69:174, 1955.

114. Kline, A. H., Blattner, R. J., and Lunin, M.: Transplacental effect of tetracyclines on teeth. J.A.M.A., 188:178, 1964.

115. Kraybill, E. N., Chaney, N. E., McCarthy, L. R.: Transplacental ampicillin: Inhibitory concentrations in neonatal serum. Am. J. Obstet. Gynecol., 138:793, 1980.

116. Kucers, A., and Bennett, N. McK.: The Use of Antibiotics. London, William Heinemann Medical Books, 1979.

117. Kutscher, A. H., Zegarelli, E. V., Tovell, H. M., et al.: Discoloration of deciduous teeth induced by administration of tetracycline ante partum. Am. J. Obstet. Gynecol., 96:291, 1966.

118. MacAulay, M. A., Berg, S. R., and Charles, D.: Placental transfer of dicloxacillin at term. Am. J. Obstet. Gynecol., 102:1162, 1968.

119. Medina, A., Fiske, N., Hjelt-Harvey, I., et al.: Absorption, diffusion, and excretion of a new antibiotic, lincomycin. Antimicrob. Agents Chemother., 3:189, 1964.

120. Monnet, P., Kalb, J. C., and Pujol, M.: Toxic influence of isoniazid on fetus. Lyon Med., 218:431, 1967.

121. Perry, J. E., and LeBlanc, A. L.: Transfer of nitrofurantoin across the human placenta. Tex. Rep. Biol. Med., 25:265, 1967.

122. Perry, J. E., Toney, J. D., and LeBlanc, A. L.: Effect of nitrofurantoin on the human fetus. Tex. Rep. Biol. Med., 25:270, 1967.

123. Philipson, A., Sabath, L. D., and Charles, D.: Transplacental passage of erythromycin and clindamycin. N. Engl. J. Med., 288:1219, 1973.

124. Posner, A. C., Prigot, A., and Konicoff, N. G.: Further observations on the use of tetracycline hydrochloride in prophylaxis and treatment of obstetric infections. Antibiot. Ann., p. 595, 1954.

125. Prigot, A., Froix, C. J., and Rubin, E.: Absorption, diffusion, and excretion of a new penicillin, oxacillin. Antimicrob. Agents Chemother., 402, 1963.

126. Remington, J. S., and Klein, J. O., (eds.): Infectious Diseases of the Fetus and Newborn Infant. Philadelphia, W. B. Saunders Co., 1976, p. 483.

127. Rubin, A., and Dvornik, D.: Placental transfer of griseofulvin. Am. J. Obstet. Gynecol., 92:882, 1965.

128. Sabath, L.: Use of antibiotics in obstetrics. In Charles, D., and Finland, M. (eds.): Obstetrics and Perinatal Infections. Philadelphia, Lea & Febiger, 1973, p. 563.

129. Schultz, J. C., Adamson, J. S., Workman, W. W., et al.: Fatal liver disease after intravenous administration of tetracycline in high dosage. N. Engl. J. Med., 269:999, 1963.

130. Sheng, K. T., Huang, N. N., and Promadhattavedi, V.: Serum concentration of cephalothin in infants and children and placental transmission of the antibiotic. Antibiot. Agents Chemother., 4:200, 1964.

131. Sutherland, J. M.: Fatal cardiovascular collapse in infants receiving large amounts of chloramphenicol. Am. J. Dis. Child., 97:761, 1959.

132. Sutherland, J. M., and Keller, W. H.: Novobiocin and neonatal hyperbilirubinemia. Am. J. Dis. Child., 101:447, 1961.

133. Varpela, E.: On the effect exerted by first-line tuberculous medicine on the fetus. Acta Tuberc. Pneumol. Belg., 45:53, 1964.

134. Wasz-Hockert, O., Nummi, S., Voopala, S., et al.: Transplacental passage of azidocillin, ampicillin, and penicillin G during early and late pregnancy. Acta Paediatr. Scand. (suppl.), 206:109, 1970.

135. Whalley, P. J., Adams, R. H., and Combes, B.: Tetracycline toxicity in pregnancy. Liver and pancreatic dysfunction. J.A.M.A., 189:357, 1964.

136. Woltz, S. H. E., and Wiley, M. M.: Transmission of streptomycin from maternal blood to the fetal circulation and the amniotic fluid. Proc. Soc. Exp. Biol. Med., 60:106, 1945.

POSTPARTUM INFECTION

137. Collins, C. G.: Suppurative pelvic thrombophlebitis. Am. J. Obstet. Gynecol., 108:681, 1970.

138. Gesner, B. M., and Jenkins, C. R.: Production of heparinase by Bacteroides. J. Bacteriol., 81:595, 1961.

139. Gibbs, R. S.: Clinical risk factors for puerperal infection. Obstet. Gynecol., 55:178S, 1980.

140. Gibbs, R. S., DeCherney, A. H., et al.: Prophylactic antibiotics in cesarean section: A double blind study. Am. J. Obstet. Gynecol., 114:1048, 1972.

141. Gibbs, R. S., Weinstein, A. J.: Bacteriologic effects of prophylactic antibiotics in cesarean section. Am. J. Obstet. Gynecol., 126:226, 1976.

142. Golde, S., and Ledger, W. J.: Necrotizing fasciitis in postpartum patients. A report of four cases. Obstet. Gynecol., 50:670, 1977.

143. Goplerud, C. P., Ohn, M. J., and Galask, R. P.: Aerobic and anaerobic flora of the cervix during pregnancy and the puerperium. Am. J. Obstet. Gynecol., 126:858, 1976.

144. Gordon, A.: A Treatise on the Epidemic Puerperal Fever of Aberdeen. London, G. G. & J. Robinson, 1795.

145. Halben, J., Kohler, R.: Die pathologische Anatomie des puerperal Prozesses. Vienna and Leipzig, 1919.

146. Hibbard, L. T., Snuder, E. N., and McVann, R. E.: Subgluteal and retropsoal infection in obstetric practice. Obstet. Gynecol., 39:172, 1972.

147. Holmes, O. W.: Contagiousness of puerperal fever. N. Engl. J. Med. Surg., 1:503, 1842.

148. Ledger, W. J., Moore, D. E., Lowensohn, R. I., et al.: A fever index evaluation of chloramphenicol or clindamycin in patients with serious pelvic infections. Obstet. Gynecol., 50:523, 1977.

149. Ledger, W. J., and Nakamura, R.: Measurement of infectious disease morbidity in obstetrics and gynecology. Clin. Obstet. Gynecol., 19:195, 1976.

150. Ledger, W. J., and Peterson, E. P.: The use of heparin in the management of pelvic thrombophlebitis. Surg. Gynecol. Obstet., 131:1115, 1970.

151. Salzman, E. W., Deykin, D., Shapiro, R. M., et al.: Management of heparin therapy. Controlled prospective trial. N. Engl. J. Med., 292:1046, 1975.

152. Schlievert, P., Johnson, W., and Galask, R. P.: Bacterial growth inhibition by amniotic fluid. V. Phosphate to zinc ratio as a predictor of bacterial growth-inhibitory activity. Am. J. Obstet. Gynecol., 125:899, 1976.

153. Semmelweis, I. P.: Die Aetiologie, der Bergriff und die Prophylaxis des Kindbettfiebers. Vienna, Hartleben, 1861. (Medical Classics, Vol. 5, translated by F. P. Murphy. Baltimore, Williams & Wilkins, 1941, pp. 350–773.)

154. Stevenson, C. S., Behney, C. A., Miller, N. F.: Maternal death from puerperal sepsis — A 16 year study in Michigan. Obstet. Gynecol., 29:181, 1967.

155. Taylor, K. J. W., de Graaff, C., Andriole, V. T., et al.: Accuracy of grey-scale ultrasound diagnosis of abdominal and pelvic abscesses in 220 patients. Lancet, 1:83, 1978.

156. Wong, R., Gee, C. L., and Ledger, W. J.: Prophylactic use of cefazolin in monitored obstetric patients undergoing cesarean section. Obstet. Gynecol., 51:407, 1978.

157. Work, B. A., Jr.: Role of preventive antibiotics in patients undergoing cesarean section. South. Med. J., 70(Suppl. 1):44, 1977.

Toxic-Shock Syndrome

158. Bergdoll, M. S., Reiser, R. F., Crass, B. A., et al.: A new staphylococcal enterotoxin, enterotoxin F, associated with toxic-shock syndrome Staphylococcus aureus isolates. Lancet, 5:1017, 1981.

159. Davis, J. P., Chesney, P. J., Wand, P. J., et al.: Toxic-shock syndrome. N. Engl. J. Med., 303:1429, 1980.

160. Morbidity and Mortality Weekly Report: Follow-up on Toxic-Shock Syndrome. 29:441, 1980.

161. Schlievert, P. M., Shands, K. N., Dan, B. B., et al.: Identification and characterization of an exotoxin from Staphylococcus aureus associated with toxic-shock syndrome. J. Infect. Dis., 143:509, 1981.

162. Shands, K. N., Schmid, G. P., Dan, B. B., et al.: Toxic-shock syndrome in menstruating women. N. Engl. J. Med., 303:1436, 1980.

163. Stevens, F. A.: The occurrence of *Staphylococcus aureus* infection with a scarlatiniform rash. J.A.M.A., *88*:1957, 1927.

164. Todd, J., Fishaut, M., Kapral, F., et al.: Toxic-shock syndrome associated with phage-group-I staphylococci. Lancet, *2*:1116, 1978.

LISTERIA INFECTIONS

165. Bojsen-Möller, J.: Human listeriosis: Diagnostic, epidemiological and clinical studies. Acta Pathol. Microbiol. Scand. (Suppl.), *229*:1, 1972.

166. Freedman, R. M., Ingram, D. L., Gross, I., et al.: A half century of neonatal sepsis at Yale. Am. J. Dis. Child., *135*:140, 1981.

167. Hoeprich, P. D.: Infection due to *Listeria monocytogenes*. Medicine, *37*:143, 1958.

168. Louria, D. B., Hensle, T., Armstrong, D., et al.: Listeriosis complicating malignant disease. Ann. Intern. Med., *67*:261, 1967.

169. Seeliger, H. P. R., and Finger, H.: Listeriosis. *In* Remington, J. S., and Klein, J. O. (eds.): Infectious Diseases of the Fetus and Newborn Infant. Philadelphia, W. B. Saunders Co., 1976, p. 333.

170. Winslow, D. L., Holloway, W. J., and Scott, E. G.: Listeria sepsis — a report of 27 cases. *In* Holloway, W. J. (ed.): Infectious Disease Reviews, Vol. VI. Mount Kisco, N.Y., Futura Publishing Co., 1981, p. 187.

Dorothy M. Horstmann, M.D.

14

VIRAL INFECTIONS

Viral infections during pregnancy are of concern not only in terms of maternal morbidity and the possibility of attendant fetal loss, but because certain agents are capable of crossing the placenta and inducing chronic perinatal infections that have serious pathogenic potential for the fetus and the newborn. The most important viruses in this connection are rubella, cytomegalovirus (CMV), and herpes simplex virus.* Less commonly, varicella zoster and hepatitis B virus infections in pregnancy also result in maternal and neonatal problems. Investigations of these and certain other agents have centered on identifying the risk factors for mother and fetus, documenting the pathogenesis of the infections and the diseases, and in the case of rubella, attempting to control the problem by immunization.

Incidence of Viral Infections in Pregnancy

By the time women reach the childbearing age they have already acquired immunity to several diseases as a result of clinical or inapparent infections. Yet there is little statistically valid information on the proportion still at risk, or on the actual incidence of various viral infections in pregnancy. Problems such as underreporting, incorrect clinical diagnoses, and the high rate of inapparent infection with certain agents all contribute to the inaccuracy of current estimates. In a 6 year prospective survey, investigators in the Collaborative Perinatal Research Study attempted to assess the frequency of viral infections in some 30,000 pregnant women.[7] Clinical information on the occurrence of various types of illnesses was collected, and paired serum specimens (taken at the first prenatal visit and at the time of delivery) were examined for the development of antibodies against a number of common

viruses. About 1600 women reported illnesses presumed viral, excluding episodes of the common cold. Most were acute influenza-like respiratory infections, herpes simplex, and a variety of nonspecific syndromes. The incidence of specific diseases was low. Serologic tests confirmed the clinical diagnoses and gave the following minimum attack rates per 10,000 persons: 10 for mumps, 8 for rubella, 5 for varicella-zoster, and 0.6 for measles.

Aspects of Pathogenesis

Maternal Infections. In general, viral diseases in adults tend to be more severe than in children, but patterns of infection and immune responses of pregnant women do not differ from those of nonpregnant women in the same age group. However, the profound physiologic changes in pregnancy have been associated with increased severity and mortality of certain diseases, such as measles and poliomyelitis. High fever and associated systemic manifestations of various acute illnesses can be responsible for abortion early in pregnancy in the absence of fetal infection. Abortion can also result from invasion of the conceptus and direct action of a lytic virus like measles. The true rate of fetal loss associated with direct and indirect effects of infection is difficult to ascertain, for in addition to other uncertainties, abortion may occur in the several weeks after fertilization, before the woman is aware of being pregnant.

Fetal Infections. The placenta has long been regarded as providing a barrier to infection of the fetus. Although the placenta does have a protective function, recent investigations indicate that this may have been overestimated. Viruses reach the fetus primarily as a consequence of maternal viremia, but it is not clear whether they may simply pass directly into the fetal circulation or whether placental infection must precede fetal infection.[4] In any event, in the course of maternal viremia, the placenta is commonly seeded

---

*Discussions of herpes and hepatitis virus infections are omitted from this chapter but can be found in Chapters 15 and 12, respectively.

333

TABLE 14-1 VIRAL INFECTIONS IN PREGNANCY

Viruses	Maternal and/or Fetal Effects
Rubella	Abortion, stillbirth; intrauterine growth retardation; congenital disease; congenital anomalies; persistent postnatal infection
Cytomegaloviruses	Prematurity; intrauterine growth retardation; congenital disease; congenital anomalies; persistent postnatal infection
Herpes simplex	Prematurity; neonatal disease, localized or disseminated
Varicella-zoster	Prematurity; congenital disease; congenital anomalies
Measles	Abortion; prematurity; congenital disease
Hepatitis	Abortion; stillbirth; prematurity; neonatal disease; persistent postnatal infection (hepatitis B)
Agents causing common respiratory illnesses	None
Influenza	Usually none; increased maternal morbidity and mortality in certain epidemics
Poliomyelitis	Increased maternal morbidity and mortality; congenital and neonatal disease
Coxsackie B	Congenital and neonatal disease
Echoviruses	Congenital and neonatal disease
Venezuelan equine encephalitis (VEE)	Abortion; congenital malformations
Western equine encephalitis (WEE)	Congenital disease

with virus, followed by development of inflammatory foci in the chorionic villi, granulomatous changes, and necrosis.[1] Vaccinia, varicella, and variola viruses produce extensive lesions in placental tissue, while the response to rubella is milder, and changes due to cytomegaloviruses are minimal. Other agents such as mumps, Coxsackie B viruses, and polioviruses cross the placenta to infect the fetus but leave no trace in terms of pathologic changes in the placenta. It seems therefore that some viruses do not affect the placenta significantly, others may infect the placenta but extend no further, while still others spread from the placenta to the fetus and may cause severe damage.

In addition to hematogenous dissemination, it is possible that certain agents infect the fetus by the ascending route. Both wild and vaccine strains of rubella virus have been recovered from the female genital tract. This is also true of cytomegaloviruses, which may be shed from the uterine cervical tissues for protracted periods, and for herpesvirus type 2.

The fate of the fetus receiving a virus inoculum via the maternal circulation is conditioned by factors such as the time in gestational development during which the infection occurs, the virus dose, and whether or not the agent is lethal to cells (e.g., measles) or, like rubella, can set up a chronic infection and multiply intracellularly without causing visible cellular damage. Depending on the balance of conditioning influences, whatever the agent, the fetus may escape infection, may suffer an acute self-limited episode without permanent damage, or may develop an acute fatal infection; it may also be involved in a chronic asymptomatic process that ultimately results in growth retardation and congenital anomalies.

For certain infections (e.g., CMV, herpes), the presence of virus in the birth canal is the most important source of exposure of the infant. Such natal infections may not become apparent until several days or more after birth. The clustering of inapparent infections with CMV manifested by viruria between 30 and 120 days of age has been shown to be associated with exposure during birth and to postnatal acquisition from the mother as a result of ingestion of virus-containing breast milk.

RUBELLA

The overall incidence of rubella in the United States has declined by 70 per cent since the introduction of vaccines in 1969, but the numbers of cases in persons over 15 years of age has changed very little. The obstetrician is therefore still frequently faced with problems arising from exposure and possible infection of the pregnant woman as well as the dilemmas posed by inadvertent rubella vaccination in early pregnancy.[18]

Clinical Aspects

After an incubation period of 14 to 21 days, rubella most commonly presents as a mild illness with rash, lymphadenopathy, and low-grade

FIGURE 14–1. Schematic diagram of clinical course, virologic findings, and immunologic responses in acute rubella.

fever (Figure 14–1). The maculopapular rash, most often the first sign of the disease in children, is not distinctive, but a helpful diagnostic feature is that it is always present on the face and is usually most prominent there. In adults, tender lymphadenopathy affecting the postauricular, posterior cervical, and subocciptal nodes is perhaps the most characteristic feature of rubella. As indicated in Figure 14–1, enlargement of lymph nodes is present a few days before the appearance of the rash. The commonest complications of rubella are arthralgia and arthritis, which occur chiefly in women over 20 years and increase sharply with age. Joint manifestations are self-limited and last only a few days to a week or more. The fingers, wrists, and knees are most frequently involved. Joint effusions may develop, and the virus (both wild and vaccine strains) has been recovered from the fluid, suggesting that joint involvement may represent direct viral action; there is also recent evidence that circulating immune complexes may be involved. Other, rare complications of rubella include encephalitis and thrombocytopenic purpura.

Viral excretion and the appearance of antibodies are shown in relation to the clinical course in the lower part of Figure 14–1. In addition to viremia, virus is shed regularly from the throat; during the acute phase it may also be recovered from stool, urine, conjunctivae, and blood leukocytes, from the skin lesions, and from cervical secretions in the female.

A point of considerable significance for the clinician is that virus excretion from the throat and viremia precede the clinical manifestations by 5 to 7 days. This means that when a pregnant woman reports that her child has developed a rash and the condition has been diagnosed as rubella, she has probably already been exposed for as long as a week and, if susceptible, may well have been infected.

The most contagious period for rubella is the 1 to 2 days prior to onset, i.e., just before the rash appears. Although not as contagious as measles, rubella spreads readily in the family setting, and all susceptible persons are usually infected. Not all infections are clinically apparent, however; investigations in various types of populations have established that there are approximately one or two silent infections to every one that is clinically expressed.

Rubella in Pregnancy

Rubella in the pregnant woman is not more severe nor is it attended by more complications than in nonpregnant women of comparable age. Inapparent maternal infection also carries a risk for the fetus. In the presence of the acute disease, there is evidence of some increase in abortion rate in the first trimester — approximately twice that in pregnant control women. The problems presented by the disease in pregnancy are thus related almost entirely to the capacity of the virus to induce chronic infection and severe congenital anomalies in the fetus. The large 1964 epidemic in the United States occurred 2 years after the virus had been finally isolated in tissue culture, and it was therefore possible to confirm the results of earlier prospective epidemiologic studies and to establish that in the event of maternal infection in the first trimester, approximately 20 per cent of infants will have abnormalities detectable at birth, while in another 10 to 15 per cent, hearing loss and other defects will become apparent later. The risk to the fetus is greatest when maternal infection occurs in the first trimester, particularly in the second month of pregnancy. This is before the placenta is a fully functioning organ and corresponds to the time of organogenesis; infants who are infected during this period are more apt to have multiple congenital anomalies. In addition, there is evidence of some risk — though much reduced — when maternal infection occurs during the second trimester, up to the 20th week of pregnancy.[23] Rubella in the weeks immediately preceding conception has also occasionally been associated with the congenital rubella syndrome. Not all infected fetuses suffer damage, however; the high rate (50 to 90 per cent) of virus recovery from tissues obtained at abortion suggests that in some instances fetal infection may be transient and may leave no permanent sequelae.[29]

INTRAUTERINE RUBELLA AND THE RUBELLA SYNDROME

Maternal viremia and infection of the placenta provide the major sources of rubella virus for the fetus. There is also evidence that infected chorionic cells may break off and act as emboli, carrying the virus to various fetal tissues such as heart, brain, and other organs.[30]

Once infection of the fetus is established, it continues until birth and persists in some infants for several years. Ten per cent may still be shedding virus from the throat at 8 months; the virus has been recovered from the lens of a child whose cataract was removed at 3 years of age.[20] The mechanism of persistence of infection is not entirely clear. Immune tolerance is not involved, since specific antibody production by the fetus begins around the 20th week of gestation, and at birth affected infants have elevated rubella IgM antibody titers in addition to maternally derived IgG antibody. Abnormalities in cellular immunity have long been postulated as contributing to the problem of virus persistence, and infants with the rubella syndrome have been shown to have impaired cell-mediated immunity.[10]

Another possible explanation for the persistence of fetal infection relates to the small size of babies with the rubella syndrome, which has been shown to be due to a reduction in the number of cells in various organs and tissues.[22] This is consistent with the hypothesis that the widely distributed infected clones of cells have a reduced life-span and gradually drop out; only when all such clones have disappeared is there clearance of the virus from the tissues.[28]

Some manifestations of the rubella syndrome are present at birth, but others — hearing loss, psychomotor retardation, retinopathy, and others — may not become apparent for months or years.[12, 23] Although single defects may be present, it is more usual to find multiple malformations in the child with the rubella syndrome. The most frequent combination seen at birth includes a cardiac lesion, cataracts, and low birth weight. Virtually any organ system may be involved, however. In the 1964 epidemic in the United States, many lesions not previously recognized or noted only rarely were documented, including petechial rash, hepatosplenomegaly, jaundice, characteristic transient long bone lesions, microphthalmia, glaucoma, and meningoencephalitis.[8]

MANAGEMENT OF THE RUBELLA PROBLEM IN PREGNANCY

The situation that arises most frequently in obstetric practice involves a woman in early pregnancy who has been exposed to rubella. Assuming that the exposure was indeed to this disease, the patient's immune status should be determined by serologic test as soon as possible. A past history of the disease is often unreliable because a number of other viruses induce "rubelliform" rashes. Furthermore, at least 50 per cent of infections are inapparent, yet they induce resistance. A variety of serologic tests are available for determining immune status to rubella, but the hemagglutination inhibition (HAI) test remains the most useful one and results can be available within 24 hours. If the test reveals the presence of antibody, and the blood specimen was drawn within a few days of exposure, the patient can be reassured that she is immune and therefore not at risk (Table 14–2). A titer of 1:16 or greater is conclusive evidence of immunity; 1:8 is also a positive result, but when this value is obtained, the test should be repeated to be certain that the titer represents specific antibody and not inadequate removal of nonspecific inhibitors present in all human sera; such inhibitors interfere with the proper conduct of the test and may give false positive results. Since a titer of 1:8 may also represent antibody that has just appeared as

TABLE 14–2 INTERPRETATION OF SEROLOGIC RESULTS IN WOMEN EXPOSED TO RUBELLA OR PRESENTING WITH POSSIBLE CLINICAL RUBELLA

History	Days after Exposure or after Onset	HAI Titer	Interpretation
Exposure to case; no clinical illness	1 24	1:32 1:64	Patient immune and not at risk; twofold difference in titer not significant and within limits of error of the test
Exposure to case; no clinical illness	2 24	<1:8 <1:8	Patient susceptible, not infected
Exposure to case; no clinical illness	18 28	1:8 1:64	Inapparent infection in a susceptible; first serum taken at the time when antibody was beginning to appear
Fever, rash; questionable case	2 10	1:16 1:16	Patient immune as result of previous infection; illness not rubella
Fever, rash, lymphadenopathy; compatible with rubella	0 10	<1:8 1:128	Clinical rubella in a susceptible confirmed

a result of inapparent infection, further confirmation should be obtained by examining a second blood specimen collected 5 to 7 days later; if there has been no change in titer *when both specimens are run in the same test*, the patient can be considered to be immune.

If the HAI test result indicates a titer of less than 1:8, the patient is susceptible and should be followed up serologically to determine whether or not she has been infected. A second blood specimen should be obtained 3 to 4 weeks after exposure and *retested along with the first specimen*. If infection has occurred, antibodies will be detected in the second sample.

Interpreting HAI results may be difficult when there has been a delay of several weeks in obtaining the first postexposure blood specimen. If HAI antibodies are present, the question arises whether they represent a recent or current infection or one that was experienced years before. This can be answered by determining the immunoglobulin class to which the antibodies belong. As in other viral infections, the first response in a primary infection is IgM antibody, which persists for 3 to 4 weeks or more, along with a rising level of IgG, which eventually represents virtually all the detectable antibody.[9]

The appearance of complement fixation (CF) antibodies, which develop later than HAI (7 to 10 days after the onset of rash in the clinical disease), may also be used to confirm current infection (see Figure 14–1).

Confirmation of Clinical Disease. Since the clinical picture of rubella is often rather nonspecific, demonstration of a rise in specific antibody is often necessary to confirm the diagnosis, particularly in sporadic cases. The HAI test is the most widely available, but simpler and more rapid tests such as the enzyme-linked immunosorbent antibody (ELISA) are coming into more general use. Others, such as CF and neutralization, are performed in certain special laboratories.

A diagnosis of rubella can also be made by recovery of the agent from a throat swab, and rarely, from the blood. Since the tissue culture techniques for virus recovery are complicated and results may not be available for 4 to 6 weeks, diagnosis by virus isolation is not commonly used.

Use of Gamma Globulin (ISG). In the pregnant woman who has been exposed to rubella, gamma globulin has frequently been given in the hope of preventing infection, should the patient be susceptible. The results have been disappointing; both rubella with rash and inapparent infection have occurred in women given gamma globulin in optimum dose soon after exposure.[23] There is some evidence that ISG may possibly modify the infection; its use might therefore be considered for women who because of religious or other reasons would not consent to termination of the pregnancy should infection occur.

PREVENTION OF RUBELLA BY IMMUNIZATION

The isolation of rubella virus in 1962 made possible the development of vaccines. By 1969, two preparations, having undergone extensive field testing to establish their safety and efficacy, were licensed in the United States: the $HPV_{77}DE_5$ strain, prepared in duck embryo tissue culture, and the Cendehill strain, grown in primary rabbit kidney cells. These two vaccines were the only ones available in the United States until 1979, when the HPV_{77} vaccine was withdrawn and replaced by a third preparation, the RA 27/3 strain, which is sold under the trade name Meruvax II.

The RA 27/3 vaccine, grown in human diploid cells, has certain advantages over the others in that it is more like naturally occurring wild virus in inducing a broader range of antibody responses, including precipitating antibodies and local IgA secretory antibody.[9, 25] The resulting immunity is thus closer to that which follows natural infection. Of particular importance is that the neutralizing antibody response, considered to be the protective one, persists at higher levels after vaccination with RA 27/3, resembling the pattern following natural infection with wild virus.[26]

Clinical, Virologic, and Serologic Responses to Vaccines. Rubella vaccines induce antibody responses in 95 per cent of susceptibles. Side reactions occur in 10 to 50 per cent or more of recipients, depending upon age and sex.[31] By and large the symptoms are minor and insignificant. Low grade fever, malaise, and sometimes rash may appear 12 to 21 days after vaccination, but such reactions are infrequent. As in the natural infection, arthralgia and arthritis may occur, particularly in women over 20 years of age, its frequency and severity increasing with age. Fingers, wrists, and knees are most commonly involved and actual joint effusion may develop, as in infection with wild virus.[15]

Although shedding from the throat in small quantities for a few days occurs in approximately 60 to 70 per cent of susceptible vaccinees, *vaccine virus infection is not communicable.* A reassuring serologic study documented the absence of infection in susceptible pregnant women exposed to their own children who had been vaccinated.[27]

Persistence of Immunity. Long-term serologic surveillance of HPV_{77}, RA 27/3, and Cendehill vaccinees have in general shown satisfactory persistence of HAI antibodies during the 7 to 9 years over which they have been followed up.[11] However, it has been observed that in those whose original antibody responses to the vaccine were low (1:8 to 1:16), a greater loss of detectable antibody has been found, so that overall, 10 per cent of HPV_{77} vaccinees were seronegative by 9 years.[19] Not only is RA 27/3 vaccine more immunogenic than the other preparations, but it

induces a greater resistance to reinfection either by intranasal challenge[14] or by exposure to natural infection.[17]

Vaccination of Women in the Childbearing Age. At the time of licensure of the vaccines in the United States, the decision was made to make prepubertal children the main target of vaccination campaigns. This course was taken because it was believed that by immunizing the childhood population a high degree of herd immunity could be achieved, circulation of wild virus would be greatly decreased or eliminated, and susceptible pregnant women would thus be protected from exposure indirectly. Furthermore, there was justifiable concern about giving a live rubella virus vaccine to postpubertal females who might be pregnant. While women in the childbearing age were recognized as the most important ones to protect, it was recommended that this be done cautiously on an individual basis, preferably only after establishing susceptibility by serologic test, and with the understanding that suitable pregnancy control measures would be followed for at least 2 months, later extended to 3 months.

Despite the explicit contraindication of rubella immunization in pregnancy, a number of women have received either HPV_{77} or Cendehill vaccine, often before the pregnancy was recognized. In 343 of these instances reviewed by the Center for Disease Control, 145 of the women had elected termination of the pregnancy.[21] Rubella virus was recovered from the products of conception from 6 of 28 (21 per cent) who were known to have been susceptible when vaccinated. As with wild strains, the infection was a chronic one, with tissues still virus positive as long as 20 weeks after vaccine administration. Virus has been recovered from placenta, decidua, and fetal eye and kidney; histologic changes in an infected fetal eye were characteristic of those seen in the rubella syndrome.[13]

Among women who carried their pregnancies to term, information is available on 84 who had been susceptible when inadvertently vaccinated shortly before conception or during the first trimester. All were delivered of infants who appeared normal at birth.[11] Nevertheless, by use of serologic tests, inapparent infection at birth has been documented, as evidenced by rubella-specific IgM in 10 per cent (3 of 30) infants, and persistent HAI levels at 6 months of age in several others, possibly indicating intrauterine infection.[16] Long-term followup will be necessary to rule out impaired hearing or other possible delayed manifestations of congenital rubella in such infants.

The presently available data on HPV$_{77}$ and Cendehill vaccines indicate that the potential damage to the fetus when they are given in early pregnancy is not accurately known, but it is clear that the risk is far less than with wild virus infection — probably under 5 per cent in contrast to the 20 per cent of infants with congenital abnormalities apparent at birth following natural infection. As yet there has been little experience in the United States with the RA 27/3 strain, but at least 12 seronegative pregnant women have received it; examination of the products of conception obtained at abortion failed to yield the virus in any instance.[24]

PRENATAL SCREENING FOR ANTIBODY AND POSTPARTUM VACCINATION. Good obstetric practice currently includes testing for immunity to rubella on the first antenatal visit. Most patients are antibody positive and can therefore be assured that they are immune to rubella. If the HAI titer is unusually high (> 128) there is often concern that the patient may have had a recent inapparent infection. In this situation the test should be repeated and the serum tested for rubella specific IgM. If there is no history of exposure, and the second result is similar to the first, no IgM being present, the findings indicate immunity as a consequence of infection sometime in the past.

The pregnant woman who is seronegative (HAI $< 1:8$) should be immunized after delivery and before leaving the hospital. Even though pregnancy is uncommon in the first postpartum months, contraception may be advisable during this period.

Is it safe to immunize mothers who plan to breast-feed their infants? Rubella vaccine virus has been transmitted to the infant through breast milk, but no ill effects have been noted, and the infection is not contagious. Breast-feeding is therefore not a contraindication to postpartum vaccination.

Prospects for Control

The main purpose of vaccination against rubella is to prevent the congenital syndrome by ensuring that women in the childbearing age are immune. This goal has not yet been reached in the United States. The expectation that concentration of vaccination programs on prepubertal children would result in a well-protected young adult population as immunized children moved into the 15–19 age group has turned out to be much slower in realization than was anticipated. Thus, serologic surveys indicate that some 15 per cent of those 15–40 years old remain susceptible, as was the case before introduction of vaccines in 1969. Although the total number of cases reported annually has decreased sharply, there has been no decline among the young adult age groups, who now account for 70 per cent of the reported cases (Figure 14–2). Attack rates in children have reached new lows, but data through 1978 indicate that in young people 15–24 years old they have actually increased as outbreaks continue to occur in high schools, colleges, and military installations. Recently there have been a number of epidemics among hospital personnel — nurses, house staff, medical students, and so on — in some instances with transmission to women in early pregnancy who were attending prenatal clinics. This situation has prompted the institution of programs in many hospitals for routine serologic screening of all personnel — men and women — and immunization of those found to be susceptible.

While continuing to emphasize immunization of infants and children, current recommendations place increased emphasis on reaching susceptible adolescents and young women with rubella vaccine. Premarital screening for antibodies is required in some states, so that susceptibles can be identified and immunized, following the usual precautions concerning avoidance of pregnancy for 3 months.

Long-term persistence of vaccine-induced immunity is of great importance, since most chil-

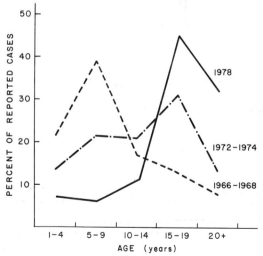

SHIFTS IN AGE OF RUBELLA CASES
1966–1978

FIGURE 14–2. Shifts in age distribution of cases of rubella reported to the Center for Disease Control. (Data from CDC Rubella Surveillance Summary, January 1976–December 1978 [issued May 1980].)

dren are now vaccinated at approximately 15 months of age. The more immunogenic RA 27/3 vaccine (Meruvax II), which has replaced the earlier HPV$_{77}$ strain in the United States, is promising in this connection, but long-term serologic surveillance is still required to ensure that over the years, women of childbearing age are well protected against rubella.

CYTOMEGALOVIRUS INFECTION

Cytomegaloviruses (CMV) are members of the herpesvirus group, which includes varicella-zoster (VZ), herpes simplex, and Epstein-Barr viruses. The characteristic cellular pathology associated with CMV — intranuclear and cytoplasmic inclusions — had been recognized for some 70 years before the responsible agent was isolated from human tissues in the mid-1950s by several groups of investigators. Cytomegaloviruses were soon shown to be widely distributed in human populations, causing both congenital and acquired infections, most of which are completely inapparent. Their importance in pregnancy is due to the capacity of the virus to induce fetal infection. Approximately 0.5 to 2 per cent of newborns are congenitally infected, as defined by the presence of viruria at birth, and approximately 10 per cent of those infected have stigmata of the disease.[38]

Acquired Infections

Cytomegaloviruses are ubiquitous agents. Serologic surveys in various parts of the world indicate that 40 to 100 per cent of adults are antibody positive.[36] Acquisition of infection is related to age and to socioeconomic factors, occurring earlier and at higher rates in populations living under crowded conditions and in poor sanitary environments. Transmission by blood transfusion is well documented, but contact infection is the usual means of spread, although the exact mechanisms involved are not well understood. The virus is shed for long periods (often several years) in saliva and urine; in infected women, CMV is present in cervical and vaginal secretions and also in breast milk, which has recently been shown to be a major source of transmission to infants in the first 6 months of life.[51] There is also suggestive evidence that CMV may be transmitted venereally.[32, 41] Cervical infections are more common in women attending venereal disease clinics; following infection in the male, the virus has been recovered from semen for many months.[43]

Like other herpesviruses, CMV remains latent in the host once primary infection has occurred, reactivation and virus excretion occurring periodically. Such recurrences are not associated with antibody rises and are asymptomatic except in immunosuppressed patients, particularly transplant recipients, in whom serious disease may result.

Clinical Features. Primary infections with CMV, whatever their source, are almost always inapparent. Rarely, a syndrome of heterophile-negative mononucleosis develops in young adults;[42] it may also occur in recipients of blood transfusions. The clinical picture differs from infectious mononucleosis in that the patient is apt to be older (>25 years), there is little lymphadenitis, sore throat is uncommon, and the heterophile antibody test is negative.[35] Rare manifestations of CMV infection include hepatitis, interstitial pneumonitis, meningoencephalitis, myocarditis, and the Guillain-Barré syndrome.[39]

Specific Laboratory Diagnosis. Laboratory diagnosis can be made by recovery of the agent from saliva, cervical swab, or liver biopsy specimen, but urine is the usual source. CMV grows slowly, and cultures may not become positive for a month or more. The presence in fresh urine or in cervical smears of the characteristic owl-eyed cells containing intranuclear inclusions establishes a presumptive diagnosis, but this is a much less sensitive method than viral culture. Serologic tests include CF, fluorescent antibody (FA), and indirect hemagglutination inhibition (IHA). CF is the most widely used, but the FA test appears to be more sensitive in identifying primary infections.[39]

CMV in Pregnancy and Congenital Infections

Infection with CMV during pregnancy is the commonest cause of congenital disease. Maternal infection rates, based on prospective studies of the excretion of virus from the cervix, are 3 to 28 per cent, depending on the population surveyed.[45, 48, 52] Apparently, virus shedding is suppressed in the early months of pregnancy; thus, isolation rates are lower in the first trimester and rise steadily to reach levels comparable with those in nonpregnant control women in the third trimester. Cervical excretion may represent primary infection but is more commonly due to reactivation of latent virus. Intrauterine transmission has been considered to occur chiefly during primary infection, but recent observations indicate that recurrent infections are associated with fetal infection more frequently than had been appreciated. Intrauterine transmission of

CMV has been documented in 7 of 208 (3.4 per cent) women known to have been seroimmune before becoming pregnant.[50] None of the 7 infected infants had any evidence of congenital disease.

While recurrence of virus shedding may occasionally be due to reinfection with a different serotype, in most instances it has been shown to represent reactivation of endogenous virus.[50] Antigenic and genetic homology between viral strains isolated from two siblings consecutively infected in utero was demonstrated, and these observations have been extended.[40]

Primary infection during pregnancy carries a known risk of congenital abnormalities, chiefly of the central nervous system. The incidence of primary infection varies greatly in different population groups, but in the United States and Great Britain it is small. Three large prospective studies indicate that among some 9800 pregnant women tested, 1909 (19 per cent) were seronegative for CMV.[36, 44, 52] Of these, 23 (1.2 per cent) experienced primary infection during gestation. Thirteen of the 23 infants were infected, as indicated by viruria at birth, but only 3 had any clinical evidence of disease.

Since maternal infections are so rarely associated with clinical disease, little is known of the effects of the virus on the fetus when infection occurs at specific times in gestation. Severe congenital disease has been documented in two infants following infection in the second trimester as well as inapparent infections in two others whose mothers seroconverted in the third trimester.[44] The virus has been recovered from the fetus at termination of a pregnancy at 22 weeks in a patient who had CMV mononucleosis in the seventh week of gestation.[33] The limited data available suggest that the outcome is more serious when infection occurs in early pregnancy, but more information is needed to confirm this.

Infants with cytomegalovirus disease present with a picture similar to that of congenital rubella. Low birth weight, hepatosplenomegaly, jaundice, and petechial eruptions are prominent. Death in the neonatal period from disseminated disease is not uncommon. In those who survive, microcephaly and various neurologic problems are frequently present. Long-term followup studies of congenitally infected children have shown that approximately 15 per cent, whether clinically abnormal or apparently normal at birth, subsequently manifest auditory or ocular defects.[49]

At birth, laboratory diagnosis of the congenital infection can be made by isolation of the virus from the urine, in which it is excreted in large quantities, or serologically, by the CMV-IgM test, using cord blood.[37] This test is estimated to be 95 per cent accurate in detecting congenital infection, but it is less reliable in diagnosing acquired infections because of cross-reactions with EBV and VZ viruses.

Postnatal infections, acquired either during passage through an infected birth canal or in the first few months of life, occur in over half of the infants exposed to infected mothers.[48] It has been shown that breast-feeding is the main source of virus transmission to the young infant, resulting in infection in 58 per cent of those whose mothers were known to be infected.[51] The presence of virus in the mother's saliva or urine was not associated with infection of the infant. Unlike intrauterine infection, postnatally acquired CMV apparently results in asymptomatic infection only in the neonate.

Prevention and Treatment

At present there is no satisfactory means of preventing infection with CMV or of treating the congenital disease. Human interferon and drugs such as 5-iodo-2-deoxyuridine (IUDR), adenine arabinoside (Ara A), and cytosine arabinoside (Ara C) have been tried therapeutically without success. Prevention of the congenital disease, which is responsible for the birth of some 4000 neurologically damaged infants in the United States each year, could be approached through vaccination, as has been done with rubella. Efforts to develop a vaccine have begun,[34, 47] but there are many problems, and much more needs to be known about the virus and the natural history of the infection before a safe and effective attenuated live virus vaccine can be achieved.[46]

CHICKENPOX (VARICELLA)

Chickenpox

Varicella and zoster are both caused by varicella-zoster virus, a member of the herpes group. Chickenpox is an uncommon disease in adults and is correspondingly rare in pregnancy. As with a number of other childhood infections, the course is usually more severe in adults, who tend to have a more extensive rash, higher fever, and more frequent complications, including the potentially fatal varicella pneumonia. The course and outcome, however, appear to be no different in pregnancy from the pattern in other adults with the disease.

Varicella is readily transmitted by direct contact with an infected person; the incubation period is 10 to 21 days, commonly 18. The period of communicability lasts between 1 to 2 days before appearance of the rash and 2 to 5 days after, when the lesions have crusted. The characteristic vesicular eruption develops in crops, is centripetally distributed, and is most prominent on the trunk. Treatment is symptomatic. Varicella pneumonia may result in severe pulmonary involvement requiring aggressive management, including mechanical ventilation. Antibiotics are not indicated unless bacterial superinfection develops.

Laboratory Diagnosis. Diagnosis can be made by recovery of the virus from the vesicles or by serologic test. The CF test is satisfactory for demonstrating a rise in antibodies, thus confirming the diagnosis, but CF antibody is not long-lasting and is therefore unreliable for identifying exposed susceptibles. For this purpose, the FAMA (fluorescence antibody membrane antigen) test is the most useful at present.[54] It is rapid and reliable but is not generally available except in medical centers.

Exposure During Pregnancy. In assessing the risks involved when a pregnant woman near term reports that she has been exposed to chickenpox, several factors are important. The disease is much more contagious when exposure is to a family member than when the contact occurs in a community setting. The likelihood of susceptibility in an adult born in the United States is only 5 to 10 per cent, but it is much higher in those who come from tropical areas, where the disease is more common in adults.[58] By use of the sensitive FAMA serologic test, it was found that among women of childbearing age in New York City, 16 per cent of those from Puerto Rico were susceptible, while only 5 per cent of those born in the United States were seronegative.[55] A history of having had the disease proved unreliable, emphasizing the importance of making rapid serologic testing for immunity more available than is currently the case.

Perinatal Infection. Viremia is apparently a regular feature of the infection, but the fetus is not necessarily involved. Only about 24 per cent of infants develop the disease when maternal infection occurs during the 3 weeks before delivery.[57] Prospective studies of large numbers of cases do not indicate significant increase in abortions or congenital defects when infection develops in the early months of gestation. Nevertheless, reports of some nine infants with a cluster

TABLE 14–3 ABNORMALITIES ASSOCIATED WITH VARICELLA INFECTION IN UTERO

Abnormality	Number of Infants Affected
Cutaneous scars (zigzag or circumferential)	9/9
Hypoplasia of limb	6/9
Low birth weight	5/9
Paralysis with muscular atrophy of a limb	5/9
Death	5/9
Rudimentary digits	4/9
Convulsions and/or psychomotor retardation	4/9
Chorioretinitis	3/9
Cortical atrophy	3/9
Cataract or other eye defects	2/9
Fresh skin ulcers	1/9
Talipes equinovarus deformity	1/9

From Andiman, W., 1979.[53] Adapted from DeNicola, L. K., and Hanshaw, J. B.: J. Pediatr., *94*:175, 1979; and Bai, P. V., and John, T. J.: J. Pediatr., *94*:65, 1979.

of similar defects have appeared (Table 14–3), suggesting the possible occurrence of a congenital varicella syndrome.[53, 56]

While anomalies are rare, *congenital chickenpox,* defined as disease with onset in the first 10 days of life, occurs more frequently. Most infections are mild, with sparse skin lesions and few systemic signs. In some instances, however, the infant suffers a severe disease with widespread visceral dissemination. The mortality is high. The severity of the infection is correlated with the time of onset of the maternal disease (Table 14–4).[57] If the onset was 5 or more days before delivery, and the infant's rash appears between 0 and 4 days of age, the course is mild and recovery is the rule. However, if the mother's onset was during the 4 days before delivery, some 17 per cent of infants develop signs of chickenpox between the fifth and tenth days of life; the disease is more severe and there is a 30 per cent mortality. This pattern indicates that the earlier the maternal infection, the more likely that there will be time for specific antibody to develop and be transferred to the fetus, thus providing some protection and modifying (or preventing) the infant's infection.

Prevention in High Risk Infants. Zoster immune globulin (ZIG) is a hyperimmune serum prepared from pooled blood of persons convalescent from zoster, and it prevents the disease if administered soon after exposure. It should be given to infants born to mothers who developed chickenpox between 4 days before and 2 days after delivery. ZIG is in short supply and in

TABLE 14-4 RELATIONSHIP BETWEEN ONSET OF MATERNAL VARICELLA AND OUTCOME IN INFANT

Maternal Onset	Age of Onset in Infant	Total	Fatal	Survived	Fatality Rate Per Cent
Five or more days before delivery	0 to 4 days	27	0	27	0
Four or fewer days before delivery	5 to 10 days	23	7	16	30
Total		50	7	43	14

From Andiman, W., 1979.[53] Adapted from Krugman, S., and Gershon, A. (eds.): Progress in Clinical and Biological Research, Vol. 3. New York, Alan R. Liss, Inc., 1975, pp. 79–95.

addition to such infants is available only for immunosuppressed hosts at high risk of severe disease. Information concerning local sources can be obtained by communicating with the Center for Disease Control, Atlanta, GA (tel: 404-329-3745).

Immune serum globulin (ISG) in a dose of 0.6 ml per kg has been used with some success to modify (but not prevent) the disease in children if given within 72 hours of exposure. Presumably the results would be similar in pregnant women, but no data are available on this point.

Isolation Procedures. A mother with chickenpox should be isolated from her infant until the lesions have crusted. Nosocomial infection in nurseries is uncommon, but isolation of the infant is indicated to prevent possible transmission to other neonates and the staff.

Immunization. An experimental live attenuated vaccine against varicella-zoster virus has recently been developed and is currently being tested in persons at high risk of severe disease. The vaccine has been shown to induce protective immunity, but concern about the unpredictable long-term effects of latent vaccine virus dictates caution in considering the vaccine for general use.[53a]

Zoster

Zoster, or shingles, occurs in pregnancy, but few cases have been reported. There seems to be no enhancement of maternal risk from the disease, and involvement of the fetus is apparently very rare.[59] The disease represents a reactivation of latent V-Z virus in dorsal root ganglia; it is almost always unilateral, and the vesicular eruption is distributed along dermatomes, usually corresponding to the areas most commonly involved in varicella. Susceptibles exposed to zoster are at risk of developing chickenpox. Since herpes simplex infection can induce zoster-like lesions, vesical fluid culture is required to establish V-Z as the etiologic agent.

INFLUENZA AND OTHER RESPIRATORY INFECTIONS

Minor viral respiratory illnesses such as the common cold, upper respiratory tract infections, pharyngitis, and bronchitis are frequent in pregnancy, but the more common agents responsible for these syndromes (coronaviruses, rhinoviruses, parainfluenza and respiratory syncytial viruses, adenoviruses, and so on) do not appear to affect the fetus. However, respiratory syncytial (as well as influenza and parainfluenza) viruses have caused outbreaks of nosocomial infections in nurseries and infants' wards during community outbreaks associated with these agents.[63, 67]

Influenza has been associated with increased severity and mortality in late pregnancy, largely as a result of pneumonia. This association has been inconstant; it was striking in the 1918 pandemic and in the Asian influenza epidemic of 1957, but it has not been observed in subsequent outbreaks, which have been generally milder.[62]

Infection with influenza may be asymptomatic, may resemble the common cold, or in the more typical form may present as a prostrating 5 to 7 day illness, characterized by sudden onset of fever, chilly sensations, headache, myalgia, sore throat, and dry cough. In some cases primary influenza virus pneumonia develops early in the course. This is a severe, often fatal manifestation, which occurs chiefly in patients who are pregnant or have pre-existing cardiac or pulmonary disease. The course is one of rapidly progressive respiratory distress and terminal vascular collapse. Antibiotics, oxygen, steroids, and all other measures are ineffective. Bacterial pneumonia, which develops later in the course, is more common and occurs in previously normal persons as well as in high risk groups. Routine prophylactic use of antibiotics to prevent bacterial superinfection is not generally indicated, but for pregnant patients and others in high risk categories, it might be considered. Penicillin should be given in full therapeutic doses for prophylaxis. If pneumonia develops, the choice of antibiotic depends on the organism cultured from sputum or tracheal aspirate.

Effects on the Fetus

Viremia is not a regular feature of influenza, and intrauterine infection is correspondingly rare. Cases of the congenital disease have been described, and the virus has been recovered from fetal tissue following a maternal death in the third trimester.[68] The congenital infection resembles neonatal sepsis; the diagnosis can be confirmed by virus isolation and serologic test.

The evidence concerning abortion, stillbirths, and congenital defects associated with maternal influenza is conflicting but predominantly negative. In a prospective study involving large numbers of cases and control subjects, no evidence of increased rates of abortion, stillbirths, or malformations was found.[65] Although a high mortality rate was associated with Asian influenza in pregnancy in the 1957–58 epidemic, one group did not document any significant differences between pregnancy outcome in survivors with serologically proved infections and control subjects who remained seronegative.[64] However, there was some suggestion that infection in the first trimester resulted in a slight increase in abortions and congenital anomalies. Anencephaly and other central nervous system malformations following maternal influenza have been reported by several investigators, but their significance has been difficult to assess.[61] The same is true of investigations of a possible association between influenza during pregnancy and subsequent development of leukemia in the child. In some studies, no correlation has been shown,[66] but in others there appears to have been an increased risk of leukemia following certain epidemics. In a cohort study, the effect was most marked in children who were in the first trimester of gestation at the time of the epidemic, the relative risk for this group being 3.4.[60]

Prevention of Influenza

The protective effect of influenza vaccine is not complete, nor is it long-lasting. Nevertheless, the approximate 70 per cent reduction in morbidity that can be achieved is substantial and attests to the value of immunization. The vaccine causes no harmful effects in mother or fetus, but it is recommended in pregnancy primarily for women in a high risk group as a result of cardiac, pulmonary, or other chronic disease. Hypersensitivity to hen's eggs is a contraindication, but it is safe to give vaccine to persons who can eat eggs or egg-containing products.

MUMPS

Mumps is primarily a disease of childhood and occurs infrequently during pregnancy.[77] The infection is transmitted by droplet nuclei, saliva, and fomites; primary virus multiplication in the upper respiratory tract is followed by viremia, during which the agent is distributed to target organs, mainly glandular tissues and the central nervous system. Most infections are accompanied by clinical signs, but approximately 30 per cent are completely inapparent. Parotitis, the most characteristic manifestation, develops after an incubation period of 14 to 18 days. The onset is with fever and malaise, followed after a day or more by swelling and tenderness of the parotid glands. The disease is usually mild, but occasionally there are complications, which may be severe. They include meningoencephalitis, orchitis, oophoritis, and pancreatitis. In general the diagnosis of mumps is obvious on clinical grounds; in questionable cases it can be confirmed by observation of a rising CF antibody titer between acute and convalescent serum specimens, or by virus isolation from the throat, urine, blood, or spinal fluid. The virus is present in the throat for 2 to 3 days before onset and up to 7 days afterward. Skin tests document immunity but are of no use in the diagnosis of the acute infection.

Pregnancy does not increase the severity or the incidence of complications associated with mumps. However, prospective studies have documented an approximately twofold increase in the abortion rate, primarily in the first trimester.[73]

Congenital Mumps. The viremia of mumps lasts approximately a week, beginning 2 days before onset and terminating by the fifth day of the disease. That intrauterine transmission can occur is supported by rare reports of the congenital disease[77] and by the immunologic responses of the fetus exposed in utero.[69] Virologic confirmation has only recently been achieved. In an investigation of three infants born to mothers who had mumps 4 to 7 days before delivery, one baby had a swollen parotid at birth, another developed severe bilateral pneumonia at 7 days of age, and a third remained asymptomatic.[71] Mumps virus was recovered from the throats of two of the infants on the day of birth.

Congenital malformations can be induced in experimental animals by mumps virus. Various reports indicate that similar effects may occur in rare instances in humans, but the studies are largely uncontrolled and interpretation is difficult. In a prospective study of 501 pregnancies complicated by mumps, no differences were observed in stillbirths or congenital abnormalities compared with matched controls.[72]

An association between intrauterine mumps and endocardial fibroelastosis (EFE) has been postulated.[74] This has not been proved, but suggestive evidence that it may occur has been presented.[70]

Prevention

Active Immunization. A safe, effective, live attenuated mumps virus vaccine prepared in chick embryo culture was licensed in the United States in 1965.[75] Its use has resulted in a marked decline in the incidence of the disease and its complications. The vaccine induces immune responses in approximately 95 per cent of recipients, and immunity appears to be long-lasting. Unless immunized in infancy, vaccination is advised for children approaching puberty, adolescents, and young adults, particularly males, with no history of the disease. It is not recommended for pregnant women, since it contains live virus. Although no adverse effects have yet been reported when it has been given inadvertently to pregnant women, the possibility has not been excluded. The virus has been recovered from the placentas of two of three seronegative women given the vaccine 10 days before the planned termination of their pregnancies.[76]

Passive Protection. Mumps immune globulin is available, but its effectiveness has not been proved. Since the maternal and fetal risk from infection is so minimal, there is little indication for its use in women exposed during pregnancy, most of whom are immune by virtue of previous infection, even though giving no history of the disease.

MEASLES

Measles is rare in pregnancy, for most adults are immune as a result of immunization or previous natural infection. However, as the incidence of the disease in childhood has declined due to widespread use of the vaccine in infants and children there has been a marked shift in the age distribution of reported cases, as in rubella. Instead of less than 5 per cent of reported cases occurring in the age group 15 and over, as was the pattern before vaccines were introduced, more than 25 per cent were in adolescents and young adults in 1977. A number of outbreaks in high schools, colleges, and among military recruits have been described. Most of the cases have been in the unimmunized, but a number have occurred in those previously vaccinated whose immunity had waned. This was common among persons given vaccine when under 1 year of age, i.e., at a time when their antibody responses were modified by persisting maternal antibody. A serologic survey of students at a university involved in an epidemic in 1977 revealed that 12 per cent who were seronegative had been vaccinated; overall, 9 per cent of the student population lacked immunity, indicating a potential pool of susceptibles in the childbearing age group.[78]

Clinical Manifestations. Measles develops after an incubation period of 10 to 12 days. The onset is with catarrhal symptoms, followed by fever, the characteristic Koplik spots, and finally the rash, which develops between days 12 and 14. The typical case is easily recognized clinically, but in mild or questionable cases, virus isolation from the throat, or serologic test of serum specimens obtained during the first few days after onset and 6 to 7 days later, may be necessary to confirm the diagnosis. Complications involve primarily the respiratory tract; in adults, pneumonia is the main problem. This may be entirely due to the virus, or bacterial superinfection may also play a part. Encephalitis is rare.

Atypical Measles. This syndrome has occurred in vaccinees exposed to wild virus and has caused diagnostic problems, particularly in young adults, in whom it is often a severe disease. The clinical picture suggests a hypersensitivity reaction, with sudden onset of high fever, myalgia, and abdominal pain, followed after several days by a rash that begins in the extremities and spreads cephalad. Besides maculopapular lesions, petechial and vesicular ones are frequent. Pneumonia is a prominent feature, and in adults pulmonary lesions may last for several months.[82] Most of the cases described have occurred in individuals who received killed measles virus vaccine, which was withdrawn in 1967, but there have been rare examples in persons who received only the live virus preparation.

Measles in Pregnancy. In general measles in pregnancy is not more severe than in nonpregnant persons of the same age.[84] Increased mortality was reported in the Greenland epidemic of 1951, which involved many pregnant women,[79] but tuberculosis was rife in the population at that time and it is possible that it also played some role.

A review has been published of 327 pregnancies complicated by measles during 10 epidemics in Greenland between 1951 and 1962.[81] Abortion occurred in 50 per cent of women infected during the first 2 months of gestation and in 20 per cent infected during the third month. Prematurity (birth weight < 2500 grams) was also relatively high (11 per cent) but was uninfluenced by the time of maternal infection during gestation. These figures are similar to those in a 1940 report[80] but are higher than indicated by a later controlled prospective study.[83]

Congenital Measles. When maternal infection occurs near term, there is a risk of approximately 30 per cent of the congenital disease in the infant.[80, 84] Koplik spots and rash may be present at birth or may develop within the first 10 days of life. The clinical picture varies from mild to severe; the mortality rate as documented on earlier reports is as high as 30 per cent, particularly in premature infants.[84]

Congenital Defects. Defects due to intrauterine infection with measles virus have been reported in scattered instances, but because of this rarity of the disease in pregnant women, the true risk — if any — is hard to ascertain. Careful investigations involving relatively large numbers provide suggestive evidence that the virus can be teratogenic.[81] Four of 28 infants born to women infected in the first 2 months of gestation had severe anomalies of various types, leading to death in 3. Taken as a whole, the available information points to the probability of some risk of malformation as a result of intrauterine infection, but this risk must be very small.

Prevention

Active immunization with live attenuated measles virus vaccine is recommended for infants at age 12 to 15 months. In populations in which the attack rates are high in the first year of life, vaccine should be given at 6 months of age and repeated a year later. Older children, adolescents, and young adults who have not previously been immunized should also receive vaccine. *Revaccination* is indicated for those who were given killed virus vaccine only or who received live virus vaccine before 12 months of age.

Immunization is contraindicated in pregnancy becaue the vaccine contains live virus. Since approximately 10 per cent of young adults may still be susceptible, however, immunization of this age group is recommended, preferably after serologic testing has identified those who are antibody-negative.[78]

Passive immunization by intramuscular injection of immune serum globulin (ISG), 0.25 ml per kg, should be considered for pregnant women with no history of measles or of immunization; it should be given as soon as possible after exposure, but even if immunization is as late as 7 days, it may prevent or modify the disease. It is desirable to obtain a blood sample before administration of ISG to establish the patient's immune status by serologic test. If she is antibody-negative, live virus vaccine should be given post partum but not until at least 8 weeks after the administration of ISG.

SMALLPOX AND VACCINIA

The dangers to pregnant women from smallpox and vaccinia no longer exist. Extensive immunization programs carried out under the auspices of the World Health Organization in all endemic areas resulted in the worldwide eradication of smallpox by 1979.

ENTEROVIRUS INFECTIONS

The enteroviruses include Coxsackie, echo, and polioviruses, all of which share biologic and epidemiologic features. They are transmitted by direct contact and can cause a variety of syndromes, including minor illnesses, aseptic meningitis, paralytic disease, respiratory disease, and myocarditis, but a high proportion of infections are inapparent. The agents circulate widely in human populations, chiefly between July and October in temperate climates, but they are present the year round in tropical areas.

Poliomyelitis, the most serious enterovirus disease, has been virtually eliminated in industrialized countries by immunization, but it still occurs in endemic and epidemic form in the developing areas of the world. Coxsackie and echovirus infections can be counted on to appear in the summer and fall every year, and in countries like the United States, localized outbreaks are common. The viruses spread primarily among young children, but infections in adults also occur and are more apt to be clinically apparent and of greater severity than in childhood.

Infections in Pregnancy. During epidemics, poliomyelitis occurs more frequently, is more severe, and has a higher mortality in pregnant women than in nonpregnant women in the same age group. It is also associated with increased rates of abortion and stillbirth. When the disease occurs near term, transmission to the fetus has occasionally resulted in congenital poliomyelitis. Coxsackie and echoviruses are less pathogenic; they have not been shown to cause abortions, and there are only rare reports of a possible relationship to congenital anomalies. There is some evidence that Coxsackie B viruses may occasionally be associated with prematurity and stillbirths.

Neonatal Infections. Viremia occurs in the course of enterovirus infections, and Coxsackie, echo, and polioviruses are all capable of crossing the placenta. Documented examples of congenital disease, however, are few. Infection of the fetus may be inapparent, or symptoms may appear shortly after birth.[86] Neonatal infection may also be a result of exposure during birth, in the course of a silent or overt maternal infection. Disease due to echoviruses is usually mild, but severe disseminated infections with hepatic necrosis, hemorrhagic manifestations, adrenal necrosis, and central nervous system involvement have occasionally been reported.[88]

Coxsackie and echoviruses have also caused a number of epidemics in newborn nurseries; the responses of infants involved have ranged from inapparent or mild to severe and fatal disease. In general, however, the infections have not had serious consequences. Earlier outbreaks due to Coxsackie B viruses have been associated with myocarditis and encephalomyocarditis and have caused many deaths in newborn nurseries[87]; in recent years fewer such epidemics have been reported. Other forms of illness due to enteroviruses often suggest a diagnosis of sepsis;[89] the nature of the syndrome is confirmed by virus isolation from stool, throat swab, or spinal fluid or by serologic test.

Prevention

Inapparent infection with Coxsackie or echoviruses in a hospital staff member can result in infection of an infant, but the commonest source of nursery epidemics appears to be contact infection from mother to infant, followed by spread to hospital staff members and other infants. Maternal infections are often inapparent, but a history of a minor febrile illness or any of the other characteristic syndromes near term should alert the obstetrician to the possibility of an enterovirus infection with potential danger for the infant. There are no specific preventive measures, but isolation of the mother and rigorous attention to aseptic technique, especially hand washing, are the most effective barriers to spread of the viruses.

Vaccination against poliomyelitis with live attenuated oral poliovirus vaccine (OPV) is recommended as part of the routine immunization of infants and children. For adults, the risk of exposure is so low in the United States that vaccination of adults is not advised except for persons who have never been immunized and who are traveling to areas where the infection is highly endemic. For such individuals, including pregnant women, inactivated poliovirus vaccine (IPV) should be given. Four doses are required: three at 3 to 4 week intervals and a fourth 6 to 12 months later.[85] If time does not permit this schedule, two doses of IPV may be given three to four weeks apart or a single dose of trivalent OPV if exposure will occur in less than three weeks.

RABIES

Human rabies is an exceedingly rare, highly fatal encephalitis, acquired as a result of contact with the saliva of an infected animal, usually a skunk, raccoon, fox, or bat. In the United States, immunization of domestic animals has greatly reduced but not eliminated the risk of dogs and particularly cats being sources of infection.

There has been little experience with the disease in pregnant women, but in experimental animals the virus has been demonstrated to cross the placenta. Rabies vaccine has been given in pregnancy without ill effect on the fetus; the serious consequences of maternal infection dictate its use whenever exposure is known to have occurred.

A greatly improved vaccine prepared in human diploid cell cultures has recently been licensed in the United States.[91] It supplants the previously used duck embryo preparation, which sometimes failed to protect and also carried a risk of local reactions and occasionally neurologic problems.

The new vaccine apparently causes no adverse reactions and induces satisfactory antibody responses in close to 100 per cent of vaccinees. It has been used successfully in the face of significant exposure to the virus.[90]

Postexposure Immunization. The nature of the bite and the circumstances surrounding it dictate the procedures to be followed. If significant exposure has occurred, the wound should be cleansed thoroughly with soap and water, and 20 IU per kg of human rabies immune globulin (HRIG) administered. Half of the dose is given intramuscularly, and half is infiltrated into the wound site. At the same time, a course of immunization with human diploid cell rabies vaccine is begun. This consists of 1 ml intramuscularly, repeated on days 3, 7, 14, and 28. Another dose at 3 months is optional. The patient's serum should be tested for antibody after 2 to 3 weeks to assure an adequate response. The testing can be arranged through state health departments.[91]

ARBOVIRUS INFECTION

Arbovirus infections are reported every year from certain parts of the United States where the mosquito vectors of the agents are present. In some years, sizable epidemics have occurred, most commonly in the western and southern regions of the country. Several case reports have dealt with infection during pregnancy with *Western equine encephalitis virus* (WEE). Congenital disease with this agent, resulting from in utero infection in the course of maternal viremia near term, develops during the first week of life. It is manifested by fever, lethargy, and seizures. No malformations have been observed.[92, 94]

Maternal infection with *Venezuelan equine encephalitis virus* (VEE) is manifested by an influenza-like illness and occasionally encephalitis. Infection in pregnancy has been associated with abortion, stillbirths, and congenital neurologic abnormalities.[93, 96] Severe damage to the central nervous system, with extensive destruction of brain tissue, has been described when maternal infections occurred in the second trimester.

Dengue is an acute febrile illness, with morbilliform rash, and severe pain in muscles and joints ("break bone fever"). The disease is widely prevalent in the Caribbean area; it has recently reappeared in the United States after a long absence, several cases being confirmed in Texas in 1980. Serologic surveys in regions of high incidence indicate that many infections have occurred in pregnant women, but congenital disease has not been described.[95]

References

GENERAL

1. Benirschke, K., and Driscoll, S. G.: Pathology of the Human Placenta. New York, Springer-Verlag, 1967.
2. Hanshaw, J. B., and Dudgeon, J. A.: Viral Diseases of the Fetus and Newborn. Philadelphia, W. B. Saunders Co., 1978.
3. Krugman, S., and Gershon, A. E. (eds.): Infections of the Fetus and the Newborn Infant. New York, Alan R. Liss, Inc., 1975.
4. Plotkin, S. A.: Routes of fetal infection and mechanisms of fetal damage. Am. J. Dis. Child., *129*:444, 1975.
5. Remington, J. S., and Klein, J. O. (eds.): Infectious Diseases of the Fetus and Newborn Infant. Philadelphia, W. B. Saunders Co., 1976.
6. Sever, J. L., Larson, J. W., Jr., and Grossman, J. H., III: Handbook of Perinatal Infections. Boston, Little, Brown and Co., 1979.
7. Sever, J., and White, L. R.: Intrauterine viral infections. Annu. Rev. Med., *19*:471, 1968.

RUBELLA

8. Alford, C. A.: Rubella. *In* Remington, J., and Klein, J. (eds.): Infectious Diseases of the Fetus and Newborn Infant. Philadelphia, W. B. Saunders Co., 1976, pp. 71–106.
9. Al-Nakib, W., Best, J. M., and Banatvala, J. E.: Rubella-specific serum and nasopharyngeal immunoglobulin responses following naturally acquired and vaccine induced infection. Lancet, *1*: 182, 1975.
10. Buimovici-Klein, E., Lang, P. B., and Ziring, P. R.: Impaired cell-mediated immume response in patients with congenital rubella: Correlation with gestational age at time of infection. Pediatrics, *64*:620, 1979.

11. Center for Disease Control: Rubella Surveillance Summary, Jan. 1976–Dec. 1978 (issued May 1980), pp. 1–32.
12. Cooper, L. Z.: Congenital rubella in the United States. Prog. Clin. Biol. Res., *3*:1, 1975.
13. Fleet, W. F., Jr., Benz, E. W., Jr., Karzon, D. T., et al.: Fetal consequences of maternal rubella immunization. J.A.M.A., *227*:621, 1974.
14. Grillner, L.: Immunity to intranasal challenge with rubella virus two years after vaccination: Comparison of three vaccines. J. Infect. Dis., *133*:637, 1976.
15. Hayden, G. F., Herrmann, K. L., Buimovici-Klein, E., Weiss, K. E., Nieberg, P. I., and Mitchell, J. E.: Subclinical congenital rubella infection associated with maternal rubella vacination in early pregnancy. J. Pediatr., *96*:869, 1980.
16. Hildebrandt, H. M., and Maassab, H. F.: Rubella synovitis in a one-year-old patient. N. Engl. J. Med., *274*:1428, 1966.
17. Hillary, I. B., and Freestone, D. S.: Persistence of antibody induced by rubella vaccine (Wistar RA 27/3 strain) after six years. J. Hyg. (Camb.), *75*:407, 1975.
18. Horstmann, D. M.: Rubella: Still a problem for obstetricians. Contemp. OB/Gyn., *13*:67, 1979.
19. Horstmann, D. M., and Schluederberg, A.: Long-term surveillance of rubella vaccinees. Acta Pathol. Microbiol. Scand. (Suppl.) #275 (in press).
20. Menser, M. A., Harley, J. D., Hertzberg, R., Dorman, D. C., and Murphy, A. M.: Persistence of virus in lens for three years after prenatal rubella. Lancet, *2*:387, 1967.
21. Modlin, J. F., Herrmann, K., Brandling-Bennett, A. D., Eddins, D. L., and Hayden, G. F.: Risk of congenital abnormality after inadvertent rubella vaccination of pregnant women. N. Engl. J. Med., *294*:972, 1976.

22. Naeye, R. L., and Blanc, W.: Pathogenesis of congenital rubella. J.A.M.A., *194*:1277, 1965.
23. Peckham, C. S.: Clinical and laboratory study of children exposed in utero to maternal rubella. Arch. Dis. Child., *47*:571, 1972.
24. Plotkin, S. A.: Rubella vaccination. Lancet, *1*:382, 1979.
25. Plotkin, S. A., Farquar, J. D., and Ogra, P. L.: Immunologic properties of RA 27/3 rubella vaccine: A comparison with strains presently licensed in the United States. J.A.M.A., *225*:585, 1973.
26. Schluederberg, A., Horstmann, D. M., Andiman, W. A., and Randolph, M. F.: Neutralizing and hemagglutination-inhibiting antibodies to rubella virus as indicators of protective immunity in vaccinees and naturally immune individuals. J. Infect. Dis., *138*:877, 1978.
27. Scott, H., and Byrne, E. B.: Exposure of susceptible pregnant women to rubella vaccinees. Serologic findings during the Rhode Island immunization campaing. J.A.M.A., *215*:609, 1971.
28. Simons, M. J.: Congenital rubella: An immunological paradox? Lancet, *2*:1275, 1968.
29. Thompson, K. M., and Tobin, J. O'H.: Isolation of rubella virus from abortion material. Br. Med. J., *2*:264, 1970.
30. Tondüry, G., and Smith, D. W.: Fetal rubella pathology. J. Pediatr., *68*:867, 1966.
31. Weibel, R. E., Stokes, J. Jr., Buynak, E. B., and Hilleman, M. R.: Influence of age on clinical response of HPV 77 duck rubella vaccine. J.A.M.A., *222*:805, 1972.

CYTOMEGALOVIRUS INFECTION

32. Chretien, J. H., McGinniss, C. G., and Muller, A.: Venereal causes of cytomegalovirus mononculeosis. J.A.M.A., *238*:1644, 1977.
33. Davis, L. E., Tweed, G. V., Stewart, J. A., Bernstein, M. T., Miller, G. L., Gravelle, C. R., and Chin, T. D. Y.: Cytomegalovirus mononucleosis in a first trimester pregnant female with transmission to the fetus. Pediatrics, *48*:200, 1971.
34. Elek, S. D., and Stern, H.: Development of vaccine against mental retardation caused by cytomegalovirus infection in utero. Lancet *1*:1, 1974.
35. Evans, A. S.: Infectious mononucleosis and related syndromes. Am. J. Med. Sci., *276*:325, 1978.
36. Gold, E., and Nankervis, G. A.: Cytomegalovirus. *In* Evans, A. S. (ed.): Viral Infections of Humans. New York, Plenum Press, 1976, pp. 143–161.
37. Hanshaw, J. B.: Congenital cytomegalovirus infection: Laboratory methods of detection. J. Pediatr., *75*:1179, 1969.
38. Hanshaw, J. B., and Dudgeon, J. A.: Viral Diseases of the Fetus and Newborn. Philadelphia, W. B. Saunders Co., 1978, pp. 97–152.
39. Ho, M.: Cytomegalovirus infections and diseases. Disease-a-Month, *14*:1, 1978.
40. Huang, E. S., Alford, C., Reynolds, D., Stagno, S., and Pass, R. F.: Molecular epidemiology of cytomegalovirus infections in women and their infants. N. Engl. J. Med., *303*:958, 1980.
41. Jordan, M. C., Rousseau, W. E., Noble, G. R., Stewart, J. A., and Chin, T. D. Y.: Association of cervical cytomegaloviruses with venereal disease. N. Engl. J. Med., *288*:932, 1973.
42. Klemola, E., and Kääriänen, L.: Cytomegalovirus as a possible cause of a disease resembling infectious mononucleosis. Br. Med. J., *2*:1099, 1965.
43. Lang, D. J., and Kummer, J. F.: Demonstration of cytomegalovirus in semen. N. Engl. J. Med., *287*:756, 1972.
44. Monif, G. R. G., Egan, E. A., Held, B., and Eitzman, D. V.: The correlation of maternal cytomegalovirus infection during varying stages in gestation and neonatal involvement. J. Pediatr., *80*:17, 1972.
45. Numazaki, Y., Yano, N., Morizuka, T., Takai, S., and Ishida, N.: Primary infection with human cytomegalovirus: Virus isolation from healthy infants and pregnant women. Am. J. Epidemiol., *91*:410, 1970.
46. Phillips, C. F.: Cytomegalovirus vaccine: A realistic appraisal. Hosp. Pract., *14*:75, 1979.
47. Plotkin, S. A., Furakawa, T., Zygraich, N., and Huygelen, C.: Candidate cytomegalovirus strain for human vaccination. Infect. Immun., *12*:521, 1975.
48. Reynolds, D. W., Stagno, S., Hosty, T. S., Tiller, M., and Alford, C. A., Jr.: Maternal cytomegalovirus excretion and perinatal infection. N. Engl. J. Med., *289*:1, 1973.
49. Stagno, S., Reynolds, D. W., Amos, C. S., Dahle, A. J.,

McCollister, F. P., Mohindra, I., Ermocilla, R., and Alford, C. A.: Auditory and visual defects resulting from symptomatic and subclinical congenital cytomegaloviral and toxoplasma infections. Pediatrics, *59*:669, 1977.
50. Stagno, S., Reynolds, D. W., Huang, E. S., Thames, S. D., Smith, R. J., and Alford, C. A., Jr.: Congenital cytomegalovirus infection: Occurrence in an immune population. N. Engl. J. Med., *296*:1254, 1977.
51. Stagno, S., Reynolds, D. W., Pass, R. F., and Alford, C. A.: Breast milk and the risk of cytomegalovirus infection. N. Engl. J. Med., *302*:1073, 1980.
52. Stern, H., and Tucker, S. M.: Prospective study of cytomegalovirus infection in pregnancy. Br. Med. J., *2*:268, 1973.

VARICELLA-ZOSTER

53. Andiman, W. A.: Congenital herpesvirus infection. Clin. Perinatol., *6*:331, 1979.
53a. Brunell, P. A.: Varicella vaccination: Where do we go from here? Hosp. Pract., *15*:91, 1980.
54. Gershon, A.: Varicella in mother and infant: Problems old and new. *In* Krugman, S., and Gershon, A. (eds.): Progress in Clinical and Biological Research, Vol. 3. New York, Alan R. Liss, Inc., 1975.
55. Gershon, A., Raker, R., Steinberg, S., Topf-Olstein, B., and Drusin, L. M.: Antibody to varicella-zoster virus in parturient women and their offspring during the first year of life. Pediatrics, *58*:692, 1976.
56. Hanshaw, J. B., and Dudgeon, J. A.: Viral Diseases of the Fetus and Newborn. Philadelphia, W. B. Saunders Co., 1978, pp. 192–208.
57. Meyers, J. D.: Congenital varicella in term infants: Risk reconsidered. J. Infect. Dis., *129*:215, 1974.
58. Weller, T.: Varicella-herpes zoster virus. *In* Evans, A. S. (ed.): Viral Infections of Humans. New York, Plenum, 1976, pp. 457–480.
59. Young, N.: Chickenpox, measles, and mumps. *In* Remington, J. S., and Klein, J. O. (eds.): Infectious Diseases of the Fetus and Newborn Infant. Philadephia, W. B. Saunders Co., 1976, pp. 521–551.

INFLUENZA

60. Austin, D. F., Karp, S., Dworsky, R., and Henderson, B. E.: Excess leukemia in cohorts of children born following influenza epidemics. Am. J. Epidemiol., *101*:77, 1975.
61. Elizan, T. S., Ajers-Froelich, L., Fabiyi, A., Ley, S., and Sever, J. L.: Viral infection in pregnancy and congenital CNS malformations in man. Arch. Neurol., *20*:115, 1969.
62. Finland, M.: Influenza complicating pregnancy. *In* Charles, D., and Finland, M. (eds.): Obstetric and Perinatal Infections. Philadelphia, Lea and Febiger, 1973, pp. 355–398.
63. Hall, C. B., Douglas, R. G., Jr., Geiman, J. M., and Messner, M. K.: Nosocomial respiratory syncytial virus infections. N. Engl. J. Med., *293*:1343, 1975.
64. Hardy, J. B., Azarowicz, E. N., Mannini, A., Medearis, D. M., Jr., and Cooke, R. E.: The effect of Asian influenza on the outcome of pregnancy. Am. J. Pub. Health, *51*:1182, 1961.
65. Manson, M. M., Logan, P. D., and Loy, R. M.: Rubella and other virus infections during pregnancy. Report on Public Health and Medical Subjects No. 101, Ministry of Health. London, Her Majesty's Stationery Office, 1960.
66. McCrea-Curnen, M. G., Varma, A. O., Christine, B. W., and Turgeon, L. R.: Childhood leukemia and maternal infectious diseases during pregnancy. J. Natl. Cancer Inst., *53*:943, 1974.
67. Meibaline, R., Sedmak, G. V., Sasidharan, P., Garg, P., and Grausz, J. P.: Outbreak of influenza in a neonatal intensive care unit. J. Pediatr., *91*:974, 1977.
68. Yawn, D. H., Pyeatte, J. C., Joseph, J. M., Eichler, S. L., and Garcia-Bunuel, R.: Transplacental transfer of influenza virua. J.A.M.A., *216*:1022, 1971.

MUMPS

69. Aase, J. M., Noren, G. R., Reddy, V., and St. Geme, J. W., Jr.: Mumps virus infection in pregnant women and the immunologic response of their offspring. N. Engl. J. Med., *286*:1379, 1972.
70. Hutchins, G. M., and Vie, S. A.: The progression of interstitial

myocarditis to idiopathic endocardial fibroelastosis. Am. J. Pathol., 66:483, 1972.

71. Jones, J. F., Ray, C. G., and Fulginiti, V. A.: Brief clinical and laboratory observations — perinatal mumps infection. J. Pediatr., 96:912, 1980.

72. Manson, M. M., Logan, W. P. D., and Loy, R. M.: Rubella and other virus infections during pregnancy. Report on Public Health and Medical Subjects No. 101, Ministry of Health. London, Her Majesty's Stationery Office, 1960.

73. Siegel, M., Fuerst, H. T., and Peress, N. S.: Comparative fetal mortality in maternal virus diseases: A prospective study in rubella, measles, mumps, chickenpox, and hepatitis. N. Engl. J. Med., 274:768, 1966.

74. St. Geme, J. W. Jr., Noren, G. R., and Adams, P. Jr.: Proposed embryopathic relation between mumps virus and primary endocardial fibroelastosis. N. Engl. J. Med., 275:339, 1966.

75. Weibel, R., Buynak, E., McLean, A., and Hilleman, M.: Persistence of antibody after administration of monovalent and combined live attenuated measles, mumps, and rubella virus vaccines. Pediatrics, 61:5, 1978.

76. Yamauchi, T., Wilson, C., and St. Geme, J. W., Jr.: Transmission of live attenuated mumps virus to the human placenta. N. Engl. J. Med., 290:710, 1974.

77. Young, N. A.: Chickenpox, measles, and mumps. In: Remington, J. S. and Klein, J. O., (eds.): Infectious Diseases of the Fetus and Newborn Infant. Philadelphia, W. B. Saunders Co., 1976, pp. 570–579.

MEASLES

78. Cherry, J. T.: The "new" epidemiology of measles and rubella. Hosp. Pract., 15:49, 1980.

79. Christensen, P. E., Schmidt, H., Ban, H. O., Anderson, V., Jordal, B., and Jensen, O.: An epidemic of measles in southern Greenland, 1951. Measles in virgin soil. II. The epidemic proper. Acta Med. Scand., 144:431, 1953.

80. Dyer, I. S.: Measles complicating pregnancy: Report of twenty-four cases with three instances of congenital measles. South. Med. J., 33:601, 1940.

81. Jespersen, C. S., Littauer, J., and Sagild, U.: Measles as a cause of fetal defects: A retrospective study of ten measles epidemics in Greenland. Acta Paediatr. Scand., 66:367, 1977.

82. Martin, D. B., Leonard, B. W., Nieburg, P. I., and Blair, D. C.: Atypical measles in adolescents and young adults. Ann. Intern. Med., 90:877, 1979.

83. Siegel, M., and Fuerst, H. T.: Low birth weight and maternal virus diseases: A prospective study of rubella, measles, mumps, chickenpox, and hepatitis. J.A.M.A., 197:88, 1966.

84. Young, N. A.: Chickenpox, measles, and mumps. In Remington, J. S., and Klein, J. O. (eds.): Infectious Diseases of the Fetus and Newborn Infant. Philadelphia, W. B. Saunders Co., 1976, pp. 551–570.

ENTEROVIRUSES

85. Center for Disease Control, U.S. Public Health Service: Poliomyelitis prevention. M.M.W.R., 28:510, 1979.

86. Cherry, J. D., Enteroviruses. In Remington, J. S., and Klein, J. O. (eds.): Infectious Diseases of the Fetus and Newborn Infant. Philadelphia, W. B. Saunders Co., 1976, pp. 366–413.

87. Gear, J. H. S., and Measrock, V.: Coxsackie infections in the newborn. Prog. Med. Virol., 15:42, 1973.

88. Katz, S. L.: Other viruses associated with infections of the fetus and newborn infant. In Krugman, S. and Gershon, A. (eds.): Progress in Clinical and Biologic Research, Vol. 3. New York, Alan R. Liss Inc., 1975, pp. 55–61.

89. Lake, A. M., Lauer, B. A., Clark, J. C., Wesenberg, R. L., and McIntosh, K.: Enterovirus infections in neonates. J. Pediatr., 89:787, 1976.

RABIES

90. Anderson, L. J., Sikes, R. K., Langkop. C. W., Mann, J. M., Smith, J. S.: Winkler, W. G., and Deitch, M. W.: Post-exposure trial of a human diploid cell strain rabies vaccine. J. Infect. Dis., 142:133, 1980.

91. Center for Disease Control, U.S. Public Health Service: Rabies prevention. M.M.W.R., 29:265, 1980.

ARBOVIRUS INFECTION

92. Copps, S., and Giddings, L.: Transplacental transmission of western equine encephalitis. Pediatrics, 24:31, 1959.

93. London, W. et al.: Congenital cerebral and ocular malformations induced in rhesus monkeys by Venezuelan equine encephalitis virus. Teratology, 16:285, 1977.

94. Schinefield, H., and Townsend, T.: Transplacental transmission of western equine encephalitis. J. Pediatr., 43:21, 1953.

95. Ventora, A., Ehrenkranz, N., and Rosenthal, D.: Placental passage of antibodies to dengue virus in persons living in a region of hyperendemic dengue virus infection. J. Infect. Dis., 131:62, 1975.

96. Wenger, F.: Venezuelan equine encephalitis. Teratology, 16:369, 1977.

15

SEXUALLY TRANSMITTED INFECTIONS

Over the past 20 years the incidence of venereal infections, especially gonorrhea, herpes simplex virus, and chlamydia, has reached the proportions of an epidemic, so that the obstetrician is obligated to search for sexually transmitted infections in every patient. Personal feelings about contemporary sexual mores should not interfere with vigorous pursuit of the diagnosis and treatment of venereal disease among sexually active people, particularly pregnant women. As with most diagnoses, suspicion is the major ingredient of success: Sexually transmitted diseases spare no group of people except perhaps the absolutely chaste, and they are not a subject for this book.

A careful medical history, physical examination, and routine screening for sexually transmitted infection are integral parts of antenatal care. Moreover, because sexual activity occurs after conception, sometimes even to the day of delivery, a thoughtful inquiry about sexually transmitted infections and appropriate screening tests must not be considered a part of only the first prenatal visit. The physician must keep in mind the potential for infections spread by sexual contact throughout the pregnancy and puerperium.

It is crucial to remember that these diseases are transmitted by a human vector. The physician must be scrupulously compulsive about inquiring into the patient's sexual history, including attitudes, behavior, and consorts. For example, optimal treatment of trichomonas vaginitis or of the asymptomatic gonococcal carrier includes contact detection and treatment in order to avert reinfection. Optimal management of the patient with reportable sexually transmitted disease includes epidemiologic investigation and treatment of contacts by state and federal preventive medicine departments. These essential public health services cannot be effective if individual cases are not reported. There is no place in good obstetric practice for avoiding the reporting of venereal diseases.

Defining sexual transmission can be difficult, and it is wise to keep an open mind. The whole of the human external surface can serve a sexual function; almost any infection can be transmitted during and by the intimate contacts of sexual relations. In this chapter the discussion is confined to infectious agents that are transmitted primarily by the skin-to-skin or secretion-to-surface contact of sexual activity, that are uniquely adapted to surviving and multiplying in the genitourinary tract, and that usually, but not always, produce symptoms or signs referable to the genitourinary tract when they cause clinical disease (Table 15–1). Many of these agents are capable of establishing asymptomatic or latent infection within the host or on the host's genitourinary mucosa. All pose some risk to the health of the pregnant woman or produce local discomfort. Some are a potential risk to the successful completion of the pregnancy because of ill effects upon the mother. Some are a hazard to the fetus as a result of in utero infection.

It is important to stress that sexually transmitted diseases are common, have no racial or socioeconomic prejudice, are frequently latent or asymptomatic or missed, and always have a source other than the patient. Effective management of these infections includes a physician who is alert to the vagaries and varieties of sexual behavior, a probing sexual history and physical examination, routine screening, followup or referral for followup of sexual contacts, and appropriate antimicrobial therapy. It is only by such alertness and vigor that the tragedy of

351

TABLE 15–1 SEXUALLY TRANSMITTED INFECTIONS

Agents	Infections
Viruses	Herpesvirus hominis, type 2
	Molluscum contagiosum venereum
	Condyloma acuminatum
Chlamydiae	Trachoma, inclusion conjunctivitis
	Lymphogranuloma venereum
Mycoplasmas	*Mycoplasma hominis* infection
	T. mycoplasma infection
Fungi	*Candida albicans* vaginitis
	Torulopsis glabrata vaginitis
Bacteria	Gonorrhea (*Neisseria gonorrhoeae*)
	Chancroid (*Hemophilus ducreyi*)
	Granuloma inguinale (*Donovania granulomatis*)
Spirochetes	Syphilis (*Treponema pallidum*)
Parasites	*Trichomonas vaginalis* vulvovaginitis
	Crab lice infestation (*Phthiris pubis*)
	Scabies (*Sarcoptes scabiei*)

congenital syphilis or serious gonococcal disease of the mother, her infant, or both can be avoided.

VAGINAL DISCHARGE

The vagina and the cervix of a healthy genital tract contain a luxuriant normal flora, which, in combination with the anatomic and physiologic milieu, contributes to fertility and fecundity. Sexually transmitted pathogens may disrupt reproduction in four ways: first, by distorting the normal cervicovaginal flora so that fertilization is impaired and infection by abnormal flora is enhanced; second, by disrupting the normal flora so that the closure of the cervical canal to infection and toxins during pregnancy is impaired; third, by producing pelvic infection with interruption of nidation; and fourth, by producing intrauterine infection of the placenta and fetus. The increase in spontaneous abortion, premature rupture of membranes, premature labor, and postpartum pelvic infection associated with venereal infections may be the result of the loss of the normal cervicovaginal flora caused by sexually transmitted pathogens and not exclusively a direct effect of the infecting organism.

During pregnancy, most women experience an increase in cervical and vaginal secretions. Vaginal discharge is regarded as a normal event, and pregnant patients rarely complain about it. In one clinic, less than 1 per cent of women complained of discharge, but one third admitted to its presence on direct questioning.[168] The vaginal discharge of the normal pregnant woman is often profuse, creamy, and white. It is highly acidic and contains many epithelial cells, few white blood cells, and a preponderance of gram-positive lactobacilli. This vaginal discharge is the response of the cervix and vagina to the hormonal stimulation of pregnancy. The discharge and local estrogen-produced changes in the cells and glands of the vagina and cervix are important host factors in preventing infectious complications during gestation and the puerperium.

The vaginal secretions in healthy, menstruating females have a pH of 4.5 or less and an almost pure growth of Döderlein's bacillus with some growth of enterococci, group B beta-hemolytic streptococci, diphtheroids, or coliforms.[165] Severe vaginitis with significant inflammation and discharge is accompanied by an alkaline pH, purulent discharge, the absence of any Döderlein's bacilli, and the emergence of several potential pathogens, including anaerobes.[155] In severe vaginitis the risk of fetal loss, serious neonatal infection, and puerperal sepsis appears to be increased.[124]

Alterations in the normal flora and vaginal discharge can be induced by broad-spectrum antibiotics, disinfectants, deodorants, and almost all sexually transmitted infectious agents. Disruption of the normal cervicovaginal environment by noninvasive local infections such as *Trichomonas vaginalis* and herpes simplex virus may predispose to more serious or invasive infection of mother and baby. Careful clinical attention to these conditions is therefore an important part of obstetric management, especially appreciated by the patient with uncomfortable vulvovaginitis.

Evaluating Vaginal Discharges and Genital Skin Lesions

Most sexually transmitted infections have vaginal discharge or genital skin lesions or both as part of the clinical presentation. In view of the superficial similarities among many of these infections, precision and care are essential in evaluating the condition of each patient.

Certain clinical features help direct the clinician's use of the laboratory (Table 15–2): the presence or absence of pain and whether the skin lesion is an ulcer (sore) or a mass (bump). Painful lesions, ulcers, or nodules suggest viral or bacterial infection. Nonpainful ulcers are almost always due to syphilis, and painless nodular lesions or lymph nodes are syphilitic until proved

TABLE 15-2 CLINICAL FEATURES OF GENITAL LESIONS RESULTING FROM SEXUAL ACTIVITY

Type of Lesion	Disease	Agent	Appearance of Lesion	Inguinal Nodes	Systemic Symptoms	Laboratory
Painful sore	Primary genital herpes	Herpes simplex Type II	Groups of vesiculopustules	Yes — painful	Yes — fever	Virus, culture Stain of scrapings
	Recurrent genital herpes	Herpes simplex Type II	Groups of vesiculopustules	No	No	Same
	Trauma	Homo sapiens	Abrasions, toothmarks, ecchymosis	Not without 2° infection	Not without 2° infection	—
	Chancroid	Hemophilus ducreyi	Ulcer with friable base, shaggy, exudate, ragged edges; not indurated; occasionally multiple	Yes — unilocular painful bubo	No	Stain and culture of pus aspirate from bubo
	Lymphogranu-loma venereum	Chlamydia trachomatis	Shallow ulcer or eroded papule; single; short duration	Yes — enlarging mass, draining fistulas, painful	Rare	Serology culture smear for cyto-plasmic inclusion
Painful bump	Granuloma inguinale	Donovania granulomatis	Ulcerating papulonodules, exuberant granulations, occasionally multiple	Rare	No	Stain of crushed tissue
	Mulluscum contagiosum	Wart-pox virus	Umbilicated papules, foreign body; reaction may produce furuncle-like lesion	Yes	No	Smear of molluscum body for cyto-plasmic inclusion
Non-painful sore	Primary syphilis	Treponema pallidum	Well-demarcated ulcer, indurated base, usually single	Yes — nonpainful	No	Darkfield Serology
Non-painful bump	Secondary syphilis	Treponema pallidum	Wet: Multiple skin-colored papules Dry: Papulosquamous papules; occasionally circinate	Yes — nonpainful	Yes — mild	Darkfield Serology
	Condyloma acuminatum	Papova virus	Fleshy, broccoli-like warts Multiple	Not without 2° infection	Not without 2° infection	
Itchy bumps	Scabies	Sarcoptes scabiei	Pruritic erythematous papular rash; raised burrows with mite at opening	Not without 2° infection	Not without 2° infection	Examine scrapings for mites
	Crab lice	Phthiris pubis	Mites, crab lice, ecchymotic bite sites	Not without 2° infection	Not without 2° infection	Catch a crab

Modified from Lee, 1980.

TABLE 15–3 EVALUATION OF VAGINAL DISCHARGES

Procedure	Purpose
Gram stain of discharge or scrapings	Assess vaginal flora and check for yeasts and gram-negative intracellular diplococci
Wet preparation of vaginal secretions	Check for motile trichomonads
Endocervical and vaginal swabs	Gonococcal, chlamydial, herpes simplex cultures
Papanicolaou smear of cervix and vaginal secretions	Check for cytologic evidence of neoplasia, herpesvirus hominis, chlamydiae, trichomonads
Serologic tests	Test for syphilis
ADDITIONAL STUDIES (IF INDICATED BY PATIENT'S HISTORY OR FINDINGS ON PHYSICAL EXAMINATION)	
Culture	Check for yeasts, trichomonads, herpesvirus hominis
Scrapings of cervical lesions for Giemsa's or Wright's stain	For intranuclear and intracytoplasmic inclusions
Bacterial and special cultures	Identification of nongonococcal bacterial pathogens (enterococci, group B beta-hemolytic streptococci, genital mycoplasmas)
Darkfield examination	For spirochetes in suspicious lesions
Additional gonococcal cultures from rectum, urethra, pharynx	For extragenital gonococcal infection

otherwise. Pruritic bumps are usually caused by bites.

As a general rule, the tests listed in Table 15–3 constitute a thorough procedure for the office evaluation of vaginal discharges.

The taking of swabs for bacterial, chlamydial, and viral culture; making a Papanicolaou smear; and obtaining material for Gram stain and wet preparation are procedures that can be performed quickly in the office with simple laboratory equipment and with minimal discomfort to the patient. Careful examination of Gram stains and wet preparations can provide ready, excellent guidance in management. These procedures are often neglected, and thus initial therapy is misguided. Supplemented by appropriate cultures, the wet preparation and Gram stain are the mainstay of the rapid office diagnosis of vulvovaginitis.

SEXUALLY TRANSMITTED VIRUSES

Many viruses have been found in the secretions and tissues of the male and female genital tracts. Some reach the genitourinary tract during viremia following infection by nonsexual transmission. Others are transmitted by kissing and other intimate contact accompanying sexual intercourse. Both cytomegalovirus (CMV) and hepatitis B antigens (HBAg) have been isolated from semen and saliva.[59, 80] Infection by these agents occurs more frequently in marital partners and among sexually promiscuous populations, such as prostitutes and homosexual men; however, nonsexual modes of transmission have not been excluded.

Herpes Simplex Virus

Herpes simplex (HSV) belongs to a group of DNA viruses whose properties include the induction of intranuclear inclusions in infected cells and the ability to produce prolonged infection, presumably throughout the life of the infected host, with recurrent episodes of clinical illness. HSV can infect a wide range of animals and tissue cultures and can be rapidly identified in the virus diagnostic lab.

There are two antigenic types of HSV.[108] HSV-1 is transmitted by nonvenereal contact and usually causes nongenital infection, and HSV-2 is sexually transmitted and usually causes genital infection.[103, 151] Sexual practices may alter the usual pattern; HSV-2 infection may occur at extragenital sites following orogenital intercourse, and HSV-1 may cause genital lesions following orogenital or oroanal contact.

The acquisition of HSV-1 infection begins and peaks in childhood; the rate of primary infection declines in adults.[17] The acquisition of HSV-2 infection begins following puberty and peaks in adolescence and early adulthood,[105] paralleling sexual activity. The presence of antibody to HSV-2 as well as clinical disease caused by HSV-2 is more common among the sexually promiscuous. There is a high risk of infection to sexual contacts of patients with genital herpes. The combined data from two separate studies demonstrate that 75 per cent of susceptible sexual partners of patients with herpetic genital lesions became infected with HSV-2.[103, 132]

Genital HSV infection is often associated with other venereal diseases. A correlation between HSV-2 antibody and positive serologic tests for syphilis has been observed among prostitutes.[132] Gonococcal infection and HSV-2 infection share epidemiologic and clinical similarities, including prolonged cervical infection and transmission to the neonate during delivery.[109]

There is a seroepidemiologic relationship of HSV-2 to invasive squamous cell carcinoma of the cervix.[19, 133, 141] Although data from different studies are not consistent, in general they suggest that women with cervical cancer have been infected with HSV-2 more frequently and at a younger age than women without cervical cancer.[72]

Clinical Features. The characteristic herpetic lesion is a vesicle surrounded by an erythematous zone. The lesions begin as a closely aggregated group of painful papules, progressing rapidly to vesicles, shallow ulcers, pustules, and crusts. Healing takes several days to several weeks (Fig. 15–1). Healing in the absence of secondary infection occurs without scar formation. The appearance and discomfort of herpetic lesions are helpful clues to the nature of a genital sore. The pain may be so severe as to require hospitalization. Primary infection is inapparent in many patients. In those with clinical signs, infection is associated with tender regional lymphadenopathy and constitutional symptoms — chills, fever, malaise, headache, myalgia, and occasionally generalized lymphadenopathy, splenomegaly, and atypical lymphocytosis.[43]

In tissue culture and in exfoliated material from lesions, HSV produces a diagnostic cytopathogenic effect manifested by multinucleated giant cells and intranuclear inclusions. This is the basis for the clinically useful Tzanck test, in which the base of a suspected herpetic lesion is scraped and the material is spread on a slide and stained with a Romanovsky-type stain (Wright or Giemsa). Finding multinucleated giant cells and intranuclear inclusions supports, but does not prove, the diagnosis of HSV infection. The cytopathogenic effects have also been usefully exploited in detection of the presence of latent or chronic infection of the uterine cervix.[108] Virologic confirmation is readily accomplished because of the rapidity with which the virus produces cytopathic effects in tissue culture. At present, virus culture laboratory techniques can easily and rapidly confirm the clinical suspicion of *Herpes simplex* virus infection; these diagnostic aids deserve greater utilization by clinicians.

In women, the cervix is the principal site of infection, which is commonly not accompanied by symptoms.[103, 105] Primary infections may be associated with severe herpetic cervicitis with necrotizing, bleeding lesions that may shed virus for as long as 3 months. Recurrent and latent

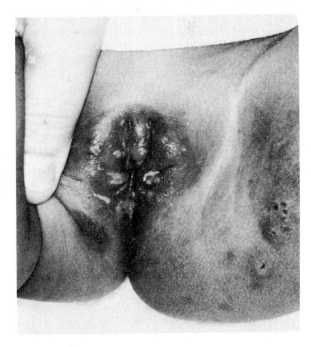

FIGURE 15–1. Sexually acquired primary herpes simplex infection in a prepubertal girl. The patient had fever, dysuria, and intense local discomfort. The vesicles have coalesced to form large shallow ulcerations on the vulva and in the vagina.

herpetic cervicitis are virtually always asymptomatic and are most often diagnosed by exfoliative cytologic studies. Recurrent external genital lesions are accompanied by cervical shedding of virus in about one third of patients.[50] Genital herpes may be about three times more common in pregnant women than in nonpregnant women.[54] The observation that herpetic cervicitis is common in pregnancy suggests that hormonal effects play some role in the disease process.[7] Only about one third of pregnant women with "herpes" have characteristic vesicular lesions, ulcerative lesions, or both. Lesions on the buttocks and thighs are infrequent. Extragenital lesions suggest extragenital sexual contact or HSV-1 infections. Genital herpes in either sex can produce urethritis and cystitis with dysuria and urinary retention. Herpetic cervicitis can be clinically confused with gonorrhea, and herpetic urethritis and cystitis can be mistaken for bacterial urinary tract infection.

Active herpes simplex virus infection during pregnancy increases the risk of fetal loss and prematurity.[106, 112] One group reported on the outcome of pregnancy in 283 women with confirmed genital herpes.[106] Of 37 patients who developed lesions during the first 20 weeks of pregnancy, 12 (34 per cent) aborted; in contrast, there was only a 10 per cent abortion rate in the control, uninfected population. There were 21 premature births among 101 patients who developed herpes genitalis after 20 weeks of gestation. This was slightly higher than the rate of 17.6 per cent of premature births in the control group, but the difference was not statistically significant. The risk of abortion and prematurity was especially high when the maternal HSV-2 infection was primary rather than recurrent.

The vast majority of neonatal HSV infections are acquired during passage through an infected birth canal or by the ascending spread of virus from the cervix through ruptured membranes.

The risk of infection is highest in infants delivered of women with primary genital herpes beginning shortly before delivery.[73] If virus is present at delivery, the risk of infection in the infant is about 40 per cent, unless delivery is by cesarean section either before or within 4 hours after the membranes rupture.[106] The risk of neonatal herpes simplex infection following maternal lesions occurring after 32 weeks of gestation is about 10 per cent.[106]

Neonatal infection may range from undetected infection without sequelae to occasionally serious, rarely fatal disseminated disease, the survivors of which usually suffer severe ocular or neurologic sequelae.[45, 54, 64, 172] Maternal antibody to HSV does not appear to play a significant role in protection of the fetus and neonate against infection.[128] The incidence of herpetic infection among premature infants is four to five times that among full-term infants and is probably related in part to inadequate development of the immune response in premature infants.[54] The incubation period of neonatal herpes simplex infection is usually 3 to 7 days after the delivery; however, disease may appear earlier if delivery was significantly delayed after rupture of membranes. External herpetic lesions of the skin, mouth, and eye occur in about 50 per cent of cases and are the most reliable clinical indicator of HSV infection of the neonate.[102] These lesions often appear first on the presenting part, and thus a careful inspection for vesicles, especially of the scalp and buttocks, may give a useful early clue to the diagnosis.[33, 101] Except for skin and corneal lesions, there is little to distinguish neonatal herpes from other viral or bacterial infections. Indeed, the review showed that a correct clinical diagnosis was made in only 44 per cent of the 148 neonatal HSV infections.[102] Early recognition is important because infected infants should be isolated.[73] There is scarce but convincing evidence that transplacental transfer of virus, although rare, can occur.[41, 104, 181] There are occasional case reports of presumed ascending herpetic infection despite intact membranes.[51] Cytologic changes in placental tissues and in the endometrium suggestive of the affects of herpes simplex virus suggest that virus may be present in utero even before nidation and may traverse the placenta by routes other than the blood stream.[5, 47] An infant with microcephaly and central nervous system calcifications has been described, in whom HSV-1 was recovered from cerebrospinal fluid.[41] The same report describes six other cases with congenital malformations associated with intrauterine HSV infection; the majority of these infections were HSV-2. Microcephaly, chorioretinitis, and intracranial calcifications were the most common abnormalities in this small group. Five of the seven cases had a vesicular rash at birth or very soon after birth, suggesting that virus has been acquired before descent through an infected birth canal.

The woman who develops clinically active genital herpes after 20 weeks of pregnancy presents a major dilemma in management (Table 15–4).[73, 106, 111] The incidence of neonatal infections in this situation, especially with clinically active maternal infection, is high, and the sequelae of neonatal infection are potentially severe. Because of the very small risk of intrauterine infection, it may be desirable to perform amnio-

TABLE 15–4 MANAGEMENT OF PREGNANCY COMPLICATED BY
MATERNAL HERPES SIMPLEX VIRUS INFECTION

	Vaginal Delivery	Cesarean Section
Mandatory	Evidence of intrauterine fetal infection confirmed by amniocentesis	Active lesions at time of labor
Recommended	Rupture of membranes for more than 4 hours, if active lesions are present, or if virus is known to have been present during last 4 weeks of gestation	Presence of virus by culture during last 4 weeks of gestation
Debatable	Evidence of maternal infection (clinical lesions or culture) during last 20 weeks of gestation	Evidence of maternal infection (clinical lesions or culture) during last 20 weeks of gestation

Viral cultures for herpes simplex are an essential part of the management of pregnancies complicated by HSV infection. A rational decision about method of delivery is dependent upon the results of viral culture.

centesis to examine the amniotic fluid for the presence of virus. If virus is present, then nothing further need be done, and the presumably infected infant can be delivered vaginally. Amniocentesis for viral culture should be done only if the clinical course or sonography suggest altered fetal growth consistent with intrauterine infection.

It is mandatory for the obstetrician to follow the patient with cervical and vaginal cultures for HSV-2 closely during the remainder of her pregnancy[8] and to examine her for active genital lesions during the last month of pregnancy. If cultures or examination reveal the presence of infective virus in the birth canal at delivery or within 2 to 4 weeks before delivery, then cesarean section is desirable. If the membranes have been ruptured for more than 4 hours, the fetus is most likely already exposed to infection by the ascending route, and abdominal delivery is not likely to prevent neonatal infection. If serial cultures do not reveal the presence of infective virus, then vaginal delivery can be undertaken with reasonable safety to the fetus.[6, 106] It has been suggested that abdominal delivery be performed before rupture of the membranes in any pregnancy in which HSV-2 is known to have been active in the last month of gestation,[106] based on the experience of one group, in which at least 50 per cent of newborns vaginally delivered of mothers with recent or active genital herpes were infected, whereas only 1 of 16 newborns delivered abdominally before or shortly after membrane rupture became infected. The available data indicate that cesarean section is mandatory when active maternal herpetic infection is present at the onset of labor.[73, 110]

Because infection with HSV-2 is a common venereal disease, and the potential harm to the fetus is great, cervical cultures for HSV-2 and screening of Papanicolaou smears for cytopathic effects should become an integral part of antenatal care. This is especially important for any patients with other sexually transmitted infections and for sexually promiscuous patients.

Treatment of genital herpes in the mother is nonspecific and not particularly satisfying. Symptomatic relief can be obtained with sitz baths, open wet dressings, or lotions. Topical antibiotics may be of benefit if superficial secondary infection supervenes. Topical anesthetics and corticosteroids are not indicated. Narcotic analgesics may be necessary when severe vulvar pain or pelvic discomfort related to pelvic lymphadenopathy is present, almost always in primary infection. Phenazopyridine (Pyridium) may be useful if dysuria is present. Hospitalization may be required if urinary retention and severe discomfort occur. Photodynamic inactivation of the virus has achieved some popularity.[36, 70, 175] The long-term effects of such therapy during pregnancy, especially upon the oncogenicity of the virus, are not clear. Phototherapy for herpes genitalis during pregnancy is therefore not recommended. Recent success with topical 2-deoxy-D-glucose[13] requires further confirmation and elaboration of risks to pregnant patients.

Molluscum Contagiosum Venereum

The usual lesions of molluscum contagiosum are umbilicated papules. Histologically, the center of the lesion is filled with a mass of loosely adherent epithelial cells (the "molluscum body"), the cytoplasm of which is virtually replaced by the molluscum contagiosum inclusion body. Electron microscopy has demonstrated a virus-like structure, believed to be a poxvirus.[129] Generally, several of these smooth-surfaced, skin-colored papules with the characteristic central umbilication are distributed randomly on the genitalia, perineum, and pubic area. The lesions are usually asymptomatic except for occasional mild pruritus or when local irritation or maceration produces inflammation. Inflamed molluscum contagiosum lesions are common in the adult perineal and paragenital areas. They often resemble furuncles and may be associated with local lymphadenopathy.[86] The inflammatory process is believed to be the result of traumatic extrusion of the central core into the surrounding dermis, which generates a foreign body reaction.[86] Diagnosis is readily accomplished by curettage of a lesion and observation, even in unstained preparations, of typical large cytoplasmic inclusion bodies. Molluscum contagiosum is uniformly a benign disease with eventual spontaneous resolution of lesions after as long as 2 years. It may last as long as 4 years, with continual development or recrudescence of molluscum contagiosum. There is reasonable evidence that venereal transmission has occurred between sexual partners.[67, 86, 87, 129] Autoinoculation, as well as person-to-person contact, occurs. When an unusual papular lesion is present in a pregnant woman, careful search for other molluscum contagiosum lesions may spare unnecessary therapy for presumed pyogenic skin infection. The recommended management of inflamed lesions is curettage of the molluscum body; uninflamed lesions may be left alone or curetted.

Condyloma Acuminatum

Condyloma acuminatum is a benign viral skin disease. Convincing epidemiologic evidence illustrating its sexual transmissibility was reported in 1954 in a study of women with vulvar condylomata.[9] All the women were wives of United States servicemen returning from Korea; their husbands were all found to have had penile warts and extramarital sexual contact while overseas. Subsequently, other authors demonstrated a high sexual infectivity; about two thirds of sexual consorts of individuals with condyloma acuminatum developed lesions, the incubation period being about 3 months.[116, 167]

Condyloma acuminatum usually begins as a single warty growth in the genital or perineal area. Satellite lesions soon appear and under suitable conditions may coalesce or become exuberantly luxuriant. Moist, warm skin folds exaggerated by poor personal hygiene or poor ventilation resulting from tight-fitting synthetic clothing are commonly associated with hyperplastic condylomata. These fleshy, cauliflower-like warts are unmistakable. Perianal lesions suggest transmission by rectal intercourse.

Genital warts in women most commonly occur on the posterior introitus, labial minora and majora, and perineum. One observer reported perianal lesions in only 18 per cent and cervical lesions in 6 per cent of 141 affected women.[116] Condylomata almost never occur outside the anogenital area. The clinical presentation and appearance of the uncomplicated genital warts are characteristic. Occasionally, when other conditions — ulceration, secondary infection, bleeding — coexist, a biopsy may be desirable, especially when there are ulcerated lesions, to exclude the possibility of vulvar carcinoma. Although condyloma acuminatum often coexists with other venereal diseases, there is no unique association between it and other sexually transmitted infections, except possibly genital candidiasis. Secondary infection can produce a malodorous, painful lesion and may facilitate the growth or spread of genital warts.

Pregnancy can provide a dramatic stimulus to hyperplasia of condyloma acuminatum.[116, 130, 184] Massive condylomata interfering with delivery, even necessitating cesarean section or surgical excision of the lesion, have been recorded. Spontaneous regression following pregnancy, even with very large lesions, does occur. The effect of hormonal contraception upon condyloma acuminatum has not been carefully explored, but personal experience does not indicate that oral contraceptives have a significant effect upon the size of lesions. Laryngeal papillomas have been reported to occur in the offspring of mothers with condyloma acuminata, and the obstetrician should alert the pediatrician to the possibility of this infection.[26]

Condyloma acuminatum can usually be treated by applying a small amount of 10 to 25 per cent podophyllin resin in tincture of benzoin. Podophyllin therapy is contraindicated during pregnancy because of reports of fetal death and premature labor following its use.[130] Some authors prefer trichloracetic acid, electrocoagulation, cryosurgery, or surgical excision. Electrocoagulation may be especially useful when large lesions have developed during pregnancy.[184] Recently, the use of autogenous vaccine, especially for patients with recurrent lesions, has been advocated.[130] Because the biology of the causative virus and its effect upon the developing fetus are unknown, this treatment is not advisable during pregnancy.

CHLAMYDIAL INFECTIONS

Chlamydiae are the causative agents of several important human and veterinary infections.[144] Strains of *Chlamydia psittaci* are the cause of abortions and arthritis in cattle and sheep, ornithosis in birds, and psittacosis in humans. Different serotypes of the human chlamydial species, *Chlamydia trachomatis,* produce trachoma, lymphogranuloma venereum, and various urogenital infections, which may be transmitted to the neonate during delivery.

All chlamydiae share common antigens, which are detectable by complement fixation techniques. Serotyping of *C. trachomatis* is done with microimmunofluorescent techniques, which have allowed the identification of certain serotypes as the cause of specific clinical syndromes.

Chlamydiae are obligate intracellular parasites and cannot grow on artificial media. They can be cultivated in laboratory animals, chicken eggs, and tissue culture. They contain both DNA and RNA and, like bacteria, possess independent enzyme systems, and can produce a cell wall. The infective particles penetrate the host cell, possibly by phagocytosis, and grow within a membrane-lined vacuole in the cytoplasm. The organism grows to about 5 microns in diameter and then subdivides into larger numbers of smaller infective particles. Completion of the cycle occurs with cell death and release of infective particles from the cytoplasmic inclusions. Chlamydiae are capable of maintaining persistent asymptomatic infection at several sites, including the uterine cervix, urethral mucosa, and conjunctivae. *Chlamydia trachomatis* is usually transmitted through skin-to-skin contact during sexual activity or during delivery. Nonvenereal transmission may result from skin carriage of infective particles between eyes and genitals and occasionally from the release of infective particles from infected secretions into inadequately chlorinated swimming pools.

Lymphogranuloma Venereum

Lymphogranuloma venereum (LGV) has a worldwide distribution but is most common in tropical and subtropical climates. About 600 cases are reported annually in the United States,

most from large metropolitan areas of the southern states such as Washington, DC.[127] The majority of cases are found among sexually promiscuous persons. As with all other sexually transmitted infections, LGV is often accompanied by other venereal diseases. Serologic or clinical manifestations of chlamydial infection are common in the sexual consorts of infected patients, which is consistent with sexual transmission of the infection. However, because chlamydial infections are so common in the sexually active population and because the chlamydia share certain common antigens, serologic tests alone should not be used as an indication for treating contacts on epidemiologic grounds.

Acute, early infection generally presents as one of two syndromes: inguinal or genitoanorectal.[1, 49] Constitutional signs and symptoms accompany the inguinal syndrome more often than the genitoanorectal syndrome and include fever, headache, meningismus, arthralgia, erythema multiforme, and erythema nodosum.[144]

The inguinal syndrome is characterized by regional lymphadenopathy and constitutional signs and symptoms. The initial lesion is usually a small erosion or indurated papule, usually single, relatively painless, and healing prior to the onset of regional lymph node involvement. Coincident with the appearance of the inguinal bubo is the appearance of an ulceration on the genitalia that is often mistaken for the primary lesion but is in fact a secondary manifestation.[49] The inguinal mass consists of many discrete, enlarged nodes held together by plastic periadenitis. The inflammatory reaction in these nodes is not uniform, hence the uneven distribution of softening and induration and, when breakdown occurs, drainage from multiple fistula tracts. This inguinal mass is very different from the firm induration of syphilitic adenitis and the unilocular abscess of chancroid. A characteristic of LGV is the formation of a groove corresponding to the inguinal ligament and separating the lymph node mass into inguinal and femoral areas. In about 20 per cent of patients, the nodes resolve spontaneously; breakdown and drainage occur in about 75 per cent; and a small minority progress to chronic indurated inguinal masses.

The genitoanorectal syndrome accounts for about one fourth of the cases. It is seen predominantly, but not exclusively, in women. This syndrome is characterized by a bloody, mucopurulent anal discharge and friable edematous hemorrhagic anorectal mucosa. Ulcerative lesions of the vulva, vagina, and urethra, usually painless, are other manifestations. These lesions may progress so that destruction of tissue produces fenestrations of the labia, destruction of the urethra, and subsequent incontinence.[158] Fibrosis of the ulcerative lesions may produce urethral or vaginal stenosis. Rectal or vulvar lesions may occur together or alone and are infrequently accompanied by inguinal buboes. In some patients the inflammation of the vulva may persist for months or years, resulting in scarring and elephantiasis (esthiomene). Following acute proctitis, there may be constipation or diarrhea, tenesmus, and abdominal pain. LGV proctitis can progress to perirectal abscesses and to rectal stricture. LGV rectal strictures almost always occur between 5 and 10 cm from the anus. About one third of women with perirectal strictures also develop rectovaginal fistulas. Many males with rectal LGV are passive homosexuals, and some women are probably infected during anal intercourse. It may be that in most women, the infection begins in the lower vagina and spreads along the tissue planes of the perineal body to invade the rectum at the area where the fascia is most thin and the vagina and the rectum are closest to each other.[158] This area, about 5 to 10 cm above the anus, is the most common site for proctitis and vaginal fistulas. These complications constitute late manifestations and do not appear until the disease has been present for months or years.

The infection can be transmitted as long as perineal, urethral, or vaginal ulcerations and drainage persist or if rectal drainage from proctitis or rectovaginal fistulas is present. Infection of the newborn by passage through an infected birth canal is a possibility, although it has not been described. The disease is not believed to be transmitted across the placenta.

The diagnosis can be aided by one or more of three diagnostic tests — cytologic stains, cultures, and serology. Skin testing with Frei skin test antigen is no longer widely used, and the skin test antigen is not commercially available in the United States. Aspiration of inguinal buboes may yield the organism on culture. Giemsa stain of aspirated material spread on a slide may reveal typical intracytoplasmic inclusions. The complement fixation test may be a more helpful diagnostic aid. It becomes positive within 4 weeks after infection and detects about 97 per cent of known cases of chlamydial infection. There is cross-reactivity with all chlamydiae and occasionally in narcotics addicts and patients with cat-scratch fever. A complement fixation titer of 1:16 or higher is considered significant, especially if clinical findings suggest the diagnosis of LGV. Complement fixation titers greater than 1:32 usually indicate recent disease.[145] Microimmunofluores-

cent serologic tests are available only in a few medical centers. This test can identify particular serotypes of *C. trachomatis*.

Treatment of early disease during pregnancy includes aspiration of large fluctuant buboes and administration of sulfonamide or erythromycin. Therapy lasts from 3 to 6 weeks, guided by the reduction in size and fluctuance of nodes, diminution of drainage from fistulas or proctitis, and healing of genitourethral ulcerations. Reconstructive surgery is often necessary in late disease to relieve rectal stricture, to close rectovaginal fistulas, and to excise elephantine changes of the vulva.

UROGENITAL CHLAMYDIAL INFECTION

For the obstetrician the importance of *Chlamydia trachomatis* resides in the organism's ability to produce salpingitis and urethritis, to produce nonsymptomatic cervical infection, and to infect infants as they descend the birth canal, resulting in neonatal ophthalmitis and pneumonia. The possibility that some infertile men may have chlamydial urogenital infection is also noteworthy.

C. trachomatis can be isolated from 30 to 40 per cent of men with nongonococcal urethritis. Approximately 70 per cent of sexual partners of men with chlamydial urethritis have evidence of endocervical infection.

The principal sites of infection in women are the cervix and endocervix. *C. trachomatis* infection often coexists with other sexually transmitted diseases; simultaneous infections with chlamydia and the gonococcus are common in women. Asymptomatic or latent infection appears to be common and may be chronic. In one study, 69 of 82 infected but untreated and asymptomatic women had intracytoplasmic inclusions on repeated vaginal smears for more than 1 year after initial detection.[11] The potential for producing more acute disease in the female genital tract is indicated by serologic or cultural evidence of chlamydial infection in 20 to 30 per cent of nonpregnant women with pelvic inflammatory disease[35, 98] and the occurrence of postpartum pelvic infection in the mothers of 37 per cent of infants developing chlamydial ophthalmitis.[134] A role for chlamydia in producing urinary tract infection is suggested by the identification of *C. trachomatis* in 10 of 16 women with pyuria and urine cultures negative for bacteria.[156]

In both sexes urogenital chlamydial infection may be associated with concurrent infection of other anatomic sites such as the rectum, throat, ear, and eye.

Chlamydiae have been cultured from 5 to 20 per cent of women attending prenatal clinics.[3, 85, 145] Most of those women had no symptoms from their infection. Among the infants of infected mothers, 40 to 50 per cent develop conjunctivitis and 10 to 20 per cent develop pneumonia.[11, 88, 145]

The identification of serious respiratory disease caused by chlamydiae in neonates has been followed by the recognition that chlamydiae colonize many mucosal sites. Otitis media and obstructive nasopharyngeal infection may be part of neonatal chlamydial infections.

There are no clinical features of chlamydial urogenital infections that distinguish them from other urogenital infections in women. Chlamydial urethritis produces the urethral syndrome and may be confused with bacterial urinary tract infection. Patients with vaginal discharge from vaginitis and cervicitis should be evaluated carefully for all of the potential pathogens causing these syndromes. Acute pelvic infection caused by chlamydiae may be accompanied by fever, pelvic cramps, and pelvic pain indistinguishable from disease caused by gonococci. Fever, right upper quadrant pain, and tenderness — the so-called Curtis-Fitzhugh syndrome, or perihepatitis — can be caused by both chlamydiae and gonococci.[182]

In general, clinical suspicion, stimulated by the knowledge that sexually transmitted infections are often multiple, is the major reason for searching further for chlamydial infection. The absence of pathogenic bacteria despite numerous polymorphonuclear leukocytes on Gram stain and the failure to recover bacteria from a purulent discharge should be important clues for the clinician to search specifically for chlamydial organisms.

As with lymphogranuloma venereum, cytology, serology, and culture are the laboratory methods available to confirm the diagnosis of chlamydial infection. Unfortunately not all of these methods, except for Giemsa staining of scrapings, are widely available. Intracytoplasmic inclusions can be demonstrated in the Giemsa stains of purulent material or scrapings. Fluorescent antibody staining has been shown to be more sensitive than the Giemsa method for identifying chlamydial inclusions in scrapings from the eye and the genital tract.[145] Antibodies to *C. trachomatis* can be detected in tears, cervical secretions, and blood by use of the microimmunofluorescent test. Diagnosis of recent infection requires the demonstration of rising antibody titers, which makes these tests useful mostly for epidemiologic studies. The complement fixation test is not of value. Isolation of the organism in tissue culture has become a routine procedure in many research laboratories.

Chlamydia trachomatis appears to have surpassed the gonococcus as the most prevalent genital pathogen. Furthermore, *Chlamydia* produces a wider spectrum of serious neonatal disease than does the gonococcus. Chlamydial cultures, therefore, should become a standard part of good antenatal care. The goal of such routine screening of high risk patients is to identify and treat infected patients in order to prevent postpartum infection of both child and mother. No data indicate that such an approach will reduce perinatal morbidity; however, identification of mothers and neonates at risk is alone worth the cost.

Chlamydiae are sensitive to a number of antibiotics. During pregnancy the most useful agents are topical and oral sulfonamides and oral erythromycin. The tetracyclines should not be used during pregnancy and infancy. Treatment for gonococcal infection with penicillin or spectinomycin will not eradicate chlamydiae. Topical sulfonamides alone for 14 days will reduce vaginal discharge and cervicitis, but whether such treatment reduces postpartum maternal and neonatal infection is unknown. Oral erythromycin or sulfonamide for 14 days can be used to treat chlamydial urethritis and pelvic inflammatory disease. Systemic sulfonamides should be used with caution close to term because of adverse effects upon bilirubin metabolism in the neonate.

SEXUALLY TRANSMITTED BACTERIA

Syphilis, gonorrhea, chancroid, and granuloma inguinale are the "classic" venereal diseases. Recent investigations into the syndrome of nonspecific vaginitis indicate that mycoplasmas, anaerobic bacteria, and *Hemophilus vaginalis* contribute to urogenital infections. Bacteria that are not residents of the genitalia may be incidentally transmitted by sexual practices. Synergistic infections caused by human bites and bacterial diarrhea may result from oral and anal sexual activities.

Genital Mycoplasmas

The role of mycoplasmas as pathogens in human genitourinary tract and perinatal infections is poorly defined.[35, 88] Mycoplasmas have long been recognized by veterinarians as causing bovine genital infections and reproductive failure.

Only two species, *Mycoplasma hominis* and *Ureaplasma urealyticum* (previously named *T. mycoplasma*), have been isolated with any regularity from the human genital tract. These organisms are acquired through sexual contact and are part of the normal genital flora of healthy, sexually active young men and women.[89, 94] Sexually inexperienced women have low rates of vaginal colonization with mycoplasmas, whereas colonization rates increase with increasing numbers of sexual partners among sexually active women. About one third of newborns have *Ureaplasma urealyticum* and a smaller number are colonized with *Mycoplasma hominis*. Mycoplasma colonization of the neonate apparently does not lead to infection and does not persist.[92] In contrast to these studies there is considerable evidence suggesting, but not proving, a pathogenic role for genital mycoplasmas in nonspecific urethritis of men and in prematurity, spontaneous and septic abortion, and puerperal infection in pregnant women.[57, 58, 79, 92, 93, 94, 166] The ubiquity of the organism in the normal flora of sexually active women precludes an uncritical assignment of pathogenicity for mycoplasmas found in pregnancies complicated by infection.

There are several reports of the isolation of ureaplasmas from spontaneously aborted fetuses and placentas. Carefully controlled and microbiologically well-documented studies are needed to further clarify the possible role of mycoplasmas in causing infertility and spontaneous abortion. An association between maternal and neonatal colonization with ureaplasmas and low birth weight has been found. Indeed, birth weight has been shown to be inversely proportional to the rate of mycoplasma colonization. Several case reports and series of patients with postpartum fever have indicated *Mycoplasma hominis* as a pathogen causing puerperal fever and postpartum infections. A large series from the Boston City Hospital, however, found no consistent relationship between the isolation of mycoplasmas from the lochia and postpartum fever.[93] The available information indicates that *Mycoplasma hominis* has the potential to invade the uterus and blood stream and is probably responsible for an as-yet-undefined proportion of puerperal fever cases. It does not seem wise, especially in view of the association between mycoplasmas and other sexually transmitted pathogens, to treat nonspecific genital symptoms blindly for mycoplasma infection.

Nonspecific Vaginitis

Nonspecific vaginitis is a rather ill-defined clinical entity consisting of an increased, malodorous, gray exudate not attributable to monilia, *Trichomonas vaginalis*, gonorrhea, *Chlamydia*, or herpes simplex virus. "Clue cells" in the vaginal discharge, large epithelial cells with granular cytoplasm covered by small gram-negative rods, were described in 1955.[42] The bacteria, a pleomorphic, facultative anaerobe that grows in thioglycolate broth or on rabbit blood agar in 10 per cent CO_2, was named *Hemophilus vaginalis*. The organism, also known as *Corynebacterium* or *Gardnerella vaginale*, has been isolated from many patients with nonspecific vaginitis; however, its causative role in this condition has not been proved.[31, 91]

Nonspecific vaginitis characteristically produces a change in vaginal flora, pH, and biochemistry. Increased acetate, succinate, and butyrate and a predominent flora, consisting of *H. vaginalis* and species of bacteroides and peptococcus, have been observed in patients with this syndrome.[155] With successful treatment, lactobacilli and lactate became the predominent organism and metabolic by-products.

The role of *H. vaginalis* in puerperal and neonatal infection is not clear except insofar as nonspecific vaginitis has a disruptive effect on the normal cervicovaginal milieu.

Treatment of nonpregnant patients with metronidazole has been recommended.[126] Although metronidazole has been used without ill effect in pregnancy, its teratogenic potential demands caution in its use. *H. vaginalis* is resistant to sulfonamides and tetracycline in vitro, and ampicillin fails to eradicate the organism in an unacceptably large number of patients despite in vitro susceptibility. In the absence of good clinical studies giving suitable alternatives to metronidazole therapy during pregnancy, and on the basis of previous reports[42] and personal experience, a trial of topical sulfonamide, after documentation of nonspecific vaginitis by smear and culture, may be worthwhile.

Chancroid

Chancroid is an acute, localized, autoinoculable infection of the genitals caused by *Hemophilus ducreyi*, a small gram-negative rod. The disease is endemic in tropical and subtropical areas and is not common in the temperate areas of North America and Europe, where the major problem with this disease follows importation by seamen and military personnel returning from endemic areas. The disease is uncommon in the United States, but the rapidity and ease of travel require the clinician to consider chancroid in the differential diagnosis of any ulcerated genital lesion. Although prostitution is a most important reservoir of chancroidal infection, there is a disproportionately low incidence of the disease in women, perhaps because of difficulties in diagnosis or the existence of an asymptomatic carrier state in females. The disease apparently does not pose a threat to the fetus or neonate, though this remains a theoretical possibility.

The incubation period is short, usually 5 days or less. The initial lesion is almost exclusively on or near the genitalia and presents as a small, inflammatory papule with a narrow circumference of erythema. There may be more than one lesion. The lesion progresses rapidly to pustules, which rupture, forming the characteristic painful, sharply circumscribed ulcer with ragged underlined edges. The lesions are shallow, usually fairly small, and tender to touch. The base is often covered with a grayish, necrotic exudate and bleeds easily with even gentle manipulation. The presence of pain and the lack of induration about and underneath the ulcer serve to distinguish chancroid from the chancre of primary syphilis.[49] Occasionally, the infection may produce rapidly enlarging ulcers, often in a linear fashion, or a progressive, necrotizing infection that may destroy the external genitalia. Spread by autoinoculation occurs anywhere in the perigenital zone, pubis, abdomen, or thighs. Extragenital chancroids are remarkably rare. Unilateral inguinal adenitis, progressing to the characteristic unilocular, painful bubo, occurs in over half the cases. Chancroidal buboes should be aspirated, not incised, because of the risk of establishing an infection along the skin margins.[49]

The disease is usually self-limiting and notable mostly for the local, painful ulcerations and tender inguinal adenitis. Recalcitrant ulcers may persist for months or years without healing, even with presumably adequate therapy. Secondary infection with superficial infections or synergistic, progressive infections can occur, especially when fusospirochetes are the secondary invaders. Twelve to 15 per cent of typical chancroid lesions are mixed infections with H. ducreyi and T. pallidum.[49] Treponemes may not be demonstrable during the initial stages of the development of the chancroidal ulcer.

Smears taken directly from chancroidal ulcers for Gram stain are difficult to interpret when superficial and secondary infections are present.

Smears prepared from aspirated pus from a bubo are more reliable and often show small gram-negative rods, which are in chains or within polymorphonuclear leukocytes. Cultures of aspirated pus are more reliable than cultures obtained from open sores. Because the organism is fastidious and requires special media, culture techniques are difficult and are not readily accessible to the clinician. Smears of aspirated pus are a more practical, though limited, diagnostic aid.

Successful management includes adequate drainage and antimicrobial drugs. Sulfonamides are the mainstay of chemotherapy and are usually effective in doses of 4 to 6 gm daily for 10 to 14 days. Long-acting sulfonamides should not be used because of the risk of Stevens-Johnson syndrome. The best prophylaxis appears to be soap and water.

Granuloma Inguinale

Granuloma inguinale is a chronic, progressive, autoinoculable, granulomatous disease of the genitalia and perineum. Its lesions contain characteristic mononuclear cells with intracytoplasmic coccobacillary organisms known as Donovan bodies. The disease is generally regarded as being a mildly contagious infection, is caused by the bacteria Calymmatobacterium (Donovania) granulomatis, and is transmitted by sexual intercourse.[49] Like lymphogranuloma venereum and chancroid, the disease is worldwide in distribution but is most commonly found in tropical and subtropical areas. The disease is rare in prostitutes and in the heterosexual consorts of infected patients. The lesions always begin on or near the genitalia and are most common in promiscuous people who often have other venereal infections. In homosexuals and heterosexuals practicing sodomy, the lesions are often perianal in location.[29] The contention that the gut may be a source of the infection and that anal intercourse or fecal contamination of the genital area is a mode of transmission is supported by the reported isolation of an organism resembling C. granulomatis from the stool[44] and the finding that the organism shares capsular antigens with Klebsiella pneumoniae and K. rhinoscleromatis.[121] The incubation period is not known. In experimental inoculations of aspirated pus into human beings, about 6 weeks elapsed before definite infection was produced.[29, 49] Early lesions are papulonodules, the skin of which breaks down to form an ulcerated lesion with a characteristic beefy red, velvety granulation tissue. Secondary infection, especially with fusospirochetes, can produce a malodorous, rapidly progressive necrotizing ulcer. Half the patients in one small series had evidence of syphilis.[29] Untreated, the disease may progress to subcutaneous granulomas (pseudobuboes) and exuberant granulomatous lesions. Inguinal adenopathy without bubo formation does occur but is not common. The lesions are usually on the external genitalia, although they may be found on the cervix. They may be spread by autoinoculation to other locations in the perineum and paragenital areas. Organisms are best seen on smears made from crushed-tissue preparations, stained with Wright-Giemsa stain, though they can be found on histologic sections stained with silver technique or Wright-Giemsa stain.

Late sequelae include striking hypertrophy and swelling of the external genitalia without sclerosis of lymphatics.[158] When the ulcers heal they have a characteristic smooth, pliable, depigmented skin covering. Granuloma inguinale must be considered in any granulating tissue lesion of the perineum and may be premalignant for squamous cell carcinoma. Congenital infection resulting from intrapartum or antepartum infection of the fetus has not been reported.

In nonpregnant patients, treatment with tetracycline and with streptomycin has been most successful. Because of adverse effects of tetracycline on pregnancy, treatment should be withheld until after delivery.

Gonorrhea

Gonorrhea is pandemic throughout the world, an estimated 150 million patients being reported annually. Transmission is almost exclusively by the skin-to-skin contact of sexual intimacy. The possibility of transmission by fomites has been suggested by earlier reports of nursery outbreaks of gonococcal disease in which rectal thermometers were believed to be the carrier[27] and by more recent evidence that, under appropriate conditions, *Neisseria gonorrhoeae* can survive outside the body for as long as 24 hours.[34]

Clinical Manifestations. The important clinical appearances of gonorrhea are summarized in Table 15–5. The classic clinical picture of gonococcal pelvic inflammatory disease, purulent vaginal discharge, and lower abdominal discomfort in a previously uninfected woman, 3 to 5 days following exposure to an infected sexual contact, is rather a rarity in clinical practice. Moreover, because the major sites of infection in women — the endocervix, urethra, anal canal, and pharynx — are also common sites of

TABLE 15–5 THE SPECTRUM OF GONOCOCCAL INFECTION

Primary genital infections
  Vulvovaginitis (prepubertal females)
  Cervicitis (prepubertal and postpubertal females)
  Urethritis (both sexes, any age)
  Asymptomatic carrier (both sexes, any age)
Extension of infection within genitourinary tract
  Females, any age, usually postpubertal
    Endometritis
    Salpingitis
    Infection of Skene's and Bartholin's glands
    Urethritis
    Cystitis
  Males, any age
    Prostatitis
    Cystitis
    Epididymitis
    Seminal vesiculitis
Extension of infection to extragenitourinary sites
  Females, usually postpubertal
    Proctitis
    Pelvic peritonitis
    Perihepatitis
Dissemination of infection via blood stream
  Males and females, any age
    Uncomplicated and asymptomatic
    Dermatitis-arthritis syndrome
      Bacteremic phase
      Skin lesions
      Tenosynovitis
      Polyarthralgia
      Positive blood cultures
      Septic joint phase
      Purulent monarticular arthritis
      Positive joint fluid cultures
    Pericarditis and myocarditis
    Hepatitis
    Endocarditis
    Meningitis
Primary extragenital infection
  Either sex, any age
    Conjunctivitis-ophthalmitis
    Skin infection: cellulitis and abscess
  Either sex, consenting adults
    Stomatitis
    Parotitis
    Pharyngitis
  Homosexual males
    Proctitis

infection with other pathogens transmitted by sexual or nonsexual contact, it is impossible to prove that the symptoms were produced solely by the gonococcus unless all other pathogens have been excluded.[62]

Symptoms of acute gonococcal infection are most frequently caused by extension of infection from the endocervix to the contiguous structures of the genitourinary tract. Infection of the urethra may extend to the bladder, producing dysuria, urgency, and frequency. Symptoms of urinary tract infection are common in symptomatic gonococcal infections in women.[62] Gonococcal urethritis or cystitis produces pyuria and occasionally hematuria. Ascent of infection to the endometrium and fallopian tubes, resulting in endometritis and salpingitis, occurs in women with patent genital tubing.

Infection of the adult female genital tract by the gonococcus is not always characterized by a profuse purulent discharge. The actual frequency of symptoms in the early stages of infection in the adult female is uncertain.

There are no reliable data on the frequency of symptomatic versus asymptomatic infection in women. It is estimated, however, that 75 to 90 per cent of infected women are asymptomatic.[37, 62, 122] The prevalence of asymptomatic infections in a study of women seen in family planning clinics was 5 per cent.[15] Among private patients 30 years of age or younger, the prevalence of asymptomatic gonorrhea was about 2 per cent.[56, 123] A major hindrance to understanding the epidemiology of venereal infections is the inadequacy in reporting these infections. It was found that in 1968, private physicians treated approximately 80 per cent of these cases but reported only 10 per cent.[40]

In North America, the reported incidence of asymptomatic cervical infection during pregnancy has ranged from 2 to 7.3 per cent.[22, 23, 78, 143] In contrast, studies from the United Kingdom and Scandinavia have reported a lower (0.02 to 0.6 per cent) prevalence of asymptomatic endocervical infection.[18, 134, 149] Since the general trend of epidemic gonorrhea has existed in all the areas studied, the discrepancies between the North American and European reports must be evaluated further. One apparent difference is the correlation of higher prevalence rates with the use of Thayer-Martin selective medium in the North American studies. On the basis of North American data from prenatal and nonpregnant patients, the obstetrician should expect asymptomatic endocervical gonorrhea in 2 to 5 per cent of prenatal patients.

While the literature has stressed the importance of asymptomatic endocervical infection, the importance of asymptomatic infection at nongenital sites and among men must also be emphasized. In one venereal disease clinic study, 40 per cent of infected women had positive rectal cultures; half of these women had negative cervical cultures. Seventy-five per cent of the patients with positive rectal cultures admitted to rectal intercourse or sexual play involving the anus and

rectum with their male partners. At this same venereal disease clinic, all infected patients were interviewed during a 7 month period and were specifically asked about the practice of fellatio. Among the 138 patients admitting to the practice of fellatio, 22 per cent had positive pharyngeal cultures for gonococci.[122] Most of these patients were asymptomatic white women who had acquired their infection through heterosexual contact. All but 4 of the 31 patients had a positive cervical or rectal culture as well. The problem of asymptomatic infection in men has been obscured because acute urethritis in males is so dramatically obvious and because the majority of asymptomatic women come to venereal disease clinics because their symptomatic male partners have named them as contacts. When the problem is approached by using the woman as the index case, a different picture emerges.[53, 99] For example, two thirds of infected male contacts of women with acute gonococcal arthritis have had asymptomatic urethral infection.[173] Forty-two per cent of the male contacts of women found to have gonorrhea on screening in prenatal and family-planning clinics had gonococcal infection; of this group, 80 per cent either had no symptoms or were not sufficiently inconvenienced by their symptoms to seek medical attention.[14]

Asymptomatic carriers of both sexes represent the reservoir of gonococcal infection, and it is asymptomatic carriers who transmit the infection to new partners. Moreover, carriage can occur at the cervix, rectum, urethra, and oropharynx.

The Effect of Gonorrhea on Pregnancy. Gonococcal infection, symptomatic or asymptomatic, may exert an adverse influence upon the course of pregnancy, causing both maternal and infant morbidity. In a study of 14 neonates with *N. gonorrhoeae* isolated from orogastric aspirates there was a higher incidence of prematurity, prolonged rupture of the fetal membranes, associated maternal peripartum fever, histologic evidence of chorioamnionitis, and a clinical diagnosis of sepsis compared with infants with no pathogenic bacteria in gastric contents.[53] Intrauterine growth retardation seems to be another adverse effect produced by symptomatic or asymptomatic gonococcal disease of the mother. These facts are the basis for the following guidelines for prenatal care in the United States:

1. All pregnant women should be screened for gonococci by history, physical examination, and routine cultures.

2. Cultures should be done on selective media and taken from the endocervix; optimally, cultures should be taken from both cervix and

rectum. When indicated, an additional culture from the oropharynx should be obtained.

3. Management of infected pregnant women includes identification and treatment of all sexual partners, asymptomatic and symptomatic. In some cases, repeated cultures for gonococci during pregnancy will be indicated, especially in the patient with frequent infections before pregnancy or with a psychosocial setting predisposing to sexual promiscuity.

4. Because other sexually transmitted organisms often accompany gonococci, management includes a careful search for their presence by obtaining syphilis serologic tests and microscopic or cultural examination for organisms such as yeasts and trichomonads.

Gonococcal Infection in the Neonate. Neonatal gonococcal infection may be produced by ascending infection during prolonged premature rupture of the membranes or during delivery through an infected birth canal. Many sites can be contaminated by *N. gonorrhoeae* — the eye, external ear canal, oropharynx, stomach, and anorectal mucosa. Gonococcal vulvovaginitis and urethritis are not known to occur in neonates, probably because maternal estrogens stimulate a well-cornified stratified squamous epithelium of the vulva and vagina. Neonatal gonococcal infections of the eye, pharynx, stomach, and anal canal have all been implicated as the source of hematogenous dissemination of gonococci with resulting meningitis and arthritis.[53, 76, 77, 161]

Gonococcal ophthalmia is less common in the neonate than other types of eye infection, such as chlamydial inclusion conjunctivitis.[62] There is an increase in the number of reported cases of gonococcal eye infection, coincident with an increase in the number of mothers with gonococcal infections. The incidence of gonococcal ophthalmia neonatorum can be reduced by approximately 90 per cent with the prophylactic use of 1 per cent silver nitrate eye drops.[152] Even though failures with Credé prophylaxis do occur because of faulty instillation of the drops or because the infection has become well established following prolonged rupture of the membranes, most authorities prefer this method to other prophylactic measures for the neonate.[10] Antibiotic preparations such as bacitracin, penicillin, or tetracycline either are of no prophylactic value or are no more effective than 1 per cent silver nitrate and may unnecessarily sensitize the infant. It has been said that the best prophylaxis for gonococcal ophthalmia neonatorum is an uninfected birth canal.

The practical difficulties of Credé prophylaxis are well known and are certainly responsible for some failures. In some cases the solution may not have been instilled, an oversight not uncommon in a busy delivery suite, especially when physicians become complacent. Holding open the eye of a slippery, wriggling neonate is a remarkably frustrating task at times, and the silver nitrate solution may not actually reach the conjunctival surface because of blepharospasm, particularly during the attempt to put the drop into the second eye. Occasionally, premature flushing with saline precipitates the silver ion, leaving an ineffective medication in the eye. Finally, the importance of the short incubation period and the ascent of infection to the fetus with premature rupture of the membranes in the failure of Credé prophylaxis should be emphasized.[152, 170] In this circumstance there may be little the physician can do to prevent the disease, as was illustrated by the Duke experience in which, after an increase in neonatal gonococcal eye infection, two cases occurred despite the use of silver nitrate drops in the delivery room and again in the nursery.[152]

Because of the speed with which the infection may injure the eye, rapid diagnosis is essential. Unfortunately, the first sign is conjunctivitis indistinguishable from that produced by a 1 per cent solution of silver nitrate. However, the drug-induced conjunctivitis usually clears within 24 hours and should not be present by the time gonorrheal conjunctivitis begins to be clinically apparent on the third or fourth postpartum day. The infected eye develops a discharge, at first watery or serosanguinous, and then within a day the discharge becomes thick and purulent. Involvement of the cornea may result in ulcerations followed by the development of hypopyon and iridocyclitis.

Gonococcal Arthritis-Dermatitis Syndrome. The most common complication of bacteremic gonococcal disease is the gonococcal arthritis-dermatitis syndrome, which has become the most common acute polyarthritis in young adults.[62]

The onset of the gonococcal arthritis-dermatitis syndrome is heralded by fever, chills, and myalgia.[1a, 7a, 62a, 71a, 177a] Within 2 to 4 days a polyarticular tenosynovitis, especially of the wrists and extensor tendons of the fingers, and the characteristic rash appear. Usually, 5 to 20 skin lesions appear on the distal extremities and around or over joints. The lesions are painful papules or petechiae with an erythematous base. They may progress through vesicular, pustular, or bullous stages, often with a hemorrhagic base (Fig. 15–2). During the early phase of the dis-

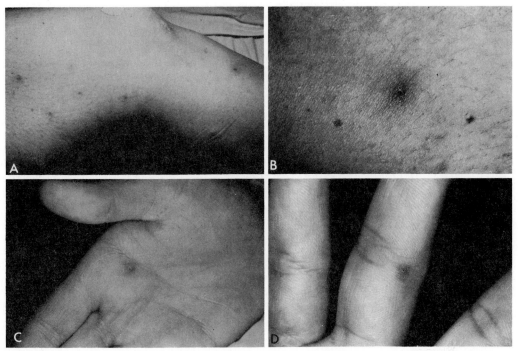

FIGURE 15–2. Skin lesions of gonococcal arthritis-dermatitis syndrome or gonococcemia. There are usually only a few lesions in juxta-articular areas. They have an erythematous base (*B*) and a hemorrhagic vesicle, which may become pustular (*C* and *D*).

ease, blood cultures are positive. Special immunofluorescent techniques may reveal the presence of gonococci in the skin lesions,[172a] but the organism is almost never found in aspirates taken from tenosynovitis or joint fluid if any is obtainable during the early stages of the disease. If the patient remains untreated, manifestations will slowly resolve, but after 8 to 10 days, some patients develop a purulent mono- or oligoarticular arthritis.[62a, 71a] A few patients present with septic arthritis without having other recognizable manifestations of gonococcemia. During this "septic joint" stage, blood cultures are negative, but culture of the joint effusion may be positive in up to 50 per cent of cases.[62] A negative culture does not exclude the diagnosis; sometimes special culture techniques may yield the organism. Suspicion of gonococcal disease should be indulged by culturing, on special media, material from the prime sites of asymptomatic infection — cervix, rectum, and oropharynx — and from other sites — eyes, urethra, prostate, and Skene's and Bartholin's glands — when appropriate. In this writer's experience, the diagnosis of disseminated gonococcal disease has been made most frequently on the basis of the clinical picture and a positive culture from the cervix, rectum, or oropharynx. Positive blood, skin le-

sion, or synovial fluid studies are gratifying confirmation but must not be relied upon as the only criteria for diagnosis and for the decision to institute antimicrobial therapy.

Other complications of gonococcemia include endocarditis, myopericarditis, meningitis, and hepatitis. These manifestations often occur concomitantly with the arthritis-dermatitis syndrome and should be carefully watched for.

Laboratory Diagnosis. The use of Gram stain for presumptive diagnosis or as a guide to initial therapy is a much neglected diagnostic aid (Fig. 15–3). Because of its poor reliability in proving the absence of *N. gonorrhoeae* in cervical or vaginal material, the use of the Gram stain in obstetrics and gynecology has been discouraged, an attitude that the author regards as a serious mistake. In urethral exudate from men, the demonstration of intracellular, gram-negative diplococci allows a presumptive diagnosis of gonorrhea. In women, examination of direct smears of endocervical material is a useful guide to initial therapy while awaiting results of cultures. A negative endocervical Gram stain is meaningless in regard to the diagnosis of gonorrhea, but even without the demonstration of intracellular gram-negative diplococci, the Gram stain allows the physician to assess the flora of

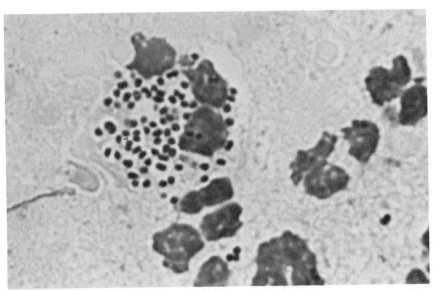

FIGURE 15–3. Gram stain of cervical material showing gram-negative intracellular diplococci. Culture was positive for *N. gonorrheae*. This finding on a cervical smear provides an adequate indication for beginning treatment while cultures are pending.

the endocervical exudate, especially for other pathogens such as yeasts. A positive Gram stain allows the physician to begin treatment with the caveat in mind that abnormal vaginal flora include other gram-negative cocci (*Mimea, Herellea*) that may be morphologically indistinguishable from gonococci. It is important to re-emphasize the value of direct microscopic examination of Gram-stained material in the evaluation of a woman's symptoms, signs, and history suggestive of gonococcal infection.[174]

While the Gram stain provides rapid information for tentative diagnosis and initial therapy, the crux of the diagnosis of gonorrhea is the culture. Among women with gonorrhea, positive cultures are obtained from the endocervix in 80 to 90 per cent, from the anal canal in 50 to 60 per cent, from the urethra in 50 to 60 per cent, and from the pharynx in about 10 per cent. The urine sediment should also be cultured for gonococci in young women with symptoms of lower urinary tract infection. Cultures of the anal canal are important in assessing the efficacy of treatment of proved gonorrhea, because gonococci persist only in the anal canal in about 30 per cent of treatment failures.[147] The importance of cultures of blood and synovial fluid has already been indicated. Selective media such as the Thayer-Martin medium, containing antibiotics to inhibit other bacteria and fungi, should be in standard use for culturing sites normally heavily colonized by a mixed flora. Selective media need not be used in routine urethral cultures and should

probably be avoided in cultures from the synovial fluid, since some gonococci may be sufficiently inhibited by the concentration of the antibiotics to give a false negative result.

The simplest and best way to handle culture specimens is to heavily inoculate the appropriate agar plate, warmed to room temperature, directly with a culture swab at the time of examination. The plates should be promptly placed in a candle jar and may then be transported to the bacteriologic laboratory with relative leisure. Various transport media can be used if there is no significant delay in plating the specimen on the appropriate medium; however, this is clearly less desirable than inoculating plates at the bedside or examining table. The use of Transgrow culture bottles, which contain Thayer-Martin medium in small bottles with a CO_2 enriched atmosphere, is a great help in remote places or where the delay in processing jeopardizes the value of culturing. The Transgrow bottles should be warmed to room temperature and should be preincubated for 24 hours before mailing.

Treatment. Antibiotic therapy of gonococcal infection during pregnancy is influenced by the epidemiology of the drug resistance of the organism and the requirement of not harming the pregnancy.[48] In some parts of the world, penicillinase-producing *Neisseria gonorrheae* (PPNG) limits the effectiveness of the least toxic, nonteratogenic antibiotic available for curing gonorrhea, penicillin. Throughout the urban, industrial areas of the world, gonococci have adapted to antibiotic usage so that relative resistance to several antibiotics has developed. It is imperative that the obstetrician keep up to date with the changing patterns of infection and antibiotic susceptibility in the environs of his or her practice.

For obstetrical practice only a small antibiotic armamentarium is needed to treat gonorrhea: penicillin or ampicillin for the majority of patients, spectinomycin for the penicillin-allergic patient and those with PPNG infections, and some of the cephalosporin and aminoglycoside antibiotics for unusual circumstances. Except for rare allergic reactions, none of these drugs, in the doses used, has been shown to have adverse effects upon the fetus or the mother.

Treatment regimens are given in Table 15–6. A management protocol for the pregnant woman with gonococcal disease is presented in Figure 15–4.

Acute uncomplicated gonorrhea is one of the few infectious diseases that is treated with a single large dose of antimicrobial drug. Single dose treatment is not always successful because of antimicrobial resistance and because the infection may be located at sites other than urogenital mucosal surfaces. In order to reduce the failure rate and to prevent the emergence of increasing penicillin resistance, the treatment of uncomplicated or asymptomatic gonorrhea should consist of 4.8 million units of aqueous procaine penicillin G, given intramuscularly one-half hour after 1 gm of probenicid has been given orally. This regimen has proved eminently successful and is the

TABLE 15–6 TREATMENT OF UNCOMPLICATED UROGENITAL, RECTAL, OR OROPHARYNGEAL GONOCOCCAL INFECTION DURING PREGNANCY

Parenteral, single-session therapy
  Procaine penicillin G, 4.8 million units intramuscularly, after probenecid, 1 gm, is given orally
  Alternative treatment for patients allergic to penicillin or probenecid:
  Spectinomycin, 2 gm intramuscularly; not effective in oropharyngeal infection
  Parenteral cephalosporin or aminoglycoside
  Alternative treatment for patients not responding to penicillin or proved to have penicillinase-producing gonococci:
  Spectinomycin, 2 gm intramuscularly
Oral, single-dose therapy
  Ampicillin, 3.5 gm, and probenecid, 1 gm, administered simultaneously

standard by which other treatment regimens are presently compared.[154]

Treatment with 4.8 million units of aqueous procaine penicillin G given in a single session prevents the development of syphilis in patients with no clinical or serologic evidence of syphilis despite exposure to infectious syphilis within the previous 30 days.[148] In patients given a placebo injection, 30 per cent developed syphilis. Only penicillin has been proved to be effective in interrupting the course of early, clinically or serologically undetectable syphilis during treatment for gonorrhea.[84, 148] Presumably, this treatment adequately prevents congenital syphilis in

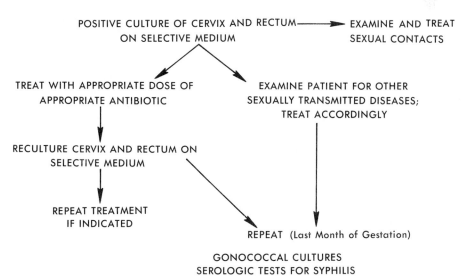

POSITIVE CULTURE OF CERVIX AND RECTUM ————▶ EXAMINE AND TREAT
ON SELECTIVE MEDIUM   SEXUAL CONTACTS

TREAT WITH APPROPRIATE DOSE OF   EXAMINE PATIENT FOR OTHER
APPROPRIATE ANTIBIOTIC   SEXUALLY TRANSMITTED DISEASES;
                                        TREAT ACCORDINGLY

RECULTURE CERVIX AND RECTUM ON
SELECTIVE MEDIUM

REPEAT TREATMENT
IF INDICATED   REPEAT (Last Month of Gestation)

GONOCOCCAL CULTURES
SEROLOGIC TESTS FOR SYPHILIS
OTHER INDICATED DIAGNOSTIC TESTS

FIGURE 15–4. Steps in the management of gonorrhea in pregnant females.

the fetus, but there are no reliable data to confirm this assumption. Following treatment for gonorrhea, therefore, the obstetrician should perform maternal serologic tests regularly throughout the pregnancy.

Considerable heat, but little light, can be generated in discussions of the best treatment for uncomplicated gonorrhea. Some physicians stress the inconvenience, pain, and risk of anaphylactic shock of treatment with parenteral penicillin. Others stress the poor compliance with a multidose oral regimen and the prevalence of pill-sharing among sexual consorts, which may predispose to the emergence of resistant strains and which usually results in inadequate therapy for the individual patient. A careful 20 year study by the Center for Disease Control showed no increase in allergic reactions among 95,000 patients treated with penicillin in venereal disease clinics.[142] This study found an adverse reaction in only 0.4 per cent and fatal anaphylaxis in 1 to 2 per 100,000 patients given parenteral penicillin. An additional point in favor of parenteral penicillin is its efficacy in curing incubating syphilis. On the basis of these facts and personal experience, this writer prefers using parenteral penicillin, particularly in pregnant patients when adequate treatment is essential for the health of both mother and fetus. If the patient has a history of adverse reaction to penicillin, spectinomycin is used. A careful history, clinical judgment, and immediate access to life-support equipment and epinephrine are mandatory accessories to using parenteral penicillin therapy for gonococcal infection. Single dose oral ampicillin-probenecid therapy has its advocates and is an acceptable alternative treatment. Physicians should use no less than the recommended doses of penicillin and ampicillin for gonorrhea.

Treatment of disseminated gonococcal disease usually requires hospitalization. When clinical evidence suggests gonococcemia, most experts use large doses of intravenous penicillin; 10 million units per day for 7 to 10 days has been the standard dosage. The success of a three day course of penicillin of 10 million units per day has been reported in 28 cases of gonococcal arthritis-dermatitis syndrome.[12] This study supports the hypothesis that in the absence of closed space infection, endocarditis, or meningitis, shorter courses of high-dose penicillin may be satisfactory in the treatment of disseminated gonococcal disease.

In all cases, treatment results must be evaluated by repeat cultures, not only of all initially infected sites but also of other sites of potential asymptomatic persistence. In most cases of un-complicated genital infection, culture of the endocervix and rectum 4 to 7 days after therapy is a reliable test for cure. Post-treatment blood cultures, examination of skin and joints, and routine careful cardiac auscultation are required in patients treated for bacteremic gonococcal infection.

Prevention and Control. Little can be done immediately to control the present epidemic of gonorrhea. The disease has a short incubation period and a high degree of transmissibility and elicits little lasting or solid immunity. The organism has shown itself adept at adapting to the antibiotic milieu. In order for an epidemic to be interrupted, infected and exposed patients must be treated with sufficient antimicrobial drugs to eradicate the organism before they can transmit the infection to others, a task that is virtually impossible in view of the vast reservoir of asymptomatic carriers. Control of gonorrhea has not been made any easier by changing sexual and social customs, armed conflicts abroad, and the remarkable increase in travel during the twentieth century. Prospects for a gonococcal vaccine do not, at the present time, encourage optimism.

Syphilis

Inoculation of *Treponema pallidum,* usually as a result of sexual contact, is followed by multiplication of spirochetes at and near the site of inoculation. Rapid invasion of lymphatics and blood vessels enables spirochetes to reach regional lymph nodes and become hematogenously disseminated to all organs of the body even before a primary lesion appears.[173] Thus, blood from the patient with incubating syphilis is infectious. The concentration of treponemes usually reaches 10^7 per gm of tissue at the site of inoculation before the appearance of a clinical lesion. At this point the local inflammatory response to the spirochetes has produced an obliterative endarteritis and periarteritis and characteristic induration. The typical primary chancre begins as an indurated, painless papule. As its blood supply becomes compromised by the inflammation and occlusion of small vessels, the lesion is eroded and develops into the classical, clean, well-demarcated ulcer with "cartilaginous" induration of the base and circumference.

Serology. Infection with treponemes elicits two types of antibodies[112a, 114a, 114b] (Fig. 15–5):

1. Antibodies to nontreponemal, lipoidal antigens.

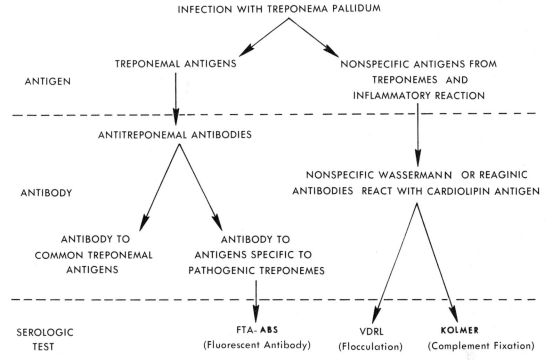

INFECTION WITH TREPONEMA PALLIDUM

FIGURE 15–5. Antigens, antibodies, and commonly used serologic tests in syphilis.

2. Antibodies to a variety of specific treponemal antigens

Antibodies to nontreponemal lipoidal antigens (cardiolipin) are the so-called Wassermann or reaginic antibodies. They should not be confused with allergy-related reagins, which are unrelated antibodies of the IgE class. Serologic tests for antibody against cardiolipin antigens were thought to be specific for syphilis, but wide application of these tests demonstrated reactivity in other diseases. There is no evidence that Wassermann antibodies confer immunity against infection by *T. pallidum*.

All treponemal infections evoke Wassermann antibodies. The quantity of Wassermann antibodies is directly proportional to the degree of inflammatory response produced by the treponemal infection. As the number of spirochetes and the inflammatory response increase, the titer of Wassermann antibody increases; as they decline, the titer of Wassermann antibody falls. Quantitative measurement of nontreponemal antibodies is, therefore, important both in diagnosis and in evaluating response to treatment. The quantity of Wassermann antibody declines during the latent and late stages of untreated disease. About one third of untreated patients with latent and late syphilis have negative tests for Wassermann antibodies, and many of the other two thirds have low titers of antibody. For

example, in a patient with untreated syphilis, the titer might be 1:8 when the primary lesion is present and could rise to 1:128 during florid secondary syphilis and decline gradually over the next several years to 1:2 or 1:4. The appearance of a gumma might be accompanied by a rise in titer to 1:16 or 1:32.

The incubation period is inversely proportional to the size of the inoculum and ranges from 10 to 90 days with a median of 21 days. Spirochetes are demonstrable intracellularly and extracellularly in the chancre and regional lymph nodes by electron or darkfield microscopy, special silver stains, or inoculation of material from the chancre or buboes into animals. The chancre heals spontaneously, usually within 4 to 6 weeks, with a range of 2 to 12 weeks. Intracellular spirochetes may persist for some time after the lesion heals.[81, 120, 162, 163]

The development of antibody and a cellular immune response begins to be measurable about 3 to 6 weeks following inoculation. It is not uncommon, therefore, for the serologic test of a patient with a chancre to be negative for syphilis. Although the immune response is not consistently present at the time the primary lesion develops, it is always well developed by the time the chancre has healed.

The manifestations of generalized or secondary syphilis begin about 6 to 12 weeks following inoculation, with a range of 4 weeks to 6 months. The time course is influenced by the size of the original inoculum, the quantity of organisms in the spirochetemia that seeded the disseminated lesions, and the developing immune response in the host. The secondary rash may appear while the primary lesion is still present or several months later. The mucocutaneous lesions of secondary syphilis are histologically similar to, but clinically different from, primary lesions. Ulceration is remarkably rare; the individual lesions tend to be smaller and have less induration. The spirochetes obtained from the lesions are structurally indistinguishable from those of primary lesions and are equally infective to other human beings and to experimental animals. The differences between primary and secondary lesions are therefore believed to be due to increased host resistance. A host response, as measured by serologic tests for antibodies and tests for lymphocyte transformation evoked by treponemal antigens, is universally present during the secondary manifestations of the disease. The secondary lesions remit over 2 to 6 weeks. About one fourth of untreated patients will experience one or more recurrences of secondary lesions at some time during the first 2 years of infection.[24] The blood remains infectious during this time because of repeated episodes of spirochetemia, which presumably are the source of recurrent crops of skin lesions. The characteristic features of this stage of the disease are the constant presence of large numbers of spirochetes and high levels of antibody.[30, 114, 121a, 153, 173]

Resolution of secondary lesions is also probably due to changes in host response. The repetitive secondary skin lesions tend to be smaller, fewer in number, and of shorter duration than the initial crop of secondary lesions. Once the lesions have healed, the patient has achieved a "balance of power" with the treponeme and is asymptomatic. In this so-called latent stage, the disease is undetectable. During this stage, the spirochete population is dramatically reduced, and about two thirds of untreated patients live the rest of their lives without further inconvenience and frequently with no pathologic manifestations of the persisting spirochetal infections.[24, 114, 121a] The remaining third develop clinically apparent late syphilitic lesions after a latent stage of 3 to 20 years.[24]

The manifestations of late syphilis are of two major types.[69, 113] The first and most common is the gumma. The second is obliterative endarteritis of small vessels, which produces a granulomatous degeneration of the media of large arteries, the prime target being the vasa vasorum of the aorta, and a perivascular granulomatous re-

sponse in the parenchyma and meninges of the central nervous system. Although few spirochetes are present in late syphilis, the untreated patient may still have spirochetemia, which is invariably unrecognized except when a pregnant woman infects her fetus.

Syphilis and Pregnancy. Pregnancy in a syphilitic woman or pregnancy complicated by the acquisition of syphilis may have one of the following outcomes: (1) a late abortion at any time after the fourth month of pregnancy, (2) a stillborn infant at term, (3) a congenitally infected infant born prematurely or at term, or (4) an uninfected live infant.

In 1972, the number of cases of congenital syphilis in the United States rose to 422.[95] Proper antenatal care and treatment could have prevented virtually all these cases.[16] The prevalence of congenital syphilis reflects not only the rising incidence of infectious syphilis among parents but also problems with the adequacy of antenatal care. The relative benignity of maternal syphilitic infection is to be contrasted with the potentially disastrous effect of syphilitic infection on the pregnancy and the fetus. This is no place for complacency.

There is some evidence to indicate that pregnancy exerts a suppressive effect upon the clinical manifestations of early syphilis in human beings and in experimental infections in rabbits. The woman who contracts syphilis during pregnancy may have few if any signs of infection except for a positive serologic test. Similarly, the untreated syphilitic woman who becomes pregnant commonly has few signs or symptoms of the disease unless late syphilitic lesions are present. However, the effect of pregnancy upon the clinical lesions is not uniform, and there is no solid evidence that pregnancy alters the natural progression of untreated spirochetal infection. It is important for the clinician to recognize that active syphilitic infection may be exceptionally difficult to detect clinically in the pregnant female and that liberal use of serologic tests is indicated.

Infection of the fetus requires maternal spirochetemia.[28, 61] The stage of maternal infection is of importance in assessing the risk to the fetus. If the mother is suffering from primary or secondary syphilis, with the attendant intense continuous spirochetemia, there is probably no chance that the infant will be uninfected and born healthy unless treatment is given. If, however, the mother has early latent syphilis with episodic spirochetemia, there is about an 80 per cent chance of fetal infection.[74a] As the maternal disease progresses the gradual reduction in the frequency and intensity of spirochetal blood stream dissemination accounts for the reduction in risk to the fetus. This explains the old clinical observation that the longer the duration of untreated syphilis in the mother, the less likely it is that the fetus will die in utero and the more likely that a live, congenitally infected infant will be born or that the fetus will be uninfected ("Kassowitz's law").

Third-generation syphilis resulting from a congenitally syphilitic woman transmitting the infection to her offspring is extremely rare.

Syphilis in the pregnant woman is diagnosed in the same way as syphilis in other individuals.[68] The major difference in the clinical approach to syphilis in pregnancy is the urgency in establishing the diagnosis and beginning treatment in order to protect the fetus. Two sound and eminently practical clinical rules have been established.[38] First, any genital lesion should be suspected of being syphilis until time and repeated examination prove otherwise. Second, if an indolent, painless lesion fails to heal within 2 weeks, regardless of location but particularly if the erotic area of the body surface is involved, syphilis should be suspected.

Any genital lesion or suggestive extragenital lesion should be evaluated by examination of appropriate material by darkfield microscopy and serial serologic tests over a 6 to 8 week period. The importance of a darkfield examination and repeated serologic tests during pregnancy is illustrated by several case reports of unsuspected congenitally infected infants.[4, 179] In a case of infant death from congenital syphilis at the Yale–New Haven Hospital the mother had had a normal antenatal examination including negative STS at 16 weeks.[82] She developed vulvar lesions believed to be herpes genitalis at 26 weeks of gestation but did not have darkfield microscopic or serologic examinations. At 35 weeks she was delivered of a severely depressed female infant, who died after a day and a half. Serologic tests for syphilis were strongly positive in both the mother and the child. Postmortem examination of the child revealed histologic changes consistent with severe neonatal syphilis.

It is foolhardy to disregard a positive serologic test for syphilis in a pregnant woman, regardless of the history and physical findings. Figure 15–6 outlines the management protocol for the pregnant patient with a positive serologic test (STS) for syphilis. There is some suggestion that preg-

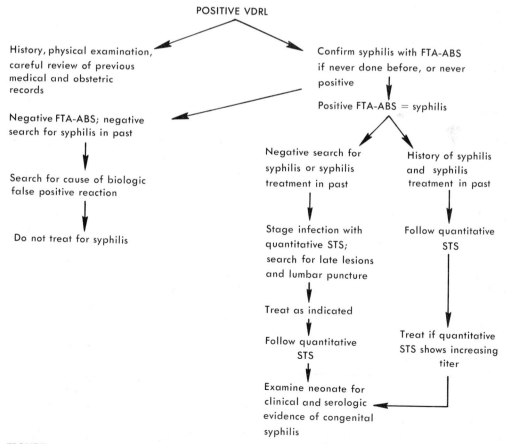

FIGURE 15–6. Steps in the management of a pregnant patient with a positive serologic test for syphilis.

nancy itself may produce biologic false positive (BFP) nontreponemal and treponemal tests; however, there is equally convincing evidence that the incidence of such results in pregnant women is no different from that in nonpregnant women. Regardless, a positive nontreponemal test should be followed up with an FTA-ABS test. If the treponemal test is positive, it is wisest to regard it as evidence of syphilis and to begin treatment. A diminution in the titer of nontreponemal antibody provides some confirmation for the diagnosis.

If the treponemal antibody test is borderline or nonreactive, the patient's condition should be evaluated with appropriate tests for conditions causing BFP tests for syphilis (including antinuclear factor, protein immunoelectrophoresis, heterophil antibodies, and viral and chlamydial serologic tests). Repeated quantitative STSs during the pregnancy are helpful; a rising titer suggests active syphilitic infection that must be rechecked with the FTA-ABS test and treated accordingly. Because the risk of acquiring syphilis during the 9 months of gestation is not insignificant, it is our policy to repeat the maternal STS just before term or at delivery.

It is not uncommon for a woman who seeks prenatal care to have had syphilis diagnosed and treated in the past. A careful review of the history and physical examination must be supplemented by documentation of the patient's diagnosis, estimated stage of syphilis at the time of treatment, the treatment given, and the patient's clinical and serologic response to treatment. The quantitative nontreponemal STS should be rechecked on the initial antenatal visit, at least once during the pregnancy (preferably more often), and at delivery. A two-tube dilution rise in titer on any test or a gradual, progressive rise in titer on several tests is indicative of reinfection or persisting, active infection and demands treatment. The FTA-ABS or other treponemal antibody tests are of little use, since they remain positive following the initial syphilitic infection. As a general rule, a pregnant patient with adequately treated syphilis in the past and a nonreactive or weakly reactive nontreponemal STS does not automatically need to be treated. If there is any question about the adequacy of treatment or if several years have passed since the last serologic test, raising the possibility of reinfection that has achieved latency with a low titer STS, it is safest to be cautious and to repeat treatment (Table 15–7).

Although five states do not require premarital STS and eight do not require prenatal STS, exclusion or neglect of these examinations in

TABLE 15–7 INDICATIONS FOR TREATMENT OF SYPHILIS IN THE PREGNANT WOMAN

Active, untreated syphilis at any stage
Previously treated patient
    Treatment judged to be inadequate by history, e.g., uncooperative patient with early syphilis
    Treatment judged to be inadequate because of unsatisfactory pattern of serologic response
    Presumed reinfection or inadequate treatment because of rising titer of nontreponemal antibody
    Previous delivery of congenitally syphilitic infant despite presumed adequate treatment

enlightened obstetric practice is to be condemned. Indeed, failure to perform a prenatal STS at some point during pregnancy should be considered a legally pursuable act of omission.

Congenital Syphilis. In congenital syphilis there is no stage analogous to the primary stage in acquired infection. Once treponemes have entered the fetal circulation, dissemination to all tissues follows immediately. The rarity of histologic evidence for syphilis in aborted fetuses of less than 16 to 20 weeks' gestational age remains unexplained. Spirochetes are infrequently found in fetal tissues prior to 18 weeks of intrauterine life, but when they are present there is little or no reaction to their presence. It is possible that the layer of cylindric Langhans' cells of the developing placenta acts as a physical barrier to spirochetal penetration. However, the inability of the fetus to generate a mononuclear cell inflammatory response eliminates the only measurable manifestation of spirochetal infection.

Experience with multiple births indicates that the effect of maternal spirochetemia and the development of congenital infection is not uniform. Both neonates of an identical twin pair, sharing the same placenta, are invariable infected, whereas with dizygotic twins, with separate placentas, only one may be infected. The same circumstance has been found in one set of triplets in which two apparently identical siblings were infected and the remaining nonidentical sibling was free of disease. A subsequent pregnancy in the same mother produced a set of fraternal twins, one being infected and the other not infected.

The most severe fetal disease is the result of the intense spirochetemia of early syphilis in the mother. In this instance, if the fetus is infected by large quantities of treponemes early in pregnancy it may be overwhelmed by the infection and die, resulting in abortion. If spirochetemia occurs later in pregnancy, the child may be stillborn or may die in the neonatal period with severe congenital syphilis. If intrauterine spirochetemia is not severe or occurs very late in pregnancy, the child may be born without any evidence, other than serologic, of congenital syphilitic infection or with relatively unpretentious signs of infection. In this instance the clinical signs of early congenital syphilis are seldom recognized at birth but usually manifest themselves 2 to 4 weeks after delivery. Occasionally the disease does not become apparent until several months have passed. It is also possible for the fetus to be infected by inoculation from contact with an infectious early syphilitic lesion during passage down an infected birth canal. The resulting disease process, however, more closely resembles that of sexually acquired syphilis, with the development of one or several primary lesions along the line of contact as the earliest manifestation.

Syphilis in the neonate may be clinically indistinguishable from other conditions, especially other congenital infections.[64] It presents as a systemic disease marked by hepatosplenomegaly, hyperbilirubinemia, evidence of hemolysis, and generalized lymphadenopathy. The characteristic cutaneous lesions may not be present initially, and the hematologic, serologic, and radiologic signs may be misinterpreted or missed. Congenital syphilis must be differentiated from erythroblastosis fetalis and from congenital infections with toxoplasma, rubella, and cytomegalovirus. The concept that the placenta contains pathognomonic gross and microscopic findings for congenital syphilis is no longer accepted.

The clinical manifestations of congenital syphilis are arbitrarily divided into three categories. Early lesions occur during the first two years of life and, like the early lesions of acquired syphilis, are infectious, teeming with spirochetes, and occasionally recurrent. Late congenital lesions begin during the third year of life or later. Some are similar to those of late acquired syphilis, such as gummas and neurosyphilis, while some are characteristic of congenital infection, such as interstitial keratitis and nerve deafness. The "stigmata" of congenital syphilis are residual scars and deformities that are no longer active; no spirochetes are present and the local cellular immune response has apparently been spent.

The diagnosis of early congenital syphilis is usually not difficult when clinical lesions are apparent. The appearance of the clinical lesions and the observation of spirochetes by darkfield microscopy establish the diagnosis. The history and serologic tests of the mother also indicate the appropriate background of the child's infection. Serologic testing of the fetus is confusing because maternal IgG, but not IgM, crosses the placenta and causes a positive reaction with nontreponemal and treponemal antibody tests of both cord and fetal blood. However, the intrauterine fetal antibody response is almost exclusively IgM. A fetus infected in utero will therefore be born with endogenous IgM antibodies and maternal IgG antibodies, whereas a noninfected fetus of a mother with a positive serologic test for syphilis will have only maternal IgG antibodies.

Antibiotic Treatment of Syphilis. The goal of antibiotic treatment is to eradicate the spirochetes by producing a sufficient level of antibiotics for a sufficient length of time.[29a, 30, 38, 114, 153] *Treponema pallidum* is exquisitely sensitive to antibiotics, especially penicillin. Prolonged exposure to antimicrobials is required because of the unusually slow rate of multiplication of the organism. Antibiotic treatment for gonococcal disease is not adequate for coexisting syphilitic infection except in the case of high dose penicillin therapy for the gonorrhea patient with incubating syphilis. Treatment of syphilis in pregnancy requires an effective antisyphilitic antibiotic that crosses the placenta in sufficient quantities to produce treponemicidal blood levels in the fetus and that does not jeopardize the pregnancy or the fetus.

The current recommendations for treatment and management are outlined in Tables 15–8 and 15–9.

A pregnant woman with sexual exposure to active, early syphilis should automatically be treated with 2.4 million units of benzathine penicillin G, even when there is no evidence of maternal spirochetal infection. Such a patient should be followed up with monthly serologic tests.

The management of latent and late syphilis differs from that of primary and secondary syphilis in that lumbar puncture is essential to detect asymptomatic or symptomatic neurosyphilis. If the cerebrospinal fluid of a patient with latent syphilis is not examined, treatment should be adequate for possible neurosyphilis. It has been claimed by some authors that lumbar puncture has a definite abortifacient effect and that it should not be performed during pregnancy. This view is not widely accepted, and it has been this writer's experience that lumbar puncture can be performed without undue risk to the pregnancy. It is extremely important to the future health and medical management of the mother found to

TABLE 15–8   RECOMMENDED TREATMENT OF SYPHILIS DURING PREGNANCY

	Benzathine Penicillin G (Bicillin) (Parenteral)	Aqueous Procaine Penicillin G (Parenteral)	Cephaloridine (Parenteral)	Erythromycin (Oral)
Acquired syphilis, early stages: primary, second-ary, and early latent	2.4 million units at 2-week intervals; total dose, 4.8 million units	600,000 units per day for 8 days; total dose, 4.8 million units	0.5 to 1.0 gm per day for 10 days	2 to 3 gm per day for 10 to 15 days; total dose, 30 gm
Acquired syphilis, late stages: late latent, gumma, cardiovascular, and neurosyphilis	2.4 million units at 1-week intervals; total dose, 6 to 20 million units	600,000 to 2 million units per day for 10 to 15 days; total dose, 6 to 20 million units	Unknown	Total dose, 80 gm (?)
Congenital syphilis, early stage	50,000 units per kg of body weight; single dose	10,000 units per kg of body weight per day for 10 days; total dose, 100,000 units	25 to 50 mg per kg of body weight per day for 10 days	Total dose, 400 mg per kg for 10 days will most likely be effective
Congenital syphilis, late stage	2.4 million units at 1-week intervals for 4 weeks; total dose, 6 to 9 million units	600,000 to 2 million units per day for 10 to 15 days; total dose, 6 to 20 million units	Unknown	2 to 3 gm per day for 15 to 20 days; total dose, 40 gm

TABLE 15–9 MANAGEMENT OF SYPHILIS

Type of Syphilis	Means of Diagnosis	Treatment	Followup
Primary and secondary	Darkfield microscopy; serologic tests for syphilis	Benzathine penicillin G or procaine penicillin, 4.8 million units	Serologic testing after treatment at 1 month, 3 months, 6 months, and 12 months
Latent	Serologic tests for syphilis; lumbar puncture to exclude asymptomatic neurosyphilis	If lumbar puncture is negative, treat as primary and secondary syphilis; if lumbar puncture is not performed or is positive for asymptomatic neurosyphilis, treatment consists of 6 to 20 million units penicillin	Same as for primary and secondary syphilis plus serologic testing every 6 months for 1 or 2 years, then once per year; if CSF is positive, repeat lumbar puncture every 3 to 6 months until cell count and protein have returned to normal
Late	Serologic tests for syphilis; lumbar puncture; biopsy; look for specific organ involvement	9 to 20 million units penicillin	Same as for latent syphilis
During pregnancy	Same as above, depending upon stage	Same as above, depending upon stage	Same as above, depending upon stage
Congenital	Same as above, depending upon stage	Same as above, depending upon stage; adjust drug dosage to weight or age	Same as above, depending upon stage

have latent syphilis during pregnancy that the status of her disease be fully evaluated in order to determine proper treatment.[68]

Good management includes repetitive quantitative measurement of nontreponemal antibodies to assess the adequacy of treatment. Because *T. pallidum* cannot be cultured in vitro, there is no clinically reliable tool for judging the efficacy of therapy other than quantitative serologic tests. Because of the difficulty in establishing the adequacy of treatment of individual patients, it is recommended that the doses of antibiotics and their routes of administration recommended here or by the United States Public Health Service be strictly adhered to and that careful followup of the patient, report of the case to the appropriate epidemiologic control center, and treatment of contacts become a standard, indeed inviolable, procedure.

ANTIBIOTICS. Penicillin remains the drug of choice. It crosses the placenta with ease. The maintenance of a penicillin blood level ranging between 0.03 and 0.2 units per ml over a period of ten days is adequate treatment for most cases of early syphilitic infection. The United States Public Health Service recommends a dose of 2.4 million units of benzathine penicillin G. There is some evidence that higher doses produce more rapid seroreversal and a higher percentage of patients who eventually become seronegative. One group has recommended a total of 6 million units of benzathine penicillin G in three doses given three to five days apart.[32] Our experience with a treatment schedule of three doses of 2.4 million units of benzathine penicillin G two weeks apart has also been satisfactory. Alternatively, the patient can be treated with 600,000 units of procaine penicillin G daily for eight to ten days. All these treatment schedules produce 95 per cent cure rates or better. Oral penicillin is not recommended for treatment.

Higher blood levels of penicillin and longer or repeated courses of therapy are necessary in late syphilis. There is sparse but distressing evidence that pathogenic treponemes may persist in the tissues of late syphilitics despite high doses of penicillin. Because of this, some authors recommend as much as 20 million units of penicillin as a total dose for late syphilis and neurosyphilis.[63]

A history of allergy to penicillin must be searched for routinely. In patients with no history of allergic reactions to penicillin, it is remarkably safe in treating syphilis. Clinical caution and epinephrine at hand are essential to proper use of the drug.

Erythromycin has been used in treatment of early syphilis with a total dose of about 30 to 40 gm. Cephaloradine, 0.5 to 1 gm intramuscularly daily for ten days, has been shown to be effective in treating early syphilis during pregnancy. There is a small risk of allergic crossover between penicillin and the cephalosporin antibiotics.

TREATMENT FAILURE. Treatment of pregnant women with all of these recommended agents has failed with distressing frequency to eradicate fetal infection in utero. Erythromycin achieves fetal plasma levels of only 6 to 20 per cent of the maternal plasma levels, and poor placental transfer of the drug is the presumed cause of treatment failure.[61] Cephaloridine, previously recommended as alternative therapy for the penicillin-allergic patient, achieves levels in cord and fetal blood of about 60 per cent of maternal blood levels.[61, 159] However, several treatment failures during pregnancy have been reported despite adequate dosage.[170] There are cases of failure of penicillin therapy in arresting congenital treponemal infection in utero and post partum.[55] Biochemical resistance of *T. pallidum* to penicillin or to cephalosporins has not been demonstrated, and the cause of these treatment failures is unknown.

Obstetricians must alert their pediatrician colleagues to the possibility of active congenital syphilis. There is never a reason to withhold repeat antisyphilitic therapy for the mother who has an unsatisfactory serologic or clinical response to initial therapy.

FUNGAL INFECTIONS

Monilial vulvovaginitis is usually a benign but bothersome disease. The most common cause is *Candida albicans,* although *Torulopsis glabrata* has been found in several studies of symptomatic and asymptomatic women. These yeastlike fungi have a wide distribution in the external and internal environment. They can be isolated from the lower genital tract of approximately one third of women of childbearing age[165] and can be found in the oral cavity and lower gastrointestinal tract as part of the normal flora in many more. They are infrequently found in prepubertal and postmenopausal women. Only about half of women, pregnant or not pregnant, with a positive vaginal culture or smear for monilia have symptomatic vulvovaginitis.[124, 171]

The pathology of infection by yeasts is not clearly defined. Exogenous estrogens, pregnancy, and diabetes mellitus are associated with the most severe and persistent monilial infections. The growth of *C. albicans* in vitro is enhanced by estrogens.[137] Clinical information suggests that the estrogen-induced increase in glycogen content of vaginal epithelium favors the growth of yeastlike organisms. Other predisposing factors to symptomatic monilial vulvovaginitis include an impaired host response, corticosteroid treatment, broad spectrum antibiotic treatment, and obesity. Since deep tissue invasion rarely occurs, it is assumed that the severe inflammation of the vulva and vaginal mucosa is caused, in part, by as yet undefined toxic products of yeast metabolism. Because these organisms are frequently asymptomatic commensals, it is not clear whether clinical disease represents sexual transmission or sexual activation of infection. The severity of monilial vulvovaginitis is also influenced by the coexistent flora. The most severe cases of vaginitis involve multiple agents, as with simultaneous infection with *C. albicans* and *T. vaginalis*.

The afflicted patient is often extremely uncomfortable because of intense pruritus, which may be accompanied by dysuria and dyspareunia. On examination, the vulva is erythematous, occasionally edematous, and frequently excoriated. Speculum examination may be impossible because of pain and introital edema. The vagina appears beefy red with scattered white plaques and has a curdlike white discharge. Examination of material from the discharge or exudate reveals pseudomycelial and budding yeast forms, easily detected and differentiated from other microbes by size and configuration. Gram-stained preparations are better than unstained material for rapid diagnosis of yeast infections. Culture is easily accomplished in the office by use of prepackaged Nickerson's medium on which *Candida* species grows dark brown or black colonies within 48 hours of incubation at room temperature. A search for trichomonads and other sexually transmitted pathogens is essential because simultaneous infection is common and requires combined therapy.

Effective treatment includes the search for and management of concurrent infections, infection in the sexual consort, and diabetes mellitus. A variety of topical antifungal agents are available: nystatin, candicydin, amphotericin B, and co-trimoxazole. The effectiveness of topical applications of 1 per cent gentian violet solutions is often ignored because of the associated mess. The use of polypharmaceutical creams containing antifungal agents, antibiotics, and corticosteroids is not recommended, especially during pregnancy.

Successful eradication of yeasts from the vagina during pregnancy is often difficult and occasionally impossible. The usual 10 to 15 day treatment with nystatin vaginal tablets, 100,000 units each, twice a day may be insufficient. Longer initial treatments lasting up to 3 or 4 weeks and continuous therapy during the latter part of the third trimester may be necessary. Simultaneous treatment of the husband and a condom or sexual abstinence are imperative to prevent reinfection. If pruritus ani is a complaint, anorectal infection is probably present, and oral nystatin, 100,000 units four times a day, should be included in the treatment regimen. Monilial vulvovaginitis in the absence of any other infecting agent does not appear to destroy the highly acidic vaginal secretions produced by the normal gram-positive bacterial flora. The likelihood of ascending infection during labor, delivery, and the puerperium in the presence of *Candida* infection alone is probably less than with other sexually transmitted infection.

SEXUALLY TRANSMITTED PARASITES

The importance of parasitic diseases during pregnancy has become better appreciated in the United States with the influx of refugee immigrants from tropical areas over the past decade.[97] Parasites having life cycles without intermediate hosts, and therefore compatible with worldwide prevalence, may be sexually transmitted. Anorectal intercourse and oroanal or orogenital sexual activity allows the transmission of *Entameba histolytica*, *Giardia lamblia*, *Enterobius vermicularis*, *Trichuris trichura*, and *Strongyloides stercoralis*. Three parasites, *Trichomonas vaginalis*, *Phthyris pubis*, and *Sarcoptes scabiei*, are spread regularly and primarily by sexual practices.

Trichomonas Vaginalis

The protozoan *Trichomonas vaginalis* is a common cause of genitourinary infection. Because infection is commonly asymptomatic in both sexes, the true incidence of the disease is unknown. The parasite is said to be present in 10 to 25 per cent of women of childbearing age and in 12 to 15 per cent of all men presenting with urethritis.[20] It is transmitted almost exclusively by sexual intercourse, but the rare finding of trichomonads in infants and abstinent women suggests that nonvenereal infection may occur. In one study, all of the female sexual consorts of 56 men with trichomonal urethritis harbored trichomonads.[21] The infection is common in prostitutes and the sexually promiscuous. It is frequently associated with other venereal infections. As many as 50 per cent of women with gonorrhea also have trichomonal vaginitis. *T. vaginalis* infection is also frequently associated with chlamydial and monilial infections.

Clinical and experimental evidence indicates that the incubation period is 4 to 28 days. However, many women are symptomless or ignore the minor symptoms produced. The parasite can infect the vagina, urethra, bladder, and Skene's and Bartholin's glands. When symptoms occur, the patient may complain of malodorous discharge, perineal discomfort, dyspareunia, and dysuria. The symptoms may resemble recurrent attacks of urinary tract infection. There is some evidence that growth of the parasite is enhanced in vitro by estrogens;[157] this may explain the recurrence of symptoms and tenacity of infection during pregnancy and estrogen administration. In the severely symptomatic woman, examination reveals a seropurulent, bubbly, greenish discharge, erythema, and edema of the vulva, sometimes with perineal excoriations and tender inguinal nodes. The vagina and cervix may be friable and inflamed and often have a characteristic speckling with small punctate hemorrhages. Occasionally, introital inflammation is severe enough to preclude speculum examination. Most commonly, however, there are few signs of infection except for a modest amount of greenish or mucoid discharge.

Careful laboratory examination is necessary for diagnosis, as there is no clinical way to distinguish between the various other genital infections. The simplest and fastest diagnostic aid — microscopic examination of a wet preparation — is eminently reliable. *T. vaginalis* is larger than a polymorphonuclear leukocyte and is readily recognized by its motility and the lashing movements of the flagella. Culture on appropriate media is also reliable and effective, but because of expense and time it is a less desirable diagnostic technique for the practitioner.[96] Because *T. vaginalis* infection is commonly a portent of concomitant venereal disease, cultures for chlamydia and gonorrhea, and serologic testing for syphilis should be obtained.

Infection and colonization with *T. vaginalis* are usually accompanied by a Grade III vaginal flora. There is conflicting evidence on the association of *T. vaginalis* with puerperal fever and neonatal infection. Unfortunately, most studies of this relationship are not recent and do not exclude multiple infections of the same patient. There is little evidence that *T. vaginalis* is an invasive organism or that it produces amnionitis or endometritis. *T. vaginalis* is so often associated with other infections that produce puerperal or neonatal infection that the clinician cannot disregard its presence in the pregnant woman.

In men, *T. vaginalis* can be found in the urethra and prostatic secretions, urine, and semen. Though most men are asymptomatic carriers, some may have a small amount of morning discharge or occasional dysuria, while others have a more profuse purulent urethral discharge. It is imperative, therefore, that the sexual partner of the pregnant woman be examined and treated simultaneously in order to prevent the infection.[39]

The introduction of metronidazole and its congeners immensely simplified treatment of trichomoniasis.[180] A decade and a half later, metronidazole was found to have potential mutagenic and carcinogenic activity in experimental conditions. Several small series have shown metronidazole to have no adverse effects upon the fetus or the pregnancy;[46, 138, 139] nevertheless, considerable anxiety presently surrounds the use of this compound during pregnancy. Fortunately, the use of a single 2 gram dose of metronidazole has been successful in about 90 per cent of cases.[39, 140, 183] Longer courses of therapy, necessary for the treatment of other protozoan diseases, are no better than single dose therapy for trichomonal vulvovaginitis. The best recommendation for using metronidazole to date is this: "It would be prudent to use metronidazole as seldom as possible and then in the lowest effective dosage for the shortest possible time."[100]

Single dose metronidazole therapy may be indicated as a reasonable choice for treatment of acute, severe trichomonal infection after the first trimester of pregnancy. It should not be used in longer courses of therapy for trichomoniasis, giardiasis, or amebiasis in the pregnant woman. During pregnancy, metronidazole should not be used for asymptomatic or minimally symptomatic infection. Treatment with less potentially hazardous drugs for coexistent sexually transmitted infections should precede the use of metronidazole in the pregnant woman. Often, the eradication of other sexually transmitted pathogens and the re-establishment of a resident bacterial flora more closely resembling the normal flora can reduce the clinical severity of vulvovaginitis. Metronidazole is well tolerated, although it may cause occasional gastrointestinal disturbances, and it has a mild disulfiram (antabuse) effect. Alcohol ingestion at the time of single dose treatment may produce unpleasant symptoms, and both patient and sexual consort should be cautioned in this regard.

Crab Lice Infection and Scabies

There has been a resurgence of skin disease caused by the pubic or crab louse, *Phthiris pubis*,[2, 75] and the mite, *Sarcoptes scabiei*.[119] The reappearance of those "old friends" as a common problem has paralleled the increase and incidence of other venereal diseases among young, sexually active people.[39] Neither of these ectoparasites is transmitted exclusively by sexual intercourse. Prolonged skin-to-skin contact, readily achieved by sharing the bed of a parasitized host, is usually required. Neither parasite can survive away from the host for more than 1 to 3 days, and transmission through bedding and clothing is uncommon. They are important to the obstetrician because they are commonly an external indication of more serious venereal infections. They can produce severe discomfort and secondary skin infection and can be transmitted from mother to child during the close contact of infant care. Neither is an arthropod vector of pathogens of human disease.

The crab louse is appropriately named; it resembles a tiny crab, 1 or 2 mm in diameter. A rather lethargic creature, it tends to remain in a restricted area, grasping a pubic hair and feeding through mouthparts adapted to piercing skin. The feeding sites are sometimes marked by small bluish hemorrhages into the skin. The life cycle is about 25 to 30 days from egg to egg. The eggs or nits are small, translucent ovals about 0.5 mm long. They attach themselves to a hair near the skin by a chitinous envelope and are difficult to remove.

Although usually found in the pubic hair, the pubic louse also can be found on any terminal hair of the body. Transfer from the pubic hair is probably mechanical, assisted by animated scratching, fingernails, towels, and other similar means rather than by self-propulsion. The perianal and axillary hairs are often infected, and the hair of the trunk, beard, scalp, and eyelashes is occasionally colonized. Even with a hand lens, pubic lice are difficult to discern and may be present in surprisingly small numbers compared with the symptoms produced. The diagnosis should be confirmed by microscopic examination of a crab or its nit or both.

P. pubis infestation elicits a variable host response, ranging from no symptoms to intolerable itching or blepharitis. Treatment with 1 per cent gamma benzene hexachloride is curative.

The cream or lotion is applied to affected areas for 4 minutes; the hair is then rinsed, dried, and combed. One application is usually sufficient, but in heavy infestations repeat application in 4 days may be needed. Lice should be removed from eyelashes by the application of 0.25 per cent physostigmine ophthalmic ointment with a cotton-tipped applicator.

It is not necessary to shave affected hairs nor is it necessary to discard or disinfect clothing and bedding. The patient should be advised to use freshly laundered undergarments and bed linens daily for a week or more. The physician's staff often needs assurance that infestation from casual contact is improbable, but this assurance does not usually prevent the itchy sensation that the thought of crab lice elicits among fastidious people.

The scabies mite burrows into the stratum corneum, deposits eggs in the tunnels it creates, and produces a characteristic pruritic skin eruption. The adult female is the culprit. As the gravid female burrows into the skin, she produces a slightly elevated, tortuous tunnel externally marked by a vesicle or a pustule. Eggs and feces are deposited in the tunnel. Larvae hatch in 3 to 4 days and reach the skin surface, where they mature in hair follicles over the next 4 to 6 days. After mating takes place on the surface, the cycle is repeated. Initial infections are often asymptomatic. However, after several weeks have passed, the number of mites has increased, and the host response to the organism is marked by eosinophilia (5 to 15 per cent) in the peripheral blood and by infiltration with lymphocytes and eosinophils around the tunnels. The rash often bears no direct relation to the number of existing mites. Occasionally, hyperinfection of the superficial skin layers produces a highly contagious, crusted lesion ("Norwegian scabies").

The eruption is most commonly located between the fingers, on the backs of the arms and legs, and in areas where clothes may be tight — the wrists, axillae, waist, and crotch. Except for intense pruritus, the rash may be difficult to distinguish clinically from syphilis. Because the patient is continuously scratching, the erythematous, papular eruption becomes excoriated and impetiginized, masking the underlying scabies infestation. The diagnosis must be made by finding the mites or eggs. The secret of finding *S. scabiei* is to search in the appropriate places with a strong hard lens. An inhabited burrow is marked by the whitish oval mite at the proximal end of the tunnel. Either the burrow may be scraped or biopsy may be performed and the material placed in saline or mineral oil for microscopic examination. Potassium hydroxide may distort the eggs or the mite and is not recommended for routine examination.

The infection spreads readily among family members. When one member has the disease, others are sure to be infected. An epidemic of scabies was reported in which evaluation of the index case, a 3 month old infant, uncovered infection of two baby-sitters as well as of the parents and the pediatrician.[66] Sarcoptes species that produce mange in animals rarely infect man, and it is best to examine other close human contacts before incriminating pets as the source.

Good medical management includes examination and treatment of family members, close contacts, and animal pets. Topical application of 1 to 10 per cent gamma benzene hexachloride or a 12.5 to 25 per cent suspension of benzyl benzoate is very effective. These agents should be applied from the head downward following a bath. Single treatment is often adequate, but this writer's personal preference is to treat again in 3 to 5 days. Small infants may absorb sufficient amounts of topically applied gamma benzene hexachloride to produce neurologic symptoms. No adverse effects upon mother or fetus are recorded, but cautious use of this agent is indicated in the second and third trimester of pregnancy.

Secondary skin infection and impetigo are not unusual with both crab lice and scabies infestations. Because of the risk of poststreptococcal glomerulonephritis, systemic antibiotic treatment with penicillin or erythromycin is indicated when streptococcal impetigo develops.

References

1. Abrams, A. J.: Lymphogranuloma venereum. J.A.M.A., 205:199, 1968.
1a. Abu-Nassar, H., Hill, N., Fred, H. L., and Yow, E. M.: Cutaneous manifestations of gonococcemia. Arch. Intern. Med., 112:731, 1963.
2. Ackerman, A. B.: Crabs — the resurgence of Phthirus pubis. N. Engl. J. Med., 278:950, 1968.
3. Alexander, E. R., Chandler, J., Pheifer, T. A., Wang, S., English, M., and Holmes, K. K.: Prospective study of perinatal Chlamydia trachomatis infection. In Hobson, D. and Holmes, K. K. (eds.): Nongonococcal Urethritis and Related Infections. Washington, D.C., American Society for Microbiology, 1977, pp. 148–152.
4. Al-Salihi, F. L., Curran, J. P., and Shteir, O. A.: Occurrence of fetal syphilis after a non-reactive early gestational serologic test. J. Pediatr., 78:121, 1971.
5. Altshuler, G.: Pathogenesis of congenital herpesvirus infection. Am. J. Dis. Child., 127:427, 1974.
6. Amstey, M. S.: Management of pregnancy complicated by genital herpes virus infection. Obstet. Gynecol., 37:515, 1971.
7. Amstey, M. S.: Effect of pregnancy hormones on herpesviruses and other deoxyribonucleic acid viruses. Am. J. Obstet. Gynecol., 129:159, 1977.
7a. Barr, J., and Danielsson, D.: Septic gonococcal dermatitis. Br. Med. J., 1:482, 1971.
8. Baker, D. A., and Plotkin, S. A.: Genital herpes simplex virus (HSV) isolation during pregnancy. Obstet. Gynecol., 53 (Suppl.):9, 1979.
9. Barrett, T. J., Silbar, J. D., and McGinley, J. P.: Genital warts — a venereal disease. J.A.M.A., 154:333, 1954.
10. Barsam, P. C.: Specific prophylaxis of gonorrheal ophthalmia neonatorum. N. Engl. J. Med., 274:731, 1966.
11. Beem, M. O., and Saxon, E. M.: Distinctive pneumonia syndrome in infants infected with Chlamydia trachomatis. In Hobson, D., and Holmes, K. K.: Nongonococcal Urethritis and Related Infections. Washington, D.C., American Society for Microbiology, 1977, pp. 153–158.
12. Blankenship, R. M., Homes, R. K., and Sanford, J. P.: Treatment of disseminated gonococcal infection. N. Engl. J. Med., 290:267, 1974.
13. Blough, H. A., and Giuntoli, R. L.: Successful treatment of human genital herpes infections with 2-deoxy-D-glucose. J.A.M.A., 241:2798, 1979.
14. Blount, J. H.: A new approach for gonorrhea epidemiology. Am. J. Public Health, 62:710, 1972.
15. Brown, W. J.: Trends and status of gonorrhea in the United States. J. Infect. Dis., 123:682, 1971.
16. Brown, W. J., and Moore, M. B.: Congenital syphilis in the United States. Clin. Pediatr., 2:220, 1963.
17. Buddingh, G. J., Schrum, D. I., Lanier, J. C., and Guidry, D. J.: Studies of the natural history of herpes simplex infections. Pediatrics, 11:595, 1953.
18. Cassie, R., and Stevenson, A.: Screening for gonorrhoea, trichomoniasis, moniliasis and syphilis in pregnancy. J. Obstet. Gynaecol. Br. Commonw., 80:48, 1973.
19. Catalano, L. W., and Johnson, L. D.: Herpes virus antibody and carcinoma in situ of the cervix. J.A.M.A., 217:447, 1971.
20. Catterall, R. D.: Trichomonal infections of the genital tract. Med. Clin. North Am., 56:1203, 1972.
21. Catterall, R. D., and Nicol, C. S.: Is trichomonal infestation a venereal disease? Br. Med. J., 1:1177, 1960.
22. Cave, V. G., Bloomfield, R. D., Hurdle, E. S., Gordon, E. W., and Hammock, D.: Gonorrhea in the obstetric and gynecologic clinic. J.A.M.A., 210:309, 1969.
23. Charles, A. G., Cohen, S., Kass, M. B., and Richman, R.: Asymptomatic gonorrhea in prenatal patients. Am. J. Obstet. Gynecol., 108:595, 1970.
24. Clark, E. G., and Danbolt, N.: The Oslo study of the natural course of untreated syphilis. Med. Clin. North Am., 48:613, 1964.
25. Cohen, P., Stout, G., and Ende, N.: Serologic reactivity in consecutive patients admitted to a general hospital. Arch. Intern. Med., 124:364, 1969.
26. Cook, T. A., Cohn, A. M., Brunschwig, J. P., Butel, J. S., and Rawls, W. E.: Wart viruses and laryngeal papillomas. Lancet, 1:782, 1973.
27. Cooperman, M. B.: Gonococcus arthritis in infancy. Am. J. Dis. Child., 33:932, 1927.
28. Curtis, A. C., and Philpott, O. S.: Prenatal syphilis. Med. Clin. North Am., 48:707, 1964.
29. Davis, C. M.: Granuloma inguinale. J.A.M.A., 211:632, 1970.
29a. Drusin, L. M.: The diagnosis and treatment of infectious and latent syphilis. Med. Clin. North Am., 56:1161, 1972.
30. Duncan, W. C., and Knox, J. M.: Modern management of syphilis and gonorrhea. In Nicholas, L. (ed.): Sexually Transmitted Diseases. Springfield, Ill., Charles C Thomas, 1973, pp. 26–42.
31. Dunkelberg, W. E.: Corynebacterium vaginale. Sex. Transm. Dis., 4:69, 1977.
32. Durst, R. D., Sibulkin, D., Trunnell, T. N., and Allyn, B.: Dose-related seroreversal in syphilis. Arch. Dermatol., 108:663, 1973.
33. Echevarria, P., Miller, G., Campbell, A. G. M., and Tucker,

G.: Scalp vesicles within the first week of life: A clue to early diagnosis of herpes neonatorum. J. Pediatr., 83:1062, 1973.

34. Elmros, T., and Larsson, P. A.: Survival of gonococci outside the body. Br. Med. J., 2:403, 1972.

35. Eschenbach, D.: Significance for the fetus of sexually acquired maternal infection with mycoplasma, chlamydia, and Neisseria gonorrheae. Semin. Perinatol., 1:11, 1977.

36. Felber, T. D., Smith, E. B., Knox, J. M., Wallis, E., and Melnick, J. L.: Photodynamic inactivation of herpes simplex. J.A.M.A., 223:289, 1973.

37. Fiumara, N. J.: The diagnosis and treatment of gonorrhea. Med. Clin. North Am., 56:1105, 1972.

38. Fiumara, N. J.: Venereal diseases. In Charles, D., and Finland, M. (eds.): Obstetric and Perinatal Infections. Philadelphia, Lea & Febiger, 1973, pp. 447–478.

39. Fiumara, N. J.: The sexually transmissable diseases. Disease-A-Month, 25:3, 1978.

40. Fleming, W. L., Brown, W. J., Donohue, J. F., and Branigan, P. W.: National survey of venereal disease treated by physicians in 1968. J.A.M.A., 211:1827, 1970.

41. Florman, A. L., Gershon, A. D., Blackett, P. R., and Nahmias, A. J.: Intrauterine infection with herpes simplex virus. J.A.M.A., 225:129, 1973.

42. Gardner, H. L., and Dukes, C. D.: Hemophilus vaginalis vaginitis: A newly defined specific infection previously classified "nonspecific" vaginitis. Am. J. Obstet. Gynecol., 69:962, 1955.

43. Gardner, H. L., and Kaufman, R. H.: Herpes genitalis: Clinical features. Clin. Obstet. Gynecol., 15:896, 1972.

44. Goldberg, J.: Studies on granuloma inguinale. V. Isolation of a bacterium resembling Donavania granulomatis from the faeces of a patient with granuloma inguinale. Br. J. Vener. Dis., 38:99, 1962.

45. Golden, B., Bell, W. E., and McKee, A. P.: Disseminated herpes simplex with encephalitis in a neonate. J.A.M.A., 209:1219, 1969.

46. Goldman, P.: Metronidazole. N. Engl. J. Med., 303:1212, 1980.

47. Goldman, R. L.: Herpetic inclusions in the endometrium. Obstet. Gynecol., 36:603, 1970.

48. Goodrich, J. J.: Treatment of gonorrhea in pregnancy. Sex. Transm. Dis., 6:168, 1979.

49. Greenblatt, R. B.: Management of Chancroid, Granuloma Inguinale, Lymphogranuloma Venereum. Public Health Service Publication No. 255. Washington, D.C., United States Government Printing Office, 1958.

50. Guinan, M. E., MacCalman, J., Kern, E. R., Overall, J. C., and Spruance, S. L.: The course of untreated recurrent genital herpes simplex infection in 27 women. N. Engl. J. Med., 304:759, 1981.

51. Hain, J., Doshi, N., and Harger, J. H.: Ascending transcervical herpes simplex infection with intact fetal membranes. Obstet. Gynecol., 56:106, 1980.

52. Handsfield, H. H., Hodson, W. A., and Holmes, K. K.: Neonatal gonococcal infection. I. Orogastric contamination with Neisseria gonorrhoeae. J.A.M.A., 225:697, 1973.

53. Handsfield, H. H., Limpman, T. O., Harnisch, J. P., Tronca, E., and Holmes, K. K.: Asymptomatic gonorrhea in men. N. Engl. J. Med., 290:117, 1974.

54. Hanshaw, J. B.: Herpesvirus hominis infections in the fetus and the newborn. Am. J. Dis. Child., 126:546, 1973.

55. Hardy, J. B., Hardy, P. H., Oppenheimer, E. H., Ryan, S. J., and Sheff, R. N.: Failure of penicillin in a newborn with congenital syphilis. J.A.M.A., 212:1345, 1970.

56. Hart, M.: Gonorrhea in women. J.A.M.A., 216:1609, 1971.

57. Harwick, H. J., Iuppa, J. B., and Fekety, F. R.: Microorganisms and amniotic fluid. Obstet. Gynecol., 33:256, 1969.

58. Harwick, H. J., Purcell, R. H., Iuppa, J. B., and Fekety, F. R.: Mycoplasma hominis and abortion. J. Infect. Dis., 121:260, 1970.

59. Heathcote, J., Cameron, C. H., and Dane, D. S.: Hepatitis-B antigen in saliva and semen. Lancet, 1:71, 1974.

60. Heyman, A., Sheldon, W. H., and Evans, L. D.: Pathogenesis of the Jarisch-Herxheimer reaction. Br. J. Vener. Dis., 28:50, 1952.

61. Holder, W. R., and Knox, J. M.: Syphilis in pregnancy. Med. Clin. North Am., 56:1151, 1972.

62. Holmes, K. K.: Gonococcal infection. Adv. Intern. Med., 19:259, 1974.

62a. Holmes, K. K., Gounts, C. W., and Beaty, H. N.: Disseminated gonococcal infection. Ann. Intern. Med., 74:979, 1971.

62b. Holmes, K. K., Gutman, L. T., Belding, M. E., and Turck, M.: Recovery of Neisseria gonorrhoeae from "sterile" synovial fluid in gonococcal arthritis. N. Engl. J. Med., 284:318, 1971.

63. Hooshmand, H., Escobar, M. R., and Kopf, S. W.: Neurosyphilis: A study of 241 patients. J.A.M.A., 219:726, 1972.

64. Hudson, A. W., and McFarland, C.: Disseminated herpes simplex in a newborn. J.A.M.A., 208:859, 1969.

65. Hunter, E. F., Deacon, W. E., and Meyer, P. E.: An improved FTA test for syphilis, the absorption procedure (FTA-ABS). Public Health Rep., 79:410, 1964.

66. Hurwitz, S.: Scabies in babies. Am. J. Dis. Child., 126:226, 1973.

67. Jacobs, P. H.: Molluscum contagiosum. Aerosp. Med., 41:1196, 1970.

68. Jones, J. E., and Harris, R. E.: Diagnostic evaluation of syphilis during pregnancy. Obstet. Gynecol., 54:611, 1979.

69. Kampmeier, R. H.: The late manifestations of syphilis: Skeletal, visceral and cardiovascular. Med. Clin. North Am., 48:667, 1964.

70. Kaufman, R. H., Gardner, H. L., Brown, D., Wallis, C., Rawls, W. E., and Melnick, J. L.: Herpes genitalis treated by photodynamic inactivation of virus. Am. J. Obstet. Gynecol., 117:1144, 1973.

71. Kaufman, R. E., Olansky, D. C., and Wiesner, P. J.: The FTA-ABS (IgM) test for neonatal congenital syphilis: A critical review. J. Am. Vener. Dis. Assoc., 1:79, 1974.

71a. Keiser, H., Ruben, F. L., Wolinsky, E., and Kushner, I.: Clinical forms of gonococcal arthritis. N. Engl. J. Med., 279:234, 1968.

72. Kibrick, S.: Herpes simplex. In Charles, D., and Finland, M. (eds.): Obstetric and Perinatal Infections. Philadelphia, Lea & Febiger, 1973, pp. 75–94.

73. Kibrick, S.: Herpes simplex infection at term. J.A.M.A., 243:157, 1980.

74. Kimball, M. W., and Knee, S.: Gonococcal perihepatitis in a male. N. Engl. J. Med., 282:1082, 1970.

74a. King, A., and Nicol, C.: Venereal Diseases. 2nd Ed. London, Bailliere, Tindall, & Cassell, 1969, p. 76.

75. Kinmont, P. D. C.: Phthiriasis pubis. Practitioner, 209:342, 1972.

76. Kleiman, M. B., and Lamb, G. A.: Gonococcal arthritis in a newborn infant. Pediatrics, 52:285, 1973.

77. Kohen, D. P.: Neonatal gonococcal arthritis: Three cases and review of the literature. Pediatrics, 53:436, 1974.

78. Kraus, G. W., and Yen, S. S. C.: Gonorrhea during pregnancy. Obstet. Gynecol., 31:258, 1968.

79. Kundsin, R. B., and Driscoll, S. G.: The role of mycoplasmas in human reproductive failure. Ann. N.Y. Acad. Sci., 174:794, 1970.

80. Lang, D. J., and Kummer, J. F.: Demonstration of cytomegalovirus in semen. N. Engl. J. Med., 287:756, 1972.

81. Lauderdale, V., and Goldman, J. N.: Serial ultrathin sectioning demonstrating the intracellularity of T. pallidum. Br. J. Vener. Dis., 48:87, 1972.

82. Lee, R. V., and Risser, W.: Fatal congenital syphilis in Connecticut. Conn. Med., 41:470, 1977.

83. Lee, R. V.: Genital skin lesions caused by sexually transmitted diseases. Infect. Control Urol. Care, 5:17, 1980.

84. Lucas, J. B.: The effects of gonorrhea therapy on incubating syphilis. In Nicholas, L. (ed.): Sexually Transmitted Diseases. Springfield, Ill., Charles C Thomas, 1973, pp. 71–83.

85. Lumicao, G. G., and Heggie, A. D.: Chlamydial infections. Pediatr. Clin. North Am., 26:269, 1979.

86. Lynch, P. J.: Molluscum contagiosum venereum. Clin. Obstet. Gynecol., 15:966, 1972.

87. Lynch, P. J., and Minkin, W.: Molluscum contagiosum of the adult. Arch. Dermatol., 98:141, 1968.

88. McCormack, W. M.: Genital infections of perinatal importance. Clin. Obstet. Gynecol., 22:313, 1979.

89. McCormack, W. M., Almeida, P. C., Bailey, P. E., Grady, E. M., and Lee, Y. H.: Sexual activity and vaginal colonization with genital mycoplasmas. J.A.M.A., 221:1375, 1972.

90. McCormack, W. M., Braun, P., Lee, Y. H., Klein, J. O., and Kass, E. H.: The genital mycoplasmas. N. Engl. J. Med., 288:78, 1973.

91. McCormack, W. M., Hayes, C. H., Rosner, B., Evrard, J. R., Crockett, V. A., Alpert, S., and Zinner, S. H.: Vaginal

colonization with *Corynebacterium vaginale* (Hemophilus vaginalis). J. Infect. Dis., *136*:740, 1977.

92. McCormack, W. M., and Lee, Y. H.: Genital mycoplasmas. *In* Charles, D. and Finland, M. (eds.): Obstetric and Perinatal Infections. Philadelphia, Lea & Febiger, 1973, pp. 95–105.

93. McCormack, W. M., Lee, Y. H., Lin, J. S., and Rankin, J. S.: Genital mycoplasmas in postpartum fever. J. Infect. Dis., *127*:193, 1973.

94. McCormack, W. M., Lee, Y. H., and Zinner, S. H.: Sexual experience and urethral colonization with genital mycoplasmas. Ann. Intern. Med., *78*:696, 1973.

95. McCracken, G. H., and Kaplan, J. M.: Penicillin treatment for congenital syphilis. J.A.M.A., *228*:855, 1974.

96. McLennan, M. T., Smith, J. M., and McLennan, C. E.: Diagnosis of vaginal mycosis and trichomoniasis. Obstet. Gynecol., *40*:231, 1972.

97. MacLeod, C. L.: Parasites and their management during pregnancy. In Press.

98. Mardh, P., Ripa, T., Svensson, L., and Westrom, L.: *Chlamydia trachomatis* infection in patients with acute salpingitis. N. Engl. J. Med., *296*:1377, 1977.

99. Marino, A. F., Pariser, H., and Wise, H.: Gonorrhea epidemiology — is it worthwhile? Am. J. Public Health, *62*:713, 1972.

100 Metronidazole (Flagyl). Med. Lett. Drug Ther., *21*:89, 1979.

101. Music, S. I., Fine, E. M., and Togo, Y.: Zoster-like disease in the newborn due to herpes simplex virus. N. Engl. J. Med., *284*:24, 1971.

102. Nahmias, A. J., Alford, C. A., and Korones, S. B.: Infection of the newborn with herpes virus hominis. Adv. Pediatr., *17*:185, 1970.

103. Nahmias, A. J., Dowdle, W. R., Naib, Z. M., Josey, W. E., McLone, D., and Domescik, G.: Genital infection with type 2 herpes virus hominis. Br. J. Vener. Dis, *45*:294, 1969.

104. Nahmias, A. J., Josey, W. E., and Naib, Z. M.: Significance of herpes simplex virus infection during pregnancy. Clin. Obstet. Gynecol., *15*:929, 1972.

105. Nahmias, A. J., Josey, W. E., and Naib, Z. M.: Venereal herpes simplex virus infections. *In* Nicholas, L. (ed.): Sexually Transmitted Diseases. Springfield, Ill., Charles C Thomas, 1973, pp. 192–205.

106. Nahmias, A. J., Josey, W. E., Naib, Z. M., Freeman, M. G., Fernandez, R. J., and Wheeler, J. H.: Perinatal risk associated with maternal genital herpes simplex virus infection. Am. J. Obstet. Gynecol., *110*:825, 1971.

107. Nahmias, A. J., Josey, W. E., Naib, Z. M., Luce, C. F., and Guest, B. A.: Antibodies to herpesvirus hominis types 1 and 2 in humans. I. Patients with genital herpetic infections. Am. J. Epidemiol., *91*:547, 1970.

108. Nahmias, A. J., and Roizman, B.: Infection with herpes simplex viruses 1 and 2. N. Engl. J. Med., *289*:667, 1973.

109. Nahmias, A. J., Von Reyn, F., Josey, W. E., Naib, Z. M., and Hutton, R. D.: Genital herpes simplex virus infection and gonorrhea. Br. J. Vener. Dis., *49*:306, 1973.

110. Nahmias, A. J., Visintine, A. M., and Josey, W. E.: Cesarean section and genital herpes. N. Engl. J. Med., *296*:1359, 1977.

111. Naib, Z. M.: Cytology of TRIC agent infection of the eye of newborn infants and their mothers' genital tracts. Acta Cytol., *14*:390, 1970.

112. Naib, Z. M., Nahmias, A. J., Josey, W. E., and Wheeler, J. H.: Association of maternal herpetic infection with spontaneous abortion. Obstet. Gynecol., *35*:260, 1970.

112a. Nicholas, L., and Beerman, H.: Present day serodiagnosis of syphilis. Am. J. Med. Sci., *249*:466, 1965.

113. Olansky, D.: Late benign syphilis (gumma). Med. Clin. North Am., *48*:653, 1964.

114. Olansky, S.: Syphilis — rediscovered. Disease-A-Month, May, 1967.

114a. Olansky, S.: Serodiagnosis of syphilis. Med. Clin. North Am., *56*:1145, 1972.

114b. Olansky, S., and Norins, L. C.: Current serodiagnosis and treatment of syphilis. J.A.M.A., *198*:165, 1966.

115. Oppenheimer, E. H., and Hardy, J. B.: Congenital syphilis in the newborn infant: Clinical and pathological observations in recent cases. Johns Hopkins Med. J., *129*:63, 1971.

116. Oriel, J. D.: Natural history of genital warts. Br. J. Vener. Dis., *47*:1, 1971.

117. Oriel, J. D., Powis, P. A., Reeve, P., Miller, A., and Nicol, C. S.: Chlamydial infections of the cervix. Br. J. Vener. Dis., *50*:11, 1974.

118. Oriel, J. D., Reeve, P., Powis, P., Miller, A., and Nicol, C. S.: Chlamydial infection. Br. J. Vener. Dis., *48*:429, 1972.

119. Orkin, M.: Resurgence of scabies. J.A.M.A., *217*:593, 1971.

120. Ovcinnikov, N. M., and Delektorskij, V. V.: Electron microscopy of phagocytosis in syphilis and yaws. Br. J. Vener. Dis., *48*:227, 1972.

121. Packer, H., and Goldberg, J.: Studies of the antigenic relationship of *D. granulomatis* to members of the tribe Eschericheae. Am. J. Syph., *34*:342, 1950.

121a. Pariser, H.: Infectious syphilis. Med. Clin. North Am., *48*:625, 1964.

122. Pariser, H.: Asymptomatic gonorrhea. Med. Clin. North Am., *56*:1127, 1972.

123. Pedersen, A. H. B., and Bonin, P.: Screening females for asymptomatic gonorrhea infection. Northwest Med., *70*:255, 1971.

124. Penza, J. F.: Moniliasis and trichomoniasis. *In* Charles, D., and Finland, M. (eds.): Obstetric and Perinatal Infections. Philadelphia, Lea & Febiger, 1973, pp. 209–224.

125. Penza, J., and Rankin, J. S.: Infectious vaginopathies in pregnancy. Clin. Obstet. Gynecol., *13*:223, 1970.

126. Pheifer, T. A., Forsyth, P. S., Durfee, M. A., Pollock, H. M., and Holmes, K. K.: Nonspecific vaginitis. N. Engl. J. Med., *298*:1429, 1978.

127. Philip, R. N., Hill, D. A., Greaves, A. B., Gordon, F. B., Quan, A. L., Gerloff, R. K., and Thomas, L. A.: Study of chlamydiae in patients with lymphogranuloma venereum and urethritis attending a venereal disease clinic. Br. J. Vener. Dis., *47*:114, 1971.

128. Poste, G., Hawkins, D. F., and Thomlinson, J.: Herpesvirus hominis infection of the female genital tract. Obstet. Gynecol., *40*:871, 1972.

129. Postlethwaite, R.: Molluscum contagiosum: A review. Arch. Environ. Health, *21*:432, 1970.

130. Powell, L. C., Jr.: Condyloma acuminatum. Clin. Obstet. Gynecol., *15*:948, 1972.

131. Putkonen, T., Sald, O. P., and Mustakallo, K. K.: Febrile Herxheimer reaction in different phases of primary and secondary syphilis. Br. J. Vener. Dis., *42*:181, 1966.

132. Rawls, W. E., and Gardner, H. L.: Herpes genitalis: Venereal aspects. Clin. Obstet. Gynecol., *15*:912, 1972.

133. Rawls, W. E., Kaufman, R. H., and Gardner, H. L.: Relation of herpes virus type 2 to carcinoma of the cervix. Clin. Obstet. Gynecol., *15*:919, 1972.

134. Rees, E. A., and Hamlett, J. D.: Screening for gonorrhea in pregnancy. J. Obstet. Gynaecol. Br. Commonw., *79*:344, 1972.

135. Rees, E., Tait, I. A., Hobson, D., and Johnson, F. W. A.: Perinatal chlamydial infection. *In* Hobson, D., and Holmes, K. K. (eds.): Nongonococcal Urethritis and Related Infections. Washington, D.C., American Society for Microbiology, 1977, pp. 140–147.

136. Reimer, C. B., Black, C. M., and Phillips, D. J.: The specificity of fetal IgM: antibody or anti-antibody? Ann. N.Y. Acad. Sci., *254*:77, 1975.

137. Reiss, F.: Steroid hormones. Arch. Dermatol. Syph., *59*:405, 1949.

138. Rodin, P., and Hass, G.: Metronidazole and pregnancy. Br. J. Vener. Dis., *42*:210, 1966.

139. Roos, R. F.: Trichomoniasis treated with a single dose of benzoylmetronidazole. S. Afr. Med. J., *2*:869, 1978.

140. Ross, S. M.: Single and triple dose treatment of trichomonas infection of the vagina. Br. J. Vener. Dis., *49*:475, 1973.

141. Royston, I., and Aurelian, L.: The association of genital herpesvirus with cervical atypia and carcinoma in situ. Am. J. Epidemiol., *91*:531, 1970.

142. Rudolph, A., and Price, E. V.: Penicillin reactions among patients in venereal disease clinics. J.A.M.A., *223*:499, 1973.

143. Sarrell, P. M., and Pruett, K. A.: Symptomatic gonorrhea during pregnancy. Obstet. Gynecol., *32*:670, 1968.

144. Schachter, J.: Lymphogranuloma venereum and other non-

ocular *Chlamydia trachomatis* infections. *In* Hobson, D., and Holmes, K. K. (eds.): Nongonococcal Urethritis and Related Infections. Washington, D.C., American Society for Microbiology, 1977, pp. 91–97.

145. Schachter, J.: Chlamydial infections. N. Engl. J. Med., *298*:428, 490, 540, 1978.

146. Schachter, J., Smith, D. E., Dawson, C. R., Anderson, W. R., Deller, J. J., Hohe, A. W., Smartt, W. H., and Meyer, K. F.: Lymphogranuloma venereum. I. Comparison of the Frei test, complement fixation test, and isolation of the agent. J. Infect. Dis., *120*:372, 1969.

147. Schroeter, A. L., and Reynolds, G.: The rectal culture as a test of cure of gonorrhea in the female. J. Infect. Dis., *125*:499, 1972.

148. Schroeter, A. L., Turner, R. H., Lucas, J. B., and Brown, W. J.: Therapy for incubating syphilis — effectiveness of gonorrhea treatment. J.A.M.A., *218*:711, 1971.

149. Silverstone, P. I., Snodgrass, C. A., and Wigfield, A. S.: Value of screening for gonorrhea in obstetrics and gynecology. Br. J. Vener. Dis., *50*:53, 1974.

150. Skog, E., and Gudjonsson, H.: On the allergic origin of the Jarisch-Herxheimer reaction. Acta Derm. Venereol., *46*:136, 1966.

151. Smith, I. W., Peutherer, J. F., and Robertson, D. H. H.: Characterization of genital strains of herpesvirus hominis. Br. J. Vener. Dis., *49*:385, 1973.

152. Snowe, R. J., and Wilfert, C. M.: Epidemic reappearance of gonococcal ophthalmia neonatorum. Pediatrics, *51*:110, 1973.

153. Sparling, P. F.: Diagnosis and treatment of syphilis. N. Engl. J. Med., *284*:642, 1971.

154. Sparling, P. F., Wiesner, P. J., Holmes, K. K., and Kass, E. H.: Treatment of gonorrhea. J. Infect. Dis., *127*:578, 1973.

155. Spiegel, C. A., Amsel, R., Eschenbach, D., Schoenknecht, F., and Holmes, K. K.: Anaerobic bacteria in nonspecific vaginitis. N. Engl. J. Med., *303*:601, 1980.

156. Stamm, W. E., Wagner, K. F., Amsel, R., Alexander, E. R., Turck, M., Counts, G. W., and Holmes, K. K.: Causes of the acute urethral syndrome in women. N. Engl. J. Med., *303*:409, 1980.

157. Stein, L. F., and Cope, E. J.: Trichomonas vaginalis. Am. J. Obstet. Gynecol., *25*:819, 1933.

158. Stewart, D. B.: The gynecological lesions of lymphogranuloma venereum and granuloma inguinale. Med. Clin. North Am., *48*:773, 1964.

159. Stewart, K. S., Shafi, M., Andrews, J., and Williams, J. D.: Distribution of parenteral ampicillin and cephalosporins in late pregnancy. J. Obstet. Gynaecol. Br. Commonw., *80*:902, 1973.

160. Swanson, J.: Studies on gonococcus infection. IV. Pili: Their role in attachment of gonococci to tissue culture cells. J. Exp. Med., *137*:571, 1973.

161. Swierczewski, J. A., Mason, E. J., Cabrera, P. B., and Liber, M.: Fulminating meningitis with Waterhouse-Friderichsen syndrome due to *Neisseria gonorrhoeae*. Am. J. Clin. Pathol., *54*:202, 1970.

162. Sykes, J. A., and Miller, J. N.: Intracellular location of *Treponema pallidum* (Nichols strain) in the rabbit testis. Infect. Immun., *4*:307, 1971.

163. Sykes, J. A., Miller, J. N., and Kalan, A. J.: *Treponema pallidum* within cells of a primary chancre from a human female. Br. J. Vener. Dis., *50*:40, 1974.

164. Taber, L. H., and Feigin, R. D.: Spirochetal infections. Pediatr. Clin. North Am., *26*:377, 1979.

165. Tashjian, J. H., Coulan, C. B., and Washington, J. A.: Vaginal flora in asymptomatic women. Mayo Clin. Proc., *51*:557, 1976.

166. Taylor-Robinson, D.: Possible role of ureaplasmas in nongonococcal urethritis. *In* Hobson, D., and Holmes, K. K. (eds.): Non-gonococcal Urethritis and Related Infections. Washington, D.C., American Society for Microbiology, 1977, pp. 30–37.

167. Teokharov, B. A.: Non-gonococcal infections of the female genitalia. Br. J. Vener. Dis., *45*:334, 1969.

168. Thin, R. N. T., and Michael, A. M.: Sexually transmitted disease in antenatal patients. Br. J. Vener. Dis., *46*:126, 1970.

169. Thompson, T. R., Swanson, R. E., and Wiesner, P. J.: Gonococcal ophthalmia neonatorum. J.A.M.A., *228*:186, 1974.

170. Thompson, S. E., III: Treatment of syphilis during pregnancy. J. Am. Vener. Dis. Assoc., *3*:158, 1976.

171. Timmonen, S., Salo, P., Meyer, B., and Haapoja, H.: Vaginal mycosis. Acta Obstet. Gynecol. Scand., *45*:232, 1966.

172. Torphy, D. E., Ray, C. G., McAlister, R., and Du, J. N. H.: Herpes simplex virus infection in infants: A spectrum of disease. J. Pediatr., *76*:405, 1970.

172a. Tronca, E., Handsfield, H. H., Wiesner, P. J., and Holmes, K. K.: Demonstration of *Neisseria gonorrhoeae* with fluorescent antibody in patients with disseminated gonococcal infection. J. Infect. Dis., *129*:583, 1974.

173. Turner, T. B.: Syphilis and the treponematoses. *In* Mudd, S. (ed.): Infectious Agents and Host Reactions. Philadelphia, W. B. Saunders Co., 1970, p. 346.

174. Wallin, J.: A clinical pattern for making an immediate presumptive diagnosis of gonococcal infection in women. Acta Derm. Venereol., *54*:157, 1974.

175. Wallis, C., Melnick, J. L., and Kaufman, R. H.: Herpes genitalis: Management — present and predicted. Clin. Obstet. Gynecol., *15*:939, 1972.

176. Ward, M. E., and Watt, P. J.: Adherence of *Neisseria gonorrhoeae* to urethral mucosal cells. An electron-microscopic study of human gonorrhea. J. Infect. Dis., *126*:601, 1972.

177. Waters, J. R., and Roulston, T. M.: Gonococcal infection in a prenatal clinic. Am. J. Obstet. Gynecol., *103*:532, 1969.

177a. Wheeler, J. K., Heffron, W. A., and Williams, R. C.: Migratory arthralgias and cutaneous lesions as confusing initial manifestations of gonorrhea. Am. J. Med. Sci., *260*:150, 1970.

178. Wiesner, P. J., Tronca, E., Bonin, P., Pedersen, A. H. B., and Holmes, K. K.: Clinical spectrum of pharyngeal gonococcal infection. N. Engl. J. Med., *288*:181, 1973.

179. Wilkinson, R. H., and Heller, R. M.: Congenital syphilis: Resurgence of an old problem. Pediatrics, *47*:27, 1971.

180. Willcox, R. R.: An imidazole derivative (Flagyl) effective orally in vaginal trichomoniasis. Br. J. Vener. Dis., *36*:175, 1960.

181. Witzleben, C. L., and Driscoll, S. G.: Possible transplacental transmission of herpes simplex infection. Pediatrics, *36*:192, 1965.

182. Wolner-Hanssen, P., Westrom, L., and Mardh, P.: Perihepatitis and chlamydial salpingitis. Lancet, *1*:901, 1980.

183. Woodcock, K. R.: Treatment of trichomonal vaginitis with a single oral dose of metronidazole. Br. J. Vener. Dis., *48*:65, 1972.

184. Young, R. L., Acosta, A. A., and Kaufman, R. H.: The treatment of large condylomata acuminata complicating pregnancy. Obstet. Gynecol., *41*:65, 1973.

16

Richard V. Lee, M.D.

PARASITIC INFESTATIONS

In the highly industrialized areas of the temperate climate zones, the prevalence of parasitic diseases during pregnancy is considerably lower and is attended with lower morbidity and mortality than in agrarian or underdeveloped parts of the world. In the tropical and subtropical climate zones, parasitic infections may pose a serious hazard to the health of the mother and the success of the pregnancy. It is not within the scope of this chapter to describe the vast array of parasitic diseases and all their various clinical manifestations. Those of particular importance to obstetricians practicing in industralized countries in temperate climates, because of either importation or endemicity, will be briefly described. More exotic parasites are referred to in tabular form; pertinent parasitologic and tropical medicine tests are listed in the references section at the end of this chapter.

The importance of a knowledge of parasitic infections to the practicing physician has been dramatically illustrated by the large number of intestinal parasites and cases of malaria in refugees coming to the United States from Southeast Asia and the Caribbean Islands. Because of the rapidity and ease of foreign travel, the chances of civilians acquiring exotic parasitic infections during a trip, the illness manifesting itself only after the return home, are considerable. More than 15 million Americans travel abroad each year and more than 3 million foreign visitors travel in the United States each year. A history of where the patient comes from and where the patient has been is an important diagnostic aid.

Emphasis on the exotic aspect of parasitic diseases should not obscure the fact that in some parts of the United States, environmental, economic, and sanitary conditions allow endemic parasitic infection. Giardiasis and amebiasis occur in epidemic form in the United States. Small outbreaks of trichinosis occur episodically. Some southern states continue to harbor

hookworm. It is possible that imported parasites may become established in the United States under appropriate circumstances of inadequate sanitation, housing, and disease detection. It must be remembered that many so-called tropical diseases — malaria, yellow fever, cholera — were endemic in the United States less than 100 years ago.

Harboring a parasite is not synonymous with disease. People may have a small number of intestinal parasites and feel well and have no adverse effects. With many parasites, especially the intestinal helminths, a quantitative assessment of the intensity of infestation is necessary before symptoms can be ascribed to the parasite. A heavy worm burden is more likely to produce illness and require treatment than is a light infection. Treatment of asymptomatic carriers may be more unpleasant or hazardous than watchful waiting. Several factors must be considered in the diagnosis and the decision to treat the individual patient: the nature and intensity of the infection, the public health risk, the patient's psychologic state, and the severity of the symptoms.

EFFECTS OF PARASITES ON REPRODUCTION

Parasitic infestation can impair a woman's reproductive capacity in three ways (Tables 16–1, 16–2, and 16–3). First, the infestation may impair fertility. Second, disease produced by the parasite may produce spontaneous interruption of the pregnancy or necessitate medical intervention for termination of the pregnancy. Third, some parasites may cross the placenta, producing fetal loss from either placental failure or fetal infection.

Parasitic Diseases Causing Impaired Fertility. Parasites that produce chronic disease may

TABLE 16–1 EFFECTS OF PROTOZOAN INFECTIONS ON REPRODUCTION

	Impaired Fertility	Failure to Carry to Term	Fetal Infection
Entamoeba histolytica	X	X	X
Giardia lamblia	X		
Leishmania species	X	X	?
Plasmodia species (Malaria)	X	X	X
Trypanosoma species	X	X	X
Toxoplasma gondii		?	X
Pneumocystis carinii			X

cause maternal debility with suppression of ovulation or cessation of sexual activity. Anemia and malnutrition are common manifestations of infection by parasites affecting the reticuloendothelial system and the gastrointestinal tract. A few parasites may cause direct damage to the genital tract and, by aberrant migration or implantation of parasites, produce anatomic abnormalities that prevent fertilization or implantation.

Parasitic Diseases Adversely Affecting Maternal Health During Pregnancy. Parasites that produce acute febrile disease may cause a pregnancy to end prematurely because of the maternal illness. The nutritional effects of some intestinal helminths can be exaggerated by the increased demands of pregnancy. Tissue-invasive parasitic diseases such as echinococcosis and filariasis may produce local lesions that obstruct vaginal delivery.

Parasitic Diseases Affecting the Fetus. Intrauterine infection of the placenta, the fetus or both almost always requires hematogenous dissemination of an invasive form of a parasite. Rarely, the uterine contents can be infected by direct spread from a genital tract reservoir of infection or by lymphatic spread. As a general rule there is an inverse relationship between

TABLE 16–2 EFFECTS OF NEMATODE INFECTIONS ON REPRODUCTION

	Impaired Fertility	Failure to Carry to Term	Fetal Infection
Ascaris lumbricoides	X		
Enterobius vermicularis (Pinworm)	X		
Trichuris trichiura (Whipworm)			
Hookworm species	X	X	
Strongyloides stercoralis	X	X	
Trichinella spiralis	X	X	X
Filaria species	X	X	X

maternal immunity and the risk of intrauterine infection of the fetus from parasitemia. Mothers reinfected by a parasite against which they have an immunity have a smaller risk of fetal infection than do nonimmune mothers acquiring infection during pregnancy.

TREATMENT OF PARASITIC INFESTATIONS DURING PREGNANCY

There are no safe antiparasitic drugs for use during pregnancy. Every effective agent has some known or theoretical adverse effect upon the fetus or the pregnancy, especially if given during the first trimester. The clinician must first decide whether treatment is warranted and then decide upon the appropriate drug. In two instances there is no choice. In the first, the mother has contracted an infection for which there is no reliable therapy — for example, Chagas' disease. In the second, the mother has contracted an infection that is life-threatening and must be treated and for which there is a limited therapeutic choice — for example, chloroquine-resistant falciparum malaria or African trypanosomiasis. The majority of parasitized pregnancies do not require treatment unless there is risk to the fetus or serious impairment of maternal health. For example, a light hookworm infection does not require antiparasitic drug therapy during pregnancy. The treatment of many parasitic diseases, such as pinworm, is best left until after delivery.

PLANNING FOR TRAVEL

The hazards of traveling are easily minimized in the excitement of planning for a trip. Advertisements emphasize the comforts and pleasures of adventurous luxury travel. In contrast, the Morbidity and Mortality Weekly Reports of the Center for Disease Control contain descriptions of fatal and nearly fatal parasitic diseases in unwary travelers. However, restricting travel during an otherwise uncomplicated pregnancy is not encouraged except when patients are close to term.

Careful medical planning should be an essential part of travel preparation for anyone — especially the pregnant woman. The physician should discourage travel that may pose serious risk to the mother. Safaris and treks almost always expose the participant to potentially hazardous climate and geography, to uncertain food and water safety, and to insect vectors. Apparently safe and cosmopolitan cities have recurrent epidemic disease during certain phases of their weather cycle. For example, mosquito-borne

TABLE 16–3 EFFECTS OF TREMATODE AND CESTODE INFECTIONS ON REPRODUCTION

	Impaired Fertility	Failure to Carry to Term	Fetal Infection
TREMATODES			
Schistosoma species	X	X	
Clonorchis sinensis	X		
Paragonimus westermanii	X		
CESTODES			
Echinococcus species	X	X	
Taenia species	X	X	

dengue fever is prevalent in Bangkok, Thailand, during the rainy season. Travel to most countries in South America and Africa requires immunization against yellow fever, a live virus vaccine, which should not be given during pregnancy.

The Center for Disease Control (CDC) in Atlanta, Georgia, provides a unique advisory and diagnostic service for physicians with questions about tropical medicine and parasitology.

The CDC publishes an annual review of the health requirements for international travel, which contains the immunization requirements for all countries and summaries and maps of epidemic and endemic diseases.[50] Obstetricians should use this publication to help their patients plan realistically for foreign travel.

Not infrequently the practitioner is asked about chemoprophylaxis for "traveler's diarrhea." In general, but especially during pregnancy, this is not a desirable practice. None of the available drugs are free of side effects or potential toxicities; all, taken in suboptimal doses, may predispose to the development of suppressed occult bacterial or parasitic infection. Moreover, the vast majority of cases of traveler's diarrhea are not caused by parasites and are not preventable by antiparasitic drugs. Nothing else surpasses personal hygiene and care in the selection of food, water, and lodging to reduce the risk of serious gastrointestinal infection when traveling. This advice, rather than a prescription for chemoprophylaxis, should be offered to the pregnant traveler by the obstetrician.

PROTOZOAN INFECTIONS

TOXOPLASMOSIS

Toxoplasma gondii is one of the widespread protozoan parasites in nature.[37] It is found in herbivorous, carnivorous, and omnivorous animals, including all orders of mammals and some birds. It is found wherever human beings and their domestic animals are found.

There are three phases in the life cycle of toxoplasma: the trophozoite, the tissue cyst, and the oocyst. The trophozoite is seen during the acute stage of infection and can invade many kinds of mammalian cells; it is not able to survive freezing and thawing, desiccation, or digestive juices. The tissue cyst is formed within host cells and may contain a few to about three thousand organisms. Tissue cysts may be found as soon as the eighth day of infection and are presumed to persist, containing viable parasites, throughout the life of the host. Brain and striated muscle are the most frequent sites of tissue cyst persistence, although tissue cysts can be found in virtually every organ. Freezing and thawing, desiccation, and cooking destroy the tissue cyst. However, when the cyst wall is destroyed by peptic digestion, the liberated parasites may be viable for several hours of exposure to digestive juices. The oocyst has been described in cats,[27] in which the sexual cycle of the organism takes place. If the cat eats toxoplasma-infected meat, the sexual cycle proceeds in the epithelium of the small intestine, producing oocysts excreted in the feces. The sporozoites formed in the oocysts after passage in the feces are infective for man and domestic animals.

Infection follows ingestion of oocysts in material contaminated by cat feces or ingestion of tissue cysts in undercooked meat. Seroepidemiologic studies indicate that *Toxoplasma gondii* infection is common but that clinical disease is uncommon. The clinical manifestations of infection are determined by the size of the inoculum, by the immune status of the host, and possibly by differences in virulence among strains of *Toxoplasma*. The most severe disease occurs in immunosuppressed or immunoimmature hosts, such as patients with malignancies or transplant and fetuses of less than five or six months of gestation.

Parasitemia has been demonstrated in animals and human beings after release of parasites from tissue cysts. The duration of parasitemia and the frequency of its occurrence are not known, but acute disease is almost always accompanied by parasitemia, and chronic disease is infrequently accompanied by parasitemia. Transplacental migration of blood-borne parasites is the primary source of intrauterine fetal infections.

In immunocompetent hosts, acquired infection is usually not clinically obvious. The most commonly recognized illness is lymphadenopathy, which is occasionally accompanied by fever, malaise, and skin rash. The adenopathy may be localized or generalized, with splenomegaly; characteristically, the posterior cervical chain is involved. Atypical lymphocytosis may occur, indistinguishable from that found in patients with mononucleosis due to Epstein-Barr virus or cytomegalovirus. The atypical lymphocytosis is usually transient, but the lymphadenopathy may persist for months. It is important to emphasize that clinical illness may be so mild as to escape detection.

The importance of toxoplasmosis to obstetricians resides in the ability of the organism to produce clinically vague or silent infection in the mother while retaining the potential of infecting the fetus in utero.[17, 23, 24, 41] A study was made of 378 pregnant women with toxoplasmosis acquired before or during pregnancy.[17] The great majority of infants born to mothers acquiring the organism during pregnancy were not infected or were infected without serious clinical effects. Among the affected infants, only a small minority had evidence of serious disease. Abortion, stillbirth, or severe congenital infection occurred almost exclusively when women had been infected early in pregnancy. However, such severe clinical effects occurred in only 10 to 15 per cent of such pregnancies. The incidence of abortion, stillbirth, or severe congenital infection when women were infected before conception was very small.

The risk to the fetus appears to be related to the time during pregnancy when maternal infection occurs. Transmission of the parasite to the fetus occurs most often when maternal infection has been acquired during the last trimester, but the disease in the neonate is almost always subclinical. If the mother is infected early in pregnancy, transmission to the fetus occurs less frequently but the disease in the neonate is more severe. Presumably, the differences in the severity of clinical disease are dependent upon the immune capacity of the fetus at the time parasitemia occurs.

There is evidence that some chronically infected mothers may have foci of toxoplasma in the uterus. Whether this circumstance may result in congenital infection of the fetus or abortion is not clear. There is no conclusive evidence from animal and human studies that toxoplasma can cause abortion in chronically infected females.[25, 37] If a causal relationship does exist, the incidence of abortion due to chronic toxoplasma infection is not very large.

The severe forms of congenital infection are associated with fever, seizures, hydrocephaly or microcephaly, chorioretinitis, cerebral calcifications, abnormal cerebrospinal fluid, hepatosple-

nomegaly, and jaundice. The manifestations of toxoplasmosis in the newborn can mimic infection by virtually any pathogen producing intrauterine disease. Many babies so affected develop serious residual medical problems — mental retardation, seizures, and severely impaired vision. At present, there is no way to predict the outcome of infants with subclinical or asymptomatic congenital toxoplasma infection.

In one case report, *Toxoplasma gondii* was isolated by mouse inoculation from amniotic fluid obtained by amniocentesis and from placenta obtained later after prostaglandin-induced abortion.[43] No organisms were seen in cytologic or histologic preparations. The patient was one of 37 people in a common source epidemic and was shown by serologic tests to have acute toxoplasmosis. Amniocentesis may be useful in identifying fetal infection if parasitologic studies, including animal inoculation, are carefully done. Further clinical studies are needed, however.

Isolation of the organism from blood or biopsy tissue by animal inoculation or by microscopic identification are the most direct diagnostic methods. Inoculation techniques are not readily available except in hospitals with active research laboratories.

Serologic techniques have become the mainstay of clinical diagnosis. The most commonly used serologic tests are the Sabin-Feldman dye test, the complement fixation test, and the indirect fluorescent antibody test. The diagnosis of acute acquired toxoplasmosis is established by the demonstration of rising serologic titers. However, titers as high as 1:1000 or 1:4000 may persist for some years after acute infection. This is particularly true of the Sabin-Feldman dye test and the indirect fluorescent antibody test. A single high serologic titer is therefore not an absolute indication that a clinical illness is toxoplasmosis. Repetitive serologic testing is necessary in order to assess the nature of the antibody response. Complement-fixing antibodies appear later than those demonstrated by the dye test and the indirect fluorescent antibody test. A negative complement fixation test that turns positive, or increasing complement fixation test titers occurring with a high but stable dye or indirect fluorescent antibody test titer, indicate active or recent infection. Because the initial antibody response to toxoplasma infection is mostly IgM, the fluorescent antibody test, modified to demonstrate IgM toxoplasma antibody, can also be used to establish acute infection, either congenital or acquired. The absence of IgM toxoplasma antibody in the presence of a positive dye test titer probably excludes the diagnosis of acute toxoplasmosis in an immunologically normal patient. A rising IgM fluorescent antibody titer or a titer of 1:512 or more appears to correlate well with recent onset of infection. Most of the serologic tests, including experimental techniques, are available through state health department laboratories and the Center for Disease Control.

The IgM fluorescent antibody test and the quantitative measurement of IgM in cord or fetal blood have proved helpful in diagnosing congenital toxoplasmosis. However, the absence of IgM antibodies in the neonatal period does not rule out congenital toxoplasma infection; repetitive testing in a suspected case is necessary.

At present there is no way to reliably detect all pregnancies at risk or all neonates at risk. Although serologic testing is of value in selected cases, the high incidence of antibody in the general population diminishes the value of a serologic screening program such as that used in syphilis detection. Mothers with clinical and serologic evidence of recently acquired infection should be carefully followed up and tested during pregnancy, and their offspring should be carefully followed up clinically and serologically.

Treatment of acquired infection in the nonpregnant patient is rarely indicated. There is no indication that a woman infected before conception requires chemotherapy or consideration of therapeutic abortion. There are no reliable guidelines to the best treatment of the woman who acquires infection during pregnancy. Since the risk of serious congenital disease is small but undeniably present, the decision to perform a therapeutic abortion depends on other factors. There are indications that the use of drugs active against toxoplasma during pregnancy may reduce the frequency of fetal infection and abortion. Until further data are available on the efficacy and safety of drugs such as spiramycin and pyrimethamine in pregnant women with toxoplasmosis, such treatment should be considered experimental and is not indicated for general use. Sulfonamides can be given safely if toxoplasmosis develops early in pregnancy; however, the results of such therapy are not clear.[26]

Because cats serve as a reservoir of toxoplasma, the obstetrician should inquire about their presence in the home. A pregnant woman with exposure to cats should be alerted to the potential risk of toxoplasma infection. It might be well for the clinician to obtain serologic tests for toxoplasmosis in such women. If the patient has not yet acquired toxoplasmosis, the physician should attempt to dissuade the patient from maintaining close contact with cats. The passionate regard many cat lovers have for their animals may preclude appropriate preventive measures.

MALARIA

Human malaria is caused by four *Plasmodium* species transmitted from man to man by anopheline mosquitoes. It remains a worldwide health problem. Infected human beings may carry the organism from endemic areas to areas where further transmission may occur by blood transfusion, shared needles among drug addicts, and native anopheline mosquito vectors. Special concern has followed the appearance of plasmodia resistant to many first-line antimalarial drugs.

Following inoculation of sporozoites from the mosquito salivary glands, the parasite multiplies in the liver. The culmination of this exoerythrocytic phase is the release of merozoites into the blood stream. Invasion of red blood cells by merozoites begins the cycle of growth and multiplication (schizogony), which results in destruction of the parasitized erythrocyte. When a sufficient concentration of parasites is reached in the blood, the clinical cycle of periodic fever begins. Each of the four human species — *P. falciparum, P. malariae, P. vivax,* and *P. ovale* — has its characteristic cycle and morphologic appearance, which are used for diagnosis. These features are well described in standard references.

Infection with *P. falciparum* is the most serious and life-threatening. Unlike the other species, *P. falciparum* parasitizes erythrocytes of any age and is able to reach extraordinarily high concentrations of parasites in the blood. Large numbers of parasitized red cells have altered rheologic and immunologic properties, which contribute to the life-threatening complications of black water fever, pulmonary edema, and cerebral malaria that occur almost exclusively with *P. falciparum* infection. In the past decade the problem caused by resistance of falciparum malaria to antimalarials has expanded. The geographic range of resistant falciparum has increased so that resistant organisms may be found in enlarging areas of Southeast Asia, Africa, South America, and the Pacific Islands. The organism has acquired resistance to an even larger number of drugs. Among the refugees of Southeast Asia, falciparum malaria has become resistant not only to chloroquine but also to sulfonamide and pyrimethamine (Bascom et al, 1980). These events have major implications for prophylaxis and therapy.

In endemic areas infection occurs in childhood, and cellular and humoral immunity is presumed to be responsible for the reduction in the severity of repeated clinical attacks. The new strains of *P. falciparum* seem to have undergone antigenic variation as well as changes in drug susceptibility. Even lifelong residents of areas where resistant falciparum species are now prevalent are susceptible to devastating clinical disease. Nonimmune travelers can be expected to have more severe clinical disease from any of the human malaria organisms than immune residents. Malaria acquired during pregnancy may be less dangerous to a mother with a high degree of immunity than to a nonimmune mother.

Some evidence suggests that pregnancy exerts a dampening effect on immunity to malaria.[22] Latent malaria is said to persist during pregnancy and to become active during parturition and lactation.[31] Clinical reports indicate that attacks of malaria during pregnancy, especially falciparum malaria, may be particularly severe.[12, 36, 40, 42] This writer's experience with stable, well-nourished refugees in Southeast Asia suggests that falciparum malaria, because of its intrinsic ability to produce overwhelming parasitemia and because of the appearance of new antigenic and resistant strains, is a serious threat to the pregnant woman, regardless of her nutritional and immune status. Premature labor, stillbirth, and transplacental infection resulting in congenital malaria have occurred only with drug-resistant falciparum malaria infection of mothers without prior exposure to the resistant strains.

There is a gradient of clinical illness caused by malaria during pregnancy. The most severe illness occurs in women not immune to the most virulent plasmodia, namely, drug-resistant *P. falciparum*. Moderately severe disease — fever, anemia, fetal growth retardation, and congenital fetal infection — occurs in nonimmune women with drug-sensitive plasmodia infection. An immune mother with reactivated latent disease can be expected to have mild illness with placental infection and no fetal infection, whereas a nonimmune mother with acquired drug-sensitive malaria may have near-fatal clinical disease with a high risk of fetal loss. The mother's immune status appears to modulate both the clinical expression of the infection with drug-sensitive organisms and the effectiveness of the placenta as a barrier to fetal infection.

In the neonate, congenital malaria infection becomes manifest 48 to 72 hours after birth with fever, hepatosplenomegaly, jaundice, anemia, seizures, and occasionally pulmonary edema.

Neonatal malaria may follow parasitemia caused by mechanical disturbances to the colonized placenta during labor and delivery.

The best prophylaxis is not to go to malarious places! Pregnancy is a contraindication to travel or residence in areas known to have drug-resistant *P. falciparum*. Conscientious chemoprophylaxis during and after travel to endemic malarious areas is mandatory if traveling cannot be postponed until after delivery. The standard chemoprophylactic regimen is 500 mg of chloroquine phosphate by mouth once a week, beginning 1 week before departure to an endemic area and continued for 8 weeks after departing from the endemic area. Chloroquine alone suppresses the erythrocytic phase of infection but does not affect the liver or tissue phase, hence the necessity for continuing chloroquine prophylaxis for 2 months after leaving a malarious area.

All antimalarial agents have potentially adverse effects upon the fetus. Chloroquine produces retinal and cochleovestibular damage, quinine is ototoxic and mildly oxytocic, and primaquine causes hemolysis in susceptible individuals as well as methemoglobinemia. Nonimmune mothers insisting upon travel to malarious places should be given chemoprophylaxis and advice about the risks of the drugs and the infection. The patient should not be allowed to overlook the need for taking precautions against mosquitoes: insect repellent and mosquito netting.

In nonimmune mothers, clinical attacks of malaria during pregnancy should be treated promptly. Except for drug-resistant *P. falciparum,* the recommended treatment is chloroquine phosphate, 1 gm initially, followed by 0.5 gm after 6 hours, and then once a day for 2 days. Because all species except *P. falciparum* have a prolonged exoerythrocytic, or hepatic, phase, primaquine phosphate, 26.3 mg by mouth daily for 14 days, should be given to prevent relapses of malaria from *P. vivax*, *P. malariae*, and *P. ovale*. However, it should be used with caution, preferably after delivery.

Antimalarial treatment during pregnancy may reduce the maternal antibody response and transplacental transfer of malaria antibody[13] as well as correct maternal anemia and fetal growth retardation.[42]

Falciparum malaria is a medical emergency. Drug-resistant *P. falciparum* should be treated with a regimen of multiple drugs including quinine. Additional drugs include pyrimethamine, sulfonamides, and dapsone. Prophylaxis for drug-resistant *P. falciparum* during pregnancy requires the use of folic acid metabolism inhibitors such as pyrimethamine, which has risks to both the mother and fetus.

Trypanosomiasis

African trypanosomiasis, caused by *Trypanosoma gambiense* and *Trypanosoma rhodesiense*, is transmitted to man by the bite of the tsetse fly. American trypanosomiasis, or Chagas' disease, caused by *Trypanosoma cruzi*, is transmitted to man by the bite of reduviid bugs *(Triatoma)*. Trypanosomes multiply locally and in regional reticuloendothelial tissue. During this early febrile phase, widespread dissemination occurs via lymphatics and the blood stream. *T. cruzi* invade cells, assuming a leishmanial form, which produces characteristic involvement of the heart and gastrointestinal tract. Infection with *T. cruzi* is followed by serious acute or chronic disease in only a small minority of the population at risk. The clinical manifestations of acute infection appear to be, in part, a manifestation of developing host immune response. Chronic Chagas' disease develops insidiously in patients with no history of acute disease. The African trypanosomes do not invade cells. These organisms undergo antigenic variations, which contributes to the relative ineffectiveness of host immune response and the variability in the inexorable clinical course.[46] West African trypanosomiasis *(T. gambiense)* is characterized by lymphadenopathy and a slow progression of neurologic disease, whereas East African trypanosomiasis *(T. rhodesiense)* has a more rapid progression of neurologic involvement, often without the helpful clinical clue of lymphadenopathy. Animal reservoirs, including man, are important aspects of their epidemiology.

All of these organisms have the potential for transplacental transmission with resulting infection of the fetus during parasitemia. Asymptomatic parasitemia derived from intracellular foci is known to occur in chronic Chagas' disease. However, the risk of intrauterine infection appears to be greater in nonimmune patients with acute *T. cruzi* infections. Infective *T. cruzi* may be found in breast milk and may infect the infant by penetration of the skin, buccal mucosa, or the gastrointestinal tract. Fortunately these events are remarkably infrequent. African trypanosomiasis usually produces such severe, progressive disease that pregnancy is not possible. If it is acquired during pregnancy, abortion, premature labor, and stillbirth may occur. East African trypanosomiasis usually kills those afflicted in a matter of weeks or months, before gestation can be completed.

The diagnosis should be suspected in patients with unexplained febrile illnesses acquired during residence or travel in areas of trypanosome endemicity. Examination of blood and lymph node tissue may demonstrate the organism. Because parasitemia is intermittent in chronic Chagas' disease, the diagnosis may be accomplished by serologic techniques.

There is no effective treatment for the intracellular leishmanial stage of chronic Chagas' disease. Acute Chagas' disease may be treated with an experimental agent, Nifurtimox (Bayer 2502), available from the Center for Disease Control. Amniocentesis, when appropriate, may indicate whether the fetus is infected. Should the nonimmune pregnant patient have evidence of myocarditis or meningoencephalitis with acute Chagas' disease, treatment should be started. The mortality of acute Chagas' disease ranges from 5 to 10 per cent. With mild clinical disease, the decision to treat may be helped by amniocentesis demonstrating infection of the fetus.

The pregnant woman unfortunate enough to acquire African trypanosomiasis should be treated with suramin or pentamidine. Since these drugs do not penetrate the central nervous system effectively, arsenicals may need to be used when the central nervous system is involved. The inexorable progression of the disease in the mother obviates consideration of withholding treatment until after pregnancy.

Trekking through African national parks where the game is the reservoir of *T. rhodesiense* has become increasingly popular. Pregnant women should be discouraged from participating in such excursions. There seems to be little to be gained by using pentamidine prophylactically.[6] If the pregnant patient must travel to an endemic area, she should exercise due caution about the bites of tsetse flies.

Leishmaniasis

Leishmaniasis has three distinct clinical forms caused by protozoans of the genus *Leishmania*. Visceral or systemic leishmaniasis (kala-azar) is caused by *L. donovani;* cutaneous leishmaniasis (Oriental sore) by *L. tropica;* and mucocutaneous leishmaniasis (American leishmaniasis) by *L. brasiliensis* and *L. mexicana*. Each clinical variety has a distribution coincident with the insect vector, species of sand flies *(Phlebotomus),* and an animal reservoir. Transmission is usually by the bite of an infected insect vector, but occasionally infection may result from venereal contact or animal bites. Only kala-azar has a well-documented parasitemia, and it is the only form of leishmaniasis reported to cause intrauterine fetal infection.[30] Infection by *L. donovani* acquired during pregnancy is said to be associated with increased fetal loss.

The appearance of fever and hepatosplenomegaly as much as two years after travel or residence in an endemic area should suggest the possibility of kala-azar. The diagnosis is established by demonstrating organisms in blood or reticuloendothelial tissue or with culture on appropriate media. Indolent ulcerations appearing on exposed skin within months of travel or residence in an endemic area should suggest the possibility of one of the cutaneous forms of leishmaniasis. Because of the effects of drug therapy with pentavalent antimonials and diamidine compounds, chemotherapy should be given with caution.

AMEBIASIS

Amebiasis is transmitted from person to person. Although the prevalence of infection with *Entameba histolytica* is higher in areas with a warm, humid climiate, amebiasis is mistakenly regarded by many health workers as a tropical disease. Infections with *E. histolytica* occur wherever human beings inhabit the earth. Because people can carry the parasite without clinical manifestations, the total number of infected people is difficult to determine. Prevalence rates of clinical disease range from 1.5 per 100,000 persons in the United States to 458 per 100,000 in Venezuela.[34]

Infection is acquired by ingestion of cysts in fecally contaminated food or liquid. Once in the gut, the cysts rupture, and the released organisms multiply as trophozoites. The trophozoites inhabit the gut lumen but may also invade the gut wall. Invasion of the large intestinal wall is the precursor of visceral amebic infection. Trophozoites are usually encysted by the time they are excreted in the feces; however, in the presence of diarrhea and mucus production, motile trophozoites can be found in the fecal material.

The clinical spectrum of intestinal amebiasis ranges from the asymptomatic infection, identified only by the detection of cysts in the stool, to fulminant dysentery. The diarrheal stool almost always contains mucus and frequently blood. Sigmoidoscopic findings depend upon the severity of the infection. In severe cases the small openings of the classical "flask-shaped" ulcerations may become extensive ulcerations covered with chronic exudate. Constitutional signs and symptoms — malaise, anorexia, weight loss, abdominal cramps — may be highly variable. Differential diagnoses include ulcerative or granulomatous colitis, nonspecific gastroenteritis, and bacterial dysentery.

Intestinal amebiasis may progress to extraintestinal involvement by perforation of the bowel wall or by metastasis of trophozoites via the portal venous system or lymphatics. Direct extension through the bowel wall is regularly preceded by clinically apparent intestinal infection. Metastasis, usually to the liver, may develop without premonitory symptoms; indeed, the patient with amebic liver abscess may have negative stool examinations for amebic trophozoites and cysts. Hematogenous dissemination of trophozoites from hepatic foci of infection is presumed to be the root of infection to the pleura, the pericardium, and the central nervous system. Visceral disease is usually accompanied by constitutional symptoms, weight loss, and fever.

The organism can be transmitted by sexual practices involving anorectal penetration or oral-anal contact. Cutaneous amebiasis is rare and results from direct contamination of the skin with trophozoites. In the female, genital amebic lesions are painful, deep ulcerations covered with necrotic debris. Local destruction may be quite severe and disfiguring.

Asymptomatic carriage with passage of cysts is the most common clinical type of amebiasis. The pathogenetic relationship between the asymptomatic carrier state and active disease is not well understood. Estimates of clinical disease occurring among asymptomatic carriers range from 10 to 50 per cent. Infected patients may be asymptomatic for long periods of time only to develop sudden, catastrophic bowel and liver disease.

Immunosuppression, malnutrition, and pregnancy have been reported to predispose to severe clinical disease and to transform the asymptomatic carrier into an ill patient. Corticosteroids and progesterone have been found to exacerbate disease in experimental animal infections. Several reports have indicated that pregnancy may increase the severity of amebic infections with a disturbingly high incidence of maternal mortality.[1, 4, 29, 38] Similarly, there is some evidence that amebiasis during pregnancy may have an adverse effect upon the fetus and the successful completion of gestation.[16] *Entamoeba histolytica* is not known to cause intrauterine and fetal infection, presumably because it rarely escapes the portal circulation. Amebic liver abscess is an unusually rare complication of pregnancy.[14] Amebic dysentery may result in pelvic adhesions or may contribute to infertility.

Demonstrating the organism in fecal material remains the only specific laboratory procedure for the diagnosis of amebiasis. Examination of freshly passed mucus allows identification of motile, hematophagous trophozoites. Stains and concentration techniques are useful for detecting cysts. Aspiration or biopsy of ulcers via the sigmoidoscope often proves a reliable method of obtaining clinically useful material for study. The importance of experienced laboratory personnel cannot be overstressed; one or two careful examinations of fecal material by reliable observers proves more effective than many examinations by inexperienced workers.

Serologic tests are not helpful in diagnosing intestinal infection without tissue invasion. Extraintestinal visceral involvement and deep intestinal wall involvements are usually accompanied by detectable antibody rises measured by hemagglutination or complement fixation tests. These tests, available through state health department laboratories and the Center for Disease Control, are reliable and readily accessible to the clinician. Radioisotope techniques have proved helpful in localizing hepatic, thoracic and central nervous system lesions; however, during pregnancy ultrasonography is an effective and less potentially hazardous technique for identifying abscesses. Aspiration or biopsy of abscesses or effusions provides material for direct microscopic visualization of trophozoites. Aspiration or biopsy should not be done without concomitant antiamebic therapy in order to prevent complications from local cutaneous spread or more widespread dissemination.

The cyst stage is resistant to many physical and chemical agents. Chemotherapy is directed against trophozoites in the intestinal lumen or mucosa and against organisms in visceral abscesses. A confusing variety of drugs is available; some are active against both intestinal and visceral infection, and some are effective only against intestinal disease. The treatment regimen must be designed for the location and severity of the patient's infection, according to three general categories: first, the asymptomatic carrier and mild intestinal infection; second, acute or chronic amebic dysentery, and third, amebic hepatitis and abscess. Pregnant patients with amebiasis should be treated during pregnancy because of the risk of the development of more severe disease.

The asymptomatic infected person passing cysts harbors trophozoites, and treatment for these patients is the same as the treatment for mild symptomatic intestinal amebiasis. The preferred agent is usually diiodohydroxyquin or diloxanide furoate. Diloxanide furoate is available only through the Center for Disease Control. Because of uncertainties about the effects of these drugs during pregnancy, the clinician should first use paromomycin (Humatin), a poorly absorbed aminoglycoside antibiotic, which is active against lumenal amebae and the gut bacteria necessary for *E. histolytica* to persist. The patient should be carefully followed up after treatment to ensure that cyst passage does not persist. If there is evidence of recurrence, the patient should be re-treated.

The patient passing mucus and blood and having symptoms of colitis is usually treated with at least two drugs, one active against trophozoites in the lumen and superficial mucosa; the other active against trophozoites invading the deeper layers of the colon and possibly other viscera. The luminal agent can be paromomycin, diiodohydroxyquin, or diloxanide. Most experts recommend metronidazole or another nitroimidazole as the extralumenal drug. Although metronidazole has been used without ill effect in a number of pregnancies, it has been shown to be mutagenic and possibly carcinogenic. The teratogenic effects, while hypothetical, are sufficient to warrant cautious deliberation before using the drug in pregnancy. Chloroquine phosphate in a dose of 1 gram daily for 2 days and then 0.5 grams daily for 2 to 3 weeks can be used instead of metronidazole. However, chloroquine may have adverse effects upon the fetal retina and cochlea. It may be wise, therefore, to treat the pregnant patient first with luminally active drugs alone. After completion of therapy, the physician should reevaluate the patient's condition. In the absence of persistent or metastatic infection, additional therapy can be withheld and the patient monitored at frequent intervals for evidence of recurrent or metastatic amebic infection. Should this occur, the patient should be re-treated with luminally active drugs and serious consideration given to using the standard recommendations for adding extraluminally active drugs.

As a rule, patients with ameboma, hepatitis, or abscess are seriously ill, and therapy with potentially harmful drugs is justifiable. Metronidazole is used in a dose of 750 mg three times a day for 7 to 10 days. Chloroquine phosphate can also be used. A third group of tissue-active drugs, emetine and dehydroemetine, possesses considerable cardiac toxicity. Visceral abscess often requires drainage as well as chemotherapy for maximally effective treatment. This should be carried out by needle aspiration.

GIARDIASIS

The flagellate *Giardia lamblia* may infect the duodenum, producing a spectrum of clinical illness ranging from no symptoms to severe diarrhea with malabsorption. Giardiasis is usually an illness with few, poorly defined symptoms (malaise, easy fatigue, and vague abdominal discomfort), occasionally with mild to moderate diarrhea characterized by bulky, foul-smelling stools. Like amebiasis, it is ubiquitous among human beings and has a resistant cyst stage, which is transmitted by the fecal-oral route. Epidemics occur; acquisition of the parasite has been particularly common in some cities in Europe and North America and in areas with poor sanitation.[5, 20, 44] Beavers have been identified as an animal reservoir in some North American outbreaks. Giardiasis is therefore one of the many causes of traveler's diarrhea. The association of giardiasis with nodular lymphoid hyperplasia of the small intestine and with IgA immunoglobulin deficiency is well documented.[2] It has been this writer's experience that chronic fatigue and vague gastrointestinal distress attributed to psychoneurosis or morning sickness may be due to giardiasis. Malabsorption may impair fertility and adversely affect the outcome of the pregnancy. When detected, giardiasis should serve as the stimulus to search for an underlying immunoglobulin disorder.

Diagnosis may be difficult. Cysts can be found in stool, but concentration techniques are usually necessary. Motile trophozoites can be found in duodenal aspirates. Occasional nonspecific abnormalities are found on barium examination of the upper gastrointestinal tract or in small bowel biopsies. There are no reliable serologic tests for *Giardia lamblia* infection.

Treatment should be individualized. Mild clinical disease may not require treatment. Quinacrine and metronidazole are about equally effective in treating giardiasis; however, they should be used in pregnancy only with great caution and clear indication. Quinacrine (Atabrine), 100 mg three times a day for 5 to 7 days, is the preferred treatment during pregnancy when clinical disease is hazardous to the pregnancy.

Pneumocystis carinii INFECTION

Pneumocystis carinii is a protozoan of uncertain taxonomy that causes a diffuse, interstitial pneumonia in premature infants and immunoincompetent hosts. It is widespread throughout nature. Epidemics of *Pneumocystis* pneumonia in nurseries have resulted from airborne spread of the organism from an asymptomatic carrier. Instances of transplacental transmission have been reported. A complement fixation test can be used to detect some carriers. In patients with pneumonia, demonstration of the organism in lung biopsy of aspirated material is the preferred diagnostic method. Therapy with trimethoprim-sulfa or Pentamidine isethionate has given satisfactory results.

HELMINTHIC INFECTIONS

Worms parasitizing human beings can be found virtually everywhere that human beings live, but there is a particular abundance of parasitic worms in the tropics. There are two important groups of parasitic worms: (1) roundworms, or Nematoda, and (2) flatworms, or Platyhelminthes. The flatworms include the trematodes, or flukes, and the cestodes, or tapeworms. Almost without exception, helminths do not multiply in the human host, in contrast to disease-producing organisms that can complete their life cycle within a single host. An increase in the number of helminthic parasites in the host is almost always impossible; reproduction requires completion of the life cycle outside the human host. The size of the infestation is dependent upon the number of infective parasites the host initially acquired and therefore upon the length and frequency of exposure to the infective stage of the worm. For the careful traveler the risk of acquiring a large number of worms is relatively small. These organisms require special conditions for survival, multiplication, and successful parasitization of the human host: appropriate temperature and humidity; particular vertebrate or invertebrate hosts, such as fish, snails, crustacea, or insects; and permissive cultural and sanitary customs. For example, the practice of using human feces for fertilizer combined with food habits such as eating raw fish, shellfish, meat, or aquatic plants provides the setting for several successful human parasitic worms. Similarly the practice of storing night soil–fertilized root vegetables in weak brine or vinegar solutions allows for transmission of *Ascaris, Trichuris,* and hookworm because the eggs are not killed by weak salt or acid solutions.

The mechanisms of disease in the human host are also complex and may not be due to the adult worm itself but rather to ova or larvae produced by the worm. For example, the disease produced by schistosomes is the result of inflammation produced by the eggs or cercaria. Some worms produce disease in the course of migration of the larvae or adult worms; others localize in the lymphatics and produce lymphatic obstruction subsequent to acute and chronic inflammation. Intestinal helminths may compete with the host for essential nutrition or may deplete the host of iron by consuming blood or inducing bleeding.

Intestinal Nematodes

Parasitic roundworms of the intestinal tract (Table 16–4) are some of the most geographically widespread helminths. Maternal infection by intestinal roundworms is almost always a benign nuisance except when there is a heavy worm burden. None of the intestinal helminths is known to have a stage that crosses the placenta and causes intrauterine infection of the fetus. Egg excretion in the feces is readily quantifiable, and quantitative evaluation is useful for estimating the number of infecting worms. Infection with many different parasites is common, and the clinician should thoroughly examine the patients infected with one nematode for other intestinal nematodes.

ENTEROBIASIS

Enterobius vermicularis, the pinworm, has a simple life cycle: ingested infective eggs hatch into larvae that mature into adults without leaving the gut lumen. The fertilized female remains in the cecum until she becomes full of eggs. After migrating from the anus, she discharges her eggs and deposits them on the perianal skin. The worms become mature 3 to 4 weeks after ingestion of eggs. The eggs are infective within a few hours of deposition, making autoinfection possible. Because the eggs can remain viable and infective for 7 to 10 days and are widely disseminated in the environment of the infected person, pinworms are usually a family affair. Infection is detected more frequently in children than in adults. There is a high incidence of asymptomatic infection. Pruritus ani and pruritus vulvae are the usual clinical manifestations of pinworm infection.

Migrant female worms may ascend the vagina to the pelvic peritoneum, producing vaginitis[18] and, rarely, acute granulomatous pelvic inflammatory disease.[11] Pregnancy may exacerbate symptoms of vaginitis and pruritus vulvae.

Mebendazole, the preferred treatment, should not be used during pregnancy. Pyrvinium pamoate and pyrantel pamoate are acceptable alternate drugs.

TRICHURIASIS

Trichuris trichiura, the whipworm, is a cosmopolitan parasite of the human large intestine, most abundant in warm, moist climates. The geographic distribution of whipworm infection coincides with that of ascariasis and hookworm infections. Infection is acquired by ingesting embryonated eggs, which are not infective until at least 10 days after passage in the feces. As with *Enterobius vermicularis,* there is no extraintestinal larval migration.

Clinical manifestations of *Trichuris* infection are related to the size of the worm burden: light infections are asymptomatic; heavy infections, especially in children, may produce diarrhea with mucus, rectal bleeding, abdominal pain, and malaise. Severe infections with dysentery and tenesmus can produce rectal prolapse. Bleeding from a heavy infection may be sufficient to produce iron deficiency anemia. Other than this

TABLE 16–4 INTESTINAL NEMATODES

Parasite	Infective Stage	Mode of Transmission	Adult Habitat	Drug of Choice and Dose in Nonpregnant Patient	Indications for Treatment During Pregnancy
Enterobius vermicularis (Pinworms)	Egg	Ingestion	Cecum	Mebendazole, 100 mg PO single dose	None
Trichuris trichiura	Egg	Ingestion	Colon	Mebendazole, 100 mg PO b.i.d. × 3	Rectal prolapse; blood loss
Ascaris lumbricoides	Mature egg	Ingestion	Small intestine	Mebendazole, 100 mg PO b.i.d. × 3	Worm obstruction; risk of neonatal infection
HOOKWORM *Necator americanus Ancylostoma duodenale*	Larvae	Skin penetration	Small intestine	Mebendazole, 100 mg PO b.i.d. × 3	Heavy infestation; anemia or malnutrition not responding to supportive therapy
Strongyloides stercoralis	Larvae	Skin or colon mucosa penetration	Small intestine	Thiabendazole, 25 mg/kg b.i.d. × 2	Presence of infection

unusual circumstance, whipworm infections pose little threat to pregnancy. The diagnosis is made by the discovery and quantifying of *Trichuris* eggs. The preferred treatment is mebendazole, which should be used after delivery.

ASCARIASIS

Ascaris lumbricoides is the largest of the intestinal nematodes, and passage of a mature worm can be an unforgettable experience for the patient. Human infection is widespread, especially in areas with considerable fecal contamination of the soil. Under appropriate conditions, the eggs become infective in about 3 weeks. Ingestion of infective embryonated eggs is followed by hatching in the intestine and penetration of the larvae through the intestinal mucosa into the portal vein radicals and intestinal lymphatics. The bloodborne phase terminates when the larvae penetrate into the alveolus, migrate up the tracheobronchial tree, and are swallowed. Maturation to the adult state occurs in the small intestine. A new generation of eggs appears in the feces 8 to 12 weeks after the ingestion of infective *Ascaris* eggs. The majority of *Ascaris* infections involve only a few worms and are not clinically apparent.[35]

Rarely, a single adult worm may migrate to an anatomically important area such as the biliary or pancreatic ducts or the appendix, or it may perforate the intestine, thus producing clinically apparent disease. With heavy infestation, the chances for migration of adult worms are commensurately increased. An unusual complication is intestinal obstruction by a bolus of several worms. When many eggs are ingested, the larval migration through the lungs may be accompanied by a spectrum of symptoms. Nocturnal cough and peripheral eosinophilia are the most frequent findings; occasionally the patient may have fever, persistent cough, rales and wheezes, and transient diffuse infiltrates on chest x-ray. Adult worms can invade the female genital tract[18] and cause tubo-ovarian abscess, pelvic pain, and menorrhagia. Infection with *Ascaris* may exacerbate nutritional deficiency in patients with marginal or inadequate nutrition.

The diagnosis is established by demonstration of the characteristic eggs in the stool, the recovery of an adult worm, or identification of larvae in sputum or gastric aspirates.

Pyrantel pamoate should be used to treat intestinal infection during pregnancy. There is no specific chemotherapy for the larval migration. Treatment during early pregnancy should be given only to mothers with heavy worm burdens.

The lightly infected mother should be treated immediately before or after delivery because of the risk of infecting her newborn.

HOOKWORM

Hookworm infection is widespread throughout the tropical and subtropical areas of the world. It is caused by infection of the small intestine by *Ancylostoma duodenale* (the old-world hookworm) or *Necator americanus* (the new-world hookworm).

Adult worms live attached to the mucosa of the small intestine. During its life, the female worm produces large numbers of eggs each day: 6000 to 11,000 for *Necator,* 15,000 to 20,000 for *Ancylostoma.* The eggs are passed in the feces, and under suitable conditions they hatch in 24 to 48 hours, liberating rhabditiform larvae. During the next 7 to 10 days the larvae undergo three molts and become infective or filariform larvae. Under ideal circumstances the filariform larvae can remain viable and infective for as long as 6 months. Man becomes infected by penetration of filariform larvae through the skin. Contact with contaminated soil for at least 5 to 10 minutes is required for skin penetration. Infection can also follow ingestion of infective larvae, which can penetrate the buccal and gastrointestinal mucosa. The larvae are carried by the blood to the lungs, where they emerge in the alveoli, ascend the tracheobronchial tree, and are swallowed. Maturation to adulthood occurs in the small intestine. Fertile eggs appear in the stool 5 weeks or more after invasion of the host by infective larvae.

The parasite's larvae flourish in climates providing warm temperatures, adequate rainfall, and well-drained soil. Heavy infections occur when people frequent the same fecally contaminated area repeatedly. *Necator* is the most prevalent in the Americas and central and southern Africa. Endemic foci persist in the southern United States, Puerto Rico, and other Caribbean islands. *Ancylostoma* is the most prevalent hookworm in Asia, the Malay Archipelago, and the Mediterranean littoral. There is overlap of the two species in many parts of the world.

The clinical manifestations of hookworm infection are dependent upon the stage of infection and the number of invading parasites. Invasion of the skin by infective larvae may be accompanied by a pruritic vesiculopapular rash on the exposed skin, the so-called ground itch. Migration of larvae from lung to gastrointestinal tract may cause cough, wheezing, symptoms of pharyngitis, fever, and eosinophilia. The attachment of larvae to the gastrointestinal mucosa may be accompanied by abdominal discomfort and gastroenteritis.

The chronic manifestations of hookworm infection are directly proportional to the number of worms and are related to the protein and blood loss caused by the parasites. Depending upon the species, each adult worm can extract 0.03 to 0.26 ml of blood per day. The host can recover less than half the iron and very little of the protein or other nutrients taken by the parasite. With light infection, for example 50 to 100 worms, there is a blood loss of about 30 ml or less per day. With heavy infection, for example 300 worms or more, the victim may sustain a blood loss of 80 ml or more per day. There is a rough correlation between the quantitative egg count and the amount of blood lost: about 2 ml of blood per day per 1000 eggs per gram of feces.[32] Only if egg counts exceed 5000 per gram of feces, roughly equivalent to five or more eggs per low power microscope field on a stool smear, is the infection likely to have clinical significance. Victims with good nutritional status and adequate intake and storage of iron tolerate a light to moderate worm burden better than marginally nourished patients. A previously asymptomatic hookworm infection may become clinically important under conditions producing increased iron needs, such as pregnancy and lactation.[28]

Other essential nutritional factors can occasionally be depleted by hookworm infection. Edema may result from hypoproteinemia if the host is unable to increase hepatic albumin production. Folic acid and vitamin B_{12} deficiency have also been reported. The clinical manifestations of severe hookworm disease are primarily those of anemia and malnutrition: weakness, malaise, anasarca, and high output cardiac failure. Vague abdominal complaints, "ground itch," and rare respiratory symptoms are unpleasant but are not of themselves dangerous to the pregnant patient.

Hookworm infection is often accompanied by other parasitic infections. The evaluation of the clinical importance of hookworm infection, therefore, requires both quantitation of the hookworm infection and careful study of the host for any other fellow travelers.

In the absence of anemia and malnutrition, hookworm infection during pregnancy should be watched and not treated. Patients with mild anemia and light to moderate worm burdens may be managed by vigorous hematinic and diet therapy during pregnancy and by withholding drug therapy until after delivery. In the pregnant patient with severe hypoproteinemia and anemia, replacement of iron, vitamins, and protein (including transfusions) is appropriate. Specific hookworm chemotherapy is indicated only if there is an inadequate response to vigorous nutritional therapy and supportive care. Mebendazole is the drug of choice; 100 mg twice a day is given for 3 days and produces a 95 per cent cure rate or reduction of egg count. Mebendazole is not well absorbed from the gastrointestinal tract and probably poses only a small hazard to the mother and fetus. However, it has been teratogenic in animals. When parenteral replacement therapy and transfusions are not available, the patient should be treated with mebendazole and vigorous oral replacement therapy. Pyrantel pamoate is a good alternative drug for the pregnant patient.

STRONGYLOIDIASIS

Stronglyloides stercoralis is the only common parasitic nematode capable of completing its life cycle in the human host. Hyperinfection with potentially fatal complications can occur, especially with alterations in the host's immune status like those that may occur in pregnancy. Strongyloidiasis is, therefore, the only intestinal roundworm for which therapy is recommended regardless of the clinical status of the patient.

Like hookworm, *Strongyloides* filariform larvae penetrate the skin, migrate via the blood stream to the lungs, escape into the alveoli, ascend to the trachea, and then are swallowed. After about 4 weeks, adult females begin to deposit eggs in the duodenum and the upper jejunum. The eggs may mature and release larvae, which metamorphose into infective filariform larvae within the gastrointestinal tract. These larvae may then penetrate the intestinal mucosa to start the life cycle again. Because of the repetitive larval migration, persistent eosinophilia is a prominent feature of the disease. The large numbers of adult worms inhabiting the proximal small intestine may produce malabsorption, protein-losing enteropathy, and iron deficiency anemia.

Strongyloidiasis is not uncommon in temperate zones, especially among institutionalized populations. The diagnosis may require duodenal aspiration for identification of *S. stercoralis* larvae, especially if the majority of eggs produce infective larvae before passage in the feces. Thiabendazole is the only effective drug and should be given in a dose of 25 mg per kg twice a day for 2 days.

TABLE 16-5 TISSUE NEMATODES

Parasite	Vector/Mode of Transmission	Distribution	Major Clinical Manifestations
Trichinella spiralis	Ingestion of infective larval cysts	Worldwide	Eosinophilia, myopathy, fever, meningoencephalitis; possible intrauterine infection
Angiostrongylus cantonensis	Ingestion of infected mollusks or crustaceans	Southeast Asia	Eosinophilia, meningitis
Dracunculus medinensis	Ingestion of infected copepods in drinking water	Africa, Middle East, India	Chronic ulcers
Dirofilaria immitis	Mosquito	Zoonotic infection of dogs, throughout USA	Pulmonary nodules
Toxocara canis *Toxocara cati*	Dog and cat ascarid; ingestion of infective eggs	Worldwide	Visceral larva migrans
Ancylostoma braziliense *Ancylostoma caninum*	Dog and cat hookworm; ingestion of infective eggs	All tropical and subtropical areas	Cutaneous larva migrans (creeping eruption)
Filarial worms			
Wuchereria bancrofti	Mosquito	Africa, South America, Pacific and Caribbean islands	Chronic lymphadenopathy, lymphatic obstruction
Brugia malayi	Mosquito	Southeast Asia	Chronic lymphadenopathy, lymphatic obstruction
Onchocerca volvulus	Black flies (Simulium)	Central and South America, Africa	Skin rash, skin nodules, keratitis progressing to blindness
Loa loa	Tabanid flies (Chrysops)	Africa	Calabar swellings (Subcutaneous nodules)

Tissue Nematodes

A large number of roundworms parasitize the extraintestinal tissues of man (Table 16–5). All of these parasites have larval, microfilarial, or adult worm migrations within the body and therefore have the potential for invading the placenta and the fetus. However, most of them are not known to pose serious problems during pregnancy except insofar as they may affect general maternal health or injure the reproductive organs. Filariasis and trichinosis are the two tissue-invasive nematodes with documented effects upon pregnancy.

FILARIASIS

The adult worms of *Wuchereria bancrofti* and *Brugia malayi* inhabit the lymphatics and regional lymph nodes. The acute and chronic inflammations elicited by the adult worms produce obstructive inflammatory disease. Edema and ultimately elephantiasis may develop. This process may affect the breast, vulva, and pelvic organs, having an adverse effect upon fertility and lactation. Elephantiasis of the vulva may obstruct labor and necessitate abdominal delivery. Other late effects include chylothorax, chylous ascites, and chyluria when lymphatics rupture into body cavities. Pregnancy may exacerbate the edema and chyluria of filariasis. It has been suggested that filariasis may be associated with hydramnios.[45]

The adult female worm discharges microfilaria into the lymphatics. Microfilaremia commonly occurs at night, when mosquitoes are most likely to be biting. The microfilaria can invade the placenta and the fetus.[10] No ill effects are known to occur as a result of fetal microfilaremia.

The diagnosis is established by finding adult worms or microfilaria in tissue or blood. Early in the course of the disease, acute lymphadenitis and impressive eosinophilia may be found.

The treatment for obstructive elephantiasis of the birth canal is surgical.

Diethylcarbamazine (Hetrazan) may reduce the number of microfilaria in the blood and may kill adult worms. Chemotherapy may precipitate a transient widespread acute inflammatory response around the adult worm. If other filarial disease such as onchocerciasis coexists, a severe reaction with fever, skin rash, and acute keratitis and iritis may occur. Chemotherapy may reduce the severity of clinical filariasis during pregnancy. However, unless there are compelling reasons it is probably best not to treat until after delivery.

TRICHINOSIS

Thirty years ago trichinosis was one of the most common infections in the United States.[47] The parasite, *Trichinella spiralis,* is widespread throughout the temperate regions of the world wherever hogs are an important source of dietary protein. The worms enter the gastrointestinal tract as larvae encysted in undercooked muscle. After leaving the cyst, the larvae penetrate the duodenal and jejunal epithelium, where they mature. Females are fertilized within 5 to 7 days and then penetrate the intestinal mucosa to begin discharging larvae. In heavy infestations, large numbers of larvae circulate in the blood. The larvae leave the blood stream and invade striated muscles, where they encyst. Larvae lodging in nonmuscular tissue will not become infective. After about 6 months the cyst calcifies, but some encysted larvae may remain viable and infective for years. The most important reservoir for *T. spiralis* is the pig. However, many flesh-eating animals, including man, can serve as reservoirs. Since the advent of restrictions on the feeding methods of commercial hog feeders, recent large epidemics of trichinosis in the United States have been traced to the meat of game animals such as bears and walruses.

The clinical manifestations vary with the stage of the disease. Nausea, vomiting, diarrhea, and abdominal pain accompany the larval invasion of the small intestinal epithelium during the first few days of infection. About one week later when larval release and circulation in the blood begin, fever and eosinophilia develop. Larval invasion of muscle starts soon afterward and is accompanied by increasing fever, myalgia, periorbital edema, splinter hemorrhages, and rash. Larval migration into the central nervous system may produce meningoencephalitis and simulate a cerebral vascular accident.

Trichinosis may temporarily disrupt the normal menstrual cycle. The infection does not usually interfere with pregnancy, although rare instances of abortion, premature labor, and stillbirth have been recorded. Conversely, there is no evidence that pregnancy exacerbates the acute disease or the chronic stage of larval cyst carriage.

Two instances of possible intrauterine infection in human beings have been reported, as well as intrauterine infection in experimental animals.[21]

The diagnosis may be difficult to make in the early gastrointestinal stage of the illness. Fever, eosinophilia, and myalgia in a patient with a history of rare or raw meat ingestion should immediately suggest the diagnosis. Serologic tests may be helpful but are often not reactive during the early and more severe stages of the disease. Intradermal skin testing with trichinella antigen is not of great help. Demonstration of encysted larvae in biopsied muscle is diagnostic; however, the patient usually has a characteristic clinical syndrome at this point, including marked eosinophilia.

Treatment includes supportive care and, when severe illness occurs, corticosteroids to suppress the inflammatory response. Thiabendazole is active against the ingested larvae and if given immediately following ingestion of contaminated meat may abort the disease or reduce its clinical severity. Once larval migration in the blood stream and invasion of muscle begins, thiabendazole is ineffective.

TREMATODES

Flatworms, or flukes, are important human parasites that have complex life cycles involving aquatic snails as intermediate hosts. The schistosomes differ from other parasitic trematodes in that they are not hermaphroditic and they infect man by free-living cercariae. As a group, the schistosomes are the most important trematodes parasitizing man.

SCHISTOSOMIASIS (BILHARZIASIS)

The geographic distribution of the three species of parasitic schistosomes most commonly infecting man is determined by the intermediate snail host. Characteristics of the individual schistosome species determine the clinical diseases produced in the human host. *Schistosoma mansoni* is geographically the most widespread. It occurs throughout Africa, the Middle East, northern South America, and some of the Caribbean islands, notably Puerto Rico. *S. haematobium* is limited to Africa and the Middle East. *S. japonicum* is found only in areas of the Far East.

Water is the medium through which humans are infected. Cercariae are often present in the water only at certain times of the day. Occasionally, with heavy cercarial invasion, a pruritic erythematous papular eruption (swimmer's itch) may appear. After the worms mature in their respective venous locations, egg production begins. *S. mansoni* localizes in the mesenteric and hemorrhoidal veins, *S. japonicum* in the mesenteric and portal veins, and *S. haematobium* in the hemorrhoidal, pelvic, and the bladder venous plexuses. The eggs secrete enzymes that facilitate their migration from veins to

TABLE 16–6 SOME PARASITIC TREMATODES

Organism and Disease	Carrier of Infective Metacercaria	Hosts and Major Areas Organism is Found	Location in Host	Effects on Host	Symptoms
Fasciolopsis buski (fasciolopsiasis)	Water plants: water chestnut, water caltrop	Pigs and man; Asia, Southeast Asia, Malay Archipelago, Taiwan	Duodenum, jejunum	Ulceration, bleeding, eosinophilia, malabsorption	Abdominal pain, diarrhea, weight loss, anasarca
Clonorchis sinensis (clonorchiasis)	Fresh-water fish	Fish-eating mammals, including man; Japan, Korea, China, Southeast Asia	Biliary tract	Obstructive jaundice, fatty liver, cirrhosis	Abdominal pain, fever, eosinophilia, jaundice, hepatomegaly, anasarca due to hepatic cirrhosis
Fasciola hepatica (fascioliasis)	Water plants: watercress	Sheep, rarely in man; found wherever sheep are prevalent	Biliary tract, liver	Hepatitis, obstructive jaundice	Fever, eosinophilia, jaundice, hepatomegaly
Paragonimus westermani (paragonimiasis)	Fresh-water crustacea	Man, carnivorous mammals	Lung	Local inflammation and necrosis; cysts may rupture into bronchi or pleural space	Cough, hemoptysis, dyspnea

gut or bladder lumen. The eggs elicit an acute inflammatory response followed by a foreign body granulomatous response. When eggs ascend the portal or systemic venous system, an inflammatory response in the receptacle organ (liver, lung, central nervous system) is evoked.

In *S. mansoni* disease, symptoms are usually due to involvement of the liver and gastrointestinal tract. With *S. haematobium* infection the bladder, pelvic organs, and lower gastrointestinal tract are most commonly affected. *S. japonicum* infection is similar to *S. mansoni* in the organs affected, but it is a more virulent infection than the other two schistosomal diseases. The chronic phase of schistosome infection represents the progression of chronic inflammatory response to the eggs, with scarring and granuloma formation.

The acute phase is heralded clinically by urticaria, fever, and malaise. *S. mansoni* and *S. japonicum* can produce diarrhea with mucus and blood, accompanied by weight loss, abdominal pain, and an enlarging liver and spleen. The chronic phase is characterized by Banti's syndrome or polyposis of the colon. The acute phase of *S. haematobium* infection is characterized by hematuria; the organism may occasionally produce hepatosplenomegaly and diarrhea with blood and mucus. The chronic phase of *S. haematobium* infection is marked by polyposis and, ultimately, malignant change in bladder. A unique association between schistosomiasis and the chronic *Salmonella* carrier state has been observed with both *S. mansoni* and *S. haematobium*.

During pregnancy schistosomiasis may predispose the patient to anemia and malnutrition. Involvement of the urinary tract can result in chronic proteinuria, episodes of hematuria, and recurrent urinary tract infection. These patients must be monitored with frequent urine cultures and promptly treated with antibiotics in order to diminish the risk of acute pyelonephritis.

Eggs of both *S. mansoni* and *S. haematobium* are often found in the reproductive organs of the infected female.[3, 15, 19] Acute and chronic inflammation of the fallopian tubes can lead to salpingitis, infertility, and tubal pregnancies.[39] Similarly, lesions of the cervix, vagina, and vulva may impede intercourse, vaginal delivery, and fertility. Abortions in women with cervicitis due to schistosome eggs have been reported.[15] Bilharzial endometritis is very rare. Although schistosomiasis may adversely effect pregnancy, there is no evidence that pregnancy accelerates the development or increases the severity of schistosomal disease.

The majority of patients are infected with only a few worms and have minimal or no clinical disease. These patients also have small numbers of eggs in their tissues or feces. The diagnosis is established by demonstrating eggs in feces, urine, vaginal discharge, and tissue from rectum, bladder, and liver. Microscopic examination of ova in fresh feces, scrapings, or crushed tissue allows for species identification according to the presence, size, and location of the spine. Examination of ova in fresh material allows the identification of viable eggs, and therefore living egg-laying adults, by observing movements of the contained larva. Finding living eggs is an indication for treatment. Finding only dead eggs implies that egg laying has ceased and that antiparasitic treatment may not be necessary.

Treatment is directed at the living adult worms and the effects of egg-induced injury. Antiparasitic drugs include the organic antimony compounds, niridazole, hycanthone, and oxamnaquin. Chemotherapy should be withheld during pregnancy because of adverse reactions and drug toxicity. Surgical excision of obstructing granulomas may be necessary.

TREMATODES OTHER THAN SCHISTOSOMES

Nonschistosome trematodes parasitic for man have general similarities in life cycle, structure, and physiology (Table 16–6). They are all hermaphrodites, and each parasitizes a snail and then encysts on aquatic vegetation or in an aquatic animal that is ingested by man. These parasites are a much smaller public health problem than the schistosomes. None have specific adverse effects upon pregnancy, but all may impair maternal well-being. The important characteristics of disease produced by some of these trematodes are given in the table.

CESTODES

Human infection with tapeworms is of two types: parasitization of the small intestine by adult tapeworms and invasions of extraintestinal tissue by larval tapeworms.

INFECTION WITH ADULT TAPEWORMS

Human infection follows ingestion of raw or undercooked meat containing the larvae of *Taenia saginata* (the beef tapeworm), *Taenia solium* (the pork tapeworm), or *Diphyllobothrium latum* (the fish tapeworm). Infections occur where sanitary customs allow for transmission of eggs passed in human feces to the intermediate hosts — cows, hogs, fish. The larvae encyst in the flesh of the intermediate host, which is then consumed by man. Of the three tapeworms, *D. latum* has the most potential for adversely effecting pregnancy. The worm has high concentrations of folic acid and vitamin B_{12}, and competition for these essential nutrients with the pregnant woman may produce megaloblastic anemia. Infections with *T. solium* and *T. saginata* are usually asymptomatic. The diagnosis is made by finding proglottids or eggs in the stool. Treatment can be with quinacrine, niclosamide, or paromomycin. However, unless there are serious medical or psychologic problems because of the tapeworm, it is safest to withhold specific treatment until after delivery. The pregnant woman with anemia due to *D. latum* should receive both vitamin B_{12} and folic acid as well as other vitamins and minerals. If the megaloblastic anemia is severe, transfusions may be necessary.

INFECTION WITH LARVAL TAPEWORMS

Occasionally, human ingestion of *T. solium* eggs can be followed by the development of larvae that invade and encyst in muscles, heart, eyes, and brain. Small numbers of cysticerci usually do not produce symptoms; the diagnosis may be made by finding calcified cysts in soft tissues with x-ray examinations. Symptoms of a mass lesion or seizures may follow cerebral invasion with cysticerci.[8] A large inoculum can produce fatal cysticercosis characterized by high fever and profound eosinophilia. There is no effective treatment.

Man may serve as a casual intermediate host for the larvae of the carnivore tapeworm, *Echinococcus granulosus*. The usual intermediate hosts are sheep, deer, moose, and caribou. The disease is common in sheep-raising areas, where soil and foodstuffs may be contaminated by eggs passed in dog feces. The United States, Canada, Australia, New Zealand, Argentina, the Mediterranean countries, and the Middle East are known to be endemic for echinococcosis. Ingestion of infective eggs is followed by larval penetration in a variety of organs. Large hydatid cysts may develop, most commonly in the liver. Echinococcal cysts of the pelvic organs may rupture during pregnancy or labor with the risk of producing anaphylaxis and peritoneal dissemination of daughter cysts. Pelvic cysts may impair fertility and impede labor and delivery.[9] The diagnosis should be suggested by observation of a cystic mass and eosinophilia in a patient from an endemic area. The Casoni skin test and serologic tests can be very helpful in confirming the diagnosis. The treatment is surgical and involves killing the germinal layer of the cyst with dilute formalin or cryosurgical techniques, followed by careful excision of the entire cyst.

References

1. Abioye, A. A.: Fetal amoebic colitis in pregnancy and puerperium. J. Trop. Med. Hyg., 76:97, 1973.
2. Ament, M. D., and Rubin, C. E.: Relation of giardiasis to abnormal intestinal structure and function in gastrointestinal immunodeficiency syndromes. Gastroenterology, 62:216, 1972.
3. Arean, V. M.: Mason's schistosomiasis of the female genital tract. Am. J. Obstet. Gynecol., 72:1038, 1956.
4. Armon, P. J.: Amoebiasis in pregnancy and the puerperium. Br. J. Obstet. Gynecol., 85:264, 1978.
5. Babb, R. R., Peck, C. D., and Vescia, F. G.: Giardiasis. J.A.M.A., 217:1359, 1971.
6. Barrett-Connor, E.: Chemoprophylaxis of amebiasis and African trypanosomiasis. Ann. Intern. Med., 77:797, 1972.
7. Bascom, S., Hanson, K., Thompson, W., Heinichen, C. L., Paulissen, J. P., et al.: *Plasmodium falciparum* malaria contracted in Thailand resistant to chloroquine and sulfonamide-pyrimethamine. M.M.W.R., 29:493, 1980.
8. Bazley, W. S.: Maternal mortality due to *Cysticercus cerebri*. Obstet. Gynecol., 39:362, 1972.
9. Bickers, W. M.: Hydatid disease of the female pelvis. Am. J. Obstet. Gynecol., 107:477, 1970.
10. Bloomfield, R. D., Suarez, J. R., and Malangit, A. C.: Transplacental transfer of bancroftian filariasis. J. Nat. Med. Assoc., 70:597, 1978.
11. Brooks, T. J., Goetz, C. C., and Plauche, W. C.: Pelvic granuloma due to *Enterobius vermicularis*. J.A.M.A., 179:492, 1962.
12. Bruce-Chwatt, L. J.: Malaria in African infants and children in southern Nigeria. Ann. Trop. Med. Parasitol., 46:173, 1952.
13. Campbell, C. C., Martinez, J. M., and Collins, W. E.: Seroepidemiological studies of malaria in pregnant women and newborns

from coastal El Salvador. Am. J. Trop. Med. Hyg., 29:151, 1980.
14. Cowan, D. B., and Houlton, M. C. C.: Rupture of an amoebic liver abscess in pregnancy. S. Afr. Med. J., 53:460, 1978.
15. Cowper, S. G.: A Synopsis of African Bilharziasis. London, H. K. Lewis & Co., 1971.
16. Czeizel, E., Hancsok, M., Palkovich, I., Janko, M., and Zoltai, N.: Possible relation between fetal death and *E. histolytica* infection of the mother. Am. J. Obstet. Gynecol., 96:264, 1966.
17. Desmonts, G., and Couvreur, J.: Congenital toxoplasmosis: A prospective study of 378 pregnancies. N. Engl. J. Med., 290:1110, 1974.
18. Garud, M. A., Saraiya, U., Paraskar, M., and Khohhawalla, J.: Vaginal parasitosis. Acta Cytolog., 24:34, 1980.
19. Gelfand, M., Ross, M. D., Blair, D. M., and Weber, M. C.: Distribution and extent of schistosomiasis in female pelvic organs, with special reference to the genital tract, as determined at autopsy. Am. J. Trop. Med. Hyg., 20:846, 1971.
20. Giardiasis (editorial). Br. Med. J., 2:347, 1974.
21. Gould, S. E. (ed.): Trichinosis in Man and Animals. Springfield, Ill., Charles C Thomas, 1970.
22. Homer, R. S., and McNall, E. G.: Natural resistance to infectious diseases during pregnancy. Am. J. Obstet. Gynecol., 81:29, 1961.
23. Hume, O. S.: Toxoplasmosis and pregnancy. Am. J. Obstet. Gynecol., 114:703, 1972.
24. Kimball, A. C., Kean, B. H., and Fuchs, F.: Congenital toxoplasmosis: A prospective study of 4048 obstetric patients. Am. J. Obstet. Gynecol., 111:211, 1971.
25. Kimball, A. C., Kean, B. H., and Fuchs, F.: The role of

toxoplasmosis in abortion. Am. J. Obstet. Gynecol., *111*:219, 1971.

26. Krick, J. A., and Remington, J. S.: Toxoplasmosis in the adult — an overview. N. Engl. J. Med., *298*:550, 1978.

27. Krogstad, D. J., Juranek, D. D., and Walls, K. W.: Toxoplasmosis. Ann. Intern. Med., *77*:773, 1972.

28. Langer, A., and Hung, C. T.: Hookworm disease in pregnancy with severe anemia. Obstet. Gynecol., *42*:564, 1973.

29. Lewis, E. A., and Antia, A. U.: Amoebic colitis: Review of 295 cases. Trans. R. Soc. Trop. Med. Hyg., *63*:633, 1969.

30. Low, G. C., and Cook, W. E.: A congenital case of kala-azar. Lancet, *211*:1209, 1926.

31. Manson-Bahr, P.: Manson's Tropical Diseases 15th ed. London, Cassell, 1960, p. 55.

32. Martinez-Torres, C., Ojeda, A., Roche, M., and Layrisse, M.: Hookworm infection and intestinal blood loss. Trans. R. Soc. Trop. Med. Hyg., *61*:373, 1967.

33. Miller, L. H., and Brown, H. W.: The serologic diagnosis of parasitic infections in medical practice. Ann. Intern. Med., *71*:983, 1969.

34. Perez-Tamayo, R., and Brandt, H.: Amebiasis. *In* Marcial-Rojas, R. A. (ed.): Pathology of Protozoal and Helminthic Diseases, Baltimore, Williams & Wilkins Co., 1971, pp. 145–188.

35. Piggott, J., Hansbarger, E. A., and Neafie, R. C.: Human ascariasis. Am. J. Clin. Pathol., *52*:223, 1970.

36. Reinhardt, M. C., Ambroise-Thomas, P., Cavallo-Serra, R., Meylan, C., and Gautier, R.: Malaria at delivery in Abidjan. Helv. Paediatr. Acta, *33* (suppl. 41):65, 1978.

37. Remington, J. S.: Toxoplasmosis. *In* Charles, D., and Finland, M. (eds.): Obstetric and Perinatal Infections. Philadelphia, Lea & Febiger, 1973, p. 27.

38. Rivera, R.: Fatal postpartum amoebic colitis with trophozoites present in peritoneal fluid. Gastroenterology, *62*:314, 1972.

39. Rosen, Y., and Kim, B.: Tubal gestation associated with *Schistosoma mansoni* salpingitis. Obstet. Gynecol., *43*:413, 1974.

40. Smith, A. M.: Malaria in pregnancy. Br. Med. J., *4*:793, 1972.

41. Stray-Pedersen, B.: A prospective study of acquired toxoplasmosis among 8043 pregnant women in the Oslo area. Am. J. Obstet. Gynecol., *136*:399, 1980.

42. Taufa, T.: Malaria and pregnancy. Papua New Guinea Med. J., *21*:197, 1978.

43. Teutsch, S. M., Sulzer, A. J., Ramsey, J. E., Murray, W. A., and Juranek, D. D.: *Toxoplasma gondii* isolated from amniotic fluid. Obstet. Gynecol., *55* (Suppl.):2, 1980.

44. Thompson, R. G., Karandikar, D. S., and Leek, J.: Giardiasis. Lancet, *1*:615, 1975.

45. Tolls, R. M.: Hydramnios and filariasis. Trop. Doct., *9*:231, 1979.

46. Weinman, D., and Ristic, M. (eds.): Infectious Blood Diseases of Man and Animals. New York, Academic Press, 1968.

47. Zimmerman, W. J., Steele, J. H., and Kagan, I. G.: Trichiniasis in the U.S. population, 1966–1970. Health Services Report, *88*:606, 1973.

GENERAL REFERENCES

48. Cahill, K. M.: Tropical Disease in Temperate Climates. Philadelphia, J. B. Lippincott Co., 1964.

49. Drugs for Parasitic Infections. Med. Lett. Drugs Ther., *20*:17, 1978.

50. Health Information for International Travel. Center for Disease Control, U.S. Department of Health and Human Services. Washington, D.C., HHS Publication No. (CDC) 80–8280, 1980.

51. Hunter, G. W., Swartzwelder, J. C., and Clyde, W. W. (eds.): Tropical Medicine. Philadelphia, W. B. Saunders Co., 1976.

52. Lawson, J. B., and Stewart, D. B. (eds.): Obstetrics and Gynecology in the Tropics. London, Edward Arnold, 1967.

53. Maegrith, B. G., and Gilles, H. M. (eds.): Management and Treatment of Tropical Diseases. Oxford, Blackwell Scientific Publications, 1971.

54. Marcial-Rojas, R. A. (ed.): Pathology of Protozoal and Helminthic Diseases. Baltimore, Williams & Wilkins Co., 1971.

55. Most, H.: Treatment of common parasitic infections of man encountered in the United States. N. Engl. J. Med., *287*:495, 1972.

56. Neva, F. A.: Parasitic diseases of the G.I. tract in the United States. Disease-A-Month, June, 1972.

57. Remington, J. S., and Klein, J. O. (eds.): Infectious Diseases of the Fetus and Newborn Infant. Philadelphia, W. B. Saunders Co., 1976.

58. Snow, K. R.: Insects and Disease. New York, John Wiley & Sons, Inc., 1974.

Steven E. Weinberger, M.D.
Scott T. Weiss, M.D.

17

PULMONARY DISEASES

Pregnancy is associated with both mechanical and biochemical changes that may affect maternal respiratory function and gas exchange. Although it is clear that dyspnea may result from these changes even in women without prior lung disease, it does not automatically follow that women with preexisting lung disease will be adversely affected by pregnancy or that the fetus will necessarily suffer from the presence of maternal lung disease. Consequently, the goal of this chapter is to analyze the effects of pregnancy on respiratory function and disease as well as the effects of lung disease on pregnancy and the fetus. In addition, the potential adverse effects of drugs used to treat lung disease and of maternal smoking will be discussed.

PHYSIOLOGIC CHANGES IN PREGNANCY AFFECTING THE RESPIRATORY SYSTEM

Both mechanical and biochemical factors interact in the pregnant woman to produce the observed changes in respiratory function and gas exchange that will subsequently be described. The most prominent of these factors appear to be the mechanical effect of the enlarging abdomen on diaphragmatic position and the effect of increased levels of circulating progesterone on ventilation. Other factors, such as alterations in corticosteroid, prostaglandin, and cyclic nucleotide levels, may also be important, particularly in women with underlying lung disease, but their role must remain speculative at present.

Mechanical Changes

The enlarging uterus, which produces obvious changes in abdominal shape and size, also alters the resting position of the diaphragm and the configuration of the thorax. In an early study of the mechanical changes during pregnancy, the diaphragm at rest rose to a level up to 4 cm above its usual resting position, while the chest en-

larged in transverse diameter by up to 2.1 cm. Simultaneously, the subcostal angle progressively increased from an average of 68.5 degrees in early pregnancy to 103.5 degrees during the latter part of gestation.[23] However, the increase in uterine size could not entirely explain the observed changes in chest wall configuration, since the increase in subcostal angle occurred before it could be satisfactorily accounted for by mechanical pressure from the enlarging uterus. The increasing abdominal size and high resting position of the diaphragm apparently do not impair diaphragmatic motion, which was actually increased in two studies quantitating diaphragmatic excursion with tidal breathing in pregnancy.[18, 19]

Biochemical Changes

Progesterone and Estrogen. It is well established that serum progesterone levels rise gradually through the course of pregnancy, from an average of 25 ng/ml at six weeks to 150 ng/ml at 37 weeks.[12, 25] There is also a corresponding increase in urinary excretion of pregnanediol, the major metabolite of progesterone found in maternal urine.

The possibility that elevated progesterone levels in pregnancy influence ventilation was suggested by workers who first demonstrated that intramuscular administration of progesterone to normal subjects resulted in increased minute ventilation.[17] The subjects also exhibited a heightened ventilatory response to hypercapnia, suggesting that progesterone enhanced the sensitivity of the respiratory center to CO_2. Pregnant women tested under the same conditions but without receiving exogenous progesterone demonstrated a similar increase in sensitivity to CO_2 inhalation, and the investigators concluded that their increased circulating level of progesterone was responsible for increased respiratory center sensitivity to CO_2.

The mechanism of action of progesterone on

ventilation is not yet entirely clear, although it appears that the effect is not indirectly mediated through either an increase in basal temperature or an increase in metabolic rate.[6] Recent work in normal subjects suggests that progesterone acts by directly stimulating the respiratory center rather than by altering its sensitivity to existing stimuli.[22]

Although a role for progesterone in modulating the ventilatory changes in pregnancy is well established, it is unclear if estrogen contributes to the response. Early studies suggested that estrogen increased the "irritability" of the respiratory center, an effect that was additive to that of progesterone, but no recent studies are available to confirm or refute this hypothesis.[10]

Prostaglandins. As interest in prostaglandins has grown over the past several years, it has become apparent that these fatty acid derivatives may influence airway tone because of their effect on smooth muscle. Specifically, prostaglandin $F_2\alpha$, by virtue of its smooth muscle stimulatory action, induces constriction of bronchial smooth muscle, while prostaglandins E_1 and E_2 exert a bronchodilator effect.[11, 21]

Changes in prostaglandin levels have recently been demonstrated during pregnancy, and a possible role for prostaglandin $F_2\alpha$ in contracting uterine smooth muscle and initiating labor has been suggested. By use of a bioassay technique, the appearance of prostaglandin $F_2\alpha$ in plasma during labor was demonstrated, whereas no detectable concentrations were present before labor.[13] However, measurements by the more recent and sensitive radioimmunoassay technique have demonstrated an increase in prostaglandin F concentrations in all trimesters of pregnancy.[24] In contrast, prostaglandin E was increased only in the third trimester.

Whether pregnancy-related changes in prostaglandin levels have any role in influencing airway tone in women with airway disease, especially asthma, is unknown at present. However, intravenous or intra-amniotic administration of prostaglandin $F_2\alpha$ to induce abortion can produce reversible bronchoconstriction and precipitate asthmatic attacks in susceptible women with underlying reactive airway disease.[9, 15] It is unlikely that such airway responses produce clinically significant effects in healthy pregnant women without asthma or other forms of obstructive airway disease.

Cyclic Nucleotides. The cyclic nucleotides, cyclic AMP and GMP, are thought to play a major role in modulating airway tone, the former producing bronchodilation and the latter bronchoconstriction. In addition, increased cyclic AMP levels decrease release of mediators that have an important pathogenetic role in asthma, while increased cyclic GMP levels have the opposite effect.

During pregnancy, plasma cyclic AMP increases from the initial nonpregnant levels to a peak at 14 weeks, followed by a fall to nonpregnant levels at 18 weeks. Thereafter follows a rise in cyclic AMP concentration to a second peak at 34 weeks.[16] Urinary cyclic AMP concentration increases in the second trimester or earlier and subsequently reaches a plateau during the third trimester. In contrast, cyclic GMP excretion increases rapidly during the first trimester and then remains relatively constant throughout the remainder of pregnancy.[14]

However, as with prostaglandins, even though cyclic nucleotides affect airway tone and have altered levels during pregnancy, it is unclear what clinical significance can be ascribed to these changes in pregnant women.

Corticosteroids. Pregnancy is associated with a rise in plasma cortisol concentration, partly because of the increased corticosteroid-binding globulin levels observed during pregnancy. However, there is also an increase in metabolically active cortisol, as demonstrated by the two- to three-fold elevation of unbound cortisol levels over those found in nonpregnant women.[8, 20]

Presumably, the increase in endogenous corticosteroids has no clinically observable respiratory effects in normal women during pregnancy. However, it has been speculated that the alteration in steroid levels may be responsible for the improvement in steroid-responsive pulmonary disease that is sometimes associated with pregnancy. It is unlikely that any proof will be forthcoming for this hypothesis, which will thus remain a theoretical consideration only.

PULMONARY FUNCTION AND GAS EXCHANGE DURING PREGNANCY

Changes in the respiratory system that occur during pregnancy can best be described by measurements of pulmonary function and gas exchange and by quantitation of ventilation. Such data are available primarily in women without underlying lung disease, and the following discussion will refer specifically to women without known respiratory disease. In situations where data for specific lung diseases during pregnancy are available, they will be discussed under the individual disease entities.

Lung Volumes

Lung volumes are routinely measured by a combination of spirometry and either gas dilution or body plethysmography. Total lung capacity (TLC) is the total volume of gas present in the lungs at the end of a maximal inspiration. When the patient exhales as completely as possible from TLC, the expired volume is the vital capacity (VC), and the volume remaining in the lungs after a maximal expiration is the residual volume (RV). At the resting position of the thorax, i.e., the position at the end of a normal expiration, the volume of gas within the lungs is called functional residual capacity (FRC). If the patient then exhales from FRC down to RV, the volume that has been expired is termed the expiratory reserve volume (ERV). A diagrammatic representation of these volumes is shown in Figure 17–1.

During pregnancy, the major factors that alter lung volumes appear to be the changes in diaphragmatic position and configuration of the chest wall. As mentioned previously, although the diaphragm during pregnancy is elevated in its resting position, diaphragmatic motion with respiration is unimpaired. In line with these roentgenographic observations, one would expect a decreased volume in the lungs at their resting position (FRC), while VC should be relatively preserved because of normal movement of the diaphragm and thoracic musculature.

Measurements of lung volumes in a number of studies have generally confirmed these predictions, even though major variations may be found from study to study. In an extensive evaluation of pulmonary function in 19 normal women during pregnancy, lung volumes were found to be unchanged until the latter half of pregnancy, at which time a decrease in ERV and RV combined to produce an 18 per cent mean decrease in FRC.[38] Vital capacity (VC) was unchanged, and therefore TLC (the sum of RV and VC) was slightly diminished at term. Other studies have found a similar decrease in ERV in late pregnancy, with a range of values between 8 and 40 per cent less than in nonpregnant control subjects. Residual volume (RV) at term was also decreased by 7 to 22 per cent, and thus the net effect of lower RV and ERV was a 9.5 to 25 per cent diminution in FRC. Although minor changes in both directions have been observed for TLC and VC, the magnitude of these changes was sufficiently small to suggest they are probably of no clinical significance. A diagrammatic summary of the altered lung volumes in pregnancy is presented in Figure 17–1.

In studies that have followed pulmonary function serially during pregnancy, the observed changes in RV and ERV were apparent after the fifth to sixth month of gestation and were progressive throughout the remainder of pregnancy.[26, 38]

Airway Function and Mechanics

Large airway function is most commonly assessed by spirometry, using the absolute values and the ratio between the volume exhaled in the first second and the total volume exhaled on a forced expiratory breath from TLC to RV; this is expressed as FEV_1/FVC, or forced expiratory volume in 1 second divided by forced vital capac-

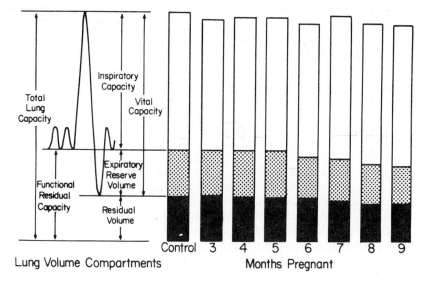

FIGURE 17–1. Serial measurements of lung volume compartments during pregnancy. (From Prowse and Gaensler: Anesthesiology, 26:381, 1965.)

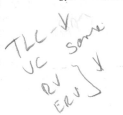

Lung Volume Compartments

Months Pregnant

ity. In numerous studies that have investigated forced expiratory flow rates during pregnancy, FEV_1 and FEV_1/FVC have been unchanged from values in nonpregnant subjects, suggesting that large airway function is preserved during pregnancy.[26, 31, 36, 38]

Measurement of airway resistance is another method for assessing airway function, but the technique requires a body plethysmograph and is less readily available. The available studies of respiratory resistance performed during pregnancy have demonstrated either a decrease in airway resistance and the expected increase in its reciprocal, airway conductance,[41, 43] or no change in airway conductance.[51] In an early study of pulmonary resistance, it was suggested that relaxation of airway smooth muscle occurs during pregnancy, possibly as a result of hormonal changes, but no direct proof is available for this theory.[54]

Lung compliance, a measurement of the "stiffness" of the lungs, can be determined by correlating changes in pleural pressure, measured indirectly by an esophageal balloon, with the associated changes in lung volume. In a study of ten normal women during pregnancy, postpartum lung compliance was unchanged from that measured during the last trimester of pregnancy.[43]

Small Airway Function

Interest has recently focused on small airways, i.e., bronchi with a diameter of 2 mm or less, as the initial site of airway obstruction in patients with various forms of obstructive lung disease. However, because of the branching of the bronchial tree, these airways constitute a small portion of resistance to airflow, and isolated disease in small airways has an insignificant effect on measurements of VC, FEV_1, and airway resistance. It has been only since the development of techniques specifically capable of assessing peripheral airway function that such disease in small airways has become appreciated as an important pathophysiologic feature of most types of obstructive airway disease.

Studies that reflect small airway dysfunction include the maximal expiratory flow volume loop, measurement of airway closure with closing volume (CV) or closing capacity (CC), and frequency dependence of dynamic compliance. Although detailed description of these techniques is beyond the scope of this discussion, a brief explanation will be given of studies that have been performed during pregnancy.

Determination of closing volume involves measurement of exhaled gas concentrations after inhalation of a specified gas (either oxygen or a labeled tracer gas such as xenon). The test is based on the theory that small airways toward the lung bases are subject to closure as the patient exhales, normally at a lung volume between RV and FRC. When disease of the peripheral airways exists, such closure occurs at a lung volume higher than normal, and the measured CV or CC is increased.

Several studies have examined airway closure during pregnancy and have reported the results as either CV or CC. In addition, the relationship between the volume in the lungs at airway closure and the FRC has been noted, since it has been postulated that changes in the usual relationship might adversely affect gas exchange. Under normal conditions, if airway closure at the lung bases occurs between RV and FRC, such airways do not close during normal tidal breathing, since FRC is the smallest volume reached. However, if CC exceeds FRC, the implication is that airway closure at the lung bases would occur during part of each respiratory cycle, i.e., whenever the volume in the lungs fell below CC. Under these circumstances, ventilation to the lung bases would decrease, ventilation-perfusion ratios in affected areas would decrease, and arterial hypoxemia would result. However, it is important to note that debate exists over the meaning of closing volume and closing capacity, and thus, using such measurements for a theoretical construct to explain abnormal gas exchange is not universally accepted.

A high incidence of airway closure above FRC during the last month of pregnancy has been reported,[33] suggesting that airway closure may occur during tidal breathing. In a subsequent study of these patients by the same group,[44] this observation was found to be due to a decrease in ERV and hence FRC, while CV remained unchanged. Measurements of CC and FRC were made in 24 pregnant women, and a reduced difference between FRC and CC was found compared with that found in postpartum studies.[37] The cause of this reduction was a 15 per cent decrease in FRC, while CC remained unchanged. However, in contrast with the other two studies, CC exceeded FRC only infrequently. In a study of 19 healthy pregnant women, no change in closing volume at the end of pregnancy was documented compared with the postpartum period.[31] These authors did not comment on airway closure relative to FRC in their patients. A recently published study shows an increase in the actual volume at which airway closure occurs; in a series of 10 patients, both CV and CC rose progressively after the 18th week of pregnancy.[41]

Another type of study that has been used to demonstrate abnormalities in small airways is the maximal expiratory flow-volume curve; its use for this purpose is based on the fact that flow rates at low lung volumes are dependent primarily on the mechanical properties of the peripheral airways. In the only available studies of maximal expiratory flow-volume curves during pregnancy,[31] no changes in maximal expiratory flow at 25 and 50 per cent of VC were found,[31] and no changes at 50 per cent of VC were found.[42]

In summary, most studies using either measurements of airway closure (CV and CC) or maximal expiratory flow-volume curves suggest that small airway dysfunction is not found during pregnancy. However, since ERV and thus FRC decrease during pregnancy, airway closure during late pregnancy occurs either above FRC or closer to FRC than it does in the nonpregnant state. Although the significance of such changes has not been clearly proved, it has been suggested that the potential consequence of airway closure near or above FRC is a lowering of arterial oxygen tension, due to a decrease in ventilation and hence ventilation-perfusion ratios to involved areas of lung.

Diffusing Capacity

The diffusing capacity of the lung for carbon monoxide ($D_{L_{CO}}$) is a nonspecific test that measures the ability of carbon monoxide to diffuse from the alveolus into pulmonary capillary blood, where it combines with hemoglobin in the circulating red blood cells. The $D_{L_{CO}}$ may be partitioned into its two separate determinants, a membrane component and a pulmonary capillary blood volume component, and abnormalities in the $D_{L_{CO}}$ can generally be attributed to qualitative or quantitative changes in either the alveolar-capillary interface or the pulmonary capillary blood. Some of the major disease categories in which diffusing capacity is found to be abnormal include emphysema, interstitial lung disease, and pulmonary vascular disease.

Early studies investigating $D_{L_{CO}}$ in pregnancy found no change from values in nonpregnant women, and there was an appropriate increase in $D_{L_{CO}}$ with exercise (over resting levels) in pregnant subjects.[32, 46] When $D_{L_{CO}}$ was partitioned into membrane and pulmonary capillary blood volume components, either no change or a slight decrease was found in the membrane component, while pulmonary capillary blood volume remained unaltered.[42, 46] Again, there was no significant net effect on overall $D_{L_{CO}}$.

In a more extensive study where serial changes were evaluated throughout pregnancy, an increase was found in single-breath $D_{L_{CO}}$ during the first trimester.[50] This was followed by a decrease until approximately 24 to 27 weeks of gestation, after which it remained constant until delivery. The postpartum diffusing capacity was slightly but significantly greater than the value measured between 36 weeks and term. There is no apparent explanation for these minor changes, which appear to be of little clinical significance. The changes could not be attributed to any alterations in hemoglobin concentration, alveolar volume, or plasma 17-β-estradiol levels during pregnancy.

In summary, $D_{L_{CO}}$ during early pregnancy is generally unchanged or increased over control values in the same patients. Subsequently, there is a frequent decrease to a plateau during the latter half of pregnancy that is equivalent to or slightly less than the control value. The relative roles of alterations in membrane diffusing capacity or pulmonary capillary blood volume in producing these changes are unclear.

Ventilation and Oxygen Consumption

In the early 1900s, several investigators observed that resting ventilation increases during pregnancy, and this finding has subsequently proved to be the most consistently demonstrated physiologic change in maternal respiration. Although both oxygen consumption and basal metabolic rate are elevated during pregnancy, the increment in minute ventilation is out of proportion to that observed in any measurements of maternal metabolism. In one specific series, minute ventilation at term was stated to increase by 48 per cent over the control level, whereas oxygen consumption and basal metabolic rate were augmented by only 21 per cent and 14 per cent, respectively (Fig. 17–2).[6] Subsequent studies have confirmed these findings, although the magnitude of change does vary to some extent in each study. In separate studies, a 30 to 35 per cent increase was found in resting oxygen consumption and an increase of approximately 50 per cent in resting minute ventilation at the end of pregnancy compared with postpartum values.[45, 52, 53] An increment in tidal volume appears to be the major factor accounting for the increase

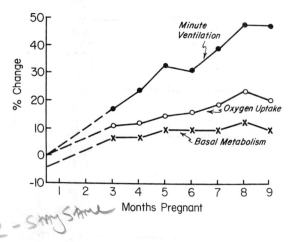

FIGURE 17–2. Time course of per cent changes in minute ventilation, oxygen uptake, and basal metabolism during pregnancy. (From Prowse and Gaensler: Anesthesiology, 26:381, 1965.)

in minute ventilation, whereas respiratory rate remains essentially unchanged throughout the course of pregnancy.[6, 38]

That the increase in minute ventilation exceeds that of either oxygen consumption or metabolic rate suggests that an additional factor must contribute to the genesis of hyperventilation in pregnancy. The currently accepted theory is based on the well-described stimulatory effect of progesterone on ventilatory drive, as discussed in a previous section of this chapter. According to this theory, the elevated progesterone levels during pregnancy are responsible to a large extent for maternal hyperpnea.

Data have also been recently accumulated by several investigators on the physiologic response of minute ventilation and oxygen consumption to exercise during pregnancy, and there is a similar augmentation of the ventilatory response compared with postpartum results. During exercise, the pregnant subjects increased ventilation and oxygen consumption by 38 per cent and 15 per cent, respectively, above the comparable levels with postpartum exercise.[52, 53] Because the increment in minute ventilation exceeded the increase in oxygen consumption, the ventilatory equivalent, which is the ratio of minute ventilation to oxygen consumption, was significantly higher with antepartum than postpartum exercise.[45]

In summary, both at rest and with exercise, minute ventilation and, to a lesser extent, oxygen consumption are increased during pregnancy over the nonpregnant control values. Although the increase in oxygen consumption may account for part of the rise in minute ventilation, the respiratory stimulating effect of progesterone is probably the major factor explaining the disproportionate increase in minute ventilation over oxygen consumption observed during pregnancy.

Arterial Blood Gases and Acid-Base Status

A fall in arterial P_{CO_2} during pregnancy is a well-documented finding and is a consequence of the progesterone-induced increase in alveolar ventilation. Numerous studies have consistently demonstrated that maternal arterial P_{CO_2} generally falls to a plateau of 27 to 32 mm Hg,[27, 34, 39, 40, 48, 49] but there is no general agreement about the time course of this change. Some investigators have observed a progressive serial decrease in alveolar and arterial P_{CO_2} starting early in pregnancy,[35, 48, 49] whereas others have noted that arterial P_{CO_2} remains at a low but constant level throughout pregnancy.[27, 55] During labor, there is a further transient fall in arterial P_{CO_2} with each contraction; by the time the cervix is fully dilated, the decrease in P_{CO_2} persists even between contractions.[28]

As a consequence of the hyperventilation and respiratory alkalosis of pregnancy, renal excretion of bicarbonate secondarily increases, and the overall pH remains relatively intact. The loss of bicarbonate appears to be a compensatory phenomenon, and attempts to document a primary metabolic acidosis have been unsuccessful.[47] In most studies, the pH resulting from the respiratory alkalosis and metabolic compensation has been approximately 7.40 to 7.45,[27, 39, 47, 48] although one series of 37 pregnant women reported a mean pH as high as 7.47.[48] Corresponding serum bicarbonate levels have decreased to 18 to 21 mEq/l, resulting in a base deficit of approximately 3 to 4 mEq/l.[27, 40, 48, 55]

In studies where maternal oxygenation has been followed serially throughout pregnancy, mean values for arterial P_{O_2} have generally been increased, ranging from 106 to 108 mm Hg in the first trimester to 101 to 104 mm Hg in the third trimester.[27, 55] It is important to note that interpretation of arterial P_{O_2} during pregnancy must include evaluation of arterial P_{CO_2}, since changes in arterial and alveolar P_{CO_2} affect alveolar and hence arterial P_{O_2}. During pregnancy, low arterial P_{CO_2} is associated with a low alveolar P_{CO_2}, and the corresponding increase in alveolar P_{O_2} should thus result in an elevation of arterial P_{O_2}.

In order to evaluate whether maternal oxygenation is deranged during pregnancy, a more meaningful value than the arterial P_{O_2} is the alveolar-arterial P_{O_2} gradient. This gradient takes into account the effect of P_{CO_2} changes on arterial P_{O_2}, and any alterations in the gradient therefore truly reflect maternal gas exchange by the respiratory system. The alveolar-arterial P_{O_2} gradient has been reported as either unchanged[55] or slightly increased[30] during pregnancy. An increase in the gradient might be explained by hypothesizing that a decrease in FRC in late pregnancy contributes to airway closure and thus a decreased P_{O_2} as closing volume approaches FRC.

Postural effects also appear to influence measured arterial P_{O_2} and the alveolar-arterial gradient during pregnancy. One group demonstrated a 13 mm decrease in capillary P_{O_2} near term on changing from the sitting to supine position,[29] while another noted an increase in the alveolar-arterial oxygen gradient from 14.3 to 20 mm Hg under similar conditions.[30] Although augmented effects of diaphragmatic pressure in the supine position may contribute to airway closure, it is not clear if an additional role is played by caval compression and hemodynamic alterations.

Summary

Alterations in respiratory physiology occur during normal pregnancy, not only because of the obvious increase in abdominal girth but also because of the changing hormonal milieu that accompanies pregnancy. Although there may be some variability in pulmonary function tests from person to person, a distinct pattern of changes during pregnancy has emerged. The most apparent change in lung volumes is a decrease in FRC, the resting position of the lungs at the end of a normal expiration, due primarily to elevation of the diaphragm by pressure from the enlarging uterus. This decrease in FRC, which occurs during the second half of pregnancy, is the net result of a decreased ERV and a lesser decrease in RV. Despite the alteration in resting diaphragmatic position, diaphragm excursion is unaffected, so that VC is preserved. Total lung capacity (TLC) is generally either unchanged or decreased by a minor amount.

Large airway function appears to be normal during pregnancy, as reflected by normal or even increased specific conductance. Peripheral airways, i.e., those with a diameter of 2 mm or less, are similarly unaffected by pregnancy; recently designed tests to assess small airway function do not show abnormalities.

Diffusing capacity is frequently unchanged, although an increase early in pregnancy and a decrease late in pregnancy have been observed in some patients.

Ventilatory changes are perhaps the most apparent alterations in respiratory physiology during pregnancy, since resting minute ventilation increases by approximately 50 per cent over postpartum control values. This hyperventilation, which is in excess of the observed changes in oxygen consumption, is presumed to be a result of the respiratory stimulant effect of progesterone and is expressed primarily as an increased tidal volume with an unchanged respiratory frequency. As a result of the hyperventilation, arterial P_{CO_2} decreases during pregnancy, but metabolic compensation by renal excretion of bicarbonate partially offsets the expected pH change. Therefore, the net effect of the respiratory alkalosis and metabolic compensation is a slightly alkalotic pH in arterial blood.

As a result of the decreased arterial and hence alveolar P_{CO_2}, alveolar P_{O_2} and therefore arterial P_{O_2} increase. However, even though arterial P_{O_2} is generally elevated, the gradient between alveolar and arterial P_{O_2} ($A_aD_{O_2}$) may be elevated, especially near term, and may partially offset the increase in P_{O_2} expected from hyperventilation. There is a further decrease in arterial P_{O_2} and an increase in the alveolar-arterial gradient in the supine compared with the sitting position in late pregnancy. However, in patients without underlying pulmonary disease, these changes in arterial P_{O_2} appear to have little clinical significance.

DYSPNEA OF PREGNANCY

It is well established that women often have dyspnea at some time during a normal pregnancy. Consequently, dyspnea may erroneously suggest the development of lung disease, even when it is merely a result of the normal physiologic changes of pregnancy.

It has been stated that dyspnea may be expressed at some time during the course of gestation by as many as 60 to 70 per cent of pregnant women.[6] In a 1953 series, the development of dyspnea did not correlate with changes in a number of pulmonary function tests, specifically maximal breathing capacity, VC, resting ventilation, breathing reserve, oxygen uptake, or subdivisions of TLC.[56]

When dyspnea occurs, it commonly commences during the first or second trimester,[57, 58] before any significant increase in abdominal girth. In a recent study of dyspnea during normal pregnancy, it was found that the frequency of dyspnea increased from 15 per cent in the first trimester to approximately 50 per cent by 19 weeks and 75 per cent by 31 weeks of gestation (Figure 17–3).[60] By the last trimester, the severity of dyspnea was generally stable.

Although several mechanisms have been postulated to explain the dyspnea of pregnancy, the underlying pathophysiology is still not entirely clear. The frequent onset in the first or second trimester suggests that mechanical factors do not play a significant role in its genesis, since abdominal girth is often not yet appreciably increased. It has been postulated that dyspnea might be due to a decrease in diffusing capacity, based on a finding that diffusing capacity differed between women who experienced dyspnea and those who did not.[59] However, the observed changes were small and are unlikely to serve as an adequate explanation for the symptom.

The most generally accepted theories to explain dyspnea of pregnancy are based on the hyperventilation that occurs with pregnancy. It was suggested in 1953 that the newness of the sensation of hyperventilation might result in dyspnea, and a gradual acclimatization might explain the frequent improvement of the symptom as pregnancy progresses.[56] In a later study, the presence of dyspnea was correlated with a low P_{CO_2} during pregnancy, but the women most likely to experience dyspnea were those who had relatively high nonpregnant values for P_{CO_2}.[58] These investigators therefore suggested that the marked change in P_{CO_2} to a particularly unfamiliar low level might account for the observed symptoms. In a later study by the same group, patients who experienced dyspnea appeared to have a greater ventilatory response to inhaled CO_2 than those who did not experience dyspnea.[57] They concluded that women with dyspnea may have an increased awareness of the physiologic hyperventilation associated with pregnancy. Finally, it has also been suggested that dyspnea of pregnancy is related to hyperventilation and might be due to a ventilatory response that is inappropriately high for the demand.[3]

SPECIFIC DISEASES

Asthma

Definition and Etiology. Asthma is one of several specific disease entities included in the general category of obstructive lung disease, which is characterized by limitation of airflow that is generally more marked during expiration than inspiration. In asthma, the obstruction is a reversible process caused by increased responsiveness of the airways to a variety of stimuli. The airway response to these stimuli includes contraction of bronchial smooth muscle, mucous hypersecretion, and mucosal edema, all of which contribute to the pathophysiology of reversible airway obstruction characteristic of this disease.

Although airway hyperirritability and reversible airway narrowing is the final common path-

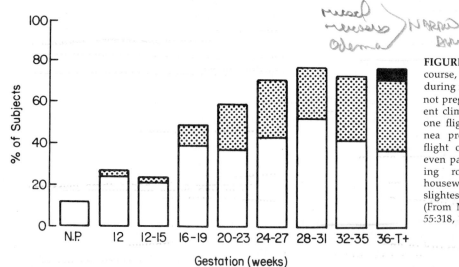

FIGURE 17–3. Incidence, time course, and severity of dyspnea during normal pregnancy. N.P. = not pregnant. □ = dyspnea present climbing hills or more than one flight of stairs. ▨ = dyspnea present on climbing one flight of stairs, walking at an even pace on level ground, during routine performance of housework. ■ = dyspnea on slightest exertion or at rest. (From Milne: Postgrad. Med. J., 55:318, 1979.)

way in patients with asthma, it is still not clear what underlying abnormality distinguishes the asthmatic patient from his or her normal counterpart. In addition, specific stimuli may trigger the airway changes by different mechanisms, again making it difficult to explain the disease by a single, unified mechanism.

In some cases, particularly in patients with a strong personal or family history of allergies, the patient has been sensitized to specific allergens and has circulating antibodies of the IgE class. Exposure to the allergen then results in an antigen-antibody complex bound primarily to mast cells, inducing release of a variety of humoral mediators including histamine, slow-reacting substance of anaphylaxis (SRS-A), eosinophilic chemotactic factor of anaphylaxis (ECF-A), and platelet-activating factor (PAF). These and other humoral mediators have several adverse effects, including stimulation of irritant receptors, constriction of bronchial smooth muscle, and increase in vascular permeability.

With other stimuli, such as respiratory tract infections, environmental pollutants, cold air, and exercise, nonallergic mechanisms are operative. In these situations, stimulation of airway irritant receptors or, in the case of cold air or exercise,[81] heat loss from the intrathoracic airways may precipitate bronchoconstriction.

Disease in the Nonpregnant State. Asthma is a relatively common disorder that affects approximately 3 per cent of the population. Although most commonly the onset is in childhood, the disease can occur at any age, and it is therefore a common problem in women of childbearing age.

The classic symptoms during an exacerbation of asthma are dyspnea, cough, and wheezing. Although specific inciting events, such as allergen exposure or a respiratory tract infection, may be identified for a particular attack, it is common for the patient to present with symptoms but no clear precipitating factor. It has recently been recognized that cough may be the sole presenting feature of asthma,[69] and the diagnosis may be missed in such patients if investigation for reversible airway obstruction is not specifically pursued.

Common physical findings during an exacerbation include diffuse wheezing and evidence of hyperinflation, such as increased anteroposterior diameter and low diaphragms. The presence of a pulsus paradoxus and the use of accessory muscles of respiration indicate severe airflow obstruction, while the amount of wheezing does not correlate with the severity of an attack. In fact, wheezing may sometimes diminish with worsening airflow obstruction if airway diameter is critically reduced and there is insufficient airflow to generate a wheeze.

Pulmonary function tests during an attack demonstrate abnormal expiratory flow rates, including depressed FEV_1, FVC, and FEV_1/FVC ratio. Arterial blood gases most frequently show hypoxemia (decreased Po_2) and respiratory alkalosis (decreased Pco_2). Normalization or elevation of the Pco_2 is an ominous finding, generally indicative of severe obstruction and an FEV_1 less than 20 per cent of the predicted value. Even when the patient improves with treatment of an asthmatic attack, the disappearance of symptoms and even signs is not a sensitive indicator of clinical status, since pulmonary function abnormalities are still frequently present at this stage.

Asthma in Pregnancy. Asthma is by far the most common form of obstructive lung disease encountered during pregnancy, with an estimated frequency of 0.4 to 1.3 per cent.[96] Several studies have investigated the natural history of asthma in pregnancy, and although there is some variation in the results, most data suggest that the course of asthma for a given patient is unpredictable. In 1946 it was stated that patients may improve considerably, remain stable, or significantly worsen during pregnancy, although the patients in that study uniformly stayed the same or improved.[71] In a 1961 series of almost 300 pregnant asthmatics, it was found that 93 per cent were subjectively unchanged during pregnancy, while the remainder were almost equally divided between those who improved and those who became worse,[87] Two other workers[78, 97] found their patients more evenly divided among those who were better (40 per cent), remained the same (35 per cent), or became worse (25 per cent). The latter study found that the severity of asthma prior to pregnancy played a role in determining the course of the disease; patients with mild asthma were unlikely to have further problems during pregnancy, whereas in 44 per cent of patients with severe asthma the disease became worse during pregnancy.[97]

In a prospective study of serial measurements of flow rates (FEV_1 and FVC) in pregnant asthmatics, no change in these parameters was documented in patients with active disease or in those with disease in remission.[90] However, only 11 patients in this series had asthma classified as "active," and the severity of disease was not discussed. In a recent study of 47 patients during pregnancy, the patients were divided into categories by severity, although objective measurements were not made.[74] Overall, 43 per cent of the patients remained unchanged, while 43 per cent were worse and 14 per cent better. Generally, those patients with severe asthma prior to pregnancy were more likely to become worse, whereas those with mild asthma tended to remain unchanged. Preliminary data from this study suggest that patients with increased or unchanged IgE levels during pregnancy tended to have exacerbations of their disease, while those with a decrease in IgE levels frequently improved.

Several interacting factors have been postulated to account for changes in the course of asthma during pregnancy, although the relative importance of any of these factors is unclear. An increase in circulating free cortisol, a decrease in bronchomotor tone and airway resistance (possibly due to progesterone), and an increase in serum levels of cyclic AMP could each contribute to improvement in the frequency and severity of asthma attacks during pregnancy.[74] Conversely, exposure to fetal antigens, alterations in cell-mediated immunity with an increase in viral upper respiratory tract infections, and hyperventilation could provoke attacks or an increase in symptoms. The unpredictable course of asthma during pregnancy makes it especially difficult to quantitate the role of these or other factors in any given patient.

The effect of asthma on the outcome of pregnancy has also been examined in some of the previously mentioned studies as well as others. No significant increase in prematurity or spontaneous abortion compared with controls was documented in one series;[87] the few patients who had severe asthmatic attacks during pregnancy did not go into premature labor. In another study, complications and fetal morbidity or mortality in 277 pregnancies were assessed in asthmatic women compared with a control group with more than 30,000 deliveries.[75] These investigators found an increased incidence of approximately twofold (5.9 per cent vs. 3.2 per cent) of perinatal mortality in infants born to asthmatic mothers compared with controls, although no significantly increased risk of prematurity was observed. Fetal morbidity and mortality were problems especially when maternal asthma was severe; in this latter group, there was a particularly high incidence of perinatal mortality or neurologic abnormality at 1 year of age.

One group compiled data from 381 patients with asthma during pregnancy, in whom an approximately twofold increased incidence of hyperemesis, vaginal hemorrhage, or toxemia was observed.[64] Similarly, complicated labor was more frequent in asthmatic mothers (14.4 per cent) than normal mothers (9.6 per cent). Although offspring of asthmatic mothers appeared to be at higher risk for stillbirth, perinatal mortality, and infant mortality, only the approximate twofold increase in neonatal mortality was statistically significant. Despite a similar overall mean gestation time in infants born to asthmatic mothers, there was a statistically significant increase from 5 per cent to 7.4 per cent in the number of infants that were premature (<37 weeks gestation). Also, low birthweight and hypoxia at birth were seen more frequently in this population.

In another study, birthweight of infants born to women with active asthma was slightly decreased.[90] Although the difference was not statistically significant, statistical analysis is limited by the small number of patients in that study.

In summary, there is no predictable effect of pregnancy on asthma, as individual patients may improve, remain unchanged, or become worse. As a general rule, the patients whose asthma becomes worse tend to be the ones with more severe disease prior to pregnancy. The major documented effect of asthma on the course of pregnancy is an approximately twofold increase in perinatal mortality, which is also a problem particularly when maternal asthma is severe. A slight increase in prematurity and in frequency of low birthweight has also been suggested but not yet definitely proved, and the magnitude of any such effect would certainly be small.

Treatment. The treatment of asthma has been discussed in detail in recent reviews,[73, 86] and only a general approach will be covered here. For outpatient treatment of mild asthma attacks or for a maintenance regimen in the patient requiring chronic therapy, oral methylxanthines, such as aminophylline or theophylline, and either oral or inhaled sympathomimetics are the mainstays of therapy. Both classes of drugs act by increasing cyclic AMP, which has both a bronchodilator effect and an inhibitory effect on release of mediators from mast cells. The methylxanthines elevate cyclic AMP levels by inhibition of phosphodiesterase, the enzyme responsible for inactivation of cyclic AMP, while sympathomimetics activate adenyl cyclase and therefore increase production of this cyclic nucleotide.

For therapy of mild asthma, treatment can be given with a methylxanthine or sympathomimetic, both drugs generally being used if a single drug is ineffective. Numerous preparations of xanthines are available, but the preferred choices are one of the more soluble salts or compounds of theophylline (such as uncoated aminophylline), anhydrous theophylline or oxtriphylline. For aminophylline, 800 to 1200 mg/day are given in divided doses; for other preparations, a dose equivalent to this amount of aminophylline is administered. Slow-release preparations of theophylline and aminophylline are also available, allowing a decreased frequency of administration. Since the half-life of xanthines varies considerably from patient to patient, it is advisable to measure serum levels in patients who require prolonged therapy, in order to achieve a concentration of 10 to 20 μg/ml. The major side effects of xanthines are gastrointestinal symptoms (nausea, vomiting, anorexia) or nervousness, whereas frankly toxic levels may result in cardiac arrhythmias or seizures.

Sympathomimetic preparations are available in both oral and inhaled form; the newer preparations, metaproterenol and terbutaline, have been specifically designed to obtain more β_2-selectivity and to increase the duration of action. Inhaled preparations may be given by a metered-dose inhaler or by either a compressed-air or hand-held nebulizer; the convenience of the metered-dose inhalers has made them the most popular route of administration. One or two puffs can generally be given, the dose being repeated at intervals of approximately 3 to 6 hours depending on the particular preparation. The oral sympathomimetics most frequently used are terbutaline, at a dose of 2.5 to 5 mg three times a day, or metaproterenol, at a dose of 10 to 20 mg 3 to 4 times a day. The major side effect of these oral preparations is tremor, whereas any of the sympathomimetics may induce tachycardia.

For more severe attacks, patients may need to be hospitalized, and parenteral administration may be more appropriate. Because of its water solubility, aminophylline is the only xanthine preparation available for intravenous administration. If the patient is not currently taking xanthines, a loading dose of 5 to 6 mg/kg should be given intravenously over 20 to 30 minutes, at which time a maintenance infusion of 0.5 to 0.9 mg/kg/hr can be started. Catecholamines can also be administered subcutaneously, either as epinephrine (1:1000) 0.3 to 0.5 cc or as terbutaline 0.25 to 0.5 mg; either can be given at the time of initial presentation, but epinephrine is usually not used for more prolonged therapy because of its short duration of action.

For severe attacks, intravenous or oral corticosteroids are also administered and then ideally are tapered over the course of the next 1 to 2 weeks. Variable doses have been recommended, but the minimum initial daily dose is generally at least the equivalent of prednisone, 60 mg/day.

For patients with refractory disease, steroids may need to be tapered more slowly or even maintained at a low or moderate dose for prolonged outpatient therapy.

Other available medications used for management of the asthmatic patient include disodium cromoglycate (cromolyn sodium) and inhaled beclomethasone. Disodium cromoglycate, which inhibits mediator release from mast cells, is given only by inhalation, and it may be useful as a maintenance therapy for prevention of attacks. It is not effective for treatment of an ongoing attack, and may actually be harmful in this setting because of an airway irritant effect. Beclomethasone has recently been introduced for inhaled administration; the advantage is that relatively little systemic absorption occurs when it is given by this route. It is generally used at a dose of two puffs (100 μg) four times a day. Although it may be given to allow tapering of systemic steroids, it may also be useful in patients who have not been receiving prolonged maintenance therapy with oral steroids. The major potential side effect is oropharyngeal candidiasis, which can frequently be prevented by gargling after each dose.

Additional treatment modalities for the patient with status asthmaticus are beyond the scope of this discussion but have been reviewed in the recent literature.[89] In particular, hydration and oxygen administration are generally beneficial, while indications for endotracheal intubation are much more difficult to define, and are dependent on clinical judgment in each particular situation.

Management in Pregnancy. The management of asthma in the pregnant woman differs little from management in the nonpregnant patient. However, it is important to be aware of certain effects of medications when treating asthma in the pregnant woman.

Xanthine bronchodilators appear to be safe for the fetus.[76] Although there is some evidence of digital malformations in laboratory animals given large doses of aminophylline parenterally,[82] no teratogenic effect has been demonstrated in human studies.[77] In nonpregnant women, aminophylline can inhibit and, in some cases, abolish uterine activity, presumably by an inhibitory effect of increased cyclic AMP on uterine smooth muscle.[70] To our knowledge, whether aminophylline alters uterine contractility at the time of labor has never been studied, but it is reasonable to expect that an inhibitory effect is possible. Xanthines are transferred across the placenta, and theophylline concentrations in cord blood are similar to those in maternal blood.[63] Tachycardia and irritability have been reported in neonates of mothers receiving xanthines, presumably as a direct effect of the drug.

Sympathomimetic bronchodilators also appear to be relatively safe during pregnancy, although some potential effects on the uterus and fetus must be considered. A radiographic study in monkeys has shown vasoconstrictive effects of epinephrine on the uteroplacental circulation,[83] but the intra-arterial mode of administration in that study makes it difficult to attribute any clinical relevance to this finding. On the other hand, uterine blood flow appears to be preserved or even enhanced after administration of terbutaline.[61, 68] No teratogenicity has been documented for ephedrine in humans or for metaproterenol in animals, but a slightly increased incidence of malformations over the expected number was found by the Collaborative Perinatal Project in women given epinephrine during pregnancy.[65, 77] No human studies of metaproterenol or terbutaline during pregnancy are available; to date, no individual problems with malformations have been reported.

By virtue of their stimulation of uterine beta receptors, sympathomimetics clearly inhibit uterine contractility at term and are useful in the management of premature labor.[92] This effect has been documented for intravenous administration of metaproterenol, terbutaline, and salbutamol.[62, 80, 98] Oral terbutaline has a similar action on uterine contractility and has therefore also been used for inhibition of premature labor.[79]

Since disodium cromoglycate is still relatively new, insufficient data are available to assure its safe use in pregnancy. To date, however, there is no evidence to suggest an increased risk to the fetus.[96]

Numerous studies have now been reported concerning potential problems with use of corticosteroids during pregnancy. The risks, although real, appear to be small, and it is generally agreed that corticosteroids should not be withheld in this setting if they are clinically indicated.

In animals, it has been demonstrated that maternal administration of glucocorticoids may be associated with cleft palate in the offspring.[72] In human studies, a few cases of cleft palate have been reported in offspring of women receiving corticosteroids during pregnancy, but a causal relationship has been difficult to prove. In a literature review of 260 pregnancies in women who had received pharmacologic doses of steroids during pregnancy, two infants were found to have been born with cleft palates.[67] In both cases, maternal exposure was prior to the 14th week of gestation; since closure of the palatal processes is usually complete by the 12th week, the time course was consistent with a causal effect, though not proof of it. On the other hand, several other more recent studies suggest that there is no risk of either cleft palate or other congenital malformations in humans as a result of prenatal administration of steroids.[77, 88, 91]

One group noted a high frequency of stillbirth or placental insufficiency in mothers receiving prednisolone during pregnancy, and they speculated that prednisolone had a deleterious effect on placental function.[94] Others have found an apparently high rate of fetal loss and perinatal mortality,[84a, 93] but because a control population was not examined in either study, it is difficult to assess the contribution of steroids compared with that of the underlying disease.[84]

A recent study did not confirm an increased risk of abortion, stillbirth, or neonatal death when mothers received an average daily dose of 8.2 mg prednisone.[8] Similarly, the occurrence of uterine hemorrhage or toxemia was not increased. A slightly increased frequency of prematurity was noted (14 per cent compared with 9.3 per cent in a historical control population), but whether this increase was due to steroids, asthma, or other factors is unknown. In another recent study, use of 10 mg prednisone per day throughout the duration of pregnancy was associated with a significantly lower birthweight in offspring, unassociated with any change in the length of gestation.[85] This finding was confirmed by a parallel experimental study in mice, in which it was clear that reduction in birthweight was due to steroid exposure and not to other maternal disease. The authors speculated that the effect of steroids could result either from placental transfer of the hormone and a direct inhibition of fetal growth, or from indirect effects on the placenta or other aspects of maternal physiology.

A potential risk of fetal adrenal suppression after maternal administration of corticosteroids has been suggested, and cases of fetal adrenal atrophy documented pathologically have been reported.[84, 93] However, clinical evidence of adrenal insufficiency in the newborn in such circumstances is unusual. In one series, there was no evidence of neonatal adrenal insufficiency in any of 71 infants born to mothers receiving an average daily dose of 8.2 mg of prednisone for variable periods of time during pregnancy.[88] The absence of clinical evidence for neonatal adrenal insufficiency has even been observed with doses as high as 40 to 60 mg of prednisone per day given throughout the entire duration of pregnancy.[95]

One possible explanation for the lack of neonatal adrenal suppression may be the relative inability of the fetal-placental unit to convert prednisone to its active form, prednisolone.[66] However, it is important to note that the use of steroids during pregnancy does suppress maternal adrenal function, and supplemental corticosteroids for the mother at the time of labor and delivery are generally indicated.

It is reasonable to expect that an inhaled steroid preparation, i.e., beclomethasone, would be potentially useful in pregnancy, since the decreased frequency of systemic side effects should be associated with fewer possible fetal complications. However, since this preparation is still relatively new, insufficient data are yet available to fully assess its usefulness and role in treating the pregnant asthmatic woman.

Other Forms of Obstructive Lung Disease

Because chronic bronchitis and emphysema are unusual in women of childbearing age, little information is available regarding interactions between pregnancy and forms of obstructive lung disease other than asthma. The only pregnant woman with emphysema reported in the literature was a patient with alpha-1-antitrypsin deficiency, a disease associated with early onset of panacinar emphysema.[99] This patient, who had significant obstructive disease, was delivered of a normal infant after normal labor at 38 weeks.

Bronchiectasis, an irreversible dilation of bronchi often associated with chronic cough, sputum production, and recurrent infections, is occasionally found in women of childbearing age. It is often the result of prior bronchial injury due to various types of infection, particularly necrotizing viral or bacterial pneumonia in childhood.

One author has reported a total of 44 pregnancies in 21 patients with bronchiectasis;[104] in only one instance could difficulty during pregnancy or the postpartum period be attributed to bronchiectasis. In another study,[101] little change was found in pulmonary function, degree of dyspnea, or volume of sputum production in each of three pregnant women with bronchiectasis, and no evidence of intrauterine growth retardation was observed. However, a patient has been reported with bronchiectasis and a prior lobectomy whose pregnancies resulted in an infant of low birth-

weight and an intrauterine fetal death at 38 weeks.[105]

The most severe obstructive functional abnormalities during pregnancy are observed in women with cystic fibrosis. In this disease, abnormal mucus results in pancreatic disease, with ductal obstruction and pancreatic insufficiency, and lung disease, with airway plugging, inflammation, bronchiectasis, and recurrent bronchopulmonary infections. The pulmonary disease that occurs with cystic fibrosis generally does not produce a pure obstructive physiologic pattern but rather a mixed picture of obstructive and restrictive disease.

The initial description of pregnancy in a woman with cystic fibrosis was reported in 1960,[103] and at least ten other cases have subsequently been reported.[100, 102] Approximately half of these patients had serious and progressive pulmonary decompensation during and after pregnancy, while the other half did not experience significant adverse effects from their pregnancy.[100] However, since the natural history of this disease involves a downhill course, it is difficult to determine how pregnancy contributed to any deterioration in clinical status. Of 13 infants in the latter report,[100] 11 were believed to be normal at birth, although 3 of these were premature. As expected from the autosomal recessive transmission of this disease, none of the infants had cystic fibrosis, although they are presumably carriers of the abnormal gene.

Sarcoidosis

Definition. Sarcoidosis is a multisystem granulomatous disease of unknown cause presenting frequently in young adults; although it most commonly affects the lungs, some of the other systems or organs that can be involved include lymph nodes, skin, eyes, heart, and liver. The characteristic pathologic finding in affected tissues is the noncaseating granuloma, but no specific etiologic agent initiating the granuloma formation has yet been identified. Immunologic abnormalities, namely impaired delayed hypersensitivity and excessive immunoglobulin production, are well described as frequent accompaniments of the disease, and current theories of pathogenesis rely heavily on immunologic mechanisms being operative.

Disease in the Nonpregnant State. The pulmonary abnormalities that may occur in sarcoidosis include bilateral hilar adenopathy, interstitial lung disease, or both, any of which may or may not be accompanied by extrathoracic involvement or systemic symptoms. The most common presentations of the disease are with respiratory symptoms, especially dyspnea and nonproductive cough, or with an abnormal chest roentgenogram but no symptoms.

Definitive diagnosis is made in the appropriate clinical setting by the finding of noncaseating granulomas in affected tissues, particularly the lung. Techniques for obtaining involved tissue within the chest include transbronchial biopsy via fiberoptic bronchoscopy, mediastinoscopy, and open lung biopsy. The first of these procedures has become a particularly popular method for diagnosing sarcoidosis, since it is relatively noninvasive and has a high yield of diagnostic findings, even when the chest roentgenogram does not show parenchymal disease.

Although the course of the disease is variable, in approximately two thirds of patients the manifestations of disease clear within two to three years, or improve, leaving minor residual chest roentgenographic abnormalities without active extrathoracic disease. Of the remaining one third of patients, most have a smoldering course over years.

Disease in Pregnancy. Several series investigating the effects of pregnancy on sarcoidosis have produced generally consistent results. One report described 16 pregnancies in 10 patients with sarcoidosis and found that pregnancy frequently ameliorated the patient's underlying disease.[110] In 8 of the 10 patients, improvement in at least some of the manifestations of sarcoidosis occurred during the antenatal period; the condition of 2 patients remained unchanged. However, the abnormal findings returned within several months in approximately one half of the patients, and some had new manifestations of sarcoidosis not previously noted.

Another author followed up 10 patients with sarcoidosis through 17 pregnancies, concluded that pregnancy had no consistent effect on the course of the disease,[112] and subsequently reported two patients who had successful pregnancies despite severe restrictive lung disease due to sarcoidosis.[113]

Several other studies each suggested that pregnancy does not adversely affect the course of sarcoidosis, since almost all patients improve or remain unchanged.[107, 108, 111] Only a rare patient seems to get worse during the antepartum period.

Scadding has perhaps best summarized the overall effects of pregnancy on sarcoidosis and has described characteristic patterns in different categories of patients.[114] When a woman's chest roentgenogram had resolved to normal or showed inactive fibrotic residua prior to pregnancy, it remained unchanged throughout gestation. When the roentgenogram was resolving prior to pregnancy, it generally continued on the course of resolution throughout the prenatal period. Finally, patients with active disease tended to have partial or complete resolution of their roentgenographic changes during pregnancy, though most patients in this group experienced an exacerbation of their disease within three to six months after delivery.

Since, as will be described, corticosteroids suppress the manifestations of sarcoidosis, it has been suggested that the elevated circulating levels of both free and total cortisol during pregnancy may explain the frequent tendency for improvement at this time. Although this seems like a reasonable explanation, there is no definite proof that changes in circulating corticosteroid levels are responsible. In fact, since sarcoidosis improves spontaneously in many patients, it is likely that improvement in some patients is coincident with, but not due to, their pregnancy.

There is no current evidence for any adverse effect of sarcoidosis on either fertility or the course of pregnancy.[114] Although a few patients have been described with either miscarriages or congenital abnormalities,[110, 112] the incidence of such problems with pregnancy or the fetus does not appear to be increased over that in mothers without sarcoidosis.[111, 114] It is also of interest that histologic examination of placental tissue has shown no evidence of granulomatous disease.[109, 113] In the single reported case of antepartum death in a patient with sarcoidosis,[109] the patient also had pre-eclampsia, and the contribution of the patient's pulmonary disease to her death is therefore not clear.

Treatment. Corticosteroids are the treatment of choice for patients with sarcoidosis. However, even though steroids clearly suppress many of the manifestations of the disease, it has not been definitely shown that they alter its overall course. Treatment decisions are further complicated by the fact that sarcoidosis often follows a course of spontaneous improvement and roentgenographic resolution, even without any therapy.[106]

Well-accepted indications for treatment include significant disease affecting a vital organ, especially with myocardial, ocular, or central nervous system involvement. Pulmonary involvement should not be treated on the basis of roentgenographic manifestations alone, since they may not correlate with functional impairment and may also spontaneously improve. Corticosteroid treatment for pulmonary sarcoidosis should rather be based on significant pulmonary functional impairment; if available, information about the course of a patient's disease, by observation over at least two time points, may also be useful in deciding whom and when to treat.

When therapy is begun, the starting dosage is often 40 to 60 mg of prednisone per day. It is usually continued for at least a six-month period but is generally tapered during this time to a lower maintenance dose.

Treatment in Pregnancy. Use of corticosteroids for treatment of sarcoidosis during pregnancy generally follows the same guidelines as treatment in the nonpregnant patient. Since sarcoidosis rarely develops or becomes worse during pregnancy, it is quite unusual for indications for treatment to develop de novo during pregnancy. In women who are already receiving steroids for sarcoidosis, the dose should be kept constant or decreased because of the frequent amelioration of the disease during pregnancy.

Potential complications of steroid use during pregnancy have been discussed in detail in a previous section of this chapter and will not be repeated here.

Tuberculosis

Disease in the Nonpregnant State. Tuberculosis, caused by infection with the acid-fast bacillus *Mycobacterium tuberculosis,* has undergone a most dramatic decline in frequency over the past 50 years, owing to improved sanitation and the development of effective chemotherapy. The organism may cause either pulmonary or extrapulmonary infection, approximately 90 per cent of patients with active disease having pulmonary involvement.

The majority of cases of pulmonary tuberculosis in the United States result from reactivation of old disease, frequently in elderly or debilitated patients. In this setting, disease often appears on chest roentgenogram as upper lobe infiltrates with or without cavitation. Patients may be asymptomatic or may present with constitutional symptoms (low-grade fever, weight loss, malaise, anorexia, night sweats) or respiratory symptoms (cough, sputum production, hemoptysis).

Primary tuberculous infection, although formerly considered mainly a childhood problem, is not uncommon in the adult population, particularly as the incidence of previous exposure during childhood has declined considerably. Patients are frequently asymptomatic at the time of infection and are often only recognized by con-

version of the tuberculin skin test. Primary infection may also result in (1) nonspecific symptoms of pneumonia (fever and cough, often nonproductive), with roentgenographic findings of parenchymal infiltrates or adenopathy, or (2) pleural effusion, with symptoms of pleuritic chest pain, fever, and cough. Patients may occasionally present with direct progression to upper lobe disease, similar to the classic "reactivation" pattern, or with extrapulmonary disease.

Diagnosis in Pregnancy. In the hope of detecting cases of active or inactive tuberculosis that might require therapeutic intervention, many clinicians have, until relatively recently, advised routine prenatal chest roentgenograms.[130, 149, 152] However, because of recent studies examining the value of routine prenatal chest roentgenograms, it has become apparent that this routine practice is no longer justified. The rationale for eliminating the routine prenatal chest roentgenogram is based not so much on potential risk to the fetus as on the low yield of the procedure now that the prevalence of tuberculosis is low. In two large series of routine prenatal chest roentgenograms, a positive history or physical examination almost always suggested the need for a roentgenogram in patients eventually found to have an abnormality.[121, 139] Thus, roentgenography should be reserved for patients with a history or findings suggestive of pulmonary disease or tuberculosis.

If a chest roentgenogram is clinically indicated, pregnancy should not be considered a contraindication to the study. The exposure to radiation from a chest roentgenogram is approximately 50 mrad to the chest and 2.5 to 5 mrad to the gonads.[121, 153, 154] In a detailed analysis of prenatal radiation exposure and subsequent occurrence of malformations or cancer, an overall risk has been estimated of 0 to 1 case per 1000 patients irradiated by 1 rad in utero during the first four months of pregnancy.[140] Given that the radiation exposure from a chest roentgenogram is much smaller than the 1 rad dose used to calculate that risk, there appears to be no measurable risk associated with a chest roentgenogram during pregnancy.[121, 153] When indicated, however, the roentgenogram should be performed with abdominal shielding and preferably after the first trimester to avoid even this small amount of exposure to rapidly dividing and differentiating fetal tissues.

The tuberculin skin test is currently an important screening test for tuberculosis, but it is well recognized that a positive test indicates only a history of tuberculous infection and not active disease. In addition, only approximately 80 per cent of patients with reactivation tuberculosis have a positive skin test, negative tests being at least partially due to anergy in some patients.

The validity of tuberculin testing during pregnancy has been questioned, partly because of the finding of decreased lymphocyte reactivity in vitro to purified protein derivative (PPD) during the course of pregnancy. However, there has been debate about the effect of pregnancy on the tuberculin skin test, which is an in vivo measure of delayed hypersensitivity. A lower prevalence of positive tuberculin tests was found in pregnant women than in control subjects,[128] but the study has been criticized because study patients did not serve as their own control subjects.[135] Other studies testing the same patients during and after pregnancy have demonstrated no effect of pregnancy on cutaneous tuberculin hypersensitivity, and it is now generally accepted that tuberculin skin testing is probably valid through the course of pregnancy.[141, 144, 157]

In consideration of the available information on chest roentgenograms and tuberculin skin testing during pregnancy, it seems reasonable to perform tuberculin skin testing early in the course of pregnancy as a screening procedure for tuberculosis. A chest roentgenogram should then be performed only in (1) tuberculin reactors with known prior negative reactions; (2) tuberculin reactors in whom the time of conversion is unknown; and (3) patients with a suggestive history or physical examination, even if the skin test is negative.[157]

Definitive diagnostic proof of tuberculosis in both the pregnant and the nonpregnant patient is dependent on demonstration of *Mycobacterium tuberculosis* by culture, especially of sputum. If a spontaneous sputum specimen cannot be obtained, sputum can frequently be induced by chest physiotherapy and inhalation of an aerosol effective in generating a productive cough, such as hypertonic saline. If necessary, specimens can always be obtained with washings and brushings via a fiberoptic bronchoscope.

In many cases, a diagnosis of tuberculosis can be made by demonstration of acid-fast bacilli on an appropriately stained smear, but culture should always be additionally performed for definitive identification and for determination of drug sensitivity.

In patients who present with a tuberculous pleural effusion, acid-fast organisms are rarely found on a smear of pleural fluid, and culture of the fluid is positive in only 30 per cent of patients. In such cases, a strong clinical suspicion of tuberculous effusion can be based on an unexplained exudative effusion with lympho-cytes predominating, in a patient with a positive tuberculin skin test. Diagnostic yield is greatest by combining culture of pleural fluid with culture and histologic examination of a pleural biopsy; the combined procedures document a tuberculous cause in approximately 80 per cent of cases. In the setting of a strong clinical suspicion of tuberculosis in the patient with a positive skin test, however, it is generally advisable to begin therapy while awaiting culture results.

Course in Pregnancy. Medical opinion about the interaction between pregnancy and tuberculosis has changed several times since antiquity. From the time of Hippocrates until the middle of the 19th century, it was thought that pregnancy had an overall beneficial effect on tuberculosis. A diametrically opposite view was taken from 1850 until the 1940s, and therapeutic abortion was frequently recommended to avert the presumed deleterious effect of pregnancy. An intermediate view was taken in 1953 by Hedvall,[133] who reached the conclusion based on a large number of patients that pregnancy and labor seldom have a harmful effect on women with tuberculosis. A comparison of the course of tuberculosis in 22 pregnant and 40 nonpregnant women of the same age also found no differences between the two groups.[129] Three criteria were used for comparison: rate of stabilization of disease, conversion of sputum and gastric washings, and cavity closure. There was no significant difference between the two groups by any of these three criteria.

Even though pregnancy itself has little effect on the natural history of tuberculous infection, several studies in the prechemotherapeutic era found an increased rate of deterioration or progressive disease during the first postpartum year. In a series of 276 women whose tuberculosis remained stable throughout the course of pregnancy, 37, or 13.4 per cent, showed deterioration during the first postpartum year.[133] In another study of 930 women with pulmonary tuberculosis, progression of disease occurred in 90 cases within the first 6 weeks after delivery, even though the antenatal course was favorable in 70 of these 90 patients.[131] Several theories have been proposed to explain this phenomenon, including rapid hormonal changes, postpartum descent of the diaphragm, the nutritional strain of lactation, and insufficient sleep because of the time demands of a newborn infant. However, it is not universally accepted that an increased risk of progression exists in the first postpartum year, compared with the potential for deterioration that exists in any untreated patient over a one-year period.[149]

Any unsettled controversy about the effect of pregnancy or the postpartum period on tuberculosis has become unimportant since the advent of effective chemotherapy. With adequate treatment for active tuberculosis, pregnant women appear to have the same excellent prognosis as their nonpregnant counterparts. In one series,[149] all 72 pregnant women with active tuberculosis showed regression and control of disease with treatment. Women with inactive tuberculosis given prophylactic isoniazid similarly had a stable course without reactivation during pregnancy and the postpartum period. Of 444 such patients in the inactive category, 442 remained stable and had no evidence of activation, while two had some progression of disease despite isoniazid prophylaxis. These latter patients required more intensive therapy to control their disease.

Several more recent studies have confirmed the excellent prognosis of treated tuberculosis in pregnant women. One review of the course of 149 pregnancies in 100 women with tuberculosis showed no adverse effect of pregnancy, birth, the postpartum period, or lactation.[127] There was no risk of relapse when the lung disease was adequately treated, even in patients with active disease or those with persistence of a post-chemotherapy cavity. The experience at New York Lying-In Hospital in 1565 patients followed between 1933 and 1972 was recently reviewed.[147] Since 1965, the incidence of tuberculosis diagnosed during pregnancy has been in the range of 0.6 to 1.0 per cent. In patients seen between 1957 and 1972 and therefore treated with antituberculous drugs, progression of disease occurred in less than 1 per cent. The comparable progression rate from 1933 to 1956 was 3 to 4 per cent.

Most series investigating the effect of tuberculosis on the course of pregnancy and on the newborn have concluded that pregnancy is not altered by the patient's tuberculosis. In one large series, 600 out of 616 pregnancies resulted in the birth of 602 normal live infants.[149] There were 7 cases of early, spontaneous abortion and 9 cases of antepartum or intrapartum fetal death. The authors did not note an effect of tuberculosis on the duration of pregnancy. One group reported no increase in prematurity and no cases of congenital tuberculosis in the 1588 infants delivered in their series.[147]

A carefully controlled series investigating the course and outcome of pregnancy in women with pulmonary tuberculosis was recently reported from Norway.[118] Based on a comparison of pregnancies in 542 women with pulmonary tuberculosis and 112,530 women without tuberculosis, these authors found an excessive occurrence of pregnancy complications, miscarriage, and difficult labor in women with tuberculosis. Among antepartum complications, the study population had a statistically significant higher frequency of toxemia (7.4 vs 4.7 per cent) and vaginal hemorrhage (4.1 vs 2.2 per cent), while hyperemesis was not significantly increased. Labor was induced more often in the study group than in controls (14.6 vs 9.1 per cent) and was more often complicated (15.1 vs 9.6 per cent), and interventions during labor were required more frequently (12.6 vs 7.7 per cent). However, the most striking difference between the two groups was in the risk of miscarriage, defined in this study as fetal death between 16 and 28 weeks. The frequency of miscarriage was approximately ninefold higher (20.1/1000 vs 2.3/1000) in the patients with tuberculosis than in controls. No differences were found in numbers of multiple births or congenital malformations. Comparison of live births showed no differences in the mean gestation period, percentage of premature infants, percentage of low birthweight infants, or mean birthweight. In interpreting this study, however, it is difficult to define which factors contributed to the greater frequency of miscarriage and pregnancy complications. In particular, since tuberculosis is more common in lower socioeconomic groups, the potential role of social or economic factors, rather than tuberculosis, must be considered.

Because of the excellent prognosis for treated tuberculosis in pregnant women, the recommendation for therapeutic abortion that was commonly given for these patients has long since been abandoned. Nevertheless, the development of chemotherapy has not entirely eradicated the complicated management problems that can occur in pregnancy. Even in the recent literature, there are reports of women who have been quite ill from meningeal,[132, 151] miliary,[151] and peritoneal[124] involvement with tuberculosis during pregnancy.

Treatment. Treatment of tuberculosis is based on the principles that (1) more than one drug must be used in order to prevent selection and growth of resistant organisms, and (2) therapy must be prolonged. Within this framework, newer regimens have been devised to simplify treatment and reduce the duration of drug administration, and these regimens are gradually being accepted as routine therapy in many instances.

Until recently, the standard regimen of therapy for pulmonary or extrapulmonary tuberculosis has consisted of two drugs, isoniazid (INH) and ethambutol, administered for 18 to 24 months. In cases of life-threatening disease, especially miliary, pericardial, or meningeal tuberculosis, or sometimes with advanced pulmonary disease, a third agent, generally either rifampin or streptomycin, should be added for 1 to 3 months to provide a more intensive initial regimen. Another alternative for advanced pulmonary disease has been the specific combination of INH and rifampin, which is as effective for advanced disease as either INH-ethambutol-streptomycin or INH-ethambutol-rifampin.[142]

Numerous British and American studies have now described the use of either intermittent or short-course chemotherapy for routine treatment of tuberculosis. These studies have shown the following regimens to be effective: (1) intermittent chemotherapy given twice weekly after an initial phase of daily therapy, which may be particularly useful for noncompliant patients in whom supervised administration of drugs is essential; and (2) short-course chemotherapy, particularly the regimen of INH and rifampin given for 9 to 12 months.

The American Thoracic Society and the Center for Disease Control have recently accepted short-course chemotherapy as an acceptable alternative to more conventional chemotherapy and have published guidelines for its use.[116] The various acceptable regimens for conventional and short-course chemotherapy are summarized in Table 17–1. According to the published guidelines, short-course chemotherapy was not recommended for patients with extrapulmonary tuberculosis, for drug-resistant cases, or for patients with complicating medical conditions. In addition, patients receiving intermittent rifampin should be regularly monitored by history for manifestations of thrombocytopenia (purpura, petechiae, hematuria) or a "flu-syndrome," and patients should remain under surveillance for 12 months after completion of therapy.

The major potential side effects of INH are hepatitis, hypersensitivity reactions, and peripheral neuropathy. Transient elevation of SGOT, occurring in 10 to 20 per cent of patients, is not necessarily an indication for discontinuing therapy; serious hepatotoxicity resembles viral hepatitis and has an increased incidence with advancing age. Based on data from a recent large study,[123] serious hepatotoxicity seems to be avoidable if SGOT is routinely monitored monthly, and INH is discontinued if SGOT elevation is greater than 5 times normal. In addition, INH should also be stopped in patients with symptoms suggestive of toxicity and any level of SGOT elevation. Peripheral neuropathy with INH can be prevented by supplemental administration of pyridoxine, 50 mg/day; although pyridoxine is not routinely necessary in the normal patient, it may be advisable to administer it to the pregnant woman receiving INH, as described later. Hypersensitivity reactions may include fever, rash, and a lupus-like syndrome, often with a positive test for antinuclear antibodies.

Although optic neuritis has been well described as a potential complication of ethambutol therapy, it is quite rare with the usual dose of 15 mg/kg/day. Rifampin may cause hepatitis, hypersensitivity reactions, and occasional hematologic toxicity. Patients should be forewarned to expect orange discoloration of urine, sweat, tears, and saliva. When given intermittently, rifampin has

TABLE 17–1 REGIMENS FOR TREATMENT OF TUBERCULOSIS*

Regimen	Drugs	Duration	Comments
Standard course	INH (300 mg/d) + ethambutol (15 mg/kg/d)	18–24 months	Standard regimen for most cases of drug-sensitive tuberculosis
	INH (300 mg/d) + ethambutol (15 mg/kg/d) + streptomycin (1 g/d)	1–3 months for all 3 drugs; then INH and ethambutol alone to complete 18–24 months	Can be used with more severe or with life-threatening disease; streptomycin best avoided during pregnancy
	INH (300 mg/d) + rifampin (600 mg/d)	18–24 months	As effective as three-drug regimen
Short course	INH (300 mg/d) + rifampin (600 mg/d)	9–12 months	None of short-course regimens yet recommended for extrapulmonary tuberculosis
	INH (300 mg/d) + rifampin (600 mg/d) followed by INH (15 mg/kg biw) + rifampin (600 mg biw)	1–3 months daily therapy followed by biweekly therapy to complete 9–12 month course	

*All regimens must be modified if drug resistance is suspected or known.

occasionally been described to cause a "flu-syndrome," abdominal pain, acute renal failure, or thrombocytopenia. Although these potential reactions were a cause of concern over the use of rifampin in intermittent chemotherapy, recent studies have not shown a clinically important frequency of these effects. Finally, the efficacy of oral contraceptives may be impaired by the concurrent administration of rifampin. At least eight cases of pregnancy in women who were taking both oral contraceptives and rifampin have now been reported, possibly related to altered hepatic metabolism of exogenous estrogens.[150]

Effect of Treatment on Pregnancy and the Fetus. Indications for chemotherapy of proven or suspected active tuberculosis and the principles of management are similar in the pregnant woman and the nonpregnant patient. The use of short-course chemotherapy in the pregnant woman has not been well described, but it seems reasonable to consider it an effective treatment alternative in the pregnant patient.

Extensive experience with the use of isoniazid in pregnancy has accumulated. Even though INH crosses the placenta, its use does not appear to be contraindicated in active tuberculous disease. Most studies have shown no teratogenic effect of INH, even when the drug was administered during the first 4 months of pregnancy.[138, 148] However, one recent series did note an approximately twofold increased risk of malformations when mothers were exposed to isoniazid.[134] Consequently, it seems advisable to limit the use of INH during pregnancy to patients for whom its use is clearly indicated, namely, those with active disease. Prophylactic therapy with isoniazid, which is normally given to patients at high risk for future development of active disease,[115] should be withheld during pregnancy and started in the postpartum period. When isoniazid is used in the pregnant patient, supplemental pyridoxine is recommended to satisfy the increased need for this vitamin during pregnancy[122] and to prevent any potential neurotoxicity in the fetus.[156]

Use of ethambutol during pregnancy has been reported in several recent series, and it does not appear to be contraindicated during pregnancy.[120, 137, 148] No relationship has been established between use of ethambutol during pregnancy and subsequent fetal abnormalities, and overall experience has not suggested any other adverse maternal or fetal effects in this setting.

Although the ability of rifampin to inhibit DNA-dependent RNA polymerase has led to some concern about its use during pregnancy, no adverse fetal effects of rifampin have yet been noted in the more than 100 reported cases.[148] The lack of reported toxicity to date suggests that the drug is safe in pregnancy, but since it can cross the placental barrier, the possibility of future reports of fetal toxicity always exists.

Streptomycin used to be given frequently for treatment of tuberculosis during pregnancy, but its potential for fetal ototoxicity suggests that other first-line drugs are preferable. Although the most frequently observed effects in offspring of treated mothers are minor vestibular impairment, auditory impairment, or both,[126] cases of severe and bilateral hearing loss and marked vestibular abnormalities have been reported.[146]

Little is known about the specific effects in pregnancy of the second-line, much less commonly used antituberculous drugs. Their usefulness is clearly limited, more by the potential side effects on the mother than by adverse effects on the fetus. In particular, the gastrointestinal effects of para-aminosalicylic acid, the central nervous system effects of cycloserine, and the potential hepatotoxicity of pyrazinamide make their use during pregnancy undesirable. A teratogenic effect has been attributed to ethionamide, and its use is therefore contraindicated in pregnancy.[143]

Neonatal Management. Management of the infant born to a mother with tuberculosis generally involves preventing or treating early infection contracted in the neonatal period. Congenital infection, transmitted either by a hematogenous route or by aspiration of infected amniotic fluid, is uncommon, and most infection is by postpartum maternal contact.[119, 145, 155] The risk of active disease during the first year of life may be as high as 50 per cent if prophylactic measures are not taken.[136] The main options for protection of the newborn without active infection involve either isoniazid chemoprophylaxis or BCG vaccination. Isoniazid chemoprophylaxis is effective in the newborn, but adequate treatment requires daily administration.[157] BCG vaccination is useful in this setting,[136] particularly since only a single administration of vaccine is necessary. Therefore, if reliability of administration of isoniazid to the baby is a concern, then BCG vaccination may be preferable, even though the value of future tuberculin testing is lost. Further consideration of these issues can be found in detail in previous articles.[117, 125, 157]

Other Infectious Diseases of the Lung

Apart from tuberculosis, the major infectious diseases that can affect the lung during pregnancy are the same as those frequently found in nonpregnant adults of childbearing age, namely those due to viruses, mycoplasma, and bacterial pathogens. This particular differential diagnosis must be considered in the otherwise healthy patient who presents with relatively acute symptoms of fever, cough (either productive or nonproductive), and infiltrates on chest roentgenogram.

In all such cases, the most important diagnostic information can be obtained from sputum examination and culture, which may be indicative of pneumonia due to a particular bacterial pathogen. If sputum is not obtainable by spontaneous expectoration, an attempt should be made to induce a sputum specimen by chest physiotherapy and inhalation of an aerosol (e.g., hypertonic saline) to promote cough and sputum production. If the patient is quite ill with a presumed but undiagnosed bacterial pneumonia, consideration must be given to either transtracheal aspiration or fiberoptic bronchoscopy for obtaining a good specimen. However, it is difficult to formalize indications for either of these procedures, and clinical judgment must be exercised in the individual case.

BACTERIAL PNEUMONIA

The most common bacterial pneumonia found in otherwise healthy women of this age group is pneumococcal pneumonia due to *Streptococcus pneumoniae*. This organism is an encapsulated gram-positive diplococcus that often inhabits the nasopharynx of normal persons. However, frequently after disruption of normal respiratory clearance mechanisms from a viral upper respiratory tract infection, pneumococci may enter and proliferate in the alveoli, evoking a vigorous inflammatory response.

The clinical presentation of pneumococcal pneumonia is generally that of abrupt onset of fever, chills, pleuritic chest pain, and cough productive of purulent or blood-tinged sputum. Patients may complain of dyspnea and characteristically are tachypneic on examination. Other physical findings include fever and often signs of localized consolidation, such as rales, dullness, and bronchial breath sounds. Early in the course, however, findings may be more nonspecific, and may include only some localized rales. The chest roentgenogram classically shows a picture of lobar consolidation with air bronchograms, but involvement may instead be either patchy or multilobar. Gram stain of sputum typically shows numerous polymorphonuclear leukocytes and gram-positive, lancet-shaped diplococci. Sputum culture is frequently negative because of the

fastidious nature of the organism, and the diagnosis therefore does not necessarily depend on identifying the organisms on culture. Bacteremia is present in approximately 30 per cent of cases; pleural effusions occur in approximately 5 per cent of patients, either as sterile parapneumonic effusions or as frank empyema.

The treatment of choice is penicillin, given either orally (penicillin VK 250 to 500 mg four times a day) or, in the more severely ill patient, parenterally (1.2 to 2.4 million units/day in divided doses). Treatment should generally be continued at least 3 to 5 days after defervescence, making a total course of 7 to 14 days of therapy, In the penicillin-allergic patient, erythromycin is an acceptable alternative; erythromycin is also useful in the patient for whom pneumococcus and mycoplasma both remain diagnostic possibilities.

Prevention of pneumococcal infection by a vaccine incorporating multiple capsular polysaccharides is now recommended for patients at particular risk for development of pneumococcal disease. However, the effect of this vaccine in pregnancy is not known, and the vaccine is currently considered to be contraindicated in the pregnant woman.[158]

Other types of bacterial pneumonia are much less common in women of this age group and will not be discussed here. However, it is important to note that viral infections, particularly influenza, may sometimes be complicated by development of a superimposed bacterial pneumonia. In these cases, the pneumococcus is still a common pathogen, but additional considerations include pneumonias due to streptococci, staphylococci, and *Hemophilus influenzae*.

Although bacterial pneumonia during pregnancy has been well described in the older literature, very little recent information is available about its course and potential complications in the pregnant woman.[164] This paucity of recent data is presumably due to the efficacy of antimicrobial drugs in treating such pneumonias. Pregnancy itself does not appear to adversely affect the response to therapy, and there are no recent data to suggest specific fetal complications from bacterial pneumonia developing during pregnancy. Further discussion of antibiotic therapy in pregnancy is found in Chapter 13.

MYCOPLASMA PNEUMONIA

Mycoplasma species, the smallest known free-living organisms, are unlike bacteria because of the absence of a rigid cell wall. Pneumonia is caused by the agent *Mycoplasma pneumoniae*, which is responsible for a large percentage of pneumonias in ambulatory patients, and is particularly common in children and young adults.

The onset of mycoplasma pneumonia is often more gradual than the bacterial pneumonias, symptoms of sore throat, nonproductive cough, headache, and fever being particularly prominent. Although patients may have rales on chest examination, pneumonia is usually diagnosed by the infiltrates on the chest roentgenogram. The infiltrates are generally patchy, and either unilateral or bilateral involvement may occur; occasionally, there is frank consolidation. Pleural effusions are seldom clinically apparent, although they may be demonstrable on lateral decubitus views in up to 20 per cent of patients. Other associated findings or complications that occasionally occur with mycoplasma pneumonia include bullous myringitis, hemolytic anemia, skin eruptions (especially erythema multiforme), and either cardiac or neurologic involvement.

Diagnosis of this disease is generally dependent upon the presence of cold agglutinins, which are suggestive but not diagnostic of mycoplasma, or the presence of complement-fixing antibodies to mycoplasma. However, these serologic tests often do not reveal significant titers until the second week of illness, and thus their value in early diagnosis is limited. In contrast to the bacterial pneumonias, patients do not generally have leukocytosis, and sputum, if obtainable, usually does not show an abundance of polymorphonuclear leukocytes.

Since diagnosis can often not be made with certainty at the time of initial presentation, a presumptive diagnosis is frequently made on the basis of the entire clinical picture. Treatment for mycoplasma is either erythromycin or tetracycline; however, since tetracycline is contraindicated during pregnancy, erythromycin is clearly the drug of choice in this setting. As mentioned earlier, erythromycin is particularly useful when pneumococcal and mycoplasma pneumonia are both possible, since it is effective against either entity. It is of interest that, although adequate treatment of mycoplasma pneumonia decreases the length of associated clinical symptoms, it does not necessarily eradicate shedding of the organism from the sputum.

To our knowledge, no clinical studies have specifically investigated the course of mycoplasma pneumonia during pregnancy. As with bacterial pneumonia, it is likely but not proved that pregnancy does not exert an adverse effect on the natural history of mycoplasma pneumonia. Similarly, no data are available to suggest any fetal complications due to maternal mycoplasma pneumonia.

VIRAL INFECTION

Discussion of influenza, the viral respiratory tract infection that has been best studied in pregnancy, is included in Chapter 14, Viral Infections.

The other virus for which respiratory tract involvement during pregnancy has been well described is varicella. At least 20 cases of varicella pneumonia have been reported during pregnancy, constituting approximately 10 per cent of all reported cases of varicella pneumonia.[163, 166, 167] In the cases reported to date, maternal mortality has been approximately 45 per cent, in comparison with the 15 to 20 per cent mortality described among nonpregnant patients. In addition to the high maternal mortality rate, only approximately one out of six pregnancies has been free of neonatal complications, including abortion, in utero death associated with maternal death, prematurity, or neonatal varicella.[163] It is presumed that maternal hypoxia due to extensive pneumonia is a prime factor resulting in maternal and fetal complications.[167]

FUNGAL INFECTIONS

A detailed analysis of the clinical aspects and diagnosis of the various fungal disorders of the lung is beyond the scope of this discussion but can be found in recent review articles.[159, 161]

Of the various fungal infections that may be encountered during pregnancy, coccidioidomycosis has generated the most interest, primarily because of its tendency to disseminate during pregnancy. Of the 50 cases of coccidioidomycosis either reported or reviewed by Harris,[162] 22 became disseminated. In patients having the onset of coccidioidomycosis before pregnancy, the risk of dissemination increased to 20 per cent from the 0.2 per cent risk expected for dissemination in the nonpregnant patient. The risk was even higher in patients who contracted the infection during pregnancy, particularly in the second or third trimester.[162]

When coccidioidomycosis remains in its benign, nondisseminated form, there appears to be no particular hazard for either the mother or the fetus. By contrast, in the untreated disseminated form, the maternal mortality rate is nearly 100 per cent, compared with the 50 per cent mortality among untreated nonpregnant patients.[162] However, it has been reported that amphotericin B therapy of the pregnant woman with disseminated disease will save a significant proportion of patients.[170]

Prognosis for the fetus depends largely on whether there is dissemination of maternal disease. It was noted that approximately three fourths of the pregnancies in patients with non-disseminated coccidioidomycosis resulted in viable term infants, compared with approximately one fourth in patients with disseminated disease.[162] In the patients with disseminated disease, prematurity occurred in almost half, and a large proportion of the premature infants died in the neonatal period. As expected, treatment of the mother with amphotericin during pregnancy does appear to improve the outlook for the fetus,[170] but further data are not available regarding the prognosis of adequately treated maternal coccidioidomycosis. Although placental involvement by coccidioidomycosis is well described, fetal infection is rare, even when there is extensive disease of the placenta.[165]

A variety of other fungi have been reported in pregnant women, but except for coccidioidomycosis, involvement appears to occur primarily in women who are immunosuppressed.[168]

The use of amphotericin B has been described during pregnancy, primarily during the second and third trimesters. Although extensive data are not available regarding its effect on the fetus, amphotericin appears not to have any detrimental effects on the fetal or the neonatal course.[160, 169] At least one case of amphotericin use during the first trimester has been reported, and no adverse effects on the fetus were observed.[160]

Pulmonary Embolic Disease

The problems of peripheral venous thrombosis, pulmonary embolism, and anticoagulation in pregnancy are discussed in detail in Chapter 7.

AMNIOTIC FLUID EMBOLISM

Amniotic fluid embolism is the one lung disease that is uniquely associated with pregnancy. Although it is not a common disorder, its high mortality rate makes it account for up to 10 to 15 per cent of maternal deaths.[179]

In this disorder, amniotic fluid enters the maternal circulation during or following labor, with resulting embolization to the pulmonary vasculature. The material that embolizes includes not only amniotic fluid but also fetal squames, lanugo hairs, meconium, fat, mucin, and bile.[174]

This syndrome does not appear to be due to embolization of amniotic fluid itself, since intravenous infusion of fresh, autologous amniotic fluid into pregnant rabbits or rhesus monkeys is innocuous.[171, 180] Rather, one of many contaminants, of either fetal or placental origin, is presumably responsible for initiating the clinical syndrome. Although the major precipitating feature of the disorder is unknown, speculation has centered on three main theories: (1) mechanical occlusion of the pulmonary vasculature by particulate material in the amniotic fluid, (2) hypersensitivity or an anaphylactoid reaction to fetal antigens or particulate matter, and (3) intravascular coagulation due to entry of thromboplastic material into the circulation.[172, 174]

There have been several postulated sites for entry of amniotic fluid into the maternal venous circulation, including (1) endocervical veins, which are lacerated even during normal labor; (2) the placental site, especially with placenta previa, uterine rupture, premature separation of the placenta, or cesarean section with an incision involving the placental implantation site; and (3) uterine veins, at sites of uterine trauma.[174] Exceptionally strong uterine contractions may often be involved in contributing to entry of amniotic fluid into the venous circulation.

Several risk factors have been identified that predispose the mother to development of amniotic fluid embolism. These include (1) tumultuous labor, (2) use of uterine stimulants, (3) meconium in the amniotic fluid, (4) advanced maternal age, (5) multiparity, and (6) intrauterine death.[172, 174, 178] It has been suggested that the association with intrauterine fetal death may be related to increased permeability and friability of fetal membranes.[175]

The clinical picture of amniotic fluid embolism consists of respiratory distress, cardiovascular collapse, and disseminated intravascular coagulation associated with or following labor and delivery. However, since the course of the illness is frequently catastrophic, the full clinical syndrome may not have time to develop. Presenting features may include dyspnea, cyanosis, profound shock, seizures, or cardiac arrest.[172, 178] Heavy bleeding is not a sole presenting feature but rather occurs along with or subsequent to other manifestations of the disorder. Pulmonary edema, brochospasm, and pulmonary hypertension are frequently clinically apparent; pathologic examination of the lungs demonstrates pulmonary edema in addition to amniotic fluid debris in the pulmonary vasculature.[178]

Diagnosis of amniotic fluid embolism has generally been done clinically, based on the constellation of findings just discussed. In particular, the dramatic appearance of dyspnea, hypoxemia, and hypotension in the early postpartum period suggests the diagnosis.[177] Since pulmonary thromboembolism may present with similar findings, the presence of disseminated intravascular coagulation (see Chapter 3) suggests amniotic fluid embolism rather than thromboembolic disease. The diagnostic use of lung scanning has been suggested,[176] but the relatively diffuse and peripheral nature of the involvement, along with the difficulty in distinguishing it from thromboembolism if there is localized disease, makes it doubtful that this will be a definitive diagnostic test. In recent case reports, diagnosis was made by demonstration of squamous cells and cellular debris in blood drawn from a central venous pressure line[179] and in a sample of pulmonary artery blood obtained through a Swan-Ganz catheter.[177] Special stains were used for these studies; in the latter case, a Papanicolaou smear was made from the buffy coat of the blood sample.

Maternal mortality exceeds 80 per cent in amniotic fluid embolism, death often occurring immediately or within the first several hours.[174] Treatment primarily revolves around circulatory and respiratory support. In the acute episode, intubation is commonly necessary for ventilatory support; addition of positive end-expiratory pressure (PEEP) may also be required to decrease the intrapulmonary shunt and assist oxygenation. Vasopressors and volume expansion are frequently required for circulatory support, but care must be given to avoid overhydration, which may aggravate the gas exchange problem. Other suggested modes of therapy have included prompt heparinization, for control of disseminated intravascular coagulation with its attendant bleeding complications,[173] and corticosteroids.[174] The potential uses of these latter two forms of therapy have yet to be well demonstrated.

Aspiration of Gastric Contents

Pulmonary aspiration of gastric contents during pregnancy is primarily a problem at the time of labor and delivery. It has been suggested that the pregnant woman may be particularly susceptible to aspiration, and the following mechanisms have been proposed:[181] (1) elevation of intragastric pressure due to compression of abdominal contents by the gravid uterus, and (2) relaxation of the gastroesophageal sphincter mechanism by progesterone. In addition, it is not uncommon for the stomach to be full at the time of labor, and any complication of labor necessitating general anesthesia may be associated with vomiting and aspiration at the time of induction. Although maternal aspiration appears to be a relatively uncommon problem, it has been suggested that

approximately 2 per cent of maternal deaths result from aspiration.[183]

Two major types of aspiration can be seen at the time of labor and delivery. In the first, inhalation of liquid gastric contents (with a pH <2.5) into the lungs can induce a chemical pneumonitis; in the second, there is airway obstruction due to aspiration of particulate material. These syndromes were originally described in 1946 in a classic paper by Mendelson.[182] Of the 66 obstetric patients with aspiration reported in this series, 5 had acute obstructive reactions from aspiration of food particles, and 61 aspirated liquid gastric contents.[182]

In the syndrome due to inhalation of acid gastric contents, aspiration is soon followed by tachypnea, cyanosis, tachycardia, and hypotension. An inflammatory pneumonitis ensues, and the clinical picture of adult respiratory distress syndrome (ARDS) may result, with leakage of fluid into the alveoli and dyspnea, hypoxemia, and noncompliant lungs. On chest roentgenogram, there are fluffy infiltrates conforming to an alveolar filling pattern; they may be generalized or may correspond to the dependent areas at the time of aspiration. Treatment is mainly supportive, with maintenance of adequate oxygenation by supplemental oxygen and, if necessary, intubation and positive pressure ventilation. The use of high-dose steroids for aspiration is quite controversial. Although they are frequently given, there is no clear evidence that they are beneficial; in fact, a recent study suggested no difference in mortality but an increase in gram-negative bacterial superinfection in patients treated with steroids.[184]

Aspiration of food particles, the other major aspiration syndrome seen in obstetric patients, may cause variable amounts of airway obstruction, depending on the size and consistency of the particles. If the particulate material is sufficiently large, the patient may actually asphyxiate. Supportive measures are again essential, with maintenance of adequate oxygenation as just described. Suctioning should be done to remove particles from the larger airways, and bronchoscopy may be necessary to further localize and remove aspirated food.

Pneumomediastinum

Pneumomediastinum, the presence of free air in the mediastinal space, is an uncommon complication of pregnancy, generally occurring at the time of labor. The pathogenesis is believed to involve rupture of marginally situated alveoli into perivascular tissue planes, with tracking of air towards the hilum and into the mediastinum.[187] Under most circumstances, air subsequently dissects through fascial planes in the neck to result in subcutaneous emphysema. This escape of air from the mediastinum into the subcutaneous tissues prevents buildup of pressure within the mediastinum, which might otherwise impede venous return to the intrathoracic veins.

Spontaneous pneumomediastinum often occurs in the setting of high intra-alveolar pressure, especially with coughing, vomiting, or a Valsalva maneuver. During labor, the intense Valsalva maneuver associated with "bearing down" induces transient marked elevations in intra-alveolar pressure, occasionally resulting in alveolar rupture and the sequence of events outlined above.

Although approximately 200 cases of pneumomediastinum or subcutaneous emphysema associated with pregnancy have been reported to date, very few of them are in the recent medical literature.[185, 186] Almost all the cases have occurred during labor, but a few have been reported at other times during pregnancy.

The main symptom of spontaneous pneumomediastinum is substernal chest pain of abrupt onset, often accompanied by dyspnea. The pain commonly radiates to the shoulders and both arms, and is generally aggravated by coughing, deep inspiration, and swallowing. On physical examination, subcutaneous emphysema is found most commonly in the neck and over the face and chest wall; however, it may require hours for a large amount of subcutaneous crepitation to develop. On auscultation, Hamman's sign, a crunching or crackling sound synchronous with the heart beat, may be heard over the precordium, particularly at the apex with the patient in the left lateral position.

Free mediastinal air on PA chest roentgenogram appears as a radiolucent stripe outlining the heart border, most prominently along the left; there may also be a longitudinal air shadow adjacent to the thoracic aorta. On the lateral projection, there is frequently retrosternal air, and the posterior mediastinal structures, particularly the aorta, may be much more clearly defined than usual.

In spontaneous pneumomediastinum there is usually resorption of air over the course of several days. Although tension pneumomediastinum with death has been reported, it is quite rare, and the development of subcutaneous emphysema almost uniformly relieves the buildup

of pressure before any significant hemodynamic sequelae.

Respiratory Insufficiency

Women with limited respiratory reserve who wish to become pregnant are not encountered frequently, since the disorders associated with chronic respiratory insufficiency generally occur in an older age group. However, occasionally the obstetrician or internist is faced with a patient with limited reserve due to pulmonary fibrosis, cystic fibrosis, or neuromuscular or chest wall disease. These cases are particularly challenging, since the paucity of available data makes it difficult to predict the outcome of pregnancy. Unfortunately, decisions to recommend abortion are therefore more often based on subjective feelings of the physician rather than on hard data regarding contraindications to pregnancy. We will attempt to review the limited data available, but it must be stressed that no reliable cutoff points regarding pulmonary function have been established.

The course of pregnancy in patients with pulmonary insufficiency was first systematically investigated in a series of seven women with 40 to 75 per cent vital capacity due to lung resection or operative collapse.[189] The patients all tolerated pregnancy well, without any diminution in ventilatory capacity; subjective dyspnea was notably infrequent in these patients. The ones with more severe impairment met the greater ventilatory requirements of pregnancy by increasing respiratory rate rather than tidal volume. It is difficult, however, to extrapolate the course in these patients with surgically induced limitation of function to patients with severe obstructive disease or to those with restriction due to diffuse parenchymal fibrosis. Nevertheless, it was suggested that an impaired respiratory system is better able to cope with the additional respiratory demands of pregnancy than is the damaged heart with the increased circulatory demands.

It is difficult to quantitate the actual vital capacity necessary to sustain a patient during pregnancy. Since normal women have little change in vital capacity with pregnancy, one might theoretically expect that an unchanged vital capacity in patients with lung disease would be sufficient to sustain them during pregnancy. Unfortunately, it is frequently those patients with the most severe disease who may have deterioration of their pulmonary function during the course of pregnancy. Although it has been said that a vital capacity of one liter is the minimum functional requirement necessary to maintain a successful pregnancy,[192] there is little objective support for this particular value, and successful pregnancy has been reported with a vital capacity as low as 800 cc.[190]

Theoretically one would expect that patients with baseline CO_2 retention or pulmonary hypertension might be unable to handle the added ventilatory and circulatory demands of pregnancy, respectively. Although insufficient data are available regarding CO_2 retention, some information exists regarding pulmonary hypertension, mainly in those patients with primary pulmonary hypertension. Maternal mortality in this disorder has been reported as greater than 50 per cent,[188, 191] but the degree of pulmonary hypertension seen as a result of chronic lung disease is generally much less than in primary pulmonary hypertension.

There is similarly little information regarding the effect of maternal hypoxemia or hypercapnia on the fetus. Whether the fetus becomes hypoxic is dependent upon numerous factors other than maternal P_{O_2}, including uterine and placental compensatory mechanisms.[192] It has been suggested that premature labor is one potential effect of hypoxemia and hypercapnia, but this hypothesis is as yet unproved.[192]

As is evident from this discussion, knowledge about pregnancy in the woman with borderline respiratory function and limited reserve is inadequate for the development of useful recommendations. Each case must clearly be considered individually, and the relevant information, including the natural history of the patient's disease during pregnancy, must all be collated and then evaluated. Results of spirometry, arterial blood gas analysis, and clinical assessment for pulmonary hypertension all form an important part of the data base, but unfortunately the relative weight that should be attached to each factor has not yet been defined.

SMOKING AND PREGNANCY

Although all physicians are aware of the major role played by cigarette smoke in the production of lung cancer and chronic airflow limitation, the impact of cigarette smoking on the health and viability of the fetus and the newborn is less well recognized. The Surgeon General's Report of 1979 on smoking and health reviewed 212 articles detailing research in this area.[209] Women of childbearing age represent a segment of the population in whom use of cigarettes is increasing. However, the indirect effect of smoking on the fetus and the rarity of cigarette-induced illness in the young mother deflect clinical attention from this extremely important problem. Maternal cigarette smoking has important health consequences in four areas: (1) fetal and infant mortality, (2) birthweight, (3) lactation and breast feeding, and (4) childhood respiratory disease.

Fetal and Infant Mortality. Perinatal mortality is greater in offspring of women who smoke than in their nonsmoking counterparts. However, controversy has existed about the magnitude of the increase in risk relative to other important patient characteristics associated with fetal loss, such as race, low socioeconomic status, increased age and parity, and anemia. The Ontario perinatal mortality study, which included 51,490 births and 1356 deaths (701 fetal and 655 neonatal), represents one of the best attempts to deal with the complex methodologic issues presented by this type of research question.[201, 202, 203, 204] The authors examined the effect of three levels of maternal cigarette smoking on infant mortality: none, less than one pack per day, and greater than one pack per day. After controlling for the above-noted maternal characteristics and numerous other factors, light smoking was found to increase the risk of fetal death by 20 per cent, and heavy smoking increased the risk by 35 per cent.[203] Thus, a statistically significant dose-response relationship between increased cigarette consumption and increased fetal mortality was demonstrated. However, when multivariate analysis was performed, cigarette smoking was found to be less important than low socioeconomic status, increased maternal age and parity, and a history of prior pregnancy loss. The effect of smoking in conjunction with one of the other risk factors led to a greater mortality than either factor alone.

The physiologic mechanism by which cigarette smoking causes an increase in fetal death is unclear. When causes of fetal death are studied, no differences have been noted between offspring of smokers and nonsmokers, which suggests that maternal problems or problems related to the pregnancy are the major factors in fetal loss.[193] This hypothesis is also supported by data from the Ontario perinatal mortality study.[203] Maternal problems specifically related to the placenta and uterus, i.e., abruptio placentae, placenta previa, bleeding during pregnancy, and premature rupture of the membranes, all exhibited a statistically significant dose-response relationship to increased levels of cigarette smoking. However, the maternal complications of toxemia and pre-eclampsia are not increased in cigarette smokers, suggesting that clinical problems related to the placenta and uterus are most important.

Prematurity is another important aspect of fetal mortality. Although preterm births account for a small percentage of total births, they account for a disproportionate number of deaths. Several studies have noted an increase in preterm births in cigarette smokers, and approximately 10 per cent of such births can be attributed to this risk factor alone.[210] The frequency of premature births rises with increased levels of cigarette smoking, thus confirming a dose-response effect.[203]

Spontaneous abortion has also been noted to be more common in cigarette smokers than in nonsmokers.[211] Case ascertainment of this condition is difficult; however, in one carefully done study an 80 per cent excess of spontaneous abortions was noted in smokers versus nonsmokers.[198]

The increase in prematurity, spontaneous abortion, and placental problems suggests that the effect of cigarette smoking on infant mortality may be indirectly mediated by placental malfunction or malformation, or by changes in uterine and placental oxygenation or blood flow.

Nicotine is known to cross the placenta of humans, leading to a reflex increase in blood pressure and respiratory rate in the fetus. However, the role of nicotine in altering human uterine and placental blood flow is unknown. More data for an effect of carbon monoxide are available.[199, 200] Carbon monoxide binds avidly to hemoglobin, thus making less hemoglobin available to carry oxygen. The net effect is to decrease the amount of oxygen carried to the fetus and other body tissues, producing a functional anemia. Oxygen consumption is increased in pregnancy, and a high carbon monoxide level can effectively diminish oxygen delivery to the fetus for its metabolic needs. In addition, a shift of the oxyhemoglobin dissociation curve to the left leads to less oxygen release at the tissue level. Carbon monoxide levels of the fetus are in equilibrium with maternal levels and after 5 to 6 hours are comparable.[200] A 10 per cent concentration of carboxyhemoglobin, readily achieved in women smoking two packs of cigarettes a day, is equivalent to a 60 per cent decrease in fetal blood flow.[199] Placentas of smoking women are also larger than those of nonsmokers and are abnormal histologically.[194] Whether these changes are related solely to hypoxia or to other effects of cigarette smoke is unknown.

Finally, several retrospective studies have noted a relationship between maternal smoking and Sudden Infant Death Syndrome (SIDS).[195, 205] SIDS mothers are more likely to have smoked excessively and smoked during pregnancy than non-SIDS mothers.[195] While it is unclear whether prenatal or postnatal exposure is most important for this relationship, it is known that maternal cigarette smoking decreases fetal breathing movements in utero.[197]

Birthweight. Cigarette smoking leads to an average reduction in birthweight of approximately 200 grams that is independent of other factors influencing birthweight. This effect is dose-related to the number of cigarettes smoked; i.e., the greater the number of cigarettes smoked, the lower the birthweight.[209] This finding is independent of gestational age, suggesting that there is a growth retardant effect of cigarette smoking. In addition, the effect is not mediated through maternal eating habits but rather seems to be a direct result of smoking.[208] The long-term implications of smoking for future growth and development of the child are unclear at the present time.

Lactation and Breast Feeding. Nicotine has been found in breast milk of smoking mothers, and the concentrations of nicotine parallel the number of cigarettes smoked.[206] An effect on the baby of nicotine in breast milk is less well demonstrated. Case reports of "nicotine poisoning" in newborns of heavy smokers are available, in which individual children with irritability, restlessness, diarrhea, and tachycardia are reported.[206] However, complicating this relationship is a general reduction in breast milk supply in heavy smokers.[206]

Respiratory Illness and Pneumonia. An increased hospitalization rate for pneumonia in children of smoking mothers has been noted; however, the study was retrospective, and no clear dose-response relationship was demonstrated.[196] Recent studies suggest that young nonsmoking children (5 to 9 years) have decreased levels of pulmonary function and increased respiratory symptoms if their parents smoke. It is unclear what relationship prenatal exposure has on these effects.[207]

Conclusion. Maternal cigarette smoking during pregnancy and during the early life of the child is associated with substantial risks of fetal death, prematurity, low birthweight, abnormal breast feeding, and respiratory disease. All physicians should advise pregnant smokers of these risks and provide assistance with smoking cessation.

References

REVIEWS

1. DeSwiet, M.: Respiratory disease in pregnancy. Postgrad. Med. J., *55*:325, 1979.
2. Fishburne, J. I.: Physiology and disease of the respiratory system in pregnancy. J. Reprod. Med., *22*:177, 1979.
3. Hytten, F. E., and Leitch, I. Respiration. *In*: The Physiology of Human Pregnancy, 2nd ed. Oxford, Blackwell, 1971, p. 111.
4. Milne, J. A.: The respiratory response to pregnancy. Postgrad. Med. J., *55*:318, 1979.
5. Novy, M. J., and Edwards, M. J.: Respiratory problems in pregnancy. Am. J. Obstet. Gynecol., *99*:1024, 1967.
6. Prowse, C. M., and Gaensler, E. A.: Respiratory and acid-base changes during pregnancy. Anesthesiology, *26*:381, 1965.
7. Weinberger, S. E., Weiss, S. T., Cohen, W. R., Weiss, J. W., and Johnson, T. S.: Pregnancy and the lung. Am. Rev. Respir. Dis., *121*:559, 1980.

PHYSIOLOGIC CHANGES IN PREGNANCY AFFECTING THE RESPIRATORY SYSTEM

8. Brien, T. G., and Dalrymple, I. J.: A longitudinal study of the free cortisol index in pregnancy. Br. J. Obstet. Gynaecol., *83*:361, 1976.
9. Fishburne, J. I., Jr., Brenner, W. E., Braaksma, J. T., and Hendricks, C. H.: Bronchospasm complicating intravenous prostaglandin $F_{2\alpha}$ for therapeutic abortion. Obstet. Gynecol., *39*:892, 1972.
10. Gaensler, E. A.: Lung displacement: Abdominal enlargement, pleural space disorders, deformities of the thoracic cage. *In*: Fenn, W. O., and Rahn, H. (eds.): Handbook of physiology: Respiration (Vol II). Washington, American Physiological Society, 1965, p. 1623.
11. Hyman, A. L., Spannhake, E. W., and Kadowitz, P. J.: Prostaglandins and the lung: State of the art. Am. Rev. Respir. Dis., *117*:111, 1978.
12. Jaffe, R. B., and Josimovich, J. B.: Endocrine physiology of pregnancy. *In*: Danforth, D. N. (ed.): Obstetrics and Gynecology. Hagerstown, Maryland, Harper & Row, 1977, p. 286,
13. Karim, S. M. M.: Appearance of prostaglandin $F_{2\alpha}$ in human blood during labour. Br. Med. J., *1*:618, 1968.
14. Kopp, L., Paradiz, G., and Tucci, J. R.: Urinary excretion of cyclic $3',5'$-adenosine monophosphate and cyclic $3',5'$-guanosine monophosphate during and after pregnancy. J. Clin. Endocrinol. Metab., *44*:590, 1977.
15. Kreisman, H., Van de Wiel, W., and Mitchell, C. A.: Respiratory function during prostaglandin-induced labor. Am. Rev. Respir. Dis., *111*:564, 1975.
16. Ling, W. Y., Marsh, J. M., and LeMaire, W. J.: Adenosine-$3',5'$-monophosphate in the plasma from human pregnancy. J. Clin. Endocrinol. Metab., *44*:514, 1977.
17. Lyons, H. A., and Antonio, R.: The sensitivity of the respiratory center in pregnancy and after the administration of progesterone. Trans. Assoc. Am. Physicians, *72*:173, 1959.
18. McGinty, A. P.: Comparative effects of pregnancy and phrenic nerve interruption on the diaphragm and their relation to pulmonary tuberculosis. Am. J. Obstet. Gynecol., *35*:237, 1938.
19. Mobius, W.: Atmung und Schwangerschaft. Med. Wschr., *103*:1389, 1961.
20. O'Connell, M., and Welsh, G. W., 3rd.: Unbound plasma cortisol in pregnant and Enovid-E treated women as determined by ultrafiltration. J. Clin. Endocrinol. Metab., *29*:563, 1969.
21. Shaw, J. O., and Moser, K. M.: The current status of prostaglandins and the lungs. Chest, *68*:75, 1975.
22. Skatrud, J. B., Dempsey, J. A., and Kaiser, D. G.: Ventilatory response to medroxyprogesterone acetate in normal subjects: Time course and mechanism. J. Appl. Physiol. Respirat. Environ. Exercise. Physiol., *44*:939, 1978.
23. Thomson, K. J., and Cohen, M. E.: Studies on the circulation in pregnancy. II. Vital capacity observations in normal pregnant women. Surg. Gynecol. Obstet., *66*:591, 1938.
24. Whalen, J. B., Clancey, C. J., Farley, D. B., and Van Orden, D. E.: Plasma prostaglandins in pregnancy. Obstet. Gynecol., *51*:52, 1978.
25. Yannone, M. E., McCurdy, J. R., and Goldfien, A.: Plasma progesterone levels in normal pregnancy, labor, and the puerperium. Am. J. Obstet. Gynecol., *101*:1058, 1968.

PULMONARY FUNCTION AND GAS EXCHANGE DURING PREGNANCY

26. Alaily, A. B., and Carrol, K. B.: Pulmonary ventilation in pregnancy. Br. J. Obstet. Gynaecol., *85*:518, 1978.
27. Andersen, G. J., James, G. B., Mathers, N. P., Smith, E. L., and Walker, J.: The maternal oxygen tension and acid-base status during pregnancy. J. Obstet. Gynaecol. Br. Commonw., *76*:16, 1969.
28. Andersen, G. J., and Walker, J.: The effect of labour on the maternal blood-gas and acid-base status. J. Obstet Gynaecol. Br. Commonw., *77*:289, 1970.
29. Ang, C. K., Tan, T. H., Walters, W. A. W., and Wood, C.: Postural influence on maternal capillary oxygen and carbon dioxide tension. Br. Med. J., *4*:201, 1969.
30. Awe, R. J., Nicotra, M. B., Newsom, T. D., and Viles, R.: Arterial oxygenation and alveolar-arterial gradients in term pregnancy. Obstet. Gynecol., *53*:182, 1979.
31. Baldwin, G. R., Moorthi, D. S., Whelton, J. A., and MacDonnell, K. F.: New lung functions and pregnancy. Am. J. Obstet. Gynecol., *127*:235, 1977.
32. Bedell, G. N., and Adams, R. W.: Pulmonary diffusing capacity during rest and exercise. A study of normal persons and persons with atrial septal defect, pregnancy, and pulmonary disease. J. Clin. Invest., *41*:1908, 1962.
33. Bevan, D. R., Holdcroft, A., Loh, L., MacGregor, W. G., O'Sullivan, J. C., and Sykes, M. K.: Closing volume and pregnancy. Br. Med. J., *1*:13, 1974.
34. Blechner, J. N., Cotter, J. R., Stenger, V. G., Hinkley, C. M., and Prystowsky, H.: Oxygen, carbon dioxide, and hydrogen ion concentrations in arterial blood during pregnancy. Am. J. Obstet. Gynecol., *100*:1, 1968.
35. Boutourline-Young H., and Boutourline-Young, E.: Alveolar carbon dioxide levels in pregnant, parturient, and lactating subjects. J. Obstet. Gynecol. Br. Emp., *63*:509, 1956.
36. Cameron, S. J., Bain, H. H., and Grant, I. W. B.: Ventilatory function in pregnancy. Scot. Med. J., *15*:243, 1970.
37. Craig, D. B., and Toole, M. A.: Airway closure in pregnancy. Canad. Anaesth. Soc. J., *22*:665, 1975.
38. Cugell, D. W., Frank, N. R., Gaensler, E. A., and Badger, T. L.: Pulmonary function in pregnancy. I. Serial observations in normal women. Am. Rev. Tuberc., *67*:568, 1953.
39. Dayal, P., Murata, Y., and Takamura, H.: Antepartum and postpartum acid-base changes in maternal blood in normal and complicated pregnancies. J. Obstet. Gynaecol. Br. Commonw., *79*:612, 1972.
40. Fadel, H. E., Northrop, G., Misenhimer, H. R., and Harp, R. J.: Normal pregnancy: A model of sustained respiratory alkalosis. J. Perinatol. Med., *3*:195, 1979.
41. Garrard, G. S., Littler, W. A., and Redman, C. W. G.: Closing volume during normal pregnancy. Thorax, *33*:488, 1978.
42. Gazioglu, K., Kaltreider, N. L., Rosen, M., and Yu, P. N.: Pulmonary function during pregnancy in normal women and in patients with cardiopulmonary disease. Thorax, *25*:445, 1970.
43. Gee, J. B. L., Packer, B. S., Millen, J. E., and Robin, E. D.: Pulmonary mechanics during pregnancy. J. Clin. Invest., *46*:945, 1967.
44. Holdcroft, A., Bevan, D. R., O'Sullivan, J. C., and Sykes, M. K.: Airway closure and pregnancy. Anaesthesia, *32*:517, 1977.
45. Knuttgen, H. G., and Emerson, K., Jr.: Physiological response to pregnancy at rest and during exercise. J. Appl. Physiol., *36*:549, 1974.
46. Krumholz, R. A., Echt, C. R., and Ross, J. C.: Pulmonary diffusing capacity, capillary blood volume, lung volumes, and mechanics of ventilation in early and late pregnancy. J. Lab. Clin. Med., *63*:648, 1964.
47. Lim, V. S., Katz, A. I., and Lindheimer, M. D.: Acid-base regulation in pregnancy. Am. J. Physiol., *231*:1764, 1976.
48. Lucius, H., Gahlenbeck, H., Klein, H.-O., Fabel, H., and Bartels, H.: Respiratory functions, buffer system, and electrolyte concentrations of blood during human pregnancy. Respir. Physiol., *9*:311, 1970.

49. MacRae, D. J., and Palavradji, D.: Maternal acid-base changes in pregnancy. J. Obstet. Gynaecol. Br. Commonw., 74:11, 1967.

50. Milne, J. A., Mills, R. J., Coutts, J. R. T., MacNaughton, M. C., Moran, F., and Pack, A. I.: The effect of human pregnancy on the pulmonary transfer factor for carbon monoxide as measured by the single-breath method. Clin. Sci. Mol. Med., 53:271, 1977.

51. Milne, J. A., Mills, R. J., Howie, A. D., and Pack, A. I.: Large airways function during normal pregnancy. Br. J. Obstet. Gynaecol., 84:448, 1977.

52. Pernoll, M. L., Metcalfe, J., Kovach, P. A., Wachtel, R., and Dunham, M. J.: Ventilation during rest and exercise in pregnancy and postpartum. Respir. Physiol., 25:295, 1975.

53. Pernoll, M. L., Metcalfe, J., Schlenker, T. L., Welch, J. E., and Matsumoto, J. A.: Oxygen consumption at rest and during exercise in pregnancy. Respir. Physiol., 25:285, 1975.

54. Rubin, A., Russo, N., and Goucher, D. The effect of pregnancy upon pulmonary function in normal women. Am. J. Obstet. Gynecol., 72:963, 1956.

55. Templeton, A., and Kelman, G. R.: Maternal blood gases, (PA_{O_2}-Pa_{O_2}), physiological shunt and V_D/V_T in normal pregnancy. Br. J. Anaesth., 48:1001, 1976.

DYSPNEA OF PREGNANCY

56. Cugell, D. W., Frank, N. R., Gaensler, E. A., and Badger, T. L.: Pulmonary function in pregnancy. I. Serial observations in normal women. Am. Rev. Tuberc., 67:568, 1953.

57. Gilbert, R., and Auchincloss, J. H., Jr.: Dyspnea of pregnancy: Clinical and physiological observations. Am. J. Med. Sci., 252:270, 1966.

58. Gilbert, R., Epifano, L., and Auchincloss, J. H., Jr.: Dyspnea of pregnancy: A syndrome of altered respiratory control. J.A.M.A., 182:1073, 1962.

59. Lehmann, V.: Dyspnea in pregnancy. J. Perinatol. Med., 3:154, 1975.

60. Milne, J. A., Howie, A. D., and Pack, A. I.: Dyspnoea during normal pregnancy. Br. J. Obstet. Gynaecol., 85:260, 1978.

ASTHMA

61. Akerlund, M., and Andersson, K-E.: Effects of terbutaline on human myometrial activity and endometrial blood flow. Obstet. Gynecol., 47:529, 1976.

62. Andersson, K-E., Bengtsson, L. P., and Ingemarsson, I.: Terbutaline inhibition of midtrimester uterine activity induced by prostaglandin $F_{2\alpha}$ and hypertonic saline. Br. J. Obstet. Gynaecol., 82:745, 1975.

63. Arwood, L. L., Dasta, J. F., and Friedman, C.: Placental transfer of theophylline: Two case reports. Pediatrics, 63:844, 1979.

64. Bahna, S. L., and Bjerkedal, T.: The course and outcome of pregnancy in women with bronchial asthma. Acta Allergol., 27:397, 1972.

65. Banerjee, B. N., and Woodard, G.: Teratologic evaluation of metaproterenol in the rhesus monkey (Macaca mulata). Toxicol. Appl. Pharmacol., 20:562, 1971.

66. Beitins, I. Z., Bayard, F., Ances, I. G., Kowarski, A., and Migeon, C. J.: The transplacental passage of prednisone and prednisolone in pregnancy near term. J. Pediatr., 81:936, 1972.

67. Bongiovanni, A. M., and McPadden, A. J.: Steroids during pregnancy and possible fetal consequences. Fertil. Steril., 2:181, 1960.

68. Caritis, S. N., Mueller-Heubach, E., Morishima, H. O., and Edelstone, D. I.: Effect of terbutaline on cardiovascular state and uterine blood flow in pregnant ewes. Obstet. Gynecol., 50:603, 1977.

69. Corrao, W. M., Braman, S. S., and Irwin, R. S.: Chronic cough as the sole presenting manifestation of bronchial asthma. N. Engl. J. Med., 300:633, 1979.

70. Coutinho, E. M., and Vieira Lopes, A. C.: Inhibition of uterine motility by aminophylline. Am. J. Obstet. Gynecol., 110:726, 1971.

71. Derbes, V. J., and Sodeman, W. A.: Reciprocal influences of bronchial asthma and pregnancy. Am. J. Med., 1:367, 1946.

72. Fainstat, T.: Cortisone-induced congenital cleft palate in rabbits. Endocrinology, 55:502, 1954.

73. Feldman, N. T., and McFadden, E. R., Jr.: Asthma: Therapy old and new. Med. Clin. North. Am., 61:1239, 1977.

74. Gluck, J. C., and Gluck, P. A.: The effects of pregnancy on asthma: A prospective study. Ann. Allergy, 37:164, 1976.

75. Gordon, M., Niswander, K. R., Berendes, H., and Kantor, A. G.: Fetal morbidity following potentially anoxigenic obstetric conditions. VII. Bronchial asthma. Am. J. Obstet. Gynecol., 106:421, 1970.

76. Greenberger, P., and Patterson, R.: Safety of therapy for allergic symptoms during pregnancy. Ann. Intern. Med., 89:234, 1978.

77. Heinonen, O. P., Slone, D., and Shapiro, S.: Birth Defects and Drugs in Pregnancy. Littleton, Massachusetts, Publishing Sciences Group, 1977.

78. Hiddlestone, H. J. H.: Bronchial asthma and pregnancy. N. Z. Med. J., 63:521, 1964.

79. Ingemarsson, I.: Effect of terbutaline on premature labor. Am. J. Obstet. Gynecol., 125:520, 1976.

80. Liggins, G. C., and Vaughan, G. S.: Intravenous infusion of salbutamol in the management of premature labour. J. Obstet. Gynaecol. Br. Commonw., 80:29, 1973.

81. McFadden, E. R., Jr., and Ingram, R. H., Jr.: Exercise-induced asthma. N. Engl. J. Med., 301:763, 1979.

82. Mintz, S.: Pregnancy and asthma. In: Weiss, E. B., Segal, M. S. (eds.): Bronchial asthma: Mechanisms and therapeutics. Boston, Little, Brown, 1976, p. 971.

83. Misenheimer, H. R., Margulies, S. I., Panigel, M., Ramsey, E. M., and Donner, M. W.: Effects of vasoconstrictive drugs on the placental circulation of the rhesus monkey. Invest. Radiol., 7:496, 1972.

84. Oppenheimer, E. H.: Lesions in the adrenals of an infant following maternal corticosteroid therapy. Bull. Johns Hopkins Hosp., 114:146, 1964.

84a. Popert, A. J.: Pregnancy and adrenocortical hormones: Some aspects of their interaction in rheumatic diseases. Br. Med. J., 1:967, 1962.

85. Reinisch, J. M., Simon, N. G., Karow, W. G., and Gandelman, R.: Prenatal exposure to prednisone in humans and animals retards intrauterine growth. Science, 202:436, 1978.

86. Saunders, N. A., and McFadden, E. R., Jr.: Asthma—an update. D.M., 24:1, 1978.

87. Schaefer, G., and Silverman, F.: Pregnancy complicated by asthma. Am. J. Obstet. Gynecol., 82:182, 1961.

88. Schatz, M., Patterson, R., Zeitz, S., O'Rourke, J., and Melam, H.: Corticosteroid therapy for the pregnant asthmatic patient. J.A.M.A., 233:804, 1975.

89. Senior, R. M., Lefrak, S. S., and Korenblat, P. E.: Status asthmaticus. J.A.M.A., 231:1277, 1975.

90. Sims, C. D., Chamberlain, C. V. P., and DeSwiet, M.: Lung function tests in bronchial asthma during and after pregnancy. Br. J. Obstet. Gynaecol., 83:434, 1976.

91. Snyder, R. D., and Snyder, D.: Corticosteroids for asthma during pregnancy. Ann. Allergy, 41:340, 1978.

92. Tepperman, H. M., Beydoun, S. N., and Abdul-Karim, R. W.: Drugs affecting myometrial contractility in pregnancy. Clin. Obstet. Gynecol., 20:423, 1977.

93. Walsh, S. D., and Clark, F. R.: Pregnancy in patients on long-term corticosteroid therapy. Scot. Med. J., 12:302, 1967.

94. Warrell, D. W., and Taylor, R.: Outcome for the foetus of mothers receiving prednisolone during pregnancy. Lancet, 1:117, 1968.

95. Weinberger, S. E., Weiss, S. T., Cohen, W. R., Weiss, J. W., and Johnson, T. S.: Pregnancy and the lung. Am. Rev. Respir. Dis., 121:559, 1980.

96. Weinstein, A. M., Dubin, B. D., Podleski, W. K., Spector, S. L., and Farr, R. S.: Asthma and pregnancy. J.A.M.A., 241:1161, 1979.

97. Williams, D. A.: Asthma and pregnancy. Acta Allergol., 22:311, 1967.

98. Zilianti, M., and Aller, J.: Action of orciprenaline on uterine contractility during labor, maternal cardiovascular system, fetal heart rate, and acid-base balance. Am. J. Obstet. Gynecol., 109:1073, 1971.

OTHER FORMS OF OBSTRUCTIVE LUNG DISEASE

99. Giesler, C. F., Buehler, J. H., and Depp, R.: Alpha$_1$-antitrypsin deficiency: Severe obstructive lung disease and pregnancy. Obstet. Gynecol., 49:31, 1977.

100. Grand, R. J., Talamo, R. C., de Sant'Agnese, P. A., and Schwartz, R. H.: Pregnancy in cystic fibrosis of the pancreas. J.A.M.A., 195:993, 1966.

101. Howie, A. D., and Milne, J. A.: Pregnancy in patients with bronchiectasis. Br. J. Obstet. Gynaecol., 85:197, 1978.
102. Larsen, J. W., Jr.: Cystic fibrosis and pregnancy. Obstet. Gynecol., 39:880, 1972.
103. Siegel, B., and Siegel, S.: Pregnancy and delivery in a patient with cystic fibrosis of the pancreas: Report of a case. Obstet. Gynecol., 16:438, 1960.
104. Teirstein, A. S.: Bronchiectasis. In: Rovinsky, J. J., Guttmacher, A. F. (eds.): Medical, Surgical, and Gynecologic Complications of Pregnancy. Baltimore, Williams & Wilkins, 1965, p. 144.
105. Templeton, A.: Intrauterine growth retardation associated with hypoxia due to bronchiectasis. Br. J. Obstet. Gynaecol., 84:389, 1977.

SARCOIDOSIS

106. DeRemee, R. A.: The present status of treatment of pulmonary sarcoidosis: A house divided. Chest, 71:388, 1977.
107. Dines, D. E., and Banner, E. A.: Sarcoidosis during pregnancy: Improvement in pulmonary function. J.A.M.A., 200:726, 1967.
108. Fried, K. H.: Sarcoidosis and pregnancy. Acta. Med. Scand., 176 (Suppl 425):218, 1964.
109. Given, F. T., Jr., and Di Benedetto, R. L.: Sarcoidosis and pregnancy: Report of 5 cases and 1 maternal death. Obstet. Gynecol., 22:355, 1963.
110. Mayock, R. L., Sullivan, R. D., Greening, R. R., and Jones, R., Jr.: Sarcoidosis and pregnancy. J.A.M.A., 164:158, 1957.
111. O'Leary, J. A.: Ten-year study of sarcoidosis and pregnancy. Am. J. Obstet. Gynecol., 84:462, 1962.
112. Reisfield, D. R.: Boeck's sarcoid and pregnancy. Am. J. Obstet. Gynecol., 75:795, 1958.
113. Reisfield, D. R., Yahia, C., and Laurenzi, G. A.: Pregnancy and cardiorespiratory failure in Boeck's sarcoid. Surg. Gynecol. Obstet., 109:412, 1959.
114. Scadding, J. G.: Sarcoidosis. London, Eyre & Spottiswoode, 1967.

TUBERCULOSIS

115. American Thoracic Society: Preventive therapy of tuberculous infection. Am. Rev. Respir. Dis., 110:371, 1974.
116. American Thoracic Society: Guidelines for short-course tuberculosis chemotherapy. Am. Rev. Respir. Dis., 121:611, 1980.
117. Avery, M. E., and Wolfsdorf, J.: Diagnosis and treatment: Approaches to newborn infants of tuberculous mothers. Pediatrics, 42:519, 1968.
118. Bjerkedal, T., Bahna, S. L., and Lehmann, E. H.: Course and outcome of pregnancy in women with pulmonary tuberculosis. Scand. J. Respir. Dis., 56:245, 1975.
119. Blackall, P. B.: Tuberculosis: Maternal infection of the newborn. Med. J. Aust., 2:1055, 1969.
120. Bobrowitz, I. D.: Ethambutol in pregnancy. Chest, 66:20, 1974.
121. Bonebrake, C. R., Noller, K. L., Loehnen, C. P., Muhm, J. R., and Fish, C. R.: Routine chest roentgenography in pregnancy. J.A.M.A., 240:2747, 1978.
122. Brummer, D. L.: Letter to the editor. Am. Rev. Respir. Dis., 106:785, 1972.
123. Byrd, R. B., Horn, B. R., Solomon, D. A., and Griggs, G. A.: Toxic effects of isoniazid in tuberculosis chemoprophylaxis. J.A.M.A., 241:1239, 1979.
124. Coden, J.: Tuberculous peritonitis in pregnancy. Br. Med. J., 3:152, 1972.
125. Committee on Drugs, American Academy of Pediatrics. Infants of tuberculous mothers: Further thoughts. Pediatrics, 42:393, 1968.
126. Conway, N., and Birt, B. D.: Streptomycin in pregnancy: Effect on the foetal ear. Br. Med. J., 2:260, 1965.
127. De March, A. P.: Tuberculosis and pregnancy: Five- to ten-year review of 215 patients in their fertile age. Chest, 68:800, 1975.
128. Finn, R., St. Hill, C. A., Govan, A. J., Ralfs, I. G., Gurney, F. J., and Denye, V.: Immunological responses in pregnancy and survival of fetal homograft. Br. Med. J., 3:150, 1972.
129. Flanagan, P., and Hensler, N. M.: The course of active tuberculosis complicated by pregnancy. J.A.M.A., 170:783, 1959.
130. Freeth, A.: Routine x-ray examination of the chest at an antenatal clinic. Lancet, 1:287, 1953.

131. Giercke, H. W.: Tuberkuloseablaufe kurz nach Schwangerschaftsbeendigung. Ztschr. Tuberk., 108:1, 1956.
132. Golditch, I. M.: Tuberculous meningitis and pregnancy. Am. J. Obstet. Gynecol., 110:1144, 1971.
133. Hedvall, E.: Pregnancy and tuberculosis. Acta Med. Scand., 147 (Suppl 286):1, 1953.
134. Heinonen, O. P., Slone, D., and Shapiro, S.: Birth defects and drugs in pregnancy. Littleton, Massachusetts, Publishing Sciences Group, 1977.
135. Jenkins, D. M., and Scott, J. S.: Immunological responses in pregnancy. Br. Med. J., 3:528, 1972.
136. Kendig, E. L., Jr.: The place of BCG vaccine in the management of infants born of tuberculous mothers. N. Engl. J. Med., 281:520, 1969.
137. Lewitt, T., Nebel, L., Terracina, S., and Karman, S.: Ethambutol in pregnancy: Observations on embryogenesis. Chest, 66:25, 1974.
138. Lowe, C. R.: Congenital defects among children born to women under supervision or treatment for pulmonary tuberculosis. Br. J. Prev. Soc. Med., 18:14, 1964.
139. Mattox, J. H.: The value of a routine prenatal chest x-ray. Obstet. Gynecol., 41:243, 1973.
140. Mole, R. H.: Radiation effects on prenatal development and their radiological significance. Br. J. Radiol., 52:89, 1979.
141. Montgomery, W. P., Young, R. C., Jr., Allen, M. P., and Harden, K. A.: The tuberculin test in pregnancy. Am. J. Obstet. Gynecol., 100:829, 1968.
142. Newman, R., Doster, B. E., Murray, F. J., and Woolpert, S. F.: Rifampin in initial treatment of pulmonary tuberculosis. Am. Rev. Respir. Dis., 109:216, 1974.
143. Potworowska, M., Sianozecka, E., and Szufladowicz, R.: Ethionamide treatment and pregnancy. Polish Med. J., 5:1152, 1966.
144. Present, P. A., and Comstock, G. W.: Tuberculin sensitivity in pregnancy. Am. Rev. Respir. Dis., 112:413, 1975.
145. Ramos, A. D., Hibbard, L. T., and Craig, J. R.: Congenital tuberculosis. Obstet. Gynecol., 43:61, 1974.
146. Robinson, G. C., and Cambon, K. G.: Hearing loss in infants of tuberculous mothers treated with streptomycin during pregnancy. N. Engl. J. Med., 271:949, 1964.
147. Schaefer, G., Zervoudakis, I. A., Fuchs, F. F., and David, S.: Pregnancy and pulmonary tuberculosis. Obstet. Gynecol., 46:706, 1975.
148. Scheinhorn, D. J., and Angelillo, V. A.: Antituberculous therapy in pregnancy: Risks to the fetus. West. J. Med., 127:195, 1977.
149. Selikoff, I. J., and Dorfmann, H. L.: Management of tuberculosis. In: Rovinsky, J. J., Guttmacher, A. F. (eds.): Medical, surgical, and gynecologic complications of pregnancy. Baltimore, Williams & Wilkins, 1965, p. 111.
150. Skolnick, J. L., Stoler, B. S., Katz, D. B., and Anderson, W. H.: Rifampin, oral contraceptives, and pregnancy. J.A.M.A., 236:1382, 1976.
151. Stands, J. W., Jowers, R. G., and Bryan, C. S.: Miliary-meningeal tuberculosis during pregnancy: Case report, and brief survey of the problem of extra-pulmonary tuberculosis. J. South Car. Med. Assoc., 73:282, 1977.
152. Stanton, S. L.: Routine radiology of the chest in antenatal care. J. Obstet. Gynaecol. Br. Commonw., 75:1161, 1968.
153. Swartz, H. M., and Reichling, B. A.: Hazards of radiation exposure for pregnant women. J.A.M.A., 239:1907, 1978.
154. Turner, A. F.: The chest radiograph in pregnancy. Clin. Obstet. Gynecol., 18:65, 1975.
155. Voyce, M. A., and Hunt, A. C.: Congenital tuberculosis. Arch. Dis. Child., 41:299, 1966.
156. Warkany, J.: Antituberculous drugs. Teratology, 20:133, 1979.
157. Weinstein, L., and Murphy, T.: The management of tuberculosis during pregnancy. Clin. Perinatol., 1:395, 1974.

OTHER INFECTIOUS DISEASES OF THE LUNG

158. Austrian, R.: Pneumococcal vaccine: Development and prospects. Am. J. Med., 67:547, 1979.
159. Drutz, D. J., and Catanzaro, A.: Coccidioidomycosis. Am. Rev. Respir. Dis., 117:559 and 727, 1978.
160. Ellinoy, B. R.: Amphotericin B usage in pregnancy complicated by cryptococcosis. Am. J. Obstet. Gynecol., 115:285, 1973.
161. Goodwin, R. A., Jr., and Des Prez, R. M.: Histoplasmosis. Am. Rev. Respir. Dis., 117:929, 1978.

162. Harris, R. E.: Coccidioidomycosis complicating pregnancy. Obstet. Gynecol., 28;401, 1966.
163. Harris, R. E., and Rhoades, E. R.: Varicella pneumonia complicating pregnancy. Obstet. Gynecol., 25:734, 1965.
164. Hopwood, H. G., Jr.: Pneumonia in pregnancy. Obstet. Gynecol., 25:875, 1965.
165. McCaffree, M. A., Altshuler, G., and Benirschke, K.: Placental coccidioidomycosis without fetal disease. Arch. Pathol. Lab. Med., 102:512, 1978.
166. Mendelow, D. A., and Lewis, G. C., Jr.: Varicella pneumonia during pregnancy. Obstet. Gynecol., 33:98, 1969.
167. Pickard, R. E.: Varicella pneumonia in pregnancy. Am. J. Obstet. Gynecol., 101:504, 1968.
168. Purtilo, D. T.: Opportunistic mycotic infections in pregnant women. Am. J. Obstet. Gynecol., 122:607, 1975.
169. Silberfarb, P. M., Sarosi, G. A., and Tosh, F. E.: Cryptococcosis and pregnancy. Am. J. Obstet. Gynecol., 112:714, 1972.
170. Smale, L. E., and Waechter, K. G.: Dissemination of coccidioidomycosis in pregnancy. Am. J. Obstet. Gynecol., 107:356, 1970.

AMNIOTIC FLUID EMBOLISM

171. Adamsons, K., Mueller-Heubach, E., and Myers, R. E.: The innocuousness of amniotic fluid infusion in the pregnant rhesus monkey. Am. J. Obstet. Gynecol., 109:977, 1971.
172. Anderson, D. G.: Amniotic fluid embolism: a re-evaluation. Am. J. Obstet. Gynecol., 98:336, 1967.
173. Chung, A. F., and Merkatz, I. R.: Survival following amniotic fluid embolism with early heparinization. Obstet. Gynecol., 42:809, 1973.
174. Courtney, L. D.: Amniotic fluid embolism. Obstet. Gynecol. Surv., 29:169, 1974.
175. Courtney, L. D., Boxall, R. R., and Child, P.: Permeability of membranes of dead fetus. Br. Med. J., 1:492, 1971.
176. Gregory, M. G., and Clayton, E. M., Jr.: Amniotic fluid embolism. Obstet. Gynecol., 42:236, 1973.
177. Masson, R. G., Ruggieri, J., and Siddiqui, M. M.: Amniotic fluid embolism: Definitive diagnosis in a survivor. Am. Rev. Respir. Dis., 120:187, 1979.
178. Peterson, E. P., and Taylor, H. B.: Amniotic fluid embolism: An analysis of 40 cases. Obstet. Gynecol., 35:787, 1970.
179. Resnik, R., Swartz, W. H., Plumer, M. H., Benirschke, K., and Stratthaus, M. E.: Amniotic fluid embolism with survival. Obstet. Gynecol., 47:295, 1976.
180. Spence, M. R., and Mason, K. G.: Experimental amniotic fluid embolism in rabbits. Am. J. Obstet. Gynecol., 119:1073, 1974.

ASPIRATION OF GASTRIC CONTENTS

181. Baggish, M. S., and Hooper, S.: Aspiration as a cause of maternal death. Obstet. Gynecol., 43:327, 1974.
182. Mendelson, C. L.: The aspiration of stomach contents into the lungs during obstetric anesthesia. Am. J. Obstet. Gynecol., 52:191, 1946.
183. Mucklow, R. G., and Larard, D. G.: The effect of the inhalation of vomitus on the lungs. Br. J. Anaesth., 35:153, 1963.
184. Wolfe, J. E., Bone, R. C., and Ruth, W. E.: Effects of corticosteroids in the treatment of patients with gastric aspiration. Am. J. Med., 63:719, 1977.

PNEUMOMEDIASTINUM

185. Bard, R., and Hassini, N.: Pneumomediastinum complicating pregnancy. Respiration, 32:185, 1975.
186. Brandfass, R. T., and Martinez, D. M.: Mediastinal and subcutaneous emphysema in labor. South. Med. J., 69:1554, 1976.
187. Munsell, W. P.: Pneumomediastinum: A report of 28 cases and review of the literature. J.A.M.A., 202:689, 1967.

RESPIRATORY INSUFFICIENCY

188. Demas, N. W.: Maternal death due to primary pulmonary hypertension. Trans. Pac. Coast. Obstet. Gynecol. Soc., 40:64, 1973.

189. Gaensler, E. A., Patton, W. E., Verstraeten, J. M., and Badger, T. L.: Pulmonary function in pregnancy. III. Serial observations in patients with pulmonary insufficiency. Am. Rev. Tuberc., 67:779, 1953.
190. Hung, C. T., Pelosi, M., Langer, A., and Harrigan, J. T.: Blood gas measurements in the kyphoscoliotic gravida and her fetus: Report of a case. Am. J. Obstet. Gynecol., 121:287, 1975.
191. McCaffrey, R. M., and Dunn, L. J.: Primary pulmonary hypertension in pregnancy. Obstet. Gynecol. Surv., 19:567, 1964.
192. Novy, M. J., and Edwards, M. J.: Respiratory problems in pregnancy. Am. J. Obstet. Gynecol., 99:1024, 1967.

SMOKING AND PREGNANCY

193. Andrews, J., and McGarry, J. M.: A community study of smoking in pregnancy. J. Obstet. Gynaecol. Br. Commonw., 79:1057, 1972.
194. Asmussen, I.: Ultrastructure of the human placenta at term. Observations on placentas from newborn children of smoking and nonsmoking mothers. Acta Obstet. Gynecol. Scand., 56:119, 1977.
195. Bergman, A. B., and Wiesner, L. A.: Relationship of passive cigarette-smoking to sudden infant death syndrome. Pediatrics, 58:665, 1976.
196. Colley, J. S.: Influence of passive smoking and parental phlegm on pneumonia and bronchitis in early childhood. Lancet, 2:1031, 1974.
197. Gennser, G., Marsal, K., and Brantmark, B.: Maternal smoking and fetal breathing movements. Am. J. Obstet. Gynecol., 123:861, 1975.
198. Kline, J., Stein, Z. A., Susser, M., and Warburton, D.: Smoking: A risk factor for spontaneous abortion. N. Engl. J. Med., 297:793, 1977.
199. Longo, L. D.: The biological effects of carbon monoxide on the pregnant woman, fetus, and newborn infant. Am. J. Obstet. Gynecol., 129:69, 1977.
200. Longo, L. D., and Hill, E. P.: Carbon monoxide uptake and elimination in fetal and maternal sheep. Am. J. Physiol., 232:H324, 1977.
201. Meyer, M. B., and Comstock, G. W.: Maternal cigarette smoking and perinatal mortality. Am. J. Epidemiol., 96:1, 1972.
202. Meyer, M. B., Jonas, B. S., and Tonascia, J. A.: Perinatal events associated with maternal smoking during pregnancy. Am. J. Epidemiol., 103:464, 1976.
203. Meyer, M. B., and Tonascia, J. A.: Maternal smoking, pregnancy complications, and perinatal mortality. Am. J. Obstet. Gynecol., 128:494, 1977.
204. Meyer, M. B., Tonascia, J. A., and Buck, C.: The interrelationship of maternal smoking and increased perinatal mortality with other risk factors. Further analysis of the Ontario perinatal mortality study, 1960–1961. Am. J. Epidemiol., 100:443, 1975.
205. Naeye, R. L., Ladis, B., and Drage, J. S.: Sudden infant death syndrome. A prospective study. Am. J. Dis. Child., 130:1207, 1976.
206. Perlman, H. H., Dannenberg, A. M., and Sokoloff, N.: The excretion of nicotine in breast milk and urine from cigaret smoking. Its effect on lactation and the nursling. J.A.M.A., 120:1003, 1942.
207. Tager, I. B., Weiss, S. T., Rosner, B., and Speizer, F. E.: Effect of parental cigarette smoking on the pulmonary function of children. Am. J. Epidemiol., 110:15, 1979.
208. Underwood, P., Hester, L. L., Laffitte, T., Jr., and Gregg, K. V.: The relationship of smoking to the outcome of pregnancy. Am. J. Obstet. Gynecol., 91:270, 1965.
209. U.S. Public Health Service: Smoking and health. A report of the Surgeon General. U.S. Department of Health, Education, and Welfare. DHEW Pub. No. (PHS) 79–50066, 1979.
210. Yerushalmy, J.: The relationship of parents' cigarette smoking to outcome of pregnancy — implications as to the problem of inferring causation from observed associations. Am. J. Epidemiol., 93:443, 1971.
211. Zabriskie, J. R.: Effect of cigaret smoking during pregnancy: Study of 2000 cases. Obstet. Gynecol., 21:405, 1963.

Donald J. Dalessio, M.D. # 18

NEUROLOGIC DISEASES

There are no specific neurologic diseases related to pregnancy, but the effects of pregnancy upon antecedent or concurrent neurologic diseases or those neurologic ills that develop during pregnancy are diverse. The instructional objectives of this chapter are as follows:

1. To review the common neurologic illnesses that may present during pregnancy.

2. To discuss the specific problems that neurologic illness and its treatment produce during pregnancy.

3. To offer suggestions for the diagnosis and treatment of neurologic illnesses that may complicate pregnancy.

DIAGNOSTIC PROCEDURES

The investigation of suspected neurologic disease in a pregnant woman may be inhibited to some extent by concern for the fetus. Standard tests, including those of eye and ear function, electroencephalography, electromyography, and echoencephalography, can all be performed without risk. Lumbar puncture is almost never contraindicated, except when increased intracranial pressure with associated papilledema is suspected. Expanding lesions in the posterior fossa are one relative contraindication to lumbar puncture. In this situation, as in others, a good general neurologic precept to follow is that when brain tumor is suspected, lumbar puncture is best avoided.

Roentgenographic studies of the nervous system are sometimes restricted because of concern about fetal damage. When considering the potential radiation hazard to the fetus produced by diagnostic medical irradiation of the mother, one should refer to the National Council on Radiation Protection Report No. 54.[1] This report makes the point that if, in the judgement of the attending physician, protection of the mother's health requires a radiologic examination to be performed at a specific time, and if the examination is carried out with adequate safety equipment and careful technique, then the potential benefit to the health of the patient, the fetus, or both will in most cases outweigh the potential deleterious effects of the radiation. This conclusion is based on the finding that fewer than 1 in 1000 of all radiographic examinations (not including fluoroscopy) will, if carried out with good equipment and careful technique, subject the fetus to radiation doses of 1 rad or more. At dose levels below 1 rad, the probability of detectable effects is so small as to be outweighed by any significant medical benefit.

Actually, for doses of less than 5 rads received at the period critical for the induction of any one specific type of maldevelopment, it is unlikely that an increase in that malformation could be measurable in human populations. The probability of inducing malformations, growth retardation, or both is greatest during the period of major organogenesis, which in humans begins one to two weeks after conception (three to four weeks after the last menstruation) and extends through the tenth week after conception (twelfth week postmenses). Not enough is currently known about the risks of leukemia and childhood cancer to draw any conclusions concerning the effects of radiation during different uterine stages.

Thus, if indicated, x-rays of the head and cervical spine, extremities, and shoulders can be done with relative safety. X-rays of the lumbar spine and pelvis are considered as belonging to a high fetal dose group and should only be done with urgent indications.

Since the previous edition of this book, the advent of computerized axial tomography (CAT) of the head has made many of the older neurologic diagnostic techniques either obsolete or infrequently used. When indicated, CAT scans of the head can be done as required, since generally the amount of radiation exposure produced by this procedure is approximately that of the normal skull series. The contrast material employed in CAT scans and in cerebral angiography is physiologically inert with respect to iodine and

435

does not produce fetal thyroid abnormalities. Hence, cerebral angiograms can also be performed when necessary, although the abdomen should be shielded. It is rarely necessary to do radioisotope brain scans during the first three months of pregnancy, given the diagnostic potency of the CAT scan.

The greatest concern for fetal radiation exposure occurs in myelography, in which there is fluoroscopic evaluation of the spinal subarachnoid space. Radiation exposure to the fetus is maximal with this procedure. Cervical myelography may be performed with adequate shielding, but thoracic and lumbar myelography should probably be avoided if at all possible. If discogenic root disease in the lumbar areas is suspected in the pregnant woman and cannot be confirmed by clinical means, electromyographic studies are the procedures of choice.

Several factors should be considered when pregnancy is discovered after medical radiation exposure of the fetus. For example, if a myelogram has already been done and then it is discovered that the patient is pregnant, the question of therapeutic abortion should be raised. The patient, with the advice of her attending physician and consultants, should make the ultimate decision. In this situation, a physician, acting with a radiologist and a radiation safety officer, should advise the patient of the risks of allowing the pregnancy to continue to term and the alternate risks of an abortion. The patient should be informed that from 4 to 6 per cent of all infants are born with varying degrees of congenital defects regardless of radiation history. For any individual case, the increased risk of such defects from doses below the 10 rad level received at any stage of pregnancy, according to the best knowledge available today, is small compared with this normal risk. Nonetheless, the decision to end the pregnancy depends upon the extent and type of radiation hazard to the fetus, the ethnic and religious background of the family, the laws of the state pertaining to legal abortion, and any other relevant considerations.

In general, when considering neurologic diagnostic procedures in pregnancy, the physician should be guided by diagnostic acumen and concern for the safety of the mother and her fetus. Pregnancy is not a contraindication to neuroradiologic diagnostic studies. However, any investigations that require radiation exposure should be ordered with care, especially if they include fluoroscopy, particularly fluoroscopy of those body regions where shielding of the abdomen is liable to provide inadequate protection for the fetus.

SEIZURE DISORDERS

Pregnancy in the epileptic provides the clinician with a therapeutic dilemma because of the attempt to maintain the mother in a seizure-free state while ameliorating, if possible, the teratogenic effects of anticonvulsants on the fetus.

Types of Seizure Disorders

The classification of seizure disorders is difficult and depends largely on the training of the observer and the observer's particular bias, be it clinical, electroencephalographic, or another. The classification proposed here is useful for collecting information, for working toward a diagnosis, for choosing proper treatment, and for determining prognosis (Table 18–1). In this symptomatic classification of seizure disorders, four classes of fits are categorized. They include generalized seizures, focal seizures, pseudoseizures, and other conditions with some features of epilepsy. A complete discussion of the various forms of epilepsy is beyond the scope of this chapter. Some brief remarks regarding seizure types are appropriate, however.

TABLE 18–1   CLASSIFICATION OF
SEIZURE DISORDERS

I. Generalized seizures
  A. Convulsive
    1. Tonic-clonic major motor without focal onset (grand mal)
    2. Clonic (myoclonic) generalized
  B. Nonconvulsive
    1. Brief typical absence (petit mal)
    2. Brief atypical absence
II. Focal seizures
  A. Simple
    1. Motor (brief focal only)
    2. Sensory (focal with Jacksonian march)
    3. Autonomic (multifocal)
    4. Other (focal continuous – epilepsy partialis continua)
  B. Complex
    1. Psychomotor predominating
    2. Psychosensory predominating
III. Pseudoseizures (hysterical seizures)
IV. Other conditions with some features of epilepsy
  A. Narcolepsy
  B. Transient ischemic attacks
  C. Fainting
  D. Nightmares
  E. Rage attacks – dyscontrol
  F. Migraine
  G. Stokes-Adams attacks

Generalized seizures may be brief and without gross motor phenomena (petit mal), or they may take various forms including characteristic tonic-clonic attacks (grand mal). Seizures may occur only at night, and a careful history may be necessary to extract this information from the patient or the family. Focal seizures imply focal or cerebral disease, especially if the seizure pattern is consistently repeated. It is important to distinguish true seizures from other disorders of consciousness and especially from hysterical reactions, hyperventilation attacks, and syncope.

For a patient in whom seizures first develop during pregnancy, a detailed neurologic history and examination is necessary. Electroencephalography, skull x-rays, and metabolic studies, including a serum calcium determination, should be done on all patients. Fasting and postprandial hypoglycemia should be ruled out. A lumbar puncture and CAT scan are often desirable. Based on these studies and evidence of other positive neurologic signs or symptoms, it may be necessary to proceed to angiography.

The physician should appreciate that many patients who faint may have movements described by lay observers as resembling tonic and clonic motions. An occasional patient who faints may even pass urine. About 20 to 30 per cent of patients with seizures have a normal resting electroencephalogram; conversely, approximately 10 per cent of normal persons have a grossly dysrhythmic record. It is wise to remember that metabolic causes of seizures are common. Serum electrolyte levels should be obtained if there is any suspicion of hyponatremia. Hypoxia should always be considered. As already mentioned, measurements of serum calcium and glucose should be made.

Seizures are often related to withdrawal from medications, particularly sedatives. Seizures that occur soon after admission to the hospital should always suggest withdrawal from barbiturates, alcohol, or similar cerebral depressants. Finally, the physician should be aware that hysterical seizures may also occur in patients with epilepsy, particularly those who have assumed the sick role. The combination of hysterical seizures, true seizures, and hysterical behavior is not infrequently seen.

Seizure Control and Pregnancy

The problems of seizure control in pregnant epileptics have been reviewed.[3] Patients are divided into two categories: women who have been identified as epileptic prior to conception and in whom a level of seizure control has been established, and women who experience a seizure disorder, not related to toxemia, for the first time during pregnancy. Fewer than one quarter of women in the latter group have seizures *only* during pregnancy, and the term "gestational epilepsy" has been applied to this condition.

The incidence of epilepsy during pregnancy is difficult to ascertain precisely. It seems likely that an increase in seizure frequency can be predicted from the history of seizure control during the several years before conception. Of patients who rarely have seizures, only a few experience an increase in seizure frequency during pregnancy. In comparison, when patients experience more than one seizure per month before pregnancy, more than half have a deterioration in seizure control during pregnancy, especially during the first trimester. Further, among women in whom seizures are first manifest during pregnancy, the seizures and associated EEG abnormalities tend to be focal, perhaps associated with physiologic changes that occur during pregnancy.

In a study of 153 pregnancies in 59 patients, it is reported that in patients with epilepsy established before pregnancy, seizure frequency is increased in 45 per cent, unaltered in 5 per cent, and decreased in 55 per cent.[4] Women who report decreased seizure frequency during pregnancy may be more attentive to the use of anticonvulsants. Suter and Klingman describe seven women, five of whom had improved seizure control during pregnancy, which was associated with more careful and assiduous use of anticonvulsants.[5]

Anticonvulsants and Pregnancy

Mygind et al., Hooper and colleagues, and Lander et al. reported a decline in the plasma level of anticonvulsants during pregnancy when the maintenance dose is constant.[8, 9, 13] These investigators have reported increased plasma clearance for diphenylhydantoin and phenobarbital, although the plasma protein binding of phenobarbital remains unchanged. Subsequent to delivery, plasma levels of diphenylhydantoin and phenobarbital increase, approaching levels obtained before gravidity.

Anticonvulsants are transferred across the placenta, and placental transfer and fetal elimination rates are known for diphenylhydantoin, phenobarbital, primidone, and carbamazepine.[9, 12, 13] Diphenylhydantoin concentrations are identical in cord and maternal serum at term. The half-life of diphenylhydantoin in the plasma of the newborn ranges from 55 to 69 hours. Elimination of the drug by the fetus is generally completed by the fifth day.

Plasma levels of diphenylhydantoin (DPH) and the 24 hour urinary excretion of DPH and its major metabolite 5-(p-hydroxyphenyl)-phenylhydantoin (HHPH), measured serially during pregnancy in five unselected epileptic patients, have been reported.[10] Plasma DPH levels fell and averaged 40 per cent lower at term than during early gestation. Two patients who regularly had plasma DPH levels below 10 μg/ml suffered puerperal seizures. Thus, there was no convincing change in the urinary excretion of either DPH or HPPH during pregnancy.

In a definitive study, plasma clearance of diphenylhydantoin (DPH), phenobarbital, and carbamazepine was assessed in 14 epileptic patients during and after pregnancy.[6] Plasma clearance showed a marked increase during pregnancy, maximum level at delivery, and then a decrease to early pregnancy values. The authors suggest a higher rate of hepatic drug metabolism to explain this phenomenon.

Phenobarbital concentrations in human umbilical cord plasma are virtually identical to those of the mother's plasma.[11] Phenobarbital is eliminated from newborns within two to seven days; infants born of epileptic mothers may be dependent on phenobarbital and may experience withdrawal symptoms, characterized by hyperexcitability, tremor, restlessness, and difficulty in sleeping, but not seizures.[7]

The half-life of carbamazepine in the newborn, ranging from eight to 28 hours, is not significantly different from the half-life of the drug in adults.[9]

Maternal Complications and Epilepsy

In epileptics, there is a twofold increase in the incidence of maternal complications during pregnancy. These complications include hyperemesis, toxemia of pregnancy, vaginal bleeding, and complications of labor including the need for induction of labor and forceps delivery.[14] In addition, there is an increase in the rates of prematurity, neonatal mortality, and morbidity in the offspring of the pregnant epileptic, reported in several reviews.[15, 16] In most of these studies, information is lacking on drug regimens used, plasma drug levels, seizure frequency, and other critical data, which makes their evaluation too difficult to interpret.

Teratogenicity of Anticonvulsants

The incidence of malformations in normal infants is less than 1 per cent. Hence, an increased malformation rate can be detected in any study group only if the population is large or the rate of malformation is considerable. It has been estimated that the risk of congenital malformations among infants exposed to anticonvulsants in utero is two to three times greater than that in the general population. The anomalies appearing most frequently include cleft palate, cleft lip, and cardiac defects. Among the risk factors for teratogenicity that must be considered are the inherent teratogenicity of the anticonvulsants, the occurrence of frequent convulsions during pregnancy, the increased incidence of complications during pregnancy, and the socioeconomic class of the pregnant epileptic.

A fetal hydantoin syndrome has been the most commonly reported defect associated with the drug diphenylhydantoin.[17, 20-22] This syndrome is characterized by craniofacial anomalies, deficient growth, mental retardation, and limb defects. Craniofacial anomalies include a low, broad nasal bridge; epicanthal folds; a short, upturned nose; hypertelorism; ptosis; strabismus; prominent, low-set, malformed ears; wide mouth with prominent lips; and variations in the size and shape of the head, with widening of the fontanels and prominent ridging of the sutures. Limb defects include hypoplasia of the distal phalanges and nails, finger-like thumbs, and variations in palmar creases and hand markings. There may be intrauterine growth failure that results in small stature despite normal growth postnatally. A degree of mental retardation, mild to moderate, occurs.

A second fetal disorder associated with a specific anticonvulsant is the trimethadione syndrome.[18, 23] Affected infants have developmental delay, low-set ears, palatal anomalies, irregular teeth, V-shaped eyebrows, and speech disturbances.[19] Some infants have intrauterine growth retardation, short stature, cardiac anomalies, ocular defects, simian creases, hypospadias, and microcephaly. There are clear relationships between the trimethadione and hydantoin syndromes.

To date, no reports of carbamazepine as a teratogenic agent have been published, but birth defects have been described in infants exposed in utero to phenobarbital and primidone.[21]

According to the American Academy of Pediatrics Select Committee on Anticonvulsants in Pregnancy, no woman should receive anticonvulsant medication unnecessarily.[2] When possible, medication should be withdrawn prior to pregnancy from a woman who has been seizure-free for "many years." When a woman who has epilepsy and requires medication asks about pregnancy, she should be advised that she has a 90 per cent chance of having a normal child but that the risk of congenital malformations and mental retardation is two to three times greater than usual because of her disease and its treatment. There is no reason to switch from diphenylhydantoin to phenobarbital or to other anticonvulsants about which even less is known with respect to congenital anomalies. If the patient is actively epileptic, discontinuation of therapy is not advised, because of the danger of prolonged seizures.

Most anticonvulsants present in therapeutic levels in the mother are present in the breast milk as well. However, their concentration is so low that there is little likelihood of demonstrable effects on the infant. Thus, there is no evidence at present to suggest that a woman who needs anticonvulsants should stop taking medications, avoid nursing, or both.

New Anticonvulsants

Three anticonvulsants have been approved by the Food and Drug Administration since 1960 including clonazepam, carbamazepine, and valproic acid. Clonazepam is a benzodiazepine related to diazepam and is useful alone or as an adjunctive drug in the treatment of petit mal variant seizures, akinetic seizures, and myoclonic seizures.[24] In patients with petit mal who have failed to respond to succinimides, clonazepam may be employed. The effects of this drug in human pregnancy and nursing infants are unknown, but the drug produces congenital abnormalities in rabbits.

Carbamazepine is indicated for partial seizures with complex symptomatology, that is, psychomotor and temporal lobe seizures, generalized tonic and clonic seizures, and mixed seizures.[26] The effects of the drug in pregnant women and nursing infants are unknown. Again, adverse effects have been observed in reproduction studies in animals given carbamazepine orally. In addition, serious and occasionally fatal abnormalities of blood cells, such as aplastic anemia, agranulocytosis, thrombocytopenia, and leukopenia, have been reported following treatment with carbamazepine. Thus, this drug should be discontinued if evidence of significant bone marrow depression occurs. Patients with a history of adverse hematologic reactions to any other drug may be particularly at risk.

Valproic acid is the newest of the anticonvulsants.[25] It has a marked effect on generalized spike-wave discharges. The medication is well tolerated and has a broad spectrum anticonvulsant activity, so that it is useful in the management of major seizures, absence seizures of the petit mal type, and myoclonic, focal, and complex partial seizures. The effects of valproic acid in pregnancy are unknown, though no human congenital anomalies have thus far been attributed to it. In animals, valproic acid is teratogenic, causing dose-related morphologic abnormalities including cleft palate and renal defects.

Complex Drug Regimens and Seizure Therapy in Pregnancy

When possible, it is preferable to treat patients adequately with one or two anticonvulsants, making sure that their *blood levels are in the therapeutic ranges.* This is particularly the case in the pregnant epileptic, given the decline in plasma antiepileptic drug levels that occurs routinely during pregnancy if the oral dose ingested is constant.

If only one seizure occurs, usually no treatment is indicated. If repetitive seizures occur, treatment should always be given.

For sustained treatment of intermittent seizures, diphenylhydantoin (DPH) is the drug of choice. The effective dose is between 300 and 400 mg daily; it may be taken in divided doses in the morning and at bedtime. After approximately two weeks, DPH blood levels should be obtained. The therapeutic range is between 10 and 20 μg/ml of serum, and the medication should be raised or lowered to maintain adequate blood levels while achieving seizure control. If seizure control cannot be obtained, then another anticonvulsant, usually phenobarbital, should be added to the regimen. Phenobarbital may also be titered to blood levels, the therapeutic level for seizure control being from 15 to 30 μg/ml of serum, but the latter blood level is more useful if phenobarbital is used alone. Phenobarbital is commonly combined with DPH, and in this situation very small doses of phenobarbital may be effective. (Table 18-2 lists the common anticonvulsants that are frequently employed in pregnancy.)

Diphenylhydantoin and phenobarbital are also used in focal seizures, which are most commonly psychomotor or temporal lobe in origin. If good control is not achieved with DPH and phenobarbital, carbamazepine may be substituted. Good control of temporal lobe or psychomotor seizures is often difficult to achieve.

TABLE 18–2 ANTICONVULSANTS USED FOR EPILEPSY

Drug	Dosage	Side Effects	Toxicity	Type of Seizure Benefited			
				Major Motor	Minor Motor	Petit Mal	Psycho-motor
Diphenylhydantoin (Dilantin, DPH, Phenytoin)	Average 0.300 gm per day; range 0.060–0.600 gm per day; therapeutic level 10–25 gm/ml serum	Ataxia, drowsiness, gum hyperplasia, hypertrichosis, nystagmus	Rash, serum sickness, pseudolymphoma, Stevens-Johnson syndrome, lupus erythematosus, macrocytic anemia, rare hepatic or marrow toxicity, cerebellar degeneration, peripheral neuropathy, possibly teratogenic	+	+	−	+
Phenobarbital	Average 0.120 gm per day; range 0.030–0.210 gm per day; therapeutic level 15–30 gm/ml serum	Drowsiness, ataxia, nystagmus	Rare; rash, possibly teratogenic	+	+	−	+
Primidone (Mysoline)	Average 1 gm per day; range 0.500–2.0 gm per day	Drowsiness, nausea, ataxia, nystagmus (tachyphylaxis usual)	Rash, adenopathy, lupus erythematosus, macrocytic anemia, arthritis, edema	+	−	−	+
Carbamazepine (Tegretol)	Average 0.600 gm per day; range 0.200–1.2 gm per day; therapeutic level 4–6 gm/ml	Drowsiness, dizziness	Blood dyscrasia	+	−	−	+
Ethosuximide (Zarontin)	Average 1 gm per day; range 0.500–2.0 gm per day	Nausea, abdominal pain, drowsiness, personality change, headache	Rash, nephropathy, marrow depression	−	+	+	−
Diazepam (Valium)	Average 0.030 gm per day; range 0.500–0.050 gm per day	Ataxia, drowsiness, nausea, dizziness	Rash, neutropenia, jaundice, hypotension	+	+	+	+
Clonazepam (Clonopin)	Average 0.004–0.008 gm per day	Drowsiness, dizziness, ataxia	Coma	−	−	+	−
Valproic Acid (Depakene)	Average 0.750 gm; range 0.25–2.1 gm per day	Nausea, vomiting, abdominal cramps	Coma	+	+	+	+

Petit mal is rare in adults but may occasionally be seen during pregnancy. Ethosuximide (Zarontin) is the drug of choice, given in amounts of 250 to 500 mg three or four times daily. Diazepam (Valium) 5 to 10 mg four times daily may also be helpful in this situation.

Treatment of grand mal status epilepticus requires immediate hospitalization. It should be ascertained that the patient's airway is open and that free respiratory exchange is taking place. Blood should be drawn immediately for assessment of anticonvulsant levels before medications are given. Thereafter, a regimen such as the following can be used: An intravenous system is placed to expedite rapid drug administration. Ten mg of diazepam (Valium) is given slowly over a period of two to three minutes. It is essential that the drug be given slowly, since rapid administration may produce respiratory arrest. Thereafter, the needle is flushed and 200 to 500 mg of diphenylhydantoin (Dilantin) is given intravenously; the variation in dose depends on the anticonvulsant blood levels. It is well to monitor the patient electroencephalographically, since EEG seizure patterns may recur before actual clinical seizures appear. Should this be the case, another intravenous diazepam administration of 10 mg can be given after one half hour has passed. If seizure patterns continue thereafter, amobarbital sodium 500 mg can be given intravenously.

Should seizures persist, other more dramatic methods are employed including use of paraldehyde and general anesthesia. If seizures persist for a prolonged period, cerebral edema occurs, and dexamethasone sodium can then be employed in doses of 8 to 10 mg every four to six hours intramuscularly or intravenously.

There is no evidence that intravenous use of anticonvulsants, which might be employed in status epilepticus, has adverse effects on the fetus when one considers the alternative injurious effects on the fetus of continuous convulsions. Status epilepticus in the pregnant woman is often related to subtherapeutic plasma levels of antiepileptic drugs because of noncompliance by the patient or inadequate maintenance dose levels.

It has been suggested that a regimen be established that provides optimal seizure control with the fewest side effects using the least possible number of drugs.[3] Trimethadione should be avoided. The patient should be seen at least monthly, and plasma drug levels should be brought within the therapeutic range. It will probably be necessary to increase oral medications during pregnancy; the doses needed for maintenance sometimes reach levels that would be toxic in the nongravid state. Further, the antiepileptic drug doses required to maintain therapeutic levels during pregnancy do not decline immediately post partum. The high doses required may be maintained for variable periods after delivery, reductions in dose depending upon plasma levels obtained subsequently in the postpartum period.

Hemorrhagic Disease of the Newborn and Anticonvulsants

In newborns exposed to diphenylhydantoin, barbiturates, or trimethadione in utero, bleeding tendencies may develop during the first day of life after delivery, related to decreased levels of vitamin K–dependent clotting factors despite normal levels in the mother.[28] This form of drug-induced vitamin K deficiency should be distinguished from the physiologic deficiency occurring in normal infants between the second and fifth days. The drug-induced bleeding disorder occurs earlier and may be life-threatening.[27] This hemorrhagic disorder can be prevented with injections of vitamin K (phytonadione) into the newborn. One mg can be routinely given to all newborns after delivery. In infants known to be exposed in utero to antiepileptic drugs, clotting studies should be obtained two hours after the vitamin K is administered. If the clotting factors continue to be abnormal, additional doses will be required and the clotting time should be observed. Should hemorrhage become a problem, fresh frozen plasma is recommended.

HEADACHE

Headache is a common phenomenon, a symptom rather than a disease, and furthermore, a symptom of many complex illnesses of pregnancy. A classification of headache is thus a worthwhile undertaking, and the following is presented to the reader as one method of clarifying this uncomfortable and often confusing complaint (see Table 18–1).

I have separated headache into three main groups rather than a series of disparate headache syndromes that may tax the memory. These groups are vascular, muscle contraction, and traction and inflammatory (Table 18–3).

Vascular headache includes classic and common migraine, hemiplegic migraine, ophthalmoplegic migraine, cluster (histamine) headache,

TABLE 18-3 CLASSIFICATION AND TREATMENT OF HEADACHE IN PREGNANCY

Vascular Headache	Classification Muscle Contraction Headache	Traction and Inflammatory Headache

Migraine
  Classic
  Common
  Hemiplegic ⎫complicated
  Ophthalmoplegic ⎰migraine
	Cervical osteoarthritis	Mass lesions (tumors, edema,
		  hematomas, cerebral
		  hemorrhage)

Cluster (histamine)	Chronic myositis	Diseases of the eye, ear, nose, throat, teeth
Toxic vascular	Depressive equivalents and conversion reactions	Allergy
Hypertensive		Infection Arteritis, phlebitis (Cranial neuralgias) Occlusive vascular disease

	Suggested Treatment	
Sedation Cyproheptadine Analgesics Antihypertensives Propranolol	Simple analgesics Sedation Amitriptyline Physical therapy	Appropriate consultation Therapy of underlying disease Allergy therapy ⎫ Antibiotics ⎪ Anticonvulsants ⎬ as Corticosteroids ⎪ indicated Miotics ⎪ Surgery ⎭

toxic vascular headache, and hypertensive head-ache. Common to all is a tendency to vascular dilation, which represents the headache phase of the migraine attack.[30] Vasoconstriction may also be evident and may be responsible for painless sensory phenomena prior to the onset of head pain. Hemiplegic and ophthalmoplegic migraine are considered more severe forms of classical migraine. Toxic vascular headache is evoked by a systemic vasodilation and may be produced by fever, alcohol, CO_2 retention, agents such as nitrites, and the like. Headache syndromes most likely to occur in pregnancy and the puerperium will be discussed here.

THE MIGRAINE SYNDROME IN PREGNANCY

Two hundred women, ages 16 to 45, all preg-nant, were interviewed by one worker.[29] There was true migraine in 25 and probable migraine in 16. There was an increase in the severity of the attacks of migraine with pregnancy in three pa-tients, and four improved with respect to mi-graine during pregnancy.

In another report of 200 pregnant women with migraine, 38 had a recent history of migraine and 31 were subject to migraine before becoming

pregnant.[36] In only seven did migraine develop for the first time during pregnancy; in five during the first trimester; in one during the second trimester; and in one during the third. Of the 31 subject to migraine before becoming pregnant, 24 showed improvement in migraine while pregnant and seven had no headaches at all.

A case of classic migraine that began during pregnancy at 27 weeks gestation has been report-ed.[34] Friedman and Merritt found that 80 per cent or more women had a decreased frequency of migraine during pregnancy, and this was more or less confirmed by Lance and Anthony, who found relief in approximately 50 per cent during pregnancy.[32, 33] They noted that those patients with migraine exacerbated by the menses were particularly liable to be relieved. In general, the rule is that most patients with migraine are improved during the gravid state.

MIGRAINE AND PRE-ECLAMPSIA

Rotton and colleagues suggest, on the basis of a retrospective study, that migraine attacks occur more frequently in patients who develop pre-eclampsia than in healthy pregnant women.[35] However, more modern surveys of patients with migraine do not confirm this observation. The seven patients described by Somerville, whose migraine headaches did not improve during pregnancy, were not eclamptic.[36] One may question whether there is in fact any relationship between migraine and pre-eclampsia. The question can only be resolved by more exacting prospective studies.

HEMIPLEGIC MIGRAINE

In hemiplegic migraine the vascular reactions of classical migraine may be exaggerated to the point at which long-lasting ischemia of brain tissue occurs. This form of migraine may be strikingly familial, suggesting that an inherited instability of vascular control is present. Whether the sequelae of this form of migraine are related to the prolongation of the vasodilator or the vasoconstrictor phases of migraine is unknown; possibly both factors are implicated. Dooling and Sweeney have described migrainous hemiplegia occurring during breast feeding.[31]

OPHTHALMOPLEGIC MIGRAINE

In ophthalmoplegic migraine, first described by Charcot, ocular palsy is associated with headache. Those structures served by the third cranial nerve are most often involved.

In patients who suffer repeated attacks, ocular palsies are usually transitory. In rare instances, however, these palsies may become persistent. It is important to differentiate between the mechanisms operative in ophthalmoplegic migraine and those that produce similar symptoms but that are related to intracranial aneurysms, particularly of the posterior communicating artery. The sudden appearance of third nerve signs in a pregnant patient not subject to migraine may be an indication for arteriography.

TOXIC VASCULAR HEADACHE

This category includes all of the diseases and conditions that produce headache of the vascular nature as part of their overall symptomatology. The most common nonmigrainous vascular headache is that produced by fever. Generalized vasodilation may occur as a consequence of any significant fever, the vasodilation usually becoming more intense as the fever rises. Particularly intense vascular headaches may occur with pneumonia, tonsillitis, septicemia, typhoid fever, tularemia, influenza, measles, mumps, poliomyelitis, infectious mononucleosis, malaria, and trichinosis. The vasodilation in these diseases is often intracranial as well as extracranial.

Nonmigrainous vascular headache may also occur in a whole series of miscellaneous disorders including such diverse entities as hangover headache and headache associated with hypoglycemia regardless of cause. In hypoxic states headache may be a persistent complaint.

HEADACHE ASSOCIATED WITH ARTERIAL HYPERTENSION AND TOXEMIA OF PREGNANCY

Several categories of headache are associated with hypertension and deserve discussion. A sudden rise in blood pressure during violent exercise, anger, or sexual excitement may be associated with bilateral pounding headache, usually short-lived or transient, which is rarely of diagnostic or therapeutic importance. Effort migraine occurring in athletes after a long race or in mountain climbers experiencing anoxia is a related phenomenon. Such an episode does not usually require specific therapy.

Sudden and extreme elevations of blood pressure may occur with toxemia of pregnancy, in the malignant state of essential hypertension, and with end-stage renal disease. The syndrome termed hypertensive encephalopathy consists of severe headache, nausea, vomiting, and convulsions, proceeding to confusion and coma. Papilledema is always present as a primary sign of increased intracranial pressure. The headache is more or less continuous, generalized, pounding, and difficult to relieve with simple analgesics. It is assumed that brain edema in some form produces the headache associated with hypertensive encephalopathy. The intravenous injection of osmotically active agents such as mannitol will reduce its intensity. Oral glycerol is also effective. These agents produce relative dehydration of the brain, subsequent to which traction and displacement of pain-sensitive structures are reduced. (See also Chapter 1.)

The neurologic signs of hypertensive encephalopathy occurring in toxemia are probably related to cerebral vasospasm, thereafter producing cerebral ischemia and cerebral edema. The primary therapeutic aim in hypertensive encephalopathy is to reduce the blood pressure, which is the only effective way to relieve the symptoms.

Vascular headache may also be associated with a paroxysmal rise in blood pressure as seen in a patient with pheochromocytoma, but other physical findings should lead rapidly to that diagnosis.

What remains are those headaches associated with essential hypertension. With this common disease, the pain is vascular and is best related to the contractile state of the extracranial and intracranial arteries. Should these arteries dilate, for whatever reason, hypertensive vascular headache will occur. Usually the pain is described as dull and aching with a pounding component, often present in the morning and improving as the patient stirs, gets up, and moves about. The pain is frequently increased by effort, stooping, and jolts to the head.

Hypertensive headache is rarely present in pregnant women unless the diastolic blood pressure exceeds 110 mm Hg.

Often the headache is relieved by bed rest or other methods of relaxation that reduce the blood pressure. A low salt diet may be helpful. Weight loss is often advised. The headache can be expected to respond to those medical measures that reduce the blood pressure to normal or near-normal levels. Though ergotamine tartrate may improve vascular headache related to hypertension, its routine use in this situation is not recommended.

Patients with minimal hypertension who complain of headache need careful evaluation. Often the tendency is to blame the headache on the hypertension, although this may not be the case. As mentioned previously, unless the diastolic blood pressure exceeds 110 mm Hg, another etiology should be sought.

MUSCLE CONTRACTION HEADACHE

Perhaps the most common form of headache in pregnancy is that related to chronic muscular contraction occurring about the head and neck. This produces dull, band-like, persistent pain, which may last for days or months. In treating this type of pain, a search should be made for tender and painful areas of the head and neck as well as significant arthritis of the spine.

If the headache is incapacitating, persistent, and not obviously vascular, a disorder of mood, thought, or behavior should be suspected. Headache may represent one form of a conversion reaction. Chronic, nonspecific headache may occur in the depressed pregnant patient.

TRACTION AND INFLAMMATORY HEADACHE

Traction and inflammatory headache includes headache evoked by organic disease of the skull or its components including the brain, meninges, arteries, veins, eyes, ears, teeth, nose, and paranasal sinuses. The term traction headache is used to describe the often nonspecific headache seen with mass lesions of the brain including tumors, hematomas, abscesses, or brain edema from whatever cause. Traction headache of a particularly intense type occurs in subarachnoid and intracerebral hemorrhage and in cortical venous thromboses. Traction headache is associated with inflammatory disease of the meninges and intracranial or extracranial arteritis or phlebitis. Inflammatory headache evoked by disease of the special sense organs and the teeth, as well as allergic headache, and the major cranial neuralgia, including tic douloureux, are included here.

Treatment of Headache

Proper therapy for headache implies that an accurate diagnosis has been made and that the etiology of the head pain has been determined, insofar as this is possible. Severe headache is only infrequently caused by organic disease. Hence, it may be inferred that for the most part headache in pregnant patients represents an inability of the woman to deal in some measure with the vicissitudes of life rather than a structural disease of the nervous system. Nonetheless, headache may also be the presenting complaint of catastrophic illness such as brain tumor, cerebral hemorrhage, or meningitis, among others, and to ignore headache in this context is to risk the life of the patient. The problem is compounded further by the difficulties of studying the brain and its appendages, which, encased in the bony fortress of the skull, resist direct methods of investigation and inspection.

TREATMENT OF ACUTE INTERMITTENT MIGRAINE OF PREGNANCY (Table 18–4)

In ordinary circumstances, the cornerstone of medical therapy for migraine is ergotamine tartrate in one of its forms. In pregnancy, ergotamine tartrate is best avoided, for reasons of emotion and tradition if not of science. The tendency of some of the natural ergot alkaloids is to increase the motor contractions of the uterus. Yet ergotamine tartrate, given by mouth, is without oxytocic effects on the human uterus. The problem is compounded by the important oxytocic properties of other ergot alkaloids. For example, ergonovine, sometimes used in migraine therapy, has prompt oxytocic activity when given orally. Hence the notion of avoiding all ergot drugs in the medical therapy of pregnant migraine patients, since the clinician may become confused about which of the various forms of ergot are, in fact, oxytocic. (It may also be noted that, for the most part, ergot drugs are not effective abortifacients, particularly in the first two trimesters of pregnancy.)

Thus, treatment of acute intermittent migraine of pregnancy depends primarily on the use of

TABLE 18–4 MIGRAINE THERAPY CHART IN PREGNANCY

Class	Type	Treatment	Route	Drug	Dosage
Vascular	Migraine	Prophylactic	Oral	Propranolol (Inderal)	40–160 mg daily as tolerated
				Cyproheptadine (Periactin)	4–16 mg daily as tolerated
		Abortive	Oral	Empirin comp. with codeine 3 mg	1 or 2 every 6–8 hours as needed
			Intramuscular	Chlorpromazine (Thorazine)	25–50 mg every 6–8 hours as needed
				Dihydroergotamine (DHE-45)	
				Hydroxyzine (Vistaril)	50–100 mg every 6–8 hours as needed
			Rectal	Chlorpromazine (Thorazine)	100 mg every 6–8 hours as needed; in some patients 50 mg will suffice
				Ergotamine, caffeine, phenacetin, and belladonna	
				Trimethobenzamide (Tigan)	200 mg three times daily as needed

analgesics and sedatives, much as any other self-limited pain syndrome. Chlorpromazine, by virtue of its analgesic and antiemetic effects, is particularly useful.

TREATMENT OF CHRONIC MIGRAINE

Chronic migraine occurs only rarely in pregnancy. If simple analgesics and sedatives fail to relieve symptoms, propranolol or cyproheptadine may be employed. Propranolol is given in an average dose of 40 mg bid or tid and is the most effective and useful drug available for the pregnant migrainous patient. Symptoms of anxiety and/or depression should be treated. Chlorpromazine 25 mg three times daily may be helpful. If depression is present, amitriptyline, 25 mg three times daily or in a single bedtime dose of 75 mg, is suggested.

DIETARY MIGRAINE

Dietary migraine may occur related to the ingestion of food containing vasoactive substances including alcohol.[37] Patients with cluster headache are notoriously sensitive to even small amounts of alcohol, and they learn to avoid alcohol during the period of cluster headache recurrence. Alcohol is a nonspecific vasodilator, which probably accounts for its precipitation of the vascular headache process. The vasodilation is assumed to be the result of depression or alteration of the central vasomotor centers, since the direct action of alcohol on blood vessels is insignificant. Moderate amounts of alcohol do not affect cerebral blood flow, but severe intoxi-

cation causes a significant increase in cerebral blood flow with diminished cerebrovascular resistance.

Foods that contain tyramine, a vasoactive amine, may precipitate headache, particularly in patients who are treated with monoamine oxidase (MAO) inhibitors.[38] Tyramine-rich foods include strong or aged cheeses, pickled herring, chicken livers, canned figs, chocolate, and the pods of broad beans. Recent studies have cast doubt on the importance of this finding, some confirming and some denying that ingestion of oral tyramine *without* MAO inhibitors may provoke headache in patients subject to migraine.[39]

Dietary Suggestions in the Therapy of Migraine of Pregnancy

1. Avoid alcohol, particularly red wines and champagne.
2. Avoid aged or strong cheese, particularly cheddar cheese.
3. Use monosodium glutamate sparingly.
4. Avoid cured meats such as hot dogs, bacon, ham, and salami if these can be demonstrated to evoke vascular headache.
5. Eat three well-balanced meals per day. Avoid skipping meals, prolonged fasting, or excessive ingestion of carbohydrates at any single sitting.

I have adopted a pragmatic approach to this problem and suggest that those foods and beverages that have been shown to have vasoactive properties be eliminated from the diet of migraineurs. I do not suggest avoidance of milk products. Large amounts of monosodium glutamate (MSG) may produce a generalized vasomotor reaction that may include headache (the "Chinese restaurant syndrome"). Use of excessive amounts of monosodium glutamate is unwise.

Hypoglycemia

A word should be said about the quality and amount of food consumed by the patient with migraine. Hypoglycemia exerts a profound effect on the tone of the cranial blood vessels. If the sugar content of the blood is reduced by insulin or by other means, conspicuous cerebral vasodilation occurs. Headache is a prominent symptom of insulin shock, for example. Furthermore, in migraine patients, the relative hypoglycemia produced by fasting may evoke typical vascular headaches. Even reactive hypoglycemia occurring after ingestion of an excessive carbohydrate load may precipitate vascular headache in a susceptible person. For these reasons I suggest that the patient with migraine eat three well-balanced meals a day and avoid an overabundance of carbohydrates at any single meal.

TREATMENT OF INTERMITTENT MUSCLE CONTRACTION (TENSION) HEADACHES OF PREGNANCY

Analgesics such as aspirin 0.6 gr, repeated in two hours if needed, are usually effective. Empirin compound with codeine can be used, provided it is not abused. If muscle complaints involving the neck are present, simple measures of physical therapy to the neck including heat, hot packs, and massage may be helpful. Local injection of trigger areas with anesthesia, corticosteroids, or both may be employed as adjunctive therapy.

TREATMENT OF CHRONIC MUSCLE CONTRACTION HEADACHES OF PREGNANCY

Tricyclic antidepressants are often given, such as amitriptyline 75 mg at bedtime, given over a prolonged period, usually 90 days and possibly longer on a lower maintenance dose. Environmental counseling, environmental manipulation, and behavioral therapy, including biofeedback training techniques, may be tried. Referral for formal psychiatric counseling is advisable. I suggest that the physician avoid administering aspirin and drugs containing phenacetin over a prolonged period. Narcotics should be used sparingly.

HEADACHE RELATED TO LUMBAR PUNCTURE

Should the pregnant patient require a lumbar puncture, for whatever reason, a headache may result. Treatment is symptomatic. Place the patient on bed rest and provide adequate fluids by mouth for hydration. Simple analgesics such as aspirin may be helpful. This is a self-limited condition that does not require specific therapy. Ergot drugs are not helpful.

TREATMENT OF TRACTION AND INFLAMMATORY HEADACHE

Treatment for this form of headache generally involves specific therapy for the associated underlying disease. Extensive investigation and consultation with other specialists may be required. Thus, the therapy for headache evoked by traction or inflammation of pain-sensitive cranial constituents is varied and may range from surgery to antibiotics. It is in this group of patients that prompt and emergency treatment may be necessary. The headache is considered a secondary phenomenon that will usually respond to alleviation of the primary disease.

CEREBROVASCULAR DISEASE

Vascular disease of the central nervous system can be conveniently divided into three aspects. Initially, a disease process affects the arteries or veins. The causes are varied and include arteriosclerosis, embolism, hypertensive change, malformation, vasospasm, arteritis, and inflammation. The vessel or series of vessels then either plug or leak. Subsequent to this alteration in the vessels, pathologic changes occur in the central nervous system related to either infarction or bleeding. Finally, neurologic disease appears, with signs and symptoms as a result of infarction or bleeding.

The etiologic factors that may lead to the development of cerebrovascular disease are outlined in Figure 18–1. Depending on the blood vessel involved, different cerebral ischemic patterns are seen. These are described in Table 18–5. The clinician can frequently recognize the site of the vascular ischemia on the basis of the clinical signs and symptoms described. CAT scans should be employed in all pregnant patients with a stroke. Often, however, arteriographic study of the vessels involved is indicated, especially if surgical intervention is contemplated.

The clinician must also distinguish between episodic cerebrovascular disease and similar conditions that may mimic ischemia including epilepsy, Stokes-Adams attacks, carotid sinus disease, and Meniere's syndrome. These distinguishing features are described in Table 18–6.

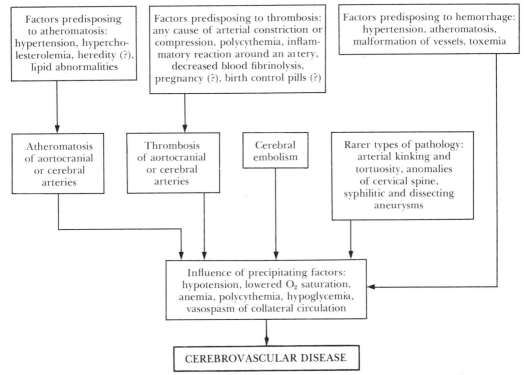

FIGURE 18–1. Etiologic factors in the development of cerebrovascular disease.

Cerebral Strokes

Thirty-one cases of ischemic cerebral stroke occurring in association with childbirth were fully investigated by Cross and associates.[42] The pathologic basis of nonhemorrhagic stroke in pregnant or puerperal women proved to be similar to that of nonpregnant women of the same age group. More than 70 per cent of cases were due to occlusive cerebral arterial disease or ischemic lesions not related to thrombosis of the intracranial venous system. Comparisons were made with other series in which only a minority of patients were thoroughly investigated with modern techniques, including angiography, and in which venous occlusion was assumed to be the primary lesion. The authors suggest that many of the patients in the older studies may also have suffered arterial rather than venous lesions.

All 31 patients had hemiplegia of varying degree. Sixteen had dysphasia. The onset of symptoms was abrupt in 23 (74 per cent). Only eight patients had a gradual onset of neurologic complaints. Paresthesias of the limbs preceding hemiplegia occurred in four women. One had a major seizure 24 hours before hemiplegia developed. One had a seizure ten weeks prior to a major stroke. There was alteration of consciousness in 19 patients. Headache occurring either before or in association with the vascular accident was present in 11 patients. Ten had visual disturbances. Three patients had hemiplegia that recurred in successive and subsequent pregnancies.

Predisposing factors could be demonstrated in 11 of the 31 patients. Five manifested pre-eclamptic toxemia with fluctuating hypertension. There were hypotensive episodes present in four patients. There was hypertension without toxemia in one, and one patient had a puerperal sepsis after a spontaneous abortion.

The authors suggest that the incidence of cerebrovascular accident is approximately one case per 20,000 births. Most of these patients were younger than 35 years. Only one cerebrovascular accident occurred in the first trimester. As many cases occur in the immediate postpartum period as in the six months prior to delivery. In this study cortical venous occlusion was rare and only one case could be demonstrated.

It may therefore be stated that the most common type of cerebrovascular accident associated with pregnancy and the puerperium is that of cerebral arterial disease. Older studies that emphasized the importance of nonseptic intracranial venous thrombosis were often collected before modern angiographic techniques were available. They should be evaluated in that light.

Middle cerebral arterial occlusion in three

TABLE 18–5 COMMONLY ENCOUNTERED CEREBRAL VASCULAR DISEASE PATTERNS

Intermittent insufficiency of the internal carotid arterial system
Unilateral signs (one or more)
1. Weakness, paralysis, or numbness (partial or complete) of the opposite side
2. Disorders of speech, often intermittent
3. Visual disturbance of the ipsilateral eye
Of 50 cases of proven carotid occlusions, 43 of which were cervical in nature, the following was found:
   a. Unilateral motor weakness, especially in arm, in 98 per cent
   b. Unilateral sensory defects in 64 per cent
   c. Visual defects in 52 per cent
   d. Aphasia in 42 per cent
   e. Recurrent symptoms in 28 per cent

Occlusion of the anterior cerebral artery
1. Weakness, sensory defects of opposite foot and leg
2. Urinary incontinence
3. Memory impairment, grasping and sucking reflexes may be observed

Middle cerebral arterial disease
As in internal carotid disease; ipsilateral blindness suggests carotid disease, and contralateral homonymous hemianopia suggests middle cerebral arterial disease

Vertebral basilar disease
1. Diplopia and other oculomotor disturbances
2. Ptosis, meiosis
3. Numbness, tingling, weakness of the face or extremities
4. Weakness of the tongue; difficulty in speaking or swallowing (hindbrain functions)
5. Vertigo, nystagmus, ataxia
6. Visual disturbances

Posterior inferior cerebellar artery (Wallenberg) (lateral area of caudal portion of brain stem—lateral medullary syndrome)
1. Dysphagia and dysarthria
2. Loss of pain and temperature sensations on homolateral side of the face
3. Horner's syndrome on the side of the lesion
4. Nystagmus
5. Cerebellar dysfunction in homolateral arm and leg
6. Impairment of pain and temperature on opposite half of the body

Cortical venous thrombosis
1. Occurs usually after delivery
2. First sign is sudden major seizure
3. Headache, generalized, is frequent occurrence
4. Papilledema may appear rapidly
5. Monoparesis or hemiparesis may occur

Cerebral hemorrhage
1. Sudden onset of severe head pain, disturbances of consciousness
2. Progressive neurologic signs including rapid onset of hemiplegia, hemianesthesia, speech disturbance, visual disturbance
3. Associated hypertension is usually present

Subarachnoid hemorrhage
1. Excruciating headache
2. Loss of consciousness
3. Rapid development of meningeal signs
4. Absence of gross lateralizing signs in many patients
5. Rarely, convulsions

TABLE 18–6 DIFFERENTIAL DIAGNOSIS OF CEREBROVASCULAR ISCHEMIC STATES

Condition	Distinguishing Features	Comment
Episodic focal ischemia	Carotid system—motor and/or sensory deficit of opposite side; visual disturbance; sometimes aphasia	The foregoing focal signs make diagnosis of ischemic attack fairly clear-cut
	Vertebral basilar system—motor and/or sensory deficit of one or more limbs; also involvement of cerebellum and cranial nerve nuclei; diplopia, dysarthria, dysphagia, facial weakness or numbness, ataxia	Loss of consciousness is rare
Epilepsy	Convulsive seizures, loss of consciousness, tongue-biting, urinary and fecal incontinence, postictal sleepiness	These features are rare or absent in focal cerebral ischemic attacks
Meniere's disease	Triad of chronic deafness, recurrent vertigo, and tinnitus	Deafness and tinnitus rare in ischemic attacks; dizziness common in vertebral basilar insufficiency; therefore, look for other evidence of brain stem ischemia
Stokes-Adams attacks and carotid sinus reflex	Syncope, confusion, but no focal neurologic signs unless there is also significant cerebrovascular pathology	Focal signs usually present in ischemic attacks

young women was described by Lavy and Kahana.[43] The authors emphasize that the differential diagnosis of arterial and venous cerebral occlusions is of great practical importance. Cerebral arterial occlusion has a better initial prognosis than venous occlusion. In venous occlusion there is often spread of the thromboembolic process, producing significant brain edema. Mortality is initially higher in cortical venous thrombosis, but those patients who recover may have no permanent neurologic residua.

Amias further describes 18 patients with occlusive vascular lesions that were associated with pregnancy and the puerperium.[41] Of these 18 patients, exactly half had arterial occlusion, with six presenting during pregnancy and three in the puerperium. The nine cases of cortical venous thrombosis all occurred in the puerperium.

Subarachnoid Hemorrhage

Subarachnoid hemorrhage is rare in childhood but increases in frequency to its greatest incidence occurring between the ages of 35 and 65. This finding suggests that the common saccular or berry aneurysm represents not a congenital abnormality of some type but a developmental defect of the arterial wall that develops slowly as the patient ages. The aneurysm takes the form of a small and thin-walled blister, which protrudes from the arteries of the circle of Willis or the major vessels that arise from that circle. The aneurysms are commonly situated at bifurcations and branchings, the result of developmental defects in the media and elastica of vessels at these sites. Eventually, owing to weakness of the arterial wall, the intima protrudes outward until gradually the outpouching enlarges and rupture occurs. Atherosclerosis probably plays no particular role in predisposition to rupture.

As maternal mortality from other serious illnesses decreases, the significance of cerebral hemorrhage in maternal mortality secondary to ruptured aneurysms has become increasingly important.[48] Miller and Hinkley surveyed the maternal deaths at a university hospital over a decade and found that ruptured aneurysms accounted for 12 per cent of these deaths.[47] They established an aneurysm rate of rupture of 1:10,400 and found that more than half the patients with ruptured berry aneurysm had had one or more pregnancies carried to term without difficulty. After comparing the mortality of pregnant and nonpregnant females with ruptured berry aneurysm, the authors advise that when rupture of an aneurysm does occur during pregnancy, the risk to the mother's life is two to three times greater than when it occurs in a nonpregnant state.

Robinson and Hall reviewed 26 cases of spontaneous subarachnoid hemorrhage that had occurred during pregnancy.[50] Of the 24 lesions demonstrated to be responsible for the hemorrhages, 13 were aneurysms and 11 were arteriovenous malformations. Eight were aneurysms of the internal carotid artery and, of these, five were operated on during pregnancy (four by a direct approach and one by carotid ligation). The remaining eight aneurysms and all the malformations were managed conservatively. Two of the malformations were subsequently treated surgically after recurrent hemorrhage. In the group there had been six previous episodes of subarachnoid hemorrhage in five patients, all with malformations. Only one of these had occurred unrelated to pregnancy. Of the 13 subsequent hemorrhages, seven occurred in seven patients with malformations and six in five patients with aneurysms.

The authors analyzed their cases in conjunction with similar series in the literature and came to the following conclusions. A cause for the hemorrhage was more likely to be demonstrable in pregnant than in nonpregnant women, and the incidences of aneurysms and malformations were about equal. The malformations were seen in younger women (ages 20 to 25) and most commonly bled between 15 and 20 weeks into the pregnancy. The aneurysms occurred in an older age group (ages 30 to 35) and caused hemorrhage usually between 30 and 40 weeks gestation but rarely in labor or in the early puerperium. Maternal prognosis was the same as in nonpregnant cases, except that the malformations seemed to have a greater propensity for recurrent hemorrhage. The fetal prognosis was related to that of the mother in the case of aneurysm but was unexpectedly poor in the malformation cases, both in the current and subsequent pregnancies.

There was no apparent fetal risk with operation under hypothermia. Vaginal delivery was done whenever possible, but the second stage of labor was modified by lumbar epidural anesthesia and forceps delivery to obviate cardiovascular stresses. Normal term delivery can be anticipated in aneurysm patients who bleed before 35 weeks gestation and are treated surgically. The same is true in patients with arteriovenous anomalies. The authors suggest that the only indication for elective cesarean section and tubal ligation is the presence of an untreated arteriovenous anomaly.

Robinson et al. have also described a retrospective survey of 146 patients with subarachnoid hemorrhage; about half of these patients were pregnant.[50] Their data indicate that pregnancy has a deleterious effect on pre-existing arteriovenous malformations (AVM), making them more likely to bleed. If a patient with an AVM does become pregnant, subarachnoid hemorrhage and some serious complication of pregnancy can be anticipated, and delivery by cesarean section with concomitant sterilization is advised by these authors.

Minielly et al. reviewed the management of eight pregnant patients who experienced subarachnoid hemorrhage from ruptured cerebral aneurysms.[48] In seven, the aneurysms were managed surgically. All of these patients survived, but one had a permanent neurologic deficit (decerebrate and institutionalized). There were seven living infants delivered, one by cesarean section and the others by vaginal delivery. There was one maternal death, in a patient whose aneurysm was inoperable (a large right vertebral aneurysm). This patient did have a successful cesarean section. The authors suggest that the prognosis for ruptured cerebral aneurysms during pregnancy is good for both mother and fetus.

Fetal heart rates were monitored by Doptone monitor during the aneurysm surgery. Clipping of the aneurysms was done under induced hypotension. The initial treatment in each case was conservative and included bed rest and sedation with diazepam and phenobarbital. Corticosteroids were administered to most patients.

Minielly et al. advise that surgery is the treatment of choice when an operable aneurysm can be demonstrated in a pregnant women with subarachnoid hemorrhage.[48]

Heron et al. report two patients who developed subarachnoid bleeding during pregnancy and the puerperium as a consequence of disseminated intravascular coagulation.[45] No demonstrable source of intracranial bleeding could be found despite bilateral carotid angiography. The authors suggest that the bleeding was the direct result of the hematologic abnormalities. Heparin, given after delivery, was useful in one patient.

Amias has reported 52 patients with intracranial hemorrhage, of whom 40 were pregnant and 12 were recently delivered.[44] Angioma was encountered more often than aneurysm in the pregnant group. There was a higher incidence of hypertension among patients with cerebral aneurysms as compared with patients with other lesions. Thus, intracranial bleeding in a hypertensive patient should always be investigated intensively. Amias states that unless labor begins during investigation, a cerebral lesion should be treated before delivery, irrespective of the stage of pregnancy, and the method of treatment should be decided primarily on neurologic and neurosurgical grounds.[44]

What if the aneurysm or arterial venous malformation is inoperable? Hunt et al. suggest that patients with inoperable aneurysms that are discovered early in gestation should be allowed to deliver vaginally.[46] If the patient begins to bleed in the third trimester, cesarean section is indicated. Similar recommendations can be given for arterial venous malformations, which frequently rebleed during delivery. If these are demonstrated and are inoperable, cesarean sections are routinely performed at 38 weeks gestation.[50]

A good rule to follow is that the neurologic and neurosurgical evaluation and treatment of a pregnant woman with a subarachnoid hemorrhage should be the same as that for a nonpregnant patient, the exception being if the patient is in active labor.

Cortical Venous Thromboses

Thrombosis of the superior sagittal sinus and cortical veins is an uncommon but well-recognized complication of pregnancy and puerperium. The reported incidence varies from 1 in 10,000 pregnancies to 1 in 600,000 consecutive births. The pathogenesis and treatment of these thromboses are controversial. During pregnancy there is increased platelet adhesiveness as well as increased levels of other clotting factors, and in those cases of puerperal venous thrombosis the levels of clotting constituents are higher than those of healthy pregnant women.

Lavin et al. describe a fatal case of intracranial venous thrombosis occurring in the first trimester of pregnancy.[52] The CAT scan showed massive cerebral venous infarct, with "decreased absorption" in both cerebral hemispheres. At necropsy, there was thrombosis of cerebral, pelvic, and ilial veins.

The treatment of cortical venous thrombosis is dictated by the circumstances. Anticonvulsants should probably be employed prophylactically. Other treatment modalities include corticosteroids and mannitol to reduce edema, therapeutic lumbar puncture, and consideration of anticoagulation therapy. Obviously anticoagulants should not be employed if the cerebrospinal fluid is bloody. Some authors have implied that anticoagulants may actually provoke intracranial hemorrhage in this situation.[51]

Treatment of Intracranial Hemorrhage and Stroke

The treatment of the various forms of intracranial hemorrhage is liable to be as varied as the hospitals or clinics in which physicians are employed. Careful attention to the vital signs including temperature, respiratory patterns, pupillary responses, and cardiac arrhythmias is mandatory. Ordinarily, unless the patient is unusually alert, parenteral fluids should be supplied. A nasal gastric tube should not be used for at least the first several days. Intake and output must be carefully recorded. A record of urine specific gravity should be correlated with serum electrolytes. Records of urine and serum osmolalities should be obtained to avoid the occurrence of diabetes insipidus or the inappropriate secretion of the antidiuretic hormone. If the patient is incontinent, a urinary catheter should be placed. Meticulous attention to joint function and protection of the skin is necessary. It is important to maintain adequate evacuation of the bowels.

Patients who bleed intracranially usually have pain and must be given medication for pain and sedation. Either diazepam or phenobarbital can be used. Convulsions should be anticipated, and the patient should be given diphenylhydantoin prophylactically. Should repeated convulsions occur, therapy described in the section on treatment of seizure disorders should be undertaken. Diazepam or diphenylhydantoin intravenously is the drug of choice.

If severe hypertension is present, precise control of the blood pressure will be necessary. If the patient can be adequately monitored, sodium nitroprusside given by an infusion pump in amounts of 0.5 to 10 μg/kg/min can be administered. Intravenous diazoxide (50 to 100 mg) is an effective alternative. Other methods of therapy include hydralazine 10 to 40 mg parenterally every four hours as needed or intravenous methyldopa 250 to 500 mg intravenously, administered over a 30 minute interval. Propranolol is also employed parenterally. Oral medication should be started as soon as possible after adequate control has been achieved.

Cerebral edema may occur in association with intracranial hemorrhage. This is best treated with dexamethasone injection, 10 mg intravenously, followed by the parenteral administration of 4 mg every six hours for the next 36 hours. Osmotic diuretics are not ordinarily used in this situation. Monitoring of intracranial pressure may be necessary.

CAT scanning of the head should be performed in all pregnant patients with intracranial hemorrhage. Consultation with a neurosurgeon is mandatory. If it is possible to demonstrate a berry aneurysm by arteriography, then ligation of the aneurysm is probably the treatment of choice. Acute evacuation of an intracerebral hematoma, conversely, is probably of no value. But evacuation of a cerebellar hematoma may be a life-saving procedure.

Treatment of occlusive cerebrovascular disease occurring during pregnancy should employ many of the guidelines set forth previously. Attention to hypertension, metabolic diseases, coagulopathies, and cardiac abnormalities is important. If cerebral edema occurs, dexamethasone can be used. Methods to improve cerebral blood flow and collateral circulation, such as the use of intravenous papaverine, have not, in my hands, been helpful. Physical therapy and rehabilitation should be started almost immediately after the occlusion has occurred. Anticoagulants are rarely indicated for the pregnant patient with occlusive cerebrovascular disease.

The treatment of patients with venous thrombosis is almost always conservative. When a cortical venous thrombosis occurs in the puerperium, as is frequently the case, anticoagulants may be used. Substances to reduce cerebral edema, including dexamethasone and oral glycerol, are also commonly employed. Anticonvulsants should be given.

SYNCOPE, HYPERVENTILATION, AND HYSTERICAL ATTACKS

Syncope (Fainting). Vasodepressor syncope, also termed vasovagal syncope and, in common language, fainting, is the most frequent cause of loss of consciousness in pregnancy. A variety of autonomic manifestations commonly precede the attack of unconsciousness including complaints of sweating, pallor, nausea, slow pulse, yawning, and overbreathing.[54] As the blood pressure falls, there may be blurring of vision, weakness, and "graying-out," and complaints of faintness may be vocalized. Eventually when the cerebral blood flow falls below critical levels, approximately 30 ml/100 gm of brain per minute, unconsciousness will occur. Electroencephalographic records made during syncope reveal high voltage, 2 to 4 cycles/second slow waves.

Syncope is a transient episode for the most part, lasting only a few seconds to several minutes. Rarely, if the unconsciousness is profound, involuntary urination may occur. Some movements may be noted during the syncopal episode, but these are not tonic-clonic in type. During the time of syncope, bradycardia is often recorded. With return of consciousness, the patient may complain of headache, weakness, and nervousness, but mental confusion is rarely seen. Sleep does not usually occur after fainting. The recovery does not suggest a postictal state.

Physiologically, syncope is initially characterized by vasodilation, particularly in the limbs. A decrease in peripheral vascular resistance is not compensated for by an increase in cardiac output, and thus, as the pulse declines, the cerebral blood flow is reduced to critical levels. Thereafter symptoms are produced. Syncope is most often associated with prolonged sitting or standing and emotional situations, particularly those associated with pain or the anticipation of pain, anxiety, or fear.

Given the tendency for venous stasis, particularly in the later stages of pregnancy, syncope or near syncope is a common complaint of the gravid woman. In the author's experience, it is most likely to occur toward the end of meals, particularly with leisurely dining, and if alcohol has been imbibed, thereby increasing the tendency to peripheral vasodilation.

Therapy for syncope is nonspecific. Inhalation of spirits of ammonia is an ancient ritual that does no harm and may hasten return to consciousness. The patient should be allowed to remain recumbent until the episode passes. Treatment of the underlying medical disorder, if any, may be indicated.

Hyperventilation. In the hyperventilation syndrome, syncope rarely occurs, although complaints of "feeling faint" and "lightheadedness" are often voiced and may last for hours. Usually the episode begins with a complaint of discomfort, such as a band-like sensation about the head or chest. Difficulty in speaking or swallowing; fullness in the abdomen, chest, or throat; and prickling sensations or numbness of the fingers or mouth may appear. If hyperventilation persists, carpopedal spasm may rarely occur. In this situation, overbreathing rapidly produces hypocapnia and a respiratory alkalosis, reducing cerebral blood flow and increasing neuromuscular irritability. There may also be slight peripheral vasodilation, and the blood pressure tends to fall, but as mentioned previously, syncope does not usually occur. The symptoms may be prolonged and are not easily relieved, although the old advice regarding breathing into a paper bag is still pertinent.

Hyperventilation is a symptom of emotional disturbance and should be treated as such. Simple sedatives may be helpful.

Hysteria. Hysterical loss of consciousness may present problems to the clinician. The episode is often recognized as a swoon ("I die, I faint, I fail"—Shelley), with a graceful descent to the floor without injury. On occasion, hysterical fainting may be extremely difficult to distinguish from a true seizure. This is especially true if atypical seizures are suspected. If it is available, an electroencephalogram will usually be normal during a hysterical attack. The subject may show little concern regarding the hysterical episodes, which almost always occur in the presence of family and friends and which suggest attempts at manipulation to focus attention upon herself. During the hysterical faint the patient may exhibit bizarre movements or may lie quiet and motionless. Blood pressure and pulse are normal, sweating does not occur, and the patient's color usually remains good. There may be waxing and waning of consciousness, and the episode may be quite prolonged. A history of previous psychiatric problems is a useful clue to correct diagnosis.

Other Causes of Loss of Consciousness. Less common medical causes of syncope deserve mention only in passing, since their incidence in pregnancy is extremely low. Stokes-Adams attacks, carotid sinus syncope, coughing, micturition syncope, cerebral arteriosclerosis, and hypoglycemia may also produce loss of consciousness. These diagnoses will be suggested by the clinical history, the examination, and certain laboratory studies, particularly the electroencephalogram and electrocardiogram. Cardiac consultation is required if a true disorder of cardiac conduction is suspected.

VERTIGO AND "DIZZINESS"

The complaint of dizziness is liable to be voiced repeatedly in the obstetrician's office, and it is important to differentiate this sensation from the symptom of vertigo. Vertigo may be defined as a sensation of motion. In objective vertigo, the subject feels that the environment is in motion ("the room is spinning"). In subjective vertigo the patient has the sensation that she herself is moving. Sometimes these sensations are described as truly rotational, and at other times they may be described as rocking, undulating, or unsteadiness without a rotary component.

The term dizziness is often used by patients to express a variety of complaints, frequently confusing to the physician.[57] It is always well to ask the patient directly about the meaning of the term dizziness. For example, the patient should be asked if she is experiencing lightheadedness, wooziness, muzziness, faintness, unsteadiness, or difficulty with her thinking.

In attempting to distinguish between vertigo and dizziness, it is important that the physician understand the patient's complaints clearly.[58] This may require a prolonged effort at history taking, with descriptions by the patient of her symptoms in the most minute detail. It is quite important to know whether the vertigo is, for example, episodic or continuous, whether it occurs with change in position, and whether it is affected by standing, sitting, or movements of the head, such as turning over in bed.[56] With true vertigo the patient must almost always lie or sit down or hold onto something to prevent falling. The physician should determine if there is true loss of balance. Have others noted that the patient is unsteady? Is the patient liable to stagger when walking down the street?

The symptoms of true vertigo can be assigned to two major groups (Table 18-7). The vertigo of central origin is due to a disease or process affecting the central nervous system. The vertigo of peripheral origin is related to abnormalities of the vestibular mechanisms.

When vertigo of central origin is present, there is usually a history of ataxia of gait between episodes of vertigo. If this history is not elicited, the vertigo is most likely of peripheral origin.

Neurologic diseases almost always produce central vertigo. The conditions that may produce central vertigo, listed in frequency of occurrence, include multiple sclerosis, head trauma, cerebrovascular insufficiency, brain tumors (especially acoustic neuromas), temporal lobe seizure disorders, vascular headaches of the migraine type, hemispheric or cerebellar tumors, and increased intracranial pressure of diverse etiology.

Peripheral vertigo is usually produced by otologic disease. In order of frequency these include Meniere's disease; benign positional vertigo; recurrent and acute infections of the middle ear, mastoid process, or inner ear; recurrent labyrinthine syndromes associated with trauma; occlusion of the eustachian tube; and wax in the outer ear.

The most common otologic disease responsible for vertigo is Meniere's disease. This is a

TABLE 18–7 PERIPHERAL AND CENTRAL VERTIGO — CONTRASTED*

Clinical Features	Peripheral	Central
Characteristic onset	Sudden	Insidious, progressive
Characteristic pattern	Episodic; paroxysmal	Continuous, occasionally paroxysmal
Sensation of rotation and spinning	Frequent	Infrequent
Severity of symptoms	Often intense	Seldom intense
Duration	Minutes to hours, rarely more than one week	Prolonged, days to months to years
Spontaneous nystagmus	May be present	May be present
Type of nystagmus	Horizontal or rotatory, never vertical	Horizontal, vertical, or rotatory
Direction of nystagmus	Unidirectional, fast phase opposite lesion	Bi- or unidirectional
Influence of head movement	Marked	Slight or none
Syncope	Absent	Rare
Seizures	Absent	Occasional
Tinnitus	Frequent	Rare
Loss of hearing	Frequent	Rare
Caloric stimulation	Nonreactive or hypoactive	Usually normal
Other cranial nerve or long tract disturbance	Rare	Common
Interim gait	Normal	Unsteady
Common causes	Infections, labyrinthitis, Meniere's syndrome, vascular, trauma	Vascular, demyelinating disease

*Modified from Rubin, 1977, and Daroff, 1970.

triad of symptoms including episodic vertigo, tinnitus, and fluctuating sensory neural hearing loss. The attack of vertigo usually appears with a sudden whirling sensation, which may be severe enough so that the patient falls to the ground. Symptoms, including nausea, vomiting, prostration, sweating, and tachycardia, almost always accompany the vertigo. A typical attack of vertigo of this type usually lasts from two to six hours. There is associated nystagmus with quick eye movements away from the affected side. Caloric testing at the time of vertigo will usually reveal hypofunction of the affected labyrinth. Not all patients have the classic triad of symptoms as described previously. Special studies, such as electronystagmography and tests of discrimination and recruitment, may be necessary to establish the diagnosis when the symptoms are atypical.

It is important to remember that diseases of the cardiovascular system may produce both central and peripheral vertigo. The vertigo is usually a manifestation of vertebral basilar ischemia or insufficiency. Cardiac arrhythmias, postural hypotension, systemic hypotension, and cerebral embolic disease from a mural thrombus must be particularly considered by the clinician concerned with this complaint.

Only rarely is disease of the ocular apparatus

responsible for true vertigo. This may occur if patients are fitted with eyeglasses for the first time, especially if they are incorrectly fitted with strong lenses. In addition, should there be a sudden loss of strength in eye muscles, producing diplopia, the patient may also complain of vertigo, but here the etiology should be obvious.

Vertigo is not more common in pregnant women than in nonpregnant women of a similar age, but exact statistics are not available. The etiology of the vertigo must be carefully sought in every case. When neurologic disease is present, treatment should be directed at the specific disease in question.

One should not leave this topic without making mention of "the vapors."[53] Besides signifying steam or gas, the vapors as defined in the dictionary are considered to be a disease of nervous disability, in which a variety of unusual images float in the brain or appear as if real. Thus, in romantic literature, the prototype of the refined woman is one who swoons. This subject is of particular interest to the obstetrician, for it was associated with the modesty and prudery that characterized the approved behavior of the female sex for so many centuries. For example, in the seventeenth century, it was not thought proper for male physicians to attend women in childbirth; when this was necessary, it was considered quite acceptable to deliver the baby under the bedclothes. Although the behavior that characterized the vapors is not identified with that term in modern times, the alert clinician should be aware that complaints of giddiness and lightheadedness, so common today, are little different from those characterized as vaporous in an earlier day. Perhaps that term should be resurrected as a substitute for dizziness. The matter is best summed up by Jane Austen in her book Love and Friendship (1790). "Beware of fainting fits. Though at times they may be refreshing and agreeable, yet believe me they will in the end, if too often repeated and at improper seasons, prove destructive."

BRAIN TUMOR AND PREGNANCY

The clinical symptoms of brain tumors are diverse and vary according to the type and location of the tumor. Tumors are especially liable to occur in children under the age of ten, and they have their peak incidence in the fifth and sixth decades of life. Primary brain tumors are uncommon during the childbearing years. Metastatic brain tumors are even less common.

There have been many attempts at classification of brain tumors. Table 18–8 represents simply another attempt at a rational classification of this subject.

The clinical manifestations of brain tumors are multiple and varied. Often the natural history of the tumor is characterized by insidious onset and slow progression of neurologic signs and symptoms, sometimes associated with evidence of increased intracranial pressure. There may be great variation in the signs and symptoms, depending on the rate of growth and the part of the brain in which the tumor is located. The primary signs and symptoms of brain tumor include headache, personality changes, papilledema and abnormalities of vision, nausea and vomiting, stiff neck, diplopias and/or hemianopias, disturbances of speech, disturbances of sensation, seizures, ataxia, and hemiplegia. The signs and symptoms of increased intracranial pressure include headache, nausea and vomiting, autonomic changes, disturbances of vision, mental changes, papilledema, and neck stiffness.

No brain tumors are specifically related to pregnancy. Some studies have suggested that the growth rate of brain tumors tends to progress under the influence of pregnancy. This is especially the case with respect to meningiomas, angiomas, and neurofibromas.[59, 60] The pituitary

TABLE 18–8 INCIDENCE OF INTRACRANIAL NEOPLASMS

I. Primary neoplasms (50 per cent of total neoplasms)
  A. Gliomas (50 per cent)
    1. Astrocytic (85 per cent)
      a. Astrocytomas (20 per cent)
      b. Glioblastoma multiforme (65 per cent)
    2. Oligodendroglial (5 per cent)   } 100 per cent of gliomas
    3. Ependymal (5 per cent)
    4. Miscellaneous (medulloblastoma, neuroblastoma, ganglioglioma) (5 per cent)
  B. Meningiomas (20 per cent)
  C. Pituitary adenomas (15 per cent)
  D. Neuromas (Schwann's cell tumors) (10 per cent — cerebellopontine tumors)
  E. Miscellaneous (pinealoma, craniopharyngioma, lymphoma, sarcoma, hemangioblastoma, teratoma, lipoma) (5 per cent)

II. Secondary (metastatic) neoplasms (50 per cent of total neoplasms)
  A. Lung (30 per cent)
  B. Breast (20 per cent)
  C. Bowel (10 per cent)
  D. Kidney (10 per cent)
  E. Other sites (30 per cent)

Note: One per cent of all autopsies reveal some type of intracranial neoplasm; 10 per cent of all neoplasms occur in the central nervous system.

also normally enlarges during pregnancy, but rapid growth of pituitary adenomas has not been reported during pregnancy.

Perhaps the most comprehensive paper on this subject is a review by Rand and Andler.[61] They collected a series of 19 brain tumors associated with pregnancy. There were 14 vaginal deliveries with 11 normal infants. Successful cesarean sections were performed in the other five patients, also with delivery of normal infants. There was no evidence that brain tumors affected pregnancy or the fetus, unless the tumor was of sufficient size or in a location that would predispose to the death of the mother. In this series symptoms of brain tumor appeared in most cases in the second and third trimesters. Headache was the most common complaint. Seizures were rare. Nausea and vomiting were prominent in five patients. Focal signs and symptoms related to the tumor were frequently found.

There were three maternal and fetal antepartum deaths. One patient had an astrocytoma of the pons. Another had an astrocytoma of the frontal lobes. A third had a sudden hemorrhage into the cerebellum related to a cystic astrocytoma. Similarly, there were three postpartum maternal deaths. One mother died one month postpartum with multiple cerebral metastases following a carcinoma of the breast. Another death occurred shortly after a normal vaginal delivery, following a second attempt at removal of a frontal astrocytoma.

Decisions regarding therapeutic abortion because of associated brain tumor must be based on the type, size, and location of the tumor. If it becomes evident that the tumor is expanding rapidly and threatening the life of the mother, then therapeutic abortion may be indicated. Therapy of the tumor itself is determined by neurologic indications. Indications for cesarean section remain primarily obstetric and related to signs and symptoms of fetal distress.

The neurologic workup of pregnant patients has been discussed in detail in another section.

The problem of metastatic brain tumors in the pregnant patient deserves brief comment. Usually the primary tumor is the focus of therapy. If necessary, radiotherapy to the pregnant mother can be given with adequate shielding of the fetus. Surgical therapy of metastatic brain tumors in the pregnant patient is almost never required. Obviously, in this situation, therapeutic abortion related to the primary disease may be indicated.

Choriocarcinoma

Choriocarcinoma is a highly invasive tumor of trophoblastic origin that occurs frequently in the tropics and the Orient but is unusual in Western countries. Most choriocarcinomas appear in the months following a hydatidiform molar pregnancy or an abortion, although a few appear after a normal full-term pregnancy. Cerebral metastases are a common neurologic manifestation of metastatic choriocarcinoma. Their appearance is frequently that of single or multiple strokes, intercranial hemorrhage, or solitary mass lesions.[62] The symptoms are those of any intracranial lesion including headaches, seizures, hemiplegia, and the like. Chorionic gonadotropin levels may be increased in serum and cerebrospinal fluid in this condition. Treatment includes whole brain radiation and, particularly, chemotherapy, which may be curative.[63]

Pituitary Tumors

If a pituitary tumor is found during pregnancy and if rapid vision loss and constriction of the visual fields develop, operative intervention is the treatment of choice. The surgery can be done during any trimester of pregnancy, but if gestation has reached the 36th week, induction of labor is indicated. The pituitary tumor may then shrink after parturition.

If a pituitary tumor is found and the patient desires to become subsequently pregnant, questions regarding methods of treatment of the tumor will invariably arise. Either radiotherapy or surgery may be employed, with the decision regarding therapy based on the best method of obliterating the tumor with the least risk to the potential mother. Successful gestation has occurred after both radiation and trans-sphenoidal surgery.[64, 65] If the neurosurgical team is experienced, trans-sphenoidal removal of the micro-adenoma is probably the procedure of choice.

Pseudotumor Cerebri in Pregnancy

Powell describes a woman who developed pseudotumor cerebri in pregnancy and reviews the available medical experience with this disease.[66] There are 21 cases in the literature, with 37 pregnancies being described. There were 23 normal births, two stillbirths, and 12 abortions, either spontaneous or therapeutic. The author suggests that the disease is a self-limited process and that the prognosis for recovery is excellent. Patients almost always improve quickly after delivery. During the course of the pregnancy the vision should be monitored carefully, with repeated visual fields. If the vision becomes compromised during the first trimester, therapeutic abortion should be seriously considered. If the vision becomes compromised during the second or third trimester, medical treatment should be instituted with bed rest, hospitalization, and the use of diuretics and corticosteroids. Rarely is surgical "decompression" of the brain necessary. On the other hand, if the disease becomes rapidly progressive close to term, cesarean section may be indicated. If the disease is stable and vision is not threatened, vaginal delivery should be accomplished.

It should be remembered that the pituitary gland enlarges during pregnancy. Some cases of asymptomatic bitemporal hemianopia will be related to this benign enlargement, which terminates after pregnancy. The diagnosis of pseudotumor cerebri of pregnancy should not be made in the absence of papilledema.

MULTIPLE SCLEROSIS IN PREGNANCY

Multiple sclerosis is a disorder of myelin, often difficult to diagnose given the absence of specific diagnostic tests. When the disease manifests itself as a well-recognized and discernible syndrome characterized by remissions and exacerbations, diagnosis is not a problem. More subtle problems characterized by sensory abnormalities in the absence of objective findings on examination may be difficult to categorize. In general, it may be stated that multiple sclerosis is a chronic and relapsing disease, but a minority of patients, perhaps 30 per cent, seem to progress relatively steadily from the onset of symptoms. The disease reflects involvement of the central white matter in the demyelinating process rather than neuronal or gray matter.

Multiple sclerosis affects males and females approximately equally. The majority of patients note the onset of symptoms between the ages of 20 and 40. Populations residing in tropical and subtropical zones have a notably low risk of being affected by multiple sclerosis. Populations that reside north of 40° latitude in North America and Europe are at a particular risk. Multiple sclerosis may cluster in communities.[68] The prevalence rate in the United States varies from 10:100,000 in the Southern states to about 50 to 75:100,000 in the Northern states. There are at any time approximately 75,000 to 100,000 persons with identifiable multiple sclerosis under treatment in the United States.[67]

Genetic studies have not clarified the etiology of multiple sclerosis. There are numerous reports in the literature of the occurrence of the disease in several members of a single family, but these fail to exclude the common effects of environmental and other factors.[71] The symptoms of multiple sclerosis are diverse and usually include weakness, difficulties with coordination, paresthesias, and visual complaints. Headache is rare. Similarly, lesions that are characteristic of involvement of gray matter, including aphasia, seizures, wasting, fasciculations, and the like, are also unusual. Often the illness begins with a complaint of weakness in one of the lower extremities associated with urinary complaints, visual phenomena, and incoordination.

The only significant and relatively consistent laboratory abnormalities are found in the cerebrospinal fluid, particularly in the globulin fractions. The determination of CSF immunoglobulin G by either electroimmunodiffusion or radioimmunodiffusion shows an elevation of this fraction, above 13 to 15 per cent of the total protein, in 40 to 60 per cent of cases of multiple sclerosis. In addition, the presence of oligoclonal bands of IgG may be confirmatory. Unfortunately, the elevation of CSF IgG is not pathognomonic of multiple sclerosis, and other neurologic conditions, such as postinfectious or postvaccinial myelinopathies, dysproteinemias, subacute sclerosing panencephalitis, lupus erythematosus, and syphilis, may also elevate this laboratory value.

There is also interest in measuring the amount of myelin basic protein in the CSF, which appears to be increased in multiple sclerosis, particularly in exacerbations of the disease. However, to reiterate, at this time there is no single absolutely reliable or completely diagnostic laboratory examination for multiple sclerosis. Alterations in visually and auditorily evoked responses, while not diagnostic, may also be helpful if they are abnormal. But obviously other neurologic conditions can affect these laboratory procedures as well. For a more complete discussion of the many and varied forms of multiple sclerosis, the reader is referred to a standard text book of neurology.

Over the years a series of presumed aggravating factors affecting the course of multiple sclerosis have been accumulated including recurrent infections of the respiratory and urinary tracts, immunizations, trauma, surgery, emotional stress, and diagnostic neurologic procedures including lumbar puncture, myelography, cerebral angiography, and pneumoencephalography. It is difficult to relate any of these factors to exacerbations of the disease. In general, it may be stated that indications for surgery in patients with multiple sclerosis should be judged entirely on their own merits. Similarly, if diagnostic procedures are necessary, they should be performed.

The question then arises regarding the relationship of multiple sclerosis to pregnancy. Since multiple sclerosis often appears during the childbearing period, it may be that the first attack of the disease occurs during pregnancy. On the other hand, pregnancy does not necessarily exert a deleterious effect on the course of the disease. Millar and colleagues have studied a group of 262 women with multiple sclerosis.[70] The relapse rates of the disease for single and married women were essentially identical. After the onset of the disease, 70 women had 170 pregnancies, during which 45 relapses occurred, 39 of these relapses occurring during the puerperium and six during the pregnancy itself.

Leibowitz and associates compared the obstetric histories of patients with multiple sclerosis and control subjects in Israel.[69] The controls were matched for age at onset, sex, and region of birth to 241 patients with multiple sclerosis seen in 1963. Of these patients, 208 were followed in 1965, and 13 new patients were evaluated at this time, for a total of 221. In 1963, 69 per cent of 131 female patients and 64 per cent of 523 controls reported having been pregnant at least once before the age of onset. The percentages of pregnancy and live births did not differ significantly between the two groups. In 1965, the incidence of pregnancy was 60 per cent in the patients and 56 per cent in the controls. Although 16 per cent of the patients and only 8 per cent of the controls became pregnant less than one year before the age at onset, the respective figures for 1 to 2 years before the age at onset were 7 and 13 per cent.

These observations do not support the view that pregnancy and delivery are directly related to the cause of multiple sclerosis, but the authors suggest that pregnancy may have a "precipitating" effect. In a woman who is "incubating" multiple sclerosis or who is in the "premorbid" stage, various factors, including pregnancy, might cause the disease to become manifest. The critical period occurs during the two years before the onset of clinical symptoms.

A significant number of nonmedical, social, and economic factors should be considered by the physician who is asked to advise on whether or not the patient with multiple sclerosis should become pregnant. Multiple sclerosis is not an indication for therapeutic abortion or sterilization. On the other hand, given the progressive nature of the disease and the possibility of progressive impairment of function in the mother, patients with active multiple sclerosis should probably be dissuaded from becoming pregnant.

There is no specific therapy for multiple sclerosis when the disease is active. A short course of ACTH or prednisone during exacerbations of optic neuritis may be helpful, but there are no other indications for the use of these drugs. There are certainly no indications for long-term or maintenance therapy of ACTH or corticosteroids. Some have suggested that immunosuppressive agents may be useful, but the potentially deleterious effects of these agents if administered over a prolonged period of time would seem to outweigh any possible usefulness in this disease.

The prognosis of multiple sclerosis is unpredictable. Approximately 50 per cent of patients are still able to be employed after ten years of illness. After 20 years, only 35 per cent are employed. Life expectancy tends to vary considerably, depending on the progressive or nonprogressive nature of the disease. The average life expectancy is from 13 to more than 25 years after onset. If death does occur related to the disease, it usually occurs in those in whom the disease has become progressive, who are incapacitated, and who suffer a terminal infection of some sort, frequently a urinary tract infection in a chronically catheterized patient.

MYASTHENIA GRAVIS AND PREGNANCY

Myasthenia gravis is a chronic disease characterized by muscular fatigability occurring after repeated use of voluntary muscles. The illness has a characteristic tendency toward exacerbations and remissions. The basic defect is an abnormal neuromuscular function similar to that produced by the drug curare. Pathologically, muscle biopsies of patients with myasthenia gravis show mixtures of atrophy and inflammatory cellular exudate, with collections of lymphocytes present among the muscle fibers (lymphorrhages). Necrosis of muscle fibers is also described. Electrical studies have demonstrated abnormalities of nerve terminals and end plates. The thymus gland may be enlarged, and thymomas may be present. Antibodies to acetylcholine receptors, muscle, and thymic epithelial cells can be demonstrated in some patients with myasthenia gravis,[72, 74] but the role of these antibodies in pathogenesis remains uncertain. Antibodies to acetylcholine receptors are presumably responsible for the partial neuromuscular blockade, although titers do not correlate with the severity of the disease.[73]

The prevalence of myasthenia gravis is approximately 3:100,000 population. The disease most commonly begins in the third decade of life and occurs more often in females than in males. However, the coincidence with thymoma is greater in males.

Congenital myasthenia gravis is rare, accounting for less than 1 per cent of the total cases of myasthenia.[76] Symptoms usually occur within the first month of life and are mild, consisting of poor sucking and weak cry. The diagnosis may not be made until several months to a year later. Reviewing the data to date concerning 22 sets of twins with myasthenia, it appears that some cases of myasthenia gravis are in fact hereditary, but it is not possible to explain all cases by one mode of inheritance. It has been estimated that familial myasthenia gravis occurs in 3 to 4 per cent of all cases and is more common in children. Almost all myasthenia of the adult variety seems to be acquired. In 1971, Namba reported 27 patients in 12 families of 702 cases of myasthenia gravis studied at the Maimonides Medical

Center.[77] He found 137 additional familial cases in the literature and estimated the familial incidence at 3.4 per cent. The younger the patient at the onset of symptoms, the greater the familial occurrence.

The cardinal symptom of myasthenia gravis is muscular fatigability. This is most frequently observed in the ocular muscles. Muscular fatigability may be generalized from the beginning of the disease. The symptoms characteristically wax and wane and often become worse as the muscles are used repeatedly, i.e., toward evening. Difficulties with swallowing and speech are common. The facial muscles are almost always affected. The disease must be differentiated from other neurologic conditions that cause ptosis, diplopia, or general fatigability. These include amyotrophic lateral sclerosis, the inflammatory myopathies, botulinus toxicity, and, occasionally, use of drugs that produce similar symptoms. The great problem in the diagnosis is to differentiate this disease from chronic fatigability associated with neurosis.

Generally, when a thymoma is present, the course of the disease is more inexorably downhill and the pattern of illness is more severe.

Given the tendency for the disease to appear during the childbearing years, the association between myasthenia gravis and pregnancy is of considerable importance to the clinician. Remissions of the disease have been described during pregnancy, although in some patients the disease may become worse, often during the early stages of pregnancy. Moderate exacerbations of the disease commonly occur following delivery of the child and especially appear in the first six weeks postpartum.

Ferguson described a group of 145 patients with myasthenia gravis, of whom 22 had a total of 34 pregnancies.[79] During their pregnancies, 14 of these patients had exacerbations of their disease, 12 were improved, and eight remained essentially unaffected during the course of the pregnancy. In only one case did the initial onset of myasthenia gravis occur during pregnancy. Osserman reports on a very large group of patients including 226 females with myasthenia followed during their childbearing years.[81] Of these, 68 (30 per cent) experienced remissions during pregnancy, 72 (32 per cent) experienced exacerbations, and 86 (38 per cent) were unchanged. Although these figures suggest that the effects of pregnancy on myasthenia gravis are not much different from those that would be found in nongravid women of the same age, Osserman reports that exacerbations or remissions during pregnancy are often dramatic, i.e., "abrupt or acute," depending on the responses of the patient.[81] It would probably be well to see the myasthenic patient at monthly intervals during the pregnancy to adjust the dosage of anticholinesterase medication (Table 18–9).

Osserman suggests that during labor, anticholinesterases be administered parenterally, particularly as labor advances.[81] He advises that patients with myasthenia gravis are particularly sensitive to curare and therefore should not be given this drug as a supplementary anesthetic relaxant. Ether and chloroform have a similar curare-like action and should be avoided.[80] Demerol may be used for pain. Myasthenia gravis does not present a contraindication if spinal or caudal anesthesia is the procedure of choice. After delivery, routine postpartum care is advisable. It is probably unwise for the patient to breast feed the child, since anticholinesterase drugs taken by the mother may be secreted in her milk. Otherwise, resumption of the usual dose of anticholinesterase may be given by mouth as soon as the mother can swallow. It is rarely necessary to readjust the therapy for myasthenia gravis during the first few days of the postpartum period.

Duff has described three cases of myasthenia gravis in pregnancy, of whom two were preeclamptic with moderately severe hypertension,

TABLE 18–9 DRUGS USED IN MEDICAL THERAPY OF MYASTHENIA GRAVIS IN PREGNANCY

Drug	Tablets	Syrup	Parenteral Solution	Average Dose
Neostigmine (Prostigmine)	15 mg	—	0.5 mg/ml 1.0 mg/ml	15 mg qid, po
Pyridostigmine (Mestinon)	60 mg	60 mg/5 ml	—	60 mg qid
Mestinon Timespan	180 mg	—	—	Orally, once a day
Ambenonium	10 mg	—	—	—
(Mytelase)	25 mg	—	—	—
Edrophonium (Tensilon)	—	—	10 mg/ml	Not available
Prednisone	5–10 mg	—	Not available	60 mg every other day

which was difficult to control.[78] This association is uncommon.

Neonatal Myasthenia Gravis. Neonatal myasthenia gravis is associated with placental transfer of antiacetylcholine receptor antibodies and can be cured by exchange transfusion.[83, 84] The antiacetylcholine receptor antibodies in the patient described by Keesey fell progressively to normal values over the first three months. In his reported case, anticholinesterase drugs were employed during the first month of life but were not required thereafter, and the infant's strength progressively improved as the receptor antibody titer fell.

Namba et al. report that approximately 12 per cent of babies at risk will develop neonatal myasthenia gravis,[77] but there is no association or relationship between neonatal illness and maternal age, the duration or severity of maternal disease, or the maternal dose of anticholinesterase. A previous maternal thymectomy does not protect the infant from neonatal myasthenia, and mothers who have delivered affected infants may subsequently produce normal infants.

It is almost always the case that neonatal myasthenia gravis will appear within the first 96 hours after birth. The vast majority of infants affected will become so within the first day of life. Thus, any infant who remains well for the first week without signs of myasthenia can be assumed to be normal.

Other Disorders of Muscle

Occasionally, a dystrophic patient will become pregnant, particularly a patient with myotonic muscular dystrophy. The disability from the weakness and myotonia increases or remains constant during pregnancy. Spontaneous abortion and premature labor are common. Prolongation of any stage of labor may be associated with the myotonic dystrophy. Uterine inertia has been described.[86]

Other rare causes of muscular weakness, such as myotonia congenita, polymyositis, and McArdle's disease, have been described during pregnancy. In general, obstetric problems were not encountered with either myotonia congenita or McArdle's syndrome, but in polymyositis, infant mortality is high.[87]

Porphyria and Pregnancy

Seckler and Rovinsky have collected reports on 55 women with porphyria, among whom 48 pregnancies occurred prior to the appearance of the clinical symptoms of porphyria and 67 pregnancies occurred thereafter.[92] Although all categories of porphyria are included in this series, the largest portion of patients exhibited acute intermittent porphyria, numbering 48 (87 per cent). Seventy-seven per cent of patients experienced an exacerbation of their porphyric complaints during pregnancy, and only 16 per cent went into remission. In 36 per cent, the initial attack of porphyria occurred during pregnancy. Subsequent to pregnancy, approximately one third of the patients had remissions, one third had exacerbations, and maternal death occurred in the puerperium in one fifth.

When the clinical manifestations of porphyria appear during pregnancy, the fetal loss is significant, in the range of 40 per cent. The spontaneous abortion rate is twice the normal rate. When pregnancy proceeds into the last trimester, however, premature delivery does not occur, unless cesarean section becomes necessary because of significant disease in the mother. The maternal mortality in pregnancy with porphyria is in the range of 22 per cent. Almost half of the maternal deaths occurred during the first attack of acute intermittent porphyria, and 15 of the 17 deaths occurred in association with first pregnancies.

Unfortunately, there is no benefit from spontaneous or therapeutic abortion early in gestation. Seckler and Rovinsky state that the stress of abortion is contraindicated in the acute stage of exacerbation of porphyria and that the wiser course is to provide supportive therapy in an attempt to carry the patient into a stage of temporary remission.[92]

In pregnancies that proceed to term, maternal porphyria has no permanent effect on the newborn. There are no fetal congenital abnormalities described in the literature. In some cases in which the infants were studied for porphyrins, a transient porphyrinuria was found during the newborn period.[89] It is assumed that this is related to passive transfer of the porphyrins across the placenta from the mother. The excretion of the abnormal porphyrin metabolites usually ceases after the first week of life, and there is usually no evidence of the disease subsequently. Since, however, porphyria is a hereditary disease, the newborn should be observed for evidence of the development of clinical porphyria in later life.

The neurologic symptoms of acute porphyria that appear during pregnancy are not different from those that appear in nonpregnant females. The rapid appearance of peripheral neuropathies, often asymmetric, with associated cranial nerve palsies is described. There are often recurrent bouts of abdominal pain. An organic mental syndrome may occur. The disease may be provoked by ingestion of barbiturates, sulfonamides, or thiopental anesthesia. Kerr has described inappropriate secretion of the antidiuretic hormone in porphyric pregnancy, with associated seizures.[90]

The treatment of acute porphyria is a medical emergency. The patient's life is in grave danger, and intensive medical and nursing care will be required. The patient should be admitted to the hospital. Respiratory failure may occur, and there should be no delay in tracheostomy and use of mechanical respiration, if respiration does in fact become embarrassed. Anticonvulsants and sedatives (but not barbiturates), including especially phenothiazines, may be advised. Hypertension can be controlled with propranolol.[88] Careful attention to serum electrolytes is necessary. Infusion of hematin will control the enzyme delta amino acid synthetase and will improve neurologic manifestations of porphyria.[91]

SPINAL CORD SYNDROMES

Spinal cord tumors are divided, according to location, into extramedullary and intramedullary groups. The extramedullary tumors may be intradural, extradural, or extravertebral. Tumors of the spinal cord are relatively infrequent but occur predominantly in young or middle-aged adults and so may appear during or coincident with the onset of pregnancy.[94, 95] Spinal tumors are more likely to occur in the thoracic region than in either the cervical or lumbar area.

Extramedullary tumors usually involve several segments of the spinal cord and produce symptoms of cord compression. Commonly, the first complaint is pain resulting from compression of spinal nerve roots. Shortly thereafter, this is associated with significant sensory loss, weakness, and signs of muscular wasting in the distribution of the affected roots. A combination of upper and lower motor neuron signs then appears, including spasticity and weakness of the muscles below the level of the lesion, loss of abdominal responses, abnormal Babinski responses, loss of bladder control, and impairment of cutaneous and proprioceptive sensation. A laterally placed tumor may produce a Brown-Séquard syndrome.

Intramedullary spinal cord tumors, which intrinsically involve the spinal cord, may extend over many segments, and for this reason their symptoms are more variable than those of extramedullary tumors. Occasionally they may be confused with the diagnostic signs of syringomyelia.

Angiomas that compress the spinal cord may be adversely affected by pregnancy.[97] Hemangiomas are usually benign extradural tumors that, as they enlarge, cause pressure on the spinal cord with resulting back pain.[96, 96a] When they are associated with pregnancy, benign extradural hemangiomas often enlarge, particularly during the third trimester, and are associated with typical symptoms of cord compression.[98-100] Usually the complaints involve the legs and the bladder but not the upper extremities. The diagnosis of cord compression is often evident on neurologic examination. Palpation of the vertebrae may reveal bone tenderness. A careful spinal fluid examination with manometric studies suggests subarachnoid block.

If the plain x-rays of the vertebrae do not show a diagnostic lesion, myelography is required. Attempts at shielding the fetus should be made, even though this may not be completely effective.

Hemangiomas usually remit to some extent with termination of the pregnancy. This being the case, the onset of spontaneous remission after delivery should be anticipated. If serious complaints of cord compression become evident toward the end of pregnancy, then induction of labor or delivery by cesarean section may be considered by the obstetrician. If the mother's condition permits, radiologic studies should be delayed until after delivery has been accomplished. Thereafter, a neurosurgical decision will have to be made regarding removal of the hemangioma. If the lesion is not removed, exacerbation may occur with subsequent pregnancies.

The enlargement of benign extradural hemangiomas during pregnancy is presumably related to weight gain and water retention associated with the pregnancy itself. The remarkable remission of some of these masses after termination of pregnancy suggests that there may be hormonal influences as well.

Garcia et al. describe a ruptured aneurysm of the spinal artery of Adamkiewicz during pregnancy.[101] They report a 34 year old pregnant woman who died within eight hours of admission to a hospital and who was found, at autopsy, to have diffuse subarachnoid hemorrhage and a fusiform aneurysmal sac arising from the artery of Adamkiewicz. These solitary aneurysms of the extramedullary arteries of the spinal cord that are not associated with arterial venous malformations are rarely reported. It is unlikely that any therapy would have been helpful in this situation.

Divers et al. report a spinal cord neurolemmoma in pregnancy, removed successfully after cesarean section.[93] Their review of the literature shows 28 cases of spinal cord tumor appearing in pregnancy; more than half (15) were angiomas.

PREGNANCY IN PARAPLEGIC PATIENTS

Automobile accidents and other diverse forms of trauma, as well as some neurologic diseases, have resulted in a significant number of paraplegic and quadriplegic women. The spinal cord lesions suffered usually do not prevent conception. Thus, women who are paraplegic may present exceptional problems in management during the course of their pregnancy.[102] They are especially prone to urinary tract infections and pressure necrosis of the skin. If the lesion producing the paraplegia is above the tenth thoracic cord level, the patient will usually experience painless labor, though she will have normal uterine contractions. Those with cord lesions below the tenth thoracic cord level will feel uterine contractions. Those patients whose paraplegia is related to anterior horn cell disease will have a normal perception of labor pains. Those with spasticity may show increased spasticity during labor. In general, however, paraplegic patients bear labor well, often have rapid and painless labors, and usually deliver normal children. The physician should be alert to episodic problems with autonomic dysreflexia, which may occur in the paraplegic patient, particularly evoked by bladder distention.

The effect of a neurogenic bladder is some degree of retention or incontinence. No other bladder symptoms are neurogenic in origin. However, retention may be associated with recurrent episodes of urinary tract infection and cystitis, thereby producing pyuria and dysuria. When such bladder dysfunction appears, consultation with a urologist is mandatory. Determinations of residual urine volume, cystoscopy, and cystometrics and evaluations of the vesicle sphincter and the tone of the bladder as well as its ability to perceive sensation all provide valuable information in the workup of a patient with bladder dysfunction.

CHOREA GRAVIDARUM

In chorea, pathologic changes are commonly found in the corpus striatum, especially in the small cell components of the putamen and the caudate nucleus. The classification of choreas into separate entities is based on age of onset, familial incidence, association with an identifiable disease, and occurrence of other neurologic abnormalities. Acute chorea (Sydenham's chorea) occurs in childhood, between the ages of five and 15, and rarely thereafter. It is often encountered as a manifestation of infection, complicating viral encephalitis, and in the encephalopathies associated with pertussis, diphtheria, and, especially, rheumatic fever. The outstanding clinical feature of chorea is involuntary movements; associated findings include muscular weakness, emotional lability, and incoordination. Often the onset of symptoms is abrupt, but occasionally the complaint may appear subtly. Initial disturbances include clumsiness, unsteady gait, irritability, and fidgets, followed by more typical choreic movements involving the body, face, tongue, hands, or limbs. Although some of these involuntary movements may appear to be coordinated, usually they will be noted to be random jerking, purposeless and aimless. They occur at rest, are increased by attempts at volitional movement, and generally disappear during sleep. Facial grimacing and difficulties with chewing, swallowing, and speaking also occur.

Chorea that occurs during pregnancy has been characterized as chorea gravidarum, implying a specific form of chorea; in fact this is a misnomer. It probably represents the occurrence of acute chorea during pregnancy.[103] When the disease does occur, it usually appears in youthful primiparas. As mentioned previously, many of these patients have a history suggestive of rheumatic fever, and in more than half, rheumatic manifestations including carditis, valvular heart disease, and arthritis will be found.

Zegart and Schwarz describe a recent episode of chorea gravidarum in a black female.[107] They note that the incidence varies greatly, but obviously this disease occurred considerably more frequently 25 years ago. Most patients with chorea gravidarum have the onset of symptoms in the first trimester, and the problem may recur in subsequent pregnancies. Twenty-five per cent of women with chorea in childhood may notice a recurrence of the chorea during pregnancy. The duration of the complaints averages two and one-half months, and usually the disease disappears when the pregnancy terminates.

The treatment for chorea gravidarum is rest and sedation. Chlorpromazine may be employed. Usually the disease is self-limited. The fetus is not affected by the disease. Therapeutic abortion is no longer indicated. The symptoms almost always stop spontaneously before the end of pregnancy or with the termination of pregnancy.

Chorea and Oral Contraceptives. Chorea is thought to be a rare complication of the use of oral contraceptive medication, but Nausieda et al. have reported five cases of chorea in young women receiving low or high dose estrogen-containing oral contraceptives.[106] All of the patients described by the authors were nulliparous and young and became symptomatic shortly after initiation of the contraceptive therapy, usually within five weeks. Two of the five patients had previously suffered an episode of Sydenham's chorea, and two had a history of congenital cyanotic heart disease without chorea. Dyskinesia resolved in all patients upon discontinuing the oral contraceptives. The authors advise that patients with pre-existing abnormalities of the basal ganglia appear more susceptible to oral contraceptive–induced chorea than normal controls. The mechanism of action of oral contraceptive–induced chorea is unknown, but the authors suggest that the contraceptives alter central dopaminergic activity. They reviewed 17 cases previously summarized in the literature[104, 105] and note that a few patients with oral contraceptive–induced chorea subsequently became pregnant without experiencing recurrent chorea.

INFECTIONS OF THE NERVOUS SYSTEM IN PREGNANCY

The pregnant woman is as subject to pyogenic infections as any other person but is not unusually predisposed to them. The routes of infection to the nervous system are (1) through hematogenous spread, directly, via the choroid plexus, or by first producing a focus in overlying bone; (2) by adjacent infection in paranasal or aural air sinuses; and (3) by traumatic disruption of normal structures by fractures through the air-containing sinuses or open cranial wounds. Both epidural and subdural infections are rarely seen today. The most common infection is that of leptomeningitis, produced by the meningococcus, the pneumococcus, and the *H. influenza* bacillus, in descending order of frequency.

The signs and symptoms of meningitis are characteristic and include malaise, headache, development of meningeal signs, fever, and leucocytosis. Treatment depends on the rapid identification of meningeal infection and the demonstration of the causative organism.

Viral infections may appear during pregnancy. Intrauterine infection with rubella and cytomega-

lic inclusion body disease are particularly serious problems, since both produce congenital abnormalities in the fetus. Maternal infection in the first trimester with rubella causes cataracts, congenital heart disease, deafness, and mental retardation. The virus may be recoverable from the infant's excreta for as long as 18 months after birth and may also be cultured from cataracts. With cytomegalic inclusion disease, prematurity, hepatitis, microcephaly, intracranial calcification, and pancytopenia are common.

Acute aseptic meningitis may occur in pregnancy. The clinical manifestations include fever, headache, irritability, and neck rigidity. This syndrome is usually caused by the enterovirus, or mumps. The Coxsackie group of viruses are also commonly implicated in this syndrome.

Encephalitis represents direct invasion of the central nervous system, producing inflammation and neuronal injury. The viruses produce degeneration and necrosis of neurons and glia and hemorrhage and necrosis of gray and white matter. Cellular infiltration of the meninges is common as well. Viruses that produce encephalitis include the arboviruses, mumps, herpes simplex, poliomyelitis, rabies, and infectious mononucleosis, among others.

Postinfectious encephalitis is characterized by diffuse demyelination, predominantly perivascular in location. The clinical manifestations are expressed by both meningeal and encephalitic signs. Viruses that produce this syndrome include measles, varicella, rubella, smallpox, and vaccinia. Obviously, these viruses may sometimes cause a primary infection of the brain as well.

Slow virus infections include subacute sclerosing panencephalitis, kuru, and some types of presenile dementias. These rarely occur during pregnancy.

Tuberculous Meningitis

Stephanopoulos has reviewed the development of tuberculous meningitis during pregnancy in Greece.[109] He describes six patients and reviews 31 additional patients. Of these, 25 lived and 12 died. In two cases, miliary tuberculosis was noted, which appeared during the postpartum period. Of the 25 patients who survived, 22 live infants were delivered. In six of the infants, tuberculosis developed after delivery, and of these, three had tuberculous meningitis. Of the six cases described by Stephanopoulos, four had tuberculous meningitis only.

Weinstein and Murphy suggest that ethambutol and isoniazid should be used in the primary treatment of tuberculous meningitis during pregnancy.[110] Rifampin may also be employed, but since the drug inhibits DNA-dependent RNA polymerase, it is a potential hazard to the fetus and probably should be reserved for those cases in which the microbacteria are resistant to other drugs. There is no evidence that the commonly used antitubercular drugs are teratogenic.

D'Acruz and Dandikar report an Indian study from Bombay.[108] The authors make the point that tuberculous meningitis in pregnant women is rare in Western countries but occurs frequently in underdeveloped nations. Eleven pregnant women with tuberculous meningitis and 21 in whom tuberculous meningitis developed within six months of termination of pregnancy are described. The signs and symptoms of the disease were typical and included fever, headache, vomiting, impairment of consciousness, and focal neurologic signs. Of these patients 19 eventually died. All seven of the pregnant patients with tuberculous meningitis died. The authors noted difficulty in following these patients, presumably for economic and social reasons.

ORGANIC MENTAL SYNDROMES ASSOCIATED WITH PREGNANCY

The nervous system is the mechanism by which the patient deals with the environment. Implicit in the examination of a patient is close observation of mood, thought, and behavior. Considerable information can be obtained by observing the patient and her movements (or lack thereof), facial expression, flow of speech, and responses.

Disorders of the cerebral cortex may produce abnormalities of thought. The examiner must decide if the patient is able to perform cognitive functions compatible with her age, education, and previous performance. At times this may be done directly by asking such questions as "Is your memory poor?" and "Is your mind clear?" Some patients may take evidence of organic mental deterioration as a threat, however, and construct elaborate defenses to hide the defects. The patient may be affronted by such direct questions. If this is the case, the examiner should proceed more cautiously and should make indirect inquiries. One should be particularly concerned with mental function, orientation, judgment, and ability to solve problems. Loss of these functions may be the first sign of organic mental disease.

Observation of the patient and her responses is extremely important. Is the patient alert and attentive? Is she reasonably neat and appropriately dressed? Does she answer questions directly or obliquely? Is the history chronological? Is she confused by questions regarding details of the history? An important clue in this regard is the arrival of the patient with the spouse. The spouse gives the history in detail and answers all the questions while the patient adds little or nothing to the discussion. This situation suggests either abnormalities of dependency needs, organic mental disease, or both.

While the history is being taken there is opportunity to examine language function. The patient's choice of words is important. Long lapses of speech may indicate blocking characteristic of schizophrenia or early organic dementia. If the examiner suspects cognitive disorders, the conversation should be steered to a discussion of issues of the day or perhaps current controversies on which an opinion may be requested. Patients with early mental disease may be able to converse quite well on a superficial plane regarding the weather and other related topics. When they are stressed with requests for direct opinions, their speech tends to break down.

Memory function should be evaluated during the history but should also be tested directly. Recent memory usually fails in organic mental disease. Remote memory may remain intact for the most minute details. It is well to ask the patient about her whereabouts today and yesterday, what she was doing one week ago, what she had for breakfast, and so on. Simple memory tests involving digits should be performed. Simple arithmetic should be tested. The patient's orientation is extremely important. She should be able to estimate the length of a brief lapse of time, such as 30 seconds to one minute, quite precisely. Some assessment of the patient's mood should be made. The chronically fatigued, complaining, insomnic, depressed patient is easily recognized. It is often well to ask directly about mood. One should distinguish between mood and affect. Affect may be evaluated by objective signs. Mood is best judged by verbal content.

When dealing with the pregnant patient, several particular forms of mental dysfunction should be considered including, especially, overuse of medications; excessive use of vitamins, particularly vitamins A and D; postictal confusion; eclampsia; cerebrovascular accidents; brain tumors; acute and chronic intoxications; and acute and chronic central nervous system infections.

The treatment for acute or chronic organic

mental syndrome is to discern the cause and act directly to relieve the problem. Neurologic evaluation is almost always required. A psychiatric opinion may be helpful.

ANTIPSYCHOTICS AND THE PREGNANT PATIENT

Phenothiazines freely cross the placenta but nevertheless are rarely associated with fetal or neonatal complications. Transient dystonic movements may occur in siblings born of schizophrenic mothers,[111] but there have been no descriptions of congenital anomalies associated with these drugs. Similarly, tricyclic antidepressants can be used during pregnancy. According to Wilson, no adverse effects have been noted among children of women taking therapeutic doses of tricyclics.[113] However, lithium is associated with cardiac malformations and should be employed with caution in the pregnant patient.[112]

WILSON'S DISEASE

Wilson's disease, or hepatolenticular degeneration, affects the liver and the central nervous system and is related to an inborn disorder of copper metabolism. Prior to the induction of d-penicillamine, women with Wilson's disease either did not usually bear children or aborted spontaneously. With treatment, the fatal course of the condition has been checked, and it is not uncommon now for women with this condition to become pregnant. Walsche and Scheinberg and Sternlieb have reported a series of infants born to 28 women with Wilson's disease who have been treated with d-penicillamine for one to 16 years.[115, 116] Almost all of these mothers took 1 gram of d-penicillamine daily by mouth during pregnancy. Walsche reports that all infants were unaffected at birth and have remained asymptomatic to the present.[116] A Swedish report described congenital connective tissue defects probably owing to d-penicillamine treatment in pregnancy.[114]

AMYOTROPHIC LATERAL SCLEROSIS

Rarely a patient will be seen who has amyotrophic lateral sclerosis that appears during pregnancy.[117] A case of this type has been reported from the Mayo Clinic. The progressive weakness characteristic of amyotrophic lateral sclerosis continued during the pregnancy. The pregnancy itself was not adversely affected, and a normal infant was delivered. There are no special indications for the termination of pregnancy. However, since the disease is progressive and it can be assumed that the mother will not survive more than several years, puerperal sterilization should probably be performed.

DISEASES OF THE CRANIAL AND PERIPHERAL NERVES

Diseases of the cranial and peripheral nerves are manifested by complaints of weakness and loss of sensation of the face, extremities, or trunk. The weakness is characteristically lower motor neuron in nature and is associated with faulty movement of individual muscles. (In upper motor neuron lesions, groups of muscles are affected.)

Lesions of the nerves may affect all forms of sensation in the distribution of the injured nerve. Pain, paresthesias, and loss of sensation frequently occur. The pain has a characteristic intense and burning quality. Paresthesias are often described as tingling or numbness by the patient. The loss of sensation may be partial or complete, most usually the former. Often in peripheral neuropathies the long axons are affected first, producing the typical stocking and glove sensory loss in the extremities.

Several neuropathic syndromes are of particular interest in pregnancy including relapsing idiopathic polyneuritis (Guillain-Barré syndrome), compression mononeuropathies, brachial neuropathy (brachialgia), discogenic root disease, and metabolic neuropathies.

RELAPSING IDIOPATHIC POLYNEURITIS

(Guillain-Barré Syndrome)

There are sporadic reports in the medical literature describing relapsing idiopathic polyneuritis in pregnancy.[122] A recent study describes 12 cases, with the onset in pregnancy occurring as early as 13 days to three weeks after gestation or as late as 36 weeks to near term.[120] Ten of the 12 cases described occurred in the third trimester. Usually the onset of the disease is rapid, with weakness of the extremities, facial palsy, and respiratory depression common findings. Of the 12 patients described, one died eight days after delivery following emergency cesarean section, respiratory failure, and convulsions. There were no obvious underlying or predisposing factors noted. A preceding, presumably viral, respiration infection was documented in seven patients. In most instances maximum neurologic impairment occurred within ten days after the onset of the disease, but two patients continued to become progressively incapacitated over three weeks. In eight patients in whom the cerebral spinal fluid was examined there was a characteristic albuminocytologic dissociation noted. Respiratory paralysis occurred in five patients, and in three patients the disease was fatal.

Pregnancy itself did not adversely affect the prognosis of the disease, since six patients improved before delivery. Three improved after delivery.

Another form of idiopathic polyneuritis, a subacute or chronic variety, has been described, which may recur or in which corticosteroid dependency may be observed.[119] The pathologic findings of the subacute or chronic form of idiopathic polyneuritis are identical to those of the acute forms, and it is uncertain if the chronic form of idiopathic polyneuritis represents a separate or distinct disease. Two cases of recurrent idiopathic polyneuritis appearing in successive pregnancies have been described.[118]

In both cases the polyneuritis seems to have been initiated in some manner by the pregnancy. The disease was more slow moving, characterized by more prominent sensory as well as motor impairments, and improvement prior to delivery was not noted. Improvement did occur rapidly after the termination of pregnancy, suggesting a cause-and-effect relationship between the pregnancy and recurrent idiopathic polyneuritis.

The differential diagnosis is not difficult to make, although occasionally the syndrome of idiopathic polyneuritis may be confused with severe porphyric neuropathy. In addition, other diseases to be ruled out include periodic paralysis, acute myasthenia gravis, acute polymyositis, poliomyelitis, other acute myelopathies, and, rarely, tick paralysis.

If a diagnosis of subacute or chronic idiopathic polyneuritis is made, hospitalization is necessary. Patients in whom the disease is progressing rapidly should be placed in an intensive care unit where their respiratory function can be monitored continuously. If the vital capacity falls as low as 1500 ml, hourly measurements should be made. Early performance of a tracheostomy is indicated in progressive respiratory embarrassment if there is difficulty in maintaining an adequate airway and if there are problems with

secretions. If the vital capacity falls to 800 ml, a tracheostomy is mandatory.

In addition, there should be frequent recordings of the blood pressure and the pulse, preferably by continuous monitoring. There may be autonomic involvement in idiopathic polyneuropathy, manifested by cardiac arrhythmias, hypotension, or both. If the disease becomes chronic, then meticulous attention to nursing care is necessary. Patients should be turned frequently if paralysis occurs. Peripheral nerve compression should be avoided. There should be passive range of motion exercising of all joints at least twice daily to preclude the appearance of contractures about affected joints.

The role of corticosteroids in this disease is uncertain. Nonetheless, there is no question but that some patients with the illness respond to corticosteroid therapy. Therefore, the author suggests a therapeutic trial on prednisone 60 mg daily for five consecutive days. If dramatic improvement does not occur, the corticosteroids may be rapidly tapered and discontinued. If improvement occurs, they should be continued at a lower maintenance dose for three to four weeks or possibly longer, depending on the course of the illness. Immunosuppressive medications are not recommended.

Acute idiopathic polyneuritis is not usually an indication for termination of pregnancy. As mentioned previously, many patients will respond and improve prior to delivery, related to either spontaneous improvement or the administration of corticosteroids. Most deliveries can be accomplished vaginally. If respiratory paralysis occurs and the patient is at term, cesarean section is recommended.

COMPRESSION NEUROPATHIES

Compression mononeuropathies appear frequently in pregnancy. Most are caused by trauma, often unsuspected, and are perhaps associated with the weight gain and fluid retention that accompany the later stages of pregnancy.

Carpal Tunnel Syndrome. This neuropathy is related to compression of the median nerve at the wrist. The carpal tunnel is formed by the flexor tendons (palmaris longus, flexor digitorum sublimis, and flexor carpi ulnaris) and the transverse carpal ligament. The nerve is compressed when the tunnel is narrowed, related to swelling of the synovial sheaths of the tendons or of the ligament or because of fractures or arthritis of the wrist joint itself. The median nerve reacts to the compression with swelling, and, if the process is not resolved, fibrosis of the nerve occurs. Often the findings are bilateral.

Symptoms include pain and tingling in the cutaneous distribution of the median nerve, including the thumb and index and middle fingers and the radial side of the ring finger at the volar aspect. The sensations are especially noted at night and may waken the patient early in the morning. Sensory loss may be described, and weakness may ensue, especially of the opponens pollicis and the abductor pollicis brevis. The hand becomes clumsy, owing to weakness of opposition of the thumb.

The diagnosis is established by the characteristic history and the physical findings and can be secured by performing motor and sensory nerve latencies across the wrist. A characteristic delay in the latency occurs if compression has occurred.

Forty-two cases of carpal tunnel syndrome during pregnancy are reported. Eight-five per cent of these cleared spontaneously.[125] Fifteen per cent required surgical decompression. All achieved complete relief of symptoms. In five patients there were multiple recurrences of carpal tunnel syndrome with subsequent pregnancies.

Nicholas et al. noted that 20 per cent of pregnant women complain of pains in the palm and hand but few have true carpal tunnel syndrome.[124]

Treatment is usually conser ative, including the use of a lightweight plastic splint, applied to the wrist dorsum in a neutral or slightly flexed position and, occasionally, the use of local injections of steroids into the carpal tunnel. Surgery rarely is required during pregnancy for carpal tunnel syndrome.

Massey agrees that the carpal tunnel syndrome that occurs during pregnancy almost invariably abates post partum.[123] Given the benign course and the excellent prognosis in most cases, splinting of the wrist is the preferred method of treatment in the pregnant patient.

Ulnar Neuropathy. This syndrome is almost always due to elbow trauma. The ulnar nerve is injured at the olecranon fossa at the elbow. The injury may be imperceptible or may occur at night. Avoidance of repeated trauma is necessary. A basketball knee guard, worn over the elbow, is helpful in reducing trauma. It is rarely necessary to transpose the ulnar nerve in pregnancy. Recovery usually occurs shortly after birth.

Meralgia Paresthetica. The lateral femoral cutaneous nerve of the thigh is compressed in this syndrome.[126] The compression may occur as the nerve emerges from the pelvis or as it passes through the fascia lata, producing pain and paresthesias in the lateral aspect of the thigh.[127] No loss of motor function occurs. Usually the complaint is minor, and reassurance of the patient is all that is required. After delivery, with its associated weight loss, improvement in symptoms can be expected.[128] Surgery, with section of Poupart's ligament or decompression of the fascia lata, is almost never advised.

Obturator Neuropathy. This condition is related to compression of the obturator nerve or its components by pressure of the fetus before or during delivery. It is characterized primarily by weakness of adduction of the thigh with minimal sensory loss over the medial aspect of the thigh. Usually the problem is self-limited and responds to conservative management including physical therapy.

Peroneal Neuropathy. In this condition the nerve is injured as it crosses the head of the fibula. The physical findings include footdrop, weakness of dorsiflexion of the foot, and, sometimes, sensory loss between the first and second toes. The disease may appear one to two days post partum and may be related to prolonged labor and pressure on the nerve by knee stirrups. Leg crossing is another common form of trauma in this condition. The prognosis for recovery is usually good. In an occasional patient with a severe footdrop, a short leg brace may be necessary and advisable.

Brachial Neuropathy (Brachialgia). This syndrome is known by various names and is also termed the thoracic outlet syndrome by many observers. The peculiar anatomic structure of the clavicle and the first rib predisposes patients to disorders of the structures that underlie them, particularly the brachial plexus and the subclavian artery. The brachial plexus and the subclavian artery are compressed by the bony scissors of the clavicle and the first rib. This is particularly liable to occur in pregnancy, when the increased weight of the breasts and abdomen may lead to sagging of the shoulders and the appearance of symptoms. In one large series, 5 per cent of pregnant patients were found to have symptoms of brachialgia.[130] Other anatomic abnormalities may complicate the problem including cervical rib, a prefixed brachial plexus, or a hypertrophied scalenus anticus muscle.

The symptoms of brachial neuropathy include especially pain, often referred to the ulnar border of the hand and forearm, with associated paresthesias. Motor symptoms are rare during pregnancy, and the reflexes almost always remain intact. Vascular symptoms also occur. These include blanching and cyanosis of the fingers. The complaints often worsen at night or when driving a car, reading a book, or working with the arms and hands extended or elevated.

It is important to differentiate this syndrome from a carpal tunnel syndrome, and indeed, both problems may occasionally appear in the same patient. The electromyogram is particularly helpful in this regard.

This syndrome is almost always self-limited, and simple measures of physical therapy are all that are required during pregnancy. Instructions in proper posture and strengthening of the shoulder suspensory muscles may be helpful. The problem usually resolves after delivery. Resection of the first rib through an axillary approach, a procedure sometimes employed in recalcitrant cases, is not indicated in pregnancy.

Taylor has described a heredofamilial branchial plexus neuropathy that affected 24 members of a family of 119 persons over five generations.[129] Manifestations include single or multiple attacks of acute brachial neuropathy with severe shoulder pain, wasting, weakness, atrophy, and sensory loss, usually unilateral. Repeated attacks may occur in the same individual. Single and recurrent attacks may be associated with pregnancy.[121] The course is usually self-limited and benign, with full recovery anticipated in four to eight months.

Postpartum Footdrop. Postpartum footdrop occurs in small women carrying a relatively large baby who have prolonged labor and midforceps rotation after a transverse arrest.[131] The footdrop, which is usually unilateral, is on the same side as the infant's brow during descent through the pelvis and is related to compression of the lumbosacral trunk (L_4,L_5) in the true pelvis.

Since identical symptoms can be produced by compression of the lateral peroneal nerve as it crosses the head of the fibula, electromyography should be done to establish the site of injury. Generally, physical therapy is indicated including the use of a spring splint or similar device and careful evaluation by a physiatrist, who should follow the patient until the footdrop is corrected. Surgery is rarely indicated in this situation.

Nutritional Neuropathy. A gestational distal polyneuropathy may occur in alcoholic women who are pregnant or in those who are unable to take an adequate diet or supplemental vitamins during pregnancy.[132, 134] This condition still occurs where malnutrition exists, particularly in underdeveloped countries characterized by continuous poverty.[133] This distal polyneuropathy may present as either a mild neuropathy with an acute onset coinciding with the development of the Wernicke-Korsakoff syndrome or as an insidiously progressive subacute neuropathy with encephalopathy as a late manifestation. The problem would appear to be a thiamine deficiency associated with other vitamin deprivations. Treatment calls for the administration of thiamine and related vitamins parenterally in large doses to provide an adequate diet and physical therapy as appropriate. There have been no recent studies of this condition in Western nations, and electromyographic techniques have not been used.

DISCOGENIC ROOT DISEASE

Herniation of the intervertebral discs in the lumbar region is a common cause of pain in the sciatic distribution. The herniation of the intervertebral disc occurs most frequently at the lumbosacral interspace, with diminishing frequency at higher levels. The herniation at the lumbosacral level will compress the first sacral nerve root, producing characteristic sciatic radiation of pain, present in the buttock, posterior thigh, calf, and lateral aspect of the foot. The pain is increased by many movements and by measures that increase intra-abdominal pressure including straining, coughing, or forward bending. It is associated with severe muscle spasm. Frequently there is flattening of the lumbar area from loss of the normal lumbar lordosis.

Signs of discogenic root disease include restricted movement of the lumbar spine, limitation of straight leg raising, and abnormalities of the deep tendon reflexes, particularly a decrease or absence of the associated ankle jerk. A footdrop may develop. The sensory findings are compatible with the involved root and include hypesthesia and hypalgesia on the lateral aspect of the foot, the back of the calf, the heel, and the toe.

The pain is almost always unilateral. Occasionally, if a large disc fragment is extruded in a midline protrusion, the findings may be bilateral.

The diagnosis is usually made on the basis of the history and physical examination. Electromyography may be helpful when signs of muscle denervation are present including increased insertion activity, fibrillation potentials at rest, and reduced or altered muscle action potentials.

In pregnancy, discogenic root disease must be differentiated from more serious illness including, especially, spinal cord tumors.[135] In the usual situation this is not difficult. Myelography is not advised in pregnancy because of difficulties in shielding the fetus.

Treatment of discogenic root disease is always conservative, with complete bed rest advised. Pelvic traction may be helpful. Simple measures of physical therapy to the low back are also advised if significant muscle spasm is present with associated pain. Surgery is almost never required during pregnancy, and frequently, after delivery, the problem is resolved.

Chronic low back pain is also a common finding in women who have had repeated pregnancies or in women with excessive weight gain and poor abdominal muscle function. Here the complaint is primarily persistent pain in the low back associated with twisting movements, and the radicular complaints previously mentioned are not so evident. A lumbosacral corset may be helpful in this situation.

Discogenic root disease during pregnancy is not an indication for abortion. In an occasional patient, severe back pain with associated radicular complaints will not respond to conservative therapy. Should this be the case, the disc may be removed surgically after the first trimester. A normal pregnancy can be maintained under these circumstances.

Frequently, little attention is paid to the mother's muscular status after delivery. If it is evident that low back pain with associated abdominal weakness has been a complication of the pregnancy, then the patient should be given specific instructions designed to strengthen the abdominal, pelvic, and gluteal muscles to reduce any tendency for chronic postpartum back symptoms to occur and progress.

BELL'S PALSY

Bell's palsy is a descriptive term for facial paralysis, related to presumed inflammation in or about the facial nerve close to its exit from the stylomastoid foramen. Usually the onset of symptoms is acute, and signs of paralysis appear and develop rapidly; complete paralysis may evolve in a few hours. The face sags, the forehead becomes unlined, the mouth drops, drooling occurs, and food and liquid may pool adjacent to the teeth on the affected side. The palpebral fissure is widened, and the eyelids cannot be closed. When attempts are made to close the lids, the unclosed eye rolls upward (Bell's phenomenon). Often patients will complain of facial heaviness or numbness, but on careful examination no abnormality of sensation is found.

Four levels of facial nerve dysfunction can be discerned clinically, as follows:

1. A lesion at or proximal to the geniculate ganglion will lead to loss of tearing of the ipsilateral eye, hyperacusis, paralysis of the facial muscles, and loss of taste of the anterior two thirds of the tongue.

2. A lesion above the origin of the muscle to the stapedius gives rise to all of the findings mentioned previously except loss of tearing of the ipsilateral eye.

3. Involvement of the facial nerve in the facial canal above the origin of the chorda tympani gives rise to the lesions previously mentioned except hyperacusis and loss of tearing of the ipsilateral eye.

4. Involvement of the facial nerve at or below the stylomastoid foramen produces weakness of the facial muscles. Taste, hearing, and tearing are unaffected.

With a suprasegmental facial paresis, the lower part of the face is more profoundly affected than the brow, since the brow is bilaterally innervated.

A study of Bell's palsy reveals that 20 per cent of patients surveyed were pregnant or in the puerperium, suggesting an increased predisposition for Bell's palsy in pregnant women.[140] Toxemia of pregnancy is suggested as a factor in the increased incidence of the disorder in this series. The authors describe a patient with Bell's palsy occurring during pregnancy who was treated with bilateral facial nerve decompressions prior to delivery.

Leibowitz has observed that Bell's palsy occurs in clusters, suggesting a common etiologic factor, perhaps of virus-infectious etiology.[139] Korczyn has examined nine pregnant women with Bell's palsy, a higher incidence than would be expected by chance in the six months before delivery.[138]

Hilsinger et al. describe a clear relationship between Bell's palsy and pregnancy.[137] Their studies suggest that the incidence of idiopathic facial paralysis in women of all ages and in those of childbearing age was 17 per 100,000 per year, whereas during pregnancy the rate increases to 57 per 100,000 per year. Three fourths of these cases occurred in the third trimester and in the first two weeks after delivery, an incidence of 118 per 100,000 per year.

Several authors have suggested that a seven to ten day course of prednisone, given 40 to 60 mg per day, increases the chances of recovery in Bell's palsy if the prednisone can be instituted within a week after the onset of paralysis.[136, 141]

Hilsinger et al. confirm these results in pregnant women, without apparent ill effects to mother or infant produced by a short burst of prednisone.[137]

However, Bell's palsy is often self-limited, and corticosteroid therapy is difficult to evaluate. If denervation is severe, as determined clinically and electromyographically, and if recovery does not promptly begin in a few days, then corticosteroids can be justified. But not all patients need such therapy. If the affected eye cannot be closed it should be patched. Despite the study by Hilsinger et al., surgical decompression of the facial nerve is rarely necessary.[137]

References

DIAGNOSTIC PROCEDURES

1. Medical Radiation Exposure of Pregnant and Potentially Pregnant Women. Washington, D.C., National Council on Radiological Protection Report No. 54, 1977.

SEIZURE DISORDERS

General References

2. American Academy of Pediatrics Commission on Drugs: Anticonvulsants in pregnancy. Pediatrics, 63:331, 1979.
3. Montouris, G. D., Fenichel, G. M., and McLain, W.: The pregnant epileptic: A review and recommendations. Arch. Neurol., 36:601, 1979.

Incidence

4. Knight, A. H., and Rhind, E. G.: Epilepsy and pregnancy: A study of 153 pregnancies in 50 patients. Epilepsia, 16:99, 1975.
5. Suter, C., and Klingman, K. O.: Seizure states and pregnancy. Neurology, 7:105, 1957.

Anticonvulsants, Plasma Levels

6. Dam, M., Christiansen, J., Munck, O., and Mygind, K.: Antiepileptic drugs: Metabolism in pregnancy. Clin. Pharmacokinet., 4:53, 1979.
7. Desmond, M. M., Schwanecke, R. P., Wilson, G. S., et al.: Maternal barbiturate utilization and neonatal withdrawal symptomatology. J. Pediatr. 80:190, 1972.
8. Hooper, W. D., Bochner, F., Eadie, M. J., et al.: Plasma protein binding of diphenylhydantoin: Effects of sex hormones, renal and hepatic disease. Clin. Pharmacol. Ther., 15:276, 1974.
9. Lander, C. M., Edwards, V. E., Eadie, M. J., et al.: Plasma anticonvulsant concentrations during pregnancy. Neurology, 27:128, 1977.
10. Landon, M. J., and Kirkley, M.: Metabolism of diphenylhydantoin (phenytoin) during pregnancy. Br. J. Obstet. Gynaecol., 86:125, 1979.
11. Melchoir, J. C., Svensmark, O., and Trolle, D.: Placental transfer of phenobarbitone in epileptic women, and elimination in newborns. Lancet, 2:1860, 1967.
12. Mirkin, B. L.: Drug distribution in pregnancy. In Borcus, L. (ed.): Fetal Pharmacology. New York, Raven Press, 1973.
13. Mygind, K. I., Dam, M., and Christiansen, J.: Phenytoin and phenobarbitone plasma clearance during pregnancy. Acta Neurol. Scand., 54:160, 1976.

Maternal Complications and Epilepsy

14. Bjerkedal, T., and Bahna, S. L.: The course and outcome of pregnancy in women with epilepsy. Acta Obstet. Gynecol. Scand. 52:245, 1973.
15. Burnett, C. W. F.: A survey of the relation between epilepsy and pregnancy. J. Obstet. Gynaecol. Br. Emp., 53:539, 1946.
16. Dimsdale, H.: The epileptic in relation to pregnancy. Br. Med. J., 2:1147, 1959.

Teratogenicity of Anticonvulsants

17. Bustamante, S. A., and Stumpff, L. C.: Fetal hydantoin syndrome in triplets: A unique experiment of nature. Am. J. Dis. Child., 132:978, 1978.

18. German, J., Ehlers, K. H., Kowal, A., et al.: Possible teratogenicity of trimethadione and paramethadione. Lancet, 2:261, 1970.
19. Goldman, A. S., and Yaffe, S. J.: Fetal trimethadione syndrome. Teratology, 17:103, 1978.
20. Hanson, J. W., and Smith, D. W.: The fetal hydantoin syndrome. J. Pediatr., 87:285, 1975.
21. Janz, D.: The teratogenic risk of antiepileptic drugs. Epilepsia, 16:159, 1975.
22. Loughnan, P. M., Gold, H., and Vance, J. C.: Phenytoin teratogenicity in man. Lancet, 1:70, 1973.
23. Zackai, E. H., Mellman, W. J., Neiderer, B., et al.: The fetal trimethadione syndrome. J. Pediatr., 87:280, 1975.

Anticonvulsants — New

24. Brown, T. R.: Clonazepam: A review of a new anticonvulsant drug. Arch. Neurol., 33:326, 1976.
25. Bruni, J., and Wilder, B. J.: Valproic acid: Review of a new antiepileptic drug. Arch. Neurol., 36:393, 1979.
26. Crill, W.: Carbamazepine. Ann. Intern. Med., 79:844, 1973.

Anticonvulsants and Hemorrhagic Disease of Newborn

27. Evans, A. R., Forrester, R. M., and Discombe, C.: Neonatal hemorrhage following maternal anticonvulsant therapy. Lancet, 1:517, 1970.
28. Mountain, K. R., Herst, J., and Gallies, A. S.: Neonatal coagulation defect due to anticonvulsant drug treatment in pregnancy. Lancet, 2:265, 1970.

HEADACHE

29. Callaghan, N.: The migraine syndrome in pregnancy. Neurology, 18:197, 1968.
30. Dalessio, D. J.: Wolff's Headache and Other Head Pain. 4th Ed. New York, Oxford University Press, 1980.
31. Dooling, E. C., and Sweeney, V. P.: Migrainous hemiplegia during breast feeding. Am. J. Obstet. Gynecol., 118:568, 1974.
32. Friedman, A. P., and Merritt, H. H.: Headache, Prognosis and Treatment. Philadelphia, F. A. Davis Co., 1959.
33. Lance, J. W., and Anthony, M. D.: Some clinical aspects of migraine. Arch. Neurol., 15:356, 1966.
34. Massey, E. W.: Migraine during pregnancy. Obstet. Gynecol. Surv., 32:693, 1977.
35. Rotton, W. N., Sachtlaben, M. R., and Friedman, E. A.: Migraine and eclampsia. Obstet. Gynecol., 14:322, 1959.
36. Somerville, B.: A study of migraine in pregnancy. Neurology, 22:824, 1972.

Dietary Migraine

37. Dalessio, D. J.: Dietary migraine. Am. Fam. Phys., 6:60, 1972.
38. Hanington, E.: Preliminary report on tyramine headache. Br. Med. J., 2:550, 1967.
39. Ryan, R. E., Jr.: A clinical study of tyramine as an etiological factor in migraine. Headache, 14:43, 1974.
40. Sandler, M., Youdim, M. B. H., and Hanington, E.: A phenylethylamine oxidising defect in migraine. Nature, 250:335, 1974.

CEREBROVASCULAR DISEASE

41. Amias, A. G.: Cerebral vascular disease in pregnancy: II. Occlusion. J. Obstet. Gynaecol. Br. Commonw., 77:312, 1970.

42. Cross, J. N., Castro, P. O., and Jennett, W. B.: Cerebral strokes associated with pregnancy and the puerperium. Br. Med. J., 3:214, 1968.
43. Lavy, S., and Kahana, E.: Cerebral arterial occlusion during pregnancy and puerperium. Report of 3 cases. Obstet. Gynecol., 35:916, 1970.

Subarachnoid Hemorrhage

44. Amias, A. G.: Cerebral vascular disease in pregnancy: I. Haemorrhage. J. Obstet. Gynaecol. Br. Emp., 77:100, 1970.
45. Heron, J. R., Hutchinson, E. C., Boyd, W. N., and Aber, G. M.: Pregnancy, subarachnoid hemorrhage, and the intravascular coagulation syndrome. J. Neurol. Neurosurg. Psychiatry, 37:521, 1974.
46. Hunt, H. B., Schifrin, B. S., and Suzuki, K.: Ruptured berry aneurysms and pregnancy. Obstet. Gynecol., 43:827, 1974.
47. Miller, H. J., and Hinkley, C. M.: Berry aneurysms in pregnancy: A 10 year report. South. Med. J., 63:279, 1970.
48. Minielly, R., Yuzpe, A. A., and Drake, C. G.: Subarachnoid hemorrhage secondary to ruptured cerebral aneurysm in pregnancy. Obstet. Gynecol., 53:64, 1979.
49. Robinson, J. L., and Hall, C. J.: Some aspects of subarachnoid hemorrhage in pregnancy. J. Neurol. Neurosurg. Psychiatry, 34:109, 1971.
50. Robinson, J. L., Hall, C. J., and Sedzimer, C. B.: Arteriovenous malformations, aneurysms, and pregnancy. J. Neurosurg., 41:63, 1974.

Cerebral Venous Thrombosis

51. Gettelfinger, D. M., and Kokmen, E.: Superior sagittal sinus thrombosis. Arch. Neurol., 34:2, 1977.
52. Lavin, P. J. M., Bone, I., Lamb, J. T., and Swinburne, L. M.: Intracranial venous thrombosis in the first trimester of pregnancy. J. Neurol. Neurosurg. Psychiatry, 41:726, 1978.

Syncope, Hyperventilation

53. Dalessio, D. J.: Hyperventilation. The vapors. Effort syndrome. Neurasthenia. J.A.M.A., 239:1401, 1979.
54. Engel, G. L.: Fainting. 2nd Ed. Springfield, Charles C Thomas, 1962, p. 196.
55. Wayne, H. H.: Syncope. Physiological considerations and an analysis of the clinical characteristics in 510 patients. Am. J. Med., 30:418, 1961.

Vertigo

56. Daroff, R. B.: Vertigo. Am. Fam. Phys., 16:143, 1977.
57. Drachman, D. A., Daroff, R. B., and Hart, C. W.: An approach to the dizzy patient. Neurology, 22:323, 1972.
58. Rubin, W.: Differential diagnosis of vertigo. Hosp. Med., 1970, p. 28.

BRAIN TUMOR AND PREGNANCY

59. Bickerstaff, E. R., Small, J. M., and Guest, I. A.: The relapsing course of certain meningiomas in relation to pregnancy and menstruation. J. Neurol. Neurosurg. Psychiatry, 21:89, 1958.
60. Michelsen, J. J., and New, P. F. J.: Brain tumour and pregnancy. J. Neurol. Neurosurg. Psychiatry, 32:305, 1969.
61. Rand, C. W., and Andler, M.: Tumors of the brain complicating pregnancy. Arch. Neurol. Psychiat., 63:1, 1950.

Choriocarcinoma

62. Aguilar, M. J., and Rabinovitch, R.: Metastatic chorionepithelioma simulating multiple strokes. Neurology, 14:933, 1964.
63. Stilip, T. J., Bucy, P. C., and Brewer, J. I.: Cure of metastatic choriocarcinoma of the brain. J.A.M.A., 221:276, 1972.

Pituitary Lesions

64. Child, D. F., Gordon, H., Mashiter, K., et al.: Pregnancy, prolactin and pituitary tumours. Br. Med. J., 4:87, 1975.

65. Falconer, M. A., and Stafford-Bell, M. A.: Visual failure from pituitary and parasellar tumours occurring with favourable outcome in pregnant women. J. Neurol. Neurosurg. Psychiatry, 38:919, 1975.

Pseudotumor Cerebri

66. Powell, J. L.: Pseudotumor cerebri in pregnancy. Obstet. Gynecol., 40:713, 1972.

MULTIPLE SCLEROSIS

General Reference

67. McAlpine, D., Lunisden, C. E., and Acheson, E. D.: Multiple Sclerosis. A Reappraisal. 2nd Ed. Baltimore, Williams & Wilkins Co., 1972.

Multiple Sclerosis in Pregnancy

68. Eastman, R., Sheridan, J., and Poskanzer, D. A.: Multiple sclerosis clustering in a small Massachusetts community. N. Engl. J. Med., 289:793, 1973.
69. Liebowitz, U., Antonovosky, A., Katz, R., et al.: Does pregnancy increase the risk of multiple sclerosis? J. Neurol. Neurosurg. Psychiatry, 30:354, 1967.
70. Millar, J. H. D., Allison, R. S., Cheeseman, E. A., et al.: Pregnancy as a factor in influencing relapse in disseminated sclerosis. Brain, 82:417, 1959.
71. Schapira, K., Poskanzer, D. C., and Miller, H.: Familial and conjugal multiple sclerosis. Brain, 86:315, 1963.

MYASTHENIA GRAVIS

General References

72. Engle, A. G., Lambert, E. H., and Howard, F. M.: Immune complexes at motor end plate in myasthenia gravis. Mayo Clin. Proc., 52:273, 1977.
73. Lennon, V.: The immunopathology of myasthenia gravis. Hum. Pathol., 9:541, 1978.
74. Lindstrom, J., Lennon, V. A., Seybold, M., and Wittingham, S.: Experimental auto-immune myasthenia and myasthenia gravis: Biochemical and immunological aspects. Ann. N.Y. Acad. Sci., 274:254, 1976.
75. Osserman, K. E.: Myasthenia Gravis. New York, Grune & Stratton, 1938, p. 296.

Congenital Myasthenia

76. McLean, W. T., and McKone, R. C.: Congenital myasthenia gravis in twins. Arch. Neurol., 29:223, 1973.
77. Namba, T.: Familial myasthenia gravis. Arch. Neurol., 25:49, 1971.

Myasthenia and Pregnancy

78. Duff, G. B.: Pre-eclampsia and the patient with myasthenia gravis. Obstet. Gynecol., 54:355, 1979.
79. Ferguson, F. R.: A critical review of the clinical features of myasthenia gravis. Proc. Roy. Soc. Med., 55:49, 1962.
80. Mathews, W. A., and Derrick, W. S.: Anesthesia in the patient with myasthenia gravis. Anesthesiology, 18:443, 1957.
81. Osserman, K. E.: Myasthenia Gravis. New York, Grune & Stratton, 1958.
82. Osserman, K. E.: Myasthenia Gravis. In Rovinsky, J. J., and Guttmacher, A. F. (eds.): Medical, Surgical and Gynecological Complications of Pregnancy. 2nd Ed. Baltimore, Williams & Wilkins Co., 1965, pp. 452–462.

Neonatal Myasthenia

83. Dunn, J. M.: Neonatal myasthenia. Am. J. Obstet. Gynecol., 125:265, 1976.
84. Keesey, J., Lindstrom, J., et al.: Anti-acetylcholine receptor antibody in neonatal myasthenia gravis. N. Engl. J. Med., 296:55, 1977.

85. Namba, T., Brown, S. B., and Grob, D.: Neonatal myasthenia gravis: Report of two cases and a review of the literature. Pediatrics, *45*:488, 1970.

OTHER DISORDERS OF MUSCLE

86. Shore, R. N., and MacLachlan, T. B.: Pregnancy with myotonic dystrophy: Course, complications and management. Obstet. Gynecol., *38*:448, 1971.
87. Tsai, A., Lindheimer, M. D., and Lamberg, S. I.: Dermatomyositis complicating pregnancy. Obstet. Gynecol., *41*:570, 1973.

PORPHYRIA

88. Beattie, A. D., Moore, M. R., Goldberg, A., et al.: Acute intermittent porphyria: Response of tachycardia and hypertension to propranolol. Br. Med. J., *3*:257, 1973.
89. James, C. W., Rudolph, S. G., and Abbott, L. D.: Delta-aminolevulinic acid, porphobilinogen, and porphyrin excretion throughout pregnancy in a patient with acute intermittent porphyria with "passive porphyria" in the infant. J. Lab. Clin. Med., *58*:437, 1961.
90. Kerr, G. D.: Acute intermittent porphyria and inappropriate secretion of antidiuretic hormone in pregnancy. Proc. Roy. Soc. Med., *66*:763, 1973.
91. Peterson, A., Bossenmaier, I., Cardinal, R., et al.: Hematin treatment of acute porphyria: Early remission of an almost fatal relapse. J.A.M.A., *235*:520, 1976.
92. Seckler, S. G., and Rovinsky, J. J.: Metabolic disorders. *In* Rovinsky, J. J., and Guttmacher, A. F. (eds.): Medical, Surgical and Gynecological Complications of Pregnancy. 2nd Ed. Baltimore, Williams & Wilkins Co., 1965, pp. 776–786.

SPINAL CORD SYNDROMES

Tumors

93. Divers, W. A., Hoxsey, R. J., and Dunnihoo, D. R.: A spinal cord neurolemmoma in pregnancy. Obstet. Gynecol., *52*:475, 1978.
94. Mealey, J., and Carter, J. E.: Spinal cord tumor during pregnancy. Obstet. Gynecol., *32*:204, 1968.
95. Smolik, E. A., Nash, F. P., and Clawson, J. W.: Neurological and neurosurgical complications associated with pregnancy and the puerperium. South. Med. J., *50*:561, 1957.

Angiomas

96. Aminoff, M. J., and Logue, V.: Clinical features of spinal vascular malformations. Brain, *97*:197, 1974.
96a. Aminoff, M. J., and Logue, V.: The prognosis of patients with spinal vascular malformations. Brain, *97*:211, 1974.
97. Fields, W. S., and Jones, J. R.: Spinal epidural in hemangioma in pregnancy. Neurology, *7*:825, 1957.
98. Lam, R. L., Roulhac, G. E., and Erwin, H. J.: Hemangioma of the spinal canal and pregnancy. J. Neurosurg., *8*:668, 1951.
99. Nelson, D. A.: Spinal cord compression due to vertebral angiomas during pregnancy. Arch. Neurol., *11*:408, 1964.
100. Newquist, R. E., and Mayfield, F. H.: Spinal angioma presenting during pregnancy. J. Neurosurg., *17*:541, 1960.

Spinal Aneurysm

101. Garcia, C., Dulcey, S., and Dulcey, J.: Ruptured aneurysm of the spinal artery of Adamkiewicz during pregnancy. Neurology, *29*:394, 1979.

Paraplegia

102. Robertson, D. N.: Pregnancy and labour in the paraplegic. Paraplegia, *10*:209, 1972.

Chorea Gravidarum

103. Beresford, O. D., and Graham, A. M.: Chorea gravidarum. J. Obstet. Gynaecol. Br. Emp., *57*:616, 1950.
104. Gamboa, E. T., Isaacs, G., and Harter, D. H.: Chorea associated with oral contraceptive therapy. Arch. Neurol., *25*:112, 1971.
105. Lewis. P. D., and Harrison, M. J. G.: Involuntary movements in patients taking oral contraceptives. Br. Med. J., *4*:404, 1969.
106. Nausieda, P., Koller, W., Weiner, W., and Klawans, H.: Chorea induced by oral contraceptives. Neurology, *29*:1605, 1979.
107. Zegart, K. N., and Schwarz, R. H.: Chorea gravidarum. Obstet. Gynecol., *32*:24, 1968.

TUBERCULOUS MENINGITIS

108. D'Acruz, I. A., and Dandikar, A. C.: Tuberculous meningitis in pregnant and puerperal women. Obstet. Gynecol., *31*:775, 1968.
109. Stephanopoulos, C.: The development of tuberculous meningitis during pregnancy. Am. Rev. Tuberculosis, *76*:1079, 1957.
110. Weinstein, L., and Murphy, T.: The management of tuberculosis during pregnancy. J. Perinatol., *1*:395, 1974.

PSYCHOTROPICS AND PREGNANCY

111. Hill, R. M., Desmond, M. M., and Kay, J. L.: Extrapyramidal dysfunction in an infant of a schizophrenic mother. J. Pediatr., *69*:589, 1966.
112. Weinstein, M. R., and Goldfield, M. D.: Cardiovascular malformations with lithium used during pregnancy. Am. J. Psychiat., *132*:529, 1975.
113. Wilson, J. G.: Environmental factors: Teratogenic drugs. *In* Prevention of Embryonic, Fetal, and Perinatal Disease. Washington, U.S. Govt. Printing Office, 1976, Ch. 7.

WILSON'S DISEASE

114. Mjølnerød, O. K., Rasmussen, K., Dommerud, S. A., et al.: Congenital connective tissue defect probably due to d-penicillamine treatment in pregnancy. Lancet, *1*:673, 1971.
115. Sternlieb, I., and Scheinberg, I. H.: Penicillamine therapy for hepatolenticular degeneration. J.A.M.A., *189*:748, 1964.
116. Walsche, J. M.: Pregnancy in Wilson's disease. Q. J. Med., *46*:73, 1977.

AMYOTROPHIC LATERAL SCLEROSIS

117. Huston, J. W., Lingenfelder, J., Mulder, D. W., and Kurland, L. T.: Pregnancy complicated by amyotrophic lateral sclerosis. Am. J. Obstet. Gynecol., *72*:93, 1956.

RELAPSING IDIOPATHIC POLYNEURITIS

118. Calderon-Gonzales, R., Gonzales-Cantu, N., and Rissi-Hernandez, H.: Recurrent polyneuropathy with pregnancy and oral contraceptives. N. Engl. J. Med., *282*:1307, 1970.
119. Matthews, W. B., Howell, D. A., and Hughes, R. C.: Relapsing cortico-steroid dependent polyneuritis. J. Neurol. Neurosurg. Psychiatry, *33*:330, 1970.
120. Novak, D. J., and Johnson, K. P.: Relapsing idiopathic polyneuritis during pregnancy. Arch. Neurol., *28*:219, 1973.
121. Poffenbarger, A. L.: Heredofamilial neuritis with brachial predilections. W. Va. Med. J., *64*:425, 1968.
122. Rudolph, J. H., Norris, F. H., Garvey, P. H., et al.: The Landry-Guillain-Barre syndrome in pregnancy. A review. Obstet. Gynecol., *26*:265, 1965.

COMPRESSION NEUROPATHIES

Carpal Tunnel

123. Massey, E. W.: Carpal tunnel syndrome in pregnancy. Obstet. Gynecol. Surv., *33*:145, 1978.
124. Nicholas, G. G., Noone, R. B., and Graham, W. P.: Carpal tunnel syndrome in pregnancy. Hand, *3*:80, 1971.
125. Tobin, S. M.: Carpal tunnel syndrome in pregnancy. Am. J. Obstet. Gynecol., *97*:493, 1967.

Meralgia Paresthetica

126. Ecker, A. D., and Woltman, H. W.: Meralgia paresthetica: A report of 150 cases. J.A.M.A., *110*:1650, 1938.
127. Jones, R. K.: Meralgia paresthetica as a cause of leg discomfort. Can. Med. Assoc. J., *111*:541, 1974.
128. Peterson, P. H.: Meralgia paresthetica related to pregnancy. Am. J. Obstet. Gynecol., *64*:690, 1952.

Brachialgia

129. Taylor, R. A.: Heredofamilial mononeuritis multiplex with brachial predilection. Brain, *83*:113, 1960.
130. Benson, R. C., and Inman, V. T.: Brachialgia statica dysesthetica in pregnancy. West. J. Surg. Obstet. Gynecol., *64*:115, 1956.

Postpartum Foot Drop

131. Brown, J. T., and McDougall, A.: Traumatic maternal birth injury. J. Obstet. Gynaecol. Br. Emp., *64*:431, 1957.

NUTRITIONAL NEUROPATHY

132. Berkowitz, N. J., and Lufkin, N. H.: Toxic neuronitis of pregnancy. Surg. Gynecol. Obstet., *54*:743, 1932.

133. Chaturachinda, K., and McGregor, E. M.: Wernicke's encephalopathy and pregnancy. J. Obstet. Gynaecol. Br. Commonw., *75*:969, 1968.
134. Strauss, M. B., and McDonald, W. J.: Polyneuritis of pregnancy: A dietary deficiency disorder. J.A.M.A., *100*:1320, 1933.

DISCOGENIC ROOT DISEASE

135. O'Connell, J. E.: Lumbar disc protrusions in pregnancy. J. Neurol. Neurosurg. Psychiatry, *23*:138, 1960.

BELL'S PALSY

136. Adour, K. K., Wingerd, J., and Bell, D. N.: Prednisone treatment for idiopathic facial paralysis (Bell's palsy). N. Engl. J. Med., *287*:1268, 1972.
137. Hilsinger, R. L., Adour, K. K., and Doty, H. E.: Idiopathic facial paralysis, pregnancy, and the menstrual cycle. Ann. Otol. Rhinol. Laryngol., *84*:433, 1975.
138. Korczyn, A. D.: Bell's palsy and pregnancy. Acta Neurol. Scand., *47*:603, 1971.
139. Leibowitz, N.: Epidemic incidence of Bell's palsy. Brain, *92*:109, 1969.
140. Robinson, J. R., and Pou, J. W.: Bell's palsy: A predisposition of pregnant women. Arch. Otolaryngol., *95*:125, 1972.
141. Thomas, M. H.: Treatment of Bell's palsy with cortisone and other measures. Neurology, *5*:882, 1955.

19 *Murray B. Urowitz, M.D.*
Dafna D. Gladman, M.D.

RHEUMATIC DISEASES

Pregnancy is of special interest to the rheumatologist because many of the diseases with which he is concerned occur more commonly in women, often during the childbearing years. Furthermore, pregnancy has a definite influence on the clinical course of certain rheumatic diseases. At the same time, some rheumatic diseases may affect the outcome of pregnancy. In addition, many of the drugs used to treat various rheumatic diseases may adversely affect the fetus or the pregnancy. It behooves the obstetrician and the internist to be aware of these interrelationships so that the proper diagnoses can be made, the patient can be effectively counseled, complications can be anticipated, and the most effective therapy with the least potential for harm to the mother and fetus can be given.

In several of the connective tissue diseases to be discussed, the pathogenic mechanisms underlying the tissue injury are immunologic in nature. Similarly, many immunologic changes occur during pregnancy and may play a role in the amelioration of some of the connective tissue diseases that may develop during pregnancy. On the other hand, the precipitation or aggravation of such diseases may occur during pregnancy. Thus, it is worthwhile to review the postulated immune mechanisms underlying the pathogenesis of the connective tissue diseases and the immune alterations that occur during pregnancy.

Immune Mechanisms of Tissue Injury in the Connective Tissue Diseases

The hallmark of a number of the connective tissue diseases is the presence of an array of circulating autoantibodies in the serum of patients with these diseases. The mechanism whereby tissue injury is induced in connective tissue disease can in some instances be correlated with the presence of these autoantibodies.

Autoantibodies may induce immune injury in connective tissue disease in two ways. First, they may react with antigens directly, e.g., the Coombs' antibody reacts with antigens on the surface of red blood cells, resulting in cell damage (cytotoxic mechanism). Alternatively, the autoantibodies can combine with the antigens to form immune complexes. When these complexes are fixed in tissues they activate the complement cascade, resulting in the release of several chemotactic factors. This leads to polymorphonuclear cell infiltration, immune complex phagocytosis, and subsequent lysosomal enzyme release into tissues, causing inflammation (immune complex mechanism).

The cause of excessive autoantibody production — the basis of both mechanisms of tissue injury — is still not clear. However, current research tends to indicate abnormal regulating mechanisms of the immune response system (Fig. 19–1). Antibody production is modulated in part by the cell-mediated immune system via helper and suppressor T lymphocytes. A deficiency of T lymphocyte suppressor cells in patients who have a connective tissue disease is believed to result in unchecked autoantibody production and, eventually, immune injury as previously discussed.

Inflammation is the end result of the immune

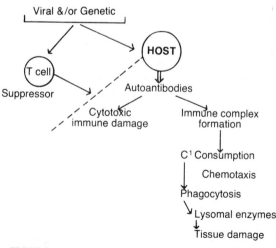

FIGURE 19–1. Pathogenesis of autoimmune disease.

474

response in most instances of immunologically mediated tissue damage. The clinical manifestations vary according to the site of inflammatory involvement, and the specific organs involved tend to vary from disease to disease, e.g., the joints in rheumatoid arthritis and many extra-articular sites in systemic lupus.

Normally during pregnancy a number of alterations occur in lymphocyte function, humoral immune response, and inflammatory response, which must be appreciated if one is investigating a suspected connective tissue disease.

Impaired T lymphocyte function during pregnancy was suggested by the demonstration of progressive atrophy in the guinea pig thymus during pregnancy[14] and by the finding of an absence of germinal centers in lymph nodes removed from pregnant women at term.[11] Impaired skin graft rejection has been demonstrated during pregnancy.[1] In vitro tests of T cell function have included cell population studies and functional assays. Although controversial results have appeared,[3, 5, 16] the majority of authors conclude that there are no changes in cell populations during pregnancy. Likewise, there is no uniform agreement among investigators regarding T cell function.[2, 6, 16] However, when the plasma effect on stimulation studies is removed, there is no significant impairment of responses in mixed leukocyte culture (MLC) and to the mitogens phytohemagglutinin (PHA) and pokeweed mitogen (PWM).[2, 3] The response of lymphocytes from pregnant women to Concanavalin A, a mitogen thought to selectively stimulate a suppressor T cell population, was recently shown to be increased toward the end of pregnancy.[4] On the other hand, response to antigenic stimulation requiring B cell response was found to be diminished in late pregnancy and increased following delivery.[4, 15] These results suggest increased T suppressor cell function and decreased B cell function, particularly in late pregnancy.[4] Specific suppressor cell assays in pregnancy have not been reported.

In addition to the reports on abnormalities of cell-mediated immunity during pregnancy, there is a growing body of evidence pointing to involvement of humoral factors in immunologic impairment. Serum and plasma from pregnant women have been found to suppress various functions of polymorphonuclear cells, such as phagocytosis and bacterial killing, and to reduce NBT reduction by leukocytes of pregnant women.[12] In addition, serum from pregnant women has been found to contain a lysosomal stabilizer.[7] This stabilizing activity in the serum continued throughout gestation and gradually decreased after delivery. Since the aforementioned factors are important mediators of inflammation, these findings are very relevant to the resolution of certain inflammatory conditions during pregnancy.

Serum taken from pregnant women also inhibited lymphocyte responses to mitogens[8] and antigens[2] as well as their ability to react in an MLC.[9] This serum suppressive effect was noted primarily with fractions of serum rich in pregnancy zone protein (PZP), a glycoprotein of a molecular weight of 364,000 with an electrophoretic mobility of alpha-2-globulin. This protein is present in very small quantities in the plasma of nonpregnant women. Its concentration rises during gestation and gradually decreases after delivery. PZP concentration increases with the administration of synthetic estrogen (BCP). Unlike other pregnancy-associated proteins, it is not synthesized by the placenta.[13]

Abnormalities of immunoglobulins have not been reported in pregnancy. There is only one investigation of rheumatoid factor during normal pregnancy in the literature, and it revealed no abnormality. There are no reports of antinuclear factors present in normal pregnancy, although some reports have been published of ANF in patients taking estrogen-progesterone preparations.[10]

Therefore, human pregnancy is associated with impaired immunologic response mediated both by cellular mechanisms thought to be increased suppressor T cells and decreased B cell function and by a humoral mechanism mediated by pregnancy zone protein.

These immunologic factors presenting during normal pregnancy may serve to ameliorate certain inflammatory conditions during pregnancy. In autoimmune disease it is postulated that there is impairment of suppressor cell activity leading to hyperactive B cell response and production of autoantibodies, which by combining with appropriate antigens activate complement cascade and phagocytic mechanisms to mediate inflammations. The opposite occurs during pregnancy, which may explain the improvement in these diseases in some patients during pregnancy.

Although there have been isolated case reports

TABLE 19–1 RHEUMATIC DISEASES THAT OCCUR DURING PREGNANCY

Rheumatoid arthritis
Systemic lupus erythematosus
Scleroderma
Gonococcal arthritis
Carpal tunnel syndrome

of pregnancy associated with some of the rarer connective tissue diseases, for practical purposes only a few rheumatic diseases present during pregnancy, and these will be stressed (Table 19–1).

RHEUMATOID ARTHRITIS

Rheumatoid arthritis is a chronic systemic inflammatory disease of unknown etiology, manifested primarily in the joints. The disease occurs worldwide and has no racial predilection. It is common, occurring in 1 to 2 per cent of the population, and affects females two to three times more frequently than males. Rheumatoid arthritis occurs at any age but in most patients presents between the ages of 20 and 60.[68]

Various infective agents, including bacteria, *Mycoplasma,* and a number of viruses, have been incriminated as the source of persistent antigenic stimulation, which is thought to cause the inflammatory manifestations.[52]

Extensive cellular and humoral immunologic phenomena have been demonstrated in rheumatoid arthritis.[25, 49, 72] Evidence to support the role of cell-mediated immune reactions in the pathogenesis of rheumatoid arthritis derives from 1) the pathologic lesions of rheumatoid arthritis, which resemble delayed hypersensitivity reactions with intense mononuclear infiltration[59]; 2) the appearance of a seronegative rheumatoid arthritis in patients with congenital agammaglobulinemia who are unable to produce gammaglobulin but have normal T cell function[30]; and 3) the improvement in rheumatoid disease activity following thoracic duct drainage and leukaphoresis and the aggravation of the condition by the reinfusion of the removed cells.[50, 62]

Many studies have indicated impaired T cell function in rheumatoid arthritis.[72] In vivo studies have shown diminished delayed hypersensitivity skin test responsiveness,[17, 66] whereas in vitro studies have demonstrated decreased response to the mitogens PHA and Con. A.[39, 42] The decreased response to Con. A. and the recent demonstration of impaired antigen specific–suppressor cell function in rheumatoid arthritis lend support to the role of immune regulation in the pathogenesis of rheumatoid arthritis.[36, 39] Mediators of cell-mediated immunity such as lymphotoxin and macrophage inhibitory factors have been found locally in the joints of patients with rheumatoid arthritis, suggesting a role for effector T cells in the tissue damage in rheumatoid arthritis.[60, 72]

There is extensive evidence for the role of humoral immunity in the pathogenesis of rheumatoid arthritis. Hypergammaglobulinemia and anti-immunoglobulins (rheumatoid factors) are common in rheumatoid arthritis. Other "autoantibodies" have also been demonstrated in the sera of patients with rheumatoid arthritis, especially those with the Felty's syndrome variant.[20] Immunoglobulins are produced by rheumatoid synovium,[49, 56] and both complement and immunoglobulins have been demonstrated in synovial cells.[26] Immune complexes containing IgG aggregates and rheumatoid factor have been found in blood, synovial fluid, and synovial membranes of patients with rheumatoid arthritis.[43, 70] These immune complexes activate the complement system to produce biologically active substances that stimulate chemotaxis, phagocytosis, and lysosomal release by polymorphonuclear cells, resulting in the inflammatory process seen in the involved areas of this disease.[49, 67, 69]

The familial occurrence of rheumatoid arthritis and studies in monozygotic twins with rheumatoid arthritis have suggested a genetic factor in its etiopathogenesis. The discovery of an association of HLA Dw4 and DR 4 and rheumatoid arthritis supports the role for hereditary factors in the development of rheumatoid arthritis.[61] The association of the disease with alleles in the HLA D region, thought to be involved in immune response functions, may explain the alterations in immune response regulation in rheumatoid arthritis.

The clinical picture of rheumatoid arthritis is one of joint inflammation, with pain, tenderness, heat, and swelling, particularly of the small and medium size joints, in a symmetric distribution. This is accompanied by morning stiffness and often by fatigue, malaise, and other constitutional symptoms. Rheumatoid arthritis may begin with an acute onset of a symmetric polyarthritis or with a more gradual onset of joint pain accompanied by significant systemic complaints. Some patients present with a monoarthritis, often thought to be the result of an injury or confused with gout, which later develops into a more symmetric polyarthritis. The course may continue to consist of acute exacerbations and remissions of joint inflammation, or it may be of a slowly progressive nature with unrelenting joint inflammation leading to gradual joint destruction. Patients with acute onset are said to have a better prognosis. Persistent joint inflammation results in joint deformity and damage as evidenced radiologically by bony erosions and joint space narrowing.[68]

In addition to joint inflammation, extra-articular manifestations have long been recog-

TABLE 19–2 EXTRA-ARTICULAR MANIFESTATIONS OF RHEUMATOID ARTHRITIS

Subcutaneous nodules	
Cardiac features	Pericarditis
	Myocarditis
	Endocarditis
	Coronary arteritis
Pulmonary features	Pleuritis
	Fibrosis
	Nodules
Ocular features	Conjunctivitis
	Scleritis
	Scleromalacia performans
Nervous system features	Polyneuritis
	Mononeuritis multiplex
	Compression neuropathy
	Cerebritis
Digital vasculitis	
Skin ulceration	
Splenomegaly	
Lymphadenopathy	

nized in rheumatoid arthritis, so that many rheumatologists prefer to speak of "rheumatoid disease." The commonest extra-articular feature (Table 19–2) is the rheumatoid nodule. Nodules occur most commonly on the extensor surface of the forearm but may appear in the lungs, heart, and sclera and along nerve sheaths, causing local manifestations. Histologically, the nodules consist of a central area of necrosis surrounded by mononuclear cells, particularly macrophages, arranged in palisades and enveloped in a layer of granulation tissue with lymphocytes and plasma cells. Extra-articular features may also result from vasculitis due to immune complex deposition in the various organs including skin, nerves, and blood vessels. The kidney is not usually affected in rheumatoid arthritis. Extra-articular features are associated with more severe disease and higher titers of rheumatoid factor.[27]

Laboratory manifestations in rheumatoid arthritis include a normochromic, normocytic anemia, elevated platelet count and sedimentation rate, and hypergammaglobulinemia. Leukopenia is seen in patients with rheumatoid arthritis and hypersplenism (Felty's syndrome). Rheumatoid factor is an anti-immunoglobulin and is detected in the sera of 75 to 80 per cent of patients with rheumatoid arthritis, usually by means of the latex fixation test. Other antibodies such as antinuclear factor occur in 20 per cent of patients

and more often in patients with Felty's syndrome, who also demonstrate positive lupus erythematosus (LE) cell preparations. Synovial fluid analysis reveals an inflammatory exudate with polymorphonuclear cells and lymphocytes. The fluid has poor viscosity and a low complement level, and rheumatoid factor may be detected. Radiographs may reveal soft tissue swelling; osteoporosis, often in a juxta-articular distribution; marginal erosions; joint space narrowing; and, in severe cases, subluxation or ankylosis. The cervical spine may be involved, showing atlantoaxial subluxation and clinically causing cord compression. Pathologic findings in the joints reveal lining cell hyperplasia and a mononuclear cell infiltrate. In more advanced disease the synovial membrane has villous projections with lymphoid "nodules" and pannus formation.[20]

The diagnosis of rheumatoid arthritis is based on the clinical and laboratory features outlined previously. The American Rheumatism Association has devised a group of criteria for the diagnosis of rheumatoid arthritis. The presence of certain criteria allows the diagnosis of classic, definite, or possible rheumatoid arthritis. A long list of exclusions helps avoid a misdiagnosis.[54]

Effect of Pregnancy on Rheumatoid Arthritis

Hench first noted the marked improvement in rheumatoid disease in 33 of 34 pregnancies occurring in 20 patients with rheumatoid arthritis.[31] There have been no prospective studies of rheumatoid arthritis during pregnancy, but the tendency of patients with rheumatoid arthritis to improve during pregnancy has been confirmed by several retrospective reports.[23] Persellin reported his own experience and reviewed the literature and concluded that 203 of 274 pregnancies in patients with rheumatoid arthritis (74 per cent) were associated with some degree of improvement.[51] In the majority of patients improvement occurred in the first trimester, and an additional group experienced improvement in the second and third trimesters. Remission in one pregnancy often indicates that a similar remission may be expected in subsequent pregnancies. Most patients who improve during pregnancy will experience a relapse between six weeks and six months post partum.[45]

There are reports of patients who show no improvement in their joint symptoms or who experience exacerbations or progression of rheumatoid arthritis during pregnancy. Furthermore, some patients experience the onset of their rheumatoid arthritis during pregnancy or in the immediate postpartum period.[21, 28, 47] A comparison between a group of 100 consecutive patients with rheumatoid arthritis during pregnancy and an equal number of nonpregnant women with a similar disease revealed no significant differences between the two groups with regard to functional capacity, disease activity, peripheral erosive arthritis, ESR, and hemoglobin. A smaller percentage of the pregnant women had a positive test for rheumatoid factor. The authors concluded that rheumatoid arthritis was not adversely affected by pregnancy and that rheumatoid arthritis was not an indication for therapeutic abortion.[48]

Effect of Rheumatoid Arthritis on Pregnancy

This aspect of the relationship between rheumatoid arthritis and pregnancy has not been thoroughly investigated. However, Kaplan and Diamond suggest that rheumatoid arthritis has no significant effect on the patient's ability to have a normal pregnancy, delivery, and infant.[35] Morris collected data on 34 pregnancies in 17 patients that indicated low abortion rates and few obstetrical complications.[44]

Mechanism of Improvement of Rheumatoid Arthritis During Pregnancy

The exact mechanism for the amelioration of rheumatoid arthritis during pregnancy is still unclear. It was initially thought that it was mediated by the increase in blood cortisol level during pregnancy.[31, 53] However, several studies have shown that steroids alone could not fully explain the improvement during pregnancy.[47, 71] There has been no correlation between the change in rheumatoid arthritis disease activity and plasma concentrations of corticosteroids.[58] Plasma cortisol levels return to normal within five days of delivery, yet the rheumatoid arthritis does not flare for four to six weeks post partum. In addition, plasma corticosteroids are for the most part transcortin bound and, therefore, not biologically active.[35] Other hormones have also been thought to play a role. Although estrogen and progesterone may be beneficial in suppressing the cell-mediated immune response, the use of the birth control pill in the treatment of rheumatoid arthritis has not been successful.[29] Infusion of plasma from pregnant women resulted in sudden improvement in 64 per cent of 28 patients with rheumatoid arthritis.[18] This was found to be nonspecific, as nonpregnant plasma infusions were equally effective.[34]

The effect of plasma focuses attention on the role of nonhormonal plasma constituents in pregnancy. As outlined earlier, pregnancy zone protein has a suppressive effect on the inflammatory activity of polymorphonuclear cells. The timing of improvement in rheumatoid arthritis parallels the rise in concentration of pregnancy zone protein during pregnancy. The lack of improvement noted in some 25 per cent of patients may be related to the women's inability to synthesize sufficient amounts of PZP.[45, 51] In addition, the cell-mediated immune response is altered during pregnancy, with increased suppressor cell function and decreased B cell response. These responses may counteract the depressed T suppressor cell function noted in rheumatoid arthritis and thus lead to decreased antibody production. This is further supported by the observation of a lower incidence of rheumatoid factor in pregnant women with rheumatoid arthritis compared with nonpregnant rheumatoid arthritis controls.[48] Further studies in this area are needed to elucidate the remission-inducing mechanism.

Treatment of Rheumatoid Arthritis

Since the cause of rheumatoid arthritis remains unknown, it is not possible to speak in terms of cure at the present time. It is, however, possible to control inflammation and thus relieve pain, restore function, and prevent deformities and damage resulting from persistent inflammation. To achieve these goals a combination of drug therapy, patient education, physiotherapy, and occupational therapy is used.[41]

The sequence of pharmacologic treatment modalities in rheumatoid arthritis is often presented schematically as a pyramid (Fig. 19–2).

SALICYLATES

The mainstay of drug therapy is salicylate. Although nonspecific, salicylates are excellent anti-inflammatory agents and serve to control rheumatoid inflammation. Regular medication in sufficient amounts is mandatory if anti-inflammatory effects are expected. Most patients require a dose of 3.6 to 4.0 gr of acetylsalicylic acid per day to achieve an adequate salicylate blood level of 20 mg %. Although a number of preparations are available, acetysalicylic acid is preferred. The fear of possible irregular or inadequate absorption when using these preparations

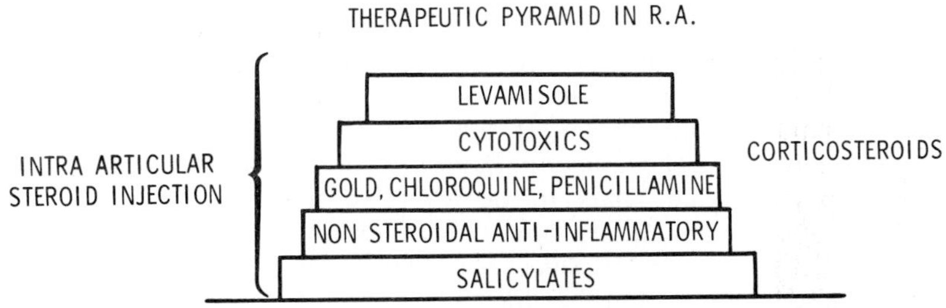

THERAPEUTIC PYRAMID IN R.A.

FIGURE 19–2. Pharmacologic treatment of rheumatoid arthritis.

INTRA ARTICULAR STEROID INJECTION

CORTICOSTEROIDS

LEVAMISOLE
CYTOTOXICS
GOLD, CHLOROQUINE, PENICILLAMINE
NON STEROIDAL ANTI-INFLAMMATORY
SALICYLATES

has been proved to be unfounded by several recent papers.[19, 24] Compared with other anti-inflammatory agents, the side effects of salicylates are minimal. Gastrointestinal complications (e.g., irritation) are common with uncoated preparations but are largely avoided by the use of enteric-coated preparations.[55] Salicylates interfere with platelet aggregation, but this rarely causes clinically significant bleeding. Salicylism (tinnitus and deafness) occurs at blood levels of around 25 mg % and is treated by decreasing the dose. These symptoms may be used as a gauge to achieve therapeutic levels when blood levels are unavailable.

Salicylates in Pregnancy. In general, aspirin is relatively safe in pregnancy. Two retrospective studies have shown an increased incidence of prolonged gestation, prematurity, longer labor, and greater blood loss during pregnancy and delivery as well as an increased incidence of anemia in women ingesting large amounts of aspirin during pregnancy. These effects are thought to result from aspirin's action as a prostaglandin inhibitor.[40] There have been reports of teratogenesis in animals but not in man.[35, 37, 57] There are rare reports of clotting defects in infants born to mothers taking salicylates during pregnancy.[22] Salicylates are known to cross the placenta and are also excreted in breast milk, but no serious effects have resulted.[53] Despite these hazards, salicylates are the drug of choice for treating arthritis during pregnancy.

Nonsteroidal Anti-Inflammatory Agents

These are the next line of agents used in arthritis when salicylates are insufficient to control inflammatory features. There are a number of medications available including the indole derivatives (indomethacin, tolmetin, sulindac) and the proprionic acid derivatives (ibuprofen, ketoprofen, naproxen).

Nonsteroidal Anti-Inflammatory Agents in Pregnancy. None of these medications have been adequately studied during pregnancy and are not recommended.

Disease-Suppressive Medications

These medications are used to control persistent joint inflammation unresponsive to salicylates and other nonsteroidal anti-inflammatory agents. In this group are included gold salts, antimalarials, and penicillamine.

Gold. Gold salts have been used for the treatment of rheumatoid arthritis since the late 1920s. There have been a number of controlled trials to show their efficacy in controlling rheumatoid inflammation.[73] The mechanism of action of gold is unclear, but there is evidence that it causes a reduction in titers of rheumatoid factor and in concentrations of other immunoglobulins. It also inhibits the phagocytic function of polymorphonuclear cells. Gold is given intramuscularly as weekly injections of 50 mg for a minimum of 20 weeks. When an improvement is noted, the frequency of injections may be reduced gradually to a maintenance dose of 50 mg once a month. Improvement is usually delayed until about 700 mg have been administered.

Gold is a potentially toxic drug. Its most common side effect is a skin rash, which is classically pruritic. Although gold has been continued in some patients with skin reactions, it should be discontinued in the face of severe reactions and particularly if mucous membranes are involved. Bone marrow suppression is an infrequent but worrisome complication, usually heralded by a drop in the platelet or hemoglobin levels or white cell count. These are, therefore, checked routinely before each injection is administered. Immune complex nephritis is another significant complication. Urinalysis is always reviewed for any evidence of proteinuria. The proteinuria is reversible upon discontinuation of the drug. Other rare reactions include colitis, lung toxicity, and hepatotoxicity. It has frequently been noted that patients who develop toxic reactions note a coincident remission of the arthritis.

Gold in Pregnancy. There have been some reports of successful treatment of pregnant women with gold without harmful effects.[21, 53] Gold is protein bound and presumably crosses the placenta poorly. Despite this apparent safe use and because rheumatoid arthritis frequently remits during pregnancy, it is safer to delay initiating gold therapy until after delivery.

Antimalarials. These agents have also been shown in controlled trials to be effective in rheumatoid arthritis and to compare favorably with gold therapy in early disease.[73] They have an advantage over gold in that they are given by mouth once a day and lack the renal and hematologic complications of gold therapy. Their major toxicity is gastrointestinal irritation and the ocular damage that results from their deposition in the retina. This appears to be dose related and is usually reversible, although there have been reports of persistent retinopathy.[73] In virtually all cases there is some chloroquine deposition in the cornea, which is of minor clinical significance and does not correlate with retinal deposits. Corneal deposits are not a contraindication to antimalarial therapy. Regular ophthalmologic examinations are recommended to detect early retinal toxicity, and antimalarial therapy should be stopped if any evidence of retinal toxicity is found. It is reported that hydroxychloroquine is associated with less toxicity than chloroquine sulfate.

Antimalarials in Pregnancy. Because chloroquine may cause chromosomal damage[46] and because there is evidence that these drugs are concentrated in the fetal uveal tract[63] and can cause retinopathy in the newborn, they are not recommended in pregnancy.

Penicillamine. This agent is a more recent addition to the armamentarium of antirheumatic medications.[33] It has recently been shown to be as effective as gold in the treatment of rheumatoid arthritis. It has a similar mode of action, with a delayed onset of response. It is thought to work by cleaving disulfide bridges and inhibiting collagen crosslinking. It has also been associated with a decrease in titers of rheumatoid factor. It is given orally as a 250 mg capsule. The initial dose is one capsule daily, to be increased slowly (at monthly intervals) to a dose of 500 to 750 mg per day. Side effects are similar to those of gold, and the same precautions apply, i.e., regular blood and urine examinations.

It has been shown that penicillamine may be effective in patients who have been gold resistant or who have had reactions to gold. Penicillamine and gold should not be administered simultaneously.

Penicillamine in Pregnancy. Although penicillamine has been used successfully in pregnancy in patients with Wilson's disease,[65] it does cross the placenta and theoretically may cause considerable harm to the fetus. In addition, because of the natural improvement in rheumatoid arthritis that may occur during pregnancy, it is advisable to withhold penicillamine until the end of gestation.

IMMUNOSUPPRESSIVE AND CYTOTOXIC MEDICATIONS

When the disease-suppressive medications either are inadequate to control disease activity or cause unacceptable side effects or toxic reactions, one may consider the next step in the therapeutic pyramid. There are basically two drugs in this group that have been extensively studied in rheumatoid arthritis, namely, azathioprine and cyclophosphamide.[64] Both have been shown to be effective in controlled trials. Cyclophosphamide appears to have more severe side effects than azathioprine. Both are bone marrow suppressive. Azathioprine has dermatologic and gastrointestinal side effects, whereas cyclophosphamide causes hemorrhagic cystitis. Both drugs predispose to infections and possibly to malignancy.

Immunosuppressive Medications in Pregnancy. These drugs should be avoided during pregnancy as they may be harmful to the fetus.

SYSTEMIC STEROIDS

Steroids are not indicated in the treatment of uncomplicated rheumatoid arthritis.[41] Although they are the best anti-inflammatory agents available, steroids have not been shown to alter the long-term course of rheumatoid arthritis. In fact, they may cause harm by masking the signs of joint inflammation, thereby allowing joint destruction to go unabated. Steroids have multiple side effects that preclude them from being used routinely in the treatment of rheumatoid arthritis. These reactions range from immediate effects, such as weight gain, "buffalo hump," thinning of the skin, striae, gastrointestinal irritation, and hypertension, to more delayed reactions such as diabetes, osteoporosis, cataracts, and predisposition to infections.

Systemic Steroids in Pregnancy. Many patients have been maintained on steroid therapy during pregnancy. However, there is a risk of adrenal suppression of the fetus, leading to hypogonadism in the newborn, and masculinization of a female infant has been described.[35] Since rheumatoid arthritis improves in most patients during pregnancy, oral steroids should rarely have to be used.

INTRA-ARTICULAR STEROIDS

This form of therapy is not associated with the severe side effects seen with systemic steroid administration and has been shown to be an effective way of controlling local joint inflammation.[32] It may be used at any phase of the disease management.

Intra-Articular Steroids in Pregnancy. Intra-articular steroid injections are a very useful therapeutic modality in pregnancy. Although some absorption into the systemic circulation does occur, this is related to the dose administered and is not of long-term duration.[38]

Delivery in Rheumatoid Arthritis

There have been no reports of particular obstetrical problems in pregnant women with rheumatoid arthritis. These may occur if there is significant hip involvement with the disease. The cervical spine may be involved, with atlantoaxial subluxation, and this may be a potential problem, with excessive flexion of the neck during anesthesia.

Family Planning

There is no evidence that rheumatoid arthritis adversely affects conception. Pregnancy in itself is not harmful to the mother or the baby, unless the added work related to the newborn and the emotional stress in the family prove to be too much for a particular patient. Therapeutic abortions are generally not indicated in pregnant women with rheumatoid arthritis.

SYSTEMIC LUPUS ERYTHEMATOSUS

Systemic lupus erythematosus (SLE) is a chronic systemic disease with diverse clinical and laboratory manifestations and a course characterized by its variability. The clinical manifestations result from inflammation of multiple organ systems, especially the joints, skin, kidneys, nervous system, and serous membranes. The disease tends to affect young women in the second, third, and fourth decades of life but may occur in any age group. Until recently, it was felt that SLE was an uncommon disease occurring in about 6 per 100,000 population. However, with the recent greater awareness of this disease, the more sensitive laboratory tests to diagnose it, and the widespread use of a number of medications known to precipitate lupus, it is now generally felt that a truer incidence is closer to 100 per 100,000. This would make SLE about one tenth as common as rheumatoid arthritis.

The current concepts of the pathogenesis of SLE suggest that it is an autoimmune disease with autoantibodies causing specific cytotoxic damage in some instances (hemolytic anemia, thrombocytopenia) and immune complexes leading to immune complex inflammation in other instances[104] (nephritis, dermatitis, central nervous system involvement) (see Table 19–3). One immune complex implicated in this mechanism is DNA anti-DNA, with the antibodies and, occasionally, the free antigen having been demonstrated in the serum[117] and anti-DNA antibody actually eluted from kidneys of patients with systemic lupus.[103]

The mechanism of excess autoantibody production and immune complex formation is not well understood, although current investigation is centered on abnormal regulator functions and the possibility of a slow virus infection[110, 114] (See Figure 19–1). In addition, certain genetic factors may be important, as indicated by a number of family and twin studies for SLE[76, 79] and the recent demonstration of an increased frequency of HLA DR 2 and 3 in patients with SLE.[96, 115] There are a number of medications that have been implicated in causing a lupuslike syndrome in some patients and inducing a number of autoantibodies without clinical disease in other patients. Drug-induced lupus is rarely associated with glomerulonephritis and frequently remits when the medication is stopped.[75] The families of drugs that have been implicated are antihypertensives (hydralazine and alpha methyldopa),[74, 99] cardiac medications (procainamide, quinidine), anticonvulsants (dilantin, phenobarbital),[123] and possibly oral contraceptive agents.

The major clinical manifestations present at some time during the course of SLE in four large series are listed in Table 19–3.

Skin lesions include a malar rash, various nonspecific erythemas, discoid lupuslike lesions, photosensitivity, and alopecia. Frank arthritis is also a very common manifestation and is generally nondeforming as compared with rheumatoid arthritis, which tends to lead to deformity. Clinical evidence of glomerulonephritis is found in over 50 per cent of cases, although if biopsies are done in all patients the incidence of some nephritis may be as high as 90 per cent. Histologically, four major types of glomerulonephritis are seen, namely, mesangial nephritis, focal proliferative nephritis, membranous nephritis, and diffuse proliferative glomerulonephritis. The prognosis

TABLE 19-3 CLINICAL MANIFESTATIONS OF SLE IN FOUR LARGE SERIES (%)

Manifestation	Lee et al. (110)	Harvey et al. (105)	Estes and Christian (150)	Dubois (520)
Skin lesions	86.3	85	81	71.5
Arthritis	61.8	90	95	91.9
Nephritis	49.0	65	53	46.1
Raynaud's phenomena	45.4	10	21	18.4
Neuropsychiatric features	40.0	—	59	25.5
Lymphadenopathy	40.0	—	36	58.6
Pleurisy	30.9	56	48	45.0
Mucous membrane ulceration	29.0	14	7	9.1
Pericarditis	24.5	45	38	30.5
Splenomegaly	10.0	15	18	9.0
Aseptic necrosis	8.2	—	7	5.0

seems to be somewhat better with mesangial and membranous glomerulonephritis and somewhat graver in the proliferative forms of glomerulonephritis. Central nervous system inflammation in SLE may present with neurologic or psychiatric manifestations or a combination of both. Neurologic manifestations include seizures, cranial neuropathies, cerebrovascular lesions, coma, intractable headache, and, occasionally, peripheral neuropathy. Psychiatric manifestations have included severe psychoneurosis, psychosis, and organic brain syndrome.

Clinical patterns of presentation are extremely varied. Patients may present with any combination of the aforementioned manifestations. Some common presenting states include the following:

1. Classic — butterfly rash, mucosal ulcers, leukopenia, etc.;
2. Pyrexia of unknown origin;
3. Arthralgia, arthritis, myositis;
4. Serositis;
5. Nephritis, nephrotic syndrome, hypertension;
6. Thrombocytopenia, leukopenia;
7. Psychosis, seizures.

Laboratory Manifestations

Patients with lupus will demonstrate evidence of hypergammaglobulinemia, the presence of a wide array of autoantibodies, and circulating immune complexes in their serum. Table 19-4 illustrates a number of the hematologic and serologic manifestations of systemic lupus in four large series. As can be seen, antinuclear antibodies are measured by the fluorescent antinuclear antibody test, and LE cells are seen in the majority of patients. Leukopenia and hypergammaglobulinemia are seen in about half the patients; rheumatoid factor, antiplatelet antibodies, Coombs' antibodies, and antibodies against cardiolipin, the Wassermann reagent, are less commonly seen.

Perhaps the most important autoantibody that presents in this disease, from a pathogenetic point of view, is anti-DNA antibody. The presence of this antibody is frequently correlated with disease activity and, specifically, with lupus nephritis. The appearance of the antibody is most specific when it is directed against native DNA rather than single-strand DNA. The test most commonly performed is a radioimmunoas-

TABLE 19-4 LABORATORY MANIFESTATIONS OF SLE IN FOUR LARGE SERIES (%)

Manifestation	Lee et al. (110)	Harvey et al. (105)	Estes and Christian (150)	Dubois (520)
ANF	88.8	—	87	—
LE cells	69.1	82	78	75.2
Leukopenia			—	—
5000	55.4	—	66	42.6
4000	41.8	—	—	—
Gammaglobulin 1.6 g %	44.2	—	77	61
RA latex	36.7	—	21	57
Thrombocytopenia	16.3	26	19	6.9
Coombs' positive anemia	13.6	—	—	—
False positive VDRL	8.3	15	24	10.9

say (Farr test), and the results are reported as a binding percentage of a given amount of radioactive DNA.

Depression of serum complement levels, measured as either total hemolytic complement or as levels of the third or fourth component of complement, is indicative of consumption by immune complexes. Again, a depressed complement level tends to correlate with disease activity, especially lupus nephritis. In the majority of patients, the presence of anti-DNA antibody and a low complement level may predict either the presence of disease activity or an impending flare.[117] However, a small number of patients may demonstrate this type of serologic activity and be clinically quiescent.[97] Only by observing the individual patient can one predict if there is concordance or discordance between serologic and clinical features. Once this is known, the appropriate therapeutic manipulation can be carried out.

American Rheumatism Association Criteria

To standardize the classification of systemic lupus among large series, a committee of the American Rheumatism Association has proposed a list of 14 criteria containing 21 items.[85] The presence of four of these manifestations of lupus correlates very highly with a clinical diagnosis of this disease state.

1. Facial erythema (butterfly rash)
2. Discoid lupus
3. Raynaud's phenomenon
4. Alopecia
5. Photosensitivity
6. Oral or nasopharyngeal ulceration
7. Arthritis without deformity
8. Positive LE preparation
9. Chronic false positive for syphilis
10. Profuse proteinuria (greater than 3.5 gm per day)
11. Cellular casts
12. Pleurisy or pericarditis
13. Psychosis or convulsions
14. Hemolytic anemia, leukopenia, or thrombocytopenia

Effect of Systemic Lupus Erythematosus on Fertility

Although SLE may influence pregnancy outcome, recent studies indicate that it does not affect the chances of conception. One large study from Mexico[92] reported that the fertility rate in patients with SLE was the same as that of the general population, confirming an earlier report in 1956.[93] In a recent study of 18 pregnancies, two women had been infertile.[122] In one woman, the infertility had preceded the diagnosis of SLE, yet, coincident with active disease, she had two subsequent pregnancies. In the second case, a normal pregnancy had ensued during active SLE and yet, after a seven year remission, secondary infertility had supervened.

In the same study failed contraception occurred in six women, in two using an intrauterine device, one after tubal ligation, one using a diaphragm alone, and two using a condom and spermicidal gel. Thus, the evidence to date would indicate that fertility rates are normal in patients with SLE.

Effect of SLE on the Pregnancy

ABORTIONS

The incidence of spontaneous abortions remains high in pregnant women with SLE, owing in part to the arteriolitis demonstrated in the decidua, perhaps causing interference with decidual-placental perfusion.[78] This was illustrated in a large review by Chesley, in which he reported on 126 spontaneous abortions in 613 uninterrupted pregnancies.[84] It has been suggested by both Chesley and Fraga et al. that it was not necessarily the presence of lupus nephritis that determined spontaneous abortions but rather the presence of active SLE.[84, 92] Thus, although SLE does not seem to significantly affect fertility, it does seem to significantly diminish the prospects of carrying a pregnancy to term.

Of course, in all large series of pregnant patients with SLE there will be a significant incidence of therapeutic abortions both for psychosocial reasons and for the treatment of an exacerbation of SLE. For example, in 24 pregnancies among 18 women in a recent study there were one spontaneous abortion and six therapeutic abortions, all for psychosocial reasons.[122]

PREMATURITY AND STILLBIRTHS

Because of the presumed decidual vasculitis with consequent compromise of maternal-fetal blood flow in pregnant women with SLE, a greater incidence of growth retardation in utero might be expected. Studies are conflicting, some indicating that the birth weight of infants born to SLE mothers was similar to that of infants born to women in the general population. In the report by Fraga et al., the mean birth weight for eight term infants was lower than normal.[92] An increased incidence of premature births in the offspring of patients with SLE has also been suggested.[125] In all large series there is a significant incidence of stillbirths.[84]

THE NEWBORN

Until recently, SLE patients were advised that if their pregnancies went to term, their newborns were at no greater risk than those of the general population for congenital abnormalities. However, this can no longer be considered universally true. Certainly, a number of offspring have been found to have transient serologic abnormalities,[81] skin lesions,[101] and congenital heart block.[82, 107, 118] So striking is the last association that it is now probably wise to evaluate all children born to mothers with SLE for congenital heart block, and, conversely, to investigate mothers of babies born with complete heart block for signs of SLE.

Effect of Pregnancy on SLE

The exacerbation of SLE by pregnancy has been reported as long ago as 1952.[89] In 1962, Garsenstein and associates reported the increased incidence of flares in SLE during the first 20 weeks of pregnancy and again in the first eight weeks post partum.[94] This could not be confirmed by Mund and colleagues in 1963.[112] However, in 1975, Zurier concluded that SLE patients frequently had exacerbations of disease activity either during pregnancy or in the early postpartum period.[125] In 1977, Grigor et al. reported an increased incidence of exacerbations, mainly in the puerperium.[98] However, in more recent reports dealing with patients both with mild disease and with disease under control before and during pregnancy, the incidence of flare-ups during and after the pregnancy has been significantly reduced. Thus, in the series by Tozman et al.[122] and Zulman et al.,[124] postpartum flare-ups were not a problem.

It has also been the experience of many[77, 124] that pregnancy sometimes leads to recrudescence of severe nephritis in lupus patients who are not sufficiently treated with steroids. However, in the review by Tozman et al.,[122] it was noted that renal disease did not recur during pregnancy in 11 of 18 patients who had had some evidence of lupus nephritis during the course of their illness. Again, the best prognosis will be found in those patients in disease remission at the onset of pregnancy.

TOXEMIA OF PREGNANCY VS. FLARE OF SLE

The onset of edema and hypertension in pregnancy in a patient with SLE gives rise to an important differential diagnosis of pre-eclampsia or flare-up of lupus nephritis. The former, of course, would be treated with very conservative means and the latter with more aggressive therapy. The occurrence of these manifestations in the absence of other signs of SLE and any serologic abnormalities would favor a diagnosis of pre-eclampsia. However, the presence of serologic abnormalities, such as a fall in serum complement, an elevated anti-DNA antibody level, or the presence of other systemic features of SLE would favor a diagnosis of lupus flare. This important clinical differentiation has recently been discussed by Zulman et al.[124]

THERAPEUTIC ABORTION

In the presteroid era it was common practice to terminate pregnancy in patients with active systemic lupus. However, with the recently reported successes of treatment of the active disease with corticosteroids, this practice has become less frequent. Patients are more apt to have inactive lupus at the onset of their pregnancy because of earlier diagnosis and more effective prepregnancy therapy. In addition, careful monitoring and early treatment of active disease during pregnancy have allowed the successful completion of the pregnancy without significant detriment to the mother or child in a larger number of cases. Another indication for therapeutic abortion in the past had been previous serious renal disease. However, as indicated previously, a recent study showed that a history of serious renal disease in the past need not be a contraindication to continuing a pregnancy.[122]

Several older reports have indicated a high incidence of disease exacerbation following a therapeutic abortion, occasionally leading to a fatal outcome.[111] In 1962, Donaldson and Alvarez reported 12 cases of therapeutic abortion, and in only one patient did the disease improve; 25 per cent died immediately after the abortion, and the others remained the same or became worse in the postabortal period.[86] The authors suggested that abortion should not be used as a therapeutic modality for systemic lupus. However, the recent study by Zulman and associates revealed no detrimental short- or long-term effects of therapeutic abortions in ten cases of pregnant women with SLE.[124]

Management of SLE and Pregnancy

PREPREGNANCY ADVICE

Ideally, the patient with SLE who is to embark on a pregnancy should be managed by both an internist-rheumatologist and an obstetrician. The consequences of the pregnancy on the lupus and of the lupus on the pregnancy and the infant should preferably be discussed in advance of the pregnancy, to a greater or lesser degree depending on the patient's interest and knowledge.

As previously stated, it is desirable that the lupus be inactive at the time that pregnancy is contemplated. The fewer drugs that are required the better in terms of the pregnancy. It would seem that prednisone has no adverse effects on the child and therefore should be used as necessary. Drugs such as chloroquine and cytotoxic agents are not recommended during pregnancy and should be discontinued several months prior to the undertaking of a pregnancy.

MONITORING DURING PREGNANCY

The pregnant patient with SLE should be seen by the internist and obstetrician with equal frequency. At these visits, signs and symptoms of an impending flare can be sought on history and physical examination, and blood samples can be drawn for serologic evaluation. As suggested previously, a rise in anti-DNA antibody titers and a fall in complement levels may predict an impending flare of SLE. It must be remembered that serum complement is an acute phase reactant and will rise somewhat in the normal pregnancy. Therefore, in a patient with SLE a falling complement may still be within the normal range but will have the same significance as a low complement in a nonpregnant patient. It is this change in complement value that must be monitored and therapy adjusted accordingly. There is currently no rationale for automatically increasing steroids in the postpartum period as prophylaxis against a postpartum flare.

SPECIFIC MEDICATIONS

Corticosteroids. Corticosteroid therapy is still the mainstay of treatment for patients with systemic lupus erythematosus. In general, the guiding principles should be to use as low a dose as necessary to control signs and symptoms of active disease and to wean the dose to the lowest possible maintenance level that does not allow a recurrence. In the past, there has been undue pressure to use very large doses of corticosteroid. Currently, when a flare is comprised primarily of nonmajor organ involvement such as rash, arthritis, and serositis one can use small to moderate doses in the range of 20 to 40 mg per day initially. With major organ involvement such as nephritis, central nervous system involvement, or vasculitis one may consider using larger doses of 40 to 80 mgs per day initially. If the patient has already been on a maintenance dose of prednisone from the onset of pregnancy, there is no need to automatically increase this dose if where are no changes in symptoms or laboratory values. In fact, on occasion, clinical disease actually improves during pregnancy and the corticosteroid dose may actually be lowered slightly. Again, it should be stressed that treatment with high dose corticosteroids during pregnancy does not seem to jeopardize the fetus.[90, 106] Prednisone has been associated with adrenal suppression in the infant of a mother who received corticosteroids during pregnancy.[113] However, in a recent study no such complication was observed.[122]

Other Nonsteroidal Anti-Inflammatory Drugs. The use of the nonsteroidal anti-inflammatory drugs may be sufficient when patients with SLE complain of arthralgias or myalgias during pregnancy. These, of course, should be used sparingly during the first trimester. These drugs have already been reviewed in the section on rheumatoid arthritis.

Antimalarials. The antimalarial drugs chloroquine and hydroxycholoroquine have been shown to be beneficial in treating some forms of skin rash in SLE and, perhaps, the systemic symptoms as well. Although these drugs have been used inadvertently during the first trimester of pregnancy with no adverse effects in some patients,[122] they are not advised during pregnancy.

Cytotoxic Drugs. The immunosuppressive cytotoxic drugs, specifically azathioprine and cyclophosphamide, have been proposed as potential steroid-sparing drugs in systemic lupus erythematosus. Although there is still controversy in the literature as to whether they have any beneficial effects their use remains widespread. Despite the known teratogenicity of these agents, there are a number of reports of patients receiving such drugs throughout a successful pregnancy.[108, 119, 121] Nevertheless, it would be advisable for these drugs to be discontinued prior to the undertaking of pregnancy. Should a patient become pregnant and require these medications for control of disease, she would have to weigh the very slight chance of teratogenicity against the desire for a baby and make an individual decision.

Delivery

In general, the decision with regard to the type of delivery should be obstetrical. Most patients with systemic lupus can deliver successfully vaginally. However, a recent paper[122] reports a high incidence of cesarean section in women with SLE. This can, in part, perhaps be explained by the fact that these patients are looked after by specialists, usually in university centers, and therefore any concern for maternal or fetal safety might more likely result in surgical delivery. Corticosteroid supplementation should be given to cover the labor or cesarean delivery in patients currently receiving steroids or who have recently been treated with these drugs.

Breast Feeding

The potential problems raised by breast feeding involve its possible effect on the systemic lupus erythematosus disease process and the possible transmission of medications through the milk to the infant. There is really no evidence that the hormonal release caused by suckling has any significant effect on the lupus disease activity; however, it is well known that postpartum flares in SLE can occur. Their correlation with breast feeding has not been studied. Breast feeding also demands time and energy of the mother, and this might lead to undue fatigue in some patients. In general, if one is considering only the effect on disease activity, the decision regarding breast feeding should be left up to the mother, giving encouragement for either decision made.

There is little evidence regarding the transmission of medication in the milk of humans. In animals there is some evidence that cortisone may be transmitted through breast milk.[109] Thus, if significant amounts of corticosteroids or cytotoxic or other disease-suppressive medications are required to control disease activity, it would probably be wise not to breast feed.

Family Planning

CONTRACEPTION

There is still significant controversy regarding the role of oral contraceptives in inducing sys-temic lupus erythematosus. The controversy was sparked in 1968 when Schleicher reported the development of a positive LE prep in ten healthy women taking oral contraceptives.[116] Some vague symptoms compatible with a systemic disease occurred as well. After discontinuation of the oral contraceptives, the tests became negative. Two women rechallenged later again developed a positive test. In the same year, however, a study of 3,014 women on "the pill" revealed the incidence of rheumatic disease to be no greater than that in the general population.[95] In the same year, Dubois and associates could not find these autoantibodies in 30 patients taking the contraceptive medication.[87] On the other hand, Bole et al. in 1969 reported rheumatic symptoms and serologic abnormalities in eight young women taking oral contraceptives.[80] All developed a positive LE prep and antinuclear antibodies, which reverted to negative when the drug was discontinued.

In 1971, Chapel and Burns reported two patients with mild systemic lupus erythematosus after taking oral contraceptives whose symptoms improved after the drug was discontinued.[83] I have seen flares in SLE in women with the disease precipitated by the use of these drugs.

Furthermore, there is evidence of increased incidence of thrombosis, vasculitis, and hypertension in women using these medications, and therefore for all of these reasons it is appropriate to encourage patients with SLE to employ other methods of contraception.

Some patients using the IUD complain of dysmenorrhea and recurrent infections, especially those taking prednisone and cytotoxic drugs. This may force discontinuation of this method of contraception and leave other methods of birth control such as the diaphragm, condom, and spermicidal preparation, preferably in combination, as the methods of choice for these women.

GENETIC COUNSELLING

Although it was initially stated that the incidence of SLE in families is no greater than the incidence in the general population, this is no longer felt to be true. Dubois, in a discussion of a paper by Stastny,[120] reported first degree relatives of patients with systemic lupus erythematosus to have an incidence of SLE of 12.8 per cent.

In addition, there is now accumulating evidence that specific HLA-D typing reveals a D locus of DR 2 or 3 as being more common in patients with SLE than in the general population.[97, 115] This again would suggest an increased familial incidence. Although it is prudent to discuss this potentially slightly increased incidence at the present time, most people would feel that this slight degree of increase is not sufficient to advise against pregnancy.

SCLERODERMA
(Progressive Systemic Sclerosis)

Progressive systemic sclerosis (PSS) is an uncommon connective tissue disease of unknown etiology, manifested by fibrosis and degenerative vascular changes in the skin, joints, and many internal organs.[136] The disease has a global distribution, with a reported incidence of 2 to 12 cases per million people per year, affecting females three to four times more frequently than males. PSS may occur at any age, but most patients present between 30 and 50 years.

The pathology of early lesions of PSS often manifests a mononuclear cell infiltrate. Serologic abnormalities are common in this disease, and there is occasionally an association with other autoimmune diseases. These factors have suggested that immunologic factors participate in the pathogenesis of PSS. On the other hand, the main pathologic lesion found in established PSS is a vascular lesion consisting of concentric proliferation of the intima and fibrosis of the adventitia of small arteries and arterioles.[134] This has led to the hypothesis that an unknown agent initiates the mononuclear inflammatory response around small arteries, leading to marked fibroblastic proliferation, which in turn results in the severe sclerosis of the small arteries and interstitium. This process leads to tissue induration and vascular insufficiency, which underlie the clinical features of this disease.[126]

The most common feature of PSS is Raynaud's phenomenon, which often precedes the other clinical features by many years. Skin involvement often presents with edema, followed by induration. The skin later becomes tight and bound down (sclerodactyly), with resultant contractures. This may be associated with hyperpigmentation and ulcerations, particularly over bony prominences. Telangiectasia (dilated blood vessels) commonly occurs on finger tips, lips, tongue, and face. Calcification in the soft tissues (calcinosis) may develop in patients with long-standing disease. Many patients present with polyarthralgia, and small effusions are occasionally detected. Tendon "rubs" have been described. Muscle involvement may develop, ranging from noninflammatory myopathy to a frank

myositis. Dysphagia is a frequent manifestation of the esophageal motility abnormality, which occurs in a large proportion of patients with PSS. Esophageal involvement may lead to esophagitis and may result in strictures. Intestinal motility disorders associated with diarrhea and malabsorption may occur. Myocardial fibrosis may lead to significant myocardial insufficiency, arrhythmias, cardiomyopathy, and sudden death. The pericardium may also be involved. Dyspnea often signifies pulmonary fibrosis or the onset of pulmonary hypertension.

Renal involvement is a major cause of death in scleroderma. It is typically manifested with the abrupt onset of malignant hypertension, leading to rapidly progressive renal insufficiency. Renal disease and pulmonary hypertension in PSS are the more ominous prognostic signs of this disease.

Laboratory manifestations of PSS include an anemia, which is usually normochromic normocytic, but in cases of rapidly progressive renal failure a microangiopathic hemolytic anemia occurs with a high frequency. Many patients have an elevated sedimentation rate, and hypergammaglobulinemia is common. Antinuclear antibodies occur in 30 to 90 per cent of patients with PSS. These commonly give a speckled pattern on subsequent staining. Elevated peripheral renin activity levels have been found in PSS patients even without clinically apparent renal disease.

The course of the disease is quite variable. Patients with the CREST variant (calcinosis, Raynaud's phenomenon, esophageal involvement, sclerodactyly, and telangiectasia) are thought to have a more benign disease with better prognosis. Pulmonary hypertension and renal disease are indicators of more severe disease and carry a grave prognosis. The diagnosis of PSS is based on the clinical manifestations. The American Rheumatism Association has recently devised preliminary criteria for the diagnosis of systemic sclerosis,[135] determining proximal scleroderma as a major criteria and sclerodactyly, digital pitting scars, and bibasilar pulmonary fibrosis as minor criteria, with one major or two minor criteria necessary for the diagnosis.

Effect of Pregnancy on Scleroderma

The association of PSS and pregnancy is unusual, first because scleroderma is a rare disease, and second because it often begins in the fourth or fifth decade, after the major childbearing years. There may be decreased fertility among patients with scleroderma.

A number of case reports suggest that scleroderma is unaffected by pregnancy.[136-139] However, Johnson et al. described onset or worsening of scleroderma in 14 of their 36 patients with concomitant scleroderma and pregnancy.[132] Analysis of an additional 18 case reports shows that eight pregnancies were associated with worsening of scleroderma.[133] Most authors agree that if scleroderma is rapidly progressive, with cardiac or renal disease, the effect of pregnancy may be serious, with sudden worsening of renal function and death.[130, 131, 139] In addition, esophagitis is often aggravated by pregnancy, and therapy including elevation of the head of the bed and ingestion of antacids is indicated.

Effect of Scleroderma on Pregnancy

Widespread sclerosis of the skin may make pregnancy difficult, but vaginal delivery can usually be accomplished without significant difficulty. Scleroderma tissue heals in a normal manner. Although Winkelman[139] and Johnson et al.[132] concluded that scleroderma had no adverse effect on pregnancy, the literature contains several reports of maternal deaths and fetal wastage.[130, 137, 138] Karlen and Cook point out that scleroderma can adversely affect the course of coexistent pregnancy.[133] Six of 17 patients had toxemia, and five perinatal deaths occurred. Most complications developed in the presence of renal scleroderma. It therefore appears that systemic sclerosis, particularly with major organ involvement (i.e., heart and kidneys), has an overall adverse effect on pregnancy and vice versa. There is no report of systemic sclerosis occurring in a newborn of a mother with this disease.

Treatment of PSS

There is no effective treatment for PSS. Current modes of therapy are aimed at suppression of the microvascular abnormalities and inhibition of the processes that give rise to overgrowth of collagen.[128, 136] Supportive measures include patient education, avoidance of exposure to cold, and the use of physical therapy designed to preserve hand function and minimize contractures.

There are a variety of pharmacologic agents used in the treatment of PSS. Antihypertensives such as reserpine and methyldopa and a variety of vasodilators have been used to control Raynaud's phenomenon. Corticosteroids have only a transient effect on the skin but may be useful in the treatment of the myositis. Other medications include para-aminobenzoate, D-penicillamine, and, more recently, colchicine. None of these medications has been uniformly beneficial. Other treatment modalities have included sympathectomy for Raynaud's phenomenon and antacids and metoclopramide for esophageal involvement. Patients with severe renal disease may require dialysis. There are promising reports on the successful use of the new antihypertensives in rapidly progressive sclerodermal renal disease and malignant hypertension.[127, 129]

TREATMENT DURING PREGNANCY

Most of the pharmacologic agents used in scleroderma have not been tried in pregnancy and should be avoided. In the presence of rapidly progressive cardiac or renal disease, immediate termination of pregnancy is recommended.[133]

GONOCOCCAL ARTHRITIS

In the past two decades there has been an alarming increase in the incidence of gonorrhea reported in both the United States and Canada. The majority of patients reported have been between the ages of 20 and 39. Concomitantly, numerous reports of gonococcal arthritis have appeared in the literature. The gonococcus seems to have a predilection for synovium, and during a septicemic phase gonococci not uncommonly settle in joints. Most cases of gonococcal arthritis occur in patients who are chronically infected, usually asymptomatically. Access to the blood stream and hence dissemination to joints seems to be facilitated by menstruation, pregnancy, pelvic surgery, and instrumentation of the urethra.

A number of different clinical forms of gonococcal arthritis have been described in the literature, and there is controversy as to whether they are distinct presentations or merely stages in the same process. A recent report by Fam et al. describes three stages of gonococcal arthritis.[140] In the first, or bacteremic, stage the patient may present with fever, chills, skin lesions, polyarthralgia, tenosynovitis, and, occasionally, conjunctivitis and electrocardiographic changes. The joint involvement is frequently only a migratory arthralgia, and may be associated with tenosynovitis, usually over the wrist or ankle region. Skin lesions may be few and may be easily missed if the patient is not thoroughly examined. They begin as erythematous papules, develop hemorrhagic centers or blisters, and occasionally break down and exude pus. During this phase of gonococcal arthritis blood cultures and cultures of the cervix are positive, but synovial fluid cultures are invariably negative.

The second stage of gonococcal arthritis, termed the septic joint stage, presents with localization of the infection in a few joints. The patient may present with pain and gross swelling in an oligoarticular pattern. During this phase blood cultures are almost invariably negative. Cervical cultures are positive, and cultures of the synovial fluid, if properly handled on appropriate media, are positive. During this phase there is a pronounced leukocytosis in the synovial fluid, and synovial fluid white counts exceeding 100,000 are occasionally seen.

The third stage of gonococcal arthritis is the stage of residual deformity and need not be seen in this day and age. Gonococcal infection left untreated will cause cartilage destruction and significant secondary degenerative arthritis.

Gonococcal Arthritis in Pregnancy

As mentioned previously, pregnancy seems to be a common predisposing factor for gonococcal arthritis. Taylor et al. reported that 30 of 103 patients with gonococcal arthritis were pregnant at the time of diagnosis.[143] In another study of 50 female patients with gonococcal arthritis, 28 per cent were pregnant at the time of onset of articular symptoms.[142] The onset of the gonococcal arthritis tends to occur in the last trimester. The reason for this apparent increased incidence of gonococcal arthritis in pregnant women with latent gonococcal infection is unclear. The increased vascularity of the genital organs may be partly responsible for dissemination.

The major differential diagnoses include acute rheumatic fever and Reiter's syndrome in the acute bacteremic phase and acute gout or septic arthritis in the septic stage of the disease. A specific diagnosis can be made by the findings of a typical clinical picture and positive blood cultures, cervical cultures, or cultures of skin lesions during the bacteremic phase and specific joint cultures during the septic joint stage.

If the clinical picture is compatible and joint fluid or other blood and cervical cultures have been taken, therapy should be instituted.

Patients should be hospitalized to receive an initial course of parenteral therapy for gonococcal arthritis. There is still some controversy as to the exact therapeutic program required to eradicate gonococcal arthritis. Classically, 8 to 10 million units per day of penicillin G given parenterally is indicated. However, Garcia-Kutzbach et al. recently showed that the administration of procaine penicillin G in divided intramuscular doses totaling 1.2 to 2.4 million units per day for 10 to 14 days appeared to be effective.[141] Fortunately, most species of gonococci remain sensitive to penicillin, and this drug remains the drug of choice.

It is seldom necessary to surgically drain an infected joint, but repeated aspirations of a joint that reaccumulates fluid are helpful in hastening the resolution. There seems to be no indication for therapeutic abortion when gonococcal arthritis is present, nor is there evidence that the fetus is adversely affected by the infection or its treatment.

THE CARPAL TUNNEL SYNDROME

The carpal tunnel syndrome is probably the commonest of the entrapment neuropathies. It is important to understand the anatomy of the carpal tunnel to understand the pathophysiology of this clinical syndrome. The palmar surface of the carpal tunnel has at its medial border the pisiform bone and the hooklike process of the hamate and at its lateral border the tubercles of the scaphoid and the trapezium. These borders are joined by the flexor retinaculum, thus creating a fibro-osseous carpal tunnel. Through this closed space traverse the median nerve and the flexor tendons as they enter the hand. The volume of the carpal tunnel is at its maximum with the wrist in a few degrees of flexion and is reduced in size at the extremes of flexion and extension.

Any factor that reduces the size of the carpal tunnel or increases the volume of its contents will increase the pressure within the canal. Common precipitating factors are strenuous or repetitive use of the wrist and a number of infiltrative conditions such as myxedema, amyloidosis, rheumatoid arthritis, and pregnancy.

Symptoms consist of numbness and tingling in the median nerve distribution in the hand and pain in the hand and wrist, occasionally radiating back up the forearm and characteristically coming on during the night. This forces the patient to sit up and shake the hands to try to relieve the discomfort.

The diagnosis is usually easy to make by history alone. On examination there may or may not be signs of neurologic impairment over the distribution of the median nerve. One can frequently aggravate the pain by performing Tinel's maneuver — that is, compressing the median nerve with a percussion hammer.

Carpal Tunnel Syndrome and Pregnancy

Because of the associated fluid retention during pregnancy, carpal tunnel symptoms do occur. When the symptoms develop during pregnancy, conservative therapy is indicated, as invariably the symptoms will abate with delivery. Conservative therapy includes wrist splints to immobilize the wrist, especially at night. Occasionally, diuretics used sparingly will be helpful. If these conservative modalities still do not give relief of discomfort, then a small dose of local steroid can be injected into the carpal tunnel. Decompression of the tunnel by surgical release is virtually never required when pregnancy is the etiologic factor.

SERONEGATIVE SPONDYLOARTHROPATHIES

The diseases included in the group of seronegative spondyloarthropathies have been distinguished from rheumatoid arthritis by the absence of rheumatoid factor, hence the term seronegative. The group includes classic ankylosing spondylitis as the prototype as well as Reiter's disease, psoriatic arthritis, the arthritis of ulcerative colitis and Crohn's disease (enterocolitic arthropathies), and Behçet's syndrome.[148] In the past two decades it has become clear that these diseases are distinct clinical entities but with closely interlinked clinical manifestations. As a group these diseases share several articular and nonarticular manifestations, although the distinction of a particular disease is possible in most cases. The common articular features of the seronegative arthropathies include sacroiliitis, spondylitis, seronegative polyarthritis, and dactylitis.

Sacroiliitis presents as low back pain of inflammatory character, that is, pain that is aggravated by rest and improves with activity, associated with significant stiffness and, often, early morning pain. Radiographs show evidence of sacroiliitis in the form of erosions, sclerosis, and, in advanced cases, total ankylosis with loss of joint contour. The involvement tends to be symmetric in classic ankylosing spondylitis and often unilateral in Reiter's disease and psoriatic arthritis.

Spondylitis, which is inflammation of the apophyseal joints of the spine, is common in this group of diseases. It is most severe in ankylosing spondylitis, presenting with low back pain of inflammatory character and leading to marked muscle spasm and, later, deformities. As the disease progresses ankylosis sets in. In ankylosing spondylitis the whole spine is affected, starting at the thoracolumbar junction and spreading up into the neck and down throughout the lumbar spine. In Reiter's disease, psoriatic arthritis, and the enterocolitic arthropathies, the spondylitis is not widespread and "skip" lesions are common. Radiographs demonstrate the classic syndesmophytes arising from the vertebral margins in ankylosing spondylitis with nonmarginal syndesmophytes in other entities.

Seronegative polyarthritis is a classically asymmetric form of inflammatory arthritis, often involving large joints as well as the distal intraphalangeal joints, which are commonly spared in rheumatoid arthritis. There is often a periosteal reaction, and ankylosis may occur.

Dactylitis is inflammation extending from the joint to involve part of or the whole digit and is a common feature among the diseases of this group.

The following extra-articular features of seronegative spondyloarthropathies may appear. A psoriasiform rash and nail changes are seen more frequently in patients with psoriatic arthritis and Reiter's disease than in those with classic ankylosing spondylitis. Ocular inflammation is one of the commonest manifestations in all seronegative diseases. The inflammation usually involves the uveal tract. Genitourinary inflammation is seen, particularly in Reiter's disease and ankylosing spondylitis. Buccal and genitourinary ulcerations are common in all entities of this group. Aortic insufficiency is seen most frequently in classic ankylosing spondylitis.

Another feature of this group of diseases is the strong familial aggregation, which occurs not only within each entity but also among the entities of the group. Further support for the distinction of these clinical entities as an interrelated group of disorders comes from the recent demonstration of a strong association between the HLA antigen B27 and several entities in this group (Table 19-5). A more appropriate designation for this group of diseases is, therefore, the B27 spondyloarthropathies. The discovery of the association with B27 may be relevant to the study of the etiology of these conditions.

One of the postulated etiologic factors in seronegative arthropathies is an infection, particularly with colonic bacteria. This has been supported in many cases by a history of a bowel or

TABLE 19–5 HLA B27 IN SERONEGATIVE
SPONDYLOARTHROPATHY

Disease Entity	B27 positive (%)
Ankylosing spondylitis	88–96
Reiter's disease	63–90
Enteropathic spondylitis	50–75
Psoriatic spondylitis	41–100

genitourinary tract infection preceding the onset of the spondyloarthropathy. Recently, there have been observations on the similarity between the molecular structures of certain colonic bacteria and certain aspects of the B27 antigen molecule.[144]

The diagnosis of seronegative arthropathy is made on the basis of the clinical features, both articular and extra-articular, and the radiologic evidence of sacroiliitis and spondylitis. Laboratory investigations are for the most part unhelpful except for the negative test for rheumatoid factor. The sedimentation rate is often not elevated, although it may be quite high in the presence of severe disease. Tissue typing may be helpful in the occasional difficult case.

With the exception of psoriatic arthritis, seronegative diseases are traditionally thought to be much more common in males than in females. The diagnosis of ankylosing spondylitis in women is often missed, perhaps because the disease is often milder in women.[146]

Seronegative Disease in Pregnancy

There are very few reports on the association of seronegative diseases and pregnancy. Hart reported on 14 pregnancies in patients with ankylosing spondylitis.[145] He concluded that, although several patients said they were either improved or worse during pregnancy, there was no apparent change in the progress of the disease. Childbirth had little effect on the course of the disease. Similarly, Wright et al. found that pregnancy had little effect on the psoriatic skin lesions or psoriatic arthritis, although individual patients occasionally developed exacerbations at that time.[149]

Although the studies are few, it appears that seronegative diseases are again distinguished from rheumatoid arthritis by the lack of improvement during pregnancy and the lack of flares post partum. With the exception of a patient with severe hip and pelvic disease, patients with spondylitis do not have any difficulties with vaginal deliveries.

Treatment of Seronegative Diseases

The treatment of early seronegative disease is similar to that of rheumatoid arthritis, namely control of inflammation. Enteric-coated salicylate is the drug of choice, but the seronegative diseases are commonly resistant to salicylate therapy. Other medications, particularly indomethacin and phenylbutazone, appear to be more specific for these conditions. As indicated earlier, phenylbutazone is not recommended for long-term use, and therefore, indomethacin becomes the drug of choice. This medication is ulcerogenic and may cause CNS manifestations when used in high doses. The use of tolmetin has recently been suggested in an attempt to overcome some of the side effects of indomethacin. It is seldom necessary to use other medications in the seronegative diseases. There have been very severe cases of Reiter's disease that required steroid therapy and immunosuppressive and/or cytotoxic therapy. Similarly, the use of gold or chloroquine therapy has been studied in severe psoriatic arthritis, with encouraging results. Methotrexate has also been used in the treatment of psoriatic arthritis,[147] particularly when severe skin involvement occurs simultaneously. The use of all these medications in pregnancy has already been discussed.

An important aspect of treatment in seronegative diseases, particularly of sacroiliitis and spondylitis, is physical therapy with the appropriate exercise program. Postural and breathing exercises are particularly important for the pregnant woman with this condition.

MECHANICAL BACK PAIN IN PREGNANCY

Back pain is a very common complaint during pregnancy. The majority of patients with back pain do not suffer from the inflammatory back disorders described previously, but rather from mechanical causes. Hyperextension of the lumbar spine is commonly associated with pregnancy. This is exaggerated by the weight gained during gestation and its distribution in the pelvis and abdomen. The diagnosis may be confirmed by assessing the distance between L_4 and S_1 spinal processes when the patient rises from full flexion to full extension of the back. If the distance between the two landmarks becomes fixed before the patient has reached full extension, then she tends to walk in hyperextension. This can be dealt with by pelvic tilt exercises.

Uterine compression on the pelvic wall may

lead to back pain, particularly in the later stages of pregnancy. Rest is of definite benefit. The patient should be instructed to lie on her side with the knees drawn up (fetal position).

Discogenic pain with or without nerve root irritation is another cause of mechanical back pain during pregnancy. This usually presents as severe pain, acute in onset, that is aggravated by coughing and sneezing as well as by standing and walking. When there is nerve root irritation the sciatic nerve is usually involved, and the pain radiates down the lateral aspect of the leg. In severe cases reflex changes may occur. Treatment should be conservative with bed rest as the mainstay of therapy. The patient should rest with the knees flexed or in the fetal position while lying. Mild analgesia may be indicated. Heat and massage may be helpful after the initial severe pain is relieved. For all these mechanical causes of pain, abdominal strengthening exercises should be done post partum.

POLYMYOSITIS/DERMATOMYOSITIS

Polymyositis is a diffuse inflammatory disease of striated muscle with an estimated incidence of 1 in 280,000. It affects females twice as often as males, with a peak incidence in the fifth and sixth decades of life. The etiology of polymyositis/-dermatomyositis (PM/DM) remains unknown, but there is evidence to support the role of immunologic factors in the pathogenesis.[55]

Clinically, PM/DM presents with symmetric proximal muscle weakness of variable intensity of either acute or gradual onset, with or without the typical dermatomyositis rash. The latter is a dusky erythematous eruption on the face, neck, and arms associated with a violaceous rash over the eyelids. Other skin manifestations include mucous membrane lesions, scaly lesions over the knuckles, bullous lesions, and exfoliative dermatitis. Raynaud's phenomenon is frequent. A mild arthritis occurs in about one third of the cases. Transient pneumonitis and pulmonary fibrosis may occur. Cardiac manifestations include rhythm and conduction disturbances. Myocardial inflammation has also been described. Dysphagia, abdominal pain, and, rarely, gastrointestinal hemorrhage may occur. Renal involvement is uncommon in PM/DM.[153, 158] Constitutional complaints may include fever, fatigue, and malaise. An association with malignancy is recognized.[152, 155, 156]

Laboratory manifestations include an elevated sedimentation rate, leukocytosis, and elevated muscle enzyme levels (creatine phosphokinase, SGOT, aldolase). Urinary creatine is elevated as well. Serologic abnormalities include positive rheumatoid factor and antinuclear factor in some patients. *Toxoplasma* antibodies have been detected in patients with polymyositis. Recently, an antinuclear antibody with a distinct specificity for polymyositis was described.[154, 159] Electromyographic studies reveal the triad of polyphasic short small motor unit potentials, fibrillation, and bizarre high frequency repetitive discharges. Muscle biopsy commonly shows primary degeneration of muscle fibers, basophilia and central positioning of the nuclei (regeneration), necrosis, and an inflammatory infiltrate.[151]

The diagnosis of polymyositis is based on the clinical features of muscle weakness with or without the rash, the enzyme elevation, and the typical EMG and biopsy findings.

There are very few reports of PM/DM occurring during pregnancy. This may be due to the rarity of this condition and to the fact that it most commonly presents after the childbearing period. There are 15 reported cases of pregnancy in patients with established PM/DM. In nine patients the disease was unaffected by pregnancy. The disease exacerbated during pregnancy in three instances and improved in another three. A high fetal mortality was noted. The two cases of PM/DM developing during the first trimester of pregnancy also resulted in fetal and neonatal death. In both cases, however, the disease remitted following delivery.[150, 157]

Although there is a paucity of cases, it appears that the disease may have an adverse effect on the pregnancy.

Treatment of PM/DM

In addition to supportive measures, including rest, physiotherapy, and analgesics, corticosteroids remain the drug of choice for this disease. The dose required is often high, 60 to 80 mg of prednisone per day. This therapy results in improvement in both the clinical and biochemical changes of this disease. The use of methotrexate and azathioprine has recently been reported and is usually reserved for refractory cases.[155] Corticosteroids have been used successfully during pregnancy.

THE VASCULITIC SYNDROMES

The group of the vasculitic syndromes comprises a broad spectrum of uncommon diseases

TABLE 19–6 CLASSIFICATION OF
VASCULITIDES

Polyarteritis nodosa group
Hypersensitivity angiitis
Wegener's granulomatosis
Giant cell arteritis
Arteritis of collagen disease or miscellaneous
  arteritis

resulting from inflammation and necrosis of blood vessels. This process may involve vessels of different types, sizes, and locations, characterized by various clinical manifestations with or without identifiable precipitating factors. Recognition and understanding of specific entities in this group have been difficult because of the confusion surrounding the classification of these disorders. The prevailing classification is still complex but is necessary not only for academic reasons but also to provide a rational basis for therapy. Table 19–6 lists the current classification of the vasculitides. Only polyarteritis nodosa and Wegener's granulomatosis will be discussed in detail, as there have been no reports of pregnancy occurring in combination with any of the other disorders.[162]

Polyarteritis Nodosa Group

The characteristic clinical manifestations are those of a systemic disease with multiple organ involvement, resulting from necrotizing angiitis of small and medium size muscular arteries, often in a segmental fashion. Patients present with fever, malaise, fatigue, myalgias, and arthralgias. Hypertension is common. Abdominal pain (resulting from intestinal infarction), mononeuritis multiplex, and evidence of coronary arteritis may be present. Hematuria and casts signifying renal involvement with either vasculitis or glomerulitis are frequent. Skin manifestations include subcutaneous nodules and purpuric rashes. Hepatitis may occur as a result of liver involvement with vasculitis or may be related to hepatitis B antigenemia. Other manifestations include epididymitis and involvement of the ovaries and other parts of the genitourinary tract.

Pathologically, the lesions consist of a leukocytic infiltrate, initially with polymorphonuclear cells and later with mononuclear cells, in the vessel wall. Intimal proliferation is followed by evidence of degeneration and necrosis of the vessel wall. Thrombosis, ischemia, and infarction give rise to the various clinical manifesta-

tions. Lesions in all stages of development are found simultaneously, and aneurysmal dilation is common. Anemia, eosinophilia, an elevated sedimentation rate, and hypergammaglobulinemia are commonly found as well as rheumatoid factor, antinuclear factor, and hepatitis B antigen and antibody. Immune complexes are thought to play a role in the pathogenesis of polyarteritis. One complex currently under investigation is the hepatitis B antigen–antibody complex.

The association of polyarteritis with pregnancy is rare, there having been only eight reported cases of polyarteritis and pregnancy.[161, 166, 167] Six of the cases resulted in maternal death, and every patient died in the postpartum period. Of the two patients who survived, one had limited disease and the other was the only one diagnosed and treated before conception. The fetal outcome, however, was good. It appears that termination of pregnancy is the precipitating event in polyarteritis. A change in hormone levels has been postulated, but no evidence is available to confirm this hypothesis. The development of polyarteritis in pregnancy may be confused with toxemia, but a fulminating diastolic hypertension in the presence of multisystem involvement should alert the clinician to the possibility of polyarteritis.

The treatment of choice of polyarteritis is high dose prednisone. There are recent reports suggesting that cytotoxic medications may be helpful, particularly in aggressive renal disease and hypertension.[163, 164] The use of both of these medications during pregnancy has been discussed. It seems that in the rare case of the association of pregnancy with polyarteritis a prompt diagnosis is important, together with prompt treatment and control of the disease. There seems to be no advantage in therapeutic termination of pregnancy.[166]

Wegener's Granulomatosis

This entity has a distinctive clinicopathologic complex of necrotizing granulomatous vasculitis of the upper and lower respiratory tracts, necrotizing glomerulonephritis, and a variable disseminated small vessel vasculitis. The clinical features include severe paranasal sinusitis, nasopharyngeal ulceration with nasal septal perforations and saddlenose deformity, and pulmonary infiltrates, occasionally with cavitation. Proteinuria, hematuria, and red cell casts with ensuing renal failure are the hallmark of generalized Wegener's granulomatosis. Skin involvement is common, with papules and ulcerations.

Coronary vasculitis and pancarditis, various ocular manifestations, and both cranial and peripheral nerve involvement occur in a large proportion of patients with this disease. Anemia, leukocytosis, hypergammaglobulinemia, and elevated sedimentation rate are characteristic laboratory features of Wegener's granulomatosis.[168]

There has been only one case report of pregnancy with Wegener's granulomatosis.[160] A 25 year old woman developed nasal symptoms; Wegener's granulomatosis was confirmed on biopsy, and she was successfully treated with radiation after initial corticosteroid therapy. Corticosteroids and azathioprine therapy were maintained through a fourth pregnancy, which resulted in the birth of a normal child. It appears that,

like polyarteritis, if the underlying disease is under control at the time of conception pregnancy has no deleterious effect on the disease and the disease has no adverse effect on the mother or the infant.

The treatment of Wegener's granulomatosis is based on adequate steroid therapy. There are several recent reports on the use of cytotoxic agents in this disease.[162, 165] Cyclophosphamide appears promising, for the renal manifestations in particular. Because of the paucity of cases, it is impossible to develop guidelines for treatment during pregnancy. However, since the disease may be otherwise fatal, the use of cytotoxic medications even during pregnancy may be indicated.

References

IMMUNE MECHANISMS

1. Anderson, R. H., and Monroe, C. W.: Experimental study of behavior of adult skin homografts during pregnancy. Am. J. Obstet. Gynecol., 84:1096, 1962.
2. Birkeland, S. A., and Kristoffersen, K.: Cellular immunity in pregnancy blast transformation and rosette formation of maternal T and B lymphocytes. A cross sectional analysis. Clin. Exp. Immunol., 30:408, 1977.
3. Birkeland, S. A., and Kristoffersen, K.: T and B lymphocytes during normal human pregnancy: A longitudinal study. Scand. J. Immunol., 10:415, 1979.
4. Birkeland, S. A., and Kristoffersen, K.: Lymphocyte transformation with mitogens and antigens during normal human pregnancy: A longitudinal study. Scand. J. Immunol., 11:321, 1980.
5. Clements, P. J., Yu, D. T. Y., Levy, J., and Pearson, C. M.: Human lymphocyte subpopulations: The effect of pregnancy. Proc. Soc. Exp. Biol. Med., 152:664, 1976.
6. Fujasaki, S., Mori, H., Sasaki, T., and Maeyama, M.: Cell mediated immunity in human pregnancy. Changes in lymphocyte reactivity during pregnancy and post partum. Microbiol. Immunol., 23:899, 1979.
7. Hemple, K. H., Fernandez, L. A., and Persellin, R. H.: Effect of pregnancy sera on isolated lymphocytes. Nature, 225:955, 1970.
8. Hsu, C. C. S.: Peripheral blood lymphocyte responses to phytohemagglutinin and pokeweed mitogen during pregnancy. Proc. Soc. Exp. Biol. Med., 145:771, 1974.
9. Jones, F., Curzon, P., and Gangas, J. M.: Suppressive activity of pregnancy plasma on MLR. J. Obstet. Gynecol. (Br.), 80:603, 1973.
10. Kay, D. R., Bole, G. G., and Ledger, W. J.: Antinuclear antibodies, rheumatoid factor and C-reactive protein in serum of normal women using oral contraceptives. Arthritis Rheum., 14:239, 1971.
11. Nelson, H. H. Jr., and Hall, J. E.: Studies on thymolymphatic system in man. I. Morphologic changes in lymph node in pregnant women at term. Am. J. Obstet. Gynecol., 90:482, 1964.
12. Persellin, R. H., and Leibfarth, J. K.: Studies on the effect of pregnancy serum on polymorphonuclear leukocyte function. Arthritis Rheum., 21:316, 1978.
13. Scultz, von B.: A qualitative study of the pregnancy zone protein in the sera of pregnant and puerperal women. Am. J. Obstet. Gynecol., 119:792, 1974.
14. Simmons, V. P.: Changes in the thymus during guinea pig estrus cycle. Ann. N.Y. Acad. Sci., 113:948, 1964.
15. Smith, J. K., Aspary, E. A., and Field, E. J.: Lymphocyte reactivity to antigens in pregnancy. Am. J. Obstet. Gynecol., 113:602, 1972.
16. Strelkauskas, A. J., Davies, I. J., and Dray, S.: Longitudinal studies showing alterations in the levels and functional response of T and B lymphocytes in human pregnancy. Clin. Exp. Immunol., 32:531, 1978.

RHEUMATOID ARTHRITIS

17. Adrianakos, A. A., Sharp, H. T., Person, D. A., Lidsky, M., and Duff, J.: Cell mediated immunity in rheumatoid arthritis. Ann. Rheum. Dis., 36:13, 1977.
18. Barsi, I.: A new treatment for rheumatoid arthritis. Br. Med. J., 2:252, 1947.
19. Baum, J.: Blood salicylate levels and clinical trials with a new form of enteric coated aspirin: Studies in rheumatoid arthritis and degenerative joint disease. J. Clin. Pharmacol., 10:132, 1970.
20. Baum, J., and Ziff, M.: Laboratory findings in rheumatoid arthritis. In McCarty, D. (ed.): Arthritis and Allied Conditions, 9th Ed. Philadelphia, Lea & Febiger, 1979, p. 491.
21. Betson, J. R., and Dorn, R. V.: Forty cases of arthritis and pregnancy. J. Int. Coll. Surg., 42:521, 1965.
22. Bleyer, W. A., and Breckenridge, R. T.: The effect of prenatal aspirin on newborn hemostasis. J.A.M.A., 213:2049, 1970.
23. Bulmash, J. M.: Rheumatoid arthritis and pregnancy. Obstet. Gynecol. Ann., 8:276, 1978.
24. Canada, A. T., Little, A. H., and Creighton, E. L.: The bioavailability of enteric coated acetylsalicylic acid. A comparison with buffered ASA in rheumatoid arthritis. Curr. Ther. Res., 19:554, 1976.
25. Christian, C. L., and Paget, S. A.: Rheumatoid arthritis. In Samter, M. (ed.): Immunological Diseases, 3rd Ed. Boston, Little, Brown and Co., 1978, p. 1061.
26. Cooke, D., Hurd, E. R., Jasin, H. E., Bienenstock, J., and Ziff, M.: Identification of immunoglobulins and complement in rheumatoid articular collagenous tissues. Arthritis Rheum., 18:541, 1975.
27. Decker, J., and Plotz, P. H.: Extra articular rheumatoid disease. In McCarty, D. (ed.): Arthritis and Allied Conditions, 9th Ed. Philadelphia, Lea & Febiger, 1979, p. 470.
28. Flebo, M., and Snorrason, E.: Pregnancy and the place of therapeutic abortion in rheumatoid arthritis. Acta Obstet. Gynecol. Scand., 40:116, 1961.
29. Gilbert, M., Rotstein, J., and Cunningham, C.: Norethynodrel with mestranol in the treatment of rheumatoid arthritis. J.A.M.A., 190:235, 1964.
30. Good, R. A., Rotstein, J., and Mozzitello, W. F.: The simultaneous occurrence of rheumatoid arthritis and aggamaglobulinemia. J. Lab. Clin. Med., 49:343, 1957.
31. Hench, P. S.: The amelioration effect of pregnancy on chronic atrophic (infectious) rheumatoid arthritis, fibrositis and intermittent hydrarthrosis. Proc. Mayo. Clin., 13:161, 1938.
32. Hollander, J. L.: Arthrocentesis and intrasynovial therapy. In

McCarty, D. (ed.): Arthritis and Allied Conditions, 9th Ed. Philadelphia, Lea & Febiger, 1979, p. 402.

33. Jaffe, A. I.: Penicillamine treatment in rheumatoid arthritis. In McCarty D. (ed.): Arthritis and Allied Conditions, 9th Ed. Philadelphia, Lea & Febiger, 1979, p. 368.

34. Josephs, C.: Observations on the treatment of rheumatoid arthritis by transfusions of blood from pregnant women. Br. Med. J., 2:134, 1954.

35. Kaplan, D., and Diamond, H.: Rheumatoid arthritis and pregnancy. Clin. Obstet. Gynecol., 8:286, 1965.

36. Keystone, E. C., Gladman, D. D., Buchanan, R., and Cane, D.: Impaired antigen specific suppressor cell activity in patients with rheumatoid arthritis. Arthritis Rheum., 23:1246, 1980.

37. Kimmel, C. A., Wilson, J. G., and Schumacher, H. J.: Studies on metabolism and identification of the causative agent in aspirin teratogenesis. Teratology, 4:15, 1971.

38. Koehler, B. E., Urowitz, M. B., and Killinger, D. W.: The systemic effect of intra-articular corticosteroid. J. Rheumatol., 1:117, 1974.

39. Lance, E. M., and Knight, S. C.: Immunologic reactivity in rheumatoid arthritis: Response to mitogens. Arthritis Rheum., 17:513, 1974.

40. Lewis, R. B., and Shulman, J. D.: Influence of acetylsalicylic acid, an inhibitor of prostaglandin synthesis, on the duration of human gestation and labour. Lancet, 2:1159, 1973.

41. Lightfoot, R. W.: Treatment of rheumatoid arthritis. In McCarty, D. (ed.): Arthritis and Allied Conditions, 9th Ed. Philadelphia, Lea & Febiger, 1979, p. 513.

42. Lockshin, M. D., Eisenberg, A. C., Kohn, R., Weksler, M., Block, S., and Mushlin, S. B.: Cell mediated immunity in rheumatic diseases. Arthritis Rheum., 18:245, 1975.

43. McDuffie, F. C.: Immune complexes in the rheumatic diseases. J. Allergy Clin. Immunol., 62:37, 1978.

44. Morris, W. K.: Pregnancy in rheumatoid arthritis and systemic lupus erythematosus. N.Z. J. Obstet. Gynecol., 9:136, 1969.

45. Neely, N. T., and Persellin, R. H.: Activity of rheumatoid arthritis during pregnancy. Texas Med., 73:59, 1977.

46. Neill, W. A., Panayi, G. S., Duthie, J. J. R., and Prescott, R. J.: Action of chloroquine sulfate in rheumatoid arthritis. II. Chromosome damaging effect. Ann. Rheum. Dis., 32:547, 1973.

47. Oka, M.: Activity of rheumatoid arthritis and plasma 17 hydroxycorticosteroids during pregnancy and following parturition. Acta Rheum. Scand., 4:243, 1958.

48. Oka, M., and Vainio, V.: Effect of pregnancy on the prognosis and serology of rheumatoid arthritis. Acta Rheum. Scand., 12:47, 1966.

49. Paget, S., and Gibofsky, A.: Immunopathogenesis of rheumatoid arthritis. Am. J. Med., 67:961, 1979.

50. Paulus, H. E., Machleder, H. I., Levine, S., Yu, D. T. Y., and MacDonald, N. S.: Lymphocyte involvement in rheumatoid arthritis. Studies during thoracic duct drainage. Arthritis Rheum., 20:1249, 1977.

51. Persellin, R. H.: The effect of pregnancy on rheumatoid arthritis. Bull. Rheum. Dis., 27:922, 1977.

52. Phillips, P. E., and Christian, C. L.: Infectious agents in chronic rheumatic disease. In McCarty, D. (ed.): Arthritis and Allied Conditions, 9th Ed. Philadelphia, Lea & Febiger, 1979, p. 320.

53. Plotz, C. M., and Goldenberg, A.: Rheumatoid arthritis. In Ravinsky, J. J., and Gutman, A. F. (eds.): Medical, Surgical and Gynecological Complications of Pregnancy. 2nd Ed. Baltimore, Williams & Wilkins Co., 1965, p. 720.

54. Rope, N. W., Bennet, G. A., Cobb, S., Jacox, R., and Jesson, R. A.: 1958 revision of diagnostic criteria for rheumatoid arthritis. Arthritis Rheum. 2:16, 1959.

55. Silvoso, G. R., Ivey, K. J., Butt, J. H., Lockard, O. O., Holt, S. D., Sisk, C., Baskin, W. N., MacKercher, P. A., and Hewett, J.: Incidence of gastric lesions in patients with rheumatic diseases on chronic aspirin therapy. Ann. Intern. Med., 91:517, 1979.

56. Sliwinski, A. J., and Zvaifler, N. J.: In vivo synthesis of IGG by rheumatoid synoviae. J. Lab. Clin. Med., 76:304, 1970.

57. Slone, D., Heinonen, O. P., Kaufman, D. W., Siskind, V., Momson, R. R., and Sharp, S.: Aspirin and congenital malformation. Lancet, 1:373, 1976.

58. Smith, W. D., and West, H. F.: Pregnancy in rheumatoid arthritis. Acta Rheum. Scand., 6:189, 1960.

59. Sokoloff, L.: Pathology of rheumatoid arthritis. In McCarty, D. (ed.): Arthritis and Allied Conditions, 9th Ed. Philadelphia, Lea & Febiger, 1979, p. 429.

60. Stastny, P., Rosenthal, M., and Andreis, M.: Lymphokines in rheumatoid synovitis. Ann. N.Y. Acad. Sci., 256:117, 1975.

61. Stastny, P.: Immunogenetic factors in rheumatoid arthritis. Clin. Rheum. Dis., 3:315, 1977.

62. Tenenbaum, J., Urowitz, M. B., Keystone, E. C., et al.: Leukapheresis in severe rheumatoid arthritis. Ann. Rheum. Dis., 38:40, 1979.

63. Ullberg, S., Lindquist, N. G., and Sjostrand, S. E.: Accumulation of chorioretinotoxic drugs in the fetal eye. Nature, 227:1257, 1970.

64. Urowitz, M. B.: Immunosuppressive therapy in rheumatoid arthritis. J. Rheumatoid., 1:364, 1974.

65. Walshe, J. M.: Pregnancy in Wilson's disease. Q. J. Med., 46:73, 1977.

66. Waxman, J., Lockshin, M. D., Schnapp, J. J., and Doneson, N.: Cellular immunity in rheumatic disease. Arthritis Rheum., 16:499, 1973.

67. Weissman, G.: Lysosomes and the mediation of tissue injury. In Muller, W., Harweth, H. G., and Fehr, K. (eds.): Arthritis, International Symposium on Rheumatoid Arthritis, Basel, 1971, Rheumatoid Arthritis Pathogenetic Mechanisms and Consequences in Therapeutics. New York, Academic Press, 1971, p. 141.

68. Williams, R. C. Jr.: Clinical picture of rheumatoid arthritis. In McCarty, D. (ed.): Arthritis and Allied Conditions, 9th Ed. Philadelphia, Lea & Febiger, 1979, p. 457.

69. Winchester, R. J., Angello, F., and Kunkel, H. G.: The joint fluid complexes and their relationship to intra-articular complement diminution. Ann. N.Y. Acad. Sci., 168:195, 1969.

70. Winchester, R. J.: Characterization of IgG complexes in patients with rheumatoid arthritis. Ann. N.Y. Acad. Sci., 256:73, 1975.

71. Wolfson, W. G., Robinson, W. D., and Duff, I. F.: Probability that increased secretion of oxysteroids does not fully explain improvement in certain systemic diseases during pregnancy. J. Mich. Med. Soc., 50:1019, 1951.

72. Yu, D. T. Y., and Peter, J. B.: Cellular immunological aspects of rheumatoid arthritis. Sem. Arthritis Rheum., 4:24, 1974.

73. Zvaifler, N. J.: Gold and antimalarial therapy. In McCarty, D. (ed.): Arthritis and Allied Conditions, 9th Ed. Philadelphia, Lea & Febiger, 1979, p. 355.

SYSTEMIC LUPUS ERYTHEMATOSUS

74. Alarcon-Segovia, D., Worthington, J. W., Ward, L. E., and Wakim, K. G.: Lupus diathesis and the hydralazine syndrome. N. Engl. J. Med., 272:462, 1965.

75. Alarcon-Segovia, D.: Drug-induced SLE and related syndromes. Clin. Rheum. Dis., 1:573, 1975.

76. Arnett, F. C., and Shulman, L. E.: Studies in familial systemic lupus erythematosus. Medicine, 55:313, 1976.

77. Bear, R.: Pregnancy and lupus nephritis. A detailed report of six cases with a review of the literature. Obstet. Gynecol., 47:715, 1976.

78. Benirschke, K., and Driscoll, S. G.: The Pathology of the Human Placenta. New York, Springer-Verlag, 1967, p. 464.

79. Block, S. R., Winfield, J. D., Lockshin, M. D., D'Angelo, W. A., and Christian, C. L.: Studies of twins with systemic lupus erythematosus. A review of the literature and presentation of 12 additional sets. Am. J. Med., 59:533, 1975.

80. Bole, G. G. Jr., Friedlander, M. H., and Smith, C. K.: Rheumatic symptoms and serological abnormalities induced by oral contraceptives. Lancet, 1:323, 1969.

81. Bridge, R. G., and Foley, F. E.: Placental transmission of the lupus erythematosus factor. Am. J. Med. Sci., 227:1, 1954.

82. Chameides, L., Truex, R. C., Vetter, V., Rashkind, W. J., Galioto, F. M., and Noonan, J. A.: Association of maternal systemic lupus erythematosus with congenital complete heart block. N. Engl. J. Med., 297:1204, 1977.

83. Chapel, T. A., and Burns, R. E.: Oral contraceptives and exacerbation of lupus erythematosus. Am. J. Obstet. Gynecol., 110:366, 1971.

84. Chesley, L. C.: Hypertensive disorders in pregnancy. New York, Appleton-Century-Crofts, 1978, p. 504.

85. Cohen, A. S., Reynolds, W. E., Franklin, E. C., Kulka, J. P., Ropes, M. W., Shulman, L. E., and Wallace, S. L.: Preliminary criteria for the classification of systemic lupus erythematosus. Bull. Rheum. Dis., 21:643, 1972.

86. Donaldson, L., and Alvarez, P. R.: Further observations on lupus erythematosus associated with pregnancy. Am. J. Obstet. Gynecol., 83:1461, 1962.

87. Dubois, E. L., Strain, L., Ehn, M., Bernstein, G., and Friou, G.: LE cells after oral contraceptives. Lancet, 2:679, 1968.

88. Dubois, E. L.: Lupus Erythematosus, A Review of the Current Status of Discoid and Systemic Lupus Erythematosus and Their Variants, 2nd Ed. Los Angeles, University of Southern California Press, 1974.

89. Ellis, F. A., and Bereston, E. S.: Lupus erythematosus associated with pregnancy and menopause. A.M.A. Arch. Dermatol. Syphilol., 65:170, 1952.

90. Estes, D., and Larson, D. L.: Systemic lupus erythematosus and pregnancy. Clin. Obstet. Gynecol., 8:307, 1965.

91. Estes, D., and Christian, C. L.: The natural history of systemic lupus erythematosus by prospective analysis. Medicine, 50:85, 1971.

92. Fraga, A., Mintz, G., Orozco, J., and Orozco, J. H.: Sterility and fertility rates, fetal wastage and maternal morbidity in systemic lupus erythematosus. J. Rheumatol., 1:293, 1974.

93. Friedman, E. A., and Rutherford, J. W.: Pregnancy and lupus erythematosus. Obstet. Gynecol., 8:601, 1956.

94. Garsenstein, M., Pollak, V. E., and Kark, R. M.: Systemic lupus erythematosus and pregnancy. N. Engl. J. Med., 267:165, 1962.

95. Gill, D.: Rheumatic complaints of women using anti-ovulatory drugs. J. Chronic Dis., 21:435, 1968.

96. Gladman, D. D., Terasaki, P. I., Park, M. S., Iwaki, Y., Louie, S., Quismorio, F. P., Barnett, E. V., and Liebling, M. R.: Increased frequency of HLA DRW 2 in SLE. Lancet, 2:902, 1979.

97. Gladman, D. D., Urowitz, M. B., and Keystone, E. C.: Serologically active, clinically quiescent SLE, a discordance between clinical and serological features of SLE. Am. J. Med., 66:210, 1979.

98. Grigor, R. R., Shervington, P. C., Hughes, G. R. V., and Hawkins, D. F.: Outcome of pregnancy in systemic lupus erythematosus. Proc. Roy. Soc. Med., 70:99, 1977.

99. Harth, M.: LE cells and positive direct Coombs' test induced by methyldopa. Can. Med. Assoc. J., 99:277, 1968.

100. Harvey, A. M., Shulman, L. E., Tumulty, A., Conley, C. L., and Schoenrich, E. H.: Systemic lupus erythematosus: Review of the literature and clinical analysis of 138 cases. Medicine, 33:291, 1954.

101. Jackson, R.: Discoid lupus erythematosus in a newborn infant of a mother with lupus erythematosus. Pediatrics, 33:425, 1964.

102. Kendall, M. J., and Hawkins, C. F.: Quinidine-induced systemic lupus erythematosus. Postgrad. Med. J., 46:729, 1970.

103. Koffler, D., Schur, P. H., and Kunkel, H. G.: Immunologic studies concerning the nephritis of systemic lupus erythematosus. J. Exp. Med., 126:607, 1967.

104. Koffler, D.: Systemic lupus erythematosus. Sci. Am., 243:52, 1980.

105. Lee, P., Urowitz, M. B., Bookman, A. A. M., Koehler, B. E., Smythe, H. A., Gordon, D. A., and Ogryzlo, M. A.: Systemic lupus erythematosus. A review of 110 cases with reference to nephritis, the nervous system, infections, aseptic necrosis and prognosis. Q. J. Med., 46:1, 1977.

106. McCombs, R. P., and Patterson, J. T.: Factors influencing the course and prognosis of systemic lupus erythematosus. N. Engl. J. Med., 260:1195, 1959.

107. McCue, C. M., Mantakas, M. E., Tingelstad, J. B., et al.: Congenital heart block in newborns of mothers with connective tissue disease. Circulation, 56:82, 1977.

108. McGee, C. D., and Makowski, E. L.: Systemic lupus erythematosus in pregnancy. Am. J. Obstet. Gynecol., 197:1008, 1970.

109. Mercier-Parot, L.: Disturbances in post-natal development of rats after maternal administration of cortisone during pregnancy or lactation. C. R. Acad. Sci., 240:2259, 1955.

110. Morimoto, C., Abe, T., and Homma, M.: Altered function of suppressor T lymphocytes in patients with active systemic lupus erythematosus — in vitro immune response to autoantigen. Clin. Immunol. Immunopathol., 13:161, 1979.

111. Morris, W. I. C.: Pregnancy in rheumatoid arthritis and systemic lupus erythematosus. Aust. N. Z. J. Obstet. Gynecol., 9:136, 1969.

112. Mund, A., Simson, J., and Rothfield, N.: Effect of pregnancy on course of systemic lupus erythematosus. J.A.M.A., 183:917, 1963.

113. Oppenheimer, E. H.: Lesions in the adrenals of an infant following maternal corticosteroid therapy. Bull. Johns Hopkins Hosp., 114:146, 1964.

114. Phillips, P. E.: Viruses and systemic lupus erythematosus. Bull. Rheum. Dis., 28:954, 1977–78.

115. Reinerstein, J. C., Klippel, J. H., Johnson, A. H., Steinberg, A. D., Decker, J. L., and Mann, D. L.: B-lymphocyte, alloantigens associated with systemic lupus erythematosus. N. Engl. J. Med., 299:515, 1978.

116. Schleicher, E. M.: LE cells after oral contraceptives. Lancet, 1:821, 1968.

117. Schur, P. H., and Sandson, J.: Immunologic factors and clinical activity in systemic lupus erythematosus. N. Engl. J. Med., 278:533, 1968.

118. Scott, J. S.: Systemic lupus erythematosus and allied disorders in pregnancy. Clin. Obstet. Gynecol., 6:461, 1979.

119. Sharon, E., Jones, J., Diamond, H., and Kaplan, D.: Pregnancy and azathioprine in systemic lupus erythematosus. Am. J. Obstet. Gynecol., 118:25, 1974.

120. Stastny, P.: HLA-D and Ia antigens in rheumatoid arthritis and systemic lupus erythematosus. Arthritis Rheum., 21:139, 1978.

121. Sztejnbok, M., Stewart, A., Diamond, H., and Kaplan, D.: Azathioprine in the treatment of systemic lupus erythematosus. Arthritis Rheum., 14:639, 1971.

122. Tozman, E. C. S., Urowitz, M. B., and Gladman, D. D.: Systemic lupus erythematosus and pregnancy. J. Rheumatol., 7:624, 1980.

123. Wilske, K. R., Shalit, I. E., Wilkens, R. F., and Decker, L.: Findings suggestive of systemic lupus erythematosus in subjects on chronic anticonvulsant therapy. Arthritis Rheum., 8:260, 1965.

124. Zulman, M. I., Talal, N., Hoffman, G. S., et al.: Problems associated with the management of pregnancies in patients with systemic lupus erythematosus. J. Rheumatol., 7:37, 1980.

125. Zurier, R. B.: Systemic lupus erythematosus and pregnancy. Clin. Rheum. Dis., 1:613, 1975.

SCLERODERMA

126. Campbell, P. M., and LeRoy, E. C.: Pathogenesis of systemic sclerosis: A vascular hypothesis. Sem. Arthritis Rheum., 4:351, 1975.

127. Clements, P., Furst, D., Zamad, E., Maxwell, M., and Paulus, H.: Clinical course of four patients with scleroderma renal crisis treated with captopril. Arthritis Rheum., 23:662, 1980.

128. D'Angelo, W. A.: Progressive systemic sclerosis: Management. Clin. Rheum. Dis., 5:263, 1979.

129. D'Angelo, W. A., Lopez-Ovejero, J. A., Saal, S. D., and Laragh, J. H.: Early versus late treatment of scleroderma renal crisis and malignant hypertension with captopril. Arthritis Rheum., 23:664, 1980.

130. Fear, R.E.: Eclampsia superimposed on renal scleroderma: A rare cause of maternal and fetal mortality. Obstet. Gynecol., 31:69, 1968.

131. Good, S. V., and Kohler, H. G.: Maternal death from systemic sclerosis. J. Obstet. Gynaecol. Br. Commonw., 77:109, 1970.

132. Johnson, T. R., Banner, E. A., and Winkelman, R. K.: Scleroderma and pregnancy. Obstet. Gynecol., 23:167, 1964.

133. Karlen, J. R., and Cook, W. A.: Renal scleroderma and pregnancy. Obstet. Gynecol., 44:349, 1974.

134. Mariq, H. R., and LeRoy, E. C.: Progressive systemic sclerosis: Disorders of the microcirculation. Clin. Rheum. Dis., 5:81, 1979.

135. Masi, A. for Subcommittee for Scleroderma Criteria of the American Rheumatism Association Diagnostic and Therapeutic Criteria Committee: Preliminary criteria for the classification of systemic sclerosis (scleroderma). Arthritis Rheum., 23:581, 1980.

136. Rodnan, G. P.: Progressive systemic sclerosis (scleroderma). In McCarty, D. (ed.): Arthritis and Allied Conditions, 9th Ed. Philadelphia, Lea & Febiger, 1979, p. 762.

137. Slate, W. G., and Graham, A. R.: Scleroderma and pregnancy. Am. J. Obstet. Gynecol., 101:335, 1968.

138. Spellacy, W. N.: Scleroderma and pregnancy. Obstet. Gynecol., 23:297, 1964.

139. Winkelman, R. K.: Scleroderma and pregnancy. Clin. Obstet. Gynecol., 8:280, 1965.

GONOCOCCAL ARTHRITIS

140. Fam, A., McGillivray, D., Stern, J., and Little, H.: Gonococcal arthritis: A report of six cases. Can. Med. Assoc. J., 108:319, 1973.

141. Garcia-Kutzbach, A., Dismuke, S. E., and Masi, A. T.: Gonococcal arthritis: Clinical features and results of penicillin therapy. J. Rheumatol., *1*:210, 1974.
142. Niles, J. H., and Lowe, E. W.: Gonococcal arthritis in pregnancy. Med. Ann. D.C., *25*:69, 1966.
143. Taylor, H. A., Bradford, S. A., and Patterson, S. P.: Gonococcal arthritis in pregnancy. Obstet. Gynecol., *27*:776, 1966.

SERONEGATIVE SPONDYLOARTHROPATHIES

144. Geczy, A. F., Seagar, K., Bashir, H. V., DeVere-Tyndall, A., and Edmonds, J.: The role of *Klebsiella* in the pathogenesis of ankylosing spondylitis. II. Evidence for a specific B27 associated marker on the lymphocyte of patients with ankylosing spondylitis. J. Clin. Lab. Immunol., *3*:23, 1980.
145. Hart, F. D.: Medical diseases in pregnancy. Proc. Roy. Soc. Med., *52*:771, 1959.
146. Hart, F. D., and Robinson, K. C.: Ankylosing spondylitis in women. Ann. Rheum. Dis., *18*:15, 1959.
147. Krammer, G. M., Soter, N. A., Gibson, D. J., and Schur, P. H.: Psoriatic arthritis: A clinical, immunological and HLA study of 100 patients. Sem. Arthritis Rheum., *9*:75, 1979.
148. Wright, V., and Moll, J. M. H.: Seronegative Polyarthritis. New York, North Holland Publishing Co., 1976.
149. Wright, V., Roberts, M. C., and Hill, A. G. S.: Dermatological manifestations in psoriatic arthritis: A follow-up study. Acta Derm. Venereol. (Stockh.), *49*:240, 1979.

POLYMYOSITIS/DERMATOMYOSITIS

150. Bauer, K. A., Siegler, M., and Lindheimer, M. A.: Polymyositis complicating pregnancy. Arch. Intern. Med., *139*:449, 1979.
151. Bohan, A., and Peter, J. B.: Polymyositis and dermatomyositis. N. Engl. J. Med., *292*:403, 1975.
152. Callen, J. F., Hyla, J. F., Bole, G. G., and Kay, D. R.: The relationship of dermatomyositis and polymyositis to internal malignancy. Arch. Dermatol., *116*:295, 1980.
153. Moutsopoulous, H., and Fye, K. H.: Lupoid nephrosis and focal glomerulonephritis in a patient with polymyositis. Lancet, *1*:1039, 1975.
154. Nishikai, M., and Reichlin, M.: Heterogenicity of precipitating

antibodies in polymyositis and dermatomyositis: Characterization of the Jo-1 antibody system. Arthritis Rheum., *23*:881, 1980.
155. Pearson, C. M.: Polymyositis and dermatomyositis. *In* McCarty, D. (ed.): Arthritis and Allied Conditions, 9th Ed. Philadelphia, Lea & Febiger, 1979, p. 940.
156. Talbott, J. H.: Acute dermatomyositis-polymyositis and malignancy. Sem. Arthritis Rheum., *6*:305, 1977.
157. Tsai, A., Lindheimer, M. D., and Lamberg, S. I.: Dermatomyositis complicating pregnancy. Obstet. Gynecol., *41*:570, 1973.
158. Walton, J. N., and Adams, R. D.: *In* Polymyositis. Livingston, E. (ed.). Baltimore, Williams & Wilkins, 1958, p. 70.
159. Wolfe, J. F., Adelstein, E., and Sharp, G. C.: Antinuclear antibody with distinct specificity for polymyositis/dermatomyositis. J. Clin. Invest,, *59*:176, 1977.

THE VASCULITIC SYNDROMES

160. Cooper, K., Stafford, J., and Turner Warwick, M.: Wegener's granuloma complicating pregnancy. J. Obstet. Gynaecol. Br. Commonw., *77*:1028, 1970.
161. DeBeukelaer, M. M., Travis, L. B., and Roberts, D. K.: Polyarteritis and pregnancy, South. Med. J., *66*:613, 1973.
162. Fauci, A. S., Haynes, B. F., and Katz, P.: The spectrum of vasculitis. Ann. Intern. Med., *89*:660, 1978.
163. Fauci, A. S., Katz, P., Haynes, B. F., and Wolff, S. M.: Cyclophosphamide therapy of severe systemic necrotizing vasculitis. N. Engl. J. Med., *301*:235, 1979.
164. Leib, E. S., Restivo, C., and Paulus, H. E.: Immunosuppressive and corticosteroid therapy of polyarteritis nodosa. Am. J. Med., *67*:941, 1979.
165. Reza, M. J., Dornfeld, L., Goldberg, L. S., Bluestone, R., and Pearson, C. M.: Wegener's granulomatosis. Longer term follow-up of patients treated with cyclophosphamide therapy. Arthritis Rheum., *18*:501, 1975.
166. Siegler, A. M., and Spain, D. M.: Polyarteritis nodosa and pregnancy. Clin. Obstet. Gynecol., *8*:322, 1965.
167. Varriale, P., Fusco, J. M., Acampora, A., and Grace, W.: Polyarteritis nodosa in pregnancy. Obstet. Gynecol., *25*:866, 1965.
168. Wolff, S. M., Fauci, A. S., Horn, R. G., and Dale, D. C.: Wegener's granulomatosis. Ann. Intern. Med., *81*:513, 1974.

Irwin M. Braverman, M.D.

THE SKIN IN PREGNANCY

The skin and its appendages are affected in a variety of ways during pregnancy. It is convenient to divide these cutaneous changes into three groups: changes in the skin, which most pregnant women exhibit and which are considered to be *normal;* dermatoses that are unique to the gravid state; and pre-existing dermatoses that are influenced in either a positive or negative way by pregnancy.

NORMAL CUTANEOUS CHANGES OF PREGNANCY

PIGMENTATION

Hyperpigmentation is a commonly recognized sign of pregnancy. Although it occurs to some degree in virtually all women, it is more common in brunettes than in blondes. Generalized hyperpigmentation may develop, but it is far more common to see localized areas of melanin hyperpigmentation on the nipples and areolae, umbilicus, linea alba (which becomes the linea nigra), axillas, and vulvar and perianal areas. Although melanocyte-stimulating hormone (MSH) can produce hyperpigmentation in these areas, estrogen and progesterone seem to be the hormones mainly responsible for the pigmentary changes in pregnancy.[50, 51] In individuals of fair complexion these pigmentary changes fade after pregnancy, but in individuals with darker skins some degree of hyperpigmentation remains permanently.

The mask of pregnancy, originally referred to as *chloasma* but now more appropriately termed *melasma,* also develops more often in brunettes than in blondes. Melasma is a splotchy and irregular melanin hyperpigmentation that characteristically develops on the forehead, cheeks, temples, and upper lip. This pigmentary disorder is most likely related to estrogen and progesterone, since identical changes are seen with the use of the contraceptive pill containing these hormones, especially in brunettes. MSH does not produce this type of hyperpigmentation. Although melasma generally lightens considerably or may even disappear completely in some women after pregnancy, it usually persists to some degree. With successive pregnancies melasma may recur or increase in extent. Although melasma is usually associated with pregnancy, it (or an identical-appearing pigmentary disorder) can also be found in nonpregnant women who have not taken birth control pills as well as in some men.

Treatment for melasma is not satisfactory. Topical hydroquinone (2%) is occasionally effective in lightening the hyperpigmentation. In general, treatment with this agent should not be started until after pregnancy and only under conditions of protection against sunlight, either with sunscreening agents or, preferably, during the winter months. Severe hyperpigmentation may be effectively disguised by cosmetics such as Covermark.

Pre-existing pigmented moles (nevi) and freckles often darken during pregnancy. Some nevi may increase in size, and new nevi may form. The increase in pigmentation and size sometimes prompts surgical excision. The increased clinical activity of the lesion is often accompanied histologically by markedly increased junctional activity of the nevus cells, and at times the pathologist may consider the possibility of an early melanoma in the differential diagnosis. However, after pregnancy the nevi usually regress to some extent, and the junctional activity reverts to a more common appearance.

HAIR

Postpartum hair loss is commonplace and is considered a minor nuisance by those who have previously experienced it and a major catastrophe by those who are experiencing it for the first time. The growing phase (anagen) of an individual hair lasts two to six years. The hair bulb eventually involutes and is retracted up into the middle of the hair follicle, where it enters the resting phase (telogen). After about three months a new hair bulb forms in the depth of the same follicle, and as the new hair shaft grows it ejects the old one. Each shed hair is replaced by a new one. Normally 15 to 20 per cent of scalp hair is in the telogen phase.[31]

Lynfield showed that in pregnancy the percentage of hairs in the telogen phase fell to 10 per cent in the second and third trimesters.[38] In the few weeks post partum more hairs entered the telogen phase than usual (30 per cent after nine weeks), thus explaining the clinical observation that postpartum hair loss is seen two to four months after childbirth. Hair loss usually continues for six to 24 weeks, but rarely it may persist for 15 months.[48]

Hair is lost diffusely from the scalp, but there is accentuation of loss along the anterior hairline. Virtually all the hair is replaced after several weeks unless some other process intervenes. The occasional woman who subsequently develops female-patterned baldness (analogous to male-patterned baldness) may connect, incorrectly, the onset of the irreversible balding process with an episode of postpartum hair loss.

Kligman coined the term telogen effluvium to describe this type of hair shedding.[31] The same mechanism operates in hair loss following febrile illnesses such as typhoid fever, scarlet fever, and pneumonia and during severe emotional stress.

Increased hair growth during pregnancy is a rare event and, when observed, has been associated with signs of virilization such as acne, deepening voice, and clitoral enlargement. In some of these cases an arrhenoblastoma was present and was removed, and in others bilateral ovarian enlargement was discovered. In one case, virilization disappeared post partum in association with a spontaneous decrease in the size of the ovaries, and in another, the ovarian enlargement was shown to be produced by hyperplasia of lutein cells.[20]

Turunen et al. reported three women (out of 33,000 successful pregnancies) who developed increased facial hair over the zygomas, jaws, arms, legs, shoulders, areolae, midline of the abdomen, and pubic area.[59] There was deepening of the voice, but no other signs of virilization were described. The hair spontaneously fell out a few days post partum. Turunen et al. found increased urinary 17-ketosteroids and androgens in association with decreased 17-β-dehydrogenase activity in the placentas.[59]

CONNECTIVE TISSUE

Striae gravidarum develops in most pregnant women. The striae appear chiefly on the lower abdomen and on the breasts. Initially, they are pink or purple but soon become white. They never disappear, and they leave white depressed irregular bands in the skin. For many years, it was believed that they were produced solely by the stretching of skin during pregnancy. Observations that striae also develop in Cushing's syndrome, in growing nonobese adolescents of both sexes, and with the use of topical steroids under occlusive dressings cast doubts on this theory. Poidevin showed that the degree of skin distention was not related to the formation of striae and that striae could develop in the absence of significant stretching.[42] It is currently believed that skin stretching and a "striae factor" are both required for the production of striae. The nature of this factor has not been determined, but adrenocortical hyperactivity is frequently proposed as a predisposing factor.

BLOOD VESSELS

Pregnancy produces its most impressive effects on the vascular system, especially of the skin. There is an increase in vascular permeability as well as vascular proliferation. The endothelial cells as well as the supporting smooth muscle and connective tissue are affected by as yet unidentified mechanisms.

Local venous congestion of the vestibule and vaginal mucosa is an early sign of pregnancy. Edema of nondependent areas unrelated to toxemia is common. Arteriolar proliferation with extensive branching of its associated capillary bed results in the formation of spider angiomas, which are commonly found as early as two months gestation and which continue to appear into the ninth month. Typically, they disappear within a few weeks after childbirth. Erythema on the midpalmar, hypothenar, and thenar areas is also common and may be splotchy or uniform. It is indistinguishable from the palmar erythema seen in hyperthyroidism and hepatic cirrhosis. Systemic lupus erythematosus (SLE) may appear for the first time during pregnancy and can also be associated with palmar erythema. However, in SLE the erythema is frequently composed of discrete macules or papules and extends to the finger tips,[6] whereas in pregnancy the palmar erythema is diffuse and usually spares the digits. The palmar erythema of pregnancy also vanishes post partum.

Venous varicosities occur in a significant number of women in both the vulvar and rectal areas. Although the pressure of the gravid uterus on large vessels is important, hereditary valvular incompetence has also been suggested as playing an important role. Saphenous vein varicosities and superficial venous telangiectasias in the shape of "starbursts" or linear patterns become more prominent during pregnancy and regress only slightly post partum.

Vascular proliferation in pregnancy reaches its greatest development with the formation of capillary hemangiomas. They occur chiefly on the head and neck and are considered to be unusual below these areas.[36, 46] The most common sites of involvement are the gingivae, where the developing angiomas are referred to as "pregnancy tumors." Small hemangiomas have been observed on the tongue, upper lip, eyelid, and other areas of the head and neck. Pre-existing hemangiomas have been seen to increase in size during pregnancy. The hemangiomas become smaller post partum but do not recede completely.

DERMATOSES UNIQUE TO PREGNANCY

Traditionally, a number of dermatoses have been related to pregnancy in a cause-and-effect relationship. The natural history of some of these entities is fairly well understood, but the underlying mechanisms are unknown.

Herpes Gestationis

Herpes gestationis is an intensely pruritic, blistering eruption of variable morphologic appearance, which usually appears during the second or third trimester and spontaneously remits within a few weeks post partum in most instances. This disorder is uncommon and is estimated to occur once in 3000 to 5000 pregnancies.[14, 47] Pruritus may precede the development of skin lesions by as much as a week, but usually they appear together. More often than not, the eruption begins periumbilically and spreads to involve the trunk and extremities, including the palms and soles. Lesions on the mucous membranes are uncommon.

CLINICAL FEATURES AND COURSE

The lesions are basically erythematous, urticarial plaques with vesicles or bullae arising on the periphery. The plaques expand by forming new vesicles and bullae along the circumference. In this configuration (Fig. 20–1), the lesions *superficially* have a herpetiform-like appearance, but closer inspection reveals that the blisters are not clustered, as in a true herpetiform grouping, but rather are peripheral in location. In some instances bullae and vesicles arise from the center of the urticarial base (Fig. 20–2). In some cases, the initial lesions are urticarial plaques that produce relatively clear centers as they expand, simulating the lesions of erythema annulare centrifugum (Fig. 20–3). The histologic appearance of the three lesions shown in Figures 20–1 to 20–3 was that of a subepidermal blister characteristic of herpes gestationis.

The eruption in this disorder tends to develop in crops, and individual lesions tend to subside spontaneously after one to two weeks. The disease may be mild with few lesions and tolerable pruritus, or it may spread rapidly with unrelenting itching. Lesions may coalesce to produce arcuate or circinate patterns. Although the itching can be severe, secondary infection with im-

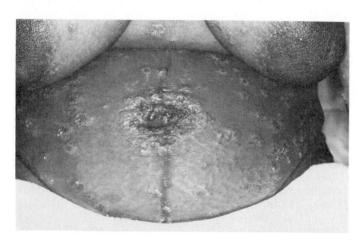

FIGURE 20–1. Herpes gestationis. Eruption began periumbilically and spread over abdomen. Individual lesions are urticarial plaques with active vesicular borders. Vesicles are not grouped in each lesion as would be expected in a true herpetiform configuration.

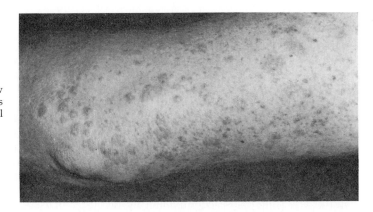

FIGURE 20–2. Herpes gestationis on elbow and extensor surface of upper arm. Lesions consist of early bullae arising from urticarial bases.

petigo and pustule formation does not occur as often as one might anticipate.

The disease usually begins in the fourth or fifth month but has been reported as early as two weeks[13] and as late as three to five days post partum.[35, 47] A fluctuating course with exacerbations and relative remissions can be seen during pregnancy. Significant flares can develop post partum. In the average case, the disorder subsides spontaneously within a few days to four weeks post partum, but it can persist for up to 16 weeks. Post partum, the disease may flare repeatedly with the menstrual cycle before spontaneously entering remission. Rarely, the disease may continue for months to years in this fashion before resolving.[33, 47] One of my patients had persistently active disease for one year post partum, requiring oral steroids for control, before she entered remission. Black reported that in three of his ten patients the disease was still persistent three to seven years post partum.[4] In these instances, the behavior of the disease is strikingly similar to that of autoimmune dermatitis.[22] Birth control pills can produce exacerba-

tions of the disease during states of remission or mild activity.[25, 35, 37]

Although the probability of recurrence with each pregnancy is high, this does not invariably happen, nor does the severity of the disease necessarily become worse with each subsequent pregnancy. One of my patients, whose first attack persisted for one year post partum, had two subsequent pregnancies, each of which was accompanied by milder and milder courses. In the second and third pregnancies corticosteroid therapy was not required, and the disease terminated promptly within a few days post partum.

DIAGNOSIS

A presumptive diagnosis is made by finding the characteristic lesions developing during pregnancy. The diagnosis becomes firmer when erythema multiforme and drug reactions are excluded. A history of a similar eruption in a previous pregnancy that cleared post partum will clinch the diagnosis.

Histologically, the cutaneous lesions in herpes

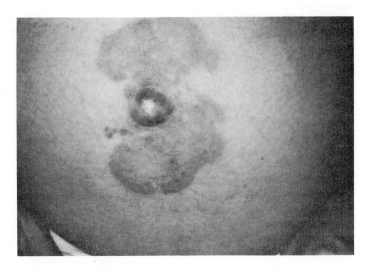

FIGURE 20–3. Herpes gestationis eruption which developed periumbilically. It began as an urticarial plaque which spread peripherally, producing an elevated edematous border and relatively inactive center. Simulates the lesion of erythema annulare centrifugum.

gestationis show a subepidermal blister with a perivascular collection of lymphohistiocytic cells and eosinophils around the upper and, sometimes, deep dermal vessels.[24] These findings had been confused with those of erythema multiforme and dermatitis herpetiformis in the past. Herpes gestationis was believed to be a manifestation of one of these entities in pregnancy. However, since 1973 it has become clear on the basis of immunofluorescent findings that herpes gestationis is a distinct entity unrelated to those disorders. Direct immunofluorescent examination of lesional and normal skin reveals a linear band of C3, sometimes accompanied by IgG, at the dermal-epidermal junction. In addition, virtually all patients have a circulating IgG, which fixes C3 to the basement membrane zone of normal skin by an in vitro complement binding technique. This IgG is referred to as the herpes gestationis (HG) factor.[28] In a minority of patients, a circulating antibody directed against the basement membrane zone is also found. These immunofluorescent findings clearly separate herpes gestationis from classic erythema multiforme.[29, 35, 44] The pattern of immunofluorescence by light and electron microscopy strongly suggests that herpes gestationis is most closely related to bullous pemphigoid.[25, 60] Some differences, however, do exist. In herpes gestationis, HG factor exists in higher titers than the circulating antibasement membrane zone antibody when the latter is present, whereas in bullous pemphigoid the converse is true.[29]

The differential diagnosis includes the bullous eruptions. Pemphigus vulgaris is characterized by flaccid bullae that arise from normal-appearing skin. Histologic examination reveals an intraepidermal blister containing acantholytic cells. The eruption of impetigo herpetiformis consists of pustules developing from an erythematous base and is usually accompanied by fever and hypocalcemia. The histopathologic appearance is that of a spongiform pustule in the epidermis. Papular dermatitis of pregnancy is a nonbullous, nonurticarial disorder in which the eruption consists of scattered individual pruritic papules that are quickly excoriated.

Herpes gestationis does not represent dermatitis herpetiformis occurring in pregnancy. Dermatitis herpetiformis is a pruritic disorder in which clusters of vesicles (rarely bullae) on an erythematous or urticarial base develop symmetrically over the scapulas, knees, elbows, buttocks, and trunk. The individual lesions never form plaques with vesicular borders or relatively clear centers. The histopathologic appearance of the blisters in dermatitis herpetiformis is that of edema of the dermal papillae associated with large numbers of neutrophils. This is the earliest phase in the formation of the fully developed subepidermal blister. The early blisters of dermatitis herpetiformis and herpes gestationis can be easily distinguished histologically. Sulfones and sulfapyridine are almost always specific therapy for dermatitis herpetiformis. Corticosteroids are relatively ineffective. The reverse is true for herpes gestationis.

Before 1973, herpes gestationis was diagnosed on the basis of cutaneous lesions that resembled erythema multiforme or dermatitis herpetiformis in association with pregnancy. Oral lesions were reported in occasional patients, suggesting that erythema multiforme might also be a manifestation of the gravid state. By applying immunofluorescent testing to all bullous eruptions developing in pregnancy, it is possible to establish whether erythema multiforme or some other as yet undefined blistering diseases can also appear during this period. Since immunologically defined herpes gestationis can exhibit iris lesions indistinguishable from those of erythema multiforme,[8] it is difficult to dismiss the possibility that such cases may represent a variant of erythema multiforme.

In 1969, on the basis of a literature review, Kolodny suggested that maternal and fetal morbidity and mortality were not increased in herpes gestationis.[33] Lawley et al. reviewed their own cases and those published since 1973 in which immunofluorescent findings were used as one of the diagnostic criteria.[35] They found that women who had circulating antibasement membrane zone antibody had a more severe clinical course and needed higher doses of steroids for effective suppression of their bullous disease. They also noted that substantial blood eosinophilia was correlated to some extent with the severity of disease activity. These two prognostic factors need to be re-evaluated in future series. Lawley et al. found that fetal morbidity and fetal mortality were increased.[35] Stillbirths occurred in 3 of 39 patients (7.7 per cent), six times higher than the rate in the general population. However, there was not an abnormally high rate of spontaneous abortions (1 of 39). Premature births occurred in 8 of 35 live births (23 per cent). The normal rate in the population is 5 to 10 per cent. Four infants were born with skin lesions compatible with herpes gestationis. In two, direct immunofluorescence showed C3 along the epidermal basement membrane zone. Indirect immunofluorescent studies of the sera in three infants showed HG factor in two and antibasement membrane zone antibody of the IgG class in one. No comment was made about the immunofluorescent markers in the mothers of the respective babies.

I have made the diagnosis of herpes gestationis in four patients in the past ten years before the immunologic markers were discovered. A fifth patient was diagnosed with immunologic confirmation. These five patients have had seven healthy babies in as many pregnancies.

TREATMENT

Corticosteroids are the drugs of choice. The disease can usually be controlled with doses of 10 to 20 mg per day (prednisone equivalent) after a higher initial dose of 40 to 60 mg per day. Fetal malformations have not been reported, since treatment rarely is necessary before the first trimester. As with all patients on steroid therapy, the patient should be observed closely, and in pregnancy special attention should be paid to excessive weight gain, fluid retention, and hypertension.

A number of patients have been successfully treated with pyridoxine (50 to 400 mg per day), thereby raising the possibility of pyridoxine deficiency as a cause of this disorder.[13, 19] Rh factor isosensitization was proposed by Cawley et al. as a causative factor in some cases, but these observations have not been confirmed.[9]

The prognosis for the disease is good, and in most cases postpartum treatment is only necessary for a few weeks.

Impetigo Herpetiformis

Impetigo herpetiformis is a rare disease, which traditionally has been classified among the unique dermatoses of pregnancy. It is a superficial sterile pustular eruption on an erythematous base that is accompanied by fever, hypocalcemia, and, sometimes, tetany. Remissions occur post partum, and recurrences in succeeding pregnancies are likely. The disease may be fatal. Only 100 cases have been reported.

CLINICAL FEATURES

Impetigo herpetiformis may appear as early as the first trimester and as late as the third. Pruritus is variable. The eruption begins as erythematous macules or large patches, which become studded with superficial but sterile pustules 1 to 2 mm in diameter (Figs. 20–4 and 20–5) within 24 hours of onset. The lesions appear in crops, and individual lesions extend by the development of erythema with pustules. As the lesions resolve, desquamation takes place. Secondary impetiginization may occur. The eruption has a predilection for the lower abdomen, inguinal areas, medial thighs, periumbilical area, and inframammary and axillary regions. The entire body can be affected. The hands and face are less frequently involved. Pustules may appear beneath the nail plate. Lesions may develop on the oral mucosa.

Each crop of lesions is usually accompanied by fever, lethargy, and prostration. Tetany and convulsions have occurred in some patients, and a few persons have died. In most instances the disease has spontaneously remitted after delivery.

Laboratory studies reveal leukocytosis with an increase in neutrophils. Hypocalcemia is often present. In some cases albuminuria and red and white blood cells in the urinary sediment have been reported, but the nature of the renal dis-

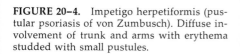

FIGURE 20–4. Impetigo herpetiformis (pustular psoriasis of von Zumbusch). Diffuse involvement of trunk and arms with erythema studded with small pustules.

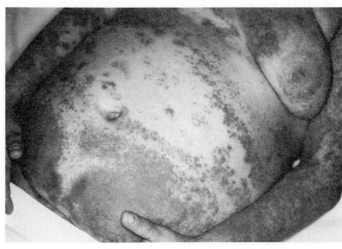

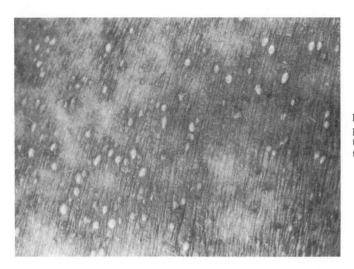

FIGURE 20–5. Impetigo herpetiformis (pustular psoriasis of von Zumbusch). Closer view of eruption shown in Figure 20–4. Small pustules scattered on an erythematous base.

order was not explained. Histologic examination of the pustules reveals collections of neutrophils beneath the stratum corneum. Neutrophils are also present as a diffuse infiltration throughout the epidermis and as a localized intraepidermal collection (spongiform pustule of Kogoj). Perivascular collections of neutrophils are present in the dermis.

Although impetigo herpetiformis was first described in pregnant women[23] or in women following thyroidectomy,[18, 26] later papers reported this condition in men, older women, and even children.[2, 30] A significant number of patients said to have impetigo herpetiformis had previously had classical psoriasis with plaques.[30, 58] Patients who developed a generalized pustular eruption and were pregnant or hypocalemic were often placed in the category of impetigo herpetiformis because of these associated findings, whereas males or females not of childbearing age were said to have pustular psoriasis of von Zumbusch. Sometimes conditions were diagnosed as impetigo herpetiformis rather than pustular psoriasis because eosinophils were present in the intraepidermal pustules.[39, 58] This distinction is controversial, however, since authorities do not agree on the significance of eosinophils in the diagnosis of impetigo herpetiformis. Careful surveys indicate that pustular psoriasis of von Zumbusch and impetigo herpetiformis cannot be separated on the basis of sex, age, pregnancy, histopathologic features, clinical course, therapeutic response, or laboratory findings.[10, 15, 27, 32, 39, 52]

Pustular psoriasis of von Zumbusch is an acute form of psoriasis that can appear any time during the natural history of psoriasis vulgaris, or it may be the sole manifestation of the psoriatic diathesis. Shelley described two patients in whom attacks of pustular psoriasis could be precipitated by the ingestion of salicylate, iodide, and progesterone.[49] There are undoubtedly many stimuli, most still unidentified, that can trigger this febrile, toxic form of psoriasis, and pregnancy may be one of them. If impetigo herpetiformis had been described for the first time in the twentieth century instead of the nineteenth, it certainly would have been classified as an instance of pustular psoriasis precipitated by pregnancy, and its reputation as a fatal disease would have been tempered by the availability of modern supportive measures.

Although hypocalcemia is traditionally associated with impetigo herpetiformis, it is also a feature of pustular psoriasis.[1, 11, 57] Some patients who developed a generalized pustular eruption diagnosed as impetigo herpetiformis following thyroidectomy were hypocalcemic because of unintentional parathyroidectomy. The mechanism of hypocalcemia in the other patients is unclear, but malabsorption has been suggested by several authors.[11, 17] Braverman et al. studied a 56 year old woman with pustular psoriasis and hypocalcemia of 14 years duration.[7] There was no evidence of malabsorption or parathyroid disease, but the patient had persistent hypoalbuminemia. It is well known that a low serum calcium is associated with hypoalbuminemia because of decreased binding. Studies with iodinated serum albumin in this patient showed that the half-life of albumin was shortened to four days (normal, 10 to 11 days), and other tests revealed that the protein was not being lost into the bowel or urine. Electron microscopic studies of the skin lesions in this patient showed gaps between the normally apposed endothelial cells of the superficial dermal capillaries. In addition, each attack of pustular psoriasis in this patient was accompanied by an elevation of alkaline phosphatase and

5'-nucleotidase enzyme activity. Liver biopsies from other patients with pustular psoriasis have shown a pericholangitis produced by a neutrophilic infiltrate,[49] which could account for the rise in the enzyme levels. Braverman et al. postulated that loss of albumin into the skin, other organs, or both with increased metabolic degradation was the most likely explanation for the shortened half-life of albumin in their patient.[7]

DIAGNOSIS

A presumptive diagnosis of impetigo herpetiformis can be made by noting the onset of generalized or flexural erythematous patches that are quickly covered with superficial sterile pustules. The patient often is febrile and appears ill. A biopsy will confirm the diagnosis by demonstrating the presence of spongiform pustules in the epidermis. Hypocalcemia is intermittently present during the course of the disease, and several samplings may be necessary to demonstrate this finding.

The differential diagnosis includes subcorneal pustular dermatosis of Sneddon and Wilkinson, which is a pustular disease arising from minimally red or normal skin. The pustules are arranged in serpiginous or polycyclic configurations, which tend to have clear centers. Histopathologic examination shows only a subcorneal collection of neutrophils and no intraepidermal abscess formation. The disease responds dramatically to sulfones and sulfapyridine and poorly to corticosteroids.

Differentiation from erythema multiforme (herpes gestationis), pemphigus, and papular dermatitis of pregnancy is easy because they are not pustular diseases at their onset.

TREATMENT

Because the disease is rare, therapeutic regimens are difficult to evaluate. Oral corticosteroids have been helpful in some patients. In nonpregnant patients long-term treatment with methotrexate and tetracycline has been reported as being effective, but these drugs should be avoided in pregnancy. General supportive measures, including appropriate antibiotics for infections, are important. Beveridge et al. reported low placental function in one patient with this disease.[3] They advocated measuring urinary pregnanediol, pregnanetriol, and dehydroepiandrosterone in the last trimester, and if levels were inadequate, they suggested that cesarean section might avoid fetal loss.

This disease requires re-evaluation. The available data are inadequate to determine whether fetal loss is normal or excessive in impetigo herptiformis. The disease is supposed to enter remissions between pregnancies, but even this point needs further confirmation. In the patient reported by Beveridge et al., the disease continued post partum for an unstated period and was still active at the time their paper was submitted for publication.[3] On the basis of current information, impetigo herpetiformis represents pustular psoriasis of von Zumbusch during pregnancy.

Papular Dermatitis of Pregnancy

Papular dermatitis of pregnancy, first described by Spangler et al., is a generalized, severely pruritic papular eruption that occurred in 0.026 per cent of births.[55] A total of 15 patients have been reported.

The eruption consists of individual erythematous papules 3 to 5 mm in diameter with a smaller papule at the apex. New lesions appear in small numbers, never in crops, and never grouped. At the time of examination, most of the papules will have been excoriated. Individual lesions heal spontaneously after seven to ten days, leaving spots of hyperpigmentation.

CLINICAL FEATURES

The disorder is limited to pregnancy and can appear as early as the first month or as late as the last. The disease disappears promptly post partum but usually recurs with successive pregnancies. No manifestations of systemic disease have been described with this disorder. In three patients reported by Spangler and Emerson, itching persisted for a few weeks after parturition.[53] Dilatation and curettage was performed with successful removal of retained placental tissue, and the pruritus promptly subsided after this procedure.

A number of placental and endocrinologic clues have been uncovered in this entity.[53, 55] Patients with this disorder exhibit inflammatory responses to intradermal injections of extracts from placentas of others with the disease but not from placentas of normal individuals. In the last trimester of pregnancy, urinary chorionic gonadotropin levels are markedly elevated, plasma cortisol levels are reduced, and plasma cortisol half-life is shortened. Urinary levels of estriol are also reduced in the last trimester. Five of the 12 patients in the original report were Rh negative.

TREATMENT

Oral corticosteroids are required for treatment. Pruritus subsided within one to two days after therapy was begun, and urinary chorionic gonadotropin levels returned to normal. Doses of prednisone ranged from 40 to 200 mg per day for control of the disorder. Sulfapyridine was not effective. Diethylstilbestrol, in a dose of 600 to 2500 mg per day, was also effective in controlling the pruritus and eruption within four to five days. However, this form of treatment has been discontinued because of the association of estrogen administration during pregnancy and the subsequent development of vaginal carcinoma during adolescence in the offspring.

FETAL LOSS

In the original report of Spangler et al., the overall fetal loss was reported as 27 per cent based on a review of 37 previous pregnancies in the 12 patients.[55] However, eight of the 11 fetal deaths — abortions and stillbirths — occurred in the absence of any skin disease in the mother. In only three fetal deaths did the mother have papular dermatitis. Whether this disorder is truly associated with a high fetal mortality remains to be determined.[41, 54]

DIAGNOSIS

The diagnosis of papular dermatitis of pregnancy is suggested by the presence of severe *intractable* pruritus, accompanied by individual papules that continually appear in a scattered distribution. High urinary chorionic gonadotropin levels and low urinary estriol and plasma cortisol levels in the last trimester would confirm the clinical diagnosis.

The differential diagnosis includes all factors capable of producing pruritus in the pregnant and nonpregnant states. They range from drug reactions, scabies, irritation from woolen and synthetic fibers, ichthyosis, xerosis (winter itch), emotional disturbances, and moniliasis of anogenital areas to underlying systemic disorders such as Hodgkin's disease. In many instances vigorous scratching produces excoriations that are erythematous and edematous and hence papular. The scratch papule must be kept in mind when evaluating pruritus. Herpes gestationis and pustular psoriasis (impetigo herpetiformis) are excluded from the differential diagnosis because they are bullous and pustular diseases.

Less easily excluded is the entity termed prurigo of pregnancy by Nurse.[40] He described 40 patients who developed pruritic papules either early (25 to 39 weeks) or late (39 weeks) in pregnancy. These lesions occurred chiefly on the proximal parts of the limbs and upper trunk (Figs. 20–6 and 20–7). Topical therapy with calamine lotion containing 1% phenol and oral trimeprazine easily controlled the pruritus. The syndrome disappeared within three to four weeks after delivery. Recurrence in subsequent pregnancies was unusual, and the fetal loss was only 1 in the 40 births. The incidence of Nurse's syndrome was 0.5 per cent. The prurigo of Besnier[12] and prurigo annularis[16] seem to be identical to the prurigo of pregnancy described by Nurse. Since Nurse performed no laboratory tests on his patients, it is not possible to state whether his syndrome is a mild variant of the entity described by Spangler et al.[55]

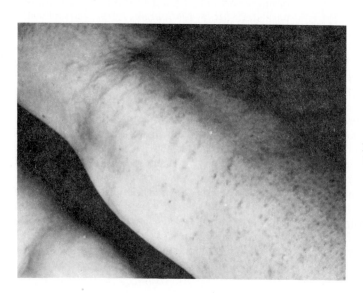

FIGURE 20–6. Prurigo of pregnancy (Nurse, 1968). Small papules on posterior thigh.

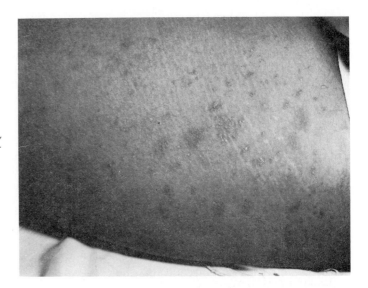

FIGURE 20–7. Prurigo of pregnancy (Nurse, 1968). Small papules on thigh. Some have become eczematous because of rubbing.

PUPPP Syndrome

Lawley et al. have delineated a syndrome that they have entitled *pruritic urticarial papules and plaques of pregnancy* (PUPPP).[34] Seven women exhibited an identical clinical syndrome of red urticarial papules and plaques that began on the abdomen and spread to involve the thighs. The buttocks, legs, and arms were less frequently affected. Truncal lesions were rarely seen above the midthorax, and the face was never affected. In spite of marked pruritus, excoriations were rare. A narrow pale halo often surrounded the papules. PUPPP developed in the last trimester (27 to 40 weeks) and promptly disappeared within two weeks after delivery. There were no abnormal hematologic or urinary findings, including serum chorionic gonadotropin levels. Direct immunofluorescent examination of lesional and normal skin was negative for immunoglobulins and complement. Histologically, the skin lesions showed perivascular collections of lymphohistiocytic cells including a few eosinophils around the superficial and, sometimes, deep vascular plexuses.

PUPPP appears to be distinct from the other pruritic papular dermatoses of pregnancy and should be able to be distinguished from them on the basis of clinical and morphologic features. The urticarial papules of PUPPP can resemble some of the early lesions of herpes gestationis, but differentiation can be made easily by direct immunofluorescent examination for immunoreactants and by routine histology. PUPPP may be identical to Bourne's toxemic rash of pregnancy based on the description of the clinical lesions and their distribution. However, the details of individual cases, histopathology, and laboratory data are lacking in Bourne's report.[5] The small number of patients in the series of Lawley et al. precludes any evaluation of possible maternal and fetal complications. Lawley et al. believe that PUPPP may be the most common variety of pruritic dermatoses of pregnancy, which has not been previously recognized because of its generally late appearance, brief duration, and excellent response to topical steroid therapy.

Intrahepatic Cholestasis of Pregnancy

Intrahepatic cholestasis of pregnancy (pruritus gravidarum) produces generalized pruritus that may or may not be eventually accompanied by jaundice. The disorder usually begins in the third trimester but may appear as early as the 20th week of pregnancy (See Chapter 12). Pruritus and jaundice, if present, promptly disappear after delivery. The pruritus usually precedes the development of jaundice by two to three weeks. The prevalence of this disorder varies from 0.06 to 0.43 per cent of all completed pregnancies.[45] The probability of recurrence in succeeding pregnancies is high; in the series of Rencoret and Aste it was 47 per cent.

This diagnosis should be considered when evaluating generalized pruritus in the absence of a specific eruption. Liver function tests reveal elevated alkaline phosphatase and bilirubin levels in the presence of normal flocculation tests and transaminase levels. Other forms of liver disease must be excluded before this diagnosis can be made.

Estrogens must play a role in the impairment of the excretory function of the liver because the syndrome can be reproduced in affected women taking oral contraceptives after pregnancy.

Cholestyramine has been used for treatment during pregnancy but has not been especially effective. No treatment is necessary post partum.

No maternal deaths due to cholestatic jaundice have been recorded. Several series have reported premature labor in as many as 30 per cent of cases. Opinions on fetal loss vary, however. In some series, there were no deaths, and in others fetal loss was as high as 37 per cent. The main causes of death were intrapartum asphyxia and respiratory distress syndrome. No obvious fetal abnormalities have been found. Because of the high incidence of fetal distress in some series, Rencoret and Aste urge fetal monitoring during labor for patients with recurrent cholestasis, particularly for those with a history of fetal loss.[45] The reasons for the variability of fetal loss in different series require further study to determine if they are directly related to cholestatic jaundice.

OTHER DERMATOSES AND PREGNANCY

Pregnancy can produce effects on other dermatoses and systemic diseases with dermatologic components. Some of these disorders, such as connective tissue disorders and condyloma acuminatum, are discussed in Chapters 19 and 11, respectively.

"Skin tags," or fibroma molle, are small pedunculated fibromas that develop on the neck and in the axillas during pregnancy. They are benign overgrowths of skin that tend to involute somewhat after delivery.

Pregnancy has an adverse effect on neurofibromatosis. Swapp and Main studied 10 women who had 24 pregnancies.[56] In five of the ten cases, the lesions of neurofibromatosis were seen for the first time during pregnancy. In the other patients, café au lait spots and neurofibromas were found to increase in size and number. After delivery, considerable regressions of the tumors occurred.

In pregnancy, about one half of patients with psoriasis enter a remission. Only a small percentage become worse.[21]

The behavior of acne vulgaris in pregnancy is unpredictable.

Condylomata acuminata frequently become larger and more numerous during pregnancy.[43, 61] In exceptional cases, the condylomata have become so large that vaginal delivery was not possible and cesarean section had to be performed.

References

1. Baker, H., and Ryan, T. J.: Generalized pustular psoriasis. Br. J. Dermatol., 80:771, 1968.
2. Beck, C. H.: On impetigo herpetiformis. Dermatologica, 102:145, 1951.
3. Beveridge, G. W., Harkness, R. A., and Livingstone, J. R. B.: Impetigo herpetiformis in two successive pregnancies. Br. J. Dermatol., 78:106, 1966.
4. Black, M. M.: The enigma of herpes gestationis. Trans. Pac. Dermatol. Assoc., 1977, p. 15.
5. Bourne, G.: Toxemic rash of pregnancy. Proc. Roy. Soc. Med., 55:462, 1962.
6. Braverman, I. M.: Skin Signs of Systemic Disease. 2nd ed. Philadelphia, W. B. Saunders Co., 1981, p. 279.
7. Braverman, I. M., Cohen, I., and O'Keefe, E.: Metabolic and ultrastructural studies in a patient with pustular psoriasis (von Zumbusch). Arch. Dermatol., 105:189, 1972.
8. Bushkell, L. L., Jordon, R. E., and Goltz, R. W.: Herpes gestationis. New immunologic findings. Arch. Dermatol., 110:65, 1974.
9. Cawley, F. P., Wheeler, C. F., and Wilhite, P. A.: Herpes gestationis and the Rh factor. South. Med. J., 45:827, 1952.
10. Champion, R. H.: Generalized pustular psoriasis. Br. J. Dermatol., 71:384, 1959.
11. Copeman, P. W. M., and Bold, A. M.: Generalized pustular psoriasis (von Zumbusch) with episodic hypocalcemia. Proc. R. Soc. Med., 58:425, 1965.
12. Costello, M. J.: Eruptions of pregnancy. N.Y. State J. Med., 41:849, 1941.
13. Coupe, R. S.: Herpes gestationis. Arch. Dermatol., 91:633, 1965.
14. Crawford, G. M., and Leeper, R. W.: Diseases of the skin in pregnancy. Arch. Dermatol., 61:753, 1950.
15. Danboldt, N.: Kasuistischer Beitrag zur Frage Psoriasis pustulo-

sa — Impetigo herpetiformis. Acta Dermatovener., 18:150, 1937.
16. Davies, J. H. T.: Prurigo annularis. Br. J. Dermatol., 53:143, 1941.
17. Feiwel, M., and Cairns, R. J.: Impetigo herpetiformis or pustular psoriasis or acrodermatitis (Hallopeau). Br. J. Dermatol., 80:125, 1968.
18. Feiwel, M., and Ferriman, D.: Impetigo herpetiformis. Proc. R. Soc. Med., 50:393, 1957.
19. Fosnaugh, R. P., Bryan, H. G., and Orders, R. L.: Pyridoxine in the treatment of herpes gestationis. Arch. Dermatol., 84:90, 1961.
20. Friedman, I. S., Mackles, A., and Daichman, I.: Development of virilization during pregnancy. J. Clin. Endocrinol. Metab., 15:1281, 1955.
21. Gruneberg, T. H.: Psoriasis und Schwangerschaft. Hautarzt, 3:155, 1952.
22. Hart, R.: Autoimmune progesterone dermatitis. Arch. Dermatol., 113:426, 1977.
23. Hebra, F.: Schwangerschaft dem Wochenbette und bei Uterinalkrankheiten der Frauen zu beobachtende Hautkrankheiten. Wien. Med. Wschr., 22:1197, 1872.
24. Hertz, K. C., Katz, S. I., Maize, J., and Ackerman, A. B.: Herpes gestationis. A clinicopathologic study. Arch. Dermatol., 112:1543, 1976.
25. Honigsmann, H., Stingl, G., Holubar, K., and Wolff, K.: Herpes gestationis: fine structural pattern of immunoglobulin deposits in the skin in vivo. J. Invest. Dermatol., 66:389, 1976.
26. Hvidberg, E.: Impetigo herpetiformis. Dermatologica, 114:337, 1957.
27. Ingram, J. T.: Pustular psoriasis. Arch. Dermatol., 77:314, 1958.
28. Jordon, R. E., Heine, K. C., Tappeiner, G., Bushkell, L. L., and

Provost, T. T.: The immunopathology of herpes gestationis. Immunofluorescence studies and characterization of "HG Factor." J. Clin. Invest., 57:1426, 1976.

29. Katz, S. I., Hertz, K. C., and Yaoita, H.: Herpes gestationis. Immunopathology and characterization of the HG factor. J. Clin. Invest., 57:1434, 1976.

30. Katzenellenbogen, I., and Feuerman, E. J.: Psoriasis pustulosa and impetigo herpetiformis — single or dual entity? Acta Dermatovener., 46:85, 1966.-

31. Kligman, A. M.: Pathological dynamics of human hair loss. Arch. Dermatol., 83:175, 1961.

32. Koch, F.: Zur Frage der Identität von Impetigo herpetiformis. Psorasis pustulosa, und Psoriasis vulgaris. Hautarzt, 3:165, 1952.

33. Kolodny, R. C.: Herpes gestationis. Am. J. Obstet. Gynecol., 104:39, 1969.

34. Lawley, T. J., Hertz, K. C., Wade, T. R., Ackerman, A. B., and Katz, S. I.: Pruritic urticarial papules and plaques of pregnancy. J. A. M. A., 241:1696, 1979.

35. Lawley, T. J., Stingl, G., and Katz, S. I.: Fetal and maternal risk factors in herpes gestationis. Arch. Dermatol., 114:552, 1978.

36. Letterman, G., and Schwiter, M.: Cutaneous hemangiomas of the face in pregnancy. Plast. Reconstruct. Surg., 29:293, 1962.

37. Lynch, F. W., and Albrecht, E. J.: Hormonal factors in herpes gestationis. Arch. Dermatol., 93:446, 1966.

38. Lynfield, Y. L.: Effect of pregnancy on the human hair cycle. J. Invest. Dermatol., 35:323, 1960.

39. Moslein, P.: Impetigo herpetiformis — Psoriasis pustulosa — Acrodermatitis continua Hallopeau. Arch. Klin. Exp. Dermatol., 208:410, 1959.

40. Nurse, D. S.: Prurigo of pregnancy. Aust. J. Dermatol., 9:258, 1968.

41. Otterson, W. N.: Diethylstilbestrol in management of papular dermatitis of pregnancy. Am. J. Obstet. Gynecol., 113:570, 1972.

42. Poidevin, L. O. S.: Striae gravidarum. Their relation to adrenal cortical hyperfunction. Lancet. 2:436, 1959.

43. Powell, L. C. Jr.: Condyloma acuminatum. Clin. Obstet. Gynecol., 15:948, 1972.

44. Provost, T. T., and Tomasi, T. B. Jr.: Evidence for complement activation via the alternate pathway in skin diseases. I. Herpes gestationis, systemic lupus erythematosus, and bullous pemphigoid. J. Clin. Invest., 52:1779, 1973.

45. Rencoret, R., and Aste, H.: Jaundice during pregnancy. Med. J. Aust., 1:167, 1973.

46. Rose, T. R.: The hemangiomata of pregnancy. J. Obstet. Gynecol. Br. Emp., 56:364, 1949.

47. Russell, B., and Thorne, N.: Herpes gestationis. Br. J. Dermatol., 69:339, 1957.

48. Schiff, B. L., and Kern, A. B.: A study of postpartum alopecia. Arch. Dermatol., 87:609, 1963.

49. Shelley, W. B.: Generalized pustular psoriasis induced by potassium iodide. J.A.M.A., 201:1009, 1967.

50. Snell, R. S.: The pigmentary changes occurring in the breast skin during pregnancy and following estrogen treatment. J. Invest. Dermatol., 43:181, 1964.

51. Snell, R. S., and Bischitz, P. G.: The effect of large doses of estrogen and estrogen and progesterone on melanin pigmentation. J. Invest. Dermatol., 35:73, 1960.

52. Soltermann, W.: Familiare Psoriasis pustulosa unter dem Bilde der Impetigo herpetiformis. Dermatologica, 116:313, 1958.

53. Spangler, A. S., and Emerson, K.: Estrogen levels and estrogen therapy in papular dermatitis of pregnancy. Am. J. Obstet. Gynecol., 110:534, 1971.

54. Spangler, A. S., and Emerson, K.: Diethylstilbesterol in management of papular dermatitis of pregnancy. Reply to Colonel Otterson. Am. J. Obstet. Gynecol., 113:571, 1972.

55. Spangler, A. S., Reddy, W., Bardawil, W. A., Roby, C. C., and Emerson, K.: Papular dermatitis of pregnancy: a new clinical entity? J.A.M.A., 181:577, 1962.

56. Swapp, G. H., and Main, R. A.: Neurofibromatosis in pregnancy. Br. J. Dermatol., 88:431, 1973.

57. Tielsch, R.: Zur differential Diagnose Impetigo herpetiformis — Psoriasis pustulosa. Dermatol. Wschr., 145:305–313, 1962.

58. Tolman, M. M., and Moschella, S. L.: Pustular psoriasis (Zumbusch). Arch. Dermatol., 81:400, 1960.

59. Turunen, A., Pesonen, S., and Ziliacus, H.: Hormone assays during recurrent excessive hair growth in pregnancy. Acta Endocrinol., 45:447, 1964.

60. Yaoita, H., Gullino, M., and Katz, S. I.: Herpes gestationis. Ultrastructure and ultrastructural localization of in vivo-bound complement. Modified tissue preparation and processing for horseradish peroxidase staining of skin. J. Invest. Derm., 66:383, 1976.

61. Young, R. L., Acosta, A. A., and Kaufman, R. H.: The treatment of large condylomata acuminata complicating pregnancy. Obstet. Gynecol., 41:65, 1973.

21

Malcolm S. Mitchell, M.D.
Robert L. Capizzi, M.D.

NEOPLASTIC DISEASES

Of all the medical illnesses complicating pregnancy, few are more ominous than cancer. Cancer threatens the life and well-being of the mother, and the therapy required may be hazardous to the fetus. Fortunately, neoplasia is not a common affliction of women in the childbearing age group, but when it is present the physician may be faced with particularly difficult therapeutic problems.

This chapter will consider several of the most common neoplastic diseases encountered in pregnant women and the special limitations that might be imposed on effective therapy. In addition, broader questions involving the interaction between neoplasia and pregnancy will be examined to put the specific diseases into perspective.

GENERAL CONSIDERATIONS

Effect of Pregnancy on Tumors

Neoplastic diseases are most common in the very young and the very old, tending to exclude those in their twenties and thirties, the age group in which pregnancy is most common. While the exact explanations for this incidence are obscure, the immunologic competence of humans may be one important factor, since data suggest that competence is strongest during young adulthood and middle age, waning during senescence. The latency of tumors after exposure to carcinogens or tumor viruses might account for the low incidence in young adulthood. Pregnant women would not be expected to have a high incidence of neoplasia unless their susceptibility were somehow increased by the pregnancy. Despite recent reports about the immunosuppressive effects of human chorionic gonadotropin (HCG) and estrogens (indicating that they are potentially damaging to tumor resistance), there is no increased incidence of malignancy in pregnant women. The acceptance by the mother of the fetus, which is a "foreign graft" bearing paternal antigens, may be dependent, in part, on a state of partial immunologic tolerance. Yet any deficiency in the mother's immunity appears to be specifically toward the fetus; there is no demonstrable deficiency in immunity to other foreign antigens such as those carried by tumor cells. In contrast, patients in the same age group receiving continuous immunosuppressive therapy to promote acceptance of renal allografts have an incidence of malignancy 100- to 1000-fold greater than age-matched controls.[51a] In other words, although profound nonspecific iatrogenic immunosuppression is capable of facilitating tumor growth in this age group, any immunosuppression intrinsically associated with pregnancy is not capable of such growth.

Earlier suggestions from small series of patients that certain neoplasms such as melanoma are increased in frequency in pregnant patients have proved unfounded. The incidence of malignancy in the 25 to 35 year old age group is approximately 0.06 per cent,[51a] and the incidence in pregnant women is virtually identical (0.07 per cent).[47] Excluding gestational neoplasms, which are specifically derived from the trophoblast, there were only 100 cases of malignancy in 153,424 women seen from 1950 to 1969 in Helsinki.[47] Of these 100, genital malignancies, especially carcinoma of the cervix, and carcinoma of the breast were common, with 33 and 23 cases, respectively. Carcinoma of the thyroid was present in nine instances and melanoma in five. The course of disease was not described in detail, but it is of interest to note that 13 of the 30 carcinomas of the cervix were in situ and apparently did not become invasive under the influence of the pregnancy.

Although we will examine several specific neoplasms in detail shortly, it is worth stating at the outset that pregnancy does not alter the course of a coexistent tumor. Such conditions as acute leukemia, Hodgkin's disease, and various solid tumors show similar five-year survival rates in nonpregnant and pregnant groups. Even when the malignancy is one that is frequently affected by changes in the hormonal milieu, such as carcinoma of the breast, the course of the disease

510

is unchanged by pregnancy despite past suggestions to the contrary. Nevertheless, if a nonpregnant patient has a tumor that may theoretically be adversely influenced by hormones, avoidance of pregnancy by the use of mechanical or surgical methods of contraception (rather than hormonal antiovulatory agents) often seems advisable during the five-year period after diagnosis, if only to err on the side of caution. The decision regarding the termination of a pregnancy requires judgment based on the natural history of the malignant disease and the stage of gestation. Two major factors that influence the decision whether to terminate pregnancy are whether the pregnancy presents a significant obstacle to effective therapy and whether the fetus will sustain significant harm as a result of therapy. Since the pregnancy itself has no effect on the course of the malignant disease, the termination of pregnancy per se does not ameliorate the disease. The natural history of the tumor should determine whether the physician can afford to wait for the fetus to become potentially viable ex utero before beginning therapy, and no rule can be applied to all situations.

Effect of the Tumor on Pregnancy and the Fetus

The influences of a tumor on the course of the pregnancy are for the most part indirect. Spontaneous abortions are not increased in pregnant women with a concomitant tumor, remaining approximately 10 per cent, as in the nontumorous group. The incidence of prematurity is also similar in the two groups. It is through involvement of the blood-forming system that tumors exert much of their harmful influence on pregnancy. Disorders such as leukemia that characteristically pre-empt the bone marrow cause thrombocytopenia, anemia, and leukopenia. This can lead to bleeding and infection at the time of delivery and can compound the problems of anemia and weakness often encountered with pregnancy. Leukemic mothers delivered of infants have not had as much of a problem as might be anticipated with infections and bleeding, judging from past reports, but the dangers must still be recognized.

Specific problems exist with tumors involving the uterine cervix when normal vaginal delivery cannot be accomplished lest there be severe bleeding of the friable cervix. Cervical incompetence does not appear to be an increased problem in women with cervical carcinoma, and the incidence of spontaneous midterm abortions is not increased above the anticipated rate.

The spread of cancer to the placenta is a possibility that is not borne out in fact. Studies have found the products of conception (placenta, fetus) to be rarely involved with metastatic tumor even when the tumor is widespread throughout the mother's body. The characteristics accounting for the uniqueness of this placental barrier have not been completely defined. The immunologic competence of the fetus, which is present from the second trimester, may also protect it from tumor. Potter and Schoeneman reviewed the totality of the world's literature and found only 24 cases of cancer that was metastatic to the products of conception.[55] Eleven instances of melanoma, four of breast carcinoma, two of stomach carcinoma, and two of lung carcinoma made up the majority of the cases, with one case each of various others. This representation of melanoma was out of proportion to its incidence in pregnant women, which is only 8 per cent of all tumors. Only eight fetuses in the 24 mothers were involved with metastatic disease. Seven of the eight had melanoma. Twelve other children survived these pregnancies without sequelae. Careful histologic observations included in a more recent study[58] have shown that all 26 patients whose placentas were examined had tumor cells in the intervillous spaces, but only six had actual invasion of the villi. Only one fetus was involved with tumor. It is also interesting that in none of 502 cases of choriocarcinoma was there involvement of the fetus.[50]

In the rare recorded instances of congenital neoplasia, such as with neuroblastoma, melanoma, or leukemia, the tumor did not spread from the fetus to the mother. The placental villus thus appears to be an effective barrier to the spread of tumor cells from the maternal to the fetal circulation as well as in the opposite direction. Failure of the tumor to afflict the mother can also be interpreted as circumstantial evidence for maternal immunocompetence, with rejection of any tumor cells that do reach her blood stream.

There is a distinct possibility that acute leukemia is an oncogenic viral disease, and it is also conceivable that the virus is transmitted at the time of conception or in early fetal life. Despite these considerations, no evidence exists that the children of a mother with leukemia contract the disease more than those whose mother does not have the disease. Leukemia and lymphoma have not been found transmissible to the fetus, with followup for as long as 20 years. One case report[15] described acute lymphocytic leukemia in a 9 month old infant whose mother may have had the same disease during pregnancy, although it was diagnosed immediately post partum.

Hazards of Diagnostic Procedures

There has been some dispute regarding the carcinogenic hazard to the fetus of diagnostic irradiation. Although numerous serial x-ray studies, such as those required for intravenous pyelography and lymphangiography, may result in substantial fetal irradiation, it is argued that most single roentgenographic procedures do not supply more than 1 to 10 rads. But is low dose irradiation a hazard, particularly in the development of tumors of long latency such as leukemia? The possible correlation between low dose irradiation and leukemia in offspring would be strengthened by the identification of a subpopulation of leukemic children who were in utero when their mother was exposed to such irradiation. Sweet and Kinzie[66] indicate that the mortality from leukemia, central nervous system tumors, and other solid tumors is 40 per cent in children whose mother received diagnostic x-ray during pregnancy. An increased incidence of hemangiomas was suggested in another study of 1,008 children exposed to diagnostic x-ray of 1.5 to 3 rads.

It is of considerable interest to note that none of 98 individuals who were exposed while in utero at a distance of 1500 meters or less from the hypocenter of an atomic bomb blast developed leukemia during a 20 year followup. At this distance a high dose (200 to 220 rads) of radiation was delivered, causing immediate congenital problems such as microcephaly and central nervous system damage. In contrast, children who were under 10 years of age during the atomic bombing of Hiroshima and Nagasaki had an incidence of leukemia that was 26 times higher than a nonexposed group.[65] The fate of children exposed in utero at a distance of *more* than 1500 meters, who thus received low dose irradiation, will provide the most important data on the effect of diagnostic x-rays. This group is currently being followed carefully.

The administration of radiolabeled compounds in the evaluation of pregnant patients with cancer may present a radiation hazard to the fetus.[85] Strontium previously used extensively in bone scanning may cross the placenta and may localize in fetal bones. One should also be aware of whether bone-seeking isotopes were used prior to conception. The negative calcium balance associated with pregnancy and lactation would cause the release of the isotope from maternal bones and thus secondarily expose the fetus. This exposure can perhaps be avoided by giving adequate calcium supplementation to the mother. [75]Selenium-methionine, used in pancreatic scanning, also crosses the placental membranes and can dangerously irradiate the fetus. However, [203]Hg- or [197]Hg-chlormerodrin used in kidney and brain scanning and colloidal materials such as colloidal gold, technetium sulfide, and macroaggregates do not significantly cross the placental barrier.

Effects of Therapy on the Fetus

TERATOGENESIS

The fetus is uniquely and exquisitely sensitive both to drugs and radiation, particularly at the neuroblast stage.[14, 28] Experimental drug effects on the fetus are influenced by the stage of gestation, the dose and duration of therapy, sex, species, and strain. Individual genetic factors are also of considerable importance. In animal teratogenicity studies, an entire spectrum of effects ranging from fetal resorptions to apparent normalcy have been seen within one litter. Furthermore, the dose that produces fetal damage may not have perceptible effects on the mother.

Death in utero can be manifested as fetal resorptions, abortions, or stillbirths with or without malformations. Delayed growth and development in utero and prematurity constitute added risks to the neonate. Those who survive the lethal effects of the drugs may have various structural malformations, which may or may not affect long-term viability. These and other considerations in teratogenesis have been reviewed in greater detail and reviews on teratology should be consulted.[21]

An area that has not received much attention is human behavioral teratology. It has been shown that the administration of various drugs to pregnant animals affected the learning potential, emotionality, sexual activity, and resistance to audiogenic seizures in the offspring without producing any gross or histologic alterations. Similarly, normal litter mates of animals with hydrocephalus did not learn a maze as well as untreated control animals and, in addition, had electroencephalographic changes. A similar relationship might be sought in human behavioral problems.

Treatment of the mother with large doses of steroids or cytotoxic drugs during the last trimester of pregnancy has produced suppression of the adrenal glands and bone marrow in the neonate.

Long-term effects of drug exposure in utero include retarded physical and/or mental growth and development, sterility, and premature aging. Subtle point mutations may occur in the developing fetus so that altered coding for certain proteins may later be manifested as disease. Most drugs useful in the treatment of leukemia or lymphoma are carcinogenic in one species or another, and, in view of the time lag for carcinogenesis, exposure in utero might be responsible for some neoplastic processes appearing later in life, as has been shown to occur in mice. Finally, a source of concern for future generations stems from studies of the effects of irradiation on mice and on the fruit fly *Drosophila melanogaster*. Evidence of deformity was shown to be delayed until the third and subsequent generations. In human beings, deformity owing to irradiation appears to be carried as a recessive trait, and although the fetus that was actually irradiated may be normal, deformity or disease may appear in a second or third generation. The increasing incidence of leukemia and Hodgkin's disease might be significant in this regard.

Adrenal steroids have produced a very high incidence of cleft palate in experimental animals. The frequency of this teratogenic effect is definitely related to the genetic strain of the animal as well as to the time during gestation that the animal was treated. A review of the literature revealed 363 pregnant women treated with steroids, mostly for non-neoplastic disease; 351 women received steroids only. Although the time of therapy during gestation was unspecified, the fetal problems included one abortion, nine stillbirths, 16 premature births, six cleft palates, masculinization of one female, and hypoadrenalism in two infants, one of whom died, although the other was effectively treated with adrenal glucocorticoids. The death of one other premature infant in this series could also have been due to unrecognized hypoadrenalism because of gland suppression by the exogenous steroids, since the mother was treated with steroids throughout pregnancy. The need for and value of steroids in these infants should always be kept in mind, especially since the deterioration of the infant, once established, is rapid and relentless. This clinical observation is supported by the experimental data, which show that cortisol passes from the maternal to the fetal circulation via the placenta in relatively constant ratios and that the developing fetus biosynthesizes essentially no cortisol.

It has long been known that the administration of the folate antagonists aminopterin and methotrexate results in a high percentage of abortions and fetal malformations. These effects are definitely dependent on the period of gestation during which these drugs are administered, since the fetus is more sensitive in early gestation than it is later in pregnancy. Nonabortifacient doses of these drugs may produce malformations in a viable fetus. Of the 36 patients described in several small series who took a folate antagonist during the first trimester, 26 aborted spontaneously within a matter of weeks. Of the six who aborted later or who had surgical evacuation of the uterus, four had malformed fetuses and two fetuses were normal on gross examination. Four patients went to term and delivered three babies with multiple congenital anomalies, two of whom lived. One patient with a diagnosis of recurrent choriocarcinoma was treated during the first trimester with methotrexate, actinomycin D, and chlorambucil. She went to term and delivered normal twins. Five patients received methotrexate or aminopterin during the second or third trimester along with steroids, 6-mercaptopurine, vincristine, or demecholine; one patient had a spontaneous abortion and four went to term and delivered normal infants.[11]

There is a case report of multiple limb abnormalities in a child who was conceived while the mother was being treated with cytosine arabinoside. Although there were no chromosomal abnormalities in peripheral blood lymphocytes of the mother or child, the child was born with bilateral microtia and bilateral atresia of the external auditory canals as well as multiple limb deformities.[66a] Similar limb deformities have been noted in mice whose mothers became pregnant during treatment with cytosine arabinoside.[32, 52]

Other case reports revealed no congenital abnormalities in fetuses exposed to cytosine arabinoside and 6-thioguanine during the tenth,[37] 25th,[51] and 26th weeks of gestation.[56] In another report trisomy C was found in a 24 week abortus exposed to cytosine arabinoside and thioguanine during the 20th week of gestation.[40]

In a recent report of nine cases of leukemia in pregnancy, four patients were treated during the first trimester with combinations of drugs including 6-mercaptopurine, methotrexate, cyclophosphamide, vincristine, prednisone, cytosine arabinoside, and doxorubicin. There were no instances of congenital abnormalities.[54] Two patients who were treated with m-AMSA and MOPP, respectively, during conception and the first trimester delivered full term, apparently normal infants.[8] In another instance, MOPP therapy during the first trimester was associated with fetal renal malformations.[43]

Other antineoplastic drugs have been administered to pregnant patients, but their effects on the fetus are obscure. These drugs include triethylenemelamine, mechlorethamine, vinblastine, and procarbazine. Asparaginase has produced fetal malformations in rabbits. The use of bleomycin, the nitrosoureas, adriamycin, and rubidomycin during pregnancy has not been reported.

Although the issue will be considered in the next section, it should be noted here that from the followup of patients treated successfully with combination chemotherapy a considerable body of evidence has accrued suggesting that chemotherapy in the female or male prior to conception does not necessarily result in later fetal abnormalities.[8, 29]

In summary, although most of the antineoplastic agents in current use have the potential to cause fetal wastage and teratogenic effects, there are a number of instances in which an apparently healthy, full term infant has been born despite active chemotherapy in the mother during conception and the first trimester. Although the possibility for teratogenesis is undeniable, the incidence is perhaps somewhat less than one would expect. It would obviously be safer to avoid such exposure, but the decision to terminate an unplanned pregnancy must also take into consideration the desire of the parents for children.

The successful use of extended field irradiation and aggressive chemotherapy programs in curing or prolonging the useful life of some patients with neoplastic diseases poses important questions in toxicology. The immediate toxicologic effects on the bone marrow and other rapidly proliferating cellular systems are well known. Of current concern is the protracted effect of therapy on fertility, since many young patients cured of lymphoma or leukemia who are otherwise in excellent health become sterile. A further consideration is the possibility that irradiation and/or chemotherapy may induce somatic mutations, thereby initiating new diseases in the host or fetus. This is supported by the occurrence of acute leukemia and other secondary neoplasms in patients with Hodgkin's disease,[1, 10] multiple myeloma, and polycythemia vera whose primary disease has been successfully controlled with chemotherapy or irradiation.

Since fertility in patients treated with chemotherapy and/or irradiation may resume months or years after the termination of therapy, genetic consequences on the offspring must be considered. Although many normal children have been born of women treated with chemotherapy and/or irradiation, their exact numbers are unknown.[8, 29] The mutagenic effects of therapy should be suspected with the appearance of diseases associated with an autosomal mode of inheritance. Similarly, the appearance of X-linked recessive mutations in the sons of treated females should be suspected of being caused by irradiation therapy. X-linked recessive mutations occurring in treated males would be less likely to be attributed to previous therapy, because the appearance of disease would skip a generation.

There is experimental and clinical precedent for the transplacental passage of carcinogens. Documentation of transplacental carcinogenesis is complicated by the fact that transplacentally induced tumors are rarely present at birth and may appear months or years after the in utero exposure to the carcinogen. The only well-documented example of transplacental carcinogenesis in human beings is the appearance of vaginal carcinoma in young women whose mothers were treated with diethylstilbestrol to prevent miscarriage. This tumor deserves further consideration here for this reason, even though it does not affect the pregnant woman herself.

ADENOCARCINOMA OF THE VAGINA AND CERVIX

This rare clear-cell adenocarcinoma of the vagina or cervix has occurred in the daughters of women who had been treated with a synthetic estrogenic steroid, usually diethylstilbestrol (DES), to sustain a difficult pregnancy. This practice was common in the early to mid 1950s. The tumor usually appears during puberty at a mean age of 19.5 years, but patients 7 to 29 years old have been recorded.[26] Approximately 60 per cent of the 346 patients reported since 1971 to a registry established to record the disease have had clear-cell adenocarcinoma of the vagina, and approximately 40 per cent have had adenocarcinoma of the cervix.[6, 26] In two thirds of the cases the mother of the patient had taken a nonsteroidal estrogenic substance to control bleeding to help protect against fetal loss.

It should be emphasized that clear-cell adenocarcinoma is rare even in those with a maternal history of ingestion of DES. Most of the changes found in the progeny have been benign, and it is estimated that although nearly two thirds of the female progeny show some degree of adenosis, no more than 0.14 to 1.4 of 1,000 exposed females have had a malignancy through age 24.[27] Furthermore, serial culposcopic examinations over several years have failed to show progression of benign adenosis to malignancy. In fact, the squamous metaplasia often found with adenosis seems to be a mechanism of healing. No squamous carcinomas have arisen.

Male progeny also show anatomic and functional abnormalities. One quarter of such boys exposed in utero have hypoplastic and/or undescended testes, epididymal cysts, or microphallus. Decreased sperm counts and poor mobility of sperm have also been noted.[6, 27] Although none has developed a carcinoma, the incidence of testicular cancer in males with cryptorchidism and hypoplastic testes is known to be increased and could be a future problem. Prostatic cancer, which arises from a müllerian duct remnant, the prostatic utricle, homologous with the female vagina, might also be increased in these male progeny, especially since it is a tumor influenced by hormonal changes.[6]

Diagnosis. Clear-cell adenocarcinoma of the vagina usually occurs where müllerian duct remnants are most often found, i.e., just below the external cervical os in the anterior wall of the upper third of the vagina. The presence of vaginal bleeding or discharge occurred as a presenting sign in 54 of 91 patients.[25] The remainder were asymptomatic, and cytology by Papanicolaou smear was frequently negative. For this reason, continued persistent followup after screening of this group of pubertal and prepubertal girls is essential. A careful vaginal examination, with acetic acid staining of the cervix and colposcopically directed biopsies, is required to rule out malignancy. The appearance of the cervix and vagina is usually far more ominous than the histology, which is only rarely indicative of malignancy. The commonest findings are of benign adenosis, including white epithelium, grape-like excrescences (seen especially well after acetic acid staining), cervical "collars," transverse ridges on the cervix and upper vagina, and hypoplastic cervix. Metaplastic squamous epithelium, which should not be confused with dysplasia, is also frequently found histologically. Clear-cell tumors with papillary or tubulocystic histologic patterns have been described, the former with the worst prognosis and the latter with the best.[26] Also, large tumors that are deeply invasive, with many mitoses, as usual have the worst prognosis.

Course and Therapy. Clear-cell adenocarcinoma is not entirely benign, since there has been a 22 per cent mortality described.[26] Moreover, 16 per cent of the patients with Stage I disease have had a recurrence of disease after surgery; 23 per cent of all patients have had a recurrence within five years. These adenocarcinomas first spread to regional lymph nodes, and recurrences have been found in the pelvis. The most common metastatic site has been the lungs. A radical operative procedure has been suggested for all cases. Radical hysterectomy with bilateral paraaortic and pelvic lymphadenectomy has been recommended for Stage I disease. A five-year survival of nearly 90 per cent is expected for this group, whereas 30 per cent of Stage III patients survive five years. Few Stage IV patients have lived even three years. The overall survival of patients with clear-cell adenocarcinoma does seem to be better than that of patients with squamous cell carcinoma of the cervix or vagina, and early diagnosis and treatment certainly effect many cures.

Surgery is useful for recurrent disease. Twelve of 58 patients with recurrent tumor treated by surgery alone survived three years or more. Radiation therapy has not been as good for producing disease-free survival, but the tumors treated by this modality have been of larger size. Chemotherapy with various single agents and combinations has been tried in disseminated disease, but no regimen has emerged as particularly effective. Eight of 34 patients have had objective responses, but none was complete; radiation therapy was also used in two of the eight.[26]

Clearly the most effective measure is prevention, i.e., avoiding the use of diethylstilbestrol or similar synthetic estrogens in pregnant women. Recent package inserts for diethylstilbestrol provided by the manufacturer have appropriately stressed this restriction. Although the use of hormones during pregnancy has virtually stopped, the number of cases reported is at a plateau of approximately 28 per year.

EFFECTS OF RADIATION

Radiation effects on the fetus depend on the stage of gestation during the exposure and the dose of irradiation. The fetus is most sensitive to irradiation in early gestation during organogenesis, and exposures as small as 1 to 5 rads in the mouse fetus at such a time have produced an increased number of anomalies.[59] A careful study of 26 subjects who had been irradiated in utero suggested a general timetable of periods of radiation risk.[16] The individuals who had several congenital abnormalities were those radiated between three and ten weeks of gestation, at which time more than half of the group developed anomalies at 250 rads. Among these were small birth size, microcephaly, mental retardation, retinal degeneration, skeletal and genital abnormalities, and cataracts. Two hundred and fifty rads given before two or three weeks gestation increased spontanous abortions but did not lead to severe congenital anomalies. At 10 to 20 weeks, effects were less severe than at three to ten weeks, with some instances of small size, microcephaly, and mental retardation. After 20 to 25 weeks gestation there were no severe abnormalities, with anemia, pigmentary changes, and dermal erythema being the only toxic effects. The effects of irradiation at this late time in utero are those that might be found after ionizing radiation at any time during postnatal life. From these data, avoidance of abdominal radiation to the mother during at least the first 16 weeks of pregnancy is suggested.[16]

Radiation to extra-abdominal sites, as in early stage Hodgkin's disease, did not result in congenital malformations, although five of the progeny died in early infancy. Twenty-two normal offspring were born who have survived into childhood, despite the fact that nine of them had mothers who received radiation at the time of conception or during the first trimester.[11] In contrast, pelvic radiation of 30 to 250 rads with radium implants or external beams caused abnormalities in 23 of 106 children, whose neurologic and skeletal problems were similar to those cited previously by Dekaban.[16]

The long-term effects of radiation constitute an important threat to the well-being of the fetus. Calculated doses of 200 to 220 rads in utero from the atomic bomb blast at Hiroshima caused one third of the children to have persistent chromosomal abnormalities. Leukemia has not (yet) shown an increased incidence, however. As we have mentioned, diagnostic doses of x-rays of 1 to 10 rads may pose a greater long-term threat. If either parent is irradiated prior to conception the rate of leukemia in the offspring is increased.[66] This risk of latent neoplasia from chromosomal damage in the hematopoietic stem cells must be considered a persistent threat to the children of therapeutically radiated mothers, including those children who are ostensibly normal at birth, until further studies prove otherwise.

The therapeutic use of short-lived radioisotopes that cross the placenta such as ^{131}I is extremely hazardous to the fetus. Beta-emitting isotopes, such as [98]Au and ^{32}P, have a short range of action and are safe since amniotic fluid absorbs most of the radioactivity. Fortunately, the transfer of radioisotopes is poorest early in gestation when the fetus is most sensitive, but their use in therapy during pregnancy should be avoided if possible.[65]

Effects of Therapy on Fertility

EFFECTS ON OOGENESIS

Unless the malignant disease directly involves the reproductive organs, there is usually no effect on fertility or reproductive capacity aside from that produced by debility or other constitutional symptoms. Impairment of reproductive function in the patient with cancer is not an uncommon result of therapy. Illustrations of this are seen following the treatment of Hodgkin's disease. Since the ovaries lie adjacent to the iliac nodes, a course of irradiation applied to these nodes for the treatment of Hodgkin's disease (usually 3500 to 4000 rads in three and one half to four weeks) would inevitably sterilize the patient, since 800 rads delivered to the ovaries in three days is usually sufficient to induce an artificial menopause. In an attempt to preserve ovarian function in patients desirous of future pregnancy, the ovaries may be transposed to a midline position prior to irradiation. Today this is conveniently performed during the laparotomy commonly used for staging. Identification of the position of the ovaries by metallic clips placed by the surgeon is helpful to the radiation therapist so that the ovaries may later be shielded as much as possible. However, even with transposition of the ovaries, the ovaries undoubtedly receive considerable radiation as a result of scattering of the beam by the tissues. Using a tissue-equivalent pelvic phantom, it has been estimated that the maximum dose delivered to the shielded ovaries during the usual pelvic irradiation for Hodgkin's disease is 500 rads over a four-week period. In a series of eight patients whose ovaries were appropriately moved and shielded from the irradiation, only two had subsequently normal menses, one had irregular menses for one year, and five were amenorrheic at one to four years postirradiation. One patient had a return of irregular menses after two years of amenorrhea; six years later she conceived and was delivered of a normal child.[3] In another series of 22 patients in whom the ovaries were moved to the midline and shielded from radiation, menses resumed in 55 per cent of the patients following a variable period of amenorrhea.[31] However, documented fertility is much less frequent.

Menstrual irregularities and amenorrhea frequently follow the systemic use of antineoplastic drugs, especially the alkylating agents. This has most commonly been reported with the use of busulfan. Histologic examination of the ovaries following prolonged treatment with busulfan has revealed ovarian fibrosis. This agent also has a propensity for producing pulmonary fibrosis following prolonged use. Ovarian function was assessed in eight women with amenorrhea who were treated with a variety of agents alone and in combination including vinblastine, vincristine, nitrogen mustard, chlorambucil, cyclophosphamide, and procarbazine. Six of these patients had high levels of FSH and LH, indicating primary ovarian failure.[63] In two other patients with oligomenorrhea, one had low gonadotropins and the other became pregnant. In addition to primary ovarian failure, the authors suggest that the menstrual dysfunction in some patients may be related to drug-induced interference with endometrial proliferation and/or disturbances in the growth of the follicles, with loss of rhythmicity without loss of function. Although reports in the literature are generally anecdotal, it appears that amenorrhea following extensive treatment with alkylating agents is usually permanent, although occasionally menses resume months or years following cessation of therapy.

Experience with the use of low doses of cyclophosphamide in the treatment of rheumatoid arthritis or systemic lupus erythematosus indicates that although amenorrhea frequently occurs, if the therapy is stopped after six to nine months, menses are more than likely to resume. Permanent sterility is thus a function of the dose and duration of therapy rather than the agent per se.[24] Amenorrhea following treatment with the vinca alkaloids or antimetabolites is more likely to be temporary, with expected restoration of menstrual function following the discontinuation of the drugs. Today the problem is compounded by the more frequent use of combinations of drugs rather than single agents. Since patients with Hodgkin's disease are surviving for longer periods of time, with a significant proportion being cured, definite attempts at preserving gonadal function are appropriate, provided there is no compromise in what is believed to be optimal therapy. This preservation of fertility has been indicated by reports of the delivery of viable, normal infants. A major unresolved question, however, is the effect of therapy on the genetic endowment of the offspring with the possible production of genetically related diseases, both neoplastic and non-neoplastic.

Significant impairment in fertility as a result of therapy is also seen in male patients. Both chemotherapy and abdominal irradiation have produced significant oligospermia or temporary or permanent sterility. Single doses of 8 to 50 rads are sufficient to produce temporary oligospermia. However, the commonly used fractionated schemes are probably more effective and efficient in reducing spermatogenesis. Such a scheme of testicular irradiation can be a concomitant of therapy for Hodgkin's disease. In a series of ten male patients receiving inverted-Y inguinal irradiation, a dosimeter was placed adjacent to the scrotal skin under the testicular shield and exposure was recorded during the course of normal treatment. These patients were found to receive a testicular dose in the range of 5 to 15 rads per day, five days a week, for a total dose in the range of 100 to 300 rads. All patients were aspermic at the completion of therapy and continued to be aspermic for the followup periods ranging from 2 to 40 months.[64] Further testicular irradiation may occur from diagnostic radiologic procedures such as intravenous pyelogram, metastatic bone survey, and lymphangiography as well as from internal scatter secondary to thoracic irradiation.

Chemotherapy also produces sterility or a significant reduction in sperm count. Eight males treated with cyclophosphamide for nephrotic syndrome developed aspermia, and testicular atrophy was seen on biopsy; two patients had evidence of regeneration at 10 and 28 months after the cessation of therapy, respectively.[34] Larger doses of cyclophosphamide may produce a more protracted aspermia or oligospermia. Oligospermia and aspermia have also been described in patients treated with chlorambucil and busulfan. In animals, procarbazine, vincristine, methotrexate, 6-mercaptopurine, nitrogen mustard, and thiotepa have been shown to have a deleterious effect on spermatogenesis. Sixteen men who were treated with one of several drug combinations for lymphoma including MOPP (nitrogen mustard, vincristine, procarbazine, and prednisone), MOMP (methotrexate substituted for procarbazine), or CVP (cyclophosphamide, vincristine, and prednisone) had an assessment of testicular function six months to seven years following the completion of therapy; ten men were azoospermic and testicular biopsy showed no germ cells, two men showed minimal evidence of spermatogenesis, and four who were in remission for two to seven years showed complete spermatogenesis. Thus, spermatogenesis may return following extensive chemotherapy after a drug-free interval of several years.[61]

SPECIFIC TUMORS

Choriocarcinoma and Other Trophoblastic Tumors

Choriocarcinoma is a disorder that is very nearly unique to pregnant women, a malignancy of the fetal trophoblastic epithelium. Although nongestational teratomatous varieties can occur in the ovary and in the male testicle, the placental choriocarcinoma is the most common type. Placental choriocarcinoma is not a common malignancy in Western nations. In this country, the estimates have ranged from an incidence of 1 in 13,850 pregnancies to 1 in

40,000 deliveries in two different surveys.[2] The disease is far more common in Asiatic countries, with an incidence ranging from 1 in 250 to 1 in 3,708 deliveries in various hospitals. Autopsy figures from Hong Kong also reveal a very high occurrence, with 1 in 114 autopsied deaths attributable to this cause.[2]

Choriocarcinoma is the most malignant of a spectrum of disorders of the trophoblast, the most benign of which is the hydatidiform mole; the invasive mole is of intermediate malignancy. Hydatidiform mole should be suspected when the uterus of a patient thought to be pregnant enlarges more rapidly than would be expected from the gestational age of the fetus. The stroma of the trophoblastic villi undergo hydropic changes, resembling the hydatid cysts seen with *Echinococcus* infestation, and there is a proliferation of trophoblastic epithelium, which points up the nature of the mole as a benign tumor rather than simply a degenerative disease. A bloody discharge is frequently the presenting symptom, beginning three to four months after the onset of pregnancy, but it is not usually profuse. Toxemia, with vomiting, albuminuria, hypertension, and edema is also frequent and occurs earlier than might be anticipated with a normal pregnancy. Human chorionic gonadotropin (HCG) titers in the urine are elevated to levels exceeding 500,000 I.U. per 24 hours, which exclude all but a few normal pregnancies (particularly with twins). Helpful diagnostic procedures also include ultrasound scanning to identify the fetus (absent with hydatidiform mole) and pelvic arteriography to outline the vascular mass.

Treatment of the hydatidiform mole usually consists of completion of the spontaneous abortion of trophoblastic material, which is occurring at the time the diagnosis is made. After evacuation is completed, HCG levels should steadily decrease, but they may not immediately fall to zero since small fragments of trophoblastic tissue often remain in the uterus, undergoing necrosis spontaneously after a few weeks or at most within two to three months. Careful followup of these patients with HCG determinations on the urine at two-week intervals at least and chest x-rays every one to two months for two years will identify those patients whose mole has evolved into a frank case of choriocarcinoma. Such monitoring is particularly necessary if the HCG is negative initially. HCG levels that are rising or that persist at high levels for more than a month may be harbingers of choriocarcinomatous degeneration of the trophoblastic epithelium and may indicate the need for further therapeutic

intervention. The longer the trophoblast remains, the greater is the risk of its degeneration.

Hysterectomy is a more definitive treatment of hydatidiform mole than simple evacuation but is not indicated as primary therapy. Chemotherapy with methotrexate and/or actinomycin D is highly successful in destroying residual trophoblastic cells of potential malignancy. Indeed, this form of therapy has been universally successful[36] and permits subsequent pregnancy. Hysterectomy is required as secondary therapy in about 10 per cent of all cases of nonmetastatic molar disease.

The invasive mole, also known as chorioadenoma destruens, also presents with profuse hemorrhage, with abdominal pain and tenderness frequently found when peritoneal extension of the disease has occurred. Embolization of villous material to the lungs may also produce dyspnea and hemoptysis, frequently with radiologic evidence of pulmonary infarction. The invasive mole usually appears within six months of evacuation of a benign mole and is indicated by uterine enlargement and masses in the vaginal vault and parametrium, together with elevation of HCG. Curettage may fail to yield definitive diagnostic information, since the disease may not have reached the surface of the endometrium. Thus, on the basis of these signs, there may be no simple way to distinguish an invasive mole from the more malignant choriocarcinoma. Hysterectomy is inappropriate and unnecessary as treatment for an invasive mole, as it is for choriocarcinoma, since the disease is usually systemic and can be cured by systemic chemotherapy.

Choriocarcinoma, also called chorionepithelioma, is extremely malignant if unchecked by chemotherapy and causes death within months. The trophoblastic villi are completely degenerated, and no villous pattern is seen. On histologic examination there is invasion of the muscles and blood vessels of the uterus. From one third to two thirds of choriocarcinomas present following a pre-existent mole. From 25 to 30 per cent occur after pregnancies ending in abortions, with an equal percentage occurring after term delivery.[2] The disorder may occur in the absence of other products of conception, during a normal pregnancy, at term, or at intervals after a pregnancy ranging from days to years. However, less than 12 months from a pregnancy is most usual, particularly if the choriocarcinoma has developed from a preceding mole. The patient may present with vaginal bleeding originating either from the uterus or from vaginal implants. As with the invasive mole, peritoneal extension and hemorrhage may occur with considerable abdominal pain. Fatal intra-abdominal hemorrhage has also been encountered. Equally frequent are symptoms arising from the metastases of the tumor, particularly to the lungs. Discrete parenchymal nodules may be found on chest x-ray examination; these are asymptomatic. A more diffuse involvement with small emboli, appearing as a fibronodular pattern on the chest x-ray, may enter the venous circulation via the pelvic veins and may cause severe dyspnea from ventilation/perfusion imbalance, as seen with pulmonary emboli from fragmented clots. Right ventricular failure may be identified by electrocardiographic and clinical criteria. Pleural effusion is less common in this diffuse variety of spread than with the single large tumor embolus, which leads to acute infarction of the lung and hemothorax. The disease usually does not spread to the bone marrow and only occasionally to the liver. The brain is involved in about 15 per cent of patients.

DIAGNOSIS

An elevation of HCG in the urine to values often exceeding several million units per day usually accompanies choriocarcinoma. The more extensive the disease, the higher the level of HCG, making this a valuable means by which to gauge the success or failure of therapy. There are a number of sensitive immunologic tests for HCG, the best of which is radioimmunoassay. Luteotrophic hormone (LH) is immunologically cross reactive with HCG, but levels of HCG greater than 150 I.U./day exceed the upper limit for LH in normal women. Immunologic identification of the beta subunit of HCG also permits highly specific discrimination of HCG.

Percutaneous pelvic arteriography is a very helpful procedure for the diagnosis of choriocarcinoma. It can demonstrate enlargement of the uterus; dilatations of the uterine, ovarian, and other arteries; increased branching of the intramural arteries; and filling of irregular vascular spaces in the tumor. A region of central hypovascularity amid a region of hypervascularity, the latter being the same sort of "tumor blush" seen with other tumors, identifies the choriocarcinoma with its neovasculature and a central region of necrosis and hemorrhage.

COURSE AND TREATMENT

If allowed to run its natural course, choriocarcinoma kills by either metastatic spread or local profuse hemorrhage, leading to death within several months to one year. Although spontaneous regressions of metastatic disease, particularly following hysterectomy, were reported in the past, these were too infrequent to be sufficient grounds for "expectant" nontherapy or for performing hysterectomy as a definitive procedure. The introduction of methotrexate, cyclophosphamide, 6-mercaptopurine, and actinomycin D into the therapeutic armamentarium against choriocarcinoma has dramatically altered the course of the disease and in fact has led to cures in at least 70 per cent of patients with metastatic involvement.

A full description of therapeutic possibilities has been provided by Goldstein,[22] according to the various categories of disease and options regarding preservation of reproductive capacity. In general, a single course of actinomycin D or methotrexate is usually sufficient to cause remission in nearly 100 per cent of patients with a hydatidiform mole or a nonmetastatic trophoblastic neoplasm after evacuation. Sequential methotrexate and actinomycin D therapy is usually sufficient to cure choriocarcinoma except in resistant cases, where triple therapy with cyclophosphamide, actinomycin D, and methotrexate is useful. Brain metastases may respond to additional whole brain irradiation.

Ross et al. treated women with sequential methotrexate and actinomycin D.[57] Complete responses were noted in all of those patients whose HCG titer was less than 100,000 I.U. per 24 hours, whose disease was confined to the pelvis and lungs, and in whom therapy was initiated within four months of apparent onset. Those patients with higher titers, longer duration, or metastases to the brain or liver were less likely to respond, so that the overall response rate for the entire series was 74 per cent. Such patients did respond, however, to a simultaneous combination of effective agents.[36] Lewis also reported that 90 per cent of those patients with metastatic disease who achieved a complete remission after treatment with chemotherapy have remained in remission without further therapy, some for more than 15 years.[36] Complete remission is defined as the disappearance of all known evidence of disease and the finding of HCG levels in the normal range on three consecutive weekly determinations.

The dose of methotrexate, after that originally reported by Hertz and collaborators, has been 0.3 to 0.4 mg/kg/day for five days, intramuscularly, and actinomycin D has been given in a single dose of 50 mcg/kg every month.[27a]

Prevention of gestational trophoblastic disease by the treatment of molar pregnancies with chemotherapy has been reported several times. In one study, 100 women were given actinomycin D (12 mg/kg/day for five days, intravenously) beginning three days before an elective evacuation. A second group of 100 nonrandomized controls were given no drug therapy. Only two women treated with actinomycin developed proliferative trophoblastic disease versus 16 in the control group. Furthermore, metastatic disease was present in four control women but in none of those who were given the single course of actinomycin D. Since early choriocarcinoma is easily cured, this "prophylactic" treatment of patients before frank malignancy should not be a substitute for a careful followup with sensitive assays for beta-HCG but could be helpful in those geographic areas where choriocarcinoma is of particularly high incidence, when the histology of the evacuated mole is suggestive or diagnostic of malignant transformation, or when sensitive assays for HCG are unavailable.[23]

Normal pregnancies have occurred after the successful eradication of choriocarcinoma by chemotherapy. More than 200 such pregnancies have been reported in women treated previously for choriocarcinoma without obvious adverse effects on the mother or the fetus. In particular, no reactivation of the trophoblastic neoplasm has been reported.

Carcinoma of the Breast

Adenocarcinoma of the breast is a disease that ordinarily afflicts women who are approaching menopausal age, with a second peak incidence in women in their sixties. One survey found only 19 per cent of all cases in women under 30[7] and no more than 8 per cent of those with breast carcinoma in women under 40. Thus it is not often found in pregnant women, with no more than 1 to 3 per cent of all cancers of the breast occurring during pregnancy or lactation. If the number of pregnancies is considered the denominator, only 1 in 3,200 pregnancies is associated with carcinoma of the breast. Yet, seen from another aspect, approximately 30 per cent of patients with carcinoma of the breast in the 30 to 36 year old age group have a coincident pregnancy because of the frequency of childbearing during those years. The pregnant patient with breast cancer is thus relatively uncommon but not rare. Women who have borne children, and particularly those who have breast fed, have a lower incidence of breast cancer than nulliparous women. Not only is pregnancy not a causal influence in breast cancer, it seems to be a protective factor against the later development of the tumor.

DIAGNOSIS IN PREGNANCY

The diagnosis of a malignant breast mass is more difficult during pregnancy than usual because of the hypervascularity, increased size, and engorgement of glandular tissue. A breast mass can always be felt best by the patient on self-examination, with the lesion being compressed by the examining hand against the chest wall. The physician can palpate only the anterior aspect of the lesion. In the enlarged breast of the pregnant woman it is difficult for either the physician or the patient to palpate small lesions, which may remain painless until they have reached considerable size. Fixation and induration of overlying skin, with subsequent ulceration, are late changes. The tumor may mimic benign mastitis, common during pregnancy, if it is associated with obstruction of lymphatics by tumor cells (inflammatory carcinoma). Yet careful serial examinations of the breasts, with special attention to the upper outer quadrant, in which 50 per cent of lesions arise, can be rewarding in the early detection of a firm nodule.

Radiography of the breast, mammography, may reveal the presence of minute calcifications, which are strongly suggestive of carcinoma. Lesions of only a few millimeters have been detected by this means in nonpregnant women. Mammography can be performed safely at low dose and with abdominal shielding and has not caused problems to the mother or fetus.[69] However, the breasts become radiodense with glandular tissue during pregnancy and lactation, sometimes obscuring the diagnosis and certainly limiting the sensitivity of mammography. We must also caution that for this reason and because of its high cost, mammography should not be used as a screening procedure, especially in a group of young women in whom the yield of positive diagnoses is so low. Mammography is a good corroborative noninvasive procedure preceding definitive biopsy of the site in clinically suspicious cases. Thermography, the recording of infrared emissions of the body on special photographic equipment, is another diagnostic procedure of perhaps the same sensitivity as mammography. Tumors are hotter than their surrounding arterial and venous blood supply and hotter than normal tissue; the hotter the tumor the more malignant it appears to be in its subsequent behavior. Mammography has generally been the diagnostic imaging procedure of choice since it is more widely available and at least of equal discriminatory capacity.

Excisional biopsy should be performed if palpation and either mammography or thermography reveal a clinically suspicious lesion. A negative biopsy does not preclude the presence of microscopic tumor cells, since some patients have developed a tumor three to five years after a positive thermogram but a negative biopsy.[16] Serial mammograms and close clinical followup are required for all suspicious lesions.

COURSE IN THE NONPREGNANT STATE

In the nonpregnant woman, carcinoma of the breast usually spreads first to regional lymph nodes of the axilla and internal mammary chain. The most common lesions, those of the upper outer quadrant, spread first to the axillary lymph nodes, whereas the less common medial lesions tend to invade the internal mammary nodes relatively earlier. Metastasis occurs to the lungs, pleural surfaces, liver, bones, brain, subcutaneous region, ovaries, and adrenal glands after a period of quiescence following initial, usually surgical, therapy. This period may be less than a year or, not uncommonly, five to ten years, and it is usually the woman whose regional lymph nodes are involved when the disease is first discovered who eventually shows metastatic disease rather than being completely cured of disease by initial surgery and/or radiotherapy. A second primary tumor in the contralateral breast arises in 5 to 10 per cent of patients and should be carefully sought at the time of diagnosis and during followup examinations.

Lesions in the lung may be blood-borne nodules in the parenchyma, but frequently lymphangitic, fibronodular infiltrates are found, causing dyspnea on mild exertion or even at rest. Bony lesions are usually osteolytic, characterized by elevated serum calcium, but may be osteoblastic, accompanied by elevated alkaline phosphatase levels in the serum. Although far less frequent than prostatic carcinoma as a cause of osteoblastic metastases, breast carcinoma is the most usual cause of that lesion in women.

COURSE DURING PREGNANCY

A pregnant woman in her first or second trimester who presents with a proved malignant breast tumor should be treated in the same way as a nonpregnant woman. Although breast cancer is sometimes responsive to hormonal manipulations, there is no conclusive evidence that the disease is deleteriously affected by the hormonal changes accompanying pregnancy. Cortisol is increased early in pregnancy, causing a decrease in thymus-dependent lymphocyte levels. However, these recover after the 20th week. Prolactin is produced in late gestation and during lactation by the pituitary and the placenta and is a possible, yet unproved, promoter of carcinogenesis in humans. The estrogens produced in pregnancy particularly include estriol, which not only is a weak estrogen but may also antagonize estrone and estradiol, thereby exerting a protective effect against carcinogenesis.[17]

Older literature had suggested that the course was accelerated and the prognosis consequently poorer when breast cancer occurred in young women and especially when it coincided with pregnancy. Birks et al. re-examined this question in their series of 58 patients followed over a period of 25 years.[7] This study did not suffer from the small numbers and variable followups of many of its predecessors and showed that the five- and ten-year survival rates of women under 30 was the same as those of the over-30 group. Thus, approximately 57 per cent lived four years and 40 per cent, ten years. The vast majority of the long-term survivors had no recurrence of disease. Moreover, a total of 23 pregnancies occurred in 16 of the patients with no adverse consequences to the disease, even though 15 pregnancies occurred within five years of diagnosis. The regional spread of breast cancer to lymph nodes at the time of diagnosis, not the coincident pregnancy, portends a poor prognosis. A delay in diagnosis because of the pregnancy and its associated changes in the breast may permit the disease to spread, and it is the difficulty of detection of breast cancer in pregnant women rather than hormonal facilitation of tumor growth that is most obviously detrimental. Overly cautious handling of the tumor is another reason why pregnant women may have fared so poorly with this disease in some instances.

TREATMENT

The best and perhaps the only reason for considering therapeutic abortion in the first or second trimester is to treat metastatic disease promptly. The removal of placental hormones and decrease of pituitary hormones by therapeutic abortion has not been found to ameliorate the course of the disease. Only about a third of nonpregnant premenopausal women respond to hormonal manipulations such as ablation of the ovaries, adrenals, and/or pituitary gland or the administration of antiestrogens or androgens.

Measurement of cytoplasmic receptors for estrogens can help considerably in predicting which patients will respond (approximately 66 per cent of receptor positives) and even more who will not respond (more than 90 per cent of receptor negatives). Younger women who are menstruating when they develop breast cancer and, paradoxically, older women more than five years postmenopasual constitute the hormonally sensitive groups. The treatment of choice for primary breast cancer is still resection in some form.

Many pregnant patients can be operated on if monitoring of the fetus is possible. Patients who are in their last trimester of pregnancy could be allowed to come to term or could be delivered shortly before term rather than having to undergo more drastic procedures to remove the large, nearly viable fetus more immediately. Therapy formerly considered standard for breast cancer is undergoing considerable re-evaluation at present by oncologists. Radical mastectomy is no longer the treatment of choice at most institutions, having been replaced by a total mastectomy, sparing the pectoralis major, with sampling of regional nodes for prognostic purposes and subsequent irradiation of the chest, axilla, and supraclavicular regions. A further modification of the procedure that has been advocated but not conclusively studied is the removal of the mass itself and some surrounding normal breast tissue without complete removal of the breast, followed by irradiation. Improvements in the technology of delivering high energy irradiation has allowed large amounts of radiation to be administered to the lesion without severely injuring surrounding and overlying normal tissue, including skin. Five- and ten-year survival rates in patients treated with radical mastectomy are no better than those in patients treated with simple mastectomy and irradiation, and tylectomy (lumpectomy or nodulectomy) appears to be as effective as the other two types of treatment for tumors less than 3 cm in diameter. The least mutilating therapy may be as effective as more mutilating procedures and certainly would be preferable cosmetically, particularly when a young woman is the victim of the disease.

Metastatic tumors that are estrogen-receptor positive are responsive to removal of the sources of endogenous estrogens, by oophorectomy initially and later by removal of adrenal sources of estrogens such as by hypophysectomy or bilateral (surgical) adrenalectomy. It should be emphasized that oophorectomy at the time of resection of the original tumor, without metastases, does not prolong survival and therefore subjects most patients to a needless procedure. It is conceivable that the estrogen-positive subgroup might benefit, since the clinical trial of adjunctive oophorectomy was done before receptors were discovered, but this remains to be determined. However, young women in the childbearing age group may want to have more children, and castration at any point in the disease, especially the early stage, should not be the treatment of choice. Oophorectomy is also a valuable guide to future endocrine manipulation therapy as performed to treat *measurable* disease. Regression of metastatic tumor implants indicates hormonal responsiveness of the tumor, which can be capitalized upon by ablative procedures later or by the administration of antiestrogens, such as tamoxifen, or androgenic steroids. Hypophysectomy has been performed occasionally during pregnancy and has not caused particular difficulties. Normal infants have been delivered after hypophysectomy, although lactation was impossible. Placental function is not affected by hypophysectomy, with chorionic gonadotropin, estrogens, and pregnanediol levels remaining within normal limits. Although the techniques for performing hypophysectomy, by the transethmoidal or trans-sphenoidal route for example, have improved significantly in recent years, there are fortunately few situations in which it is required during pregnancy. Hypophysectomy should probably be restricted to those cases in which the survival of the fetus is an overriding consideration, i.e., in a woman early in pregnancy with advancing metastatic breast carcinoma. Good medical judgment may decree that it might be more prudent in such an instance to end the pregnancy and treat the lesion with chemotherapy to avoid imminent disastrous consequences to the mother from rapidly progressive malignancy.

An important new agent that influences the course of metastatic breast cancer is tamoxifen. This compound has antiestrogenic and direct antitumor effects and is useful in both premenopausal and postmenopausal patients. Even after hypophysectomy, or oophorectomy and adrenalectomy, some patients respond to tamoxifen, indicating that it is more than simply an estrogen antagonist, but it is best used early in the course of endocrine manipulation for estrogen receptor positive tumors.

Chemotherapy with such agents as 5-fluorouracil, methotrexate, cyclophosphamide, prednisone, vincristine, or adriamycin should be administered to patients whose metastatic disease is unresponsive (no longer responsive) to hormones. Despite theoretical objections, chemotherapy can be used successfully in the pregnant woman without harm to the fetus, except when given during the first trimester. The long-term hazards to the fetus of cytotoxic agents, particularly alkylating agents such as cyclophosphamide, must be considered a possibility, but data thus far indicate significant latent effects. Chemotherapy with combinations of two or more effective agents has produced responses in 50 to 70 per cent of the patients. Unfortunately, the median duration of response is usually less than one year. The tumoricidal antibiotic adriamycin has caused remission in approximately 40 per cent of patients with metastatic disease and is now being explored in combination with other agents such as cyclophosphamide and 5-fluorouracil. Soft tissue and visceral disease usually respond well to hormonal manipulations, whereas metastases to bone often do not respond as predictably. It would not be unreasonable to institute chemotherapy as the first mode of therapy if metastases to bone are the predominant lesions. Significant palliation for bone pain can be obtained rapidly with radiation therapy. Radiation is also indicated for metastases to the brain, which are highly responsive to x-rays and may sometimes be controlled for many years.

A major advance in the approach to breast cancer has been the adjunctive therapy of Stage II disease, involving regional lymph nodes, with chemotherapy after treatment of the primary tumor by surgery and/or irradiation. In both pre- and postmenopausal patients, various combinations, such as cyclophosphamide, methotrexate, and fluorouracil, or Adriamycin and cyclophosphamide, have effected such prolongations of disease-free survival as to suggest cures of many women. Adequate treatment with any regimen is required, meaning that aggressive, somewhat toxic courses, at standard therapeutic dosage, should be given rather than sparing the patient by administering near-homeopathic doses that may be better tolerated.

COMPLICATIONS AND PROGNOSIS

According to the most recent data from careful studies done from 1968 on, the course of breast cancer arising in a pregnant or lactating woman is no different from that in a nonpregnant woman of the same age or even older.[18] At each clinical stage, the five- and ten-year survival rates are similar for the pregnant and nonpregnant patient.[53] Scattered reports had suggested that a breast cancer discovered and treated late in pregnancy had a poorer prognosis than one of the same stage discovered and treated early in pregnancy. Donegan suggested that aggressive, rapidly growing tumors were selectively discovered and treated immediately in the last trimester, whereas slow-growing and small tumors were probably treated after delivery.[17] Also, understaging was likely to occur late in pregnancy, when the breasts were larger and the tumor more difficult to define exactly. Tumors discovered late in pregnancy would actually have to be larger than those discovered in early pregnancy to be noticed. They might well be thought erroneously to be the same size as the more easily defined breast masses in the early pregnant woman.

Women who become pregnant after mastectomy have survived better than those who do not, with a prolonged disease-free survival as well.[17, 53] Patients who become pregnant within six months of mastectomy were included, eliminating the bias of early deaths in the nonpregnant group. Far from increasing the risk of recurrence, pregnancy seems to decrease it. By no means does it guarantee that there will be no recurrence, since many instances of recurrence have been reported even after several pregnancies. The risk of recurrence within the first few years (especially 18 to 24 months) and the risk of a second primary breast tumor, constant at 1 per cent per year, are the principal reasons one might counsel a patient to wait three to five years before becoming pregnant. As always, the difficult decision about family planning must be hers and her husband's, aided by the physician, based on these somewhat conflicting pieces of information on the tumor's biological behavior in the pregnant and nonpregnant host. It should also be noted that breast feeding by a mother with cancer may not be desirable since prolactin secretion is prolonged and since there may be a tumorigenic virus in the breast milk, which could transfer the potential for development of the cancer to the offspring. Although data are inconclusive in humans, mouse breast cancer viruses can be transferred by this means.

Since breast cancer is one of the most responsive of the solid tumors to therapy, a useful, pain-free existence is entirely possible, even for many patients with incurable widespread metastatic disease, after remission is attained. With combinations of chemotherapeutic agents response rates are nearly double those achieved with single agents. Although the duration of survival of such women is still suboptimal, a great deal can be done to ameliorate the disease if it is treated vigorously.

Carcinoma of the Uterine Cervix

Squamous cell carcinoma of the uterine cervix is a disease of the late childbearing years, with a median age at incidence of 50. Gynecologic malignancies as a group, and carcinoma of the cervix in particular, are nearly as commonly found in pregnant women as carcinoma of the breast.[47] Nearly 80 per cent of such gynecologic malignancies are carcinomas of the cervix.

It is important to distinguish between a premalignant lesion of a carcinoma in situ and a frankly invasive carcinoma. Ordinarily in a *nonpregnant* woman, an abnormal cytology suggestive of neoplasia, with moderate to severe dysplasia of the cells or with cells clearly having neoplastic characteristics, biopsy of the cervix is performed in short order. Punch biopsies of several quadrants may be very helpful, particularly when there is no gross abnormality of the cervix on direct clinical examination. A cone biopsy is still more useful to establish the diagnosis of invasive carcinoma, since the amount of material available for careful histologic study is greatly increased by this technique. Yet, it is precisely this sort of biopsy that is contraindicated in pregnant women regardless of the need to establish the diagnosis. Although conization has its advocates, there is considerable evidence that conization is not indispensable in diagnosis and that there are many hazards to the pregnant mother and the fetus from the procedure. Hemorrhage is often considerable following cone biopsy, and perinatal complications occur in nearly one fifth of all patients, with a fetal loss of 5 to 10 per cent. Colposcopically directed punch biopsies performed when careful cytologies have indicated probable carcinoma are most likely to yield important diagnostic information with the least morbidity to mother and fetus. No spontaneous abortions were caused by this procedure in a recent series of 131 patients when punch biopsy was compared with more extensive procedures.[38]

Marshall and Latour clearly outline a plan and a logical defense for conservative management of the patient with an abnormal cervical cytology discovered on routine screening.[39] This management must be accomplished at specialized gynecologic clinics where first-rate cytologic back-up is available, as the authors duly emphasize. Unless the patient has severe dysplasia, biopsy is not performed. Those with cytologic evidence of chronic cervicitis or mild or moderate dysplasia without clinical lesions are allowed to continue in their pregnancy, with re-evaluation by cytology once at four weeks for the mildest conditions

and three times at four-week intervals for the most severe. If no more serious disease is found, they are allowed to deliver normally and are re-evaluated post partum. Patients with severe dysplasia or carcinoma in situ (clinically apparent) are evaluated by repeat cytologies every four weeks until term, together with selected punch biopsies of suspicious areas, with a re-evaluation post partum if a cesarean hysterectomy was not performed. Only in frankly invasive carcinoma of the cervix are diagnostic cone biopsies performed and then not only to confirm the diagnosis but to judge the depth of invasion. Marshall and Latour feel that a carcinoma penetrating less than 3 mm in depth should still be managed conservatively, without necessarily terminating the pregnancy at that time.[39] Thus, diagnosis of the depth as well as the presence of invasive carcinoma is important as a guide to future management of the condition.

Carcinoma of the cervix in the nonpregnant woman is a very treatable condition, yielding ten-year survival rates of 45 to 50 per cent. If discovered before the onset of metastasis, carcinoma of the cervix can be cured by radiotherapy, with radioactive needles inserted directly, by external beam irradiation, or by a combination of the two. Surgery (hysterectomy) is also effective as an alternative to radiotherapy, but most centers now prefer radiotherapy to an invasive procedure. If the patient has not had Papanicolaou ("Pap") smears regularly and is discovered to have invasive carcinoma with metastasis, the rate of cure diminishes nearly to zero. Regional lymph nodes are first involved, and subsequent masses in the pelvis frequently obstruct the ureter, leading to azotemia and urinary tract infection. Later in the disease there is dissemination via the blood to the lung, liver, and bones, with death resulting from inanition or from the consequences of obstructive uropathy. Chemotherapy at this stage has not been consistently effective, despite trials with a variety of newer investigational agents and a host of older established drugs.

DIAGNOSIS IN PREGNANCY

As in nonpregnant women, the Pap smear is the mainstay of diagnosis during pregnancy. All patients should receive a screening Pap smear at least once during their pregnancy. Any patient whose Pap smear shows cytologic abnormalities in any way suggestive of carcinoma should be followed carefully by repeated cytologies and cervical examination, preferably with the application of Lugol's iodine (to identify any dysplastic region failing to take up iodine) if the cervix is clinically normal. Since management of the various dysplastic conditions of the cervix differs considerably, it is important to distinguish among them cytologically from the outset, as we have described.

LABORATORY VALUES

There are no changes in the serum characteristic of locally invasive cervical cancer, but the blood urea nitrogen and serum creatinine should be monitored when regionally invasive disease of the pelvis is suspected. Liver function abnormalities may likewise be observed when that organ is involved, particularly with an elevation of the serum alkaline phosphatase level.

COURSE IN PREGNANCY

As with the other malignancies discussed, there is no difference in the manner in which cancer of the cervix behaves during pregnancy from that in nonpregnant women. There is no evidence that invasiveness or metastatic spread is more rapid, nor is the survival of this group of patients any different with various modalities of therapy from matched nonpregnant subjects.[4, 20] Fogh commented that the age distribution of his pregnant patients with carcinoma of the cervix was the same as that of nonpregnant patients with the disease but that early stages were represented in younger patients in the pregnant group.[20] Although both groups had metrorrhagia, the pregnant group had a higher incidence of postcoital bleeding and presented earlier in their disease. Aside from these relatively minor differences, the course was the same, and rate of cure with radiotherapy was similar in the two groups, yielding nearly 46 per cent survival at ten years.

TREATMENT

The treatment selected depends on the stage of the disease and the age of the fetus. If the cervical cytology and clinical examination indicate conditions more benign than invasive carcinoma, including carcinoma in situ, the pregnancy should be allowed to go to term, with definitive measures postponed until the postpartum period. Carcinoma of the cervix is relatively slow moving and would not be expected to progress rapidly from carcinoma in situ to deeply invasive disease. If the carcinoma has invaded more than 3 or 4 mm into the stroma of the uterus when discovered, however, the pregnancy should be aborted immediately and therapy instituted. During the first trimester, irradiation with radium and external beam therapy, followed by evacuation of the uterus, may be most useful. In the second trimester, hysterectomy with the fetus in utero or a cesarean delivery followed by subtotal hysterectomy has been successful.[20] In the third trimester, the fetus should be allowed to come almost to term, to be delivered by cesarean section, with perhaps a subtotal hysterectomy followed by irradiation. Vaginal delivery of an infant in the presence of carcinoma of the cervix leads to severe hemorrhage and should be discouraged.

Management of the patient with a carcinoma invading less than 3 mm into the cervix is less well defined. Marshall and Latour emphasize that patients with carcinoma invading less than 3 mm into the cervix have been effectively treated by a simple hysterectomy, although this point is controversial.[39] Cesarean delivery of the fetus followed by hysterectomy or a hysterectomy with the fetus in utero at term, or one to two weeks before, appears to be as effective as more extensive surgery.

TREATMENT POST PARTUM

If the disease is discovered in the puerperium, irradiation is the treatment of choice. For carcinoma of the cervix treated during pregnancy, followup examinations should be performed at three- to six-month intervals to detect residual or metastatic disease. Unfortunately, the therapeutic choices available are not extensive, but it may be possible to prolong effective life by irradiation or resection of pelvic masses, even though metastatic disease is incurable. One half of the patients given definitive treatment early in the course of the disease will have no further difficulty from it and will live a normal life.

Melanoma

Melanoma is a disease of malignant melanocytes, arising in the basal layer of the epidermis or in the pigmented portion of the retina. The disease is not necessarily *malignant* melanoma but may remain quiescent locally for many years in an ostensible stalemate with the host, after which it may spread unpredictably and extensively throughout the body. Removal of a mole that has become malignant but has not yet invaded the deepest portion of the dermis and that has not yet spread to regional lymph nodes may result in cure of the tumor in 50 to 80 per cent of cases. The exact rate of cure within this range depends on the depth of invasion, relative both to the layers of the dermis penetrated and to the absolute depth of the excision as measured in millimeters. If the tumor has already spread to the lymph nodes or already involves the lowest third of the dermis, its curability is no more than 20 per cent. Therefore, early recognition of the signs of melanoma can enable the alert physician to institute treatment and cure the tumor. An atlas of early changes in a pigmented nevus that are indicative of malignant change is recommended for reference.[42] In particular, darkening, irregularity of outline, and elevation of a mole are ominous signs. Bleeding and ulceration are relatively late signs, and resection may not be possible. Metastatic melanoma may involve the viscera, especially the liver and lungs, the bones, the brain, and even the serosal membranes such as pericardium and pleura. In some patients the disease spreads subcutaneously almost exclusively, and in others black intradermal nodules of several millimeters to over a centimeter in diameter may be present in profusion for many months before deeper portions of the body are involved. In the latter situation, intralesional injection of bacille Calmette-Guérin (BCG) has frequently been helpful, but this therapy does not seem to alter the ultimate course of the disease. Death within six to 12 months of the appearance of metastatic disease is common.

Older literature seemed to indicate that the general darkening of the skin that occurred during pregnancy led to pathologic darkening and malignant changes in quiescent nevi. As with other tumors, more recent studies now indicate that pregnancy does not alter either the incidence or the degree of malignancy of the disease. Only 12 of 1000 patients with melanoma in the series of Pack and Scharnagel were pregnant when first seen, and only 32 cases of melanoma were associated with pregnancy or lactation.[49] There does not appear to be control exerted by HCG, although pituitary hormones such as melanocyte stimulating hormone (MSH) and the chemically related adrenocorticotropic hormone (ACTH) seem to alter pigment in the melanoma as they do in normal melanocytes.

The controversy over the role of estrogens in the development or exacerbation of melanomas has continued for years and has currently been reported by anecdotal reports of three women whose quiescent disease was apparently exacerbated by pregnancy or oral contraceptives.[35] The binding of estrogens by some melanoma cells is incontestable, but whether that binding represents the presence of true receptors with a con-

sistent binding affinity is unproved. Moreover, limited trials with pharmacologic doses of synthetic estrogens or with the antiestrogen tamoxifen have not shown significant benefit to patients with melanoma. Whether to consider melanoma a tumor influenced, favorably or adversely, by sex steroids or any other hormones must await the results of more extensive clinical trials and preclinical investigations now in progress.

There are no definitive laboratory tests that unequivocally establish the diagnosis of melanoma, but determination of urinary melanogens is an investigational study that may soon be available to permit better monitoring of the extent of the disease before and after therapy. Urinary melanin is usually absent unless the disease is extremely widespread. Liver function tests and liver and bone scanning are helpful in defining the extent of involvement. A lymphangiogram should also be considered as part of the workup of primary melanoma of the lower extremities as a supplement to limited node dissection to determine the presence or absence of positive nodes, and thus, prognosis.

COURSE DURING PREGNANCY

The course of melanoma in pregnancy is the same as in the nonpregnant woman. Similarly, the disease in pregnancy is as controllable when localized to the dermal-epidermal junction or upper dermis as is melanoma of the same extent in the nonpregnant woman. In both cases resection with a wide margin is usually performed. Radical lymph node dissection of superficial and deep regional nodes is sometimes carried out with the primary resection or at the time of a palpable lymph node recurrence shortly thereafter. The data accumulated thus far are conflicting and certainly do not convincingly support radical prophylactic dissections as a preventive measure against recurrence and dissemination. A superficial dissection of regional nodes allows the physician to know whether the nodes are involved microscopically with disease to judge prognosis. Since regional spread lowers the rate of cure that can be achieved from 80 to 20 or 30 per cent, such prognostically important information justifies the procedure.

There has been considerable unresolved debate as to whether removal of regional nodes lowers the host's immunologic resistance to the spread of the tumor in melanoma and in many carcinomas. Lymph nodes involved with tumor are clearly no longer of value in resistance since the tumor should have been destroyed by lymphocytes and macrophages in the node. A "positive" node is one that might have resisted the tumor earlier by killing any cells that reached it but changed from "negative" to "positive" when its resistance was overcome, perhaps by an excess of soluble tumor antigens or suppressor cells induced by antigen-antibody complexes. Removal of grossly positive nodes is certainly defensible by this reasoning, and even involved superficial nodes could be removed with impunity since more proximal secondary chains of nodes remain. This subject is considered in more detail elsewhere.[44]

Immunity mediated by lymphoid cells and macrophages is certainly of potential importance in control of the melanoma but has not yet been sufficiently understood to be utilized therapeutically with consistent success. Immunologic adjuvants such as BCG have been injected intradermally or by multipuncture vaccination into patients with resected primary melanoma whose lymph nodes or whose extent of local disease classified them as patients with a high risk of recurrence in the future. Although some data indicate that the disease-free interval after surgery may be increased by such "immunoprophylaxis," cure has not been effected. There is always a danger of enhancing the growth of melanoma, or any malignancy, by injecting stimulants of immunity, such as BCG, since suppressor cells that inhibit disease can be stimulated by these nonspecific agents. Patients without proved residual disease but who have presumed microscopic involvement on the basis of tumor-positive lymph nodes are reasonable subjects for the investigational use of biomodulators of various types, used according to protocol with the informed consent of the subject. Patients with macroscopic foci of disease are probably unsuitable for most immunotherapeutic maneuvers unless the immunotherapeutic agents have additional direct antitumor effects.

Intralesional injection of BCG causes an intense localized mononuclear exudate, which in nearly 50 per cent of patients leads to rejection of the injection lesion. Intradermal nodules can be treated in this way, but subcutaneous nodules often do not resolve completely since the immunologically nonspecific inflammatory response is usually localized to the region in which the BCG was injected and it is difficult to inject all portions of a deeply situated nodule. In perhaps 15 per cent of patients, a regional rejection of several intradermal nodules will occur after injecting one or two of them, but there is no way of predicting this easily.

Chemotherapy with such agents as dimethyl-triazenoimidazole carboxamide (DTIC) or nitro-soureas such as chloroethyl cyclohexyl nitro-sourea (CCNU) has led to regression of metastatic disease in 18 to 25 per cent of patients. Responses may be nearly complete, with relief of such symptoms as pain from large nodules, but are often short lived and fail to alter the prognosis significantly. Regional perfusion with DTIC or alkylating agents such as phenylalanine mustard (melphalan) has had some success in controlling local disease of the extremities, sometimes when a systemic therapy has not been effective. In general, however, the median lifespan of a patient with widespread visceral melanoma is approximately six months, with double that expectancy for those with exclusively intradermal disease. Brain involvement portends a survival of three months or less.

It is important to treat the primary lesion surgically as soon as it is discovered, making therapeutic abortion a consideration only in the first and second trimesters and then only if curative surgery would otherwise be prevented. Usually, however, definitive resection can be performed safely even under these circumstances. Early delivery of the fetus is often possible if the melanoma is found in the third trimester. Chemotherapy of metastatic disease usually cannot be accomplished with the fetus in utero. If it is possible to salvage a viable fetus by preterm delivery while still providing early therapy for the mother, this should be done. The salvaging of the fetus is an especially strong consideration in this disease since only palliation is possible for the mother if metastatic melanoma is present. Since transplacental spread of melanoma is uncommon, the fetus is in no imminent danger and this need not be a consideration in deciding whether to allow the pregnancy to proceed.

PROGNOSIS

The five-year survival figures for pregnant and nonpregnant women are similar for those with Stage I disease (i.e., without involvement of lymph nodes).[62] Two hundred and fifty-one surgically treated patients were studied, of whom 34 were diagnosed and treated during pregnancy, comprising 20 Stage I and 14 Stage II patients. There was, however, a difference in the five-year survival rate of the women with nodal disease who were pregnant compared with that of a nulliparous group (29 per cent versus 55 per cent). Nonpregnant parous women who had had an activation of a previously quiescent mole during a previous pregnancy had a 22 per cent five-year survival versus 51 per cent for parous women without such a history. The small numbers of pregnant patients (24) and of parous women who had a history of activation of a mole during pregnancy (26 of 170) make firm conclusions impossible, but the trends are interesting. There may be a subpopulation of women with hormonally sensitive melanomas for whom pregnancy is deleterious, which estrogen receptors or other hormone receptors may soon help to define but which for the moment are indicated by darkening or enlargement of a mole. Alternative forms of contraception to birth control pills might reasonably be suggested for women with a history of resected melanoma, especially Stage II disease, as a corollary to these findings and others we have noted previously. Interdicting a pregnancy solely to prevent possible recrudescence of melanoma cannot be firmly supported by the evidence, unless perhaps the original lesion arose during a pregnancy.

The influence of estrogenic substances on melanoma may not be entirely harmful, because their five-year survival rate for women aged 25 to 44 years is 86 per cent for localized (Stage I) disease and 73 per cent for all stages, compared with 80 and 64 per cent for men of that age.[62]

Leukemia

Since the pathologic components of the acute leukemias include anemia, neutropenia, and thrombocytopenia, significant management problems may occur in the pregnant leukemic patient. Leukemia may be defined as a state of uncontrolled and generalized proliferation of any member of the hematopoietic series, usually associated with the presence of abnormal numbers and/or cells in the peripheral blood.

The incidence of leukemia in females during pregnancy is the same as that for the nonpregnant population. The estimate of the annual death rate from acute leukemia in the entire female population is 2 per 100,000, with an incidence of 1 per 100,000 in the 15 to 45 year old age group. Thus, the occurrence of two cases of acute leukemia among 75,000 pregnant women in one report and of one case in 40,000 in another is what would be expected in age-matched control groups. The average age at onset of acute leukemia in pregnancy also does not differ significantly from that in the general population. In 126 pregnant patients the average age was 28 years, whereas the average age for 1000 cases of acute leukemia of all diagnostic types in both sexes was 26.8 years.[68]

The classification of the leukemias is based on the cellular morphologic characteristics, histochemistry, surface markers, cytogenetics, and clinical course. In general, the acute leukemias are composed of a predominance of poorly differentiated or undifferentiated cells and are associated with a relatively brief and fulminant clinical course. The chronic leukemias, on the other hand, are composed of well-differentiated cells, and the clinical course may be protracted over several years. All the morphologic types of acute leukemia may be seen in a pregnant patient with the exception of chronic lymphocytic leukemia, which has a peak incidence beyond the childbearing years.

The relative frequency of occurrence of the types of leukemia affecting the pregnant population is similar to that in the nonpregnant population, a comparison of which is shown in Table 21-1. The reviews of pregnant leukemic patients that appeared in 1943 and 1958 compare favorably with regard to diagnostic categories. However, the series reported in 1964 showed a decrease in the incidence of chronic granulocytic leukemia and an increase in acute granulocytic leukemia. In comparison, the figures for 102 nonpregnant females between the ages of 15 and 45 were intermediate between the earlier and later reports for pregnant patients. Yet, if one averages the figures for the 1958 and 1964 reports, the diagnostic breakdown compares favorably with that for the nonpregnant group. This would indicate that the diagnostic types affecting pregnant and nonpregnant patients do not differ. These changes in the relative proportions of each cell type are also consistent with recent epidemiologic studies.[11]

ACUTE LEUKEMIA

Diagnosis. The development of acute leukemia is usually insidious, and the presenting symptoms are related to bone marrow failure, i.e., the consequences of anemia, leukopenia, and thrombocytopenia. Patients may complain of several months of easy fatigability, a bleeding diathesis, and/or recurrent infection. The physical examination is usually nonspecific with the exception of sternal tenderness, skin pallor, and, perhaps, petechiae, ecchymoses, and hepatosplenomegaly. Lymphadenopathy is usually not prominent in the adult. In the acute lymphocytic, myelocytic, or monocytic leukemias, the laboratory evaluation usually reveals a normochromic normocytic anemia, mild to marked thrombocytopenia, and a leukocytosis; however, the white blood cell count may be low or normal. Eosinophilic splinter-shaped cytoplasmic infu-

TABLE 21–1 COMPARISON OF LEUKEMIC CELL TYPE IN PREGNANT AND NONPREGNANT WOMEN*

Period	CGL	CLL	ALL	AGL	AML	Unclassified or Blast Cell	Erythro-myelogenous	Mixed	Total
Pregnant									
Up to 1943 (McGoldrick & Lapp[41])	41 (54.7)	3 (4.0)	9 (12.0)	17 (22.7)	2 (2.7)	3 (4.0)	0	0	75
Up to 1958 (Sheehy[60])	89 (58.2)	4 (2.6)	16 (10.4)	37 (24.1)	7 (4.6)	0	0	0	153
1957–1963 (Moloney[45])	22 (31.9)	0	8 (11.5)	28 (40.0)	6 (8.6)	4 (5.8)	2 (2.9)	1 (1.4)	71
Average of 1958 and 1964 reports	(45)	(1.3)	(10.8)	(35.8)					
Nonpregnant									
1962 (Boggs et al.[9])	46 (45)	8 (7.8)	12 (11.8)	36 (35.2)					102

*Numbers in parentheses indicate percentages.
Notes: CGL = chronic granulocytic.
CLL = chronic lymphocytic.
ALL = acute lymphocytic.
AGL = acute granulocytic.
AML = acute monocytic.

sions, Auer rods, may be seen in myeloblasts and may help to differentiate the acute myeloblastic leukemias from the acute lymphoblastic leukemias. Markedly elevated serum and urinary lysozyme levels help to differentiate acute monoblastic leukemia from the other varieties. Examination of the bone marrow aspirate usually confirms the clinical impression, and histochemical stains are useful in confirming a diagnostic impression, with the myeloblasts being peroxidase positive and PAS (periodic acid–Schiff) negative; the reverse is true of the lymphoblasts. In the untreated or unresponsive patient, the acute leukemias often have a rapidly fatal course, the patients succumbing to infection or bleeding within a few months.

Course During Pregnancy. Although pregnancy does not affect the course of leukemias, these diseases may have a distinct effect on the course of gestation.[8, 11, 30, 45, 47a, 54, 60] In general, antineoplastic chemotherapy and radiation therapy, along with improved supportive therapy with whole blood, blood products, and antibiotics, have significantly lessened morbidity and prolonged survival. Parturient patients with decreased fibrinogen levels and increased fibrinolytic activity have been reported. Fibrinogen levels should, therefore, be monitored in the pregnant patient with acute leukemia, especially the pro-

myelocytic variety in which disseminated intravascular coagulation is more common. Lilleyman et al. reviewed 32 cases of leukemia occurring in the first 20 weeks of pregnancy.[37] The outcome of these 32 cases included 13 live healthy babies, six of whom were premature. A spontaneous abortion, stillbirth, or live baby surviving less than 24 hours occurred in 15 cases. Three of four pregnancies that were aborted could possibly have gone to term, with delivery of a normal-appearing infant. Of 18 cases treated with cytotoxic drugs, only one fetal abnormality was recorded. The effects of therapy during successive eras on maternal and fetal survival in acute and chronic leukemia are shown in Tables 21–2 and 21–3.

Complications. Complications of the acute leukemias include the sequelae of anemia, neutropenia, and thrombocytopenia. Severe infections with organisms of usually low virulence and overwhelming infections with opportunistic organisms are not uncommon. Central nervous system leukemia may present with signs of increased cerebrospinal fluid pressure, isolated cranial nerve dysfunction, or personality change. This can be effectively treated with whole-brain irradiation plus intrathecal methotrexate or cytosine arabinoside. Patients with white blood cell counts in excess of 100,000 cells per cu mm may

TABLE 21–2 EFFECT OF ACUTE LEUKEMIA ON PREGNANCY

Therapy	Number of Patients	Maternal Survival to Delivery (%)	Fetal Survival (%)
Before 1943 (McGoldrick and Lapp[41]), supportive	34	70	41
1943 to 1956 (Yahia et al.[68]), steroids or antimetabolites	30	80	62
1954 to 1964 (Hoover and Schumacher[30]), steroids and/or antimetabolites	59	93	64
1970 to present, combination chemotherapy (see Table 21–3)	23	100	87

have the unusual complication of leukostasis in the cerebral arteries. This constitutes a medical emergency and can be effectively treated by rapidly lowering the white blood cell count with hydroxyurea or cyclophosphamide in addition to whole-brain irradiation. All patients with organomegaly and high white blood cell counts should be treated with allopurinol to reduce complications secondary to hyperuricemia.[67]

Treatment and Prognosis. While chemotherapy has definitely altered the course of acute lymphoblastic leukemia (ALL) of childhood (approximately 50 per cent survival at ten years),

acute leukemia in adults is considerably less responsive. Approximately 50 to 80 per cent of the adults with ALL may achieve complete remission with various combinations of drugs. However, the median duration of remission is approximately one year. With relapse, other drugs are frequently useful in reinducing and maintaining another remission. Effective agents include prednisone, vincristine, asparaginase, daunorubicin, Adriamycin, 6-mercaptopurine, methotrexate, cyclophosphamide, and cytosine arabinoside. At the present time the prophylactic treatment of ALL involving the central nervous

TABLE 21–3 COMBINATION CHEMOTHERAPY IN PREGNANT PATIENTS WITH ACUTE LEUKEMIA

Author	Number of Patients	Trimester First Exposed to Drugs 1 2 3	Drugs	Maternal Survival to Delivery (No.)	Fetal Survival to Delivery (No.)	Fetal Deformities or Complications
Pizzuto et al.[54]	9*	4 2 1	Pred, 6-MP, MTX, CTX, Vcr, Ara-C, Adr	9	8	1 stillborn 1 pancytopenic
Okun et al.[47a]	1	1	Vcr, Pred, AsNase, CTX, DNR, 6-MP	1	1	1 pancytopenic
Lilleyman et al.[37]	1	1	Ara-C, 6-TG	1	—	Abortion at 20 weeks (normal fetus)
Raich & Curet[56]	1	1	Ara-C, 6-TG	1	1	
Maurer et al.[40]	1	1	Ara-C, 6-TG	1	—	Abortion at 24th week (normal fetus, trisomy C)
Pawliger et al.[51]		1	Ara-C, 6-TG	1	1	
Durie & Giles[18]	1	1	Ara-C, Vcr, Pred	1	1	Normal karyotype
Coopland et al.[13]	1	1	Pred, 6-MP, MTX, Vcr	1	1	Eclampsia
Krueger et al.[33]	1	1	Vcr, Pred, CTX, Ara-C, MTX	1	1	
Newcomb et al.[46]	2	2	Ara-C, VCR, Pred, Adr	2	2	Normal karyotype
Blatt et al.[8]	4	2 1 1	CTX, Adr, Vcr, Pred, ASNase, Ara-C, DNR, MTX, 6-MP, 6-TG	4	4	1 with pilonidal dimples

*Trimester during which exposure occurred was not specified in two patients.

system with cranial irradiation and intrathecal methotrexate has not been shown to prolong the remission in adults as it has in children.

Progress in the treatment of acute myelocytic leukemias has lagged behind that of acute lymphoblastic leukemia. Recent experimental protocols using combinations of drugs have induced remission in approximately 50 to 80 per cent of patients. However, these remissions have been relatively short; the median survival time for those patients responding to therapy was approximately one year compared with 3.5 months for the nonresponders. .

The current management of acute leukemia has clearly improved both maternal and fetal survival (see Tables 21–2 and 21–3). With supportive therapy alone, i.e., blood products and antibiotics or with single agent chemotherapy, approximately 20 to 30 per cent of women studied did not survive the gestational period and fetal mortality was approximately 50 per cent. With the advent of more vigorous supportive care measures and combination chemotherapy, most mothers survive through delivery with a concomitant improvement in fetal survival. Of 23 patients treated with a variety of drug combinations, all survived to delivery; there was one stillborn infant and the incidence of congenital abnormalities was less than 10 to 15 per cent (See Table 21–3). This is in spite of the fact that seven of the fetuses were exposed to drugs during the first trimester.

CHRONIC LEUKEMIA

Chronic myelocytic leukemia may also have an insidious onset with the development of a progressive fatigability and the complaint of a dull ache or heavy sensation in the left upper quadrant of the abdomen due to the presence of an enlarged spleen. At the initial presentation the only hematologic abnormality may be a leukocytosis with a basophilia or eosinophilia. With time the white blood cell count may increase to unusual proportions, not uncommonly to several hundred thousand cells per cu mm. The differential count consists predominantly of mature polymorphonuclear leukocytes, bands, metamyelocytes, and myelocytes. Platelets are usually normal or slightly increased and may be somewhat enlarged and functionally abnormal. Examination of the bone marrow reveals hypercellularity with an approximately five- to tenfold increase in the more mature elements of the granulocytic series; myeloblasts and promyelocytes are only slightly increased.

A distinction between chronic myelocytic leukemia and other myeloproliferative diseases such as polycythemia vera and myeloid metaplasia or a leukemoid reaction to a severe inflammatory stimulus can be made by cytogenetic analyses and histochemical staining of the white blood cells for alkaline phosphatase. Characteristically, in chronic myelocytic leukemia the cells contain an abnormal chromosome, the Philadelphia (Ph[1]) chromosome, which is a 9:22 translocation. This is present in approximately 85 per cent of the patients. Those patients lacking the Ph[1] chromosome usually have a poorer response to therapy and a shorter median survival time. In chronic myelocytic leukemia the cells also have a low leukocyte alkaline phosphatase score in comparison with the high values in cells of patients with polycythemia vera, myeloid metaplasia, or leukemoid reactions. The serum vitamin B_{12} and transcobalamin I levels are usually increased. As with acute leukemias, pregnancy has not affected the course of the disease; however, the disease has had a significant effect on maternal and fetal survival.

Control of the disease with therapy has permitted 96.5 per cent of the mothers to survive to delivery, with an 84 per cent fetal survival rate through gestation. The major drugs useful in the control of chronic myelocytic leukemia include busulfan, hydroxyurea, dibromomannitol, and cyclophosphamide. Local irradiation to the spleen may be useful in reducing spleen size and thus decreasing left upper quadrant discomfort. The chronic stage of the disease usually lasts several years, then almost abruptly transforms into an acute blastic crisis wherein the numbers of myeloblasts and promyelocytes increase in the peripheral blood and bone marrow. The Ph[1] chromosome persists, however, the serum vitamin B_{12} level decreases, and the leukocyte alkaline phosphatase level increases toward normal. This stage of the disease very closely resembles acute myeloblastic leukemia, and the results of therapy are equally poor. The median survival time after the onset of the blastic crisis is usually less than one year.

Lymphoma

The malignant lymphomas present a special problem in pregnancy because of the frequent occurrence of the disease in the pelvis and the necessary therapy that includes irradiation and drugs, both of which are potentially abortifacient, teratogenic, mutagenic, or carcinogenic. The malignant lymphomas are a group of heterogeneous disorders characterized by the uncontrolled proliferation of cells of the lymphoreticular system. They may be conveniently classified into two major categories: Hodgkin's disease and the non-Hodgkin's lymphomas.

HODGKIN'S DISEASE

Hodgkin's disease constitutes approximately 40 per cent of the malignant lymphomas and has a slight male predominance (35 per million population in males; 26 per million in females). Since 50 per cent of the cases occur in women between the ages of 20 and 40, its concurrence with pregnancy is not rare. Conversely, the non-Hodgkin's lymphomas have their peak incidence beyond the childbearing age (i.e., beyond 50 years of age), so that their concurrence with pregnancy is rare. Similarly, most of the cases of multiple myeloma occur after 40 years of age; this is reflected by the existence of only three case reports in the world's literature of the association of multiple myeloma with pregnancy.

The malignant cell in Hodgkin's disease is the Reed-Sternberg (R-S) cell, probably a dedifferentiated histiocyte. Although most commonly associated with Hodgkin's disease, the R-S cell or R-S–like cell may be seen in other conditions that may occur in the pregnant female. These include cancer of the breast and lung, malignant melanoma, and non-neoplastic conditions such as measles, myositis, infectious mononucleosis, and diphenylhydantoin therapy. Although the exact cause of Hodgkin's disease is unknown, speculation has included an infectious agent, possibly a virus. This etiology has been suggested by the frequent initial symptoms such as chills, fever, and leukocytosis; by the finding of elevated antibody titers to herpes-like virus (perhaps analogous to Epstein-Barr virus in Burkitt's lymphoma) and by the occasional affliction of several members of a household.

Approximately 90 per cent of the patients present with peripheral adenopathy: 60 to 80 per cent have involvement of the cervical nodes; 6 to 20 per cent, involvement of the axillary; and 6 to 12 per cent, involvement of the inguinal nodes. Six to 11 per cent of the patients present with primary mediastinal disease. Twenty-five per cent of the patients at presentation have retroperitoneal disease. The patient may be totally asymptomatic or may present with a variable history of fever, night sweats, weight loss, malaise, and pruritus. An unusual but pathognomonic presenting complaint is a pain occurring shortly after the ingestion of alcoholic beverages, localized to areas involved by the disease. Clinicopathologic studies have indicated that in more than 90 per cent of the patients the disease apparently spreads by contiguity to adjacent lymph node chains. This finding has an important bearing on the therapeutic approach. Those patients in whom spread appears to be noncontiguous usually have the mixed cellularity or lymphocyte depletion histology.

Although the diagnosis may be strongly suspected with the history and physical examination, definitive diagnosis can only be established by histologic demonstration of the R-S cell. This is best obtained by biopsy of an enlarged cervical node. If possible, one should not rely on inguinal or axillary node histology because of the frequent chronic inflammatory nature of nodes in these regions. Needle biopsies should be avoided. In the presence of mediastinal adenopathy without significant peripheral adenopathy, biopsy of the right supraclavicular nodes may be useful. If this is unrewarding, then biopsy of the mediastinal nodes may be useful. If this is unrewarding, then biopsy of the mediastinal nodes via mediastinoscopy should be considered.

The histologic subtype of Hodgkin's disease has important prognostic importance. The most frequent histologic type, especially in females, is nodular sclerosis (20 to 50 per cent of cases). This is composed of a pleomorphic infiltrate in a nodular pattern with wide, doubly refractile collagen bands. R-S cells are scattered throughout. The atypical lacunar cells characteristic of this subtype may be artifacts of histologic preparation. Twenty to 40 per cent of the cases are of the mixed cellularity type. This is characterized by a pleomorphic infiltrate consisting of eosinophils, plasma cells, fibroblasts, and necrotic foci with numerous R-S cells. Ten to 15 per cent are of the lymphocyte-predominant type, consisting of mature lymphocytes and histiocytes with sparse R-S cells. Five to 15 per cent are of the lymphocyte-depletion type. In these cases the lymph node is replaced by diffuse nonrefractile fibrous tissue with areas of necrosis, few lymphocytes, and abundant R-S cells.

The histologic subtype provides clues as to the probable pattern or stage of the disease and is of paramount importance with regard to prognosis and possible complications. Nodular sclerosing histology is common in young females, and a frequent pattern of presentation is right supraclavicular adenopathy along with mediastinal disease. With this histology one should suspect disease in a triangular fashion involving the neck, supraclavicular regions, and the anterior and superior mediastinum. Lung involvement is almost always associated with hilar disease and is most often seen in the nodular sclerosing or lymphocyte depletion variety. Lung involvement is almost never found with lymphocyte-predominant Hodgkin's disease. The lymphocyte predominance histology carries the best prognosis and frequently involves a single node or group of nodes, most often in the cervical region.

With the exception of adenopathy, the initial clinical status of the patient may be totally within normal limits, especially with the lymphocyte-predominant and nodular-sclerosing histologies. Alternatively, the patient may present with a history of fever, night sweats, anorexia, weight loss, malaise, and pruritus. Physical examination should place special emphasis on lymph node regions and hepatosplenomegaly. The initial workup should include a complete blood count, platelet count, and urinalysis. A normochromic, normocytic anemia may be present, along with a leukocytosis with an increased number of polymorphonuclear leukocytes. Eosinophilia and/or lymphopenia may be seen. Evaluation of the marrow is not complete without a biopsy, since the yield of positive findings in the marrow is much greater with biopsy than with an aspirate alone. Chemistries should include blood urea nitrogen, serum glutamic oxaloacetic transaminase (SGOT), alkaline phosphatase, bilirubin, and uric acid. An anemia with an elevation of the alkaline phosphatase level may suggest bone marrow involvement. Alkaline phosphatase may be elevated in the absence of liver or bone involvement and may be a tumor-associated enzyme similar to placental alkaline phosphatase (Regan isoenzyme). Serum protein electrophoresis may reveal hypergammaglobulinemia in early disease, with hypogammaglobulinemia developing in advanced disease.

Radiologic examination should include a chest x-ray, excretory urogram, and lymphangiogram. Lymphangiography may reveal retroperitoneal adenopathy in 30 per cent of clinical Stages I and IIA and 88 per cent of clinical Stage IIB. Bone films and tomography should be done in selected cases. Bone and liver scans are also useful as part of the overall staging procedure. Cutaneous anergy is of prognostic significance. Skin tests may be performed with a battery of common antigens such as tuberculin, mumps, candidin, trichophyton, and streptokinase-streptodornase (SKSD). Cutaneous anergy has been found in approximately 50 per cent of the patients with disease beyond Stage I, especially in patients with lymphopenia or lymphocyte-depletion histology. A beneficial therapeutic response has been associated with a return of cutaneous reactivity.

The Ann Arbor staging system is as follows: Stage I, disease localized to a single anatomic lymph node chain; Stage II, disease in two or more groups, either above or below the diaphragm; Stage III, disease confined to the spleen and/or Waldeyer's ring and lymph nodes above and below the diaphragm; Stage IV, disseminated disease involving lymph nodes and nonlymphoid organs (usually lung, bone and/or liver). However, the isolated involvement of a single nonlymphatic focus (e.g., lung) or the contiguous involvement of nonlymphatic tissue with lymph node involvement (e.g., hilar node plus contiguous lung) does not necessarily place the patient in the Stage IV category. In these instances the patient may be staged as a I_E (E for extralymphatic) or II_E. Further stage designation depends on the absence or presence of constitutional symptoms, e.g., fever, night sweats, weight loss, these being designated as A or B, respectively. Thus, a patient presenting with fever, night sweats, and a 10 per cent weight loss who is found to have cervical, supraclavicular, mediastinal, and hilar nodes with involvement of contiguous lung tissue would be designated as stage IIB_E. The stage of the disease has a distinct bearing on the choice of initial therapy. The treatment of choice for Stages I and II disease is radiation therapy. The reported five-year survival figures are 89 and 67 per cent for Stages I and II, respectively. These figures are for all histologic types grouped together.

The initial choice of therapy for Stage IIIA is dependent on the histology. Most centers are currently treating Stage IIIA lymphocyte-predominant or nodular-sclerosing Hodgkin's disease with irradiation only, whereas Stage IIIA patients with other histologic types have received a combination of drugs and irradiation. Stages IIIB and IV are usually treated with chemotherapy as the primary modality, with adjunctive irradiation. The results of chemotherapy with combinations of drugs have been distinctly superior to those achieved with any of the components used singly.

One of the most popular drug combinations in current use is MOPP, a combination of Mustargen (nitrogen mustard), Oncovin (vincristine), procarbazine, and prednisone. This combination has produced therapeutic results with tolerable and reversible host toxicity. In the initial reported series from the National Cancer Institute, 81 per cent of untreated Stages III and IV patients achieved complete and prolonged remission status when treated with only six-month courses. Other combinations and schedules are under current and active investigation, and preliminary results indicate significant prolongation of active and useful life (if not cure) in patients with advanced Hodgkin's disease. Other useful drugs include cyclophosphamide, vinblastine, bleomycin, Adriamycin, and bis-chloroethylnitrosourea (BCNU) and its related congeners. All these drugs, with the exception of bleomycin, vincristine, and corticosteroids, have bone marrow suppressive effects. Thus, drug-induced leukopenia or thrombocytopenia can present special hazards to the pregnant female during the course of gestation and during parturition.[31]

After the diagnosis of Hodgkin's disease is established in a pregnant patient who is near term and in whom the disease is confined to supradiaphragmatic regions, radiation therapy can be administered with appropriate uterine shielding; the remainder of the workup and subdiaphragmatic therapy, if necessary, can be administered post partum. However, if the disease is diagnosed in the first trimester and the patient's condition warrants it, full evaluation may very well present a significant hazard to the fetus. Further indications for therapeutic abortion include cases in which Hodgkin's disease is localized to the inguinal or abdominal region and adequate radiation therapy cannot be applied without risk of producing an abnormal fetus. The anecdotal experiences of the utilization of anticancer drugs in early pregnancy have suggested variable degrees of fetal damage, as will be discussed in detail.

The differential diagnosis of Hodgkin's disease includes hydantoin-induced pseudolymphoma, infectious mononucleosis, dermatopathic lymphadenopathy, toxoplasmosis, rheumatoid lymphadenitis, secondary syphilis, herpes zoster, post-vaccinial lymphadenitis, and allergic granulomatosis.

Course During Pregnancy. The effect of pregnancy on the course of Hodgkin's disease has been well documented by Barry et al.[5]: 84 of 347 females with Hodgkin's disease between the ages of 18 and 40 became pregnant one or more times for a total of 112 pregnancies during the course of their disease. The most common tissue diagnosis in the pregnant and nonpregnant groups was Hodgkin's granuloma. The median survival time for the pregnant group was 90 months compared with 52 months for the nonpregnant group. Of 50 ten-year survivors, 22 were of the pregnant group and 28 were of the nonpregnant group. The survival of 16 patients who underwent therapeutic abortion was approximately equal to those who went to term. In the series reported by Hennessy and Rottino,[24] the five- to 15-year survival time of Hodgkin's disease was no different whether or not the woman had undergone a pregnancy during the course of her disease; the survival time was 42

per cent at five years and 39 per cent at 15 years. These authors and others have concluded that pregnancy does not affect the course and prognosis of Hodgkin's disease.

The presence of Hodgkin's disease has not exerted a significant effect on the course of 430 pregnancies occurring in 342 women. The reported incidence of spontaneous abortions for patients with Hodgkin's disease is approximately the same as that reported for all pregnancies (7 to 8 per cent versus 10 per cent, respectively).

Whereas the presence of Hodgkin's disease per se affects neither the course of pregnancy nor the course of labor and the puerperium, therapy for the disease may present significant fetal complications. Therefore, patients should receive counseling regarding marriage and pregnancy. It has generally been accepted that the patient should be in remission for at least two years before pregnancy is contemplated, since recurrent disease during the first two years generally indicates a relatively poor prognosis with the probability of short remissions and frequent relapses. This advice may not be difficult to carry out because of the frequent effects of therapy on fertility.

An aggressive therapeutic approach to Hodgkin's disease has been of distinct benefit. Certain complications of radiation therapy should be recognized since their occurrence may be temporally removed from actual therapy by months or years and thus may be confused with recurrent or other diseases. Radiation pneumonitis may occur two to three months after therapy. On chest x-ray this appears as shaggy, irregular, dense strands in the paramediastinal pulmonary parenchyma. It may be totally asymptomatic or it may produce symptomatic, restrictive lung disease. It may be effectively treated with corticosteroids, which should be continued over a protracted period with slow tapering off over months. A more rapid tapering off may lead to exacerbation of the process.

Advanced Hodgkin's disease frequently involves the lungs and may have a varied roentgenographic appearance. Thus, the appearance of pulmonary density requires the usual diagnostic workup. Radiation pericarditis may appear within five to 48 months after irradiation and should be treated similarly to radiation pneumonitis. Cardiac involvement by Hodgkin's disease should be ruled out since this would be an indication for radiation therapy. Such involvement may produce sinus tachycardia, murmur, and congestive heart failure. Paraspinal nodal irradiation may produce neurologic complications, which could be confused with spinal disease. Spinal Hodgkin's disease may produce vertebral collapse with cord compression or occlusion of the blood supply, producing infarction of the cord. Extensive radiation therapy in the cervical region may produce Lhermitte and McAlpine syndrome, manifested as numbness, tingling, or an "electric sensation" in the upper and/or lower extremities or lower back which may be either continuous or precipitated by flexion of the head and neck. Usually there is no associated motor weakness or disability. It may appear within two to four months after therapy and then disappear within two to six months, leaving no residual neurologic deformity. Cervical and mediastinal irradiation may produce hypothyroidism. Radiation to the kidneys may produce a nephritis and extensive irradiation to bone, i.e., more than 4400 rads may produce necrosis.[31]

In summary, neither the occurrence of Hodgkin's disease during pregnancy nor the occurrence of pregnancy during the course of Hodgkin's disease significantly affects the other. The major considerations are the effects of therapy on the fetus. Doses of irradiation in excess of 10 rads delivered to the pelvis or full doses of chemotherapy during the first trimester can produce deleterious fetal effects. When therapy is required late in pregnancy, temporizing measures such as low to moderate doses of irradiation to extrapelvic sites are to be advocated whenever possible.

NON-HODGKIN'S LYMPHOMA

There are fewer than 20 case reports of non-Hodgkin's lymphoma during pregnancy. The diffuse non-Hodgkin's lymphomas may have a more aggressive course compared with Hodgkin's disease, and therefore one may not have the opportunity to temporize and wait to begin therapy after a term pregnancy. There are only two instances of successful therapy using relatively recently developed combinations of drugs. Both reports used the combination of cyclophosphamide, vincristine, prednisone, and bleomycin with the successful treatment of the mother and the delivery of a full term, normal-appearing baby.[19, 48]

GENERAL COMMENTS ON MANAGEMENT

It should be apparent that there are no rules that can be universally applied to all situations when a tumor is discovered during pregnancy. Slow-growing tumors or those in which the preinvasive phase may take years to proceed to the invasive phase (such as in carcinoma of the cervix) clearly do not require hasty action and allow both a viable pregnancy and satisfactory treatment of the mother. Therapeutic abortion should not be a "reflex action" when a tumor is diagnosed but should be a last resort when the nature of the tumor and the necessity for its rapid therapy dictate such an extreme procedure. Chemotherapy carries considerable risks of teratogenesis and carcinogenesis, if it does not cause abortion, and generally should be avoided when the fetus is in utero. Yet the evidence for latent deleterious effects in humans is far less compelling than in animal models, making chemotherapy for a pregnant woman an option in situations in which maintenance of the pregnancy is the paramount consideration. Extra-abdominal radiotherapy can be fairly well shielded from the uterus, and only pelvic tumors absolutely require termination of the pregnancy.

Hysterectomy is a therapeutic option in the treatment of cervical carcinoma, or perhaps choriocarcinoma, but is not obligatory in either of these conditions. This permits the physician to preserve the reproductive capacity of the patient after eradication of a highly responsive tumor. If irradiation or chemotherapy is capable of abrogating a tumor, as in the two examples mentioned, there is no need for extirpative procedures, and the same noninvasive approach that now characterizes the treatment of these tumors in nonpregnant women is of even greater importance in pregnancy.

Judgment and some caution are required in decisions concerning subsequent pregnancy in a woman who has a tumor or who has achieved remission from a tumor, even though the evidence does not substantiate a poorer prognosis because of the pregnant state. Women who are cured of choriocarcinoma can and should be allowed to have subsequent pregnancies, but with many other tumors in which a complete cure is less likely the potential risk should be made clear to the patient by her physician and an informed decision made appropriately. Here the principal risk is that recurrent metastatic tumor could leave the new baby without a mother, not that the altered hormonal environment in pregnancy will cause a recurrence. Information gathered in a controlled, prospective manner will permit more informed judgment about the factors that influence tumors in general and pregnancy specifically. The small numbers of pregnant patients with a tumor may mandate that in vitro studies of hormone receptors and hormonal alterations on cultured tumor cells be the methods of determining their influence on a tumor rather than deductions through case-control analysis. Since the data cited here were not usually gathered in a prospective manner, our conclusions are all subject to revision. Nevertheless, the information presented here may form a basis of action, for the present, in these difficult, emotionally charged situations in which a life-threatening disease coincides with the felicitous event of childbearing.

References

1. Arseneau, J. C., Sponzo, R. W., Levin, D. L., Schnipper, L. E., Bonner, H., Young, R. C., Canellos, G. P., Johnson, R. E., and DeVita, V. T.: Nonlymphomatous malignant tumors complicating Hodgkin's disease. N. Engl. J. Med., 287:1119, 1972.
2. Bagshawe, K. D.: Choriocarcinoma. The clinical biology of the trophoblast and its tumours. Baltimore, Williams & Wilkins, 1969.
3. Baker, J. W., Peckman, M. J., Morgan, R. L., and Smithers, D. W.: Preservation of ovarian function in patients requiring radiotherapy for para-aortic and pelvic Hodgkin's disease. Lancet, 1:1307, 1972.
4. Barber, H. R. K., and Brunschwig, A.: Gynecological cancer complicating pregnancy. Am. J. Obstet. Gynecol., 85:156, 1963.
5. Barry, R. M., Diamond, H. D., and Craver, L. F.: Influence of pregnancy on the course of Hodgkin's disease. Am. J. Obstet. Gynecol., 84:445, 1962.
6. Bibbo, M.: Transplacental effects of diethylstilbestrol. Curr. Top. Pathol., 66:191, 1979.
7. Birks, D. M., Crawford, G. M., Ellison, L. G., and Johnstone, F. R. C.: Cancer of the breast in women 30 years of age or less. Surg. Gynecol. Obstet., 137:21, 1973.
8. Blatt, J., Mulvihill, J. J., Ziegler, J. L., Young, R. C., and Poplack, D. G.: Pregnancy outcome following cancer chemotherapy. Am. J. Med., 69:828, 1980.
9. Boggs, D. R., Wintrobe, M. M., and Cartwright, G. E.: The acute leukemias: analysis of 322 cases and a review of the literature. Medicine, 41:163, 1962
10. Cadman, E. C., Capizzi, R. L., and Bertino, J. R.: Acute non-lymphocytic leukemia: a delayed complication of Hodgkin's disease: Analysis of 109 cases. Cancer, 40:1280, 1977.
11. Capizzi, R. L.: Hematologic neoplasms during pregnancy. In Brodsky, I., Kahn, S. B., and Moyer, J. H. (eds.): Cancer Chemotherapy II, The Twenty-Second Hahnemann Symposium. New York. Grune & Stratton, 1972, p. 131.
12. Clark, R. M.: An approach to the detection and management of early breast cancer. Can. Med. Assoc. J., 108:599, 1973.
13. Coopland, A. T., Freisen, W. J., and Galbraith, P. A.: Acute leukemia in pregnancy. Am. J. Obstet. Gynecol., 105:1288, 1969.
14. Cowen, D., and Geller, M. L.: Long-term pathological effects of prenatal x-irradiation on the central nervous system of the rat. J. Neuropathol. Exp. Neurol., 19:488, 1960.
15. Cramblett, H. G., Friedman, J. L., and Najjar, S.: Leukemia in an infant born of a mother with leukemia. N. Engl. J. Med., 259:727, 1958.
16. Dekaban, A.: Abnormalities in children exposed to x-irradiation during various stages of gestation: tentative timetable of radiation injury to the human fetus, Part I. J. Nucl. Med., 9:471, 1968.
17. Donegan, W. L.: Breast cancer and pregnancy. Obstet. Gynecol., 50:244, 1977.
18. Durie, B. G. M., and Giles, H. R.: Successful treatment of acute leukemia during pregnancy. Arch. Intern. Med., 137:90, 1977.
19. Falkson, H. C., Simson, I. W., and Falkson, G.: Non-Hodgkin's lymphoma in pregnancy. Cancer, 45:1679, 1980.
20. Fogh, I. B.: Cancer colli uteri and pregnancy. Cancer, 129:114, 1972.
21. Fraumeni, J. F.: Chemicals in human teratogenesis and transplacental carcinogenesis. Pediatrics, 53:807, 1974.
22. Goldstein, D. P.: The chemotherapy of gestational trophoblastic disease. Principles of clinical management. J.A.M.A., 220:209, 1972.
23. Goldstein, D. P.: Prevention of gestational trophoblastic disease by actinomycin D in molar pregnancies. Obstet. Gynecol., 43:475, 1974.
24. Hennessy, J. P., and Rottino, A.: Hodgkin's disease in pregnancy. Am. J. Obstet. Gynecol., 87:851, 1963.
25. Herbst, A. L., Kurman, R. J., Scully, R. E., and Poskanzer, D. C.: Clear-cell adenocarcinoma of the genital tract in young females. N. Engl. J. Med., 287:1259, 1972.
26. Herbst, A. L., Norusis, M. J., Rosenow, P. J., Welch, W. R., and Scully, R. E.: An analysis of 346 cases of clear cell adenocarcinoma of the vagina and cervix with emphasis on recurrence and survival. Gynecol. Oncol., 1:111, 1979.
27. Herbst, A. L., Scully, R. E., Robboy, S. J., and Welch, W. R.: Complications of prenatal therapy with diethylstilbestrol. Pediatrics, 62(6 Pt 2):1151, 1978.
27a. Hertz, R., Lewis, J., Jr., and Lipsett, M. B.: Five years' experience with the chemotherapy of metastatic choriocarcinoma and related trophoblastic tumors in women. Am. J. Obstet. Gynecol., 82:671, 1961.
28. Hicks, S. P.: Developmental malformations produced by radiation. Am. J. Roentgenol., 69:272, 1953.
29. Holmes, G. E., and Holmes, F. F.: Pregnancy outcome of patients treated for Hodgkin's disease. Cancer, 41:1317, 1978.
30. Hoover, B. A., and Schumacher, H. R.: Acute leukemia in pregnancy. Am. J. Obstet. Gynecol., 96:316, 1966.
31. Kaplan, H. S.: Hodgkin's disease. Cambridge, Harvard University Press, 1972.
32. Kochbar, D. M., and Narsingh, D. A.: "Chemical surgery" as an approach to study morphogenetic events in embryonic mouse limb. Devel. Biol., 61:308, 1977.
33. Kreuger, J. A., Davis, R. B., and Field, C.: Multiple drug chemotherapy in the management of acute leukemia during pregnancy. Obstet. Gynecol., 48:324, 1976.
34. Kumar, R., Biggart, J. D., McEvoy, J., and McGeown, M. G.: Cyclophosphamide and reproductive function. Lancet, 1:1212, 1972.
35. Lerner, A. B., Nordlund, J. J., and Kirkwood, J. M.: Effects of oral contraceptives and pregnancy on melanomas (letter). N. Engl. J. Med., 301:47, 1979.
36. Lewis, J. L.: Chemotherapy of gestational choriocarcinoma. Cancer, 30:1517, 1972.
37. Lilleyman, J. S., Hill, A. S., and Anderton, K. J.: Consequences of acute myelogenous leukemia in early pregnancy. Cancer, 40:1300, 1977.
38. Lurain, J. R., and Gallup, D. G.: Management of abnormal papanicolaou smears in pregnancy. Obstet. Gynecol., 53:485, 1979.
39. Marshall, K. G., and Latour, J. P.: The conservative management of pregnant patients displaying abnormal cervical cytology. Can. Med. Assoc. J., 105:1307, 1971.
40. Maurer, L. H., Jackson-Forcier, R., McIntyre, O. R., and Benirschke, K.: Fetal group C trisomy after cytosine arabinoside and thioguanine. Ann. Intern. Med., 75:809, 1971.
41. McGoldrick, J. L., and Lapp, W. A.: Leukemia and pregnancy; case report and review of the literature. Am. J. Obstet. Gynecol., 46:711, 1943.
42. Mihm, M. C., Fitzpatrick, T. B., Brown, M. M. L., Raker, J. W., Malt, R. A., and Kaiser, J. S.: Early detection of primary cutaneous malignant melanoma: A color atlas. N. Engl. J. Med., 289:989, 1973.
43. Minutti, M. R., Shepard, T. H., and Mellman, W. J.: Fetal renal malformation following Hodgkin's disease during pregnancy. Obstet. Gynecol., 46:194, 1975.
44. Mitchell, M. S.: A note on the lymph node as an immunological barrier. In Weiss, L., Gilbert, H. A., and Ballon, S. C. (eds.): Lymphatic System Metastasis. Boston, G. K. Hall, 1980, p. 74.
45. Moloney, W. C.: Management of leukemia in pregnancy. Ann. N. Y. Acad. Sci., 144:857, 1964.
46. Newcomb, M., Balducci, L., Thigpen, J. T., and Morrison, F. S.: Acute leukemia in pregnancy. J.A.M.A. 239:2691, 1978.
47. Nieminen, N., and Remes, N.: Malignancy during pregnancy. Acta Obstet. Gynecol. Scand., 49:315, 1970.
47a. Okun, D. B., Groncy, P. K., Sieger, L., and Tanaka, K. R.:

Acute leukemia in pregnancy: Transient neonatal myelosuppression after combination chemotherapy in the mother. Med. Ped. Oncol., 7:315, 1979.

48. Ortega, J.: Multiple agent chemotherapy including bleomycin in non-Hodgkin's lymphoma during pregnancy. Cancer, 40:2829, 1977.

49. Pack, G. T., and Scharnagel, I.: Prognosis of malignant melanoma in the pregnant woman. Cancer, 4:324, 1951.

50. Park, W. W., and Lees, J. C.: Choriocarcinoma; general review, with analysis of 516 cases. Arch. Pathol., 49:73, 1950.

51. Pawliger, D. F., McLean, F. W., and Noyes, W. D.: Normal fetus after cytosine arabinoside therapy. Ann. Intern. Med., 74:1012, 1971.

51a. Penn, I., Halgrimson, C. G., and Starzl, T. E.: De novo malignant tumors in organ transplant recipients. Transplant. Proc., 3:773, 1971.

52. Percy, D. H.: Teratogenic effects of the pyrimidine analogues 5-iododeoxyuridine and cytosine arabinoside in late fetal mice and rats. Teratology, 11:1103, 1975.

53. Peters, N. V.: The effect of pregnancy in breast cancer. In Forrest, A. P. M., and Kunkler, P. B. (eds.): Prognostic Factors in Breast Cancer. Baltimore, Williams & Wilkins, 1968, pp. 65–80.

54. Pizzuto, J., Avives, A., Noriega, L., Niz, J., Morales, M., and Romero, F.: Treatment of acute leukemia during pregnancy: presentation of nine cases. Cancer Treat. Reps. 64:679, 1980.

55. Potter, J. F., and Schoeneman, M.: Metastasis of maternal cancer to the placenta and fetus. Cancer, 25:380, 1970.

56. Raich, P. C., and Curet, L. B.: Treatment of acute leukemia during pregnancy. Cancer, 36:861, 1975.

57. Ross, G. T., Goldstein, D. P., Hertz, R., Lipsett, M. B., and Odell, W. D.: Sequential use of methotrexate and actinomycin D in the treatment of metastatic choriocarcinoma and related trophoblastic diseases in women. Am. J. Obstet. Gynecol., 93:223, 1965.

58. Rothman, L. A., Cohen, C. J., and Astarloa, J.: Placental and fetal involvement by maternal malignancy: a report of rectal carcinoma and review of the literature. Am. J. Obstet. Gynecol., 116:1023, 1973.

59. Rugh, R.: Low levels of x-irradiation and the early mammalian embryo. Am. J. Roentgenol., 87:559, 1972.

60. Sheehy, T. W.: An evaluation of the effect of pregnancy on chronic granulocytic leukemia. Am. J. Obstet. Gynecol., 75:788, 1958.

61. Sherins, R. J.: Effect of drug treatment for lymphoma on male reproductive capacity. Ann. Intern Med., 71:216, 1973.

62. Shiu, M. H., Schottenfield, D., Maclean, B., and Fortner, J. G.: Adverse effect of pregnancy on melanoma, a reappraisal. Cancer, 37:181, 1976.

63. Sobrinho, L. G., Levine, R. A., and De Conti, R. C.: Amenorrhea in patients with Hodgkin's disease treated with antineoplastic agents. Am. J. Obstet. Gynecol., 109:135, 1971.

64. Speiser, B., Rubin, P., and Casarett, G.: Aspermia following lower truncal irradiation in Hodgkin's disease. Cancer, 32:692, 1973.

65. Sternberg, J.: Irradiation and radiocontamination during pregnancy. Am. J. Obstet. Gynecol., 108:490, 1970.

66. Sweet, D. L., and Kinzie, J.: Consequences of radiotherapy and antineoplastic therapy for the fetus. J. Reprod. Med., 17:241, 1976.

66a. Wagner, V. M., Hill, J. S., Weaver, D., and Baehner, R. L.: Congenital abnormalities in baby born to cytarabine-treated mother. Lancet, 2:98, 1980.

67. Williams, W. J., Beutler, E., Erslev, A. J., and Rundles, R. W.: Hematology. New York, McGraw-Hill, 1972.

68. Yahia, C., Hyman, G. A., and Phillips, L. L.: Acute leukemia and pregnancy. Obstet. Gynecol. Surv., 13:1, 1958.

69. Zinns, J. S.: The association of pregnancy and breast cancer. J. Reprod. Med., 22:297, 1979.

22

Richard V. Lee, M.D.

DRUG ABUSE

The use of chemicals to affect consciousness or mood is a very old and widespread custom among humans. The excessive self-administration of chemicals to change the user's perception of his or her status is a workable definition of drug abuse. The key word is excessive, which allows for consideration of the multifactorial genesis of drug abuse. For example, the average healthy person's daily use of coffee or tea could be considered drug abuse except that several cups of coffee each day is not considered excessive by our society nor would it be considered excessive or medically unwise for a healthy adult. Because our society considers even a single intravenous injection of heroin or methamphetamine excessive, sporadic intravenous administration of these drugs is considered drug abuse. The definition of drug abuse must be individualized for the drug, the person using the drug, and the psychosocial setting in which the drug is used. The identification of teratogenicity of some commonly consumed chemicals also contributes to a redefinition of drug abuse.

It is my contention that for the pregnant woman, particularly during the first few months of pregnancy, the indiscriminate use of any drug, regardless of its ubiquity or social status, constitutes drug abuse. The risk to the fetus of such drug usage is clear, and although maternal ill effects are tolerable, the effect on the fetus may be devastating. The thalidomide incident over a decade ago should serve as a constant reminder. This chapter will be confined to a few of the "drugs of abuse" and their impact on pregnancy (Table 22–1).

Ethyl alcohol, amphetamines, barbiturates and other sedatives, cannabis, hallucinogens, and heroin are the most common drugs of abuse. The most important effect that abuse of these drugs has upon pregnancy is impairment of general maternal health as measured by inadequate nutrition and prenatal care, the incidence of serious infectious disease, and serious psychosocial stress. Because many drug-abusing mothers support their drug habit with prostitution, there is a concomitant high incidence of sexually transmitted diseases. These factors contribute as much as or more than the specific effects of the abused drugs to the clinical complications of drug use during pregnancy. The specific effects of the abused drug often affect the neonate most severely by the appearance of a withdrawal syndrome, congenital malformations, or growth retardation.

Although alcohol and sedative abuse is prevalent throughout the adult population, the abuse of heroin, amphetamines, hallucinogens, and newer sedative agents such as methaqualone is

TABLE 22–1 PREGNANCY AND DRUGS OF ABUSE

Agent	Routes	Teratogenic	Impaired Fetal Growth	Withdrawal Syndrome	
				MATERNAL	FETAL
Ethyl alcohol	oral	yes	yes	yes	yes
Barbiturates	oral	no	no	yes	yes
Benzodiazapines	oral	no	no	rare	rare
Heroin	IV; subcutaneous	no	yes	yes	yes
Methadone	oral	no	yes	yes	yes
Amphetamines	oral; IV	no	no	yes	?
Hallucinogens (LSD, PCP, etc.)	oral	presumed	no	no	no
Tobacco	inhalation	no	yes	yes	?

538

TABLE 22–2 EFFECT OF ADDICTIONS ON PREGNANCY

	Mother	Fetus
DRUG EFFECT	Tolerance Withdrawal	Tolerance Withdrawal Growth retardation Congenital anomalies
ECOLOGICAL EFFECT	Infections Malnutrition Toxemia	Growth retardation Premature delivery Infections

principally confined to teen-agers and young adults. A large number of drug abusers use more than one agent for long periods of time; others use only one agent at a time but continue to abuse at least one drug. For example, there is a distressing incidence of chronic alcoholism among ex-heroin addicts successfully withdrawn from narcotics in methadone programs.

The effects of drug addiction on pregnancy can be divided into two broad categories (Table 22–2). One category is the pharmacologic effects of the drug on mother and fetus. The other reflects the ecology of the addicted patient and includes the adverse effects of dirty needles, the economic necessities of supporting a habit by prostitution or thievery, and the psychosocial isolation dictated by the drug-dependent existence. The pharmacologic effects of a drug may be tolerable if the ecology of the addict is managed effectively. In fact, the best management of the pregnant addict may be continuation of the addiction under controlled circumstances. This is especially true with narcotic addiction, in which maternal withdrawal is primarily a risk for the fetus. In contrast, barbiturate withdrawal can be fatal for the mother and should be accomplished before delivery if possible. Drug detoxification is best carried out in the second trimester when the risks of withdrawal-induced abortion or premature labor are reportedly less than in the first or third trimester.

The majority of medical complications of parenteral drug abuse are not associated with the drug itself but with the conditions under which the drug is taken, i.e., the complications of unsterile and contaminated injections.[5, 17] The organisms causing infection are usually indigenous flora; the drug mixture with its adulterants, and diluents and the injection paraphernalia may be sources of other bacteria. The most commonly isolated organisms are staphylococci, streptococci, aerobic gram-negative rods, and those of the *Bacteroides, Clostridium,* and *Candida* species. Septic thrombophlebitis, superficial celluli-

tis, and abscess formation are common. Local repositories of quinine produced by subcutaneous injection ("skin popping") or infiltration of intravenous injections have a sufficiently low redox potential to allow the growth of *Clostridium tetani*. Using quinine as an adulterant has apparently reduced the incidence of needle-transmitted malaria. Serious bacterial infections result from bacteremia accompanying or following unsterile intravenous injection, including pyrogen reactions, septicemia, metastatic abscesses of bone and cartilage, and endocarditis. The infectious endocarditis seen in intravenous drug addicts may be right sided, with septic pulmonary emboli, and is often caused by *Staphylococcus aureus* and *Candida albicans*. Hepatitis B is particularly common among such patients. The repeated injection of inert but particulate material such as talc, contained in tablets or capsule powder, can produce obstructive pulmonary vascular disease and hyperglobulinemia with false positive serologic tests for syphilis. The intravenous drug user is therefore subject to a variety of recurrent, chronic, or potentially fatal infections and inflammatory diseases.

The evaluation and management of the drug-abusing patient presents unique problems for the clinician (Table 22–3). The conventional patient is motivated to seek out medical assistance. The drug abuser, on the other hand, is engaged in an activity that is considered undesirable and is often associated with illegal actions. Moreover, the drug abuser may not consider herself ill and may not want to give up taking drugs. Indeed, many are afraid of drug withdrawal and are compelled to continue their drug habit at almost any cost. Unless the patient becomes sick from drug intoxication or the medical complications of drug abuse, she may not seek medical attention. Because pregnancy is not considered an illness and because prenatal care may be regarded as unimportant and even potentially harmful because of fear of detection and punishment for

TABLE 22–3 MANAGEMENT OF DRUG ABUSE IN PREGNANCY

Nutrition:
    Prevent deficiency states
    Prevent maternal ketosis

Infection:
    Examine for and treat sexually transmitted disease
    Examine for hepatitis B
    Watch for and treat intercurrent illness

Psychosocial:
    Establish contact with support services
    Watch for suicidal depression
    Hospitalize without delay

Drug management:
    Watch for multiple drug use
    Controlled withdrawal:
        barbiturates
        alcohol
    Supportive withdrawal:
        minor tranquilizers and sedatives
        amphetamines
        tobacco
    Maintenance therapy for narcotics: methadone

drug abuse, many pregnant drug abusers do not seek prenatal care. If they do request prenatal care, they may attempt to obscure their drug habit. The clinician must, therefore, be alert to the psychosocial clues to drug abuse and to the clinical manifestations and complications of drug abuse. The appearance of needle tracks or tattoos used to cover needle tracks, unusual infections in unusual locations, and unexplained indifference to the need for careful prenatal nutrition and care are all clues to potential drug abuse. Chemical tests for drugs in the urine and blood are essential to the diagnosis.

There is evidence from methadone maintenance programs that good prenatal care will obviate many of the adverse effects on the mother's health despite continued use of a drug.[1, 23, 28] There does not appear to be a significant reduction in the incidence of small-for-date babies in this group, but the incidence of perinatal mortality is reduced and the management of the infant withdrawal syndrome is facilitated.[1] The greatest incidence of prematurity and perinatal morbidity occurs in women who use drugs throughout pregnancy.[26] There is much good to be gained by achieving a mutual trust that ensures good prenatal care even though drug abuse continues. Attempts to stop drug abuse before such a relationship is established may be harmful to the pregnancy by causing the patient's retreat from continuous care.

ALCOHOL

Ethyl alcohol is the most commonly abused drug in the United States and many industrialized countries. Alcohol abuse undermines maternal health by producing malnutrition, especially folic acid and thiamine deficiencies, hepatic disease, bone marrow suppression, and infectious complications such as pneumonia. Acute and chronic alcohol intoxication contribute to an enormous toll of death and disability from related accidents. Alcohol is almost always one of several sedatives abused by multiple drug abusers. Many suicides are attempted while under the influence of alcohol.

Ethyl alcohol crosses the placenta. Fetal blood levels approximate those of the mother. Fetal intoxication is known to occur. The neonate of a mother inebriated during delivery, including mothers given alcohol to halt premature labor, may be intoxicated as well. Lethargy, gastritis, and hypoglycemia with low Apgar scores are manifestations of neonatal acute alcohol toxicity.

Because of the tendency to fasting hypoglycemia and ketosis during pregnancy, the drinking mother has heightened susceptibility to the alcoholic ketoacidosis syndrome. The adverse effects of maternal ketosis on the child's neuropsychologic development may contribute to the high incidence of mental retardation among the children of alcoholic mothers.

Over the past decade, attention has been focused on a pattern of abnormalities, chiefly, central nervous system anomalies, dysmorphic facies, growth deficiency, and mental retardation, in the children of alcohol-using mothers.[12-14, 24, 25] The clinical expression of the so-called fetal alcohol syndrome is, however, variable, and the clinician must be alert to subtle fetal abnormalities.[6] The risk of fetal abnormalities and the severity of fetal involvement are related to the quantity of alcohol ingested and the time during gestation that fetal exposure to alcohol occurs. Daily alcohol consumption in excess of 5 ounces of absolute alcohol (10 oz of 100 proof whiskey) during the first trimester is associated with a 20 to 40 per cent risk of producing a clinically abnormal child. Smaller amounts of alcohol consumed on a daily basis during pregnancy may result in intrauterine growth retardation and/or impaired mental development without clinically detectable anatomic anomalies. Tobacco use combined with alcohol use may have adverse synergistic effects on the physical and mental growth of the fetus.

Although moderate to excessive alcohol intake during pregnancy is harmful, the effects of occasional, social use of alcohol on the fetus are not known. The obstetrician should be alert to the possibilities of excessive alcohol use and should discourage mothers from drinking, especially during the first trimester. The recommendation that serious consideration be given to termination of pregnancy in chronic alcoholic mothers[13] requires further documentation.

Alcohol abuse can be remarkably difficult to detect. Accident proneness, macrocytic anemia, ketosis or ketoacidosis without hyperglycemia, and unreliability in prenatal care, often with excessive explanations, are clinical clues to the alcohol-abusing mother. Questioning of other family members may confirm the clinical suspicion. Blood alcohol levels may prove alcohol usage and intoxication if blood is drawn when the patient presents with an injury or an alcohol odor. Because of the effects on the mother and the fetus and because of the risk of withdrawal syndromes in both mother and neonate, controlled detoxification during pregnancy is recommended. This task, however, may be almost impossible on a voluntary basis and may require enforced hospitalization under certain circumstances. Even after detoxification, sobriety may be difficult to maintain. Disulfiram (Antabuse) should not be used during pregnancy. A diet with added protein and vitamins, especially folic acid and thiamine, helps prevent nutritional deficiency but does not protect against the direct toxic effects of alcohol on the liver, pancreas, bone marrow, and fetus.

There are three clinical manifestations of alcohol withdrawal. The most common, "the shakes," is tremulousness and irritability, which begins within 48 hours after termination of drinking and usually subsides within a few days. Sedation with hydroxyzine or a benzodiazepine may be helpful and may retard the development of full-blown delirium tremens. The "DTs" remain a life-threatening metabolic disease characterized by marked sympathetic overactivity, fever, and encephalopathy with terrifying visual hallucinations and confabulation. About 15 per cent of patients with delirium tremens die; premature labor may occur during severe alcohol withdrawal. Alcohol withdrawal seizures, "rum fits," begin within 12 to 48 hours after cessation of drinking. Usually only one or two of these grand mal seizures occur, and anticonvulsant drugs are not needed. Multiple seizures should raise the suspicion of a pre-existing seizure focus, head trauma, or central nervous system infection. The alcohol withdrawal syndrome in the neonate includes irritability and seizures. There is no clear-cut correlation between maternal and fetal withdrawal symptoms.

Any of these withdrawal phenomena may occur in the labor and delivery suite. Management during labor and delivery must be cautious. Alcoholics may have a surprising tolerance for sedation and analgesics, and high doses of these drugs may be given with the risk of severe respiratory depression in the neonate.

NARCOTICS

Heroin and methadone are the two narcotics most commonly used — heroin illegally and often irregularly and methadone usually under medical supervision with some regularity. Illegal narcotic use continues to be a widespread problem; however, public attention to the problem and public support for treatment centers for narcotic addicts has declined since the first edition of this book (1975).

The pharmacologic effects of narcotics used during pregnancy include the development of dependence in both mother and fetus with the consequent appearance of symptoms when the drug is not taken, retardation of fetal growth, and the risks of overdosage. The ecology of the heroin addict includes the dirty needle and criminal behavior. In one series of heroin abusing mothers, 49 per cent had fever and skin or urinary tract infection; 34 per cent had evidence of inflammation or infection of the placenta, chorion, and amnion.[22] This series also documented the well-recognized problem of premature labor and low birth weight infants in heroin-addicted mothers.[29] The incidence of toxemia and hemorrhage is increased but has not proved to be a consistent complication of maternal heroin addiction. There does appear to be a definite trend toward higher perinatal morbidity and mortality among the infants of these mothers.[7, 22, 31]

Narcotic dependence develops in the majority of women and fetuses when the drugs are used on a regular basis. Some patients use heroin irregularly, and, because the content of heroin in "street bags" is highly variable, no dependence develops. It is among these less tolerant users that serious narcotic overdosage usually occurs. The overdosed patient is comatose with pinpoint pupils and should be given naloxone, a narcotic antagonist without respiratory depressant properties. The dose is 0.01 mg/kg given intravenously. Pulmonary edema that is not responsive to narcotics may occur with heroin overdosage. Chronic lung changes may follow repetitive injury to the pulmonary vasculature from particulate matter contained in the injected lung.

The use of a narcotic antagonist may precipitate the narcotic abstinence syndrome: agitation, lacrimation, rhinorrhea, perspiration, yawning, piloerection, and mydriasis. Prolonged narcotic withdrawal in the addict may produce abdominal and uterine cramps, orgasm, diarrhea, myalgias, and muscular irritability. Although profoundly uncomfortable, the narcotic abstinence syndrome is rarely injurious to the mother. Maternal withdrawal is, however, potentially fatal to the fetus. The fetus may be expelled if severe withdrawal occurs during the first trimester. Later in pregnancy, fetal withdrawal produces hyperactivity, hypoxia, and the passage of meconium. Intrauterine fetal death may occur. Because of the risk to the fetus, narcotic withdrawal is not encouraged during pregnancy, and narcotic antagonists, such as pentazocine (Talwin) and naloxone (Narcan), should be used with great caution.

Pentazocine abuse poses a clinical dilemma for the obstetrician. This drug has addictive potential but is a mild narcotic antagonist. Methadone does not block all of the effects of pentazocine. Moreover, the risk of pentazocine-induced narcotic withdrawal symptoms, while small, is sufficient to preclude the substitution of other narcotics for maintenance. Pentazocine-abusing mothers should be withdrawn gradually during the second trimester and should not be placed on methadone maintenance.

Pregnant heroin addicts are best served by enrollment in methadone maintenance programs. Methadone is a long-acting, synthetic opiate that can be taken by mouth, thereby reducing the risk of needle complications. Methadone blocks the euphoria produced by heroin and blunts the appetite for "shooting up." Methadone has the same properties as heroin; it is not a narcotic antagonist.

Over a decade of experience with methadone maintenance during pregnancy has demonstrated its value in reducing the ecology-related adverse effects of drug use during pregnancy. Detection and treatment of infections, improved nutrition, and improved prenatal and psychosocial care contribute to the improved pregnancy outcome. It is also clear that medication without psychosocial support and prenatal care is much less effective. The infant withdrawal syndrome in children born of methadone-maintained mothers tends to be less severe, although this depends in part on the mother's dosage of methadone, and tends to occur later than heroin withdrawal in infants.[15] Acute withdrawal from methadone in adults is no different from that following heroin withdrawal. Despite good prenatal care, about one third of neonates of methadone-maintained mothers are undersized, suggesting a direct negative effect of narcotics on fetal growth.

Any woman who admits to an opium habit should be designated a high risk patient and should be encouraged to enter a program for drug rehabilitation. Because detoxification of the pregnant narcotics addict is hazardous, the clinician should refer the patient to the nearest methadone maintenance program even if long distances are involved. The isolated existence of the narcotics addict allows for geographic mobility not usually possible during pregnancy. Narcotic detoxification has not been especially successful[2, 7]; the majority of patients resume their drug habit after being released from the hospital. An additional reason for prompt referral to a high risk obstetrical and neonatal center with a methadone maintenance program is that infants born to opiate addicts should be cared for in an intensive care nursery where staff can evaluate and treat the infant withdrawal syndrome.

BARBITURATES

Barbiturates are commonly prescribed and commonly abused drugs. Pregnant patients are prescribed barbiturates for control of seizures and for sedation; maternal health and nutrition are generally maintained and retarded fetal growth does not occur in these pregnancies. When barbiturates are used illegally in a nontherapeutic setting, maternal health and nutrition are usually not well maintained and often other substances are used as well. In these circumstances fetal growth and development can be impaired.

Prolonged maternal consumption of barbiturates may lead to tolerance and dependence in the mother and fetus, after which withdrawal may produce an abstinence syndrome. Barbiturate withdrawal in adults may progress beyond restlessness, irritability, insomnia, and autonomic stimulation to delirium, psychosis, and seizures. Barbiturate withdrawal, untreated, may end fatally, unlike narcotics withdrawal. Abrupt withdrawal before delivery may be accompanied by intrauterine fetal withdrawal and risk of fetal death. The neonatal withdrawal syndrome is similar to the withdrawal seen in children of narcotics addicts. There is, however, a higher incidence of seizures with barbiturate withdrawal. Neonatal withdrawal may follow maternal treatment with phenobarbital in doses appropriate for seizure control as well as illicit use of large amounts of short-acting barbiturates.[8]

Blood levels of barbiturates should be measured to help confirm the diagnosis. When the pregnant barbiturate addict can be identified and hospitalized, the drug dosage can be regulated and maternal health improved with a good diet, identification and treatment of intercurrent infections, and establishing contact with psychosocial support services. Controlled decremental doses of pentobarbital can be used to withdraw the patient without risk of a serious abstinence syndrome. The real problems are the failure to recognize the barbiturate addict before the onset of withdrawal and the failure to recognize and treat barbiturate withdrawal when it occurs. This may, of course, be exceptionally difficult during labor and delivery. Usually these patients have not received prenatal care, and their clinical presentations should suggest the likelihood of substance abuse. Obtaining blood and urine samples for drug toxicology screening is an important diagnostic aid. Barbiturate withdrawal symptoms should be treated with decremental doses of pentobarbital.

TRANQUILIZERS AND NONBARBITURATE SEDATIVES

These ubiquitous agents—benzodiazepines (diazepam, chlordiazepoxide, etc.), glutethimide, ethchlorvynol — are not known to have direct toxic effects on the fetus. Tolerance and the abstinence syndrome in both mother and neonate occur in patients who use large amounts over an extended period of time. The major risks to pregnancy that the tranquilizers and nonbarbiturate sedatives pose are overdosage, with prolonged hypoxia during coma, and maternal malnutrition. Most of these drugs are used concurrently with alcohol, and the clinician should look for the more serious effects of alcohol on the mother and fetus in patients suspected of tranquilizer or sedative abuse.

The tranquilizer withdrawal syndrome is not as severe as that seen with barbiturate withdrawal. The risk of intrauterine fetal death occurring because of abrupt withdrawal before delivery is very slight. It is probably desirable, therefore, to attempt withdrawal from these agents before delivery if it is possible to maintain the patient in a controlled environment.

AMPHETAMINES AND COCAINE

Over the past decade the availability of amphetamines for quasi-medical indications has been dramatically reduced. However, because of their euphoric, sympathomimetic properties these drugs continue to be popular among drug users and experimenters. Amphetamines are taken by the oral or intravenous route. Tremendous tolerance can develop with regular use. Patients actively abusing amphetamines are hyperactive, often are paranoid and have hallucinations, and, because of the lack of appetite and insomnia, are usually badly malnourished.[30] Amphetamines may be used in cycles following a binge of regular use of sedatives and alcohol. Patients who use amphetamines intravenously are subject to all the complications of intravenous drug abuse. The autonomic instability produced by amphetamine usage may produce serious arrhythmias and may increase the risk of serious arrhythmias, including ventricular tachycardia and asystole, during obstetrical anesthesia.[27] Withdrawal is accompanied by an abstinence syndrome of lethargy and profound depression. Neonatal withdrawal syndrome has been documented.

Amphetamine abuse may be accompanied by a progressive vasculitis in a very small number of patients. The renal, cerebral, and pulmonary vasculature may all be involved, and the sequelae of the vasculitis can be severe. No similar syndrome has been described in neonates. A few instances of cleft palate have been described; however, the major fetal problems have been retarded intrauterine growth, which may reflect poor maternal nutrition and multiple drug abuse rather than direct amphetamine toxicity.[10, 16, 18]

Active amphetamine use may be suspected by the clinical presentation of the patient and confirmed by finding amphetamines in the urine. Detoxification and good nutrition are the main components of management and probably should be carried out before delivery, if possible. However, serious amphetamine abusers often do not seek out prenatal care, abuse multiple drugs, and are resistant to social rehabilitation.

Cocaine is an expensive stimulant except in areas of South America where cocoa plants are grown. Cocaine abuse has many clinical similarities to amphetamine abuse. Vasculitis has not been described. However, cocaine is a potent vasoconstrictor. Local and intravenous use may produce local and regional ischemia. For example, atrophic rhinitis and ischemic perforation of the nasal septum may result from "snorting" cocaine. Intravenous use is attended by all the risks of dirty needles. In addition, because of local ischemia, anaerobic infections including tetanus may occur. Cocaine is not known to have direct deleterious effects on the fetus. The clinician should keep in mind that the anorexigenic effects of amphetamines and cocaine increase the risk of ketosis during pregnancy.

CANNABIS

Despite widespread usage of marijuana, there is little evidence to indicate that either marijuana or hashish has serious adverse effects on the fetus. Smoking marijuana regularly may have effects similar to tobacco on fetal growth. Adulterants, such as herbicides, contained in the smoking mixture may produce lung injury.

HALLUCINOGENS

The major risk of hallucinogenic drug abuse is psychiatric. Phencyclidine (PCP, "angel dust") and lysergic acid diethylamide (LSD, "acid") are two commonly used agents. There is suggestive but not conclusive evidence that illicit or "street" LSD can produce chromosomal anomalies in fetal tissue if taken during the first trimester of pregnancy.[26] Others are more skeptical about the possibility of small infrequent doses of LSD being teratogenic.[9] A recent case report describes an infant with dysmorphic facies and spastic quadriparesis born to a mother using PCP throughout pregnancy.[11] However, other agents in the "street" drug and the frequent use of other drugs by individuals using hallucinogens could produce the described abnormalities in children of LSD- and PCP-using mothers.

TOBACCO

Cigarette smoking is, like alcohol, very prevalent in industrialized countries. Tobacco smoking is not generally regarded as a form of drug abuse, but increasing knowledge about the detrimental effects of cigarette smoking on health is forcing a reconsideration of attitudes towards tobacco use. The association of cigarette smoking with chronic bronchitis, myocardial infarction, and cancer of the lung has received the most attention from public health and education authorities, whereas the association of cigarette smoking with increased pregnancy wastage and low birth weight has received less emphasis. Despite adverse publicity, cigarette smoking in the United States, as measured by the yearly consumption of cigarettes, has been increasing. This increase has been especially marked in young women.

Several studies have shown a mean reduction in birth weight varying between 115 and 400 grams among the offspring of mothers who smoked cigarettes during pregnancy.[4, 19, 20] Other studies have demonstrated an association between maternal smoking and an increase in abortions and stillbirths.[4, 21] The adverse effects of smoking on birth weight and perinatal mortality are independent of maternal age, parity, and socioeconomic factors. Mothers who smoke five or more cigarettes per day are at much greater risk than women who smoke four or less per day; this dose effect seems to be most important beginning in the fourth month of pregnancy. There is recent evidence that children of smoking mothers continue to exhibit some retardation of growth up to 11 years of age.[3] It should be emphasized that the data on the adverse effects of smoking on pregnancy in the fetus are derived almost exclusively from epidemiologic studies; the mechanisms by which smoking produces these effects is entirely speculative at the present time. Nevertheless, the clinician would be wise to caution mothers about the effects of smoking on maternal and fetal health, to encourage smoking mothers to stop, and to discourage nonsmoking women from starting to smoke during the reproductive years.

References

1. Blinick, G., Jerez, E., and Wallach, R. C.: Methadone maintenance, pregnancy and progeny. J.A.M.A., 225:477, 1973.
2. Blinick, G., Wallach, R. C., and Jerez, E.: Pregnancy in narcotic addicts treated by medical withdrawal. Am. J. Obstet. Gynecol., 105:997, 1969.
3. Butler, N. R., and Goldstein, H.: Smoking in pregnancy and subsequent child development. Br. Med. J., 4:573, 1973.
4. Butler, N. R., Goldstein, H., and Ross, E. M.: Cigarette smoking in pregnancy: its influence on birthweight and perinatal mortality. Br. Med. J., 2:127, 1972.
5. Cherubin, C. E.: The medical sequelae of narcotic addiction. Ann. Intern. Med., 67:23, 1967.
6. Clarren, S. K., and Smith, D. W.: The fetal alcohol syndrome. N. Engl. J. Med., 298:1063, 1978.
7. Connaughton, J. F., Jr., Reeser, D., and Finnegan, L. P.:

Pregnancy complicated by drug addiction. In Bolognese, R. J., and Schwarz, R. H. (eds.): Perinatal Medicine. Baltimore, Williams & Wilkins, 1977, pp. 265–276.
8. Desmond, M. M., Schwanecke, R. P., Wilson, G. S., Yasunaga, S., and Burgdorf, I.: Maternal barbiturate utilization and neonatal withdrawal symptomatology. J. Pediatr., 80:190, 1972.
9. Dishotsky, N. I., Loughman, W. D., Mogar, R. E., and Lipscomb, W. R.: LSD and genetic damage. Science, 172:431, 1971.
10. Eriksson, M., Larsson, G., Winbladh, B., and Zetterstrom, R.: The influence of amphetamine addiction on pregnancy and the newborn infant. Acta Pediatr. Scand., 67:95, 1978.
11. Golden, N. L., Sokol, R. J., and Rubin, I. L.: Angel dust: Possible effects on the fetus. Pediatrics, 65:18, 1980.
12. Hanson, J. W., Streissguth, A. P., and Smith, D. W.: The effects

of moderate alcohol consumption during pregnancy on fetal growth and morphogenesis. J. Pediatr., *92*:457, 1978.

13. Jones, K. L., Smith, D. W., Streissguth, A. P., and Myriantho-poulos, N. C.: Outcome of offspring of chronic alcoholic women. Lancet, *1*:1076, 1974.

14. Jones, K. L., Smith, D. W., Ulleland, C. N., and Streissguth, A. P.: Pattern of malformation in offspring of chronic alcoholic mothers. Lancet, *1*:1267, 1973.

15. Kandall, S. R., and Gartner, L. M.: Late presentation of drug withdrawal symptoms in newborns. Am. J. Dis. Child., *127*:58, 1974.

16. Larsson, G.: The amphetamine addicted mother and her child. Acta Pediatr. Scand., *278*(Suppl.):6, 1980.

17. Louria, D. B., Hensle, T., and Rose, J.: The major medical complications of heroin addiction. Ann. Intern. Med., *67*:1, 1967.

18. Milkovich, L., and van den Berg, B. J.: Effects of antenatal exposure to anorectic drugs. Am. J. Obstet. Gynecol., *129*:637, 1977.

19. Mulcahy, R., Murphy, J., and Martin, F.: Placental changes and maternal weight in smoking and nonsmoking mothers. Am. J. Obstet. Gynecol., *106*:703, 1970.

20. Murphy, J. F., and Mulcahy, R.: The effect of age, parity, and cigarette smoking on baby weight. Am. J. Obstet. Gynecol., *111*:22, 1971.

21. Murphy, J. F., and Mulcahy, R.: The effects of cigarette smoking, maternal age, and parity on the outcome of pregnancy. J. Irish Med. Assoc., *67*:309, 1974.

22. Naeye, R. L., Blanc, W., LeBlanc, W., and Khatamee, M. A.: Fetal complications of maternal heroin addiction: Abnormal growth, infections, and episodes of stress. J. Pediatr., *83*:1055, 1973.

23. Newman, R. G.: Pregnancies of methadone patients. N.Y. State J. Med., *74*:52, 1974.

24. Olegard, R., Sabel, K. G., Aronsson, M., Sandin, B., Johansson, P. R., Carlsson, C., Kyllerman, M., Iversen, K., and Hrbek, A.: Effects on the child of alcohol abuse during pregnancy. Acta Pediatr. Scand., *275*(Suppl.):112, 1979.

25. Ouellette, E. M., Rossett, H. L., Rosman, N. P., and Weiner, L.: Adverse effects on offspring of maternal alcohol abuse during pregnancy. N. Engl. J. Med., *297*:528, 1977.

26. Poland, B. J., Wogan, L., and Calvin, J.: Teenagers, illicit drugs, and pregnancy. Can. Med. Assoc. J., *107*:955, 1972.

27. Samuels, S. I., Maze, A., and Albright, G.: Cardiac arrest during cesarean section in a chronic amphetamine abuser. Anesth. Analg., *58*:528, 1979.

28. Statzer, D. E., and Wardell, J. N.: Heroin addiction during pregnancy. Am. J. Obstet. Gynecol., *113*:273, 1972.

29. Stone, M. L., Salerno, L. J., Green, M., and Zelson, C.: Narcotic addiction in pregnancy. Am. J. Obstet. Gynecol., *109*:716, 1971.

30. Sussman, S.: Narcotic and methamphetamine use during pregnancy. Am. J. Dis. Child., *106*:457, 1973.

31. Wilson, G. S., Desmond, M. M., and Verniand, W. M.: Early development of infants of heroin addicted mothers. Am. J. Dis. Child., *126*:457, 1973.

Dorothy Reycroft Hollingsworth, M.D.

23

THE PREGNANT ADOLESCENT: A SOCIOLOGIC PROBLEM WITH MEDICAL CONSEQUENCES

"I would there were no age between ten and three and twenty; or that youth would sleep out the rest: for there is nothing in the between but getting wenches with child, wronging the ancientry, stealing, fighting." Shakespeare, Shepherd in A Winter's Tale, Act III, Scene 3.

Adolescent mores and sexual activity have changed markedly in the past two decades. Earlier sexual maturation, peer pressure in junior and senior high schools, and national commercial and film emphasis on the pleasures of sex have not unexpectedly resulted in initiation of sexual intercourse at earlier ages. These well-documented sociologic and behavioral changes have presented pediatricians, internists, family physicians, and obstetricians with a new array of sexually related diseases and reproductive problems. Recognizing the awesome fact that 17 to 20 per cent

of our next generation will consist of infants of mothers of age 11 to 18, it is of critical importance to find reasonable ways of ameliorating this difficult national problem.

The teenage birth rate increased in 1977 for the first time in seven years, despite increasing availabilty and use of contraceptives by teenagers,[91] increasing federal expenditures for family planning services,[79] and an increasing abortion rate.[11]

The 570,609 births to adolescents in 1977 in the face of a declining national birth rate occurred as a result of an increase in sexual activity at an earlier age. Figure 23–1 depicts the reported 30.2 per cent increase in sexual activity among unmarried women 15 to 19 years of age from 1971 to 1976.

During the past two decades interesting trends

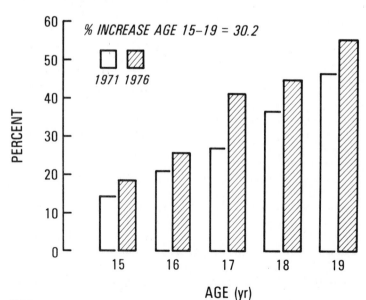

FIGURE 23–1. Per cent unmarried women aged 15 to 19 years experiencing sexual intercourse in 1971 and 1976. (Drawn from data by Zelnik et al: Fam. Plann. Perspect., *11*:177, 1979.)

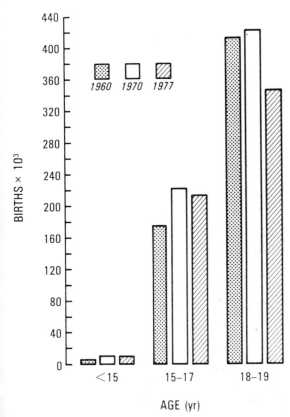

FIGURE 23–2. Total number of births to teenagers (in thousands) in 1960 (stippled bars), 1970 (open bars), and 1977 (hatched bars). (Drawn from data from National Center for Health Statistics, 1976, and monthly Vital Statistics Report: Final Natality Statistics, 1977, Vol. 27, No. 11, Supplement, February 5, 1979.)

in childbearing have been noted in teenagers. The total number of births to teenagers in 1977 is not appreciably different than in 1976 (570,609 versus 570,642) and only slightly higher than the 609,000 births to teenagers observed in 1961. However, the pattern of childbearing has changed. Figure 23–2 depicts the change in pattern of number of births to young women less than 15 years old, 15 to 17, and 18 to 19 in the years 1960, 1970, and 1977. These time periods correspond with the introduction of oral contraceptives and intrauterine devices in the 1960s and the widespread prevalence of legalized abortions since 1973. In women under age 15, births increased from 7,462 in 1960 to 11,752 in 1970. There was a slight decrease to 11,455 in 1977. There are now more abortions than live births in this age group.

In women age 15 to 17, births increased from 177,904 in 1960 to 223,590 in 1970. Despite easy access to both contraceptive counseling and abortions, there has been almost no change in

births to this group from 1970 to 1977 (213,788). Women of high school age constitute an increasingly sexually active group at high risk of becoming pregnant. Birth rates for women under 18 are now at about the highest levels ever recorded in the United States.

At age 18, young women reach the legal age of maturity and begin to make independent personal decisions regarding marriage, employment, or further education. As noted in Figure 23–2, there has been a drop in births in this older age group.

An enlightening view of teenage pregnancy emerges when the birth rate for all women 14 to 19 years of age is plotted for the United States from 1920 to 1977. Figure 23–3 shows the fluctuations in teenage births in relation to events known to affect birth rates.

In 1920, the birth rate (births per 1000 women) for women 17 to 19 years of age was higher than in 1977, whereas during the same period (1920 to 1977) the birth rate increased in women age 14 (3.6 to 6.7), age 15 (11.9 to 18.2), and age 16 (28.6 to 34.5).

The Depression years coincided with a perceptible drop in birth rate, most obvious in teenagers 17 to 19 years of age. World War II and the first postwar decade were associated with the greatest increase in birth rate for women age 15 to 19 in this century. This upward trend reached a peak in 1955, when a sharp downward deflection coincided with the introduction of oral contraceptives and intrauterine devices (IUD). The decline continued with the passage of legislation in 1973 permitting legalized abortion. Thus, viewed in perspective, teenage childbearing reflects economic, psychosocial, behavioral, and technological developments in the nation as a whole.

In the years 1976 to 1980, there was a 6.7 per cent decline in the number of 14 to 17 year olds, but the number of sexually active adolescents is expected to continue to increase. Thus, the key issues for the coming decades are the direction of adolescent reproductive behavior and the encouragement of a change in emphasis to steer peer pressure toward responsible reproduction.

DIAGNOSIS AND DECISION MAKING

In our highly technological and more mobile post World War II society, early childbearing creates difficult personal and sociologic problems. In the 1950s and 1960s, great efforts were made by many young pregnant women and their families to conceal pregnancy occurring outside

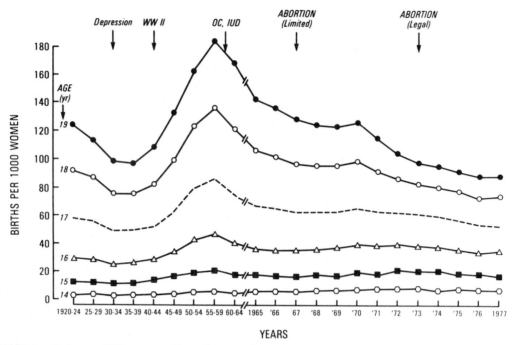

FIGURE 23–3. Births per 1000 women, 14 to 19 years of age, by single years of age for all women: United States, 1920–1977. (Drawn from data from National Center for Health Statistics. Fertility Tables for Birth Cohorts by Color: United States, 1917–1973. DHEW Publication No. (HRA) 76–1152, U.S. Government Printing Office, 1976, p. 37; and National Center for Health Statistics, Monthly Vital Statistics Report, Final Natality Statistics, 1977, Vol. 27, No. 11, Supplement, February 5, 1979.)

of marriage. In more extreme instances, pregnant adolescents were sent to other states to reside with family members or friends or in homes for unwed mothers. The severe social stigma of illegitimacy in some families, and poverty in others, resulted in a marked delay in seeking prenatal care[46] and tended to cause emotionally difficult first pregnancies.

In the 1960s, when many prenatal programs for young mothers were established, society was much more punitive and far less helpful in searching for solutions to early childbearing. This was especially true in public schools, where there was a general reluctance to permit pregnant girls to attend regular classes. Published studies focused on high risk adolescent pregnancies of urban blacks.[3, 37, 61, 70]

During the 1970s, it came to be recognized that teenage pregnancy is primarily a sociologic problem with medical consequences. It also became apparent that teenage pregnancy is common in all social, economic, and racial groups in all parts of the nation. High obstetric risk in older teenagers was found to be associated with poverty, inadequate nutrition, and poor prepregnancy health and not with maternal age.[19, 35, 46, 54, 62]

The diagnosis of pregnancy in teenagers is frequently delayed because they conceal or deny the facts. It is common for them to present initially to pediatric clinics with complaints such as earache, unexplained nausea and vomiting, afternoon somnolence, emotional lability, or "school phobia."

During the 1970s the specialty of pediatrics expanded to include adolescents. Diagnostic acuity improved and a high index of suspicion resulted in much earlier diagnosis of pregnancy. The medical evaluation of pediatric patients age 11 and older should now routinely include a menstrual and sexual history as well as a notation of stage of sexual maturation.[53]

An increase in services is resulting in earlier diagnosis of adolescent pregnancy. All clinics and most doctors' offices have rapid pregnancy tests available, which can be performed in a few minutes by the office nurse. Sexually active junior and senior high school students are aware of the signs and symptoms of early pregnancy as well as the significance of a missed menstrual period. Pregnancy tests are available with confidentiality at health departments, free neighborhood clinics, and Planned Parenthood offices.

A positive diagnosis of pregnancy in a teenager immediately changes her family and social relationships. Her first reaction is often disbelief, which is the same reaction of women of all ages upon first learning that they are pregnant. The teenager must focus rather acutely on a change in emotional setting with the baby's father if the couple have a serious and continuing relationship. A marked alteration in her relationships with her family, teachers, counselors, and friends is also likely.

An acute awareness of the need for decision making develops. Should she seek an abortion? Does she wish to continue the pregnancy, and, if so, will she try to keep the baby or place it in foster or adoptive care? These decisions are often made easily and quickly by older teenagers (age 18 to 19) and by those who are much more mature than their chronologic age. For many, however, these are agonizing questions marked by ambivalence and sometimes severe societal and family pressures. Hours of patient and skillful counseling may be needed to work out a solution for each set of circumstances. The answers that evolve depend on whether the pregnancy was wanted (consciously or unconsciously) or unwanted, stage of gestation, and availability of funds for abortion. The role of the infant's father is often critical in the final decision. Personal, educational, and career goals; pressure from prospective grandparents; and economic support systems may be key factors.

pregnancy. The important medical issues for adolescents are: (1) What abortion procedures are available and at what stage of gestation? (2) What are the medical risks of abortion? and (3) What do long-term followup studies show about women who have received abortions?

Pregnant teenagers requesting an abortion should be seen as promptly as possible for evaluation after they learn they are pregnant. A careful history and physical examination (and often a pregnancy test) are required to confirm the diagnosis of pregnancy. Counseling is a mandatory part of abortion services for adolescents. The counselor must have a sensitive understanding of young women, and a great deal of time is focused on the special circumstances of each young pregnant woman and her family. In adolescent medicine clinics, the approach of Kreutner and Langhorst has been found to be especially helpful.[47] As a consequence of extensive experience, they have developed a sound approach to the problem pregnancy as a crisis within the adolescent period. They stress that abortion counseling should include a presentation of all options and that the counselor should be able to distinguish between normal ambivalence about pregnancy

ABORTION

Abortion, or voluntary interruption of pregnancy before fetal viability, has been permitted in the United States since the historic Supreme Court decision in 1973. The original decision (Roe vs. Wade and Doe vs. Bolton) dealt with the issue of privacy and ruled that abortion was a matter between the patient and her physician in the first 12 weeks of pregnancy. Abortion services for pregnant teenagers, however, have been threatened by a Supreme Court decision made in 1980 that restricts the use of public funds for abortion. In some states, conditions have been imposed under which abortions can be performed.[12]

The subject of abortion raises profound ethical questions, which will not be dealt with in this chapter. Since 1970, abortion in some states has been an option for teenage women. Cates has stated that more is known about the epidemiology of induced abortion than any other surgical procedure.[10] Although the data, gathered from the Abortion Surveillance Branch of the Center for Disease Control and other groups, do not pertain to emotional or political questions, they do provide an excellent background of information for women struggling with the choice of continuation or termination of an unplanned

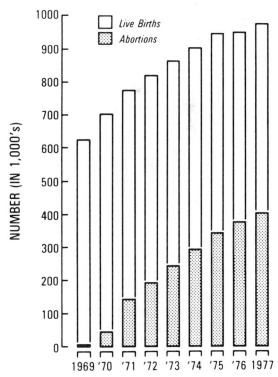

FIGURE 23–4. Live births and abortions to teenagers in the United States, 1969–1977. (Figure reproduced with permission from Cates: J. Adol. Health Care, 1:18, 1980, and Elsevier North Holland, Inc.)

and more serious underlying psychological problems. Some patients requesting abortion may be mature and sure of their decison (80 per cent); other young women are strikingly ignorant regarding details of conception and extremely frightened about both abortion and childbirth. Kreutner and Langhorst feel that the primary goal of such counseling is to help the teenager see the pregnancy and its resolution and future contraception as *her* problems.[47] If she can do this with positive help and support for a decision with which she is emotionally comfortable, she will play an active role in solving her problem. In this way the pregnancy experience becomes one of emotional growth.

The counselor of adolescents must have a basic understanding of their psychosexual maturation and be able to communicate with them. When possible and feasible, important family members and the boyfriend should be included in the counseling effort. It is our feeling, and that of Cates,[10] that information concerning teenage pregnancy should be presented in a neutral manner without overtones favoring either termination or continuation. The extra time spent in careful decision making and working through of the immediate emotional problem has critical long-term implications for the future coping ability, sexuality, and emotional stability of the young pregnant women. No teenager should be persuaded to have an abortion if she does not want one; neither should she be persuaded to continue her pregnancy if she would rather ter-

TABLE 23–1 REPORTED LEGAL ABORTIONS OBTAINED BY TEENAGERS; PER CENT DISTRIBUTION AND ABORTION RATIO, UNITED STATES, 1977*

Age	Per Cent Distribution SEPARATE	Per Cent Distribution CUMULATIVE	Abortion Ratio†
13	0.7	0.7 ⎫	1,070
14	3.1	3.8 ⎭	
15	7.2	11.0	718
16	13.8	24.8	612
17	19.1	43.9	529
18	28.5	72.4	581
19	27.6	100.0	457

*Data from Center for Disease Control: Abortion Surveillance, 1977. Issued September, 1979.

†Abortions per 1000 live births.

minate it. Bracken et al. have reported that the decision regarding abortion or delivery will depend on circumstances surrounding the specific pregnancy rather than characteristics of the mother.[7]

Teenagers comprise about 17 per cent of the population of childbearing women. Since 1973, they have accounted for 33 per cent of all abortions.[15] Figure 23–4 depicts the rate of live births and abortions to teenagers in the United States since 1969. The percentage of teenage abortions increases with each year of age, as noted in Table 23–1. This trend parallels that of sexual activity.

Teenagers have higher abortion ratios

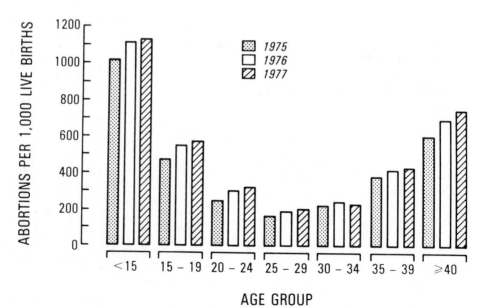

FIGURE 23–5. Legal abortions by age in the United States, 1975–1977. (Used with permission by Willard Cates, Jr., M.D., Center for Disease Control, Atlanta, Georgia, 1980.)

TABLE 23–2 ESTIMATED PER CENT DISTRIBUTION OF LEGAL ABORTIONS OBTAINED BY TEENAGERS BY RACE AND GESTATIONAL AGE*

	Age	
	≤ 19	≥ 20
RACE		
White	72.9	73.5
Black and other	27.1	26.5
WEEKS GESTATION		
≤ 8	33.7	44.8
9–12	47.7	44.3
13–15	7.3	4.4
≥ 16	11.3	5.5

*Data from Tietze (1977) and Cates and Tietze (1978).

(abortions/live births) than older women, except for those women 40 years of age or over, as shown on Figure 23–5.[11] These data also document that since 1975 women 15 years of age and younger have had more terminations of pregnancy by planned abortion than by live birth.[55]

Table 23–2 shows that the proportion of abortions obtained by teenage women of white, black, or other races is similar to those obtained by older women of the same races.[14, 76] Adolescents consistently request abortions at later ges-tational ages than older women (See Table 23–2). Almost half of all abortions performed beyond 12 weeks gestation involve teenagers.[14] This tendency is exaggerated as pregnancy advances; compared with older women, teenagers have 70 per cent more abortions in the 13 to 15 week–gestational age interval and twice as many at 16 weeks or later.[11] Younger teenagers are the most likely to have later abortions. In 1977 (in states with available data), 23 per cent of all abortions in women younger than 14 years of age were beyond 12 weeks versus 12 per cent in women 15 to 19 years of age, and 8 per cent in women age 20 and older.[11] These data have important medical implications, because gestational age is the most important determinant of abortion complications.[13] Thus, delay in requesting abortion has the largest single effect on the risk of complications and death for adolescents.

Abortion Techniques

Figure 23–6 shows the most common techniques now being performed for teenage abortions and the time during gestation when each method is appropriate.[23, 58]

Three methods are in common use during the first trimester. Menstrual regulation (menstrual extraction, "mini abortion") consists of suction

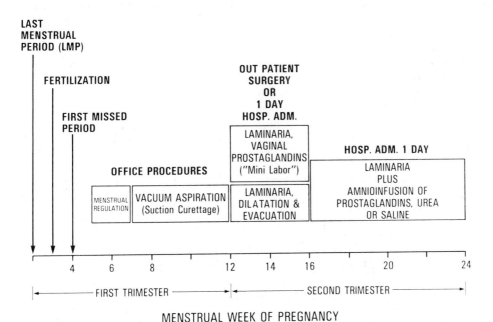

FIGURE 23–6. Abortion techniques commonly used in adolescent women. (Adapted from Kreutner and Langhorst, Abortion and abortion counseling. *In* Kreutner, A. K. K., and Hollingsworth, D. R. (eds.): Adolescent Obstetrics and Gynecology. Copyright © 1978 by Year Book Medical Publishers, Inc., Chicago. Used with permission.)

aspiration of uterine contents within two to three weeks of a missed menstrual period. Menstrual regulation is performed on an outpatient basis with minimal local or no anesthesia. Controversy exists whether a pregnancy test should be obtained before performing the procedure. Conventional pregnancy tests are not positive until day 40 of the cycle. Immunologic slide tests for human chorionic gonadotropin may yield false positive or false negative results early in pregnancy. A radioimmunoassay procedure to detect the presence of the beta subunit of HCG permits a positive diagnosis of pregnancy within a few days of implantation, but this test is costly and is not available in all clinics.

Menstrual extraction should be performed within seven weeks of the last menstrual period, because the complication rate slowly rises with increasing gestation. The procedure is sometimes performed immediately if the patient is exceptionally anxious or if a pregnancy test is declined by the patient for religious or other reasons. Informed consent should be obtained, explaining the possibility of continuing a pregnancy that might require a conventional curettage abortion later. The patient should be evaluated, including history, physical examination, and appropriate laboratory procedures, and should be counseled.

Edström, in an abortion review for the World Health Organization, reported that menstrual regulation during the fifth to seventh week of pregnancy is not always as free from risk as has sometimes been claimed.[23] In particular, this procedure has a higher failure rate in terms of continued pregnancy or retained products of conception than abortion by vacuum aspiration at 7 to 12 weeks gestation.

Vacuum aspiration (suction curettage) is the procedure of choice for pregnancy termination at 6 to 12 weeks because of its relative simplicity and safety.[2, 31, 78] Although the overall risk of serious morbidity with suction curettage is no higher for teenagers than for older women, teenagers may be more susceptible to cervical injury than older women. In nulliparous teenagers with small cervices, dilatation should be done gradually. *Laminaria* should be used only in reliable adolescents who will return for the procedure the following day, because complications such as infection can occur if the abortion is not performed. In adolescents beyond ten weeks gestation, general anesthesia may be preferable because of increased anxiety as well as increased pain associated with larger caliber dilatations, although general anesthesia increases the cost and morbidity of the procedure. Paracervical block is the most widely used anesthetic technique for suction curettage.

Dilatation and sharp curettage (D & C), when compared with vacuum aspiration, is associated with a longer operating time and higher complication rates. Sharp curettage is no longer the primary method of first trimester abortions but is sometimes used to complete a vacuum aspiration, especially if a perforation has occurred or if there are retained products of conception.

Early second trimester abortions (13 to 16 weeks) are often accomplished by dilatation of the cervix and evacuation (D & E). This method includes any combination of vacuum aspiration, conventional curettage, and use of ring forceps. Late midtrimester abortions (17 to 24 weeks) are performed by intraamniotic instillation of saline, urea, or prostaglandin (PGF_{2a}).

Medical Risks of Abortion

In considering abortion versus continuation of pregnancy, teenagers and their families need to know the risks of morbidity and mortality. The data from the Center for Disease Control show that teenagers are at no greater risk of complications or death than older women (Table 23–3). For suction curettage procedures performed at or before 12 weeks gestation, the risk of short-term major complicatons is the same in teenagers as in older women. For saline instillation procedures in the second trimester, teenagers had the lowest major complication rate of any age group (see Table 23–3). The same trend generally held with two other procedures performed after 12 weeks (D & E and prostaglandin F_{2a} instillation), but the numbers are small.

Short-term complications in teenagers are af-

TABLE 23–3 SHORT-TERM COMPLICATION RATES AND DEATH-TO-CASE RATES FOR LEGAL ABORTION BY AGE AND ABORTION METHOD*

| | Complication Rates† | | Death-to-Case Rates‡ |
Age	SUCTION CURETTAGE	SALINE INSTILLATION	
17	0.3	1.4	
18–19	0.4	1.4	1.8
20–24	0.3	1.9	4.0
25–29	0.4	2.2	3.1
≥30	0.4	3.3	5.1

*Data from Joint Program for the Study of Abortion/Center for Disease Control, Cates (1980).
†Major complications per 100 procedures.
‡Deaths per 100,000 abortions.

fected by the choice of abortion method after 12 weeks. D & E abortions had significantly lower short-term major complications (0.6/100 procedures) than those following saline (1.1/100) or prostaglandin F_{2a} instillation (2.0/100). Reports concerning complications of abortion are hampered by wide variations among clinics, level of skill of the staff, and techniques used.

The death rate following legally induced abortion is less for teenagers than for older women. Table 23–3 presents the short-term complication and death-to-case rates for legal abortions by age and method. Cates and Tietze have compared the risks of pregnancy termination for teenagers against those of pregnancy continuation.[14] They contrasted the standardized death-to-case rates for legally induced abortion with the standardized rates for death from other pregnancy-related causes. In the years 1972 to 1975, they found that teenagers who continued their pregnancy had a standardized death-to-case rate of 9.5/100,000 live births compared with a 1.8/100,000 death-to-case rate for legally induced abortions. Thus, for teenagers, the risk of dying of pregnancy continuation was fivefold higher than that of pregnancy termination. Cates and Tietze further point out that the fivefold risk for pregnancy continuation may be a *minimum* estimate.[14] Their birth-related mortalities include only deaths attributed to complications of pregnancy, childbirth, and the puerperium; they do not include deaths *associated* with delivery that are attributed to other causes such as cardiovascular disease (such associated deaths *are* included in abortion-related deaths). Furthermore, the abortion deaths to teenagers include four cases in which pregnancy was planned but was terminated because of medical indications. The abortion group includes some of the highest risk patients in whom abortion was performed *because* continuing the pregnancy was life threatening. Thus, these comparisons undercount pregnancy-related deaths to teenagers compared with abortion-related deaths in the same age group.

Followup studies of teenagers who have selected abortion to terminate their pregnancy have shown that severe psychiatric complications are extremely rare and that most adolescents are relieved to have terminated an unwanted pregnancy.[7, 36] In Lipper's study of middle- and lower-class pregnant teenage Canadian white women, 80 per cent were found to be well adjusted and stable without psychopathologic symptoms and satisfied with their decision to abort.[50] The investigators recognized that there is no psychologically painless way to deal with an unwanted pregnancy and that mild sadness or regret is an appropriate and normal reaction. Twenty per cent of women showed evidence of unstable behavior both before and after abortion. Generally, emotional status before abortion was a good predictor of postabortion mental health. In contrast to continuation of pregnancy, abortion did not significantly change a young woman's lifestyle or emotional adjustment. The crisis did, however, test her relationships.

Evans et al. studied 333 unwed teenagers ages 13 to 19, of whom 184 aborted, 113 continued pregnancy, and 36 had negative pregnancy tests.[24] Those who had abortions were more likely to remain in school. Twenty per cent of women in the abortion group expressed regret at the six-month followup. These individuals were younger, from a lower socioeconomic class, and were poorer students. It is of interest to note that most of those women who regretted the abortion were initially ambivalent or opposed to the procedure.

In Bracken's study, teenagers were shown to be at higher risk than older women for short-term sequelae following induced abortion.[7] They experienced more anxiety, depression, sadness, guilt, and regret. The most important factor affecting a woman's reaction to her abortion was the level of support from significant others including parents, partners, and peer group members. The choice of abortion procedure also affects psychological sequelae. Uterine curettage procedures are associated with more favorable postabortion reactions than labor-like instillation procedures.[67] Since teenagers are more likely to delay abortion until the later gestational ages when instillation procedures may be used, clinicians should be aware of the emotional complications of the particular method they select.

Reports of long-term complications of abortion in teenagers have provided conflicting information.[10, 88] In teenagers, the long-range abortion outcome is influenced by the procedure and skill of the physician performing the abortion. Procedures done late in gestation and repeated abortions increase the possibility of short- and long-term complications. Wide dilatations should be avoided in adolescents, as they are associated with a wider cervical os at six-week followup.[41] Sharp curettage (D & C) procedures have been reported to be associated with increased risks of midtrimester spontaneous abortion and low birth weight infants in subsequent pregnancies.[29, 88] These findings indicate a difference from the long-range outcome with suction curettage procedures, which have not been reported to have adverse sequelae in later pregnancies.

For those teenagers who choose continuation

of pregnancy rather than abortion, the potential future of the young mother must be carefully assessed in terms of her physical, emotional, educational, and vocational well-being over the ensuing 60 years of expected life. Present studies indicate that young parents acquire less education than their contemporaries and have less stable marriages and more children than they want.[80]

CONTINUATION OF PREGNANCY

The teenage woman who elects to continue her pregnancy assumes the risks of complications of pregnancy, labor, and delivery as well as the long-term risks for herself and her infant. Precise estimates of risk factors in women who continue their pregnancy are not always possible. They depend on maternal age (younger than 15 years versus 16 to 18 years), antecedent health, socioeconomic status, and access to good prenatal care. Figure 23–7 depicts the outcome of pregnancy in 406 consecutive teenagers at the University of Kentucky who were followed from 1971 to 1974. One third of all pregnancies were abnormal, and this breakdown into usual categories of outcome of pregnancy did not include infections, anemia, or maternal complications related to labor, delivery, or the immediate postpartum period.

In the McAnarney study at the University of Rochester, a high incidence of hypertension, toxemia, and abrupt or prolonged labors was not observed in a comprehensive maternity project, a community health center, and a hospital obstetrics clinic.[54] All three settings offered similar obstetric services. There were no stillborn infants, but 8 to 14 per cent of the infants were of low birth weight (less than 2500 gm). A fetal distress rate (meconium-stained amniotic fluid and/or fetal cardiac irregularity during delivery) of 16 to 38 per cent was observed, but there were no significant differences among the three study groups. Most recent national studies have concluded that adolescents who receive adequate prepartum care have good obstetric outcomes despite their age.[21]

Perkins et al. have reported on the first two years of an intensive and individual approach to dealing with pregnant women under age 17.[62] A total of 135 women, ages 13 to 16, were followed in a young mothers clinic at Colorado General Hospital and were compared with 100 women, ages 13 to 17, followed routinely in the hospital and 100 older women, ages 19 to 24. Despite differences in racial composition and social status (more blacks in the young mothers clinic group and more Chicanos in the young non–young mothers clinic group), few, if any, medical differences were noted among the three groups.

Klein studied a group of mostly black and clearly indigent patients of the same ages in Atlanta, Georgia.[43] She reported an increase in premature births, fetal deaths, and neonatal and perinatal deaths. Coates also found that poor black women under age 15 had an increased prevalence of toxemia, uterine dysfunction, one-day fever, and congenital heart disease in their infants when compared with older controls.[16] Klerman and Jekel followed pregnancies that occurred subsequent to deliveries in mothers

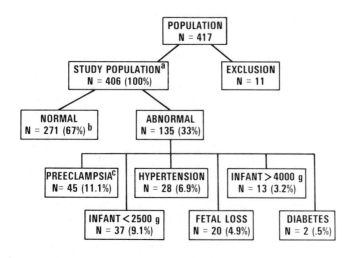

FIGURE 23–7. Outcome of pregnancy in the University of Kentucky Young Mothers' Program for primiparous adolescents, ages 12 to 18, 1971–1974. (From Kreutner, A. K. K., and Hollingsworth, D. R. (eds.): Adolescent Obstetrics and Gynecology. Copyright © 1978 by Year Book Medical Publishers, Inc., Chicago. Used with permission.)

a The study population contained 219 black (54%) and 187 white (46%) patients
b All percentages based on study population
c Abnormal subgroups are not always mutually exclusive

who participated in their young mothers program.[44] In this longer term followup, they found very high prematurity and perinatal loss rates. The consensus of medical studies on young pregnant teenagers during the 1970s indicates that maternal and infant risks are more clearly related to prepregnancy health and socioeconomic factors than to the mother's age.

Furstenberg addressed the social consequences of teenage parenthood in his six-year study of 400 young adolescent mothers and their partners, progeny, and parents.[26] He has also compared the experiences of young mothers with those of members of a peer group who terminated their pregnancy. The study participants were urban blacks who registered for prenatal care at Sinai Hospital in Baltimore between 1966 and 1968. The comparison group consisted of former classmates of the adolescent mothers. Both groups were from lower-class homes. The adolescent mothers consistently experienced great difficulty in realizing life plans when compared with their classmates. Complications of premature, unscheduled childbearing included marital instability (three out of five marriages broke up within six years), school disruption, economic problems, and difficulty in family size regulation and childrearing.

In a later report, Furstenberg and Crawford were able to show that some teenage parents do overcome the handicaps imposed by adolescent childbearing.[27] In those who continued to live with their parents or who benefited from parental assistance (financial, psychological, and child care), the outlook was much better than that for women who had to depend on their own resources. Assistance rendered by family members significantly altered the life chances of the young mother, enhancing her prospects of educational achievement and economic advancement. Further studies are urgently needed on the impact of early childbearing on the family units of all social and racial groups in America. These studies are important, as they will provide data to serve as guidelines for appropriate use of federal, state, and local funds for provision of child care facilities and educational and vocational programs for both young mothers and fathers.

ACUTE AND CHRONIC MEDICAL PROBLEMS OF TEENAGE PREGNANCY

The approach to medical care for pregnant adolescents differs in some respects from that for older women. Many young patients have not previously had a complete history and physical examination. They may not understand the signs and symptoms of normal pregnancy and are often distraught because of emotional and financial problems. They may or may not have the sympathy and support of the father of the infant and their own family.

Chronic medical problems that antedate pregnancy, such as hypertension, renal disease, diabetes, or seizure disorders, must be carefully re-evaluated during gestation and care coordinated with a perinatologist and the mother's personal physician. The approach to specific medical problems complicating pregnancy is discussed in detail elsewhere in the book and does not differ in this age group.

In teenagers, there is a somewhat different distribution of acute medical problems. When pregnancy occurs in the transitional period between childhood and adulthood, an unusual pattern of infections, which includes otitis media, chicken pox, mumps, pertussis, and viral illnesses, is seen. Cystitis and urinary tract infections are more common, and there is an increased incidence of herpes vaginitis (HVH-2), gonorrhea, and other sexually transmitted diseases.

In evaluating medical risks in adolescent women, it is often difficult to separate the influence of poor socioeconomic factors from that of age. In our prospective study at the University of Kentucky involving 406 poor black (54 per cent) and white (46 per cent) women, ages 12 to 18, followed during their first pregnancy,[32] we found hypertension (6.9 per cent) and pre-eclampsia (11.1 per cent) to be the most common medical problems of pregnant teenagers (see Fig. 23–7). The management of hypertensive disorders of pregnancy is described in Chapter 1.

Adolescents less than 15 years of age run the greatest risk of obtaining inadequate or insufficient health services and of incurring health problems related to pregnancy, educational impairment, and dire economic need.[38] In 1974, there were 30,000 pregnancies among very young teenagers (younger than 15). This is an alarming number, considering that sexual activity in this age group is thought to be sporadic and that anovulatory cycles occur frequently. Many of the 30,000 pregnancies in adolescents younger than 15 years of age end in abortion (13,500 by legal abortion and an estimated 4,000 by spontaneous abortion), with the remaining 12,000 terminating in live birth (80 per cent out of wedlock). The 1974 birth rate of 26.9 births per thousand in women age 15 and under has dropped only slightly to 24.9 per thousand in

1977, despite widespread provision of both contraceptive and abortion services. This is felt to represent increasing sexual acivity among younger adolescents.

Dott and Fort analyzed 414 births to teenagers under 15 years of age in Louisiana and found higher prematurity and infant mortality rates when compared with births to older teenagers.[19] The infants at greatest risk were those whose mothers were poor, white, married, and with minimal prenatal care. The primary medical problems of pregnant indigent adolescents 15 years of age and under include greatly increased risks for anemia, abnormal bleeding, toxemia, difficult labor, and cephalopelvic disproportion.[3, 40, 57, 74]

Fielding has reported that the number of low birth weight infants (less than 2500 gm) born to women under age 15 is double (13.5 per cent) the rate for women 20 to 24 years of age (6.9 per cent).[24a] This has not been true in some settings, and Duenhoelter has reported no difference in cesarean section rate, infant weight, or perinatal mortality in women 15 years of age or younger.[21] He did note an increase in the incidence of toxemia and small pelvic inlet. In all adolescents at the present time, but particularly in those in the youngest age group, it is not possible to separate biologic risks related to a low gynecologic age (age at conception minus age at menarche) from medical problems secondary to poverty, lack of prenatal care, and inadequate nutrition.

NEW PATTERNS OF ADOLESCENT PRENATAL CARE

In order to provide good adolescent prenatal care, specific, practical guidelines need to be established to identify high risk patients and to ensure prenatal medical supervision for chronic medical problems such as hypertension, renal disease, obesity, and carbohydrate intolerance detected during pregnancy.[32a] The following recommendations have been proposed.

1. Staffing of prenatal clinics by professional personnel who have had experience and training in obstetric problems of the very young. Ideal care involves the team effort of midwives, nurses, physicians, social workers, health educators, psychologists, and nutritionists.
2. Definition and early recognition of high risk pregnancies. These include:
   a. Adolescents 15 years of age or younger.
   b. Pregnancies complicated by chronic medical problems antedating pregnancy as well as pregnancy associated with hypertension, heart disease, abnormal bleeding, intrauterine growth retardation, twins, drug abuse (including nicotine and alcohol), chronic urinary tract or other infections, and diabetes and other metabolic or endocrine disorders.
   c. Teenagers who are below normal weight before pregnancy. They are at risk for increased complications, small birth weight infants, and high rates of fetal and neonatal loss.
3. Access to a medical center with perinatal services and a special care nursery and establishment of a close working relationship with personnel.
4. Availability of Lamaze-prepared childbirth classes as part of routine prenatal care.
5. Antenatal and postdelivery lactation instruction.
6. Coordination of community resources to provide continuing education during pregnancy in regular or special schools with postpartum assistance for infant day care, maternal and paternal education, and vocational training.

These recommendations have evolved from our experience in directing teenage pregnancy clinics over the past ten years. Obstetric solutions for prenatal care rely on a team approach that coordinates community based and medical center resources. Regionalization of adolescent prenatal care is a practical approach, as it enables patients to attend clinics near their home or school. However, there must be careful assessment of the quality of care and easy access to sophisticated perinatology services and high risk intensive care nurseries. Lamaze-prepared childbirth classes, which have proven so successful in older women, have been heavily relied upon at the University of California, San Diego.[33] This method has been helpful even in teenagers less than 15 years of age. The classes are attended by the pregnant girl and the ''most significant other'' as coparticipant. This is the father of the infant, when possible, but it may also be the patient's mother, grandmother, or friend. Four San Diego high schools have special programs for pregnant girls with child care preparation classes also available for the fathers. In both San Diego and Charleston, South Carolina, it has been possible to gain acceptance of breastfeeding by many teenagers, particularly those attending schools with day care or nursery facilities.

All teenage pregnancy programs need skillful, experienced nurses, social service workers, and health educators. They focus on support systems, childbirth preparation, attendance at regular or special schools until delivery, resumption of school or vocational training postpartum, and contraceptive counseling.

ADOPTION AND TEENAGE MOTHERS

Very little information is available at the present time about the social and emotional consequences of placing the infant of a teenage mother for adoption. This is a rarely selected option among today's adolescents with most programs reporting that 90 to 100 per cent of infants born are kept by the mother. Several reasons account for low adoption rates. Society is more tolerant of pregnancy occurring outside of marriage. There is often great pressure placed upon adolescents by both the father of the infant and the prospective grandparents to keep the baby. Young mothers are increasingly unwilling to face separation from their infant after having carried it for nine months. Finally, peer pressure is strong for young mothers to keep their babies. When adoption is chosen as an option, long-term emotional support and counseling are critical, as these young women experience the same grief and sense of loss as a woman losing a child by death.

No studies have been done on the long-term outcome and emotional health of adopted children. Many are known to experience difficult identity crises and a strong drive to find or learn about their biologic parents. No prospective long-term studies on the medical, emotional, and economic status or marital stability of adoptive parents have been published. It is tempting for lawmakers and health planners to envision that the solution to teenage pregnancy is to give the babies to infertile couples. In reality, there is no assurance, based on carefully conducted prospective studies, that this solution is *necessarily* a happy or beneficial one for young mothers, infants, or adoptive parents.

The total number of adoptions peaked in America in 1970 at 175,000. By 1977, the number was down to 104,000, and only about 25,000 of those cases involved infants adopted by unrelated couples.[64] The demand for adoptable babies is strong, since 5 to 10 per cent of all married couples in this country are involuntarily infertile. Adoption has become an intensely controversial subject. There is, at present, no agreement on

how to resolve the conflicts based on the rights of adoptees, adoptive parents, biologic parents, agencies, and taxpayers.[64]

CONTRACEPTION: RISKS AND EFFECTIVENESS FOR ADOLESCENTS

There is no ideal contraceptive for women or men at any age. Complete reproductive freedom with a temporary method of preventing conception effectively during adolescence would require a safe, cheap, easily reversible contraceptive without side effects that is not used concomitantly with sexual intercourse. Since present means of contraception do not achieve this goal and no better methods of contraception are likely to appear in the near future, a careful assessment of risk/benefit ratios for teenagers (as well as men and women of all ages) must be examined. In addition, the risks and various forms of contraception have to be weighed against the risks associated with pregnancy.

There have been few controlled investigations of teenage use of contraceptives. Akpom et al. and Settlage et al. have reported data from family planning clinics that show that teenage women are likely to be sexually active one to two years before seeking professional birth control instruction.[1, 71] Zabin et al. examined the risk of adolescent pregnancy in the first months of intercourse and found that *half* of all premarital teenage pregnancies occur in the first six months of sexual activity and more than one fifth in the first month.[90] They also showed that the first month of exposure to intercourse selects out the most fecund women (22 per cent), who become pregnant most rapidly, leaving behind a less fecund, less accident-prone group who have a lower rate of conception. Women who conceive soon after initiation of intercourse are at risk of having additional pregnancies. In these studies, second pregnancies occurred in 64 per cent of whites and 44 per cent of blacks who conceived in the first six months after first coitus. These women are at the highest pregnancy risk and account for a disproportionate share of adolescent pregnancies.

It is difficult to provide birth control information and services to teenagers early in their sexual careers, as sexual encounters tend to be impulsive and unplanned as well as sporadic. Many teenage women feel that certain periods of the month are "safe" and that pregnancy could not happen to them. Physicians and health organizations are ambivalent about or reluctant to provide contraceptive instruction and materials to young people who are not yet sexually active.

Oral Contraceptives

The combined oral contraceptive (estrogen and progestin) is the most effective reversible method of birth control (method effectiveness 99.3 per cent; use effectiveness 75 to 96 per cent). Effectiveness decreases when the medication is taken incorrectly or when discontinuation rates are high. The minipill, which contains only a small dose of progestin, is less effective in preventing pregnancy, and its use is more often accompanied by menorrhagia, irregular cycles, and amenorrhea. Adolescents find these symptoms confusing and difficult to deal with. Table 23–4 lists the oral contraceptives currently available in the United States.

It is estimated that ten million American women use oral contraceptives and that 50 million have used them in the past.[65] Evaluation of the safety of oral contraceptives has been complicated by alterations in hormone composition over the years, frequent changes in type and duration of medication prescribed for each patient, and, more recently, patient reluctance to use oral contraceptives and a tendency to curtail the duration of use. Extensive reviews have been published that summarize current data concerning risks of hormonal contraception.[1a, 4-6, 17, 18, 20, 22, 25, 28, 30, 39, 42, 45, 52, 56, 59, 63, 66, 69, 72, 73, 75, 77, 83-85]

Table 23–5 summarizes the side effects that have been associated with oral contraceptives.

In reaching a decision concerning the risks of oral contraceptives versus the risks of conception in teenagers, careful explanations as well as special education in regard to birth control techniques must be provided to the patient. If the patient has an ongoing sexual relationship, is

TABLE 23–4 ORAL CONTRACEPTIVES AVAILABLE IN THE UNITED STATES*

Trade Name	Manufacturer	Estrogen	Dose (mg)	Progestin	Dose (mg)
COMBINED					
Brevicon (21 day)	Syntex	Ethinyl estradiol	0.035	Norethindrone	0.5
Brevicon (28 day)	Syntex	Ethinyl estradiol	0.035	Norethindrone	0.5
Demulen (21 day)	Searle	Ethinyl estradiol	0.05	Ethynodiol diacetate	1.0
Demulen (28 day)	Searle	Ethinyl estradiol	0.05	Ethynodiol diacetate	1.0
Enovid E (20 day)	Searle	Mestranol	0.10	Norethynodrel	2.5
Enovid 5 (20 day)	Searle	Mestranol	0.075	Norethynodrel	5.0
Loestrin 1.5/30 (21 day)	Parke-Davis	Ethinyl estradiol	0.030	Norethindrone acetate	1.5
Loestrin 1/20 (21 day)	Parke-Davis	Ethinyl estradiol	0.020	Norethindrone acetate	1.0
Modicon (21 day)	Ortho	Ethinyl estradiol	0.035	Norethindrone	0.5
Modicon (28 day)	Ortho	Ethinyl estradiol	0.035	Norethindrone	0.5
Norinyl-1/50 (21 day)	Syntex	Mestranol	0.05	Norethindrone	1.0
Norinyl-1/50 (28 day)	Syntex	Mestranol	0.05	Norethindrone	1.0
Norinyl-1/80 (21 day)	Syntex	Mestranol	0.08	Norethindrone	1.0
Norinyl-1/80 (28 day)	Syntex	Mestranol	0.08	Norethindrone	1.0
Norinyl-2	Syntex	Mestranol	0.10	Norethindrone	2.0
Norlestrin-1 (21 day)	Parke-Davis	Ethinyl estradiol	0.05	Norethindrone acetate	1.0
Norlestrin-1 (28 day)	Parke-Davis	Ethinyl estradiol	0.05	Norethindrone acetate	1.0
Norlestrin-1(Fe) (28 day)	Parke-Davis	Ethinyl estradiol	0.05	Norethindrone acetate	1.0
Norlestrin 2.5 (21 day)	Parke-Davis	Ethinyl estradiol	0.05	Norethindrone acetate	2.5
Norlestrin (Fe) 2.5 (28 day)	Parke-Davis	Ethinyl estradiol	0.05	Norethindrone acetate	2.5
Ortho-Novum 1/50 (20 day)	Ortho	Mestranol	0.05	Norethindrone	1.0
Ortho-Novum 1/50 (21 day)	Ortho	Mestranol	0.05	Norethindrone	1.0
Ortho-Novum 1/80 (21 day)	Ortho	Mestranol	0.08	Norethindrone	1.0
Ortho-Novum-2 (20 day)	Ortho	Mestranol	0.10	Norethindrone	2.0
Ortho-Novum 10 (20 day)	Ortho	Mestranol	0.06	Norethindrone	10.0
Ovral (21 day)	Wyeth	Ethinyl estradiol	0.05	Norgestrel	0.5
Ovulen (20 day)	Searle	Mestranol	0.10	Ethynodiol diacetate	1.0
Ovulen (21 day)	Searle	Mestranol	0.10	Ethynodiol diacetate	1.0
Zorane 1/50 (21 day)	Lederle	Ethinyl estradiol	0.050	Norethindrone acetate	1.0
Zorane 1.5/30 (21 day)	Lederle	Ethinyl estradiol	0.030	Norethindrone acetate	1.5
Zorane 1/20 (21 day)	Lederle	Ethinyl estradiol	0.020	Norethindrone acetate	1.0
MINIPILL					
Micronor (35 day)	Ortho			Norethindrone	0.35
Nor-Q.D. (42 day)	Syntex			Norethindrone	0.35
Ovrette (28 day)	Wyeth			D-1-Norgestrel	0.075

*Reproduced with permission from Connell: Update on oral contraceptives. Curr. Probl. Obstet. Gynecol. Copyright © 1979 by Year Book Medical Publishers, Inc., Chicago.

TABLE 23–5 SIDE EFFECTS AND MEDICAL COMPLICATIONS OF ORAL CONTRACEPTIVES*

Minor Problems

SIDE EFFECTS	SYMPTOMS	TREATMENT
Menstrual change	Breakthrough bleeding or heavier periods	Change to pill with higher estrogen level
Vaginal moniliasis	Itching, burning, and vaginal discharge	Miconazole nitrate (Monistat 7); Clotrimazole (Gyne-Lotrimin)
Chloasma	Darkening of facial skin	Use sunscreen or discontinue OC
Migraine headaches	May worsen or improve with OC	Discontinue OC if headaches worsen
Depression	May occur or worsen in women with previous history	Take OC at night or discontinue
Nausea	More common in first few months of medication	Take OC at night or discontinue
Fluid retention	Mild puffiness	Limit salt intake (carefully observe patients who have severe cardiac disease or who are on anticonvulsant drugs)

Major Problems

Thromboembolic disease	Chest pain, thrombophlebitis	Discontinue OC; treat complication
Subarachnoid hemorrhage	Stroke	Discontinue OC; treat complication
Hypertension	Usually none	Discontinue OC
Diabetes	Worsening glucose tolerance	Increase insulin dosage or discontinue OC
Hypertriglyceridemia	None reported in adolescents	Discontinue OC
Hepatocellular adenoma	Right upper quadrant pain and hepatomegaly	Discontinue OC; remove tumor surgically
Gall bladder disease	Right upper quadrant pain	Discontinue OC; treat gall bladder disease
Pituitary microadenoma (?)	Amenorrhea, galactorrhea	Medical or surgical therapy; discontinue OC
Fetal side effects from in utero exposure (?)	VACTEL anomalies (vertebral, anal, cardiac, tracheal, esophageal, and limb syndrome (?)	HORMONAL TESTS OF PREGNANCY ARE CONTRAINDICATED; instruct adolescent in correct pill usage

*Specific risks to adolescents are difficult to ascertain in epidemiologic studies, as data are often reported for women ages 15–44. See extensive recent bibliography cited in chapter for details of published data concerning relationship of oral contraceptives to the above major complications.

Note: OC = oral contraceptives.

having intercourse daily or at least once a week, is in good health with a normal history and physical examination, and does not smoke, she can be given a combined low dose oral contraceptive with minimal risk. Most clinics are currently using a combination pill that contains 50 μg of estrogen. Table 23–6 lists the specific FDA contraindications to the use of oral contraceptives. Follow-up appointments should be arranged three months after starting medication. For adolescents, open telephone communication should be available with the clinic staff or a physician for early problems, clarification of instructions, or questions.

TABLE 23–6 FOOD AND DRUG ADMINISTRATION SPECIFIC AND RELATIVE CONTRAINDICATIONS TO USE OF ORAL CONTRACEPTIVES

Specific	Relative
Thrombophlebitis, thromboembolic disorders, cerebrovascular disease, pulmonary artery disease, or past history of these disorders	Hypertension
	Diabetes
	Cigarette smoking
Known or suspected breast cancer	Migraine
Impaired liver function	Hypercholesterolemia or hypertriglyceridemia
Known or suspected estrogen-dependent neoplasm	Cardiac or renal disease
Undiagnosed abnormal vaginal bleeding	Epilepsy
Known or suspected pregnancy	Mental depression
	Fibroid tumors of uterus
	Gall bladder disease
	Family history of breast cancer

TABLE 23–7 SIDE EFFECTS AND COMPLICATIONS OF IUD USE IN ADOLESCENTS

Side Effect	Symptom	Treatment
Expulsion	Loss of IUD	Try different IUD; with two expulsions change method of contraception
Loss of IUD string	Anxiety	Gynecologic check to recover string or confirm expulsion
Bleeding	Increased menstrual flow	$FeSO_4$; IUD with progestin
Severe dysmenorrhea	Increased uterine cramping with period	Remove IUD
Perforation of uterus or cervix	Usually none	Remove IUD by hysteroscopy or surgery
Infection	Fever, pain, vaginal discharge	Remove IUD; confirm with bacteriologic diagnosis and administer appropriate antibiotics
Pregnancy (uterine or tubal)	Missed period, breast tenderness, nausea, vomiting	Remove IUD if possible

Intrauterine Devices (IUD)

Among reversible methods of contraception, IUD use is exceeded only by oral contraceptives and condoms.[86] This method has one of the highest continuation rates of any of the medically prescribed methods of reversible contraception (75 per cent versus 65 per cent for oral contraceptives at one year).[65] The pregnancy rate among average IUD users (use effectiveness) is 4 per 100 woman years of use and includes pregnancies with unnoticed expulsions. The net pregnancy rate varies from one to six per 100 users at the end of the first year. Expulsion rates range from 4 to 18 per 100 users, and removals for medical reasons range from 12 to 16 per 100 users within one year.[82]

The mechanism of action of plastic IUDs is related to the sterile inflammation produced by a foreign body in the uterus. IUDs currently in use contain copper or progesterone, which enhances the local contraceptive action without causing systemic side effects. Tyrer has reviewed details of IUD usage, indications, contraindications, and complications and their management.[81] Problems associated with the IUD and management recommendations are summarized in Table 23–7.

The most dangerous IUD risk is pelvic infection. This complication has the highest frequency in women under the age of 25, those who have had previous pelvic infections, those who are nulligravid, and those who have multiple partners.[87]

Ory, in a review of six controlled studies, reported a three- to fivefold increase in pelvic inflammatory disease in IUD users.[60] Tyrer described an IUD-related syndrome of chronic low-grade pelvic infection occurring months after insertion of the device.[81] These infections may result in the development of tubo-ovarian abscesses, which sometimes require definitive surgery that may result in sterility. Unusual and rare pelvic infections have been reported in IUD users. Pelvic actinomycosis has been recognized in association with the IUD, and Luff reported that 25 per cent of symptomatic IUD users had *Actinomyces* organisms in fast Papanicolaou smears.[51] In one small series,[20] 80 per cent of asymptomatic women with IUDs and *Actinomyces* identified on Pap smears subsequently developed symptoms including vaginitis, abnormal bleeding, and acute pelvic inflammatory disease. The risk of future infertility in women who use the IUD is unknown.[81] The possibility of ectopic pregnancy must also be considered in adolescent women with an IUD who present with pelvic pain, as there is an increased risk of this complication in IUD users.

Kulig et al. reported their experience with the Copper-7 IUD in adolescents in a retrospective study of 120 consecutive patients from 1974 to 1978.[48] This study was unique because 81 per cent of the patients were nulliparous and follow-up information was obtained in 97 per cent of patients. The pregnancy rate was low (2.0/100 woman years), and continuation rate was 70 per cent at one year, 49 per cent at two years, and 39 per cent at three years. The Cu-7 IUD was felt to be a comparatively safe, well-tolerated contraceptive in adolescent women. Eight per cent of the study group developed pelvic inflammatory disease.

In considering IUD insertion in teenagers, several advantages are apparent. Contraception is independent of intercourse, insertion is easy and requires little patient motivation, and replacement is performed only every three years. In this age group, the use effectiveness of the IUD may exceed that of oral contraceptives.[34] When complications occur, the device is easily removed. In adolescents this method offers a minimal risk of mortality when compared with pregnancy and childbirth.[68]

Barrier Contraceptives

Teenage women and their partners have become more reluctant to use oral contraceptives, particularly for long periods of time. Physicians and family planning agencies are increasingly concerned about pelvic infections and implications for future fertility in very young sexually active women with IUDs and multiple partners. Moreover, there are many women with frank contraindications to these forms of birth control or with complications arising from their use. Thus, in the past several years, many clinics have begun to reassess the effectiveness of the diaphragm. This method is without complications and is especially well suited to women who have intercourse rarely or sporadically. The disadvantage of the method is the nuisance and negative psychological effect of proper placement of the diaphragm before intercourse. A higher level of motivation is necessary even if placement is routinely accomplished many hours before coitus. Some physicians trained in the oral contraceptive era have had little experience in fitting diaphragms. Despite these problems, Lane reported an encouraging study in teenagers who were taught to use the diaphragm.[49] He found an unintended pregnancy rate of only 1.9 per 100 diaphragm users, ages 13 to 17, with only 3.5 per cent of women lost to followup. Overall, the theoretical effectiveness of the diaphragm is 2 per 100 woman years in highly motivated individuals but 12 to 18 per 100 woman years in large-scale investigations. Similarly, condom barriers for male partners have a theoretical effectiveness of 3 per 100 woman years and a use effectiveness of 12 to 20 per 100 woman years.

In all studies of contraceptive methods for adolescents, patient and partner acceptability and compliance have been found to be essential for pregnancy prevention. The best results are obtained when extensive counseling is readily available for both young men and women by a patient educator (in public schools, Planned Parenthood Offices, and adolescent medicine clinics). Couples with steady sexual relationships need and appreciate factual, nonjudgmental information to prevent early or unwanted pregnancies. In many secondary schools, films, group sessions, and education in human sexuality are beginning to create peer pressure for responsible reproduction.

New Strategies for Prevention of Pregnancy in Adolescents

Although reproductive decisions in adolescents are personal and emotional, just as they are in every other decade during the childbearing years, specific practical suggestions are evolving to prevent early childbirth. These include

1. Encouragement of peer pressure to delay pregnancy until later, which has already occurred in 18 and 19 year olds.

2. Provision of sensitive, well-informed contraceptive counseling and readily available contraceptives. The risks and benefits of each method must be carefully explained and weighed against the risk of pregnancy. These contraceptive services should be encouraged before teenagers become sexually active because of the risk of adolescent pregnancy in the first months of intercourse.

3. Easy access to first trimester abortion. Many adolescents select this solution as the most reasonable for their particular set of circumstances. Bracken et al. showed that the choice between abortion and delivery depends upon circumstances surrounding specific pregnancies rather than characteristics of the mother.[8]

4. Encouragement of the *rarely* selected option of adoption for teenage pregnant women of all races and social classes. In these instances (1 to 5 per cent), in-depth counseling and long-term emotional support are critical.

Brann et al. reviewed strategies for prevention of pregnancy in adolescents.[9] Since federal funding and interest in programs for preventing unintended pregnancy in adolescents are growing, they felt it was important to identify successful program models and evaluate cost effectiveness. Four of the centers investigated showed an impressive decline in pregnancy or childbearing rates of their target population. These studies are relevant to future planning because of the significant increase in the percentage of unmarried teenage (15 to 19 years old) women who are sexually active. The successful programs for pregnancy prevention all involved a great deal of outreach. An intensive one-to-one, find-them-where-they-are approach in St. Paul, Minnesota, was able to demonstrate a 56 per cent reduction in student fertility rate over the first three years of operation. The cost of the program for two high schools in 1976 to 1977 was $42,000. A San Bernardino, California, county health department program involved 27 schools and employed four full-time social workers in one-to-one counseling sessions for adolescents who came to the health department for pregnancy tests. The cost of the program in 1976 was $62,000. In Maryland, the State Department of Health and Mental Hygiene funded a program in education and human sexuality in two rural areas. Six counties were involved, and there appears to have been a 33 per cent drop in pregnancy rate for 15 to 19 year olds (84 births per 1000 in 1972 versus 56 per 1000 in 1975). For the 15 to 17 year old group, there was a 36 per cent drop. The program cost $57,000 per year. Some communities have combined outreach with easy access to abortion. The city of Hackensack, New Jersey, and Bergen County noted a rapid decline in fertility among teenagers in 1975 to 1976 compared with 1970 to 1971 (48 and 53 per cent, respectively). Their programs included easy access to contraceptive services, a large outreach service, and readily available abortions. These results are encouraging, and the programs have been relatively inexpensive.

CONCLUSION

Early childbearing creates many sociologic, emotional, medical, and economic problems. Our current view of teenage pregnancy has been modified by careful studies in varied social settings and different geographic areas. Teenage pregnancy is common in all social, economic, and racial groups in all parts of the nation. In older teenagers the medical complications of early pregnancy are related to prepregnancy health status, poverty, and lack of access to high quality prenatal care. For the younger teenager (15 years of age and less), there appear to be higher risks for pregnancy-induced hypertension (toxemia), preterm births with low birth weight infants, and repeat pregnancies in a short period of time.

The critical areas for clinical investigation and implementation of services to adolescent women in the 1980s are (1) new approaches for adolescent women and men for prevention of unplanned and/or unwanted pregnancies, (2) prospective studies to assess the long-term outcomes of pregnant adolescents who choose abortion over pregnancy completion with the intention of either keeping the baby or placing it for adoption, and (3) longitudinal studies of infants born to teenage mothers.

For young women with planned pregnancies and those with unplanned pregnancies who wish to continue them, solutions must be found to provide optimum pre- and postnatal care, reasonable support systems, continuing maternal and paternal education, and vocational training and child care. Since federal funds are being allocated to the care of adolescent pregnant women, sensible guidelines are essential to ensure competent and sympathetic regionalized medical care to teenagers with wanted pregnancies, whether planned or unplanned. Prevention of unwanted pregnancies remains a high priority, requiring more experience with the practical suggestions described previously. Although the emotional, medical, social, and economic problems of adolescent pregnancy seemed hopelessly discouraging a brief decade ago, reasonable approaches are beginning to be made.

References

1. Akpom, C. A., Akpom, K. L., and Davis, M.: Prior sexual behavior in teenagers attending rap sessions for the first time. Fam. Plann. Perspect., 8:203, 1976.
1a. American College of Obstetricians and Gynecologists: Oral Contraception. Technical Bulletin No. 41, 1976.
2. Andolsek, L.: The Ljubljana abortion study: 1971–73. Bethesda (USA), National Institute of Health. Center for Population Research, 1974.
3. Battaglia, F. C., Frazier, T. M., and Hellegers, A. E.: Obstetric and pediatric complications of juvenile pregnancy. Pediatrics, 32:902, 1963.
4. Belsey, M. A., Russell, Y., and Kinnear, K.: Cardiovascular disease and oral hormonal contraceptives: A reappraisal of vital statistics data. Fam. Plann. Perspect., 112:84, 1979.
5. Beral, V.: Cardiovascular disease mortality trends and oral contraceptives use in young women. Lancet, 2:1047, 1976.
6. Boston Collaborative Drug Surveillance Program: Oral contraceptives and venous thromboembolic disease, surgically confirmed gallbladder disease and breast tumors. Lancet, 1:1399, 1973.
7. Bracken, M. B., Hachamovitch, M., and Grossman, G.: The decision to abort and psychological sequelae. J. Nerv. Ment. Dis., 158:154, 1974.
8. Bracken, M. B., Klerman, L. V., and Bracken, M.: Abortion, adoption or motherhood: An empirical study of decision-making during pregnancy. Am. J. Obstet. Gynecol., 130:251, 1978.

9. Brann, E. A., Edwards, L., Callicott, T., Story, E. S., Berg, P. A., Mahoney, J. E., Stine, J. L., and Hixson, A.: Strategies for the prevention of pregnancy in adolescents. Adv. Planned Parenthood, 14:68, 1979.
10. Cates, W. Jr.: Late effects of induced abortion: Hypothesis or knowledge? J. Reprod. Med., 22:207, 1979.
11. Cates, W. Jr.: Adolescent abortions in the United States. J. Adol. Health Care, 1:18, 1980.
12. Cates, W. Jr., Gold, J., and Selik, R. M.: Sounding board. Regulation of abortion services — For better or worse? N. Engl. J. Med., 301:720, 1979.
13. Cates, W. Jr., Schulz, K. F., Grimes, D. A., and Tyler, C. W. Jr.: The effect of delay and choice of method on the risk of abortion morbidity. Fam. Plann. Perspect., 9:266, 1977.
14. Cates, W. Jr., and Tietze, C.: Standardized mortality rates associated with legal abortion. United States, 1972–1975. Fam. Plann. Perspect., 10:109, 1978.
15. Center for Disease Control: Abortion Surveillance, 1977. United States Department of Health, Education and Welfare. Public Health Service, September, 1979.
16. Coates, J. B. III: Obstetrics in the very young adolescent. Am. J. Obstet. Gynecol., 108:68, 1970.
17. Collaborative Group for the Study of Stroke in Young Women: Oral contraceptives and stroke in young women. J.A.M.A., 231:718, 1975.

18. Connell, E. B.: Update on oral contraceptives. Curr. Probl. Obstet. Gynecol. 3, 1979.

19. Dott, A. B., and Fort, A. T.: Medical and social factors affecting early teenage pregnancy. Am. J. Obstet. Gynecol., *125*:532, 1976.

20. Droegemueller, W., and Bressler, R.: Effectiveness and risks of contraception. Ann. Rev. Med., *31*:329, 1980.

21. Duenhoelter, J. H., Jimenez, J. M., and Baumann, G.: Pregnancy performance of patients under fifteen years of age. Obstet. Gynecol., *46*:49, 1975.

22. Edmondson, H. A., Henderson, B., and Benton, B.: Liver-cell adenomas associated with the use of oral contraceptives. N. Engl. J. Med., *294*:470, 1976.

23. Edström, K.: Techniques of induced abortion; their health implications and service aspects: A review of the literature. Bull. W.H.O., *57*:481, 1979.

24. Evans, J. R., Selstad, G., and Welcher, W. H.: Teenagers: Fertility control behavior and attitudes before and after abortion, childbearing or negative pregnancy test. Fam. Plann. Perspect., *8*:192, 1976.

24a. Fielding, J. E.: Adolescent pregnancy revisited. N. Engl. J. Med., *299*:893, 1978.

25. Fisch, I. R., and Frank, J.: Oral contraceptives and blood pressure. J.A.M.A., *237*:2499, 1977.

26. Furstenberg, F. F. Jr.: The social consequences of teenage parenthood. Fam. Plann. Perspect., *8*:148, 1976.

27. Furstenberg, F. F. Jr., and Crawford, A. G.: Family support: Helping teenage mothers to cope. Fam. Plann. Perspect., *10*:322, 1978.

27a. Grimes, D. A., and Cates, W. Jr.: Complications from legally induced abortion: A review. Obstet. Gynecol., *34*:177, 1979.

28. Haesslein, H. C., and Lamb, E. J.: Pituitary tumors in patients with secondary amenorrhea. Am. J. Obstet. Gynecol., *125*:759, 1976.

29. Harlap, S., Shiono, P., Pellegrin, F., Golbus, M., Bachman, R., Mann, J., Schmidt, L., and Lewis, J. P.: Chromosome abnormalities in oral contraceptive breakthrough pregnancies (letter). Lancet, *1*:1342, 1979.

30. Heinonen, O. P., Slone, D., Monson, R. R., Hook, E. B., and Shapiro, M. B.: Cardiovascular birth defects and antenatal exposure to female sex hormones. N. Engl. J. Med., *296*:67, 1977.

31. Hodgson, J. E., and Portmann, K. C.: Complications of 10,453 consecutive first trimester abortions: A prospective study. Am. J. Obstet. Gynecol., *120*:802, 1974.

32. Hollingsworth, D. R., and Kreutner, A. K. K.: Outcome of adolescent pregnancy. *In* Kreutner, A. K. K., and Hollingsworth, D. R. (eds.): Adolescent Obstetrics and Gynecology. Chicago, Year Book Medical Publishers, 1978, pp. 249–275.

32a. Hollingsworth, D. R., and Kreutner, A. K. K.: Teenage pregnancy: Solutions are evolving. N. Engl. J. Med., *303*:516, 1980.

33. Hughey, M. J., McElin, T. W., and Young, T.: Maternal and fetal outcome of Lamaze-prepared patients. Obstet. Gynecol., *51*:643, 1978.

34. Hunt, W. B.: Adolescent fertility: Risks and consequences. Population Reports, Series J, No. 10, 1976.

35. Hutchins, F. L. Jr., Kendall, N., and Rubino, J.: Experience with teenage pregnancy. Obstet. Gynecol, *54*:1, 1979.

36. Institute of Medicine: Legalized abortion and the public health. Washington, D.C., National Academy of Sciences, 1975.

37. Israel, S. L., and Woutersz, T. B.: Teenage obstetrics. Am. J. Obstet. Gynecol., *85*:659, 1963.

38. Jaffe, F. S., and Dryfoos, J. G.: Fertility control services for adolescents: Access and utilization. Fam. Plann. Perspect., *8*:167, 1976.

39. Jick, H., Porter, J., and Rothman, K. J.: Oral contraceptives and nonfatal stroke in healthy young women. Ann. Intern. Med., *89*:58, 1978.

40. Johnson, C. L.: Adolescent pregnancy: Intervention into the poverty circle. Adolescence, *9*:391, 1974.

41. Johnstone, F. D., Beard, R. J., Boyd, I. E., and McCarthy, T. G.: Cervical diameter after suction termination of pregnancy. Br. Med. J., *1*:68, 1976.

42. Kaplan, N. M.: Cardiovascular complications of oral contraceptives. Ann. Rev. Med., *29*:31, 1978.

43. Klein, L.: Early teenage pregnancy, contraception and repeat pregnancy. Am. J. Obstet. Gynecol., *120*:249, 1974.

44. Klerman, L., and Jekel, J.: School-Age Mothers: Problems, Programs and Policy. Hamden, Connecticut, The Shoestring Press, 1973.

45. Krauss, R. M., Lindgren, F. T., Silvers, A., Jutagir, R., and Bradley, D. D.: Changes in serum high density lipoproteins in women on oral contraceptive drugs. Clin. Chim. Acta, *80*:465, 1977.

46. Kreutner, A. K. K., and Hollingsworth, D. R.: Adolescent Obstetrics and Gynecology. Chicago, Year Book Medical Publishers, 1978.

47. Kreutner, A. K. K., and Langhorst, D. M.: Abortion and abortion counseling. *In* Kreutner, A. K. K., and Hollingsworth, D. R. (eds.): Adolescent Obstetrics and Gynecology. Chicago, Year Book Medical Publishers, 1978, pp. 79–119.

48. Kulig, J. W., Rauh, J. L., Burket, R. L., Cabot, H. M., and Brookman, R. R.: Experience with the copper 7 intrauterine device in an adolescent population. J. Pediatr., *96*:746, 1980.

49. Lane, M. E., Arces, R., and Sobrers, A.: Successful use of the diaphragm and jelly by a young population: Report of a clinical study. Fam. Plann. Perspect., *8*:81, 1976.

50. Lipper, I., Cvejic, H., Benjamin, P., and Kinch, R. A.: Abortion and the pregnant teenager. Can. Med. Assoc. J., *109*:852, 1973.

51. Luff, R. D., Gupta, P. K., Spence, M. R., and Frost, J. K.: Pelvic actinomycosis and the intrauterine contraceptive device. A cytohistomorphologic study. Am. J. Clin. Pathol., *69*:581, 1978.

52. Mann, J. I., Vessey, M. P., Thorogood, M., and Doll, R.: Myocardial infarction in young women with special reference to oral contraceptive practice. Br. Med. J., *2*:241, 1975.

53. Marshall, W. A., and Tanner, J. M.: Variations in pattern of pubertal changes in girls. Arch. Dis. Child., *44*:291, 1961.

54. McAnarney, E. R., Roghmann, K. J., Adams, B. M., Tatelbaum, R. C., Kash, C., Coulter, M., Plume, M., and Charney, E.: Obstetric, neonatal and psychosocial outcome of pregnant adolescents. Pediatrics, *61*:199, 1978.

55. National Center for Health Statistics, Monthly Vital Statistics Report: Final Natality Statistics, 1977, Vol. 27, No. 11, Supplement, February 5, 1979.

56. Nora, J. J., Nora, A. H., Blu, J., Ingram, J., Fountain, A., Peterson, M., Lortscher, R. H., and Kimberling, W. J.: Exogenous progestogen and estrogen implicated in birth defects. J.A.M.A., *240*:837, 1978.

57. Nortman, D.: Parental age as a factor in pregnancy outcome and child development. Reports on Population/Family Planning, No. 16, 1974.

58. Obel, E. B.: Pregnancy complications following legally induced abortion: An analysis of the population with special reference to prematurity. Dan. Med. Bull., *27*:192, 1979.

59. Ory, H. W.: Association between oral contraceptives and myocardial infarction: A review. J.A.M.A., *237*:2619, 1977.

60. Ory, H. W.: A review of the association between intrauterine devices and acute pelvic inflammatory disease. J. Reprod. Med., *20*:200, 1978.

61. Osofsky, H. F., Hagen, J. H., and Wood, P. W.: A program for pregnant schoolgirls. Am. J. Obstet. Gynecol., *100*:1020, 1968.

62. Perkins, R. P., Nakashima, I. I., Mullin, M., Dubansky, L. S., and Chin, M. L.: Intensive care in adolescent pregnancy. Obstet. Gynecol., *52*:179, 1978.

63. Petitti, D. B., and Wingerd, J.: Use of oral contraceptives, cigarette smoking and risk of subarachnoid hemorrhage. Lancet, *2*:234, 1978.

64. Plumez, J. H.: Adoption: Where have all the babies gone? The New York Times Magazine, April 13, 1980.

65. Population Information Program, The Johns Hopkins University: OC's — Update on usage, safety and side effects. Population Reports, Oral Contraceptives, Series A, No. 5, Hampton House, Baltimore, 1979.

66. Robertson, Y. R., and Johnson, E. S.: Interactions between oral contraceptives and other drugs. A review. Curr. Med. Res. Opin., *3*:647, 1976.

67. Rooks, J. B., and Cates, W. Jr.: Emotional impact of D and E versus instillation. Fam. Plann. Perspect., *9*:287, 1977.

68. Rosenfield, A.: Oral and intrauterine contraception: A 1978 risk assessment. Am. J. Obstet. Gynecol., *132*:92, 1978.

69. Royal College of General Practitioners: Oral Contraception and Health: An Interim Report from the Oral Contraception Study of the Royal College of General Practitioners. New York, Pitman, 1974.

70. Sarrel, P. M., and Klerman, L. V.: The young unwed mother. Am. J. Obstet. Gynecol., *105*:575, 1969.

71. Settlage, D. S. F., Baroff, S., and Copper, D.: Sexual experience of younger teenage girls seeking contraceptive assistance for the first time. Fam. Plann. Perspect., *5*:223, 1973.

72. Steel, J. M., and Duncan, L. J. P.: Serious complications of oral contraception in insulin-dependent diabetics. Contraception, *17*:291, 1978.

73. Stern, E., Forsythe, A. B., Youkeles, L., and Coffelt, C. F.: Steroid contraceptive use and cervical dysplasia: Increased risk of progression. Science, *196*:1460, 1977.

74. Stickle, G., and Ma, P.: Pregnancy in adolescents: Scope of the problem. Contemp. Obstet. Gynecol., *5*:85, 1975.

75. Stolley, P. D., Tonascia, J. A., Tockman, M. S., Sartwell, P. E., Rutlege, A. H., and Jacobs, M. P.: Thrombosis with low estrogen oral contraceptives. Am. J. Epidemiol., *102*:197, 1975.

76. Tietze, C.: Legal abortions in the United States: Rates and ratios by race and age, 1972–1974. Fam. Plann. Perspect., *9*:12, 1977.

77. Tietze, C.: The pill and mortality from cardiovascular disease: Another look. Fam. Plann. Perspect., *112*:80, 1979.

78. Tietze, C., and Lewit, S.: Joint Program for the Study of Abortion (JPSA): Early medical complications of legal abortions. Stud. Fam. Plann., *3*:97, 1972.

79. Torres, A.: Organized family planning services in the United States, 1976–1977. Fam. Plann. Perspect., *11*:342, 1979.

80. Trussell, J., and Menken, J.: Early childbearing and subsequent fertility. Fam. Plann. Perspect., *10*:209, 1978.

81. Tyrer, L. B.: Update on intrauterine devices. Curr. Probl. Obstet. Gynecol., *2*:3, 1979.

82. U.S. Department of Health, Education and Welfare, Food and Drug Administration, Medical Device and Drug Advisory Committees on Obstetrics and Gynecology: Second Report on Intrauterine contraceptive devices. Washington, D.C.: U.S. Government Printing Office, 1978.

83. Vessey, M. P., and Doll, R.: Evaluation of existing techniques. Is "the pill" safe enough to continue using? Proc. R. Soc. Lond. (Biol.), *195*:69, 1976.

84. Vessey, M. P., McPherson, K., and Johnson, B.: Mortality among women participating in the Oxford/family planning association contraceptive study. Lancet, *2*:731, 1977.

85. von Kaulla, E., Droegemueller, W., Aoki, N., and von Kaulla, K. N.: Antithrombin III depression and thrombin generation acceleration in women taking oral contraceptives. Am. J. Obstet. Gynecol., *109*:868, 1971.

86. Westoff, C. F., and Jones, E. F.: Contraception and sterilization in the United States, 1965–1975. Fam. Plann. Perspect., *9*:4, 1977.

87. Westrom, L., Bengtsson, L. P., and Mardh, P. A.: The risk of pelvic inflammatory disease in women using intrauterine devices as compared to non-users. Lancet, *2*:221, 1976.

88. World Health Organization: Eighth Annual Report, Human Reproduction, 1979.

89. World Health Organization Task Force on the Sequelae of Abortion: Gestation, birth weight and spontaneous abortion in pregnancy after induced abortion. Lancet, *1*:142, 1979.

90. Zabin, L. S., Kanter, J. F., and Zelnik, M.: The risk of adolescent pregnancy in the first months of intercourse. Fam. Plann. Perspect., *11*:215, 1979.

91. Zelnik, M., and Kantner, J. F.: First pregnancies to women aged 15–19: 1976 and 1977. Fam. Plann. Perspect., *10*:11, 1978.

92. Zelnik, M., Kim, Y. J., and Kantner, J. F.: Probabilities of intercourse and conception among U.S. teenage women, 1971 and 1976. Fam. Plann. Perspect., *11*, 177, 1979.

INDEX